a LANGE medical book

CURRENT
Diagnosis & Treatment Cardiology

SIXTH EDITION

T0200680

Michael H. Crawford, MD
Professor of Medicine, *Emeritus*
University of California, San Francisco
Consulting Physician, Heart & Vascular Center
UCSF Medical Center
San Francisco, California

Mc Graw Hill

New York Chicago San Francisco Athens London Madrid Mexico City
Milan New Delhi Singapore Sydney Toronto

Current Diagnosis & Treatment: Cardiology, Sixth Edition

1 2 3 4 5 6 7 8 9 LCR 28 27 26 25 24 23

ISBN 978-1-264-64357-8
MHID 1-264-64357-8
ISSN 1079-1051

Notice

Medicine is an ever-changing science. As new research and clinical experience broaden our knowledge, changes in treatment and drug therapy are required. The authors and the publisher of this work have checked with sources believed to be reliable in their efforts to provide information that is complete and generally in accord with the standards accepted at the time of publication. However, in view of the possibility of human error or changes in medical sciences, neither the authors nor the publisher nor any other party who has been involved in the preparation or publication of this work warrants that the information contained herein is in every respect accurate or complete, and they disclaim all responsibility for any errors or omissions or for the results obtained from use of the information contained in this work. Readers are encouraged to confirm the information contained herein with other sources. For example and in particular, readers are advised to check the product information sheet included in the package of each drug they plan to administer to be certain that the information contained in this work is accurate and that changes have not been made in the recommended dose or in the contraindications for administration. This recommendation is of particular importance in connection with new or infrequently used drugs.

This book was set in Minion Pro Regular by KnowledgeWorks Global Ltd.
The editors were Timothy Y. Hiscock and Christina M. Thomas.
The production supervisor was Catherine Saggese.
Project management was provided by Tasneem Kauser, KnowledgeWorks Global Ltd.
This book is printed on acid-free paper.

Contents

Section III. Arrhythmias

Authors

Amir E. Abbas, MD
Associate Professor of Medicine
Oakland University-William Beaumont School of Medicine
Co-Director Echocardiography Laboratory
Beaumont Hospital
Royal Oak, Michigan

Karthik Ananthasubramaniam, MD
Professor of Medicine
Wayne State University
Director, Nuclear Cardiology and Cardiac PET
Senior Staff Physician, Heart and Vascular Institute
Department of Internal Medicine
Henry Ford West Bloomfield Hospital
West Bloomfield, Michigan

Mandar Aras, MD, PhD
Assistant Professor of Medicine
Division of Cardiology
University of California, San Francisco
San Francisco, California

Su Aung, MD, MPH
Assistant Professor of Medicine
Division of Infectious Diseases
University of California, San Francisco
San Francisco, California

Nitish Badhwar, MD
Professor of Medicine
Division of CV Medicine
Stanford University School of Medicine
Stanford, California

Christopher F. Barnett, MD, MPH
Professor of Medicine
Chief, Section of Critical Care Cardiology
Director, Cardiac Intensive Care Unit Service
Director, Inpatient Cardiology Service
University of California, San Francisco
San Francisco, California

René Baudrand, MD
Associate Professor of Medicine
Department of Endocrinology
Faculty of Medicine
Pontificia Universidad Católica de Chile
Santiago, Chile

Vishal Birk, MD
Clinical Cardiology Fellow
Department of Cardiology
William Beaumont University Hospital
Royal Oak, Michigan

Andrew J. Boyle, MBBS, PhD
Professor of Cardiovascular Medicine
Department of Cardiovascular Medicine
University of Newcastle
Newcastle, Australia

Michelle D. Carlson, MD
Assistant Professor of Medicine
University of Minnesota
Division of Cardiology
Hennepin Healthcare
Minneapolis, Minnesota

Richard Cheng, MD
Assistant Clinical Professor of Medicine
Division of Cardiology
University of California, San Francisco
San Francisco, California

Kuang-Yuh Chyu, MD, PhD
Associate Director, Coronary Intensive Care Unit
Department of Cardiology, Smidt Heart Institute
Cedars-Sinai Medical Center
Health Sciences Clinical Professor
Department of Medicine
University of California, Los Angeles
Los Angeles, California

Michael H. Crawford, MD
Professor of Medicine, *Emeritus*
University of California, San Francisco
Consulting Physician, Heart & Vascular Center
UCSF Medical Center
San Francisco, California

Jonathan D. Davis, MD, MPHS
Director, San Francisco Health Network Heart Failure Program
Division of Cardiology, San Francisco General Hospital
Associate Clinical Professor of Medicine, Department of Medicine, University of California, San Francisco
San Francisco, California

Teresa De Marco, MD
Professor of Medicine
Division of Cardiology
University of California, San Francisco
San Francisco, California

Yaanik B. Desai, MD
Stanford University School of Medicine
Department of Medicine
Division of Cardiovascular Medicine
San Francisco, California

Shalini Dixit, MD
Cardiology Fellow
Division of Cardiology
University of California, San Francisco
San Francisco, California

John A. Elefteriades, MD
William W.L. Glenn Professor of Surgery
Founding Director, Aortic Institute at Yale New Haven
Yale University School of Medicine
New Haven, Connecticut

Pamela Fazio, DO
Division of Cardiology
Deborah Heart and Lung Center
Brown Mills, New Jersey

Antonio B. Fernandez, MD
Assistant Professor of Medicine
University of Connecticut
Director, Cardiac Intensive Care Unit
Hartford Hospital
Athletes' Heart Program, Hartford Hospital
Hartford, Connecticut

Nora F. Goldschlager, MD
Professor of Clinical Medicine, Emerita
University of California, San Francisco
Consulting Cardiologist
San Francisco General Hospital
San Francisco, California

James A. Goldstein, MD
Director of Research and Education
Department of Cardiovascular Medicine
Beaumont Health System
Royal Oak, Michigan

Saurabh Gupta, MD
Chief of Cardiology
St. Charles Health System
Oregon Health and Science University
Bend, Oregon

Ian S. Harris, MD
Professor of Medicine
Director, Adult Congenital Cardiology Program
Division of Cardiology
University of California, San Francisco
San Francisco, California

Brian D. Hoit, MD
Professor of Medicine and Physiology and Biophysics
Case Western Reserve University
University Hospitals Cleveland Medical Center and Harrington Heart and Vascular Institute
Cleveland, Ohio

Richard H. Hongo, MD
Director, Cardiovascular Fellowship Program
Lead, Electrophysiology Service Line
California Pacific Medical Center
San Francisco, California

Jonathan Hsu, MD, MAS
Assistant Professor of Medicine
Section of Cardiac Electrophysiology
Division of Cardiology
University of California, San Diego
San Diego, California

Massimo Imazio, MD
Chief of Cardiology, Contract Professor of Cardiology
Cardiothoracic Department
University Hospital Santa Maria della Misericordia and University of Udine
Udine, Italy

Liviu Klein, MD, MS
Professor of Medicine
University of California, San Francisco
Director, Advanced Heart Failure Comprehensive Care Center
UCSF Medical Center
San Francisco, California

D. Elizabeth Le, MD
Associate Professor of Medicine
Knight Cardiovascular Institute, Oregon Health and Science University
Staff Physician
VA Portland Health Care System
Portland, Oregon

Byron K. Lee, MD
Professor of Medicine
Director of the Electrophysiology Laboratories and Clinics
Division of Cardiology
University of California, San Francisco
San Francisco, California

Ashvarya Mangla, MD
Structural and Interventional Cardiologist
Clinical Assistant Professor of Medicine
OSF Saint Francis Medical Center
University of Illinois College of Medicine
Peoria, Illinois

Carlos A. Morillo, MD
Professor Department of Cardiac Science
Cumming School of Medicine
Section Chief Division of Cardiology, Libin Cardiovascular Institute
University of Calgary
Zone Head Cardiology Calgary & Southeastern Alberta Region
Alberta Health Services
Calgary, Alberta, Canada

Joyce N. Njoroge, MD
Advanced Heart Failure, Transplant and MCS Clinical Fellow
Division of Cardiology
Stanford University
Stanford, California

Connor O'Brien, MD
Associate Director, Section of Critical Care Cardiology
Assistant Professor of Medicine
University of California, San Francisco
San Francisco, California

Eveline Oestreicher Stock, MD
Assistant Professor of Medicine
Division of Cardiology
University of California, San Francisco
San Francisco, California

Rita F. Redberg, MD, MSc
Professor of Medicine
University of California, San Francisco
Core Faculty, Philip R Lee Institute for Health Policy Studies
Director, FAMRI Bland Lane Center of Excellence in Secondhand Smoke at UCSF
UCSF Division of Cardiology
San Francisco, California

Carlos A. Roldan, MD
Professor of Medicine
University of New Mexico School of Medicine
Director, Echocardiography Laboratory
New Mexico VA Health Care Center
Albuquerque, New Mexico

Aarthi Sabanayagam, MD
Associate Professor of Medicine
Division of Cardiology
University of California, San Francisco
San Francisco, California

James Salazar, MD, MAS
Cardiology Fellow
Division of Cardiology
University of California, San Francisco
San Francisco, California

Stephanie Saucier, MD
Division of Preventive Cardiology
Hartford Hospital
Hartford, Connecticut

Melvin M. Scheinman, MD
Professor of Medicine
Division of Cardiology
University of California, San Francisco
San Francisco, California

Prediman K. Shah, MD
Shapell and Webb Professor and Director
Atherosclerosis Prevention and Treatment Center
Director, Oppenheimer Atherosclerosis Research Center
Cedars Sinai Heart Institute, Los Angeles
Professor of Medicine, University of California, Los Angeles
Los Angeles, California

Sanjiv J. Shah, MD
Professor of Medicine
Division of Cardiology, Department of Medicine
Northwestern University Feinberg School of Medicine
Chicago, Illinois

Gautam R. Shroff, MBBS
Associate Professor of Medicine
University of Minnesota Medical School
Director, Division of Cardiology
Sr. Medical Director, Heart and Vascular Service Line
Hennepin Healthcare
Minneapolis, Minnesota

Sara Sirna, MD
Professor of Medicine
Loyola University Medical Center
Maywood, Illinois

Kirsten Tolstrup, MD
Professor of Medicine
University of California, San Francisco
Associate Chief of Cardiology for Ambulatory Operations
UCSF Medical Center
San Francisco, California

Zian H. Tseng, MD, MAS
Professor of Medicine in Residence
Murray Davis Endowed Professor
Cardiac Electrophysiology Section, Cardiology Division
University of California, San Francisco
San Francisco, California

Thomas Uslar, MD
Instructor of Medicine
Department of Endocrinology
Pontificia Universidad Católica de Chile
Santiago, Chile

Bert Vandenberk, MD, PhD
Staff Cardiac Electrophysiologist
University Hospitals Leuven
Belgium

Wanpen Vongpatanasin, MD
Professor of Medicine
Norman & Audrey Kaplan Chair in Hypertension
Fredric L. Coe Professorship in Nephrolithiasis and Mineral Metabolism Research
Director, Hypertension Section
Cardiology Division
University of Texas, Southwestern Medical Center
Dallas, Texas

Sarah Westcott, MD
Resident Physician
Department of Medicine
University of California, San Francisco
San Francisco, California

Preface

Current Diagnosis & Treatment: Cardiology is a concise discussion of the knowledge needed to diagnose and manage most cardiovascular diseases. It is designed for trainees to review the essentials of specific conditions and to check the suggested literature included in each section. The experienced clinician will find it a source for quick reference. It is an excellent review for Board examinations. Nurses, technicians, and other health care professionals who help manage cardiology patients will find it a valuable resource for all aspects of cardiovascular disease care.

The 37 chapters in *Current Diagnosis & Treatment: Cardiology* cover the major disease entities and therapeutic challenges in cardiology. Also, there are chapters on major management issues such as pregnancy and heart disease, the use of anticoagulants in heart disease, and the perioperative evaluation of heart disease patients. Each section is written by experts in the particular area, but it has been extensively edited to ensure a consistent approach throughout the book and the kind of readability found in single-author texts. It is organized into six sections: Prevention of Cardiovascular Disease, Ischemic Heart Disease, Arrhythmias, Valvular Disease, Cardiomyopathy & Heart Failure, and Systemic Diseases & the Heart. Since the fifth edition, new content has been added to every chapter. Certain new content themes permeate multiple chapters such as the increased use of cardiac MRI, CT, PET, and radionuclide imaging in valve, myocardial, pericardial, and ischemic heart disease; the increased application of genetic information in cardiomyopathies, adult congenital heart disease, aortic disease, primary pulmonary arterial hypertension, and valvular heart disease: and new biologic drugs for dyslipidemia, recurrent pericarditis, and cardiac disease associated with connective tissue diseases. Also, recent pharmacologic treatment trial results of several agents used to treat the growing problem of heart failure with preserved left ventricular ejection fraction are detailed. In addition, there is new content on COVID-19 myocarditis and new antineoplastic drugs toxic to the heart such as immune checkpoint inhibitors. Finally, the issue of return to play recommendations for athletes who contract COVID-19 is discussed.

My hope is that the book is found to be useful and improves patient care. Also, I hope it is an educational tool that increases the reader's knowledge and understanding of cardiovascular disease. Finally, I hope it stimulates clinical research in areas where our knowledge is incomplete.

Michael H. Crawford, MD

Lipid Disorders

1

Pamela Fazio, DO
Sara Sirna, MD

ESSENTIALS OF DIAGNOSIS

- ► Elevated plasma levels of low-density lipoprotein cholesterol, non–high-density lipoprotein cholesterol, lipoprotein(a), and apolipoprotein (apo) B-100.
- ► Reduced plasma levels of high-density lipoprotein and apo A-I.
- ► Elevated plasma levels of triglycerides.
- ► Skin xanthomas.

General Considerations

Multiple epidemiologic studies have demonstrated a direct relationship between cardiovascular mortality and elevated plasma cholesterol levels. Lipoprotein disorders are a major modifiable cardiovascular risk factor. Lipid-lowering therapy, including but not limited to diet, exercise, and pharmacologic therapies, has demonstrated survival benefit in both primary prevention (patients without evidence of atherosclerotic cardiovascular disease [ASCVD]) and secondary prevention (patients with evidence of ASCVD). As a result, screening, risk stratifying, and treating dyslipidemia have become integral parts of preventive cardiovascular medicine and a necessary step in improving the health of individuals.

A. Lipoproteins and Apolipoproteins

Cholesterol, cholesteryl esters, and triglycerides are the major lipids found in plasma. Cholesterol is an integral component of the cell membrane. It also serves a role in steroid hormone and bile acid synthesis. Triglycerides consist of fatty acid chains and phospholipids. Fatty acid chains are a primary source of energy in humans; phospholipids are key elements of all cell membranes. Cholesterol and triglycerides are insoluble in water and are transported in plasma by lipoproteins, classified as high-density lipoprotein (HDL) cholesterol, low-density lipoprotein (LDL) cholesterol, very-low-density lipoprotein (VLDL) cholesterol, intermediate-density lipoprotein (IDL) cholesterol, and chylomicrons. Lipoproteins consist of a lipid core and a water-soluble phospholipid outer layer that carry apolipoproteins, which are specific proteins that serve as coenzymes, receptor ligands, or regulators of lipoprotein metabolism. Apolipoprotein (apo) A-I is present in HDL and promotes cholesterol efflux from tissues. Apo B, present as either apo B-100 (VLDL, IDL, LDL) or apo B-48 (chylomicron), serves as the LDL receptor ligand. Apo C-I, apo C-II, and apo C-III participate in triglyceride metabolism, and apo E is present on chylomicrons.

Lipoprotein(a) [Lp(a)] highly correlates with cardiovascular disease (CVD) and consists of an LDL particle and a specific apo A. The structure of Lp(a) is similar to plasminogen and is thought to increase thrombogenesis. It is known to predict early atherosclerotic risk independent of other risk factors. Figure 1–1 illustrates the classes of lipoproteins and their characteristics.

B. Metabolism

Transportation of dietary lipids to peripheral tissues and the liver is known as the *exogenous metabolic pathway*. Here, triglycerides are hydrolyzed by pancreatic lipases and are emulsified by bile acids, leading to micelle formation. Micelle uptake occurs in the intestinal brush border where fatty acids are re-esterified and packaged together with apo B-48, phospholipids, and cholesterol to form chylomicrons. Chylomicrons then reach the portal circulation where they are hydrolyzed to release fatty acids by lipoprotein lipase (LPL). LPL activity is regulated through apo C-II, which activates LPL, and apo C-III, which inhibits LPL. The free fatty acids are used by muscles or stored as fat in an insulin-regulated process. As the particles get smaller, the cholesterol and apolipoproteins are transferred to HDL, creating a chylomicron remnant that is then taken up by the liver for degradation in an apo E–mediated process.

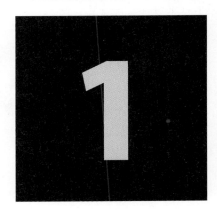

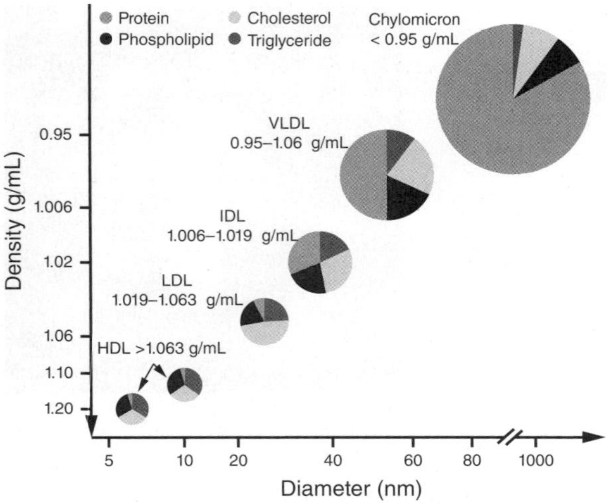

▲ **Figure 1–1.** Lipoprotein characteristics. HDL, high-density lipoproteins; IDL, intermediate-density lipoproteins; LDL, low-density lipoproteins; VLDL, very-low-density lipoproteins.

The *endogenous metabolic pathway* refers to the transport of hepatic lipoproteins to peripheral tissues via LDL. It ensures a steady supply of substrate given that food supply varies. Here VLDL, a triglyceride-rich lipoprotein, serves a similar role to the chylomicron in the exogenous pathway. VLDL is derived from esterified long-chain fatty acids in the liver. Its triglyceride component is also hydrolyzed by LPL. VLDL acquires apolipoproteins (B-100, C-I, C-II, C-III, and E) from HDL and also exchanges triglycerides for cholesteryl esters in a process mediated by cholesteryl ester transfer protein (CETP). This mechanism allows cholesterol transfer from HDL to VLDL, allowing reverse cholesterol transport. Following hydrolysis, up to 40% of the resulting VLDL remnant, known as IDL, is taken up by the liver in an apo E–mediated transfer, and the remainder is converted to LDL by hepatic lipase. LDL particles mostly contain cholesteryl esters together with apo B-100 and are the main carriers of cholesterol. Figure 1–2 illustrates the endogenous and exogenous lipid metabolism pathways.

1. LDL—LDL predominantly contains cholesteryl esters with apo B-100 and 4–8% of triglycerides. LDL is the

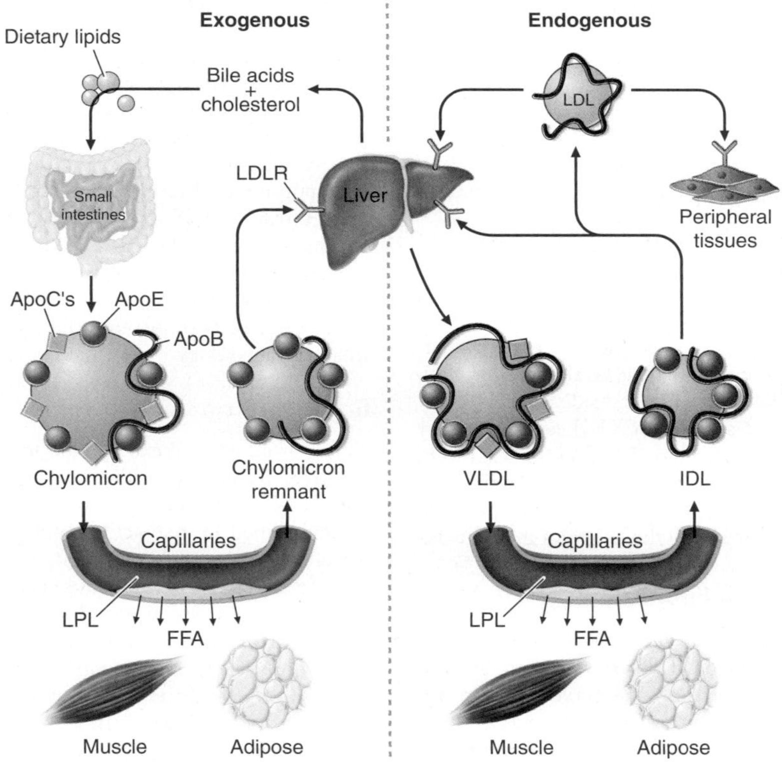

▲ **Figure 1–2.** Endogenous and exogenous pathways of lipid metabolism. FFA, free fatty acids; IDL, intermediate-density lipoproteins; LDL, low-density lipoproteins; LDLR, low-density lipoprotein receptor; LPL, lipoprotein lipase; VLDL, very-low-density lipoproteins. (Reproduced with permission from Kasper D, et al., eds. *Harrison's Principles of Internal Medicine*, 19th ed. New York: McGraw-Hill; 2015.)

major cholesterol transporter in humans. Cell cholesterol content is tightly regulated by several mechanisms. LDL is internalized through apo B-100, which binds to LDL receptors present on the cell surface. Once internalized, there is degradation of apo B-100 and release of cholesterol. LDL receptor numbers are also tightly regulated by the phosphoprotein proprotein convertase subtilisin/kexin 9 (PCSK9). PCSK9 binds to LDL receptors on the cell surface, and the PCSK9-LDL complex, including both LDL and LDL receptors, gets internalized and degraded. This leads to a decrease of LDL receptors that disrupts LDL clearances and causes accumulation of cholesterol-rich LDL particles in the blood. Inhibiting PCSK9 can help individuals reach their LDL goals. Within cells, cholesterol can be synthesized in the smooth endoplasmic reticulum through a rate-limiting step that uses hydroxymethylglutaryl–coenzyme A (HMG-CoA) reductase.

2. Lp(a)—Lp(a) is an LDL particle with an added apo(a) attached to the apo(b) component. Lp(a) is a new biomarker in the field of lipidology. Early research data suggest a link between Lp(a) and both ASCVD and valvular aortic stenosis (VAS), but the exact mechanism is not clear. Hypothetical mechanisms include thrombosis at arterial plaques, intimal cholesterol deposition, endothelial dysfunction, inflammation, and calcification in vasculature. Initial clinical trials support a link between Lp(a) levels and increased risk of myocardial infarction, coronary artery stenosis, ischemic stroke, and cardiovascular mortality. Future research needs to be completed to determine how to measure, target, and treat Lp(a) levels to reduce cardiovascular risk in individuals.

Wilson DP, Jacobson TA, Jones PH, et al. Use of Lipoprotein(a) in clinical practice: a biomarker whose time has come. A scientific statement from the National Lipid Association. *J Clin Lipidol.* 2019;13:374–392. [PMID: 31147269]

3. HDL—Epidemiologic studies have shown an inverse relationship between HDL levels and atherosclerotic coronary artery disease (CAD). HDL is responsible for reverse cholesterol transport. It inhibits lipoprotein oxidation and maintains endothelial integrity. Synthesized mostly in the liver but also in the intestine, the nascent HDL molecule consists of apo A-I, phospholipids, and cholesterol. HDL acquires cholesterol in an apo A-I–mediated process, which is then esterified by lecithin-cholesterol acyltransferase (LCAT) within the HDL particle forming mature HDL-containing cholesteryl esters, which can be taken up by the liver. Cholesterol and triglycerides can also be transferred from HDL to VLDL and chylomicrons via CETP, a process that allows HDL to transport cholesterol between cells, VLDL and chylomicrons, and the liver.

C. Atherosclerosis

Dyslipidemia is a major predisposing factor in the development of atherosclerosis and ASCVD. LDL is one of the most important causal factors for CVD. Elevated plasma LDL concentrations can indirectly and directly contribute to atherogenesis. Oxidized LDL accumulates in subintimal macrophages through active scavenger receptor–mediated uptake that leads to cellular dysfunction, apoptosis, and necrosis. Unlike the LDL receptor–mediated endocytosis, this process is not regulated by cholesterol content. These macrophages are termed foam cells and form subintimal fatty streaks. This culminates in the release of proinflammatory and prothrombotic molecules, which causes endothelial injury. Oxidized LDL can also directly cause endothelial injury through interaction with the cell surface. Endothelial injury results in platelet aggregation and smooth muscle proliferation, which initiates atherosclerotic plaque formation. HDL serves a protective role in atherogenesis. Its antiatherogenic effects are exerted through maintenance of endothelial function, apo A-I–mediated reverse transport of macrophage cholesterol, antioxidant effects, and antithrombotic effects.

Clinical Findings

Patients with dyslipidemia are asymptomatic with the exception of those who present with acute pancreatitis in the setting of severe hypertriglyceridemia. The clinical findings depend on the cause of dyslipidemia.

The most severe forms of hyperlipidemia are caused by genetic disorders of lipoprotein metabolism such as familial hypercholesterolemia (FH). FH is an autosomal dominant disease with defects in the gene for the LDL receptor. The mutant gene prevents the LDL receptor from removing LDLs from the blood. LDL cholesterol levels are typically in excess of 300 mg/dL. Common manifestations include fatty skin deposits called xanthomas over parts of the hands, elbows, knees, ankles, and around the corner of the eye (xanthelasmas). It frequently presents as premature CAD with chest pain (angina) or acute myocardial infarction. Other common primary causes of dyslipidemia are familial combined hyperlipidemia (both high LDL and triglyceride levels) and pure hypertriglyceridemia (very high triglyceride levels). In addition, elevated LDL levels are associated with the development of peripheral arterial disease with impaired functional ability. In extreme cases, major adverse limb events including acute limb ischemia may occur.

Table 1–1 summarizes the most common primary causes of dyslipidemia.

A. Secondary Causes of Dyslipidemia

Dyslipidemia develops in many patients as a result of an underlying metabolic abnormality rather than a primary dyslipidemia. Metabolic syndrome is characterized by abdominal obesity, hypertension, insulin resistance (± glucose intolerance), prothrombotic state, elevated triglycerides, small LDL particles, and low HDL levels.

Obesity affects more than 40% of adults in the United States and the incidence continues to rise each year. Obesity represents a significant secondary cause of dyslipidemia due to lack of physical activity and increased caloric intake

Table 1–1. Primary Gene Defects

Genetic Disorder	Protein (Gene) Defect	Lipoproteins Elevated	Clinical Findings	Genetic Transmission	Estimated Incidence
Lipoprotein lipase deficiency	LPL	Chylomicrons	Eruptive xanthomas, hepatosplenomegaly, pancreatitis	AR	1 in 1,000,000
Familial apolipoprotein C-II deficiency	Ape-CII	Chylomicrons	Eruptive xanthomas, hepatosplenomegaly, pancreatitis	AR	< 1 in 1,000,000
Apo A-V deficiency	ApeA-V	Chylomicrons, VLDL	Eruptive xanthomas, hepatosplenomegaly, pancreatitis	AD	< 1 in 1,000,000
GP1HBP1 deficiency	GP1HBP1	Chylomicrons	Eruptive xanthomas, pancreatitis	AD	< 1 in 1,000,000
Familial hepatic lipase deficiency	Hepatic lipase	VLDL remnants	Pancreatitis, CHD	AR	< 1 in 1,000,000
Familial dysbetalipoproteinemia	ApoE	Chylomicrons, VLDL remnants	Palmar and tuboeruptive xanthomas, CHD, PVD	AR, AD	1 in 10,000
Familial hypercholesterolemia	LDL receptor	LDL	Tendon xanthomas, CHD	AD	1 in 500
Familial defective apo B-100	Apo B-100	LDL	Tendon xanthomas, CHD	AD	< 1 in 1000
Autosomal dominant hypercholesterolemia	PCSK9	LDL	Tendon xanthomas, CHD	AD	< 1 in 1,000,000
Autosomal recessive hypercholesterolemia	LDLRAP	LDL	Tendon xanthomas, CHD	AR	< 1 in 1,000,000
Sitosterolemia	ABCG5 or ABCG8	LDL	Tendon xanthomas, CHD	AR	< 1 in 1,000,000

AD, autosomal dominant; AR, autosomal recessive; ARH, autosomal recessive hypercholesterolemia; CHD, coronary heart disease; LDL, low-density lipoprotein; LPL, lipoprotein lipase; PVD, peripheral vascular disease; VLDL, very-low-density lipoprotein.
Reproduced with permission from Kasper D, et al., eds. *Harrison's Principles of Internal Medicine*, 19th ed. New York: McGraw-Hill; 2015.

mostly derived from saturated fat and sugar. Decreased insulin sensitivity and increased carbohydrate intake cause an increase in triglyceride formation, which then enters the circulation in the form of VLDL. HDL levels are decreased in obesity. Similarly, patients with type 2 diabetes mellitus develop dyslipidemia due to insulin resistance and subsequent insulin excess. This causes an increase in free fatty acid formation in the periphery and in the liver that translates to an increase in VLDL production and hypertriglyceridemia. Lipoprotein catabolism is downregulated due to decreased LPL activity, resulting in further increases in plasma VLDL.

Hypothyroidism commonly results in dyslipidemia due to a decrease in hepatic LDL receptor activity and consequent delayed clearance of LDL. The severity of the dyslipidemia directly correlates with the degree of hypothyroidism, and correction reverses the dyslipidemia.

Liver disease can affect plasma lipid concentrations. Hepatitis is associated with increased VLDL production, and not surprisingly, severe disease and liver failure result in low plasma lipoprotein levels as synthetic function progressively decreases. Cholestatic liver disease results in significant hypercholesterolemia through the accumulation of lipoprotein-X, the deposition of which leads to the appearance of xanthomata in the skin.

Chronic kidney disease is associated with elevation of VLDL as a result of decreased lipolysis and clearance. Nephrotic syndrome results in marked hypercholesterolemia as a result of increased hepatic production of LDL and decreased clearance of VLDL, induced as a result of low plasma oncotic pressure.

Several medications can alter lipoproteins. Thiazide diuretics can increase plasma triglyceride levels. Beta-blockers can increase triglycerides and lower HDL levels. Estrogen, anabolic steroids, and corticosteroids can all increase triglycerides. Antiretroviral agents, particularly protease inhibitors, are associated with lipodystrophy syndrome. Antipsychotics are also potential causative agents that are associated with weight gain and insulin resistance.

Other secondary causes to consider include cigarette smoking, which decreases plasma HDL concentration. Dyslipidemia is a result of underlying genetics, comorbidities, age, lifestyle, and environmental effects. All aspects need to be taken into consideration when treating individuals with dyslipidemia.

Diagnosis

The 2019 American College of Cardiology (ACC)/American Heart Association (AHA) Guideline on the Treatment of Blood Cholesterol to Reduce Atherosclerotic Cardiovascular Risk in Adults recommends checking a fasting lipid panel on initial evaluation of all adult patients older than 40 years. However, after the age of 20, it is reasonable to measure traditional risk factors at least every 4–6 years. The U.S. Preventive Services Task Force (USPSTF) advocates for routine screening of men and women 40–75 years old. The USPSTF also recommends screening at an earlier age if risk factors for ASCVD are present. When lipid abnormalities are discovered, a thorough history should be performed, assessing for symptomatic CVD, as well as attempts to identify potential secondary causes of dyslipidemia. A thorough family history should be obtained, and risk factors such as sedentary lifestyle, obesity, poor diet, and cigarette smoking should be addressed. Physical examination may reveal xanthomas and xanthelasmas, which may aid in the diagnosis of a primary dyslipidemia. Basic metabolic panel, creatinine, thyroid and liver function tests should be obtained to exclude any secondary causes of hyperlipidemia.

Treatment

A. LDL Cholesterol

The ACC/AHA Task Force has identified four distinct groups of patients who would benefit from statin therapy based exclusively on evidence from available randomized controlled trials. These four groups are as follows: (1) patients with clinical ASCVD, (2) patients with LDL levels greater than 190 mg/dL (suggestive of FH), (3) diabetic patients aged 40–75 years without ASCVD and LDL levels between 70 and 189 mg/dL, and (4) nondiabetics without ASCVD who are aged 40–75 years, have LDL levels between 70 and 189 mg/dL, and have a 10-year absolute CVD risk of greater than 7.5% derived from a new pooled cohort equation. The decision to commence drug therapy is determined by the degree of cardiovascular risk and represents a move away from the use of LDL targets.

By contrast, the National Lipid Association (NLA) guidelines incorporate randomized controlled trials, subgroup analyses, observational studies, and meta-analyses. They align with international societal guidelines, which recommend LDL as well as non-HDL treatment targets. Patients can be classified as low, moderate, high, or very high risk based on the presence of ASCVD, several risk factors for ASCVD, chronic kidney disease, and diabetes, which determines the LDL and non-HDL treatment goals (Table 1–2).

U.S. guidelines emphasize the importance of identifying patients at a very high cardiovascular risk and treating them to achieve an LDL level as low as possible. The Cholesterol Treatment Trialists' Collaboration has shown that the reduction in risk for major cardiovascular events is proportional to absolute LDL reduction. Early aggressive reduction of LDL in patients with acute coronary syndrome has shown a significant reduction in plaque volume at 6 months measured by intravascular ultrasound.

Table 1–2. LDL and Non-HDL Treatment Goals

Risk Category	Treatment Goal	Consider Drug Therapy
Low		
Non-HDL (mg/dL)	< 130	≥ 190
LDL (mg/dL)	< 100	≥ 160
Moderate		
Non-HDL (mg/dL)	< 130	≥ 160
LDL (mg/dL)	< 100	≥ 130
High		
Non-HDL (mg/dL)	< 130	≥ 130
LDL (mg/dL)	< 100	≥ 100
Very high		
Non-HDL (mg/dL)	< 100	≥ 100
LDL (mg/dL)	< 70	≥ 70
Risk category	**Criteria**	
Low	0–1 major ASCVD risk factors Consider other risk indicators, if known	
Moderate	2 major ASCVD risk factors Consider quantitative risk scoring Consider other risk indicators, if known	
High	≥ 3 major ASCVD risk factors Diabetes mellitus (type 1 or 2) - 0–1 other major ASCVD risk factors and - No evidence of end-organ damage Chronic kidney disease stage 3B or 4 LDL of ≥ 190 mg/dL (severe hypercholesterolemia) Quantitative risk score suggesting high risk	
Very high	ASCVD Diabetes mellitus (type 1 or 2) - ≥ 2 other major ASCVD risk factors or - Evidence of end-organ damage	

It should be emphasized that treating LDL reduces the risk of coronary events but does not eliminate it completely. Patients on targeted therapy who are at intermediate risk may benefit from further testing to define their "residual risk" of coronary events. Levels of HDL, high-sensitivity C-reactive protein, and Lp(a); particle sizes/numbers; coronary artery calcium scoring; and vascular intima imaging are useful tools in assessing this residual risk.

It may be reasonable to test serum Lp(a) in those with premature CAD, with a strong family history of premature

CAD, or with recurrent disease despite statin treatment. Statins and PCSK9 inhibitors have a very modest impact on Lp(a) levels to reduce major adverse cardiovascular events. Therefore, Lp(a) is a therapeutic target to lower cholesterol and is in clinical development.

B. HDL Cholesterol

Low HDL is an independent risk factor for increased CVD and mortality, although a causal relationship has not been established. High HDL levels and cholesterol efflux capacity are inversely associated with ASCVD and are associated with a longevity syndrome. Low HDL levels can be caused by genetic mutations, as is the case with familial hypoalphalipoproteinemia, familial HDL deficiency, and Tangier disease. Acquired and often reversible causes include obesity, sedentary lifestyle, cigarette smoking, metabolic syndrome, hypertriglyceridemia, and certain drugs (β-blockers and steroids). Compounds that increase HDL by inhibiting CETP have been disappointing in clinical trials to date, and further trials with these agents are ongoing to define their role in lipoprotein management.

C. Hypertriglyceridemia and Non-HDL Cholesterol

Hypertriglyceridemia is common and is often associated with obesity, physical inactivity, high-carbohydrate diet, alcohol consumption, and cigarette smoking. Other conditions such as diabetes, metabolic syndrome, and renal disease, as well as drugs (particularly estrogens and protease inhibitors), are also contributory. Patients with hypertriglyceridemia are at increased risk of developing ASCVD. As with low HDL levels, it is unclear whether a causal relationship exists. Current ACC/AHA and NLA treatment guidelines recommend reducing serum triglyceride levels below 500 mg/dL given the risk of pancreatitis. Therapeutic lifestyle changes should be the major treatment goal given the constellation of risk factors that contribute to the hypertriglyceridemic state.

In addition to aerobic exercise, dietary management should focus on carbohydrate reduction as well as restricting foods that have a high glycemic index. No dietary fat restriction is required, but the correct type of fat consumption should always be emphasized. Patients with extremely high triglyceride levels (> 1000 mg/dL) are at risk of developing acute pancreatitis due to high levels of circulating chylomicrons. In this subgroup of patients, all types of dietary fat should be restricted to reduce this risk. Fibrates, nicotinic acid, and fish oils are pharmacologic agents that can reduce triglyceride levels and are discussed separately.

Non-HDL cholesterol is calculated by subtracting HDL from total cholesterol (TC − HDL). This amount includes all apo B–containing (and therefore atherogenic) lipoprotein particles: LDL, Lp(a), IDL, and VLDL. This measure is useful in the setting of a raised triglyceride level (200–499 mg/dL).

Grundy SM, Stone NJ, Bailey AL, et al. 2018 AHA/ACC/AACVPR/AAPA/ABC/ACPM/ADA/AGS/APhA/ASPC/NLA/PCNA Guideline on the Management of Blood Cholesterol: A Report of the American College of Cardiology/American Heart Association Task Force on Clinical Practice Guidelines. *J Am Coll Cardiol.* 2019;73:e285–e350. [PMID: 30423393]

Jacobson TA, Ito MK, Maki KC, et al. National Lipid Association recommendations for patient-centered management of dyslipidemia; part 1—full report. *J Clin Lipidol.* 2015;9(2):129–169. [PMID: 25911072]

D. Nonpharmacologic Treatment: Lifestyle Changes, Diet, and Exercise

Despite significant advances in medical treatment, ASCVD remains the leading cause of death worldwide. This is likely due to the increasing rates of obesity, diabetes, and metabolic syndrome. Therefore, any successful strategy to reduce ASCVD risk should emphasize weight loss, regular exercise, and a heart-healthy diet.

Dietary fats can be categorized into cholesterol, saturated fatty acids (SFAs), monounsaturated fatty acids (MUFAs), polyunsaturated fatty acids (PUFAs), and trans-fatty acids. SFAs are mostly derived from animal products that raise both total and LDL cholesterol levels and are strongly associated with increased CVD. Trans-fatty acids result from commercial hydrogenation of PUFAs and decrease HDL levels and elevate LDL levels. Conversely, MUFAs and PUFAs have favorable effects on the lipid profile and may also delay atherosclerosis by limiting the oxidization of LDL.

Every individual with dyslipidemia should always be counseled on diet and exercise. A diet should consist of three objectives: (1) allow patients to reach and maintain ideal body weight; (2) provide a well-balanced diet with fruits, vegetables, nuts, whole grains, and lean protein; and (3) have restriction on sodium, saturated fats, and refined carbohydrates. Dietitians, weight loss programs, and diabetic outpatient centers can be helpful in weight loss. The AHA-advocated dietary recommendation emphasizes varied consumption of fruits, vegetables, whole grains, low-fat dairy products, poultry, fish, nuts, legumes, and nontropical vegetable oils such as the Dietary Approaches to Stop Hypertension (DASH) diet.

Another highly successful dietary intervention is the modified Mediterranean diet (MMD). Rich in whole grains, beans, fish, and olive oil, the MMD has shown high adherence rates and a sustainable reduction of coronary events. The PREDIMED trial exhibited a significant reduction in cardiovascular events with a Mediterranean diet compared to a low-fat control diet.

Increased physical activity is a key component in improving cardiovascular health. Studies on exercise and physical fitness have consistently exhibited reductions in cardiovascular events. Per week, adults should engage in at least 150 minutes of accumulated moderate-intensity activity or 75 minutes of vigorous-intensity physical activity per week. In addition, the ACC guidelines recommend a reduction in sedentary behavior—defined as less than 1.5 metabolic equivalents while awake, such as standing or sitting at a desk to improve overall cardiovascular health.

Physical activity and nutrition remain the foundation of any successful lipid management program.

Arnett DK, Blumenthal RS, Albert MA, et al. 2019 ACC/AHA guideline on the primary prevention of cardiovascular disease. *J Am Coll Cardiol.* 2019;74:e177–e232. [PMID: 30894318]

Ferraro RA, Fischer NM, Xun H, Michos ED. Nutrition and physical activity recommendations from the United States and European cardiovascular guidelines: a comparative review. *Curr Opin Cardiol.* 2020;35:508–516. [PMID: 32649350]

E. Pharmacologic Treatment

Most patients with dyslipidemia will require targeted pharmacologic therapy to address their dyslipidemia (Table 1–3). Statins are the cornerstone in treating dyslipidemia and lowering LDL. Other drugs, however, are beneficial as an adjunctive or sole therapy in certain populations.

1. HMG-CoA reductase inhibitors (statins)—Statins (simvastatin, atorvastatin, pravastatin, rosuvastatin, fluvastatin, pitavastatin, and lovastatin) are the most commonly used drugs in treating dyslipidemia. They are competitive inhibitors of HMG-CoA reductase, which is required for cholesterol biosynthesis. The decrease in intrahepatic cholesterol

Table 1–3. Pharmacologic Therapy for Dyslipidemia

Medication	Indication	Mechanism of Action	Percent Decrease in LDL	Side Effects
Statins	First line in treating dyslipidemia	Inhibits HMG-CoA reductase	30–50% depending on the dose prescribed	Myalgia, myositis, reversible transaminitis, and rarely rhabdomyolysis
Ezetimibe	Normally used in combination with statins	Inhibits the protein Niemann-Pick C1-like 1 and inhibits intestinal absorption of cholesterol	15–20%	Diarrhea, fatigue, and joint pain
Fibrates (Gemfibrozil and fenofibrates)	Used in secondary prevention of ASCVD with elevated triglycerides	Activation of nuclear peroxisome proliferator-activated receptor alpha (PPARa)	N/A	Gastrointestinal upset, myalgias, and elevated liver enzymes
Bile acid sequestrants (Resins)	Normally used in combination with statins	Interrupts enterohepatic circulation by binding bile acids and preventing reuptake in the ileum	Can indirectly reduce LDL levels by 15–30%	Bloating and constipation
Niacin	No longer recommended	Increases HDL levels	Does not reduce LDL levels	Flushing, hyperglycemia, gastritis, and elevated liver enzymes
Omega-3 fatty acids (Fish oils)	Hypertriglyceridemia	Unknown	N/A	Can prolong bleeding time
PCSK9 inhibitors (Alirocumab, evolocumab, and bococizumab)	High-risk patients, statin-intolerant patients, and patients unable to reach target LDL goal with conventional medications	Inhibits PCSK9 from binding to LDL receptor which prevents LDL-receptor degradation	More than 60% in high-risk patients	Hypersensitivity reaction and vasculitis
Mipomersen	FDA approved for homozygous familial hypercholesterolemia	Subcutaneously administered antisense oligonucleotide that inhibits apo B-100 synthesis in the liver	N/A	Elevated liver enzymes
Bempedoic Acid	Statin-intolerant patients and high-risk patients	Inhibits adenosine triphosphate citrate lyase	20%	Increase incidence of gout and acute kidney injury
Inclisiran	High-risk patients and patients unable to reach target LDL goals with conventional medications	RNA molecule that targets the PCSK9 enzyme	By at least 50% Remains in clinical trials	Pain at the injection site, loose stools, and shortness of breath

levels through this mechanism leads to an increase in LDL receptor expression and increased clearance of plasma LDL and decreased hepatic synthesis of VLDL and LDL. In addition, there is a modest increase in HDL levels. There is a synergistic effect when used in combination with either a cholesterol absorption inhibitor or a bile acid sequestrant, which can be helpful in optimizing LDL levels. Statins also appear to exert LDL-independent anti-inflammatory effects on the endothelium and atherosclerotic plaques. For the most part, statins are well tolerated. Commonly reported side effects include myalgia, myositis, reversible transaminitis, and rarely rhabdomyolysis.

Given their efficacy, potency, and tolerability, statins have been the focus of several large-scale prospective randomized studies over the past three decades, which have demonstrated relative cardiovascular risk reduction in primary prevention when compared to placebo. Secondary prevention has also been assessed in major trials (A-to-Z, IDEAL, IMPROVE-IT, PROVE-IT, TNT, and SEARCH) and has formed the basis of the current guidelines. Statin monotherapy reduces LDL levels by approximately 30–50% depending on the dose strength prescribed. Statin medication can be used as monotherapy or in combination with nonstatin drugs to allow individuals to reach their LDL goal.

2. Cholesterol absorption inhibitors—Ezetimibe binds to and inhibits the protein Niemann-Pick C1-like 1 (NPC1L1) to decrease intestinal absorption of cholesterol. The net effect is a decrease in cholesterol reaching the liver and a subsequent increase in hepatocyte LDL receptor expression, thereby decreasing plasma LDL with no effect on HDL or triglyceride levels. Ezetimibe, the first drug in this class, decreases plasma cholesterol by 15–20% and has a synergistic effect when used in combination with a statin, as demonstrated by the IMPROVE-IT trial, which concluded that, when used in combination with simvastatin, adverse cardiovascular outcomes improved in patients with known ASCVD. Major side effects are rare, even when used together with a statin, but liver function should be monitored.

3. PCSK9 inhibitors—The subcutaneously administered monoclonal antibodies alirocumab, evolocumab, and bococizumab prevent PCSK9 from binding to LDL receptors and initiating a cascade of receptor degradation. This in turn maintains LDL receptors on the surface of hepatocytes, allowing for reduction in plasma LDL. Alirocumab and evolocumab reduced LDL levels by more than 60% in patients with heterozygous FH and patients at high risk for ASCVD and have been approved for use in treating these conditions by the U.S. Food and Drug Administration (FDA). PCSK9 inhibitors are useful in high-risk patients, statin-intolerant patients, or patients unable to reach target LDL goals with conventional treatments. Recent data from many clinical trials (ODYSSEY OUTCOMES [alirocumab], FOURIER [evolocumab], and SPIRE 1 + 2 [bococizumab]), report that the use of PCSK9 inhibitor versus lipid-lowering medication or placebo resulted in a significantly lower risk of myocardial infarction, ischemic stroke, and coronary revascularization. This medication class is commonly used in addition to statin medications and ezetimibe. Major side effects are rare, with hypersensitivity reactions and vasculitis being the most common causes of hospitalization. Longer term follow-up is underway to monitor safety outcomes with this therapeutic class of drugs.

4. Fibric acid derivatives (fibrates)—The major effects of the fibrate class of drugs (gemfibrozil and fenofibrate) are to reduce serum triglyceride levels and raise HDL levels. This effect is mediated by the activation of nuclear peroxisome proliferator-activated receptor alpha (PPARα), which results in increased LPL activity and increased VLDL clearance. The elevation of HDL levels is mediated through PPARα-mediated synthesis of apo A-I and apo A-II. Gemfibrozil is indicated in secondary prevention of ASCVD in the setting of hypertriglyceridemia, low HDL, and normal LDL based on the Veterans Administration HDL Intervention Trial (VA-HIT). Common side effects include cholelithiasis, myalgias, and elevated transaminase levels. Combination therapy with statins is effective in treating elevated LDL as well as hypertriglyceridemia; however, fibrates, especially gemfibrozil, can decrease statin elimination and increase the risk of significant myositis and rhabdomyolysis.

5. Bile acid sequestrants (resins)—Bile acid sequestrants interrupt the enterohepatic circulation through binding bile acids and preventing reuptake in the ileum. This results in a decrease in total body and intrahepatic cholesterol, leading to subsequent increase in LDL (apo B and apo E) receptor expression. The LDL receptors (apo B and apo E) then bind LDL cholesterol from the plasma, leading to further decrease in LDL levels. Bile acid sequestrants can indirectly reduce LDL levels by 15–30%. Resins are more effective when used together with a statin. Resins can increase VLDL levels and are therefore restricted to patients with relatively normal triglyceride levels.

Bile acid sequestrants are not absorbed from the gastrointestinal tract, and this reflects their side effect profile. Bloating and constipation are common and dose dependent, which affects compliance. Bile acid sequestrants can also bind to and impair the absorption of other drugs such as digoxin, warfarin, β-blockers, thiazide diuretics, and fat-soluble vitamins. This effect can be minimized by administering other drugs 1 hour before or 4 hours after the bile acid sequestrant, but this can also affect compliance.

The available bile acid sequestrants, cholestyramine, colestipol, and colesevelam, are not systemically absorbed and thus can be used safely in pregnant patients, lactating patients, and children.

6. Nicotinic acid (niacin)—The predominant effect of niacin is to substantially increase HDL levels and decrease triglyceride levels. The mechanism by which niacin increases HDL levels remains unclear. Its effects on plasma triglyceride levels are mediated through enhanced LPL activity as well as inhibition of free fatty acid release from peripheral fat.

The main obstacle with niacin therapy has been its tolerability. Common side effects include elevated transaminases, hyperglycemia, gastritis, and flushing. Taking aspirin 30 minutes prior to each dose may reduce flushing. Close monitoring of liver function is warranted due to the risk of niacin-induced hepatitis, which warrants discontinuation of therapy. An escalating dosing schedule can improve tolerability and compliance. Overall, randomized controlled trials found that niacin added to a statin did not reduce morbidity or mortality from CVD. The ACC/AHA does not recommend niacin to prevent or treat heart disease.

7. Omega-3 fatty acids (fish oils)—Omega-3 polyunsaturated fatty acids are used in the treatment of hypertriglyceridemia. Eicosapentaenoic acid (EPA) and docosahexaenoic acid (DHA) are the active compounds and are available over the counter and by prescription. They act through an uncertain mechanism to lower triglyceride levels at doses of 3–4 g/day. Recent studies revealed a reduced risk of cardiovascular total events by 25% and anti-inflammatory effects with patients on a statin medication and omega-3 fatty acid combined. Fish oils are well tolerated at these doses but can prolong the bleeding time. Studies have shown morbidity and mortality benefit in secondary prevention with ingestion of 1 g of fish oil daily. Future studies are addressing the effects of fish oil on primary prevention. Consuming one to two servings of oily fish per week has been shown to reduce the risk of ASCVD in adult patients.

8. Mipomersen—Mipomersen is a subcutaneously administered antisense oligonucleotide that inhibits apo B-100 synthesis in the liver. This in turn reduces levels of circulating VLDL and LDL, and on this basis, mipomersen has been approved by the FDA to treat patients with homozygous FH. Hepatic steatosis and elevated aminotransferase levels have been observed in clinical trials assessing safety.

9. Bempedoic acid—Bempedoic acid inhibits adenosine triphosphate citrate lyase, an enzyme in the cholesterol biosynthesis pathway, to decrease LDL. In statin-intolerant patients, bempedoic acid significantly reduced LDL by 20%. In high-risk CVD patients, bempedoic acid can be used in combination with ezetimibe and statins to further reduced LDL. Adverse side effects of bempedoic acid include effects on serum uric acid, creatinine level, and the incidence of gout. At present, bempedoic acid has no known effect on cardiac outcome.

10. Inclisiran—Inclisiran is an RNA molecule that targets the PCSK9 enzyme. This drug is administered twice a year subcutaneously and has not only shown a reduction in LDL level but also significant reductions in atherogenic lipoproteins and VLDL. A large trial is currently analyzing the effect of inclisiran for preventing major cardiovascular events in patients with ASCVD (ORION-4).

11. LDL apheresis—Despite maximum therapy with a combination of different lipid-lowering drugs, sometimes cholesterol goals cannot be reached. In such patients, treatment with LDL apheresis is indicated. This extracorporeal treatment for LDL-cholesterol elimination can be used in individuals with primary and secondary dyslipoproteinemia. One session of LDL apheresis can drop cholesterol by 50–60% on average but interval treatments are recommended every 7–14 days. Major disadvantages are high costs and increased infection rates. Current research data supports LDL apheresis as an effective treatment option in patients suffering from severe hyperlipidemia refractory of maximum conservative therapy.

F. Treatment in Specific Patient Populations

1. Familial hypercholesterolemia—Those who inherit only one copy of the defective gene (heterozygous FH) may respond well to high-dose statin therapy and diet and lifestyle modification. Newer agents, such as PCSK9 inhibitors and mipomersen, have demonstrated excellent reduction in atherogenic cholesterol subfractions in patients with both homozygous and heterozygous FH. Those with severe forms of the disease may require apheresis.

2. Diabetics—The insulin-resistant state observed in type 2 diabetes mellitus is associated with hypertriglyceridemia as a result of increased circulating free fatty acids and decreased lipolysis. Increases in VLDL, IDL, and LDL levels are observed, in addition to a decrease in HDL levels. Aggressive LDL reduction confers significant improvements in all-cause mortality in patients with type 2 diabetes mellitus as evidenced by the results from the CARE trial, the Heart Protection Study, and the CARDS study. CVD is the most important cause of morbidity and mortality in individuals with type 2 diabetes mellitus. ACC/AHA guidelines emphasize aggressively treating dyslipidemia to achieve an LDL as low as possible to reduce cardiovascular risk in patients with type 2 diabetes mellitus.

3. Stroke—Although an established risk factor for ASCVD, the link between dyslipidemia and cerebrovascular disease and stroke (cerebrovascular accident [CVA]) remains less clear. Regardless, statin therapy has been shown to be beneficial in both primary and secondary prevention. The HPS, CARE, and ASCOT-LLA trials all demonstrated CVA reduction with statin therapy, even in patients with cholesterol levels in the "normal" range. In addition, the SPARCL trial demonstrated that atorvastatin 80 mg daily reduced recurrent ischemic CVA in patients with a prior history of stroke or transient ischemic attack. It appears that the non–cholesterol-lowering benefits of statin therapy play a significant role in CVA reduction. This may explain why other lipid-lowering therapies have not shown CVA risk reduction benefits.

4. Hypothyroidism—Hypothyroidism is commonly associated with hyperlipidemia due to decreased LDL receptor activity and with hypertriglyceridemia due to decreased LPL activity. Patients with dyslipidemia should have their thyroid function assessed. If hypothyroidism is diagnosed, treatment with thyroid replacement therapy will result in improvement in the lipid profile.

Prognosis

Hyperlipidemia remains a strong and treatable risk factor for ASCVD. Major trials have demonstrated the enormous benefit of statin therapy in reducing LDL cholesterol and preventing cardiac events. Current research reveals new lipid targets to lower LDL levels and reduce cardiovascular morbidity. PCSK9 inhibitors have been shown to lower LDL levels by 40–60% and reduce major adverse cardiovascular events in selected high-risk patients. Early findings from the PAC-MAN-AMI trial, have found regression of coronary plaque in patients with a recent myocardial infarction requiring a stent when they receive alirocumab with high-intensity statin.

Effective treatment for elevated triglyceride levels has improved the prognosis for patients with hypertriglyceridemia. Therapies that increase HDL levels are also being studied. CETP inhibitors cannot raise HDL levels, but early trials were halted due to an increase in adverse cardiovascular events. Other agents are currently being studied with promising results. However, although high levels of HDL have been demonstrated to reduce mortality, there is currently no treatment for low HDL levels.

There are active clinical trials to identify additional targets to lower lipids to improve the outcomes of individuals. APOLLO is a phase 1 trial that analyzes a short interfering RNA that reduces Lipoprotein(a) via one subcutaneous injection. Early findings indicate a reduction in Lp(a) levels from 70 to 96%% in the first 5 months and reduction in LDL by 20–25%. Further research needs to be completed to understand the benefits and safety of this class of medication.

Nissen SE, Wolski K, Balog C, et al. Single ascending dose study of a short interfering RNA targeting lipoprotein(a) production in individuals with elevated plasma lipoprotein(a) levels. *JAMA*. 2022;237(17):1679–1687. [PMID: 35368052]. doi:10.1001/jama.2022.5050

Raber L, Ueki Y, Otsuka T, et al. Effect of alirocumb added to high-intensity statin therapy on coronary atherosclerosis in patients with acute myocardial infarction: The PACMAN-AMI Randomized Clinical Trial. *JAMA*. 2022;327(18):1771–1781. [PMID: 35368058]. doi:10.1001/jama.2022.5218

Systemic Hypertension

Wanpen Vongpatanasin, MD

2

ESSENTIALS OF DIAGNOSIS

- Home setting: systolic pressure of ≥ 130 or diastolic pressure of ≥ 80 mm Hg
- 24-hour ambulatory setting:
  - Average 24-hour systolic pressure of ≥ 125 or diastolic pressure of ≥ 75 mm Hg or
  - Average daytime systolic pressure of ≥ 130 or diastolic pressure of ≥ 80 mm Hg
- Office setting:
  - Stage 1 hypertension: systolic pressure of 130–139 mm Hg or diastolic pressure of 80–89 mm Hg
  - Stage 2 hypertension: systolic pressure of at least 140 mm Hg or diastolic pressure of at least 90 mm Hg

General Considerations

Hypertension is a major public health problem in the United States and many countries worldwide. Since the American Heart Association/American College of Cardiology has reduced threshold for diagnosis of hypertension and treatment targets to systolic blood pressure (BP) of 130 mm Hg and diastolic BP of 80 mm Hg, prevalence of hypertension in the United States has risen to at 47%. Similarly, prevalence of resistant hypertension (failure to achieve BP control despite three or more medications that included inhibitors of renin-angiotensin system, calcium channel blockers, and a diuretic) has increased to 20% among treated population. When the risk is calculated over lifetime, the burden of hypertension in middle-aged men and women is enormous. Eight to nine out of 10 normotensive women or men older than 55 years are expected to develop hypertension in the next 20 years. Thus, complete understanding of basic pathophysiologic mechanisms and treatment strategies is one crucial step in improving hypertension control.

Pathophysiology & Etiology

Pathophysiology of primary hypertension is complex and heterogeneous. At least one or more of the mechanisms involved in BP regulation, such as vascular, neural, renal, and hormonal mechanisms, contribute to development of primary hypertension. Accordingly, therapy often requires more than one antihypertensive agent or approach to tackle hypertension in the majority of patients.

Systemic vascular resistance and cardiac output are two major determinants of BP. Thus, augmented peripheral vasoconstriction at the level of resistance vessels may lead to hypertension in the presence of normal cardiac output. More recently, large arterial stiffness has been shown to contribute to elevated systolic BP. In many epidemiologic studies, systolic BP increases with age both in men and women. However, after the fifth decade of life, systolic BP continues to increase while diastolic BP starts to fall, causing the pulse pressure to widen. Normally, elasticity of aorta helps absorb pressure during systole, and the elastic recoil of the aorta helps maintain BP during diastole. The loss of aortic elasticity causes BP to rise excessively during systole and decrease markedly during diastole. Furthermore, the aortic pulse wave travels at much faster speed in the stiff artery, and the reflected wave from the peripheral sites further amplifies the systolic BP in the central aorta. Although diastolic BP is traditionally thought to be the most important predictor of cardiovascular risk, it is an important risk factor only for the younger population. For hypertensive patients above the age of 60, systolic BP and pulse pressures are much more important in predicting long-term cardiovascular outcomes.

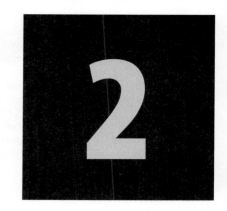

Neural control of BP also plays an important role in development of hypertension. Overactivity of the sympathetic nervous system has been identified in patients with uncomplicated essential hypertension, and many conditions predispose to hypertension such as obesity, renal failure, and obstructive sleep apnea. Sympathetic overactivity contributes to hypertension by stimulating increase in cardiac output while producing peripheral vasoconstriction. Activation of β_1-adrenergic receptor by norepinephrine released from the sympathetic nerve terminals further increases BP by increasing renin release, causing renal sodium retention. The major hormones that contribute to hypertension include the renin-angiotensin-aldosterone system (RAAS), which will be discussed later in the section on secondary causes of hypertension. Although RAAS triggers hypertension by promoting renal sodium absorption, a large body of evidence from animal experiments suggests that its direct action on the vascular system and the central nervous system further augments hypertension.

Clinical Findings

A. BP Measurement

Proper BP measurement is essential in the diagnosis and treatment of hypertension. BP monitoring should be done both at home and in the clinic.

1. Clinic BP—In the clinical setting, BP measurement should be performed after patients are sitting quietly for at least 5 minutes with the arm supported at the heart level. The bladder of the cuff should encircle more than 80% of the arm, and the width should be about 40% of the arm length. Medical personnel who perform the measurement should avoid talking to the patients during BP measurement because mental stimulation may inadvertently increase BP up to 10–15 mm Hg. Cuff should be inflated 20 mm Hg above systolic BP before deflation, and a minimum of two readings should be obtained at an interval of at least 1 minute. If BP differs by more than 5 mm Hg between the two readings, an additional one or two readings should be taken. During the initial visit, BP should be taken from both arms to exclude subtle stenosis in the subclavian or brachial artery, which could lead to underestimation of actual BP and undertreatment of hypertension. In patients with early onset of hypertension prior to the age of 40, BP should also be obtained from at least one leg to screen for aortic coarctation. In elderly patients and patients with diabetes mellitus or other conditions that predispose to autonomic failure such as Parkinson disease, BP should also be taken after 3 minutes of standing to exclude presence of orthostatic hypotension.

2. Home and ambulatory BP monitoring—Home BP measurement should be encouraged in all hypertensive patients because it may reveal different values from the clinic BP measurement. *White-coat effect* (WCE) is defined as presence of elevated office BP but normal out-of-office BP in treated hypertensive patients, whereas the term *white-coat hypertension* is restricted to the same phenomenon observed in the untreated population.

By contrast, presence of elevated home BP but normal clinic BP (< 130/80 mm Hg) is the phenomenon observed in *masked hypertension*, which has been identified in 20–25% of the general U.S. population. Both masked hypertension and white-coat hypertension are associated with cardiovascular complications compared to the population with normal BP both at home and in the clinic. Because out-of-office BP consistently predicts cardiovascular events independent of clinic BP, most hypertension guidelines have now recommended obtaining measurements of either home or 24-hour BP monitoring to confirm diagnosis of hypertension before initiating drug treatment. Home BP monitoring (HBPM) is more widely available than 24-hour BP monitoring. However, accurate device selection is an important part of HBPM. The list of validated BP devices can be obtained from several sources, including validatebp.org or stridebp.org.

Tientcheu D, Ayers C, Das SR, et al. Target organ complications and cardiovascular events associated with masked hypertension and white-coat hypertension: analysis from the Dallas Heart Study. *J Am Coll Cardiol.* 2015;66:2159–2169. [PMID: 26564592]

Whelton P, Carey RM, Aronow WS, et al. Guideline for the Prevention, Detection, Evaluation, and Management of High Blood Pressure in Adults: Executive Summary: a report of the American College of Cardiology/American Heart Association Task Force on Clinical Practice Guidelines. *Circulation.* 2018; 138:e426–e483. [PMID: 30354655]

B. Symptoms & Signs

Hypertension is well known as a silent killer because most patients remain asymptomatic until development of target organ damage. However, some patients may have symptoms that could be related to a secondary cause of hypertension. Snoring and daytime somnolence may signify presence of obstructive sleep apnea, whereas episodes of palpitation and paroxysmal hypertension may suggest pheochromocytoma. Presence of muscle weakness, polyuria, and polydipsia might be related to hypokalemia from primary aldosteronism (PA) or hypercortisolism. Other symptoms of target organ damage and other coronary risk factors should be assessed because they help to define BP threshold for treatment of hypertension. History taking should also include the onset of hypertension and prior antihypertensive treatment as well as history of side effects from previous medications. The concomitant use of other prescription or nonprescription drugs, such as herbal products, nonsteroidal anti-inflammatory drugs, or decongestant use, stimulant drugs for treatment of attention-deficit hyperactivity disorder, which can directly increase BP or interfere with efficacy of antihypertensive medications, should be obtained. In young premenopausal women, method of contraception should be documented because certain antihypertensive medications, such as angiotensin-converting enzyme inhibitors (ACEIs) or angiotensin receptor blockers (ARBs), are teratogenic or fetotoxic. Furthermore, oral contraceptives could cause hypertension in a small number of patients, although the absolute risk is lower than 0.1% with low-dose estrogen preparation. Detailed family history with specific attention to both hypertension and stroke should be obtained because early stroke could be a presenting feature in certain genetic forms of hypertension.

High sodium intake is also a major contributor for uncontrolled hypertension. The major source of dietary sodium is processed foods rather than table salt. Accordingly, a detailed dietary assessment should be obtained in patients who fail to achieve BP goals despite multiple medications. Nonadherence to medications is the major cause of apparently resistant hypertension and should be considered in patients on a complex multidrug regimen. Questions related to adherence should not be asked in the manner that sounds judgmental or critical to the patients; otherwise, accurate assessment may not be obtained. Instead of asking, "Do you take medications regularly as the doctors prescribe?", asking patients if they feel that taking multiple medications is difficult or if they have forgotten to take medications in the past 7 days is more likely to uncover a history of nonadherence.

C. Physical Examination

Physical examination should focus on signs of target organ damage such as presence of volume overload, laterally displaced apical impulses, S_3 and/or S_4 gallops, and hypertensive retinopathy. Particular attention should be paid to physical signs that may indicate underlying secondary hypertension. Abdominal bruit may indicate presence of renal artery stenosis. Truncal obesity, dorsocervical fat pads, hirsutism, and abdominal striae may represent cortisol excess. BP gradient between arms and legs and femoral-radial pulse delay may signify coarctation of aorta.

D. Diagnostic Studies

For patients with mild uncomplicated hypertension, serum electrolytes, urinalysis, and complete blood cell count should be obtained during the initial visit to assess renal function and exclude subtle target organ damage. Electrocardiogram should be obtained to screen for left ventricular hypertrophy and presence of conduction system disturbances, which may prohibit the use of β-blockers or nondihydropyridine calcium channel blockers. Echocardiography should be limited to patients with symptoms and signs of congestive heart failure or patients with syncope to exclude presence of dynamic left ventricular outflow tract obstruction, which has been identified in a subset of hypertensive patients with concentric left ventricular hypertrophy. Fasting lipid panel and plasma glucose should also be obtained to assess overall cardiovascular risks. Microalbuminuria should be tested in diabetic patients and patients with severe hypertension. Serum levels of antihypertensive drugs should be considered in patients who appear to be resistant to antihypertensive medications, but are also suspected to be nonadherent to medications, particularly when the pill count and pharmacy data are inconclusive. In the United States, the assays for most antihypertensive drugs are now available in clinical practice and covered by most health insurance plans.

Choudhry NK, Kronish IM, Vongpatanasin W, et al. Medication adherence and blood pressure control: a scientific statement from the American Heart Association. *Hypertension*. 2022 Jan; 79(1):e1–e14. [PMID: 34615363]

Differential Diagnosis

In most patients with hypertension, specific etiology cannot be identified, and patients are often labeled as having essential or primary hypertension. However, in approximately 5–10% of unselected patients with hypertension and 10–20% of all resistant hypertensive cases, causes of hypertension are identifiable and/or potentially reversible. Screening for secondary causes of hypertension is not indicated in every patient with hypertension. Indications for additional workup are as follows:

- Abrupt onset after the age of 55 or before the age of 30
- Accelerated or malignant hypertension with grade 3–4 retinopathy
- Previously, but not presently, controlled hypertension
- Poorly controlled hypertension on three or more drugs
- Recurrent flash pulmonary edema
- Hypertension with unexplained renal insufficiency
- Suspected clinical features of secondary causes such as hypokalemia, renal bruits, and truncal obesity

Common secondary causes of resistant hypertension include obstructive sleep apnea, PA, renal parenchymal diseases, and renal artery stenosis. Pheochromocytoma and other endocrine disorders are much less common causes of resistant hypertension.

A. Obstructive Sleep Apnea

Obstructive sleep apnea (OSA) is a well-established independent risk factor for the development of hypertension. Because the majority of the population in the United States is overweight or obese, OSA is now a common condition, affecting 10–20% of the population in the United States. Prevalence of OSA in drug-resistant hypertension is much greater, as high as 83% in some studies. Activation of the sympathetic nervous system via activation of chemoreceptor via repetitive hypoxia and hypercapnia is thought to play an important role in the pathogenesis of hypertension. Patients with a history of loud snoring, insomnia, and/or daytime fatigue should undergo polysomnography. Treatment with continuous positive airway pressure (CPAP) has been shown to reduce BP in hypertensive patients with OSA. However, long-term compliance is poor; less than 50% of patients continue to use CPAP after 6 months. Therefore, target BP is rarely achieved with CPAP alone, and further adjustment of antihypertensive medications is often needed to reach target goals. Hypoglossal nerve stimulation via an implantable neurostimulator device is a treatment option for OSA patients who are unable to tolerate OSA but its efficacy on BP reduction is less well established.

B. Primary Aldosteronism

Aldosterone excess, either from idiopathic bilateral adrenal hyperplasia or aldosterone-producing adenoma, is a common cause of resistant hypertension. PA has been identified in 5–10% of unselected patients with hypertension in the primary care setting, and up to 20% of patients with resistant hypertension referred to a hypertension clinic or a tertiary care center. Aldosterone induces hypertension not only by increasing renal sodium retention, but also by activation of the sympathetic nervous system. Patients with PA experienced higher cardiovascular event rates than those with essential hypertension that is out of proportion to the degree of BP elevation. This is likely to be related to direct cardiovascular toxicity of aldosterone. To screen for PA, plasma renin activity (PRA) or levels and serum aldosterone levels should be obtained. A screening test may be performed during treatment with thiazide diuretics, ACEIs, and ARBs but not during treatment with direct renin inhibitors or mineralocorticoid receptor antagonists (MRAs). However, all these agents should be discontinued for at least 3 weeks during confirmatory test with either oral salt loading test or intravenous saline suppression test. During the workup period, patients need to be on other antihypertensive agents such as α-blockers or calcium channel blockers. If needed, β-blockers or central sympatholytic drugs may be added, but this may potentially reduce PRA. If screening tests reveal suppressed renin levels or activity in the presence of elevated serum aldosterone levels of at least 15 ng/dL, a confirmatory test (oral salt loading test or intravenous saline suppression test) is warranted. Confirmatory tests may be omitted in some patients with severe elevation in serum aldosterone level of more than 20 ng/dL in the setting of renin suppression and hypokalemia since this laboratory pattern is not present in other conditions other than PA. Patients who have insuppressible aldosterone levels after salt loading should undergo adrenal vein sampling because imaging of adrenal glands is not reliable in separating patients with idiopathic hyperplasia from those with aldosterone-producing adenoma. Treatment includes surgical resection of tumor for patients with aldosterone-producing adenoma, which can cure hypertension in 20–60% of patients, depending on duration of hypertension and presence of target organ complications. MRAs (spironolactone or eplerenone) should be used in patients with bilateral hyperplasia or patients with unilateral adenoma in whom surgical risks are prohibitive.

C. Renal Parenchymal Disease

Renal parenchymal disease could be a cause or a consequence of hypertension. Hypertension is very common in chronic kidney disease (CKD) and is much more difficult to control. Despite the requirement for larger numbers of antihypertensive medications, the hypertension control rate in the United States in CKD patients is less than 30% compared with 50% in non-CKD patients. Hypertension related to renal parenchymal disease has traditionally been viewed as being largely volume-dependent due to the failing kidney's inability to excrete salt and water. However, increased systemic vascular resistance from overactivation of the sympathetic nervous system has also been identified in most patients.

D. Renovascular Hypertension

Renovascular hypertension is another common cause of secondary hypertension, accounting for 5–7% of hypertension in patients older than 60 years. Atherosclerosis is the major form of renal artery pathology in the elderly, as fibromuscular dysplasia is seen predominantly in young adults. Screening for renovascular hypertension should be considered in patients with (1) onset of hypertension at less than 30 years of age or abrupt onset of hypertension after 55 years of age; (2) accelerated or malignant hypertension; (3) unexplained atrophic kidney or size discrepancy of more than 1.5 cm between each kidney; (4) sudden, unexplained pulmonary edema; (5) unexplained renal dysfunction, including individuals starting renal replacement therapy; and (6) development of new azotemia or worsening renal function after administration of an ACEI or ARB. Imaging of renal arteries with computed tomography (CT) angiography or magnetic resonance angiography should also be obtained in patients with suspected renal artery stenosis. Unfortunately, no currently available invasive or noninvasive studies are sufficiently sensitive or specific in assessing functional significance of a given stenotic lesion or in predicting BP pressure control after revascularization. Renal artery revascularization leads to significant and sustained reduction in BP in patients with fibromuscular dysplasia but has minimal effect on BP control (< 2 mm Hg) and progression of renal disease in patients with atherosclerotic renal artery stenosis. Therefore, revascularization should be considered in most patients with fibromuscular dysplasia and selected patients with atherosclerotic renal artery stenosis plus one or more of the following features: (1) bilateral disease or stenosis of the unilateral functioning kidney; (2) rapid decline in renal function; (3) resistant hypertension despite three or more antihypertensive medications; or (4) recurrent pulmonary edema.

Cooper CJ, Murphy TP, Cutlip DE, et al. Stenting and medical therapy for atherosclerotic renal-artery stenosis. *N Engl J Med.* 2014;370:13–22. [PMID: 24245566]

E. Pheochromocytoma

Although a screening test for pheochromocytoma is often done in patients with labile hypertension or resistant hypertension, it accounts for less than 1% of patients with unselected hypertension. Patients may present with paroxysmal hypertension, palpitation from sinus tachycardia or supraventricular arrhythmia, and panic/anxiety sensation from catecholamine excess. Myocardial infarction, congestive heart failure, and Takotsubo-like cardiomyopathy may be the presenting symptoms, along with hypertension in some patients. Diagnosis requires demonstration of elevated plasma/urinary metanephrines (metanephrine and/or normetanephrine) above 3–4 times the upper limit of normal without other identifiable causes. Patients with paraganglioma or extra-adrenal tumor may have isolated elevation in plasma dopamine, and thus, a plasma catecholamines panel (epinephrine, norepinephrine, and dopamine) should be obtained in patients with suspected pheochromocytoma in the absence of adrenal mass. Borderline elevation in plasma metanephrines or catecholamines is common in hypertensive patients with underlying conditions that cause sympathetic overactivity such as OSA, congestive heart failure, or CKD. These levels may return to normal after correction of the underlying problems. A clonidine suppression test should be obtained in patients with persistent but borderline (less than twofold) elevation in plasma metanephrines or catecholamines to confirm diagnosis. CT or magnetic resonance imaging (MRI) of the abdomen should be used to localize tumor after biochemical confirmation. Metaiodobenzylguanidine scan should be used when CT or MRI fails to reveal tumor.

Lenders JWM, Kerstens MN, Amar L, et al. Genetics, diagnosis, management and future directions of research of phaeochromocytoma and paraganglioma: a position statement and consensus of the Working Group on Endocrine Hypertension of the European Society of Hypertension. *J Hypertens.* 2020; 38(8):1443–1456.

Treatment

A. Lifestyle Modification

Lifestyle modifications include sodium restriction to less than 1.5–2 g/day. The major source of sodium consumed in the United States comes from processed food including bread and rolls, pasta, cured meat, and snacks. Table salt contributes to only 20% of total sodium consumed. Avoiding table salt alone will not be an effective strategy in limiting sodium intake, and educating patients to read nutritional labels is a key to success. A diet rich in fruits and vegetables also reduces BP independent of sodium content. Replacing salt with salt substitute is another effective strategy in reducing BP and risk of stroke.

B. Pharmacologic Intervention

Antihypertensive treatment should be initiated in patients with stage 1 uncomplicated hypertension who fail a trial of lifestyle modification alone. Pharmacologic intervention should be offered promptly without any delay for patients with stage 2 hypertension or those with stage 1 hypertension in the presence of target organ complication, diabetes mellitus, renal failure, or high cardiovascular risks in conjunction with lifestyle modification. The list of antihypertensive drugs available in the United States is shown in Table 2–1.

1. Diuretics—Thiazide diuretics are the first-line drug therapy for hypertension by many hypertension guidelines due to their efficacy in reducing BP and low cost. Thiazide diuretics promote natriuresis by inhibiting sodium chloride cotransport at the distal convoluted tubule. Among thiazide diuretics, chlorthalidone has the longest half-life of between 40 and 60 hours compared to 8–15 hours for hydrochlorothiazide. Head-to-head comparison studies showed that chlorthalidone is at least two times more potent than hydrochlorothiazide in reducing BP. Chlorthalidone is effective in reducing BP even among patients with stage IV CKD (eGFR 15–30 mL/min/1.73 m^2). Thiazide diuretics are known to cause several metabolic side effects such as hypokalemia, elevated uric acid, increased fasting triglyceride, and, most importantly, increased risk of diabetes mellitus. Thiazide-induced dysglycemia or insulin resistance is mediated both by hypokalemia and potassium-independent mechanisms, which can be minimized by concomitant administration of the mineralocorticoid receptor (MR) antagonist spironolactone and inhibition of the epithelial sodium channels by amiloride (see later).

Loop diuretics promote diuresis by inhibiting $Na^+/K^+/Cl^-$ cotransport at the thick ascending limb of Henle's loop. Although loop diuretics are more potent as diuretic agents than thiazide diuretics, the short half-life limits their efficacy in reducing BP. Furosemide has a half-life of only 1.5–2.5 hours and should be given every 6 hours to have sustained effects on BP; hence the brand name "Lasix." Thus, it is not recommended for treatment of hypertensive patients with normal renal function. However, it is useful for patients with fluid retention from congestive heart failure, renal failure, or nephrotic syndrome. Among loop diuretics, furosemide has the least predictable absorption, whereas torsemide has the longest half-life.

MR antagonists, such as spironolactone and eplerenone, are known to reduce BP by inhibiting MR-dependent activation of the epithelial sodium channel in the cortical collecting duct. Furthermore, inhibition of the sympathetic nervous system and improvement in vascular endothelial function are thought to contribute to the BP-lowering effects of this class of drugs. MR antagonists are effective in lowering BP when either used alone or as add-on therapy for resistant hypertension despite use of three or more drugs. On a milligram-to-milligram basis, eplerenone is less potent than spironolactone in reducing BP in both patients with primary hypertension and patients with PA, and thus, at least a twofold higher dose is often required to achieve BP control. However, spironolactone carries antiandrogenic side effects, including gynecomastia and testicular atrophy, and long-term use at the dose of more than 25 mg/day should be avoided in men. In these patients, the use of eplerenone, which has more than 100-fold lower affinity to androgen receptors than MRs, is preferable. Hyperkalemia

Table 2–1. Antihypertensive Drugs Available in the United States

Drug	Dose Range, Total mg/day (doses per day)
Diuretics	
Thiazide diuretics	
Hydrochlorothiazide (HCTZ)	6.25–50 (1)
Chlorthalidone	6.25–25 (1)
Indapamide	1.25–5 (1)
Metolazone	2.5–10 (1)
Loop diuretics	
Furosemide	20–160 (2)
Torsemide	2.5–80 (1–2)
Bumetanide	0.5–2 (2)
Ethacrynic acid	25–100 (2)
Potassium-sparing diuretics	
Amiloride	5–20 (1)
Triamterene	25–100 (1)
Spironolactone	12.5–400 (1–2)
Eplerenone	25–100 (1–2)
β-Blockers	
Acebutolol	200–800 (2)
Atenolol	25–100 (1)
Betaxolol	5–20 (1)
Bisoprolol	2.5–20 (1)
Carteolol	2.5–10 (1)
Metoprolol	50–450 (2)
Metoprolol XL	50–200 (1–2)
Nadolol	20–320 (1)
Nebivolol	5–20 (1)
Penbutolol	10–80 (1)
Pindolol	10–60 (2)
Propranolol	40–180 (2)
Propranolol LA	60–180 (1–2)
Timolol	20–60 (2)
β/α-Blockers	
Labetalol	200–2400 (2)
Carvedilol	6.25–50 (2)
Calcium Channel Blockers	
Dihydropyridines	
Amlodipine	2.5–10 (1)
Felodipine	2.5–20 (1–2)
Isradipine CR	2.5–20 (2)
Nicardipine SR	30–120 (2)
Nifedipine XL	30–120 (1)
Nisoldipine	10–40 (1–2)
Nondihydropyridines	
Diltiazem CD	120–540 (1)
Verapamil HS	120–480 (1)
Angiotensin-Converting Enzyme Inhibitors	
Benazepril	10–80 (1–2)
Captopril	25–150 (2)
Enalapril	2.5–40 (2)
Fosinopril	10–80 (1–2)
Lisinopril	5–80 (1–2)
Moexipril	7.5–30 (1)
Perindopril	4–16 (1)
Quinapril	5–80 (1–2)
Ramipril	2.5–20 (1)
Trandolapril	1–8 (1)
Angiotensin Receptor Blockers	
Azilsartan	40–80 (1)
Candesartan	8–32 (1)
Eprosartan	400–800 (1–2)
Irbesartan	150–300 (1–2)
Losartan	25–100 (2)
Olmesartan	5–40 (1)
Telmisartan	20–80 (1)
Valsartan	80–320 (1–2)
Direct Renin Inhibitors	
Aliskiren	75–300 (1)
α-Blockers	
Doxazosin	1–16 (1)
Prazosin	1–40 (2–3)
Terazosin	1–20 (1)
Phenoxybenzamine	20–120 (2) for pheochromocytoma
Central Sympatholytics	
Clonidine	0.2–1.2 (2–3)
Clonidine patch	0.1–0.6 (weekly)
Guanabenz	2–32 (2)
Guanfacine	1–3 (1) (q hs)
Methyldopa	250–1000 (2)
Reserpine	0.05–0.25 (1)
Direct Vasodilators	
Hydralazine	10–200 (2)
Minoxidil	2.5–100 (1)
Fixed-Dose Combinations	
Aliskiren/HCTZ	75–300/12.5–25 (1)
Aliskiren/valsartan	150–300/160–320 (1)
Amiloride/HCTZ	5/50 (1)
Amlodipine/benazepril	2.5–5/10–20 (1)
Amlodipine/olmesartan	5–10/20–40 (1)
Amlodipine/valsartan	5–10/160–320 (1)
Amlodipine/valsartan/HCTZ	5–10/160–320/12.5–25
Atenolol/chlorthalidone	50–100/25 (1)
Azilsartan/chlorthalidone	40–80/25 (1)
Benazepril/HCTZ	5–20/6.25–25 (1)
Bisoprolol/HCTZ	2.5–10/6.25 (1)
Candesartan/HCTZ	16–32/12.5–25 (1)
Enalapril/HCTZ	5–10/25 (1–2)
Eprosartan/HCTZ	600/12.5–25 (1)
Fosinopril/HCTZ	10–20/12.5 (1)
Irbesartan/HCTZ	15–30/12.5–25 (1)
Losartan/HCTZ	50–100/12.5–25 (1)
Olmesartan/HCTZ	20–40/12.5 (1)
Spironolactone/HCTZ	25/25 (0.5–1)
Telmisartan/HCTZ	40–80/12.5–25 (1)
Trandolapril/verapamil	2–4/180–240 (1)
Triamterene/HCTZ	37.5/25 (0.5–1)
Valsartan/HCTZ	80–160/12.5–25 (1)

is the main side effect of both agents, and serum potassium should be closely monitored in patients with CKD, diabetic patients with hyporeninemic hypoaldosteronism, or those on concomitant treatment with ACEIs, ARBs, or nonsteroidal anti-inflammatory agents. MR antagonists have been shown to reduce mortality in patients with systolic heart failure even with mild symptoms, and they should be considered in treatment of hypertension in patients with impaired ventricular function.

In addition to MR antagonists, direct inhibitors of the epithelial sodium channels (ENaCs), such as amiloride and triamterene, are also effective in lowering BP in patients with low-renin essential hypertension. They are particularly useful in patients with gain-in-function mutation in the ENaC, causing excessive renal sodium absorption and renal potassium wasting, known as Liddle syndrome. Amiloride is also useful in patients with PA who cannot tolerate MR antagonists. Both amiloride and triamterene are often used in a combination pill formulation with hydrochlorothiazide (see Table 2–1).

Brown MJ, Williams B, Morant SV, et al. Effect of amiloride, or amiloride plus hydrochlorothiazide, versus hydrochlorothiazide on glucose tolerance and blood pressure (PATHWAY-3): a parallel-group, double-blind randomised phase 4 trial. *Lancet Diabetes Endocrinol.* 2016;4(2):136–147. [PMID: 26489809]

Vongpatanasin W. Hydrochlorothiazide is not the most useful nor versatile thiazide diuretic. *Curr Opin Cardiol.* 2015;30(4): 361–365. [PMID: 26049382]

2. ACEIs—ACEIs reduce BP by inhibiting conversion of angiotensin (Ang) I to potent vasoconstrictor Ang II. ACEIs also prevent degradation of the vasodilator bradykinin, which further contributes to BP reduction. ACEIs are particularly effective in reducing BP in younger patients and Caucasians and tend to be less effective in the setting of the low-renin form of hypertension frequently observed in the elderly and Black populations. However, the combination of ACEIs with diuretics eliminates racial and age differences in BP response to ACEIs. In addition to BP reduction, ACEIs reduce mortality in patients with congestive heart failure and improve cardiovascular outcomes in high-risk hypertensive patients without heart failure. ACEIs also slow the decline in renal function in patients with diabetic and nondiabetic kidney disease. Thus, they should be used in hypertensive patients with these comorbid conditions. The main side effects of this class of drugs are cough and angioedema from presumably excessive bradykinin accumulation. Hyperkalemia is another side effect, which may limit its use in some patients with severe CKD or bilateral renal artery stenosis.

3. ARBs—ARBs reduce BP by blocking the vasoconstrictor effects of Ang II on angiotensin receptor subtype 1 (AT1R) in the vascular smooth muscle. This class of drugs has remarkably minimal side effects and is generally well tolerated. It avoids side effects of cough and angioedema associated with ACEIs. In placebo-controlled clinical trials, ARBs reduced mortality in patients with systolic heart failure who were intolerant to ACEIs and offered renal protection in patients with diabetic nephropathy. Thus, they should be considered as part of regimen in hypertensive patients with these clinical features. The combination of ARBs with maximal doses of ACEIs usually yields minimal additional BP reduction and is generally not helpful in improving cardiovascular mortality. Although combination therapy offers synergistic or additive effect in reducing proteinuria, dual renin-angiotensin system blockade is associated with more renal dysfunction than either class of drugs alone. Therefore, it is not recommended as a strategy to control BP in hypertensive patients and should be reserved only for patients with proteinuria from primary renal disease such as immunoglobulin A nephropathy.

4. Calcium channel blockers (CCBs)—CCBs are divided into two major classes: the dihydropyridine (DHP) and nondihydropyridine (non-DHP) CCBs. DHP CCBs include amlodipine, felodipine, nisoldipine, and nicardipine and cause peripheral vasodilation with minimal effects on the heart rate or myocardial contractility. By contrast, non-DHP CCBs (diltiazem and verapamil) exert negative inotropic and chronotropic effects. Non-DHP CCBs are contraindicated in patients with systolic heart failure because of increased cardiovascular mortality and should be avoided in patients with symptomatic bradyarrhythmias or advanced heart block. DHP CCBs have neutral effect on survival in congestive heart failure and may be considered if BP remains elevated despite ACEIs or ARBs in systolic heart failure. All CCBs increase myocardial blood flow and are antianginal. Meta-analysis of clinical trials showed that CCBs are more effective than ACEIs in preventing stroke beyond BP reduction, but less effective than ACEIs and ARBs in preventing coronary heart disease or heart failure. DHP CCBs preferentially dilate afferent arterioles, causing an increase in intraglomerular hypertension, and are not as effective as ACEIs or ARBs in preventing decline in renal function in diabetic or nondiabetic kidney diseases. Therefore, they should not be used without RAAS blockade in hypertensive patients with CKD.

5. β-Adrenergic receptor blockers (BBs)—BBs reduce BP by decreasing heart rate and myocardial contractility, leading to decreased cardiac output at least initially via inhibition of β_1-adrenergic receptors (AR). Inhibition of renin release from the juxtaglomerular cells via β_1-AR and reduction of norepinephrine release from sympathetic nerve terminals via inhibition of presynaptic β_2-AR also contribute to BP reduction. BBs are divided into two major classes: selective (β_1-specific) and nonselective (β_1- and β_2-AR blockers), as shown in Table 2–2. Activation of β_2-AR leads to peripheral vasodilation and bronchodilation. Thus, nonselective BBs should not be used in patients with asthma or in the setting of sympathetic overactivity, such as clonidine withdrawal or cocaine intoxication because of unopposed α-AR–mediated vasoconstriction. However, selectivity to β_1 versus β_2 is dose-dependent and not an all-or-none phenomenon. At higher

Table 2–2. Selective Versus Nonselective β-Adrenergic Receptor Blockers

Nonselective (ratio β_1:β_2 selectivity)	Selective (ratio β_1:β_2 selectivity)
Propranolol (1:8)	Atenolol (5–10:1)
Carvedilol (1:4–5)	Acebutolol (2:1)
Labetalol (1:2–3)	Metoprolol (2–4:1)
Nadolol (1:23)	Bisoprolol (14:1)
	Esmolol (76:1)
	Nebivolol (320:1)

doses, even selective BBs such as metoprolol, bisoprolol, atenolol, or esmolol may cause bronchospasm and should be used with caution. Certain BBs exert direct vasodilating effects, which enhance antihypertensive efficacy independent of β-AR blockade. For example, labetalol and carvedilol exert α-AR–blocking properties, whereas nebivolol promotes nitric oxide release and possesses antioxidant properties. Although BBs reduce mortality in patients with systolic heart failure and myocardial infarction, older generation BBs, particularly atenolol, are not as effective as other classes of drugs in preventing stroke or all-cause mortality in hypertensive patients with cardiovascular diseases. Thus, atenolol should not be used as initial therapy in patients with uncomplicated essential hypertension, particularly in patients with low-renin hypertension, elderly patients, or Blacks.

6. α-AR blockers—α-AR blockers exert antihypertensive effect by inhibiting postsynaptic α_1-ARs in the vascular smooth muscle. α-AR blockers that selectively inhibit α_1-AR antagonists include prazosin, terazosin, and doxazosin, whereas the nonselective blockers, which inhibit both α_1- and α_2-ARs, include phentolamine and phenoxybenzamine. Side effects of α-blockers are orthostatic hypotension, nasal congestion, and volume expansion. Nonselective α-blockers tend to cause more tachycardia because of inhibition of presynaptic α_2-ARs, which normally exert inhibitory influence on norepinephrine release from sympathetic nerve terminals. α-Blockers should not be used as first-line therapy for hypertension because of increased risk of congestive heart failure. However, they are useful as an adjunctive treatment as the fourth- or fifth-line agent when BP fails to reach target goal. They should be considered as the first line of treatment in the setting of pheochromocytoma and are also useful in patients with hypertension related to cocaine intoxication or conditions associated with sympathetic overactivity such as drug or alcohol withdrawal.

7. Central sympatholytic drugs—Central sympatholytic drugs reduce BP mainly by stimulating presynaptic α_2-ARs in the brainstem centers and sympathetic nerve terminals, thereby inhibiting sympathetic nerve discharge and neuronal release of norepinephrine to the heart and peripheral circulation. Drugs in this class include methyldopa, clonidine, guanfacine, and guanabenz. Moxonidine and rilmenidine are also centrally acting drugs used in England and other European countries but are not available in the United States. α-Methyldopa is converted to α-methylnorepinephrine to activate central α_2-ARs in the brainstem, whereas clonidine, guanfacine, and guanabenz are direct α_2-AR agonists. In contrast, moxonidine and rilmenidine predominantly reduce sympathetic nerve activity and BP by stimulating the imidazoline-1 (I_1) receptor, rather than α_2-AR. Because of several major side effects, including fatigue, sedation, and dry mouth, as well as lack of clear-cut cardiovascular benefit, these drugs should be used as fourth-line drug therapy for hypertension. Central sympatholytic drug use should be avoided in patients who are nonadherent to treatment because of precipitation of withdrawal symptoms on abrupt drug discontinuation. Their use on an as-needed basis for treatment of episodes of asymptomatic BP surge in patients who are not on regular dosing of central α_2-AR agonists should also be discouraged due to rebound hypertension.

8. Direct renin inhibitors (DRIs)—DRIs block catalytic action of circulating renin, thereby preventing formation of Ang I from angiotensinogen. DRIs also inhibit activity of the proenzyme prorenin, which can also cleave angiotensinogen into Ang I on binding to the prorenin receptors. Inhibitory action of DRIs on renin and prorenin activity results in decreased production of Ang II and BP. Aliskiren is the only drug approved for clinical use in this class so far. Addition of aliskiren to ARBs reduces proteinuria in hypertensive patients with type 2 diabetes mellitus when compared to placebo. However, addition of aliskiren to ARBs or ACEIs is not more effective in reducing left ventricular (LV) mass in hypertensive patients or improving LV remodeling in patients after myocardial infarction than monotherapy with ARBs or ACEIs alone. Furthermore, a recent clinical trial showed that addition of aliskiren to ACEIs or ARBs in patients with diabetes mellitus and established cardiovascular disease failed to improve cardiovascular outcomes and even increased the risk of nonfatal stroke. Thus, the future role of DRIs in the treatment of hypertension is likely to be limited.

9. Direct vasodilators—Hydralazine and minoxidil are the two main drugs in this class; they reduce BP by dilating resistant arterioles with minimal or no effect on the venous circulation. Hydralazine has short plasma half-life of 90 minutes, but its antihypertensive action lasts much longer than its plasma level. Thus, for the ease of administration, hydralazine should be given twice daily in hypertensive patients rather than three times a day, which is the schedule typically used in patients with heart failure. Side effects of hydralazine include lupus-like syndrome, particularly at the higher doses, reflex tachycardia, nausea, vomiting, and diarrhea. Minoxidil promotes vasodilation by activating adenosine triphosphate–sensitive potassium channels in the vascular smooth muscle. Like hydralazine, minoxidil-induced BP reduction is usually accompanied by reflex tachycardia and palpitation, and the addition of BBs is often needed to mitigate these side effects. Peripheral edema and volume expansion frequently occur, requiring concomitant diuretic treatment. Less common side effects include hirsutism and pericardial effusion.

Oral nitrates are nitric oxide donors, which produce venodilating effects at low doses and arterial vasodilating effects at higher doses. In elderly patients with resistant systolic hypertension, isosorbide mononitrate predominantly reduces systolic BP without affecting diastolic BP. However, isosorbide mononitrate should be avoided in hypertensive patients with heart failure and preserved ejection because of its modest antihypertensive effect (< 5 mm Hg) and increased side effect of reduced daily activity.

C. Management of Uncomplicated Hypertension

In most patients, the goal BP should be less than 140/90 mm Hg. Tight control of systolic BP below 120 mm Hg reduces the risk of stroke by 40% in patients with diabetes mellitus. Tight control of systolic BP below 120 mm Hg also reduces cardiovascular death and all-cause mortality in hypertensive patients with high cardiovascular risks or CKD. The benefit of lower target systolic BP is observed even in elderly patients older than 75 years with high cardiovascular risks or CKD. In patients with mild uncomplicated hypertension, thiazide-type diuretics should be considered in patients who tend to be salt sensitive, such as older patients and Black patients. For younger patients, ACEIs, ARBs, and CCBs may be more suitable. The use of BBs, particularly older generation BBs such as atenolol, should be avoided in young patients with active lifestyle due to fatiguing side effects and modest efficacy in improving cardiovascular outcomes. BBs are more suitable for patients with compelling indication such as coronary artery disease or congestive heart failure. In elderly patients with isolated systolic hypertension, chlorthalidone or a DHP CCB such as amlodipine should be part of the regimen given the proven benefit in reducing stroke and adverse cardiovascular events.

For patients with BP at least 20/10 mm Hg above the goal, the use of combination therapy is preferred over monotherapy to avoid side effects related to the use of a single agent at the high dose that is often needed to control BP. In patients with high cardiovascular risks, the combination of an ACEI and DHP CCB is superior for reducing adverse cardiovascular outcomes than the combination of an ACEI with thiazide-type diuretics. Thus, the addition of DHP CCBs should be considered in such patients whose BP reduction is not adequate with ACEIs alone.

D. Management of Hypertensive Crisis

Hypertensive crisis is a common condition encountered in the emergency department that can be classified as hypertensive emergency or hypertensive urgency. Hypertensive emergency is defined as a severe elevation in BP (often > 180/120 mm Hg) in the presence of acute target organ damage involving heart, brain, kidneys, or the vascular system. Hypertensive urgency is defined as severe hypertension associated with symptoms, such as headache or chest pain, in the absence of any objective evidence of acute target organ damage. Thus, distinction between hypertensive emergency versus urgency is dependent of clinical presentation rather than severity of hypertension alone.

Once patients are identified to have hypertensive crisis, choice of therapy and rapidity of BP reduction are dependent on clinical presentation. In normotensive subjects, cerebral blood flow is maintained at a constant level despite variation in mean arterial BP between 60 and 120 mm Hg by a process known as *cerebral autoregulation*. At the lower end of this range, cerebral vessels dilate to maintain normal perfusion. Only when the mean BP is lower than 50–60 mm Hg does cerebral perfusion become pressure-dependent. Similarly, when BP rises to a higher level, myogenic vasoconstriction of the resistant arterioles prevents excessive increase in blood flow and cerebral edema. Patients with well-controlled hypertension have autoregulatory adjustment at the normal BP range similar to normotensives. However, in patients with severe hypertension, this BP range is shifted to the right between 110 and 180 mm Hg (Figure 2–1). Thus, BP lowering in patients with hypertensive encephalopathy should be done cautiously by aiming for reduction by 20–25% in the first few hours but not below 140/90 mm Hg (mean BP around 107 mm Hg) in the first 24 hours. Patients with hypertensive urgency could be treated with oral antihypertensive medications in the emergency department and discharged home with close follow-up for titration of BP medications within a few days. Rapid normalization of BP

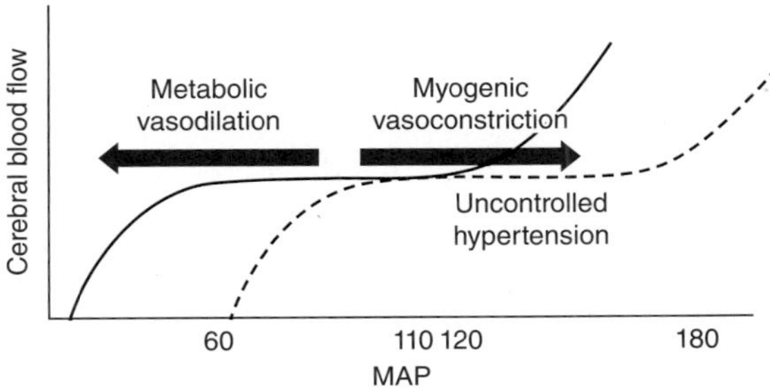

▲ **Figure 2–1.** Relationship between cerebral blood flow (CBF) and mean arterial pressure (MAP) in normotensive subjects (*solid line*). Normally, CBF is maintained constant at a MAP between 60 and 120 mm Hg. However, in patients with uncontrolled hypertension, this relationship is shifted to the right. Therefore, precipitous reductions in blood pressure in these individuals to the normal range (MAP < 11 mm Hg in the first 24 hours) may lead to cerebral hypoperfusion.

Table 2–3. Treatment of Hypertensive Emergency in Special Populations

Clinical Setting	Rapidity of BP Reduction and Target BP	Antihypertensive Drugs
Hypertensive encephalopathy without stroke	Reduce mean arterial pressure (MAP) by 20–25% over 2–3 hours	Labetalol Nitroprusside Nicardipine
Acute ischemic stroke with indication for thrombolysis and BP > 185/110 mm Hg	Reduce MAP by 15% over 1 hour	Labetalol Nicardipine Nitroprusside
Acute ischemic stroke, not a candidate for thrombolysis, with BP > 220/120 mm Hg	Reduce MAP by 15% over 1 hour	Labetalol Nicardipine Nitroprusside
Intracerebral hemorrhage, with systolic blood pressure (SBP) > 200 mm Hg or MAP > 150 mm Hg	Reduce MAP by 15% over 1 hour. For SBP 150–220 mm Hg, acute lowering of SBP to 140 mm Hg appears safe (*Stroke* 2010;41:2108–2129).	Labetalol Nicardipine *(Avoid nitroprusside or nitroglycerin if intracranial pressure is increased.)*
Aortic dissection	Reduce BP to < 120/80 mm Hg immediately	Labetalol Esmolol plus nitroprusside
Acute pulmonary edema	Reduce MAP to 60–100 mm Hg immediately	Nitroglycerin Nitroprusside
Acute coronary syndrome	Reduce MAP to 60–100 mm Hg immediately	Nitroglycerin Labetalol Nicardipine
Adrenergic crisis (pheochromocytoma, clonidine withdrawal, drug or alcohol withdrawal)	Reduce MAP by 20–25% over 2–3 hours	Phentolamine Nicardipine Labetalol
Cocaine overdose	Reduce MAP by 20–25% over 2–3 hours	Phentolamine Labetalol Nicardipine Nitroprusside

with oral agents in the doctor's office or emergency department in patients with asymptomatic severe hypertension without any target organ damage may provoke hypoperfusion of the vital organs, such as brain and kidneys, and should be avoided.

In contrast to hypertensive encephalopathy, BP should be reduced to less than 120/80 mm Hg as soon as possible in patients with hypertensive emergency in the setting of aortic dissection, because delay in BP reduction may cause the dissection plane and false lumen to expand, which may jeopardize blood flow to the vital organs. Patients with acute pulmonary edema and acute coronary syndrome should also have more rapid BP reduction to less than 140/90 mm Hg as soon as possible to decrease LV wall stress, a major determinant of myocardial oxygen demand. Thrombolytic therapy should not be given in patients with ST elevation myocardial infarction until BP is reduced below 180/110 mm Hg to avoid the risk of intracranial hemorrhage. Patients who present with primary intracranial hemorrhage pose a challenge in management because cerebral perfusion pressure is determined both by systemic BP and intracranial pressure. Similarly, for patients with ischemic stroke, rigorous reduction in BP could further compromise the flow to the infarct area and, more importantly, the border zone. More conservative reduction in BP with the goal for BP reduction of approximately 15% within the first hour is generally recommended in these two neurologic emergencies. Treatment of hypertensive emergency in specific clinical settings is summarized in Table 2–3.

Selection of antihypertensive agents in hypertensive emergency also depends on the clinical presentation (Table 2–4). Patients with hypertensive encephalopathy or ischemic stroke should be treated with labetalol, nitroprusside, or nicardipine. Nitroprusside and nitroglycerin should be avoided in patients with intracranial hemorrhage because they may increase intracranial pressure. Phentolamine should be considered in patients with pheochromocytoma or adrenergic crisis such as cocaine intoxication. However, this drug may not be available in many countries, including the United States, on a regular basis. Nicardipine is an alternative

Table 2–4. Intravenous Antihypertensive Drugs for Hypertensive Emergencies

Drug	Dose	Contraindications and Side Effects
Nitroprusside	Start at 0.25–1.0 mcg/kg/min, increase by 0.5 mcg/kg/min every 5 minutes until goal BP or maximal dose of 10 mcg/kg/min	Renal failure, cyanide toxicity, reflex tachycardia, methemoglobin
Nitroglycerin	Start at 10–20 mcg/min, increase by 5 mcg/min every 5 minutes until goal BP or maximal dose of 200 mcg/min	Headache
Nicardipine	Start at 5 mg/h, increase by 2.5 mg/h every 15–30 minutes until goal BP or maximal dose of 15 mg/h; thereafter decrease to 3 mg/h maintenance	
Clevidipine	Start at 1–2 mg/h, titrate every 90 seconds to 10-minute intervals up to 32 mg/h	Defective lipid metabolism such as pathologic hyperlipemia or acute pancreatitis
Labetalol	Start at 0.25–0.5 mg/kg at 2–4 mg/min until goal BP, then 5–20 mg/h maintenance	Bradycardia, second- or third-degree atrioventricular (AV) block, bronchospasm, systolic heart failure
Esmolol	0.5–1 mg/kg as bolus; 50–300 mcg/kg/min as continuous infusion plus sodium nitroprusside intravenous gtt; start at 0.25–1.0 mcg/kg/min, increase by 0.5 mcg/kg/min every 5 minutes until goal BP or maximal dose of 10 mcg/kg/min	Bradycardia, second- or third-degree AV block, bronchospasm, systolic heart failure
Phentolamine	1–5 mg, repeat after 5–15 minutes until goal BP is reached; 0.5–1.0 mg/h as continuous infusion	Reflex tachycardia
Fenoldopam	Start at 0.03–0.1 mcg/kg/min, titrated at the increment of 0.05–0.1 mcg/kg/min up to 1.6 mcg/kg/min	Increased intraocular pressure, reflex tachycardia

therapy for pheochromocytoma. Labetalol, although effective in reversing cocaine-induced increase in BP, should be used with caution in pheochromocytoma because it is still a predominant BB (β-AR to α-AR blockade ratio of 4:1) and may precipitate an unopposed α-AR–mediated vasoconstriction. Nitroprusside is a potent vasodilator but should be used with caution in patients with renal failure given its propensity to cause cyanide toxicity. Nitroglycerin is suitable for use in patients with acute pulmonary edema and acute coronary syndrome because of its antianginal property and ability to relieve pulmonary congestion. Nitrate tolerance may develop quickly with continuous infusion and limit its antihypertensive efficacy. Fenoldopam is a dopamine D_1-like receptor agonist, which reduces BP by promoting peripheral vasodilation. Clevidipine is a newer CCB available in intravenous form with shorter half-life (1 minute) than nicardipine (30–40 minutes). The relatively high cost of these newer agents limits routine use in clinical practice.

E. Management of Resistant Hypertension

Resistant hypertension is defined as failure to achieve BP target goal despite three or more drugs, one of which should be a diuretic. The first simple step in managing resistant hypertension, after excluding WCE, nonadherence to medications, and secondary hypertension, is to determine whether patients are on an appropriate class of diuretics based on renal function. Patients with estimated glomerular filtration rate (eGFR) greater than 50 mL/min/1.73 m^2 should be treated with thiazide diuretics, particularly chlorthalidone, rather than loop diuretics because of longer half-life and proven efficacy in lowering BP. Patients with an eGFR of less than 15 mL/min/1.73 m^2 or less should be on loop diuretics because the ability of thiazide diuretics to promote diuresis diminishes with impaired renal function. The use of an appropriate drug combination that provides synergistic effect on BP could minimize the number of medications needed to control hypertension. Assessment of hemodynamic variables is also helpful in deciding appropriate drug combination. For example, the use of BBs and a central sympatholytic drug generally yields minimal incremental benefit and is prohibited in patients with bradycardia or heart block. These patients should be treated with vasodilators such as DHP CCBs, ACEIs, ARBs, or hydralazine (Figure 2–2). Patients with elevated resting heart rate are more likely to derive large BP reduction with BBs, diltiazem, or verapamil because elevated heart rate is usually a good indicator for hyperkinetic circulation in hypertensive patients.

Addition of spironolactone should also be considered in patients with resistant hypertension despite adjustment of medications, as mentioned earlier. An increasing body of evidence suggests that low-dose spironolactone between 12.5 and 25 mg/day, which is not likely to produce a major diuretic effect, causes a dramatic fall in BP on average of 25/12 mm Hg, when used as add-on therapy in patients with

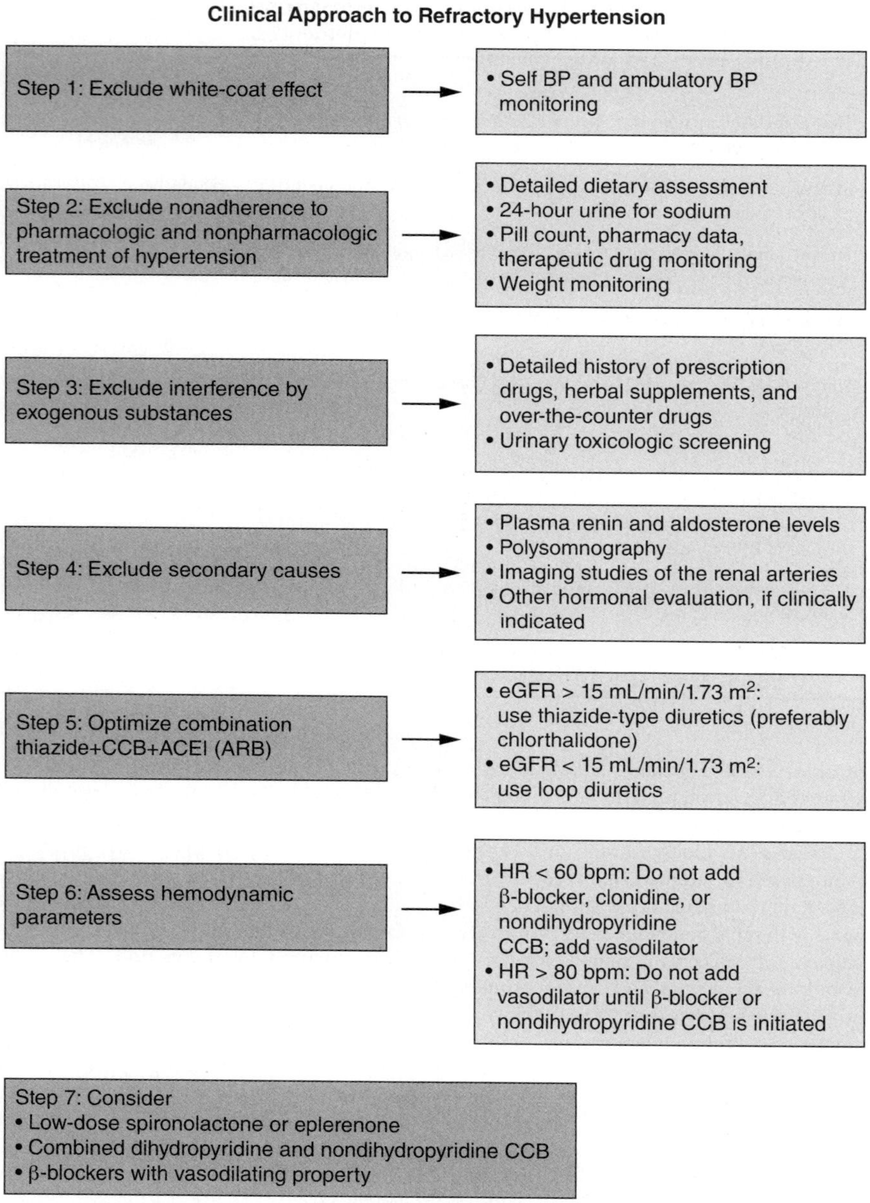
Clinical Approach to Refractory Hypertension
Step 1: Exclude white-coat effect
• Self BP and ambulatory BP monitoring
Step 2: Exclude nonadherence to pharmacologic and nonpharmacologic treatment of hypertension
• Detailed dietary assessment
• 24-hour urine for sodium
• Pill count, pharmacy data, therapeutic drug monitoring
• Weight monitoring
Step 3: Exclude interference by exogenous substances
• Detailed history of prescription drugs, herbal supplements, and over-the-counter drugs
• Urinary toxicologic screening
Step 4: Exclude secondary causes
• Plasma renin and aldosterone levels
• Polysomnography
• Imaging studies of the renal arteries
• Other hormonal evaluation, if clinically indicated
Step 5: Optimize combination thiazide+CCB+ACEI (ARB)
• eGFR > 15 mL/min/1.73 m^2: use thiazide-type diuretics (preferably chlorthalidone)
• eGFR < 15 mL/min/1.73 m^2: use loop diuretics
Step 6: Assess hemodynamic parameters
• HR < 60 bpm: Do not add β-blocker, clonidine, or nondihydropyridine CCB; add vasodilator
• HR > 80 bpm: Do not add vasodilator until β-blocker or nondihydropyridine CCB is initiated
Step 7: Consider
• Low-dose spironolactone or eplerenone
• Combined dihydropyridine and nondihydropyridine CCB
• β-blockers with vasodilating property

▲ **Figure 2–2.** Algorithm in management of resistant hypertension. ACEI, angiotensin-converting enzyme inhibitor; ARB, angiotensin receptor blocker; BP, blood pressure; CCB, calcium channel blocker; eGFR, estimated glomerular filtration rate; HR, heart rate.

uncontrolled hypertension. Spironolactone is more effective than BBs and α-blockers in lowering BP when used as the fourth-line drug therapy in patients with resistant hypertension despite a three-drug regimen including ACEI (or ARB) plus CCB plus thiazide diuretics. The antihypertensive effect of spironolactone is inversely related to PRA, suggesting benefit via reducing intravascular volume. Combination of DHP and non-DHP CCBs appears to have additive effects on peripheral vasodilation and BP, possibly due to binding to different sites of the receptors and should also be considered for these patients. By contrast, addition of an ARB to ACEI has modest effects on BP (on average, only 5/3 mm Hg).

Other than pharmacologic treatment of hypertension, several device-based therapies are designed to reduce activity of the sympathetic nervous system and BP, including catheter-based renal sympathetic denervation and carotid baroreceptor stimulation. Although initial unblinded studies showed large antihypertensive effects, subsequent randomized controlled studies showed modest results. Further studies are still needed to clarify the role of these devices.

SPRINT Research Group, et al. A randomized trial of intensive versus standard blood-pressure control. *N Engl J Med.* 2015; 373:2103–2116. [PMID: 26551272]

Vongpatanasin W. Resistant hypertension: a review of diagnosis and management. *JAMA.* 2014;311:2216–2224. [PMID: 24893089]

Williams B, MacDonald TM, Morant S, et al. Spironolactone versus placebo, bisoprolol, and doxazosin to determine the optimal treatment for drug-resistant hypertension (PATHWAY-2): a randomised, double-blind, crossover trial. *Lancet.* 2015;386: 2059–2068. [PMID: 26414968]

Zhang W, Zhang S, Deng Y, et al. Trial of intensive blood-pressure control in older patients with hypertension. *N Engl J Med.* 2021; 385:1268–1279. [PMID: 34491661]

Prognosis

Hypertension is a major risk factor for cardiovascular mortality, accounting for 50% of deaths from stroke and 45% from coronary heart disease worldwide. In addition, hypertension is a major risk factor for congestive heart failure, CKD, peripheral arterial disease, and the age-related decline in cognitive function. Presence of either persistent or new-onset LV hypertrophy or renal dysfunction during treatment contributes to poor prognosis. Patients with resistant hypertension experience a 20–25% higher risk of stroke and a 40–50% increase in risk of hospitalization from heart failure than hypertensive patients who achieve BP control with treatment. Thus, prompt evaluation of the underlying causes and intensification of pharmacologic and nonpharmacologic treatment is necessary to prevent target organ complications. Selection of appropriate antihypertensive medications that suit the patient characteristics and risk profile is the key to achieve BP goal. In addition to BP reduction, management of other cardiovascular risk factors is also essential in optimizing overall cardiovascular outcomes in hypertensive patients.

3 Antiplatelet Therapy

Ashvarya Mangla, MD
Saurabh Gupta, MD

General Considerations

Atherosclerosis is a leading cause of cardiovascular disease. Atherosclerotic plaques can acutely rupture, exposing a necrotic core that sets off the coagulation cascade, culminating in vascular occlusion. Activation of platelets is the initial event in this cascade and, depending on the vascular bed involved, can cause acute coronary syndromes, ischemic stroke, mesenteric ischemia, or acute limb ischemia. Antiplatelet therapy forms the core of acute and chronic atherosclerotic disease treatment. In this chapter, we will discuss antiplatelet therapy for the treatment of cardiovascular disease.

Role of Platelets in Thrombosis

After vascular injury, platelets bind to exposed collagen and von Willebrand factor (vWF) and are activated. Activated platelets then secrete thromboxane A_2 (TXA_2) and adenosine diphosphate (ADP), which leads to platelet aggregation and recruitment of more platelets. The final common pathway of platelet aggregation is mediated by glycoprotein (GP) II_bIII_a receptors that bind to fibrinogen and vWF, leading to platelet plug and clot formation. Antiplatelet agents target different pathways in this cascade (Figure 3–1).

Classification of Antiplatelet Drugs (Figure 3–2)

A. Cyclooxygenase Inhibitors: Aspirin

1. Mechanism of action—Acetylsalicylic acid (ASA, aspirin) in low doses irreversibly inhibits cyclooxygenase-1 (COX-1), which is required to synthesize TXA_2, a vasoconstrictor necessary for platelet aggregation. At higher doses, ASA also inhibits COX-2, which is needed for prostacyclin production; prostacyclins are platelet aggregation inhibitors and vasodilators. Thus, an ASA dose between 75 and 325 mg is recommended for optimal antiplatelet effect. For rapid onset of action, in ASA-naïve patients, an initial dose of at least 162 mg should be used.

2. Contraindications—ASA is contraindicated in patients with a history of bronchospasm or anaphylactic reaction.

3. Side effects—Dyspepsia, peptic ulcer, erosive gastritis, and upper gastrointestinal bleeding are dose-related side effects. Some patients may develop bronchospasm, urticaria, and rarely anaphylactic reactions. Complex acid-base abnormalities can occur in the setting of aspirin overdose. Some younger patients may have aspirin hypersensitivity with associated nasal polyps, allergic rhinitis, and bronchospasm (Samter's triad). These patients and others with a history of anaphylactic reactions may benefit from aspirin desensitization. Hypo-responsiveness to ASA is defined as the inability of ASA to produce expected inhibitory effects on platelet function. Clinically, this is associated with increased vascular events. There is no consensus on treatment, although empirically, an ADP receptor antagonist may be added.

4. Uses

A. Acute coronary syndromes—All patients who present with chest pain and cardiac biomarker evidence of myocardial infarction (MI), with or without electrocardiographic ST-segment elevation, or unstable angina, should be treated with non–enteric-coated aspirin 162–325 mg (preferably crushed and chewed to enable rapid onset of action). Aspirin should be continued indefinitely in all patients who are not allergic at a dose of 75–162 mg/day, once daily. Clopidogrel (or another $P2Y_{12}$ receptor antagonist) is a reasonable alternative for patients allergic to aspirin.

B. Chronic stable angina—Aspirin 75–162 mg is a standard component of routine management of patients with chronic stable angina and has been demonstrated to reduce morbidity and mortality.

C. Peripheral arterial disease—Patients with symptomatic lower extremity peripheral arterial disease have

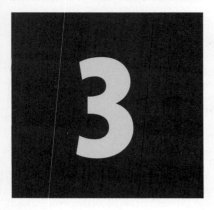

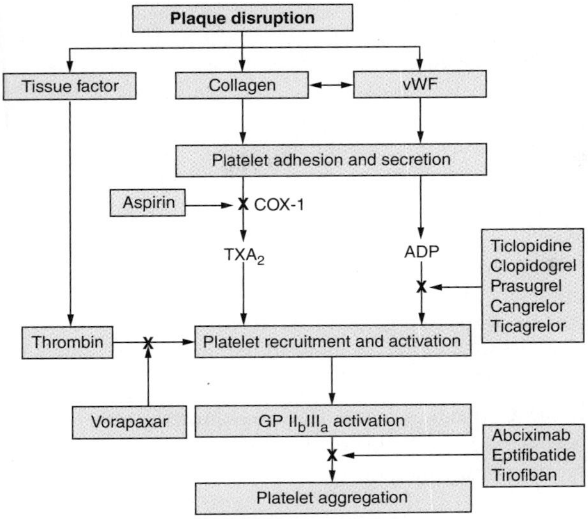

▲ **Figure 3–1.** Site of action of antiplatelet drugs. Aspirin inhibits the synthesis of thromboxane A_2 (TXA_2) by irreversibly acetylating cyclooxygenase-1 (COX-1). Reduced TXA_2 release attenuates platelet activation and recruitment to the site of vascular injury. Ticlopidine, clopidogrel, and prasugrel irreversibly block $P2Y_{12}$, a key adenosine diphosphate (ADP) receptor on the platelet surface; cangrelor and ticagrelor are reversible inhibitors of $P2Y_{12}$. Abciximab, eptifibatide, and tirofiban inhibit the final common pathway of platelet aggregation by blocking fibrinogen and von Willebrand factor (vWF) binding to activated glycoprotein (GP) II_b/III_a. Vorapaxar inhibits thrombin-mediated platelet activation by targeting protease-activated receptor-1 (PAR-1), the major thrombin receptor on human platelets. (Reproduced with permission from Kasper D, et al., eds. *Harrison's Principles of Internal Medicine*, 19th ed. New York: McGraw-Hill; 2015.)

a high likelihood of disease in other vascular beds. They should be treated with aspirin to reduce the risk of MI, stroke, or vascular death.

D. Stroke/transient ischemic attack (TIA)—Patients with prior ischemic stroke or TIA should receive aspirin 325 mg within 48 hours of the onset of symptoms. In patients who have received thrombolytic therapy for ischemic stroke, antiplatelet therapy can be started after 24 hours. Treatment should be continued indefinitely at a dose of 75 or 81 mg orally once daily.

E. Primary prevention—Based on the current United States Preventive Services Task Force guidelines, low-dose aspirin can be considered for primary prevention in adults 40–59 years of age who have low bleeding risk and ≥ 10% 10-year risk of ASCVD risk. Patients older than 60 years should not be initiated on aspirin for primary prevention as the benefits do not outweigh the risks. Aspirin 75–162 mg/day may also be considered in patients aged 50–70 years with type 1 and type 2 diabetes if they have additional risk factors such as a family history of premature ASCVD, hypertension, dyslipidemia, smoking, or chronic kidney disease/albuminuria and who are not at high risk for bleeding.

B. $P2Y_{12}$ Receptor Blockers

Commercially available products include the irreversible inhibitors ticlopidine, clopidogrel, and prasugrel and reversible inhibitors cangrelor and ticagrelor.

1. Mechanism of action—These agents inhibit the $P2Y_{12}$ receptor (required for binding ADP with a resultant increase in platelet aggregation and activation of GP II_bIII_a receptors on platelet surface). Inhibition of these receptors leads to decreased platelet activation and aggregation.

2. Contraindications—Active bleeding and a previous anaphylactic reaction are contraindications to therapy. Prasugrel

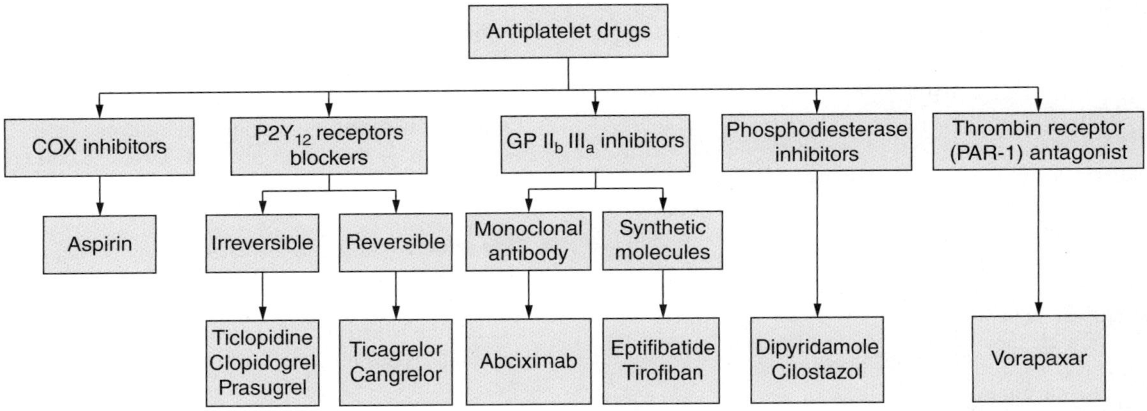

▲ **Figure 3–2.** Classification of antiplatelet drugs based on mechanism of action. PAR-1, protease-activated receptor-1

is contraindicated in patients with a prior history of TIA or stroke. It should be used with extreme caution in the elderly (≥ 75 years) or patients with low body weight (< 60 kg) due to an increased risk of bleeding events. Maintenance doses of aspirin above 100 mg appear to reduce the effectiveness of ticagrelor and should be avoided.

3. Side effects—Bleeding and purpuric lesions rarely occur. Ticlopidine can cause hematologic side effects such as bone marrow suppression, thrombocytopenia, thrombotic thrombocytopenic purpuras, and neutropenia, and regular blood count monitoring is recommended. Alternatives with more favorable risk-benefit ratios have primarily supplanted this drug. Hematologic side effects are significantly less common with clopidogrel and prasugrel. Skin rashes have been reported with clopidogrel. Ticagrelor may cause dyspnea in some patients, although it is generally not severe.

4. Clinically relevant pharmacology—Ticlopidine, clopidogrel, and prasugrel are prodrugs that require metabolism by the liver to convert them into active drugs. After a loading dose, platelet inhibition starts in 4–6 hours. Prasugrel is absorbed more completely and has a relatively rapid onset of action. Nonthienopyridines, such as ticagrelor and cangrelor, are absorbed faster, have a more rapid onset, and have a shorter duration of action. In the setting of acute MI (ST-segment elevation MI [STEMI] or non–ST-segment elevation MI [NSTEMI]), when rapid inhibition of platelets is required, a loading dose of all antiplatelet agents is recommended.

5. Thienopyridine resistance/hypo-responsiveness—Some patients treated with adequate doses of clopidogrel still have thrombotic events despite medication compliance. This variability could partially be from genetic polymorphisms in the CYP isoenzymes involved in the activation of clopidogrel. The prevalence of polymorphism is as high as 30–50% in specific populations. These genetic polymorphisms do not affect the activity of prasugrel or ticagrelor, and these potent antiplatelet agents are reasonable alternatives in populations suspected of having a genetic predisposition to clopidogrel resistance. So far, there is limited evidence that platelet testing for clopidogrel responsiveness improves clinical outcomes. In the future, there may be a role for genetic testing before initiating clopidogrel.

6. Uses

A. Acute coronary syndromes—For patients with STEMI, in whom primary percutaneous coronary intervention (PCI) is planned, $P2Y_{12}$ blockers should be administered as a loading dose before or at the time of PCI (clopidogrel 300–600 mg, prasugrel 60 mg, or ticagrelor 180 mg). In patients under 75 years of age who receive fibrinolytic therapy or who do not receive reperfusion therapy, it is reasonable to administer an oral loading dose of clopidogrel 300 mg and continue long-term maintenance therapy (1 year). Prasugrel can be considered once coronary anatomy is known (typically after coronary angiography). Patients with NSTEMI/unstable angina selected for early invasive strategy should receive aspirin and either clopidogrel or ticagrelor if a decision is made to preload with a $P2Y_{12}$ inhibitor. Prasugrel should not be administered till coronary anatomy is known. Dual antiplatelet therapy (DAPT) should be continued for 12 months in patients with an acceptably low risk of bleeding.

B. After PCI—Patients who undergo PCI should be on DAPT with aspirin and any of the three $P2Y_{12}$ inhibitors (clopidogrel, prasugrel, or ticagrelor) for 1 year. $P2Y_{12}$ inhibitors should be continued for at least 6 months for patients who undergo PCI for stable ischemic heart disease. A shorter (3 months) vs. longer duration of DAPT should be individualized based on ischemic and bleeding risk.

C. ASA allergy—Patients with chronic stable angina, peripheral arterial disease, or a stroke or TIA who are allergic to aspirin can be treated with clopidogrel. DAPT with aspirin and $P2Y_{12}$ receptor antagonists is not indicated in patients without antecedent PCI. In addition, DAPT with aspirin and clopidogrel is not superior to either agent alone in patients with strokes or TIA. In patients with a compelling indication for ASA, desensitization therapy (in the inpatient setting) can be considered and is generally successful.

C. GP II_bIII_a Inhibitors

The monoclonal antibody abciximab and the synthetic compounds eptifibatide and tirofiban are intravenous GP II_bIII_a inhibitors. Oral GP II_bIII_a receptor antagonists have not been demonstrated to be effective and currently have no role in clinical care.

1. Mechanism of action—These drugs block the GP II_bIII_a receptors on the platelet surface. These are the most abundant receptors on the platelet surface and are the final common pathway of platelet aggregation and platelet plug formation.

2. Dosage—These agents are typically administered as an intravenous loading dose followed by a continuous infusion. The dose of abciximab does not need to be adjusted for patients with renal disease; however, tirofiban and eptifibatide are renally excreted and require dose adjustments in patients with renal disease.

3. Contraindications—Abciximab should not be used in patients in whom PCI is not planned. Tirofiban and eptifibatide are contraindicated in patients with end-stage renal disease.

4. Side effects—Immune-mediated thrombocytopenia and bleeding are the common side effects. Thrombocytopenia is more common with the monoclonal antibody and relatively less common with synthetic agents. Daily monitoring of blood counts is recommended for patients treated with these agents.

5. Uses: Acute coronary syndromes—Patients who present with STEMI and are candidates for primary PCI (with or without stenting) are often treated with a strategy of heparin and a loading dose of a $P2Y_{12}$ receptor inhibitor as early as possible or at the time of primary PCI. The adjunctive use of GP II_bIII_a agents may be considered in patients with a significant thrombus burden or inadequate $P2Y_{12}$ receptor antagonist loading. In patients receiving bivalirudin (instead of heparin) as the primary anticoagulant, routine use of GP II_bIII_a inhibitors is not recommended but may be considered for "bailout" in selected cases as adjunctive therapy. There is no role for GP II_bIII_a inhibitors after fibrinolytic therapy (regardless of whether fibrinolysis was successful) due to the significantly increased risk for minor and major bleeding events. Patients with NSTEMI or unstable angina who are candidates for an early invasive strategy can be treated with GP II_bIII_a inhibitors in addition to aspirin either at the time of presentation or just before PCI if they have high-risk features. The agents of choice in this setting are eptifibatide and tirofiban. Patients for whom an early conservative strategy is chosen and who continue to have symptoms despite optimal medical therapy can also be considered for GP II_bIII_a inhibitors until the time of PCI. In addition, patients in whom a planned invasive strategy is delayed can be treated with GP II_bIII_a inhibitors until PCI.

D. Phosphodiesterase Inhibitors

Dipyridamole and cilostazol are phosphodiesterase inhibitors.

1. Mechanism of action—These agents inhibit the enzyme phosphodiesterase, thus increasing the cyclic adenosine monophosphate (cAMP) concentration in platelets, inhibiting platelet aggregation.

2. Uses

A. STROKE—Dipyridamole in combination with aspirin is superior to aspirin alone in secondary stroke prevention.

B. PERIPHERAL ARTERIAL DISEASE—Patients with symptomatic lower extremity peripheral arterial disease and intermittent claudication in the absence of heart failure benefit from the addition of cilostazol, with improvement in symptoms and an increase in exercise tolerance.

C. CARDIAC STRESS TESTING—Due to its vasodilatory properties, dipyridamole is used in chemical stress testing, although newer agents have largely supplanted its use in this setting.

E. Thrombin Receptor Antagonists

Vorapaxar is an orally active protease-activated receptor-1 (PAR-1) antagonist approved for clinical use in the United States in 2014. Vorapaxar has been shown to decrease combined cardiovascular events in patients with prior MIs or peripheral artery disease but at the cost of increased risk of bleeding.

1. Mechanism of action—Vorapaxar is a competitive antagonist of PAR-1, a major thrombin receptor on human platelets. Due to its long half-life (200 hours), it is effectively an irreversible antagonist.

2. Dosage—The dosage for oral vorapaxar is 2.08 mg daily.

3. Contraindications—Contraindications include a history of stroke, transient ischemic attack, intracranial bleeding, and active pathologic bleeding.

4. Uses—Uses include secondary prevention in patients with a history of MI, secondary prevention in patients with peripheral artery disease, and as a substitute for patients with aspirin allergy or clopidogrel intolerance and no contraindications for vorapaxar. However, there is limited experience with thrombin receptor antagonists, and the exact role of this class of medications continues to evolve.

Treatment

A. Special Issues with Antiplatelet Therapy

1. Gastrointestinal bleeding—If antiplatelet therapy is indicated in patients with a history of or those at increased risk for gastrointestinal bleeding (advanced age, concomitant warfarin, steroid, or nonsteroidal anti-inflammatory drug use), proton pump inhibitors should be used for prophylaxis or to prevent a recurrence. Earlier concerns about the diminished efficacy of clopidogrel with concomitant use of proton pump inhibitors have not been validated in randomized clinical trials.

2. Management of patients receiving antiplatelet therapy who require a surgical procedure—The decision to withhold antiplatelet treatment should be individualized based on shared decision-making with the patient and in close consultation with the cardiovascular subspecialist depending on the risk of bleeding and the clinical indication for which the antiplatelet therapy is used. For patients receiving ASA and a $P2Y_{12}$ receptor antagonist for a bare-metal stent (BMS) who require urgent surgery within 1 month of placement, DAPT should be continued in the perioperative period. For patients receiving ASA and clopidogrel after a drug-eluting stent (DES) and requiring urgent surgery within 12 months of placement, therapy should be continued in the perioperative period. However, newer stent platforms may allow for earlier discontinuation of DAPT. Elective surgery in patients receiving ASA and $P2Y_{12}$ inhibitor secondary to coronary stent implantation should be deferred for at least 6 weeks after BMS placement and 6–12 months after DES placement.

3. Combined antiplatelet and anticoagulant therapy—Optimal management of patients with CAD who are on anticoagulant therapy for atrial fibrillation, prosthetic heart valve, or venous thromboembolism (VTE) and undergo PCI remains challenging, with no clear consensus on the ideal regimen. The antithrombotic/antiplatelet regimen for these patients should be individualized with the help of subspecialty consultation with interventional cardiology.

Based on current evidence, when feasible direct oral anticoagulants (DOACs) should be preferred over warfarin for anticoagulation, and clopidogrel should be the preferred $P2Y_{12}$ inhibitor. After PCI, maintenance therapy for most patients should consist of $P2Y_{12}$ inhibitor and anticoagulant only, unless the thrombotic risk is high and bleeding risk is low, in which case triple therapy with aspirin (75–100 mg), $P2Y_{12}$ inhibitor (clopidogrel preferred), and anticoagulant (DOAC preferred) can be considered in select cases. If triple therapy is chosen, it should be limited to 1-month post PCI. Duration of $P2Y_{12}$ inhibitor should be 6 months for stable ischemic heart disease and 12 months for acute coronary syndromes, after which anticoagulant alone should be continued. If the indication for anticoagulation is provoked VTE and anticoagulation is no longer required, aspirin should be added to the $P2Y_{12}$ inhibitor to complete 6 months of DAPT for stable ischemic heart disease and 12 months post-acute coronary syndrome. The dose intensity must be carefully monitored when warfarin is administered in conjunction with clopidogrel or low-dose ASA. The addition of proton pump inhibitors or histamine 2 (H2) blockers can lower the risk of gastrointestinal bleeding while patients are on combined antiplatelet and anticoagulant therapy.

B. Special Populations

1. Antiplatelet therapy in atrial arrhythmias—In patients with nonvalvular atrial fibrillation or atrial flutter, the risk for thromboembolic events should be assessed using the CHA_2DS_2-VASc score (congestive heart failure or reduced ejection fraction ≤ 35%, hypertension, age [≥ 65 = 1, ≥ 75 = 2], diabetes mellitus, prior stroke or TIA [score = 2], vascular disease [including MI, peripheral artery disease, and aortic plaque], and female sex). For patients with a CHA_2DS_2-VASc score of ≥ 2, unless contraindicated, oral anticoagulants (warfarin, dabigatran, rivaroxaban, or apixaban) are recommended. For those with a CHA_2DS_2-VASc score of 1, it is reasonable to use either ASA or an oral anticoagulant.

2. Coronary artery bypass grafting (CABG)—When possible, ASA should be administered preoperatively to patients in whom CABG is planned; if not initiated preoperatively, it should be started within 6 hours of surgery and continued indefinitely to prevent graft occlusion. Clopidogrel 75 mg orally once daily can be substituted in patients intolerant or allergic to aspirin. Patients on DAPT with aspirin and $P2Y_{12}$ receptor blockers scheduled to undergo elective CABG should discontinue clopidogrel and ticagrelor for at least 5 days and prasugrel at least 7 days before surgery. These agents should preferably be discontinued at least 24 hours before urgent surgery to reduce the risk of major bleeding. The GP II_bIII_a inhibitors eptifibatide and tirofiban should be discontinued at least 2–4 hours before surgery.

3. Pregnancy—Antiplatelet agents can be considered in pregnancy or breastfeeding if maternal benefits clearly outweigh potential fetal risks. Low-dose ASA (75–162 mg daily) is likely safe for use during the first trimester of pregnancy; however, it should be avoided during the third trimester and while breastfeeding. The use of agents other than low-dose ASA should only be considered after weighing maternal benefits with potential risks for the newborn. $P2Y_{12}$ receptor antagonists should be used during pregnancy or breastfeeding only if clearly indicated.

4. Patients with prosthetic heart valves

A. SURGICAL PROSTHETIC VALVES—The addition of daily ASA (75–100 mg) to therapeutic warfarin is recommended for all patients with mechanical heart valves. For patients with an aortic or mitral bioprosthesis and no other risk factors, lifelong aspirin is indicated at 75–100 mg/day.

B. TRANSCATHETER PROSTHETIC VALVES—After transcatheter aortic valve replacement or transcatheter edge to edge mitral valve repair, patients should be on DAPT (usually with ASA and clopidogrel) for 3–6 months, followed by low-dose ASA indefinitely. In addition, aspirin and warfarin should be considered for 3-6 months post transcatheter mitral valve replacements and transcatheter aortic valve in valve replacement (ViV TAVR), followed by long-term aspirin alone.

5. PCI—After PCI for acute coronary syndrome, low-dose ASA should be continued indefinitely. Typically a $P2Y_{12}$ inhibitor is indicated for 12 months regardless of the stent type. Options for $P2Y_{12}$ inhibitors include clopidogrel 75 mg daily, prasugrel 10 mg daily, or ticagrelor 90 mg twice daily. After BMS implantation and increased risk of bleeding, DAPT may be discontinued in select patients after 1 month. With certain newer DES platforms, single oral antiplatelet therapy can be considered in high bleeding risk patients after 1 month of DAPT. After PCI for stable ischemic heart disease, DAPT should be continued for 6 months. Earlier discontinuation (after 3 months) of DAPT can be considered in certain high bleeding risk patients, and longer (> 6–12 months) of DAPT can be considered in certain patients with low bleeding and high thrombotic/ischemic risk.

Kumbhani D, Cannon C, Beavers C, et al. 2020 ACC Expert Consensus Decision Pathway for Anticoagulant and Antiplatelet Therapy in Patients With Atrial Fibrillation or Venous Thromboembolism Undergoing Percutaneous Coronary Intervention or With Atherosclerotic Cardiovascular Disease. *J Am Coll Cardiol.* 2021 Feb;77(5):629–658. [PMID: 33250267]

Levine G, Bates E, Bittl J, et al. 2016 ACC/AHA Guideline Focused Update on Duration of Dual Antiplatelet Therapy in Patients With Coronary Artery Disease. *J Am Coll Cardiol.* 2016 Sep;68(10): 1082–1115. [PMID: 27036918]

Valgimigli M, Bueno H, Byrne RA, et al. 2017 ESC focused update on dual antiplatelet therapy in coronary artery disease developed in collaboration with EACTS: The Task Force for dual antiplatelet therapy in coronary artery disease of the European Society of Cardiology (ESC) and of the European Association for Cardio-Thoracic Surgery (EACTS). *Eur Heart J.* 2018;39(3): 213–260. [PMID: 28886622]

Long-Term Anticoagulation for Cardiac Conditions

4

Gautam R. Shroff, MBBS
Michelle D. Carlson, MD

General Considerations

Intracardiac thrombosis can complicate a variety of conditions and lead to devastating consequences as a result of peripheral embolization. Long-term therapeutic oral anticoagulation (OAC) is effective for the prevention of thromboembolism in these conditions but carries attendant risks including major bleeding. Understanding the risks and benefits of long-term oral anticoagulant therapy for various cardiac conditions is essential for ensuring the best clinical outcomes.

A. Anticoagulants

These agents affect the coagulation protein cascade to reduce thrombosis.

1. Unfractionated heparin—Unfractionated heparin (UFH) binds to antithrombin (AT), markedly increasing the effect of AT in neutralizing thrombin and activating factor X (factor Xa). The effectiveness of UFH varies greatly from person to person due to its interactions with several plasma proteins and the endothelium, making monitoring the effects of full-dose UFH on hemostasis imperative. Monitoring of anti-factor Xa (anti-Xa) levels is recommended for accurate determination of the anticoagulant effects of UFH, and is considered more reliable compared to the previous use of activated partial thromboplastin time (aPTT). In certain dynamic situations where a higher level of anticoagulation is needed (e.g., during coronary interventions), the activated clotting time (ACT) is used to monitor its effect, and the dose of UFH is adjusted to keep the ACT at 250–300 seconds or greater. When given intravenously, the effects of UFH are immediate. It is usually administered as a bolus, followed by a continuous intravenous infusion, but may also be administered in divided therapeutic doses subcutaneously. The effects of UFH usually dissipate within 6 hours and its effects can be reversed almost completely with the use of protamine, which makes its use attractive in situations where bleeding risk is perceived to be high.

2. Low-molecular-weight heparin—Low-molecular-weight heparins (LMWHs) are breakdown products of UFH and have a selective effect on factor Xa. They bind more selectively to plasma proteins compared to UFH, so the dosing is more predictable. They are associated with lower bleeding risk, and laboratory monitoring is usually not necessary when dosage is based on body weight. Factor Xa levels, but not aPTT or ACT, can be used to monitor their effects. LMWHs are usually administered subcutaneously twice daily, and their effects are not easily reversed by protamine. They are contraindicated in the context of advanced chronic kidney disease (CKD). Since the dosing is weight based, the effects are less reliable among those with a very high body mass index.

3. Intravenous direct thrombin inhibitors—Bivalirudin and argatroban inhibit thrombin formation and are useful when UFH and LMWH are contraindicated in conditions such as heparin-induced thrombocytopenia (HIT). These agents are administered by bolus followed by a continuous infusion and inactivate both free and fibrin-bound thrombin. They do not bind to plasma proteins and, therefore, have a more predictable pharmacologic response, but their therapeutic window is narrow, and monitoring is necessary to ensure therapeutic effect, though there is no universal agreement on which assay is preferable (options include aPTT, ACT, direct thrombin inhibitor assays, or chromogenic factor Xa assay). The international normalized ratio (INR) is also affected by these agents, making transition to warfarin more difficult. The bleeding risk with the direct thrombin inhibitors may be greater than with UFH. Due to the short half-life of these drugs, bleeding complications can usually be controlled by stopping the infusion. Argatroban is the preferred thrombin inhibitor for patients with CKD. Bivalirudin has been extensively studied for its role in acute myocardial infarction (AMI) and is recommended by the American Heart Association (AHA)/American College of Cardiology (ACC) guidelines and the European Society of Cardiology (ESC) in the management of non–ST-segment elevation myocardial infarction (NSTEMI) and ST-segment elevation myocardial infarction (STEMI).

4. Fondaparinux—Fondaparinux is an analog of pentasaccharides found in UFH and LMWH that increases the effect of AT and inhibits factor Xa. It has a half-life of 17 hours when used subcutaneously and is administered once daily according to the patient's weight. It should not be used if the creatinine clearance (CrCl) is less than 30 mL/min. It is used for primary prevention of DVT, for treatment of DVT and pulmonary embolus, and treatment of HIT (though this is not an FDA-approved indication). Fondaparinux is also recommended by the AHA/ACC and ESC guidelines for use in NSTEMI, though additional anticoagulation must be added if the patient undergoes percutaneous coronary intervention (PCI).

5. Oral vitamin K antagonists—Coumarins, or vitamin K antagonists (VKA), have been the mainstay of long-term OAC for more than 70 years. Warfarin, the most used oral VKA, blocks the conversion of vitamin K to the active moiety, vitamin K epoxide, which is necessary for the synthesis of factors II, VII, IX, and X and proteins C and S. The half-life of warfarin ranges from 20 to 60 hours (mean plasma half-life 40 hours). It is nearly completely absorbed when given orally, binds strongly to albumin, and is metabolized in the liver, predominately by the CYP2C9 enzyme of the cytochrome P450 system. Its effect on hemostasis is quite variable from person to person and, sometimes, for the same person at different times. Warfarin's effect can be influenced by dietary factors, liver disease, congestive heart failure, hypermetabolic states, and numerous drug interactions, making it necessary to monitor the anticoagulant effect of warfarin with a prothrombin time (PT), which is standardized to an international thromboplastin reagent and reported as the INR. Serial INRs are used to monitor warfarin effects and adjust its dose. During initiation of therapy, there may be a brief paradoxical hypercoagulable state due to the inhibition of proteins C and S (anticoagulant factors) before the inhibition of the coagulant factors, so parenteral anticoagulation is typically used as a bridge until a therapeutic INR is achieved. During initiation of warfarin therapy, the INR should be checked frequently until a stable dose is found. Subsequently, the INR should be monitored by an individual care provider or through an anticoagulation clinic at least monthly and more frequently if the dose needs to be adjusted. Point-of-care testing is now available, allowing at-home monitoring of INR. If warfarin needs to be stopped, the INR will normalize in about 3–4 days or can be corrected in 1–2 days if vitamin K is given. If it is necessary to reverse the effects of warfarin more quickly, four-factor prothrombin complex concentrate (4f-PCC), or fresh frozen plasma is recommended.

6. Direct oral anticoagulants (DOACs)—These long-term oral anticoagulants, in distinction to warfarin, target only a single component of the coagulation cascade, either thrombin or activated factor Xa. Because of their wide therapeutic window, a fixed dosage is given for specific conditions, and there is no need for routine anticoagulant monitoring. Several clinical factors must be considered when determining the most appropriate drug and dosage for an individual patient, including renal and hepatic function, which should be tested prior to initiation of a DOAC and annually thereafter. Cost continues to be an issue for many patients as none of these medications are generic yet.

A. Direct thrombin inhibitor—Dabigatran is the only oral direct thrombin inhibitor available in the United States and is approved for prevention of stroke and systemic embolism (SSE) in those with nonvalvular atrial fibrillation (NVAF). It was compared with adjusted-dose warfarin (INR 2.0–3.0) in a large noninferiority trial. It is excreted primarily through the kidneys and is recommended at 150 mg bid for those with CrCl more than 30 mL/min. Based on pharmacodynamics data, a reduced dose of 75 mg bid has been approved by the U.S. Food and Drug Administration (FDA) for those with CrCl of 15–30 mL/min, although there are no clinical data for efficacy at this dose. It is not recommended for those with a CrCl less than 15 mL/min. Dabigatran is not metabolized by the cytochrome P450 system, but P-glycoprotein inhibitors, including verapamil and dronedarone, can increase its concentration. Potent P-glycoprotein inducers, including St. John's wort, rifampin, carbamazepine, and phenytoin, reduce dabigatran concentration and should not be given in combination with dabigatran. Various coagulation tests can be used to measure its anticoagulant effect, including the aPTT, the ACT, and the dilute thrombin time (dilute TT), which is the most sensitive assay. Dabigatran is renally excreted and hemodialysis can reduce its concentration in cases of severe bleeding. A specific monoclonal antibody, idarucizumab, is FDA-approved for reversal of the anticoagulant effect in urgent situations such as major bleeding. If idarucizumab is not available in the case of a life-threatening bleed, PCC or activated PCC can be used. In accidental overdose, activated charcoal may be used to absorb it from the stomach. In addition to prevention of SSE in NVAF, dabigatran is approved for venous thromboembolism (VTE) treatment and VTE prophylaxis in the setting of total hip arthroplasty (THA).

B. Factor Xa inhibitors—Rivaroxaban, apixaban, and edoxaban are highly selective, reversible, direct factor Xa inhibitors approved for prevention of SSE in NVAF. Approval of each was based on single, large, noninferiority-designed, randomized, phase 3 clinical trial compared with adjusted-dose warfarin (target INR 2.0–3.0). The anticoagulant effect of each factor Xa inhibitor can be measured using an anti-factor Xa activity calibrated for the specific drug. If this is not available, a prolonged PT is most helpful in identifying clinically relevant drug levels. All factor Xa inhibitors are highly protein bound, so hemodialysis is not effective in reducing their concentration. Accidental overdose may be treated with activated charcoal to absorb the drug from the stomach. Andexanet alfa is FDA-approved for life-threatening bleedings associated with anti-Xa agents. If andexanet alfa is not available, it is reasonable to use 4-factor PCC.

Rivaroxaban is a once-a-day drug that is excreted primarily through the kidneys. The dose for reduction of SSE in NVAF is 20 mg once daily with the largest meal. A decreased dose of 15 mg is recommended for those with a CrCl less than 51 mL/min, including those on hemodialysis, though there are few data on its safety and efficacy in those with CrCl less than 30 mL/min. Although drug and diet interactions are minimal, it is metabolized in the liver through cytochrome P450 (CYP)–dependent and –independent mechanisms. It is not recommended for those receiving inhibitors of both CYP3A4 and P-glycoprotein, including azole antifungals and human immunodeficiency virus (HIV) protease inhibitors. In addition to prevention of SSE in NVAF, it is also approved for VTE treatment; VTE prevention after THA, total knee arthroplasty (TKA), or in acutely ill patients; and stable coronary artery disease (CAD) and stable peripheral artery disease (PAD) at a dose of 2.5 mg bid in conjunction with aspirin 81 mg daily.

Apixaban is a twice-a-day drug that is metabolized in the liver by CYP3A4–dependent and –independent mechanisms, and about one-quarter is excreted in the urine. It is approved in the United States for stage 5 CKD patients on hemodialysis based on pharmacodynamic and pharmacokinetic studies. The usual dose is 5 mg bid; the dose should be decreased to 2.5 mg bid if the patient has two of the following: age ≥ 80 years, weight less than 60 kg, or serum creatinine more than 1.5 mg/dL. In addition to prevention of SSE in NVAF, it is also approved for VTE treatment, and VTE prophylaxis in the setting of THA or TKA, and post-PCI in the setting of NVAF.

Edoxaban is a once-a-day drug that is metabolized in the liver by CYP3A4–dependent and P-glycoprotein mechanisms and excreted in the urine. It is not recommended for those receiving inhibitors of both CYP3A4 and P-glycoprotein, including azole antimycotics and HIV protease inhibitors. A dose of 60 mg is recommended for NVAF patients with an estimated glomerular filtration rate (eGFR) of 50–94 mL/min, and 30 mg is recommended for those with an eGFR of 15–50 mL/min. It is not recommended for those with an eGFR less than 15 or more than 95 mL/min. In addition to prevention of SSE in NVAF, it is also approved for the treatment of VTE and after PCI in the setting of NVAF.

B. Risks of Anticoagulant Therapy

Bleeding is the most common adverse effect seen with the use of anticoagulant agents. Bleeding complications are more likely to occur in patients who are older than 65 years; have a history of previous stroke, gastrointestinal tract bleeding, recent myocardial infarction (MI), anemia, kidney disease, serious concurrent illness, or diabetes; drink alcohol excessively; or take nonsteroidal anti-inflammatory or antiplatelet agents including aspirin. Intracranial hemorrhage (ICH) is the most feared complication and can be devastating in the setting of anticoagulant therapy, with continued bleeding and progressive neurologic deterioration. In such situations, reversal of the anticoagulant effect is necessary as soon as possible. Of the anticoagulants available, the incidence of ICH in patients with NVAF is highest in those prescribed warfarin when the INR is more than 4.0. For those taking dabigatran or factor Xa inhibitors for NVAF, the incidence of ICH is significantly lower, only one-third the incidence seen with adjusted-dose warfarin. Although measuring drug activity is not easily available on a routine clinical basis, there are reversal agents readily available for the NOACs, including idarucizumab, which is FDA-approved for reversal of dabigatran, and andexanet alfa, which is FDA-approved for reversal of factor Xa inhibitors.

Thrombocytopenia can complicate the use of UFH and LMWH in two ways. A dose-dependent lowering of the platelet count is usually not serious and does not necessarily require stopping these agents. The second type of thrombocytopenia, *heparin-induced thrombocytopenia* (HIT), is an immune-mediated response that can be life-threatening due to arterial and venous thrombus formation. An antibody to heparin interacts with a heparin–platelet factor-4 complex on the platelet surface, resulting in platelet destruction. HIT usually starts at least 4 days after heparin initiation unless there has been previous heparin exposure, is not dose-dependent, and usually results in at least a 50% reduction in the platelet count. The diagnosis of HIT can be confirmed with an enzyme-linked immunosorbent assay (ELISA) for the antibody–heparin–platelet factor 4 complex or a functional serotonin release assay (considered the gold standard) for situations where the ELISA immunoassay is indeterminate. HIT is much less common with LMWH than with UFH, occurring about one-tenth as frequently. The treatment for HIT is immediate discontinuation of all forms of heparin, including low doses used to maintain intravenous access. A direct thrombin inhibitor, such as bivalirudin or argatroban, or a factor Xa inhibitor, such as fondaparinux, rivaroxaban, apixaban, or edoxaban, should be substituted. Of these therapies, only argatroban is FDA-approved for use in HIT. Additional rare complications seen with UFH and LMWH include hyperkalemia (due to hyperaldosteronism), osteoporosis, skin necrosis, and alopecia.

Adverse effects seen with warfarin include skin necrosis and teratogenic effects. Skin necrosis due to warfarin is a rare complication seen within the first few days of treatment. It is due to a prothrombotic milieu and is most likely to occur in patients with protein C and S deficiencies. Because of its teratogenic effects, warfarin should be used cautiously during pregnancy, especially in the first trimester and specifically between weeks 6 and 12 of gestation, and never at a dose more than 5 mg.

January C, Wann L, Alpert J, et al. 2014 AHA/ACC/HRS Guideline for the Management of Patients With Atrial Fibrillation. *J Am Coll Cardiol.* 2014 Dec;64(21):e1–e76. [PMID: 24685669] https://doi.org/10.1016/j.jacc.2014.03.022

January C, Wann L, Calkins H, et al. 2019 AHA/ACC/HRS Focused Update of the 2014 AHA/ACC/HRS Guideline for the Management of Patients With Atrial Fibrillation. *J Am Coll Cardiol.* 2019 Jul;74(1):104–132. [PMID: 30703431] https://doi.org/10.1016/j.jacc.2019.01.011

Shroff GR, Stoecker R, Hart A. Non-vitamin K-dependent oral anticoagulants for nonvalvular atrial fibrillation in patients with CKD: pragmatic considerations for the clinician. *Am J Kidney Dis.* 2018 Nov;72(5):717–727. [PMID: 29728318] doi: 10.1053/j.ajkd.2018.02.360.

Tomaselli G, Mahaffey K, Cuker A, et al. 2020 ACC Expert Consensus Decision Pathway on Management of Bleeding in Patients on Oral Anticoagulants. *J Am Coll Cardiol.* 2020 Aug;76(5):594–622. [PMID: 32680646] https://doi.org/10.1016/j.jacc.2020.04.053

Pathophysiology & Etiology

A. Pathogenesis of Cardiac Thrombi

In the nineteenth century, Virchow theorized that stasis of intravascular blood flow, endocardial injury, and a hypercoagulable state were necessary for the formation of intravascular thrombi. Intracardiac thrombosis may develop in cardiac chambers that are enlarged or have low flow. Left atrial thrombi develop in persons with atrial fibrillation (AF) with or without coexisting valvular heart disease, and there is a developing evidence that atrial cardiomyopathy is associated with mechanical dysfunction, which can lead to stasis even in the absence of atrial enlargement or AF.

Left ventricular thrombi (LVT) develops in with the setting of AMI, left ventricular aneurysm, and dilated cardiomyopathy. AMI causes stasis of intracavitary blood (secondary to regional and/or global dysfunction of the left ventricle) in the setting of a hypercoagulable state and endocardial injury; LVT were especially common before coronary reperfusion therapy was developed. Severe apical wall motion abnormalities due to anterior STEMI (i.e., akinesis or dyskinesis) or severe stunning with apical stress (Takotsubo) cardiomyopathy usually precede thrombus formation, which develop at the apex of the left ventricle 2–7 days after the index event.

Inflammatory processes such as myocarditis or noninfectious endocarditis may result in endocardial injury. A similar pathophysiology occurs in atrial cardiomyopathy, including atrial inflammation and fibrosis. These endocardial abnormalities may lead to thrombus formation, particularly when associated with decreased left ventricular systolic performance, left atrial enlargement or dysfunction, or a coexistent hypercoagulable state. Eosinophils presumably cause endothelial injury with Löeffler endocarditis leading to thrombus formation. The introduction of a foreign material, such as a prosthetic valve, can also provide a nidus for thrombus formation.

The final prerequisite for intracardiac thrombosis is a hypercoagulable state. Activation of the coagulation system and platelets can be found in conditions associated with intracardiac thrombi, including AMI, atrial cardiomyopathy, and AF. Rare cases of intracardiac thrombi have been reported even with normal function and blood flow in the setting of hypercoagulable states such as factor V Leiden mutation, prothrombin gene mutation, antithrombin deficiency, protein C and S deficiencies, homocysteine deficiency, and antiphospholipid antibody syndrome.

Although all three of Virchow's prerequisites are operative in specific settings, most clinical data indicate that a complex interaction exists, with stasis being the most easily demonstrated clinical factor leading to intracardiac thrombosis.

B. Embolization of Thrombi

The major risk of intracardiac thrombi is end-organ ischemia/infarction due to embolization. Factors that result in embolization of intracardiac thrombi are poorly understood, but restoration of mechanical function to an area of the heart where thrombosis developed because of stasis may result in embolization. LVT usually embolize 5–21 days following infarction (days to weeks after initial thrombus formation), when regional and global left ventricular function may be improving, decreasing stasis and expelling the thrombus. Improved myocardial function at the margins of a thrombus could theoretically dislodge the thrombus or change the shape of a thrombus from mural to protruding, increasing the likelihood of embolization.

Recovery of the mechanical function of the left atrium following conversion from atrial flutter or fibrillation to sinus rhythm has also been implicated in embolization of left atrial thrombi. Following conversion of AF to sinus rhythm by any means, the left atrium and/or appendage may be stunned, creating a low-flow state that leads to thrombus formation. As atrial function recovery begins, embolization may occur, which happens on average 48 hours after conversion, and the risk persists for the ensuing 4–6 weeks.

Endogenous or pharmacologic thrombolysis could also result in embolization of existing thrombus. Embolization is more likely for certain intracardiac thrombi, especially if they are large, protruding, or mobile. Although any organ system may experience peripheral embolism from an intracardiac thrombus, the most feared complication is stroke.

Diagnostic Studies

Transthoracic echocardiography (TTE) is sensitive and specific for detecting LVT (Figures 4–1 and 4–2). Intravenous ultrasound-enhancing agents (UEA) may help in accurate identification of cardiac masses, especially thrombi (see Figure 4–1). Transesophageal echocardiography (TEE) is required to reliably detect left atrial thrombi (Figure 4–3) as well as atherothrombotic material in the ascending,

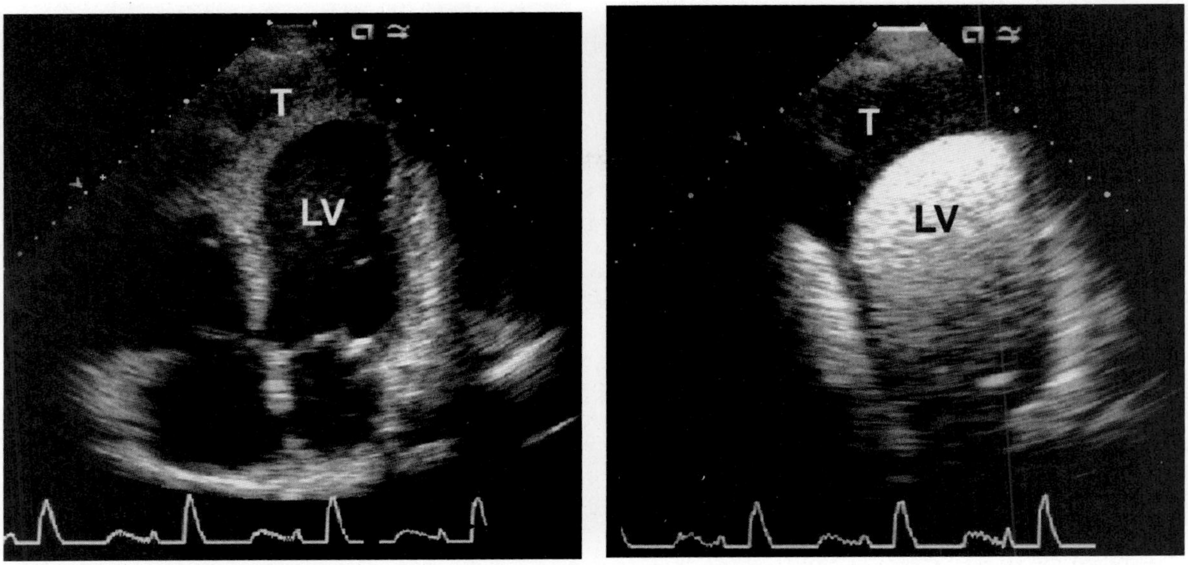

▲ **Figure 4–1.** Mural thrombus (T) in the left ventricle (LV) of a patient with a left ventricular aneurysm following anterior MI. Left panel is an apical four-chamber echocardiogram with second harmonic imaging. The thrombus is well imaged, but delineation of the underlying wall motion abnormality is difficult to appreciate. Right panel is the same view with a lipid-based echo contrast agent; note the clearer definition of the thrombus and aneurysm.

transverse, and descending thoracic aorta, another potential embolic source (Figure 4–4).

Spontaneous echo contrast ("smoke") detected in a cardiac chamber represents low-flow and early rouleaux formation and is frequently associated with thromboembolism. Patients with spontaneous echo contrast or low flow in the left atrial appendage (LAA) have a higher incidence of left atrial thrombi and thromboembolism.

Gated cardiac CT and cardiac magnetic resonance imaging (CMR; Figure 4–5) can also detect intracardiac thrombus. Contrast-enhanced CMR (using gadolinium) is highly sensitive and specific and is the gold standard for detection of LVT. It is particularly useful if TTE with UEA is indeterminate or of poor quality or in the context of imaging ambiguity. Gated cardiac CT including acquisition of a delayed phase can be a useful modality for detection of left

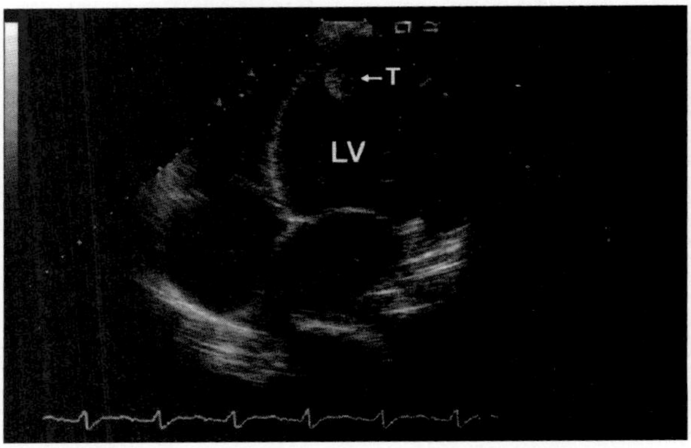

▲ **Figure 4–2.** Apical four-chamber, two-dimensional echocardiogram of a patient with dilated cardiomyopathy showing a protruding thrombus (T) at the apex of the left ventricle (LV).

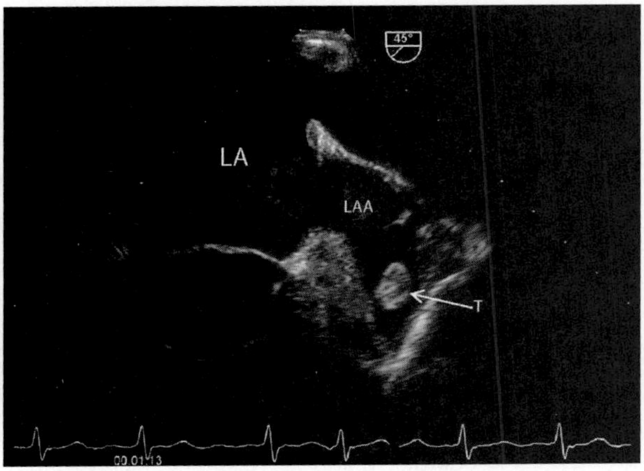

▲ **Figure 4–3.** Transesophageal echocardiogram demonstrating the left atrium (LA) with a thrombus (T) in the left atrial appendage (LAA). *Arrow* points to thrombus.

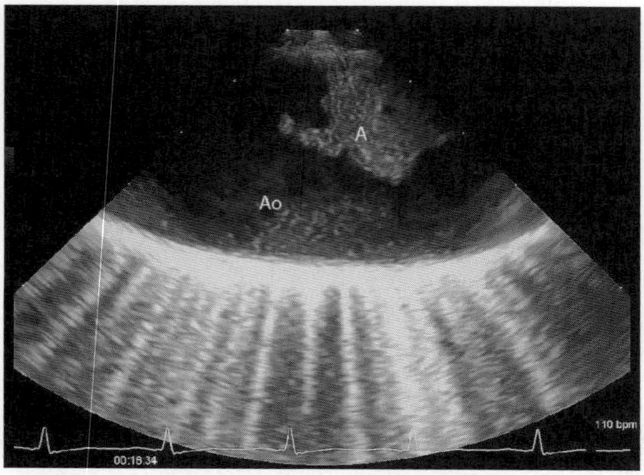

▲ **Figure 4–4.** Transesophageal echocardiogram demonstrating a large atheroma (A) in the transverse thoracic aorta (Ao).

atrial thrombi, including in the appendage, particularly if TEE is not feasible.

Although intracardiac thrombi are the most common cardiac cause of systemic embolization, there are other causes, including valvular vegetations due to infectious or noninfectious endocarditis, calcific emboli due to degenerative aortic and mitral valve disease, tumor emboli from left-sided myxoma, and atheroemboli from friable or mobile plaque in the aorta or great vessels (see Figure 4–4). In addition, embolic events can occur due to paradoxical emboli from thrombus that originates in the peripheral venous system, embolizes to the heart, and transverses an intracardiac communication (most commonly a patent foramen ovale) (Figure 4–6). These conditions can be identified by TTE and/or TEE.

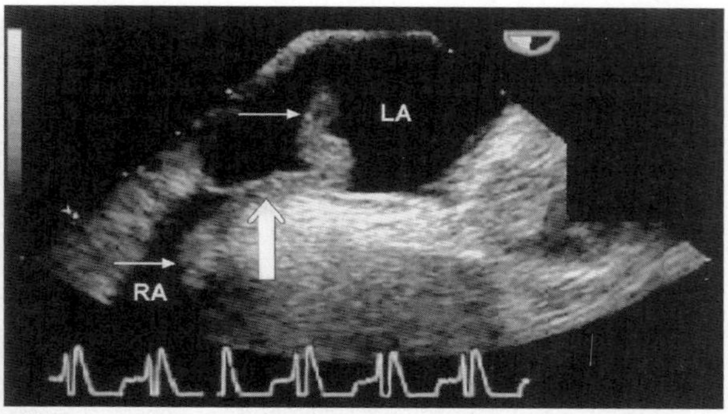

▲ **Figure 4–6.** Transesophageal echocardiogram demonstrating a systemic venous thrombus that has embolized to the heart and lodged in a patent foramen ovale. LA, left atrium; RA, right atrium. *Small arrows* indicate the thrombus; the *large arrow* indicates the patent foramen ovale.

Ning Y, Tse G, Luo G, Li G. Atrial cardiomyopathy: an emerging cause of the embolic stroke of undetermined source. *Front Cardiovasc Med.* 2021 Aug 9;8:674612. [PMID: 34434973]

Treatment of Cardiac Conditions Requiring Anticoagulation

Short-term and long-term anticoagulation is integral to the management of many cardiovascular conditions such as

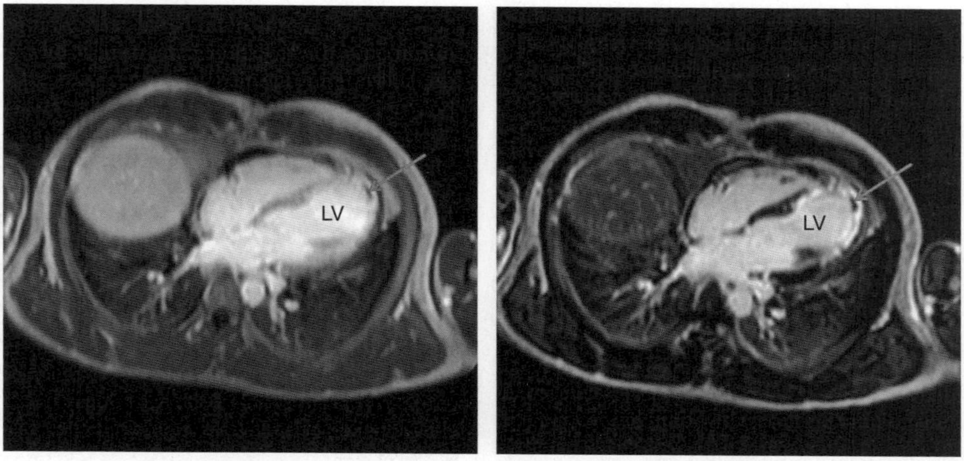

Panel A Panel B

▲ **Figure 4–5.** Cardiac magnetic resonance imaging in the detection of left ventricular (LV) thrombus. **A:** High-TI (inversion time) sequence demonstrating a small apical LV thrombus. **B:** In the same patient is a delayed hyperenhancement sequence demonstrating an area of myocardial scar involving the distal septal, apical, and distal anterolateral walls with presence of a small LV thrombus. *Arrow* points to thrombus.

acute coronary syndromes, stroke, PAD, and VTE, which will be discussed in other chapters. Long-term anticoagulation will be discussed in this chapter for the following cardiovascular conditions: AF, native valvular heart disease, prosthetic heart valves, LVT, atherosclerotic sources of emboli, paradoxical emboli associated with a patent foramen ovale (PFO), and intracardiac devices.

A. Atrial Fibrillation

AF is the most common sustained cardiac arrhythmia encountered in clinical practice and is also the most frequent cause of cardioembolic stroke by embolization of left atrial or LAA thrombus. Therapeutic anticoagulation can reduce the hazard of cardioembolic stroke with NVAF by nearly two-thirds. The risk of stroke in patients with AF is very high in the presence of rheumatic mitral stenosis, but even when not related to rheumatic mitral valve disease or a mechanical heart valve (NVAF), the incidence of stroke is 4–5 times greater than in similar patients without AF.

NVAF is categorized as (1) first episode, (2) paroxysmal, (3) persistent, and (4) permanent (see Chapter 12 for more details). The risk of stroke is generally considered equivalent for all four categories of clinically detected AF and can be calculated based on risk stratification schemes. Subclinical AF may be detected by extended monitoring techniques; there is conflicting data on the risk of stroke for such patients. Atrial flutter is much less common than AF, however, these two arrhythmias often coexist in the same individual. Patients with atrial flutter are also at risk for thromboembolism, and therefore, the two arrhythmias are treated similarly with regard to anticoagulation.

1. Chronic atrial fibrillation (nonvalvular)—The efficacy of long-term therapy with OAC for primary and secondary prevention of stroke in patients with NVAF has been repeatedly shown in randomized, placebo-controlled trials. Randomized studies have shown that aspirin has little effect in reducing the incidence of stroke in patients with NVAF, much less than with adjusted-dose warfarin or apixaban. The combination of aspirin and fixed, low-dose warfarin was not as effective in lowering the incidence of stroke when compared with adjusted-dose warfarin. Aspirin plus clopidogrel was more efficacious than aspirin alone for stroke prevention in NVAF patients, but inferior to adjusted-dose warfarin despite a similar risk of bleeding. Antiplatelet agents should not be used for prevention of SSE in AF.

Therapeutic OAC reduces the incidence of stroke by more than 60%. For warfarin, the target INR is 2.0–3.0, and the time in therapeutic range is predictive of the efficacy of anticoagulation: The most optimal results are obtained when the patient's INRs are maintained in the target range more than 65% of the time. With DOACs, there is no need for routine monitoring and the risk of medication interactions is much lower. Given these factors and the decreased risk of serious bleeding in multiple trials, DOACs are now recommended as first-line therapy over warfarin in patients with NVAF.

Table 4–1. $CHADS_2$ and $CHA2DS_2$-VASc Risk Assessment for Anticoagulation in Nonvalvular Atrial Fibrillation

$CHADS_2$		CHA_2DS_2-VASc	
CHF	1	CHF	1
Hypertension	1	Hypertension	1
Age > 75	1	Age	
Diabetes	1	65–74	1
Stroke or TIA	2	> 75	2
		Diabetes	1
		Stroke or TIA	2
		Vascular disease	1
		Sex	
		Female	1

CHF, congestive heart failure; TIA, transient ischemic attack.

2. Balancing the risk of stroke and anticoagulation in patients with nonvalvular atrial fibrillation—Identified clinical risk factors for stroke in NVAF were incorporated into the $CHADS_2$ stroke risk classification scheme (Table 4–1, left column). Risk factors included are congestive heart failure (C), history of hypertension (H), age ≥ 75 years (A), and diabetes (D), which are each assigned 1 point. Patients with previous stroke, TIA, or thromboembolism (S) are assigned 2 points. The $CHADS_2$ risk score assists in determining the approach to anticoagulation treatment, but even the lowest risk patients with a score of 0 have nearly a 2% incidence of stroke if not anticoagulated.

A revised stroke risk classification scheme, CHA_2DS_2-VASc, was developed to take into account two additional risk factors, vascular disease and female sex, and to allow additional risk stratification based on age (see Table 4–1, right column, and Table 4–2). Risk factors are congestive heart failure or left ventricular dysfunction (C), history of hypertension (H), age ≥ 75 years (A_2), diabetes mellitus (D), previous stroke, TIA, or thromboembolism (S), vascular disease (PAD, CAD, or aortic plaque) (V), age 65–74 years (A), and sex category (1 point for female, 0 points for male) (Sc). Age ≥ 75 years and history of embolic event are each assigned 2 points; the rest are assigned 1 point each. An advantage of this scheme is that those with a CHA_2DS_2-VASc of 0 have a very low incidence of stroke without anticoagulation compared to a $CHADS_2$ of 0. If the CHA_2DS_2-VASc score is 0 for men or 1 for women, it is reasonable to not use anticoagulation; if 1 for men or 2 for women, OAC should be considered; if 2 for men or 3 for women, OAC is recommended. In patients with end-stage kidney disease, who are at increased risk of both bleeding and stroke, and who have

Table 4–2. Anticoagulation for Chronic Nonvalvular Atrial Fibrillation by $CHADS_2$ and CHA_2DS_2-VASc Risk

$CHADS_2$		CHA_2DS_2-VASc	
Score	TE Rate/Year	Score	TE Rate/Year
0	1.9	0	0.5
1	2.8	1	1.5
2	4.0	2	2.5
3	5.9	3	5.0
4	8.5	4	6.0
5	12.5	5	7.0
6	18.2	6	7.0

TE, thromboembolism.

Table 4–3. Bleeding Risk in Chronic Nonvalvular Atrial Fibrillation by the HAS-BLED Score

HAS-BLED	Points
Hypertension (uncontrolled)	1
Renal disease (Cr > 2.6 mg/dL)	1
Liver disease (bilirubin 2× normal)	1
Stroke history	1
Prior major bleeding	1
Labile INR	1
Age ≥ 65	1
Medications (NSAIDs)	1
Alcohol usage	1

Cr, creatinine; INR, international normalized ratio; NSAIDs, nonsteroidal anti-inflammatory drugs.

not been well-studied in clinical trials, it is reasonable to use warfarin or apixaban for anticoagulation in patients with a CHA_2DS_2-VASc score of 2 for men or 3 for women.

Both $CHADS_2$ and CHA_2DS_2-VASc have moderate predictive value at best, and both were derived and validated in the past. Epidemiologic trends since development of these schemes indicate a decline in the absolute population incidence of stroke with NVAF, so the calculated risk from the original derivation may overestimate contemporary risk. Both schemes serve to guide therapy rather than offering mandates. In all situations, the risks and benefits of anticoagulation should be carefully considered in a shared decision-making approach with the patient before embarking on long-term anticoagulation.

It is important to remember the risk of stroke is considered similar for clinical paroxysmal, persistent, and permanent AF based on stratification schemes. Furthermore, risk classification schemes do not apply to all patients: In addition to patients with valvular AF (discussed later), patients with hypertrophic cardiomyopathy and cardiac amyloidosis are at significantly increased risk for SSE with AF, and anticoagulation is recommended even if the CHA_2DS_2-VASc is 0.

Risk stratification has also been developed for bleeding on anticoagulant therapy with warfarin. Several schemas ($HEMORR_2HAGES$, HAS-BLED, and ATRIA) were derived from NVAF patients. The definitions of clinical risk factors and of major bleeding vary for these schemes, and their predictive value is also modest. The HAS-BLED score (hypertension, abnormal renal/liver function, stroke, bleeding history or predisposition, labile INR, elderly, drugs/alcohol concomitantly) has been endorsed by some professional organizations (Table 4–3).

Unfortunately, many of the clinical risks for stroke are the same as those for bleeding, leading to a conundrum regarding anticoagulation for the clinicians. The development of a cardioembolic stroke can be devastating, and this frequently justifies acceptance of the bleeding risk for many patients. DOACs are associated with a lower risk of bleeding than warfarin, predominately due to a lower risk for ICH (Figure 4–7).

An attractive theoretical strategy for stroke prevention in NVAF is rhythm control (i.e., electrical or chemical cardioversion and maintenance of normal sinus rhythm with the aim of eliminating AF and hence stroke risk). Cohort studies show that the risk of SSE remains higher in patients with "resolved" AF than in those without AF. This may be due to subclinical (asymptomatic) AF, but atrial cardiomyopathy may also be playing a role, as it is associated with an increased risk of SSE even in the absence of AF. Guidelines recommend that decisions about long-term anticoagulation be based on the thromboembolic risk profile, rather than monitoring for recurrent AF.

Catheter ablation is increasingly used in the treatment of symptomatic patients with paroxysmal AF and in selected patients with symptomatic persistent AF. Whether ablation lowers future thromboembolic risk and hence modifies the conventional indications for long-term anticoagulation has not been determined. This technique should not, therefore, be considered for the purpose of avoiding anticoagulation in patients with NVAF. Despite guidelines recommending the use of anticoagulation after ablation based on thromboembolic risk vs. bleeding risk rather than ablation success, analysis of the ORBIT-AF registries showed that about one quarter of patients had anticoagulation discontinued after ablation.

LAA occlusion, either surgical or percutaneous, is being used with increasing frequency to decrease the risk of thromboembolic events. Percutaneous implantation of

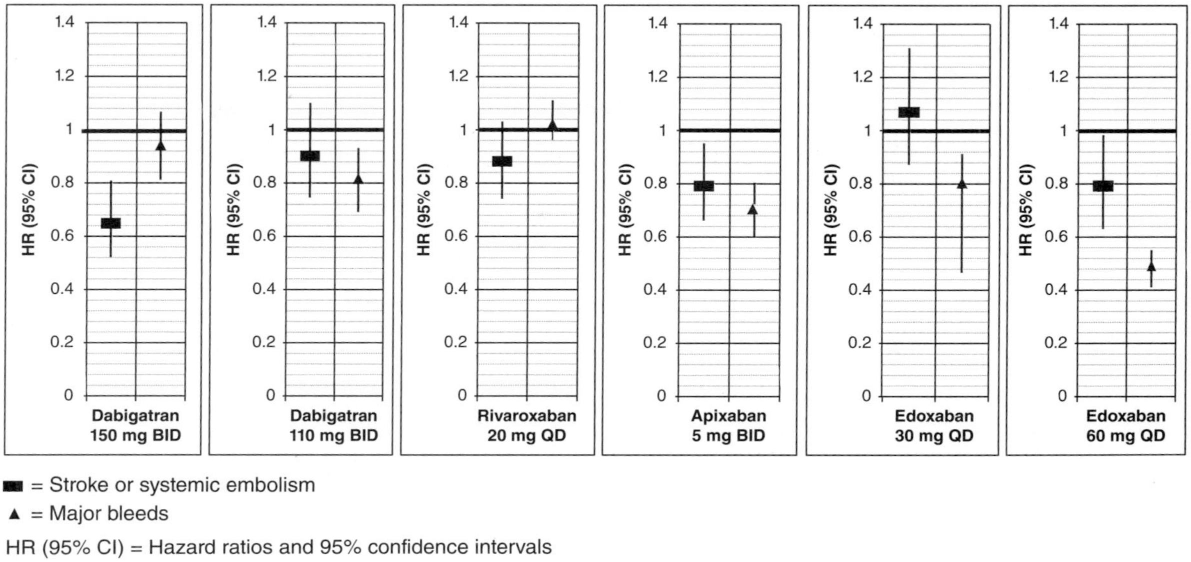

▲ **Figure 4–7.** Primary efficacy of stroke or systemic embolism and safety of major bleeding end points for direct oral anticoagulants compared with adjusted-dose warfarin.

the Watchman LAA closure device may be considered in patients at increased risk of SSE with reasons to avoid long-term anticoagulation. In addition to the original Watchman device, the Watchman FLX LAA closure device and the Amplatzer Amulet LAA occluder have also received FDA approval. There is a small periprocedural increase in the risk of ischemic stroke immediately after device implantation, but a larger long-term decrease in the risk of hemorrhagic stroke. The optimal peri-procedural antithrombotic strategy (including whether OAC or antiplatelet therapy is used) is not yet clear. Based on a multicenter randomized controlled trial, surgical LAA occlusion decreases the risk of SSE and should therefore be considered in patients with AF who are undergoing cardiac surgery. It should be noted that in this trial, those undergoing LAA occlusion had ongoing antithrombotic therapy after surgery.

3. Cardioversion for atrial fibrillation—Restoration of sinus rhythm can occur spontaneously or with chemical or electrical cardioversion. Conversion to sinus rhythm can lead to systemic embolism through either embolization of existing LAA thrombus with return of left atrial mechanical function or development of LAA thrombus during the postconversion period, when the atrium is mechanically stunned. There are two approaches to elective cardioversion to minimize stroke risk: the conventional approach and the TEE-guided approach (Figure 4–8). In the conventional approach, patients with AF of unknown duration or greater than 48 hours in duration are treated with warfarin to achieve an INR of 2.0–3.0 or one of the DOACs for at least 3 weeks before and at least 4 weeks after successful cardioversion. This recommendation applies regardless of stroke risk (CHA_2DS_2-VASc score). Continuation of anticoagulation beyond 4 weeks depends, however, on stroke and bleeding risk factors. In the TEE-guided approach, patients with AF of unknown duration or greater than 48 hours in duration are therapeutically anticoagulated with therapeutic LMWH, UFH, warfarin at an INR of 2.0–3.0, or a DOAC based on the time required to reach maximum effect after at least a single dose and then undergo a TEE. If no left atrial or LAA thrombus is seen, cardioversion is performed. If sinus rhythm is restored, anticoagulation with warfarin or DOAC should be continued for at least 4 weeks or longer, depending on stroke risk. If a left atrial thrombus is seen on TEE, cardioversion should not be performed. These patients should be treated with therapeutic oral anticoagulant for 3–4 weeks. TEE can then be repeated, and, if no thrombus is seen, cardioversion is performed followed by at least another 4 weeks of OAC.

For patients with AF of known duration less than 48 hours and a CHA_2DS_2-VASc score of 0 for men or 1 for women, anticoagulation is optional prior to and following cardioversion. If the CHA_2DS_2-VASc score is 2 for men or 3 for women, anticoagulation with heparin or OAC should be started as soon as possible before cardioversion and should be continued long-term.

4. Atrial fibrillation and coronary artery disease—For patients with AF and CAD who have undergone PCI, antiplatelet drugs must be added to chronic anticoagulation. When dual antiplatelet therapy (DAPT), including aspirin and a $P2Y_{12}$ inhibitor, is added to OAC, it is referred to as

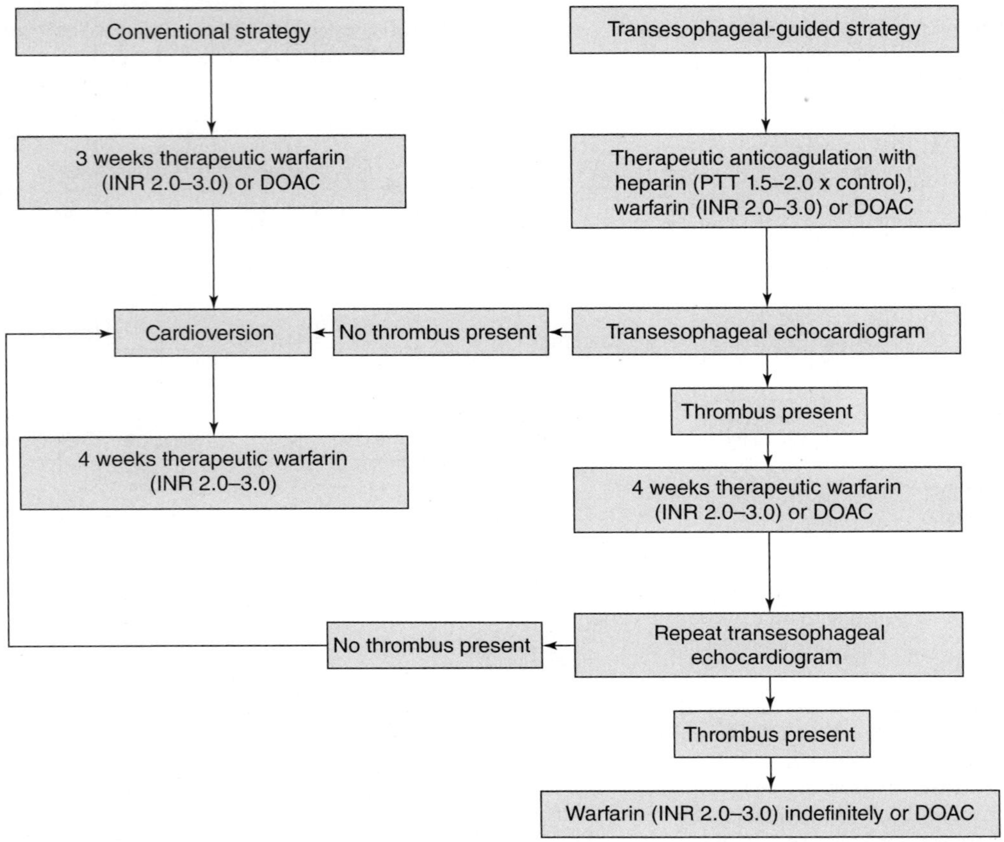

▲ **Figure 4–8.** Anticoagulation strategies for elective cardioversion of AF of unknown duration or lasting longer than 48 hours. IDOAC, new oral anticoagulant; INR, international normalized ratio; PTT, partial thromboplastin time.

triple antithrombotic therapy. Usually, clopidogrel is the preferred $P2Y_{12}$ agent in this situation. The duration of triple therapy continues to decline based on clinical trials; multiple studies have demonstrated the safety and efficacy of transitioning to dual therapy with a DOAC and a $P2Y_{12}$ inhibitor within 1 week of PCI compared to triple therapy with warfarin and DAPT. About 50% of patients in these studies had acute coronary syndrome; the remainder had stable CAD. Apixaban and edoxaban have been FDA approved for use after PCI in conjunction with clopidogrel; in clinical practice any DOAC is acceptable. Even in patients felt to merit triple therapy for longer than 1 week, it is reasonable to consider transition to dual therapy (with OAC and a $P2Y_{12}$ inhibitor) at 4 weeks, when the risk of stent thrombosis decreases dramatically with contemporary drug eluting stents. Implantation of a bare metal stent (rather than a drug-eluting stent) to limit the duration of antiplatelet therapy is no longer an appropriate consideration, as the duration of triple therapy can be safely abbreviated with new generation drug-eluting stents. When antiplatelet and anticoagulation are combined, concomitant proton pump inhibitors are recommended to decrease the risk of gastrointestinal bleeding.

In patients with stable CAD (i.e., more than 1 year after MI or revascularization), clinical data to guide selection of anticoagulant and antiplatelet therapies are limited. Meta-analysis shows that monotherapy with OAC has a similar risk of thrombotic events but a lower risk of bleeding events than dual therapy with OAC and an antiplatelet agent. If a patient with stable CAD and AF has an indication for anticoagulation based on CHA_2DS_2-VASc score, monotherapy with OAC is a reasonable consideration. Of course, each patient's risk of bleeding, risk of coronary thrombosis, and risk of SSE must be considered individually. Recent data from the AFIRE trial showed that monotherapy with rivaroxaban was non-inferior to rivaroxaban + antiplatelet therapy for ischemic outcomes and superior for bleeding. However, the generalizability of this study is unclear, since it was open label, the dose of rivaroxaban was atypical, and the trial was terminated early. Additional studies on this topic are needed.

B. Native Valvular Heart Disease

Thromboembolic complications may occur with several valvular conditions. Rheumatic mitral valve disease, particularly when accompanied by AF, has a very high incidence of embolic events. In contrast, patients with mitral valve prolapse and calcific aortic and/or mitral annular valve disease (except when AF is also present) are at low risk for embolic events.

1. Rheumatic mitral valve disease—The risk of thromboembolism with mitral stenosis and AF was reported to be 18 times greater than matched controls. Thromboembolic complications, however, can also occur in patients with rheumatic mitral stenosis who are in sinus rhythm. Patients with rheumatic mitral valve disease and AF or a previous embolic event should receive warfarin with a target INR of 2.0–3.0. If an embolic event occurs while a patient is receiving therapeutic anticoagulant therapy, the INR goal needs to be increased and an antiplatelet agent should be considered. Patients with rheumatic mitral stenosis undergoing balloon valvuloplasty should have left atrial/appendage thrombus ruled out with TEE before the procedure.

Patients with pure rheumatic mitral regurgitation may be at lower risk for thromboembolism than those with mitral stenosis because flow through the left atrium is increased, decreasing the likelihood of thrombus formation. There are no specific recommendations for anticoagulation of patients with rheumatic mitral regurgitation in sinus rhythm. Most patients with rheumatic mitral regurgitation, however, also have some degree of mitral stenosis, and recommendations for anticoagulation for mitral stenosis apply to these patients.

2. Nonrheumatic mitral regurgitation—The routine use of antithrombotic therapy for primary prevention of stroke or systemic embolus in nonrheumatic mitral regurgitation is not recommended. Secondary prevention with warfarin at a target INR of 2.0–3.0 is, however, recommended for those with previous thromboembolism or AF.

3. Mitral valve prolapse—Stroke or transient ischemic attack with no other identifiable cause is uncommon with mitral valve prolapse. The mechanism for thromboembolism in mitral valve prolapse is thought to be fibrinous exudates on the myxomatous valve itself or in the left atrium at the angle formed by the posterior mitral valve leaflet and left atrial wall. No antithrombotic measures are recommended for primary prevention of thromboembolism. Secondary prevention, however, is recommended. Those with mitral valve prolapse who have had documented but unexplained transient ischemic attack or stroke receive long-term treatment with aspirin (50–162 mg daily). For patients with mitral valve prolapse who have had systemic emboli or recurrent transient ischemic attacks despite aspirin therapy, long-term treatment with warfarin, with a target INR of 2.0–3.0, is recommended.

4. Calcific mitral and aortic valve conditions—Calcification of the mitral valve annulus and aortic valve occurs commonly with advanced age. The incidence of stroke with mitral annular calcification is increased and may be secondary to coexisting atherosclerotic disease or direct embolization of fibrocalcific material. Calcification of the mitral annulus occurs at a younger age in those with CKD in whom the calcium and phosphorous metabolism are abnormal and in those with Marfan syndrome. It may not be possible to identify thromboembolism from calcific emboli, although occasionally, calcific emboli may be seen on funduscopic examination. Patients with mitral annular calcification but without AF, complicated by systemic emboli not documented to be due to calcific emboli, should be treated with aspirin 50–100 mg/day. If recurrent thromboembolism is documented on aspirin therapy, adjusted-dose warfarin with a target INR of 2.0–3.0 is recommended. For documented systemic calcific embolism, no specific recommendation is given, although it would seem reasonable to consider aspirin 50–100 mg daily and statin therapy.

Individuals with calcified aortic valves even with mild aortic stenosis do not have an increased incidence of strokes compared to controls, although they may be at risk for calcific emboli. They should not receive warfarin unless they have other indications such as AF. For documented calcific embolism, therapy with aspirin 50–100 mg daily and statin therapy should be considered.

5. Endocarditis—The incidence of embolic events in infective endocarditis is quite high. In the pre-antibiotic era, clinically detected emboli occurred in 70–90% of patients, but the rate is lower now. Anticoagulant therapy was used in the past to improve penetration of antibiotics into the infected structures but resulted in a high incidence of cerebral hemorrhage, so the routine use of anticoagulants was abandoned. Neither anticoagulant nor antiplatelet therapy is indicated for routine use in infective endocarditis to prevent thromboembolic complications.

Infective endocarditis may, however, occur in patients who have been receiving long-term anticoagulant therapy. If endocarditis develops in a patient with a mechanical prosthetic valve, warfarin should be stopped at the time of initial presentation, until it is clear that invasive procedures will not be required and there are no signs of central nervous system (CNS) involvement.

Nonbacterial thrombotic endocarditis (marantic and Libman-Sacks endocarditis) is a condition in which fibrin thrombi are deposited superficially on normal or degenerated cardiac valves. This usually occurs in malignancies, chronic debilitating conditions, and acute fulminant diseases such as septicemia and disseminated intravascular coagulation. The reported incidence of systemic emboli in this condition varies from 14% to 91%. Treatment of nonbacterial thrombotic endocarditis should be directed at the underlying condition. The ACCP recommends UFH for patients with nonbacterial endocarditis with systemic or pulmonary emboli.

C. Prosthetic Heart Valves

Prosthetic heart valves may be either mechanical or bioprosthetic. Mechanical valves require lifelong anticoagulation to reduce risk of valve thrombosis and peripheral thromboembolism. Although warfarin is the most commonly studied agent, alternative VKA have been used worldwide. DOACs are contraindicated for mechanical valves based on a clinical study that demonstrated higher hazards with the use of dabigatran in patients with mechanical protheses. Bioprosthetic valves usually do not require long-term anticoagulation, particularly beyond 3–6 months of surgery. Mechanical valve prostheses are more durable than bioprostheses and therefore less likely to require repeat valve surgery relative to bioprosthetic valves. Therefore, it is important to carefully evaluate patients for hemorrhagic risk and likelihood for repeat surgery when choosing the type of prosthetic valve. For older patients, the risk of anticoagulation may be greater than the risk of another operation to replace a bioprosthetic valve. For women of childbearing age, the risks of anticoagulation during pregnancy should be considered in selecting the type of prosthetic heart valve. The technique of transvalvular aortic valve replacement (TAVR) is widespread and has changed the landscape among patients with aortic stenosis. In the contemporary era, the option for "valve-in-valve" prosthesis has also become available, suggesting that the previously described paradigms will likely need reexamination. Ultimately, a shared decision-making format is recommended by the 2020 AHA/ACC guidelines in the choice of a prosthesis for every patient, with careful consideration of pros and cons of the above variables with the patient.

Table 4–4. Anticoagulation for Mechanical Prosthetic Valves

Type of Mechanical Prosthetic Valve	Goal of Anticoagulation[1]
Aortic bileaflet tilting-disk or current generation single-disk prosthesis and no additional risk factors for thromboembolism	INR 2.5 (2.0–3.0)
Aortic mechanical prosthesis with any additional risk factors for thromboembolism such as atrial fibrillation, left ventricular dysfunction, hypercoagulable state, or previous thromboembolism	INR 3.0 (2.5–3.5)
Aortic mechanical On-X valve without thromboembolic risk factors	INR 2.5 (2.0–3.0) for the first 3 months after surgery and INR 1.5–2.0 starting ≥ 3 months following surgery. Continue low dose aspirin (75–100 mg) at all times.
Aortic caged-ball prosthesis	INR 3.0 (2.5–3.5)
Mitral prosthesis	INR 3.0 (2.5–3.5)

[1]Additional low-dose aspirin recommended by American Heart Association/American College of Cardiology guidelines as a class 2b recommendation for those with mechanical aortic and mitral prosthesis who have an indication for antiplatelet therapy and the risk of bleeding is judged to be low. INR, international normalized ratio.

1. Mechanical prosthetic heart valves—Currently implanted mechanical prosthetic heart valves include unileaflet tilting-disk, bileaflet tilting-disk prostheses as well as On-X valves. Caged-ball prosthetic valves are no longer implanted, and patients with these valves are rarely seen. Although flow characteristics vary, all prosthetic valves are foreign material (the sewing ring and the mechanical portions of the prosthesis) placed in the central circulation, providing a potential nidus for thrombus formation. The underlying pathologic process, AF, and decreased systolic performance of the left ventricle are important risk factors for postimplant thromboembolism. The risk of thromboembolism varies for the different types of mechanical prosthetic valves. The lowest risk is for the On-X valves followed by bileaflet tilting-disk valves and the highest risk is for caged-ball valves.

Anticoagulation with UFH for mechanical prosthesis should be initiated in the postoperative period when adequate hemostasis is achieved and continued until therapy with warfarin is in the therapeutic range for the specific mechanical prosthesis implanted. The AHA/ACC guidelines for anticoagulation in the context of mechanical prosthetic valves have recommended transitioning to a single INR goal (with an acceptable range of variation) to help better guide clinicians. According to the guidelines, for patients with a mechanical aortic valve replacement (AVR) with a bileaflet or current generation single tilting-disk valve, an INR goal of 2.5 (range 2.0–3.0) is recommended in patients without risk factors for thromboembolism. For patients with other risk factors for thromboembolism (e.g., AF, prior thromboembolism, LV dysfunction, hypercoagulable state) or for older generation AVRs (e.g., ball-in-cage), a higher INR goal of 3.0 (range, 2.5–3.5) is recommended instead. For patients with a mechanical On-X AVR and no thromboembolic risk factors, VKA to target lower INR (1.5–2) is reasonable 3 months following surgery (INR goal of 2–3 in the first 3 months) along with ASA 75–100 mg daily. For patients undergoing mechanical mitral valve replacement (MVR), an INR goal of 3.0 (range, 2.5–3.5) is recommended by the guidelines. In patients with mechanical valves, in addition to VKAs, the AHA/ACC guidelines recommend concomitant use of low-dose aspirin therapy (75–100 mg) for all patients with a low bleeding risk and indication for antiplatelet therapy. Table 4–4 summarizes anticoagulation recommendations for mechanical prosthetic heart valves. It should be noted that the newer DOACs (both direct thrombin inhibitors and anti-Xa agents) are specifically contraindicated in patients with mechanical prosthesis.

2. Bioprosthetic heart valves—Despite the advantages of bioprosthetic valves in terms of central flow and less thrombogenic valve material, thromboembolic complications do occur, particularly in the early postoperative period. The presumed mechanism in this setting is thrombus formation on the sewing ring. For patients with bioprosthetic surgical valve replacement or TAVR and bioprosthetic mitral replacement, low-dose aspirin therapy (75–100 mg daily) is considered reasonable per the 2020 AHA/ACC guidelines. In addition, among patient with bioprosthetic TAVR and low risk of bleeding, in addition to low-dose aspirin, either clopidogrel 75 mg daily or VKA (INR goal 2.5) is considered reasonable for 3 months. In the first 3–6 months following mitral or aortic bioprosthetic valve replacement, warfarin is reasonable with a target INR of 2.5 (range, 2.0–3.0) for patients at low risk of bleeding according to AHA/ACC guidelines. Heparin is usually initiated as soon as the bleeding risk is acceptable postoperatively until the INR is therapeutic, with an overlap of 3–5 days. Long-term anticoagulation treatment with warfarin (beyond 6 months) is not necessary following bioprosthetic mitral valve replacement in the absence of other thromboembolic factors such as AF, previous thromboembolism, or hypercoagulable state. Following TAVR, low-dose aspirin and clopidogrel 75 mg daily are reasonable for the first 3–6 months following implant, and lifelong aspirin is usually recommended subsequently. For patients with low risk of bleeding following TAVR, anticoagulation with VKA for INR goal of 2.5 is also considered reasonable for at least 3 months following implantation per AHA/ACC guidelines. Table 4–5 summarizes general recommendations for anticoagulants with bioprosthetic valves.

3. Prosthetic valve thrombosis—An embolic event is the most common adverse consequence seen as a result of thrombosis of a mechanical prosthetic heart valve; hemodynamic compromise can also occur which can be insidious or acute and life-threatening. Thrombi affecting mechanical prosthetic valves can either obstruct or prevent closure of the valve, and urgent imaging is indicated to make a diagnosis. Fluoroscopic imaging of prosthetic valve motion can be useful for detecting obstruction by showing reduction in excursion of prosthetic valve leaflet(s). Similarly, CT imaging is helpful in three-dimensional visualization of the valve and can often detect pannus or thrombus. However, TTE and TEE are the most sensitive and specific diagnostic tests for detecting thrombus complicating a prosthetic valve and measuring the hemodynamic consequences thereof. According to 2020 AHA/ACC guidelines, emergency surgery or urgent treatment with slow-infusion, low-dose fibrinolysis is recommended for patients with a thrombosed left-sided prosthetic valve with symptoms of valve obstruction. Fibrinolytic therapy may be considered as first-line therapy for patients with a thrombosed left-sided prosthetic valve and functional class I–II symptoms, and if emergency surgery is too high-risk or is not available. Fibrinolytic therapy is usually preferable over surgery for a thrombosed right-sided prosthetic heart valve in a patient with functional class III–IV symptoms. Emergent surgery is usually favored when patients have functional class IV symptoms, large clot burden, recurrent valve thrombosis, especially in centers with ready surgical expertise and when the overall risk is deemed to be low. Pannus formation on the sewing ring of the prosthetic valve can cause similar hemodynamic compromise and may be a nidus for thrombus. When embolic events occur despite therapeutic INR levels, the INR goal needs to be increased to prevent future events for any mechanical prosthesis.

Although bioprosthetic valves are less thrombogenic than mechanical valves, bioprosthetic valve thrombosis have been described in the first 3 months after implantation, and also more sub-acutely in the first 1–2 years following implantation; transcatheter valves are more predisposed compared to surgical valves. Echocardiography can provide initial diagnostic suspicion for this condition, but TEE or CT imaging is usually necessary to confirm the diagnosis of valve thrombosis, or leaflet hypoattenuation. This condition is usually amenable and responsive to treatment with oral VKA.

Table 4–5. Anticoagulation for Bioprosthetic Valves

Postoperative Criteria	Anticoagulation
For first 3–6 months after surgery	Warfarin INR 2.5 (2.0–3.0)
After 3 months	
No atrial fibrillation	Aspirin, 75–100 mg
Aortic bioprosthesis + atrial fibrillation, previous thromboembolism, or hypercoagulable state	Warfarin, INR 2.5 (2.0–3.0)[1]
Mitral bioprosthesis + atrial fibrillation, previous thromboembolism, or hypercoagulable state	Warfarin, INR 2.5 (2.0–3.0)[1]
Transcatheter aortic valve replacement	Aspirin 75–100 mg lifelong and clopidogrel 75 mg daily for first 3 months

[1]Add antiplatelet agent for additional risk factors.
INR, international normalized ratio.

D. Left Ventricular Thrombus

LVT can complicate MI (either acute or remote) and nonischemic dilated cardiomyopathy. Absence of or ineffective reperfusion for acute anterior MI is the most significant risk factor in the acute setting; other risk factors for LVT include anterior MI, apical wall motion abnormality, and left ventricular ejection fraction (EF) less than 40%. In dilated cardiomyopathy, EF less than 35% is the most important risk factor for LVT. Morphologic risk factors for embolization of the thrombus include protrusion into the left ventricle and mobility.

1. Acute myocardial infarction—The most effective means to prevent LVT and subsequent embolization is prompt, effective reperfusion therapy during the acute infarct. The incidence of LVT after acute MI has decreased due to current reperfusion strategies (early primary PCI) and adjunctive anti-thrombotic therapy, but LVT is still a potential complication of anterior STEMI.

A reasonable approach is patients at risk for LVT is to obtain imaging with TTE with UEA within 24 hours after acute MI (Figure 4–9). If there is no LVT, but there are features that increase the risk of LVT (particularly anterior/apical akinesis/dyskinesis), repeat imaging with TTE plus UEA or gadolinium-enhanced CMR 4–7 days after MI is reasonable to screen for interim development of LVT. The risk for LVT formation is highest in the first 2 weeks, so repeat TTE with UEA 2 weeks after the index event could also be considered.

If LVT is present, OAC is recommended for a period of at least 3 months following AMI. If repeat echocardiography shows resolution of the thrombus at 3–6 months, OAC can be stopped, particularly if the regional wall motion abnormality has improved, and DAPT should be resumed. If dyskinesis is still present, a patient-centered discussion of the risks vs benefits of long-term anticoagulation should occur. There are limited and contradictory data regarding the selection of DOAC vs VKA for anticoagulation. It is reasonable to consider VKA (to goal INR of 2.0–3.0) as first-line therapy for LVT after AMI. In patients who cannot tolerate VKA, DOAC should be used. Whenever OAC is used in the context of AMI, in most situations, a single antiplatelet agent (usually $P2Y_{12}$ inhibitor) is used to avoid the heightened risk of bleeding from "triple" anticoagulation with the use of concomitant aspirin.

The incidence of ischemic stroke is low in patients receiving prompt and effective reperfusion therapy, either with thrombolytics or direct PCI; hence anticoagulation should not be routinely prescribed post-MI. Older guidelines suggest consideration of a VKA in addition to DAPT for patients with STEMI and anterior/apical akinesis or dyskinesis, but this is based on studies performed before modern PCI. The most recent ESC STEMI guidelines do not suggest routine use of anticoagulation after AMI. There is some rationale to consider OAC following anterior MI in patients who did not receive reperfusion therapy.

2. Remote infarction with thrombus—LVT detected at least 3 months following infarction still carries a risk for embolism. If detected in the setting of a cardioembolic event, treatment with anticoagulation is obviously recommended. A repeat echocardiogram at 3 months should be performed to determine whether anticoagulation should be continued further. If LVT is detected when undergoing echocardiography or another diagnostic study in the absence of a clinical cardioembolic event, therapeutic anticoagulation is also recommended with follow-up study at 3 months.

3. Left ventricular aneurysm—Although an uncommon complication of MI in the reperfusion era, left ventricular aneurysm still occurs, and many contain thrombus, but systemic embolization is unusual. It is hypothesized that the low incidence of systemic emboli noted when LVT is flat or "mural" and contained within a discrete aneurysm (see Figure 4–1) relates to a smaller surface area of the clot being exposed to circulating blood. It is unclear whether patients with left ventricular aneurysm warrant long-term anticoagulant

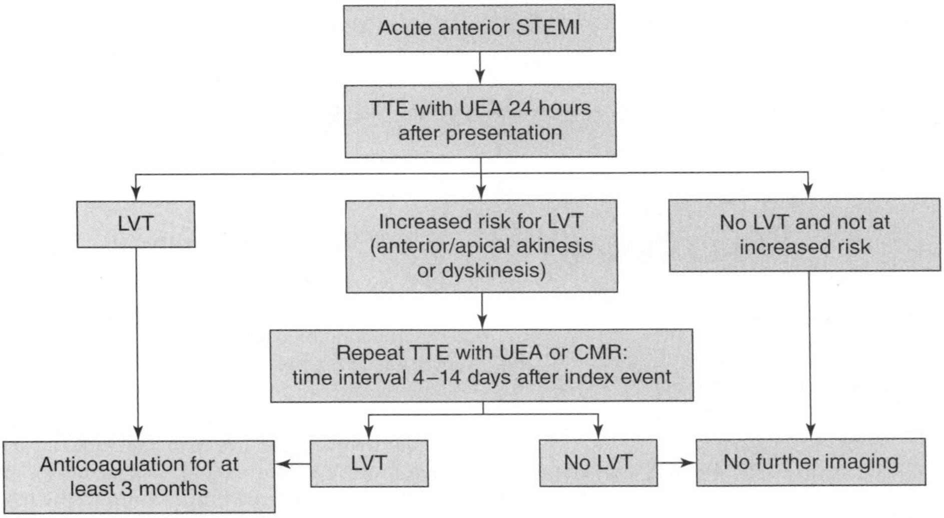

CMR: cardiac magnetic resonance imaging; LVT: left ventricular thrombus; STEMI: ST-elevation myocardial infarction; TTE: transthoracic echocardiogram; UEA: ultrasound-enhancing agent

▲ **Figure 4–9.** Sequential imaging and anticoagulant recommendations following acute anterior STEMI.

therapy for prevention of embolization if mural thrombus is contained within the aneurysm. Documented systemic embolization in patients with left ventricular aneurysm and thrombus, however, should prompt therapeutic anticoagulation for secondary prevention. Recurrent embolization despite therapeutic anticoagulation in this setting can be considered an indication for surgical left ventricular aneurysmectomy.

4. Dilated cardiomyopathy—Dilated cardiomyopathy may result from many different types of heart disease. Characteristically, generalized cardiac enlargement is present with right and left ventricular dysfunction that can cause stasis in any cardiac chamber. These patients may develop intracardiac thrombi, particularly in the left ventricle, followed by systemic embolization. For patients with clinical heart failure and reduced left ventricular systolic performance (EF < 35%), the routine use of therapeutic anticoagulation for primary prevention of stroke with warfarin reduces the incidence of stroke but increases the risk of major bleeding and is therefore not recommended. For patients with clinical heart failure and AF, previous thromboembolism, or LVT, therapeutic anticoagulation is recommended.

E. Aortic Atheroma

TEE is often performed in evaluation for a source of cardioembolism in the setting of stroke or transient ischemic attack and visualizes the ascending, transverse, and descending thoracic aorta. Aortic atheroma detected by this technique (see Figure 4–4) may be a cause of systemic embolus, including stroke. In the Stroke Prevention in Atrial Fibrillation Trial, patients who underwent TEE had a 35% incidence of complex aortic plaque greater than 4 mm in thickness. The risk of stroke at 1 year in these patients was 12–20%. The risk of stroke in patients with AF without complex aortic plaque was 1.2%. Studies have shown that plaque size greater than 4 mm in thickness increase the risk of ischemic events.

Treatment of complex aortic plaque for the primary and secondary prevention of embolic stroke is controversial. While aspirin is generally recommended, warfarin has been reported to be efficacious in some series, particularly for secondary prevention. Patients with complex aortic plaques and embolic events treated with statins have a significantly lower risk of embolic events than those taking warfarin or aspirin, and statins are therefore indicated for secondary prevention. In general, there is currently insufficient evidence for recommendation of routine anticoagulant therapy for this indication.

F. Paradoxical Emboli Associated with Patent Foramen Ovale

Intracardiac shunts are usually left to right, but there may also be right-to-left shunting under certain circumstances, such as cough or Valsalva maneuver, with the potential to permit paradoxical embolization (see Figure 4–6) that is, thrombus on the right side of the circulation embolizing to the left side of the circulation. PFO is common, occurring in up to 25% of the population, and can be detected by TTE using contrast echocardiography performed using a "bubble study" to detect right-to-left shunting. The presence of a PFO can be confirmed by TEE, and specific anatomical characteristics (e.g., presence of atrial septal aneurysm, higher size of shunt, etc.) can be further delineated. Several randomized controlled trials have now evaluated the role of antiplatelet therapy vs. anticoagulant therapy vs. PFO closure among patients with cryptogenic stroke. The SCAI guidelines in 2022 address the nuanced decision-making of choice between OAC and PFO closure in select subgroups with prior stroke. In general, the guidelines suggest a paradigm shift toward percutaneous PFO closure rather than long-term OAC. Although the discussion about management of the various subcategories of this population is beyond the scope of this book chapter, readers are encouraged to review the SCAI guidelines for more detail. A specific but rare condition called the platypnea-orthodeoxia syndrome (POS) warrants consideration of PFO closure if other causes of hypoxia have been excluded but does not have a specific indication for anticoagulation.

G. Pacemakers, Implantable Cardioverter-Defibrillators, and Other Intracardiac Devices

Thromboembolic complications occur infrequently in patients with pacemakers and implantable cardioverter-defibrillators (ICDs). The intravascular and intracardiac leads can act as a nidus for thrombus formation. On rare occasions, swelling of the ipsilateral arm may develop; venous ultrasound can assist identifying thrombus of the subclavian vein. The treatment for subclavian vein thrombosis is OAC. The duration of treatment with anticoagulants varies but is usually for at least 3 months and is longer in those with other predisposing procoagulant factors. For extreme swelling and pain of the effected extremity, interventional procedures to restore flow in the subclavian vein should be considered. Thrombolytic therapy cannot be used in the immediate post-pacemaker implant period because of the risk of bleeding into the pacemaker pocket.

TEE performed for unrelated indications has demonstrated a high incidence of incidentally detected thrombi on pacemaker and ICD leads, which can be highly mobile. Differentiation from infective endocarditis is mandatory since the clinical approach and treatment is markedly different. The risk for embolization to the pulmonary artery or systemically if there is a PFO is unknown; there are no guidelines for treating these thrombi with anticoagulation or for removal of the device. If embolic events have occurred or there are other high-risk factors for thromboembolism, it seems reasonable to initially treat with oral anticoagulants.

Technologic advances are leading to the implantation of additional intracardiac devices. Since these devices are foreign bodies, they can act as a nidus for thrombus formation. Percutaneous closure devices for atrial septal defects are available. Current anticoagulation recommendations are for aspirin and clopidogrel for 3 months following the procedure. OAC is not typically recommended. Devices for percutaneous occlusion of the LAA have been approved for use in NVAF for patients who are high-risk candidates for anticoagulation. Although anticoagulation is required for this procedure in the short term, the strategy behind these devices is to avoid long-term anticoagulation.

Asinger RW, Shroff GR, Simegn MA, Herzog CA. Anticoagulation for nonvalvular atrial fibrillation: influence of epidemiologic trends and clinical practice patterns on risk stratification and net clinical benefit. *Circ Cardiovasc Qual Outcomes*. 2017 Sep;10(9): e003669. [PMID: 28893833]

Camaj A, Fuster V, Giustino G, et al. Left ventricular thrombus following acute myocardial infarction. *J Am Coll Cardiol*. 2022 Mar;79(10):1010–1022.

Collado FMS, Poulin MF, Murphy JJ, et al. Patent foramen ovale closure for stroke prevention and other disorders. *J Am Heart Assoc*. 2018; 7(12):e007146. [PMID: 29910192]

Khan F, Fiorilli P, Messe SR, et al. Clinicians' approach to patent formne ovale closure after stroke: comparing cardioloists and neurologists. *J Am Heart Assoc*. 2022 Jul 19;11(14):e025598. doi: 10.1161/JAHA.122.025598. Epub 2022 Jul 5. [PMID: 35861812]

Otto C, Nishimura RA, Bonow RO, et al. 2020 ACC/AHA Guideline for the Management of Patients With Valvular Heart Disease: Executive Summary: A Report of the American College of Cardiology/American Heart Association Joint Committee on Clinical Practice Guidelines. *Circulation*. 2021 Feb 2; 143(5):e35–e71. [PMID: 33332149]

Whitlock RP, Belley-Cote EP, Paparella D, et al; LAAOS III Investigators. Left atrial appendage occlusion during cardiac surgery to prevent stroke. *N Engl J Med*. 2021 Jun 3;384(22):2081–2091. [PMID: 33999547]

Special Considerations

A. Pregnancy

Management of severe valve disease in female patients of child-bearing age is particularly challenging because warfarin use during pregnancy carries a significant risk for both maternal and fetal complications. Warfarin crosses the placenta and can cause an embryopathy, especially when used between weeks 6 and 12 of gestation. Fetal CNS abnormalities may occur with maternal warfarin use in any trimester. There is also a higher risk of fetal ICH if mother is fully anticoagulated at the time of delivery. UFH and LMWH do not cross the placenta, and therefore, their use in pregnancy may be safer for the fetus. However, both are expensive, difficult to administer, and associated with risks of bleeding, osteoporosis, and HIT (less likely with LMWH). Low-dose aspirin (< 150 mg/day) is considered safe in the second and third trimesters. Warfarin, UFH, and LMWH can safely be administered to the nursing mother because they do not have an anticoagulant effect in breastfed infants.

The most common cardiac condition requiring anticoagulation during pregnancy is mechanical prosthetic heart valves. Pregnancy is a hypercoagulable state, the risk of valve thrombosis is estimated to be nearly 5% during pregnancy, and maternal mortality is over 1%. Anticoagulant strategies can have several pros and cons that need to be carefully considered to make shared decisions with the patient to identify the most optimal strategy. It has been shown that warfarin is the most efficacious in preventing maternal complications such as valve thrombosis compared to UFH or fixed-dose LMWH during pregnancy; but has the highest likelihood of miscarriage, fetal congenital abnormalities, particularly if dose of warfarin exceeds 5 mg/day. The AHA/ACC 2020 guidelines recommend continuing maintenance warfarin in the first trimester of pregnancy if the warfarin dose is ≤ 5 mg/day. If the required maintenance warfarin dose is more than 5 mg/day, dose-adjusted LMWH or UFH is recommended in the first trimester followed by warfarin during the second and third trimesters. LMWH is administered twice a day in doses adjusted to keep the 4–6 hour post injection anti-Xa level at approximately 0.8–1.2 units/mL. If UFH is used, it is recommended to keep the aPTT at least two times higher than control. Warfarin in therapeutic doses is recommended for the second and third trimesters. For those needing warfarin dose more than 5 mg/day it is also considered reasonable to use LMWH with anti-Xa throughout all three trimesters, albeit this is a much more expensive strategy. Low-dose aspirin is recommended throughout pregnancy except during the week prior to delivery. Anticoagulation may be interrupted briefly for delivery and resumed postpartum using dose-adjusted UFH or LMWH as a bridge to therapeutic anticoagulation with warfarin.

Women of childbearing age who need to have a prosthetic heart valve should consider their desire to become pregnant when deciding about the type of valve to be implanted. A bioprosthetic valve or native valve repair do not require lifelong anticoagulation and would therefore be safer in terms of anticoagulation and pregnancy risks but with a long-term risk of reoperation due to bioprosthetic valve degeneration. Because of the complexities, the AHA/ACC guidelines recommend careful management of pregnant patients with mechanical valves by a heart valve team.

B. Interruption of Anticoagulation for Surgery and Invasive Procedures

At times, anticoagulant therapy needs to be interrupted because of surgery or other invasive procedures and certain endoscopic procedures. The anticoagulant effects of warfarin persist for several days. Toward the end of this period, there may be inadequate protection from thromboembolism, necessitating consideration of short-term anticoagulation with UFH or LMWH. The anticoagulant effects of the DOACs dissipate more quickly; this is an important difference compared to warfarin.

Elective and planned surgery/procedures mandate a systematic approach to dealing with anticoagulation issues with a working knowledge of accurate pharmacokinetics. Urgent or emergent procedures or surgeries on patients receiving anticoagulation require a thoughtful approach to reduce the risk of bleeding and thromboembolic complications.

The risk of bleeding for different procedures and surgeries varies and determines the need for the interruption of anticoagulation therapy. Procedures with a low risk for bleeding include cataract surgery or dental extractions. These procedures can be usually performed without interruption of OAC. Procedures with a high bleeding risk include open-heart surgery, abdominal vascular surgery, intracranial and spinal procedures, major cancer surgeries, and urologic procedures. These procedures require interruption of OAC aiming for a return of normal coagulation prior to surgery due to higher risk of bleeding complications.

The risk of thromboembolism when warfarin or any of the new anticoagulants is discontinued varies for different cardiac conditions. After the discontinuation of anticoagulant, the annual risk of thrombotic complications is as follows: 1% for "lone" AF; 5% for NVAF (low risk); 12% for high-risk AF, 10–12% for St. Jude prosthetic aortic valve (intermediate risk); 22% for a mitral mechanical prosthetic valve; and up to 91% for multiple mechanical prosthetic valves (high risk).

The period for interruption of warfarin therapy preceding surgery depends on the INR goal being achieved, the risk of bleeding from the surgery (low risk vs. high risk) as well as type of valve prosthesis. Usually, warfarin needs to be stopped four to five doses prior to surgery. For the DOACs, the period of interruption depends on the specific agent and the estimated CrCl (eCrCl). Dabigatran can be discontinued 24–48 hours prior to procedure with an eCrCl more than 50 mL/min but needs interruption for 3–5 days prior to procedure with an eCrCl less than 50 mL/min. Similarly, the factor Xa inhibitors can be usually stopped 24 hours prior to procedure for higher eCrCl values and 48 hours prior to procedure for lower eCrCl values or higher bleeding risk. Resumption of these agents following surgery should only occur after hemostasis has been achieved, noting that their onset of action is only 2–3 hours, which is very different compared to warfarin, which takes several days for therapeutic effects to be reached. Premature restarting of DOACs can increase risk of postoperative bleeding.

For patients with a higher risk of thromboembolism, bridging therapy is usually considered with heparin (UFH or LMWH) when the anticoagulant effects of warfarin are subtherapeutic before and after surgery. For patients on DOACs, bridging with heparin is not typically required due to rapid onset and offset of anticoagulant action. Among patients with AF (without mechanical valvular prosthesis and with mean $CHADS_2$ score of 2.3) in the BRIDGE trial, the strategy of foregoing bridging was found to be noninferior to bridging with LMWH with a reduced risk of major bleeding in the context of elective surgery. These findings do not support routine bridging of patients with AF undergoing temporary interruption of anticoagulation for elective surgeries due to a very low risk of systemic embolic events (Table 4–6).

Table 4–6. Interruption of Anticoagulation for Surgery or Invasive Procedures

Condition	Recommendation
Atrial fibrillation and aortic bileaflet prosthesis without high-risk features[1]	Stop warfarin 5 days before procedure Stop DOACs 24–48 hours prior to procedure depending on estimated creatinine clearance Restart oral anticoagulation after the procedure as soon as it is safe keeping in mind that DOACs have onset of action within a few hours, whereas warfarin has onset of action after several days Bridging with UFH or LMWH not typically necessary
All other mechanical valve prostheses[2]	Stop warfarin 4–5 days before the procedure Start UFH or LMWH when INR < 2.0 Stop UFH 4–6 hours or LMWH 12 hours before procedure Restart UFH or LMWH and warfarin after the procedure as soon as it is safe

[1]High-risk features include atrial fibrillation, previous thromboembolism, hypercoagulable state, and left ventricular dysfunction.
[2]Mitral bileaflet prosthesis, aortic and mitral unileaflet prosthesis, and aortic and mitral ball-cage prosthesis.
DOACs, direct oral anticoagulants; INR, international normalized ratio; LMWH, low-molecular-weight heparin; UFH, unfractionated heparin.

The 2020 AHA/ACC guidelines recommend that temporary interruption of anticoagulation without bridging is reasonable for patients with bileaflet mechanical aortic prosthesis without risk factors for thromboembolism undergoing invasive procedures. However, bridging anticoagulation is considered reasonable for those with mechanical aortic prosthesis with thromboembolic risk factors, older generation mechanical aortic prosthesis as well as mechanical mitral prosthesis. Ultimately, the decision about bridging anticoagulation must be individualized in all patients with a careful assessment of risks of bleeding vs. thrombotic events.

Emergent surgery and procedures require a different approach. For those on warfarin, immediate reversal with fresh frozen plasma or prothrombin concentrate complex (does not require a large-volume load) is recommended; anticoagulants can be restarted when the bleeding risk is acceptably low. The use of high doses of vitamin K is discouraged in the milieu of mechanical prosthesis due to long-standing inhibition of vitamin K–dependent receptors and difficulty in getting a target INR subsequently, but low doses of oral vitamin K are felt to be acceptable. Acute reversal of DOACs for emergency surgery is problematic because the precise anticoagulant effect cannot be easily determined clinically. Dialysis is an option for reversal of dabigatran but can be time consuming to accomplish. For reversal of effects of both the direct thrombin inhibitors and oral Xa inhibitors, prothrombin concentrate complex can be used. Idarucizumab (Praxbind) has been approved by the FDA for reversal of dabigatran, and andexanet alfa has been shown to rapidly reverse the effects of apixaban and rivaroxaban.

ACKNOWLEDGEMENT

The authors would like to acknowledge the contributions of Dr. Richard W. Asinger toward the earlier versions of this chapter in prior editions.

Approach to Cardiac Disease Diagnosis

5

Michael H. Crawford, MD

General Considerations

The patient's history is a critical feature in the evaluation of suspected or overt heart disease. It includes information about the present illness, past illnesses, and the patient's family. From this information, a chronology of the patient's disease process should be constructed. Determining what information in the history is useful requires a detailed knowledge of the pathophysiology of cardiac disease. The effort spent on listening to the patient is time well invested because the cause of cardiac disease is often discernible from the history.

A. Common Symptoms

1. Chest pain—Chest pain is one of the cardinal symptoms (Table 5–1) of ischemic heart disease, but it can also occur with other forms of heart disease. The five characteristics of ischemic chest pain, or angina pectoris, are as follows:

- Anginal pain usually has a substernal location but may extend to the left or right chest, shoulders, neck, jaw, arms, epigastrium, and, occasionally, upper back.
- The pain is deep, visceral, and intense; it makes the patient pay attention, but is not excruciating. Many patients describe it as a pressure-like sensation or a tightness.
- The duration of the pain is minutes, not seconds.
- The pain tends to be precipitated by exercise or emotional stress.
- The pain is relieved by resting or taking sublingual nitroglycerin.

2. Dyspnea—A frequent complaint of patients with a variety of cardiac diseases, dyspnea is ordinarily one of four types. The most common is exertional dyspnea, which usually means that the underlying condition is mild because it requires the increased demand of exertion to precipitate symptoms. The next most common is paroxysmal nocturnal dyspnea, characterized by the patient awakening after being asleep or recumbent for an hour or more. This symptom is caused by the redistribution of body fluids from the lower extremities into the vascular space and back to the heart, resulting in volume overload; it suggests a more severe condition. Third is orthopnea, a dyspnea that occurs immediately on assuming the recumbent position. The mild increase in venous return (caused by lying down) before any fluid is mobilized from interstitial spaces in the lower extremities is responsible for the symptom, which suggests even more severe disease. Finally, dyspnea at rest suggests severe cardiac disease.

Dyspnea is not specific for heart disease, however. Exertional dyspnea, for example, can be due to pulmonary disease, anemia, or deconditioning. Orthopnea is a frequent complaint in patients with chronic obstructive pulmonary disease and postnasal drip. A history of "two-pillow orthopnea" is of little value unless the reason for the use of two pillows is discerned. Resting dyspnea is also a sign of pulmonary disease. Paroxysmal nocturnal dyspnea is perhaps the most specific for cardiac disease because few other conditions cause this symptom.

3. Syncope and presyncope—Lightheadedness, dizziness, presyncope, and syncope are important indications of a reduction in cerebral blood flow. These symptoms are nonspecific and can be due to primary central nervous system disease, metabolic conditions, dehydration, or inner-ear problems. Because bradyarrhythmias and tachyarrhythmias are important cardiac causes, a history of palpitations preceding the event is significant.

4. Transient central nervous system deficits—Deficits such as transient ischemic attacks (TIAs) suggest emboli from the heart or great vessels or, rarely, from the venous circulation through an intracardiac shunt. A TIA should prompt the search for cardiovascular disease. Any sudden loss of blood flow to a limb also suggests a cardioembolic event.

5. Fluid retention—These symptoms are not specific for heart disease but may be due to reduced cardiac function.

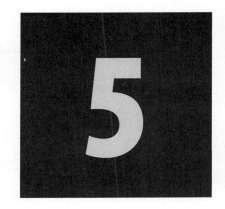

Table 5–1. Common Symptoms of Potential Cardiac Origin

Chest pain or pressure
Dyspnea on exertion
Paroxysmal nocturnal dyspnea
Orthopnea
Syncope or near syncope
Transient neurologic defects
Edema
Palpitation
Cough

Typical symptoms are peripheral edema, bloating, weight gain, and abdominal pain from an enlarged liver or spleen. Decreased appetite, diarrhea, jaundice, and nausea and vomiting can also occur from gut and hepatic dysfunction due to fluid engorgement.

6. Palpitation—Normal resting cardiac activity usually cannot be appreciated by the individual. Awareness of heart activity is often referred to by patients as palpitation. Among patients, there is no standard definition for the type of sensation represented by palpitation, so the physician must explore the sensation further with the patient. It is frequently useful to have the patient tap the perceived heartbeat out by hand. Commonly, unusually forceful heart activity at a normal rate (60–100 bpm) is perceived as palpitation. More forceful contractions are usually the result of endogenous catecholamine excretion that does not elevate the heart rate out of the normal range. A common cause of this phenomenon is anxiety. Another common sensation is that of the heart stopping transiently or of the occurrence of isolated forceful beats or both. This sensation is usually caused by premature ventricular contractions, and the patient either feels the compensatory pause or the resultant more forceful subsequent beat or both. Occasionally, the individual refers to this phenomenon as "skipped" beats. The least common sensation reported by individuals, but the one most linked to the term "palpitation" is rapid heart rate that may be regular or irregular and is usually supraventricular in origin.

7. Cough—Although cough is usually associated with pulmonary disease processes, cardiac conditions that lead to pulmonary abnormalities may be the root cause of the cough. A cardiac cough is usually dry or nonproductive. Pulmonary fluid engorgement from conditions such as heart failure may present as cough. Pulmonary hypertension from any cause can result in cough. Finally, angiotensin-converting enzyme inhibitors, which are frequently used in cardiac conditions, can cause cough.

B. History

1. The present illness—This is a chronology of the events leading up to the patient's current complaints. Usually, physicians start with the chief complaint and explore the patient's symptoms. It is especially important to determine the frequency, intensity, severity, and duration of all symptoms; their precipitating causes; what relieves them; and what aggravates them. Although information about previous related diseases and opinions from other physicians are often valuable, it is essential to explore the basis of any prior diagnosis and ask the patient about objective testing and the results of such testing. A history of prior treatment is often revealing because medications or surgery may indicate the nature of the original problem. A list of all the patient's current medications should be reviewed, confirming the dosages, the frequency of administration, and whether they are helping the patient, and noting any side effects.

2. Antecedent conditions—Several systemic diseases may have cardiac involvement. It is therefore useful to search for a history of rheumatic fever, which may manifest as Sydenham chorea, joint pain and swelling, or merely frequent sore throats. Other important diseases that affect the heart include metastatic cancer, thyroid disorders, diabetes mellitus, and inflammatory diseases such as rheumatoid arthritis and systemic lupus erythematosus. Certain events during childhood are suggestive of congenital or acquired heart disease; these include a history of cyanosis, reduced exercise tolerance, or long periods of restricted activities or school absence. Exposure to toxins, infectious agents, and other noxious substances may also be relevant. In addition, blunt chest trauma and radiation therapy can injure the heart and vasculature.

3. Atherosclerotic risk factors—Atherosclerotic cardiovascular disease is the most common form of heart disease in industrialized nations. The presenting symptoms of this ubiquitous disorder may be unimpressive and minimal, or as impressive as sudden death. It is therefore important to determine from the history whether any risk factors for this disease are present. The most important is a family history of atherosclerotic disease, especially at a young age; diabetes mellitus; lipid disorders such as a high low-density lipoprotein cholesterol level; hypertension; and smoking. Less important factors include a lack of exercise, high stress levels, lower socioeconomic status, and truncal obesity. There are formulae available online to calculate the risk of a cardiovascular event based on some of these factors.

4. Family history—A family history is important for determining the risk for not only atherosclerotic cardiovascular disease, but also for many other cardiac diseases. Congenital heart disease, for example, is more common in the offspring of parents with this condition, and a history of the disorder in the antecedent family or siblings is significant. Other genetic diseases, such as neuromuscular disorders or connective tissue disorders (eg, Marfan syndrome), can affect the heart. Acquired diseases, such as rheumatic valve disease, can cluster in families because of the spread of the streptococcal infection among family members. The lack of a history of hypertension in the family might prompt a more intensive search for a secondary cause. A history of atherosclerotic disease sequelae, such as limb loss, strokes, and heart attacks, may provide a clue to the aggressiveness of an atherosclerotic tendency in a particular family group.

Physical Findings

A. Physical Examination

The physical examination is less important than the history in patients with ischemic heart disease, but it is of critical value in patients with congenital and valvular heart disease. In the latter two categories, the physician can often make specific anatomic and etiologic diagnoses based on the physical examination. Certain abnormal murmurs and heart sounds are specific for structural abnormalities of the heart. The physical examination is also important for confirming the diagnosis and establishing the severity of heart failure, and it is the only way to diagnose systemic hypertension because this diagnosis is based on elevated blood pressure recordings.

1. Blood pressure—Proper measurement of the **systemic arterial pressure** by cuff sphygmomanometry is one of the keystones of the cardiovascular physical examination. It is recommended that the brachial artery be palpated, and the diaphragm of the stethoscope be placed over it, rather than merely sticking the stethoscope in the antecubital fossa. Current methodologic standards dictate that the onset and disappearance of the Korotkoff sounds define the systolic and diastolic pressures, respectively. Although this is the best approach in most cases, there are exceptions. For example, in patients in whom the diastolic pressure drops to near zero, the point of muffling of the sounds is usually recorded as the diastolic pressure. Because the diagnosis of systemic hypertension involves repeated measures under the same conditions, the operator should measure blood pressure under the same standard conditions each time. It is recommended that the patient be seated with their arm supported at heart level for 5 minutes before the pressure is measured.

Orthostatic changes in blood pressure are a very important physical finding, especially in patients complaining of transient central nervous system symptoms, weakness, or unstable gait. The technique involves having the patient assume the upright position for at least 90 seconds before taking the pressure to be sure that the maximum orthostatic effect is measured. Although measuring the pressure in other extremities may be of value in certain vascular diseases, it provides little information in a routine examination beyond palpating pulses in all the extremities. Keep in mind, in general, that the pulse pressure (the difference between systolic and diastolic blood pressures) is a crude measure of left ventricular stroke volume. A widened pulse pressure suggests that the stroke volume is large; a narrowed pressure suggests that the stroke volume is small.

2. Peripheral pulses—When examining the peripheral pulses, the physician is really conducting three examinations. The first is an examination of the cardiac rate and rhythm, the second is an assessment of the characteristics of the pulse as a reflection of cardiac activity, and the third is an assessment of the adequacy of the arterial conduit being examined. The pulse rate and rhythm are usually determined in a convenient peripheral artery, such as the radial. If a pulse is irregular, it is better to auscultate the heart; some cardiac contractions during rhythm disturbances do not generate a stroke volume sufficient to cause a palpable peripheral pulse. In many ways, the heart rate reflects the health of the circulatory system. A rapid pulse suggests increased catecholamine levels, which may be due to cardiac disease, such as heart failure; a slow pulse represents an excess of vagal tone, which may be due to disease or athletic training.

To assess the characteristics of the cardiac contraction through the pulse, it is usually best to select an artery close to the heart, such as the carotid. Bounding high-amplitude carotid pulses suggest an increase in stroke volume and should be accompanied by a wide pulse pressure on the blood pressure measurement. A weak carotid pulse suggests a reduced stroke volume. Usually, the strength of the pulse is graded on a scale of 1–4, where 2 is a normal pulse amplitude, 3–4 is a hyperdynamic pulse, and 1 is a weak pulse. A low-amplitude, slow-rising pulse, which may be associated with a palpable vibration (thrill), suggests aortic stenosis. A bifid pulse (beating twice in systole) can be a sign of hypertrophic obstructive cardiomyopathy, severe aortic regurgitation, or the combination of moderately severe aortic stenosis and regurgitation. A dicrotic pulse (an exaggerated, early, diastolic wave) is found in severe heart failure. Pulsus alternans (alternate strong and weak pulses) is also a sign of severe heart failure. When evaluating the adequacy of the arterial conduits, all palpable pulses can be assessed and graded on a scale of 0–4, where 4 is a fully normal conduit, and anything below that is reduced, including 0, which indicates an absent pulse. The major pulses routinely palpated on physical examination are the radial, brachial, carotid, abdominal aorta, femoral, dorsalis pedis, and posterior tibial. In special situations, the ulnar, subclavian, popliteal, axillary, temporal, and intercostal arteries are palpated. In assessing the abdominal aorta, it is important to make a note of the width of the aorta because an increase suggests an abdominal aortic aneurysm. It is particularly important to palpate the abdominal aorta in older individuals because abdominal aortic aneurysms are more prevalent in those older than 70. An audible bruit is a clue to significantly obstructed large arteries. During a routine examination, bruits are sought with the stethoscope head placed over the carotids, abdominal aorta, and femorals at the groin. Other arteries may be auscultated under special circumstances, such as suspected renal artery stenosis (flank bruit).

3. Jugular venous pulse—Assessment of the jugular venous pulse can provide information about the central venous pressure and right-heart function. Examination of the right internal jugular vein is ideal for assessing central venous pressure because it is attached directly to the superior vena cava without intervening valves. The patient is positioned in the semi-upright posture that permits visualization of the top of the right internal jugular venous blood column. The height of this column of blood, vertically from the sternal angle, is added to 5 cm of blood (the presumed distance to the center of the right atrium from the sternal angle) to obtain an estimate of central venous pressure in centimeters of blood. This can be converted to millimeters of mercury (mm Hg) with the formula:

$$\text{mm Hg} = \text{cm blood} \times 0.736$$

Examining the characteristics of the right internal jugular pulse is valuable for assessing right-heart function and rhythm disturbances. The normal jugular venous pulse has two distinct waves: *a* and *v*; the former coincides with atrial contraction and the latter with late ventricular systole. An absent *a* wave and an irregular pulse suggest atrial fibrillation. A large and early *v* wave suggests tricuspid regurgitation. The dips after the *a* and *v* waves are the *x* and *y* descents; the former coincide with atrial relaxation and the latter with early ventricular filling. In tricuspid stenosis, the *y* descent is prolonged. Other applications of the jugular pulse examination are discussed in the chapters dealing with specific disorders.

4. Lungs—Evaluation of the lungs is an important part of the physical examination. Diseases of the lung can affect the heart, just as diseases of the heart can affect the lungs. The major finding of importance is crackles at the pulmonary bases, indicating alveolar fluid collection. Although this is a significant finding in patients with congestive heart failure, it is not always possible to distinguish crackles caused by heart failure from those caused by pulmonary disease. The presence of pleural fluid, although useful in the diagnosis of heart failure, can be due to other causes. Heart failure most commonly causes a right pleural effusion; it can cause effusions on both sides but is least likely to cause isolated left pleural effusion. The specific constellation of dullness at the left base with bronchial breath sounds suggests an increase in heart size from pericardial effusion (Ewart sign) or another cause of cardiac enlargement; it is thought to be due to compression by the heart of a left lower lobe bronchus.

When right-heart failure develops or venous return is restricted from entering the heart, venous pressure in the abdomen increases, leading to hepatosplenomegaly and eventually ascites. None of these physical findings is specific for heart disease; they do, however, help establish the diagnosis. Heart failure also leads to generalized fluid retention, usually manifested as lower extremity edema or, in severe heart failure, anasarca.

5. Cardiac auscultation—Heart sounds are caused by the acceleration and deceleration of blood and the subsequent vibration of the cardiac structures during the phases of the cardiac cycle. To hear cardiac sounds, use a stethoscope with a bell and a taut diaphragm. Low-frequency sounds are associated with ventricular filling and are heard best with the bell. Medium-frequency sounds are associated with valve opening and closing; they are heard best with the diaphragm. Cardiac murmurs are due to turbulent blood flow, are usually high to medium frequency, and are heard best with the diaphragm. However, low-frequency atrioventricular valve inflow murmurs, such as that produced by mitral stenosis, are best heard with the bell. Auscultation should take place in areas that correspond to the location of the heart and great vessels. Such placement will, of course, need to be modified for patients with unusual body habitus or an unusual cardiac position. When no cardiac sounds can be heard over the precordium, they can often be heard in either the subxiphoid area or the right supraclavicular area.

Auscultation in various positions is recommended because low-frequency filling sounds are best heard with the patient in the left lateral decubitus position, and high-frequency murmurs, such as that of aortic regurgitation, are best heard with the patient sitting.

A. HEART SOUNDS—The **first heart sound** is coincident with mitral and tricuspid valve closure and has two components in up to 40% of normal individuals. There is little change in the intensity of this sound with respiration or position. The major determinant of the intensity of the first heart sound is the electrocardiographic (ECG) PR interval, which determines the time delay between atrial and ventricular contraction and thus the position of the mitral valve when ventricular systole begins. With a short PR interval, the mitral valve is widely open when systole begins, and its closure increases the intensity of the first sound, as compared to a long PR-interval beat when the valve partially closes prior to the onset of ventricular systole. Certain disease states, such as mitral stenosis, also can increase the intensity of the first sound.

The **second heart sound** is coincident with closure of the aortic and pulmonic valves. Normally, this sound is single in expiration and split during inspiration, permitting the aortic and pulmonic components to be distinguished. The inspiratory split is due to a delay in the occurrence of the pulmonic component because of a decrease in pulmonary vascular resistance, which prolongs pulmonary flow beyond the end of right ventricular systole. Variations in this normal splitting of the second heart sound are useful in determining certain disease states. For example, in atrial septal defect, the second sound is usually split throughout the respiratory cycle because of the constant increase in pulmonary flow. In patients with left bundle branch block, a delay occurs in the aortic component of the second heart sound, which results in reversed respiratory splitting; single with inspiration, split with expiration.

A **third heart sound** occurs during early rapid filling of the left ventricle; it can be produced by any condition that causes left ventricular volume overload or dilatation. Therefore, it can be heard in such disparate conditions as congestive heart failure and normal pregnancy. A **fourth heart sound** is due to a vigorous atrial contraction into a stiffened left ventricle and can be heard in left ventricular hypertrophy of any cause or in diseases that reduce compliance of the left ventricle, such as myocardial infarction.

Although third and fourth heart sounds can occasionally occur in normal individuals, all other extra sounds are signs of cardiac disease. Early ejection sounds are due to abnormalities of the semilunar valves, from restriction of their motion, thickening, or both (eg, a bicuspid aortic valve, pulmonic or aortic stenosis). A midsystolic click is often due to mitral valve prolapse and is caused by sudden tensing in midsystole of the redundant prolapsing segment of the mitral leaflet. The opening of a thickened atrioventricular valve leaflet, as in mitral stenosis, will cause a loud opening sound (snap) in early diastole. A lower frequency (more of a knock) sound at the time of rapid filling may be an indication of constrictive pericarditis. These early diastolic sounds must be distinguished from a third heart sound.

B. MURMURS—**Systolic murmurs** are very common and do not always imply cardiac disease. They are usually rated on a scale of 1 to 6, where grade 1 is barely audible, grade 4 is associated with palpable vibrations (thrill), grade 5 can be heard with the edge of the stethoscope, and grade 6 can be heard without a stethoscope. Most murmurs fall in the 1–3 range, and murmurs in the 4–6 range are almost always due to pathologic conditions; severe disease can exist with grades 1–3 or no cardiac murmurs, however. The most common systolic murmur is the crescendo/decrescendo murmur that increases in intensity as blood flows early in systole and diminishes in intensity through the second half of systole. This murmur can be due to vigorous flow in a normal heart or to obstructions in flow, as occurs with aortic stenosis, pulmonic stenosis, or hypertrophic cardiomyopathy. The so-called innocent flow murmurs are usually grades 1–2 and occur very early in systole; they may have a vibratory quality and are usually less apparent when the patient is in the sitting position (when venous return is less). If an ejection sound is heard, there is usually some abnormality of the semilunar valves. Although louder murmurs may be due to pathologic cardiac conditions, this is not always so. Distinguishing benign from pathologic systolic flow murmurs is one of the major challenges of clinical cardiology. Benign flow murmurs can be heard in 80% of children; the incidence declines with age but may be prominent during pregnancy or in adults who are thin or physically well trained. The murmur is usually benign in a patient with a soft-flow murmur that diminishes in intensity in the sitting position and neither a history of cardiovascular disease nor other cardiac findings.

The **holosystolic,** or **pansystolic,** murmur is almost always associated with cardiac pathology. The most common cause of this murmur is atrioventricular valve regurgitation, but it can also be observed in conditions such as ventricular septal defect, in which an abnormal communication exists between two chambers of markedly different systolic pressures. Although it is relatively easy to determine that these murmurs represent an abnormality, it is more of a challenge to determine their origins. Keep in mind that such conditions as mitral regurgitation, which usually produce holosystolic murmurs, may produce crescendo/decrescendo murmurs, adding to the difficulty in differentiating benign from pathologic systolic flow murmurs.

Diastolic murmurs are always abnormal and are usually graded on a 1 to 4 scale. The most frequently heard diastolic murmur is the high-frequency decrescendo early diastolic murmur of aortic regurgitation. This is usually heard best at the upper left sternal border or in the aortic area (upper right sternal border) and may radiate to the lower left sternal border and the apex. This murmur is usually very high frequency and may be difficult to hear. Although the murmur of pulmonic regurgitation may sound like that of aortic regurgitation when pulmonary artery pressures are high, if structural disease of the valve is present with normal pulmonary pressures, the murmur usually has a midrange frequency and begins with a slight delay after the pulmonic second heart sound. Pulmonic regurgitation is usually best heard in the pulmonic area (left second intercostal space parasternally). Mitral stenosis produces a low-frequency rumbling diastolic murmur that is decrescendo in early diastole, but may become crescendo up to the first heart sound with moderately severe mitral stenosis and sinus rhythm. The murmur is best heard at the apex in the left lateral decubitus position with the bell of the stethoscope. Similar findings are heard in tricuspid stenosis, but the murmur is loudest at the lower left sternal border.

A **continuous murmur** implies a connection between a high- and a low-pressure chamber throughout the cardiac cycle, such as occurs with a fistula between the aorta and the pulmonary artery. If the connection is a patent ductus arteriosus, the murmur is heard best under the left clavicle; it has a machine-like quality. Continuous murmurs must be distinguished from the combination of systolic and diastolic murmurs in patients with combined lesions (eg, aortic stenosis and regurgitation).

Traditionally, the origin of heart murmurs was based on five factors: (1) their timing in the cardiac cycle, (2) where on the chest they were heard, (3) their characteristics, (4) their intensity, and (5) their duration. Unfortunately, this traditional classification system is unreliable in predicting the underlying pathology. A more accurate method, **dynamic auscultation**, changes the intensity, duration, and characteristics of the murmur by bedside maneuvers that alter hemodynamics.

The simplest of these maneuvers is observation of any changes in murmur intensity with normal respiration because all right-sided cardiac murmurs should increase in intensity with normal inspiration. Although some exceptions exist, the method is very reliable for detecting such murmurs. Inspiration is associated with reductions in intrathoracic pressure that increase venous return from the abdomen and the head, leading to an increased flow through the right heart chambers. The consequent increase in pressure increases the intensity of right-sided murmurs. These changes are best observed in the sitting position, where venous return is smallest, and changes in intrathoracic pressure can produce their greatest effect on venous return. In a patient in the supine position, when venous return is near maximum, there may be little change observed with respiration. The ejection sound caused by pulmonic stenosis does not routinely increase in intensity with inspiration. The increased blood in the right heart accentuates atrial contraction, which increases late diastolic pressure in the right ventricle, partially opening the stenotic pulmonary valve and thus diminishing the opening sound of this valve with the subsequent systole.

Changes in position are an important part of normal auscultation; they can also be of great value in determining the origin of cardiac murmurs (Table 5–2). Murmurs dependent on venous return, such as innocent flow murmurs, are softer or absent in upright positions; others, such as the murmur associated with hypertrophic obstructive cardiomyopathy, are accentuated by reduced left ventricular volume associated with the upright position. In physically capable individuals, a rapid squat from the standing position is often diagnostically valuable because it suddenly increases venous return and left ventricular volume and accentuates flow murmurs but diminishes the murmur of hypertrophic obstructive cardiomyopathy. The stand-squat maneuver is also useful for altering the timing of the midsystolic click caused by mitral valve prolapse during systole. When the ventricle is small during standing, the prolapse occurs earlier in systole, moving the midsystolic click to early systole. During squatting, the ventricle dilates and the prolapse is delayed in systole, resulting in a late midsystolic click.

The **Valsalva maneuver** is also frequently used. The patient bears down and expires against a closed glottis, increasing intrathoracic pressure and markedly reducing venous return to the heart. Although almost all cardiac murmurs decrease in intensity during this maneuver, there are two exceptions: (1) The murmur of hypertrophic obstructive cardiomyopathy may become louder because of the diminished left ventricular volume and (2) The murmur associated with mitral regurgitation from mitral valve prolapse may become longer and louder because of the earlier occurrence of prolapse during systole. When the maneuver is very vigorous and prolonged, even these two murmurs may eventually diminish in intensity. Therefore, the Valsalva maneuver should be held for only about 10 seconds, so as not to cause prolonged diminution of the cerebral and coronary blood flow.

Isometric hand grip exercises have been used to increase arterial and left ventricular pressure. These maneuvers increase the flow gradient for mitral regurgitation, ventricular septal defect, and aortic regurgitation; the murmurs should then increase in intensity. Increasing arterial and left ventricular pressure increases left ventricular volume, thereby decreasing the murmur of hypertrophic obstructive cardiomyopathy.

Noting the changes in murmur intensity in the heartbeat following a premature ventricular contraction, and comparing these to a beat that does not, can be extremely useful. The premature ventricular contraction interrupts the cardiac cycle, and during the subsequent compensatory pause, an extra-long diastole occurs, leading to increased left ventricular filling. Therefore, murmurs caused by the flow of blood out of the left ventricle (eg, aortic stenosis) increase in intensity. There is usually no change in the intensity of the murmur of typical mitral regurgitation because blood pressure falls during the long pause and increases the gradient between the left ventricle and the aorta, allowing more forward flow. This results in the same amount of mitral regurgitant flow as on a normal beat with a higher aortic pressure and less forward flow. The increased volume during the long pause goes out of the aorta rather than back into the left atrium. Also, some of the increased blood volume in

Table 5–2. Differentiation of Systolic Murmurs Based on Changes in Their Intensity from Physiologic Maneuvers

	Origin of Murmur					
Maneuver	Flow	TR	AS	MR/VSD	MVP	HOCM
Inspiration	– or ↑	↑	–	–	–	–
Stand	↓	–	–	–	↑	↑
Squat	↑	–	–	–	↓	↓
Valsalva	↓	↓	↓	↓	↑	↑
Handgrip/TAO	↓	–	–	↑	↑	↓
Post–PVC	↑	–	↑	–	–	↑

AS, aortic stenosis; Flow, innocent flow murmur; HOCM, hypertrophic obstructive cardiomyopathy; MR, mitral regurgitation; MVP, mitral valve prolapse; PVC, premature ventricular contraction; TAO, transient arterial occlusion; TR, tricuspid regurgitation; VSD, ventricular septal defect; ↑ or ↓, change in intensity of murmur; –, no consistent change the left ventricle moves into the left atrium during isometric contraction before the aortic valve opens but does not change murmur intensity significantly. Unfortunately, there is no reliable way of inducing a premature ventricular contraction in most patients; it is fortuitous when a physician is present for one. Atrial fibrillation with markedly varying cycle lengths produces the same phenomenon and can be very helpful in determining the origin of murmurs.

Marbach JA, Almufleh A, Santo PD, et al. Comparative accuracy of focused cardiac ultrasonography and clinical examination for left ventricular dysfunction and valvular heart disease: a systematic review and meta-analysis. *Ann Intern Med.* 2019;171:264–272. [PMID: 31382273]

Qaseem A, Ikobaltzeta IE, Mustafa RA, et al. Appropriate use of point-of-care ultrasonography in patients with acute dyspnea in emergency department or inpatient settings: a clinical guideline from the American College of Physicians. *Ann Intern Med.* 2021;174:985–993. [PMID: 33900792]

B. Diagnostic Studies

1. Electrocardiography—ECG is perhaps the least expensive of all cardiac diagnostic tests, providing considerable value for the money. Modern ECG-reading computers do an excellent job of measuring the various intervals between waveforms and calculating the heart rate and the left ventricular axis. These programs fall short, however, when it comes to diagnosing complex ECG patterns and rhythm disturbances, and the test results must be read by a physician skilled at ECG interpretation.

Analysis of cardiac rhythm is perhaps the ECG's most widely used feature; it is used to clarify the mechanism of an irregular heart rhythm detected on physical examination or that of an extremely rapid or slow rhythm. The ECG is also used to monitor cardiac rate and rhythm; ambulatory ECG monitoring devices allow assessment of cardiac rate and rhythm on an ambulatory basis. ECG radio telemetry is also often used on hospital wards and between ambulances and emergency departments to assess and monitor rhythm disturbances. There are two types of ambulatory ECG recorders: continuous recorders that record all heart beats over 1–21 days and intermittent recorders that can be attached to the patient or implanted subcutaneously for weeks or months and then activated to provide brief recordings of infrequent events. In addition to analysis of cardiac rhythm, ambulatory ECG recordings can be used to detect ST-wave transients indicative of myocardial ischemia and certain electrophysiologic parameters of diagnostic and prognostic value. The most common use of ambulatory ECG monitoring is the evaluation of symptoms such as syncope, near-syncope, or palpitation for which there is no obvious cause, but cardiac rhythm disturbances are suspected.

The ECG is an important tool for rapidly assessing **metabolic and toxic disorders** of the heart. Characteristic changes in the ST-T waves indicate imbalances of potassium and calcium. Drugs such as tricyclic antidepressants have characteristic effects on the QT and QRS intervals at toxic levels. Such observations on the ECG can be lifesaving in emergency situations with comatose patients or cardiac arrest victims.

Chamber enlargement can be assessed through the characteristic changes of left or right ventricular and atrial enlargement. Evidence of chamber enlargement on the ECG usually signifies an advanced stage of disease with a poorer prognosis than that of patients with the same disease but no discernible enlargement.

The ECG is an important tool in managing suspected **acute coronary syndromes.** In patients with chest pain that is compatible with myocardial ischemia, the characteristic ST-T–wave elevations that do not resolve with nitroglycerin (and are unlikely to be the result of an old infarction) become the basis for thrombolytic therapy or a primary percutaneous intervention. Rapid resolution of the ECG changes of myocardial infarction after reperfusion therapy has prognostic value and identifies patients with reperfused coronary arteries.

Evidence of **conduction abnormalities** may help explain the mechanism of bradyarrhythmias and the likelihood of the need for a pacemaker. Conduction abnormalities may also aid in determining the cause of heart disease. For example, right bundle branch block and left anterior fascicular block are often seen in Chagas cardiomyopathy, and left-axis deviation occurs in patients with a primum atrial septal defect.

2. Echocardiography—Another frequently ordered cardiac diagnostic test, echocardiography is based on the use of ultrasound directed at the heart to create images of cardiac anatomy and display them in real time on a monitor screen. Two-dimensional echocardiography is usually accomplished by placing an ultrasound transducer in various positions on the anterior chest and obtaining cross-sectional images of the heart and great vessels in a variety of standard planes. In general, two-dimensional echocardiography is excellent for detecting any anatomic abnormality of the heart and great vessels. With two-dimensional echocardiographic imaging of dynamic left ventricular cross-sectional anatomy ventricular wall motion can be interrogated in multiple planes and left ventricular wall thickening during systole (an important measure of myocardial viability) can be assessed. In addition to demonstrating segmental wall motion abnormalities, echocardiography can estimate left ventricular volumes and ejection fraction.

Transesophageal echocardiography (TEE) involves the placement of smaller ultrasound probes on a gastroscopic device for placement in the esophagus behind the heart; it produces much higher resolution images of posterior cardiac structures. TEE has made it possible to detect left atrial thrombi, small mitral valve vegetations, and thoracic aortic dissection with a high degree of accuracy. Recent advances in image processing of multiplanar images have permitted real-time three-dimensional echocardiography, which is especially useful for evaluating structural valve pathology and guiding repair or replacement decisions. In addition, three-dimensional images are more accurate at determining chamber volumes.

The older analog echocardiographic display, referred to as M-mode, motion-mode, or time-motion mode, is currently used for its high axial and temporal resolution. It is superior to two-dimensional echocardiography for measuring the dimensions of structures in its axial direction, and its very high sampling rate allows for the resolution of complex cardiac motion patterns. Its many disadvantages, including poor lateral resolution and the inability to distinguish whole heart motion from the motion of individual cardiac structures, have relegated it to a supporting role.

Doppler ultrasound can be combined with two-dimensional imaging to investigate blood flow in the heart and great vessels. It is based on determining the change in frequency (caused by the movement of blood in the given structure) of the reflected ultrasound compared with the transmitted ultrasound and converting this difference into flow velocity. In the color-flow Doppler echocardiography technique, frequency shifts in each pixel of a selected area of the two-dimensional image are measured and converted into a color, depending on the direction of flow velocity, and the presence or absence of turbulence. When these color images are superimposed on the two-dimensional echocardiographic image, a moving color image of blood flow in the heart is created in real time. This is extremely useful for detecting regurgitant blood flow across cardiac valves and any abnormal communications in the heart.

Tissue Doppler imaging is similar to color-flow Doppler except that myocardial tissue movement velocity is interrogated. This allows for the quantitation of the rate of tissue contraction and relaxation, which is a measure of myocardial performance that can be applied to systole and diastole. Tissue Doppler images can be used to evaluate myocardial strain regionally or globally. Reduced left ventricular systolic strain is an early sign of myocardial weakness that can occur before other measures, such as left ventricular ejection fraction, are reduced. Global left ventricular strain is currently being used to detect early drug toxicity to the heart.

Because color-flow imaging cannot resolve very high velocities, another Doppler mode must be used to quantitate the exact velocity and estimate the pressure gradient of the flow when high velocities are suspected. Continuous wave Doppler, which almost continuously sends and receives ultrasound along a beam that can be aligned through the heart, is extremely accurate at resolving very high velocities such as those encountered with valvular aortic stenosis. The disadvantage of this technique is that the source of the high velocity within the beam cannot always be determined but must be assumed, based on the anatomy through which the beam passes. When there is ambiguity about the source of the high velocity, pulsed wave Doppler is more useful. This technique is range-gated such that specific areas along the beam (sample volumes) can be investigated. One or more sample volumes can be examined, and determinations made concerning the exact location of areas of high-velocity flow.

Doppler echocardiography has now largely replaced cardiac catheterization for deriving hemodynamics to estimate the severity of valve stenosis. Recorded Doppler velocities across a valve can be converted to pressure gradients by the use of the simplified Bernoulli equation (pressure gradient = 4 × velocity^2). Cardiac output can be measured by Doppler from the velocity recorded at cardiac anatomic sites of known size visualized on the two-dimensional echocardiographic image. Cardiac output and pressure gradient data can be used to calculate the stenotic valve area with remarkable accuracy. A complete echocardiographic examination including two-dimensional and M-mode anatomic and functional visualization and color, pulsed, and continuous wave Doppler examination of blood flow provides a considerable amount of information about cardiac structure and function. A full discussion of the usefulness of this technique is beyond the scope of this chapter, but individual uses of echocardiography will be discussed in later chapters.

Unfortunately, echocardiography is not without its technical difficulties and pitfalls. Like any noninvasive technique, it is not 100% accurate. Furthermore, it is impossible to obtain high-quality images or Doppler signals in as many as 5% of patients, especially those with emphysema, chest wall deformities, and obesity. Although TEE has made the examination of such patients easier, it does not solve all the problems of echocardiography. Despite these limitations, the technique is so powerful that it has moved out of the noninvasive laboratory and is now frequently being used in the operating room, the clinic, the emergency department, and even the cardiac catheterization laboratory, to help guide procedures without the use of fluoroscopy. New hand-held echocardiographic machines may soon rival the cardiac physical examination at the bedside. Some of these small new devices use the physician's smart phone to display the echocardiographic images.

3. Nuclear cardiac imaging—Nuclear cardiac imaging involves the injection of tracer amounts of radioactive elements attached to larger molecules or to the patient's own blood cells. The tracer-labeled blood is concentrated in certain areas of the heart, and a gamma ray detection camera is used to collect the radioactive emissions and form an image of the distribution of the tracer in the particular area. The single-crystal gamma camera produces planar images of the heart, depending on the relationship of the camera to the body. Multiple-head gamma cameras, which rotate around the patient, can produce single-photon emission computed tomography (SPECT) images, displaying the cardiac anatomy in slices, each about 1-cm thick. Positron emission tomography scanning requires special isotopes and imaging equipment, but positrons are less susceptible to attenuation by the chest wall and can detect cellular metabolism as well as perfusion. The presence of metabolism in a malfunctioning or poorly perfused wall suggests myocardial viability.

A. Myocardial perfusion imaging—The most common tracers used for imaging regional myocardial blood flow distribution are thallium-201 and the technetium-99m–based agents, such as sestamibi. Thallium-201, a potassium analog that is efficiently extracted from the bloodstream by viable myocardial cells, is concentrated in the myocardium in areas of adequate blood flow and living myocardial cells. Thallium perfusion images show defects (a lower tracer concentration) in areas where blood flow is relatively reduced and in areas of damaged myocardial cells. If the damage is from frank necrosis or scar tissue formation, very little thallium will be taken up; ischemic cells may take up thallium more slowly or incompletely, producing relative defects in the image.

Myocardial perfusion problems are separated from non-viable myocardium by the fact that thallium eventually washes out of the myocardial cells and back into the circulation. If a defect detected on initial thallium imaging disappears over a period of 3–24 hours, the area is presumably viable. A persistent defect suggests a myocardial scar. In addition to detecting viable myocardium and assessing the extent of new and old myocardial infarctions, thallium-201 imaging can also be used to detect myocardial ischemia during stress testing (see later section on stress testing) as well as marked enlargement of the heart or dysfunction. The major problem with thallium imaging is photon attenuation because of chest wall structures, which can give an artifactual appearance of defects in the myocardium.

The technetium-99m–based agents take advantage of the shorter half-life of technetium (6 hours; the half-life of thallium-201 is 73 hours); this allows for use of a larger dose, which results in higher energy emissions and higher quality images. Technetium-99m's higher energy emissions scatter less and are attenuated less by chest wall structures, reducing the number of artifacts. Because sestamibi undergoes considerably less washout after the initial myocardial uptake than thallium does, the evaluation of perfusion versus tissue damage requires two separate injections.

In addition to detecting perfusion deficits, myocardial imaging with the SPECT system allows for a three-dimensional reconstruction of the heart, which can be displayed in any projection on a monitor screen. Such images can be formed at intervals during the cardiac cycle to create an image of the beating heart, which can be used to detect wall motion abnormalities and derive left ventricular volumes and ejection fraction. Matching wall motion abnormalities with perfusion defects provides additional confirmation that the perfusion defects visualized are true and not artifacts of photon attenuation. Also, extensive perfusion defects and wall motion abnormalities should be accompanied by decreases in ejection fraction.

B. Positron emission tomography—Positron emission tomography (PET) is a technique using tracers that simultaneously emit two high-energy photons. A circular array of detectors around the patient can detect these simultaneous events and accurately identify their origin in the heart. This results in improved spatial resolution compared with SPECT. It also allows for correction of tissue photon attenuation, resulting in the ability to accurately quantify radioactivity in the heart. PET can be used to assess myocardial perfusion and myocardial metabolic activity separately by using different tracers coupled to different molecules. Most of the tracers developed for clinical use require a cyclotron for their generation; the cyclotron must be near the PET imager because of the short half-life of the agents. Agents in clinical use include oxygen-15 (half-life 2 minutes), nitrogen-13 (half-life 10 minutes), carbon-11 (half-life 20 minutes), and fluorene-18 (half-life 110 minutes). These tracers can be coupled to many physiologically active molecules for assessing various functions of the myocardium. Because rubidium-82, with a half-life of 75 seconds, does not require a cyclotron and can be generated on site, it is frequently used with PET scanning, especially for perfusion images. Ammonia containing nitrogen-13 and water containing oxygen-15 are also used as perfusion agents. Carbon-11–labeled fatty acids and ^{18}F-fluorodeoxyglucose are common metabolic tracers used to assess myocardial viability, and acetate containing carbon-11 is often used to assess oxidative metabolism.

The main clinical uses of PET scanning involve the evaluation of coronary artery disease. It is used in perfusion studies at rest and during pharmacologic stress (exercise studies are less feasible). In addition to a qualitative assessment of perfusion defects, PET allows for a calculation of absolute regional myocardial blood flow or blood-flow reserve. PET also assesses myocardial viability, using the metabolic tracers to detect metabolically active myocardium in areas of reduced perfusion. The presence of viability implies that returning perfusion to these areas would result in improved function of the ischemic myocardium. Although many authorities consider PET scanning the gold standard for determining myocardial viability, it has not been found to be 100% accurate. Thallium reuptake techniques and echocardiographic and magnetic resonance imaging (MRI) of delayed myocardial enhancement have proved equally valuable for detecting myocardial viability in clinical studies.

C. Radionuclide angiography—Radionuclide angiography is based on visualizing radioactive tracers in the cavities of the heart over time. Radionuclide angiography is usually done with a single gamma camera in a single plane, and only one view of the heart is obtained. The most common technique is to record the amount of radioactivity received by the gamma camera over time. Although volume estimates by radionuclide angiography are not as accurate as those obtained by other methods, the ejection fraction is quite accurate. Wall motion can be assessed in the one plane imaged, but the technique is not as sensitive as other imaging modalities for detecting wall motion abnormalities.

Although still used by some to follow ejection fraction serially, it has largely been replaced by echocardiography.

D. 99mTc-PYP IMAGING—99mtechnetium-pyrophosphate imaging was originally used to detect myocardial infarction but has evolved as simple, diagnostic test for the rare cardiac disease amyloidosis which causes heart failure. Tc-PYP radioisotope is injected intravenously, and non-gated cardiac SPECT and planar images are obtained 1 hour post injection. There is increased myocardial uptake of 99mTc-PYP in cardiac amyloidosis. Planar and SPECT images are used for visual interpretation, semiquantitative and quantitative assessment of myocardial uptake in comparison to rib uptake and lung uptake. PYP imaging has ability to specifically identify and differentiate the types of amyloidosis noninvasively.

4. Other cardiac imaging

A. CHEST RADIOGRAPHY—Chest radiography is used infrequently now for evaluating cardiac structural abnormalities because of the superiority of echocardiography in this regard. The chest radiograph, however, is a rapid, inexpensive way to assess pulmonary anatomy and is very useful for evaluating pulmonary venous congestion and hypoperfusion or hyperperfusion. In addition, abnormalities of the thoracic skeleton are found in certain cardiac disorders, and radiographic corroboration may help with the diagnosis. Detection of intracardiac calcium deposits by the radiograph or fluoroscopy is of some value in finding coronary artery, valvular, or pericardial disease. Chest X-ray (CXR) also helps in identification and location of cardiac devices, implants, and monitors. It can provide useful information about cardiac devices like pacemakers and ICDs, assessing position, number of cardiac leads, dislodgement of leads, and also immediate post-procedure complications. CXR also helps in identification of prosthetic heart valves, valve rings, clips and in some cases, vascular stents.

B. COMPUTED TOMOGRAPHIC SCANNING—Cardiac computed tomographic (CT) scanning is a noninvasive cardiac imaging technique that uses X-ray radiation to image the heart and associated blood vessels. Cardiac CT has been in use since late 1990s but the advances in CT technology and robust data from multiple randomized clinical trials has increased its use in clinical practice dramatically in the past two decades. With the latest CT technology, cardiac CT can provide images with high spatial and temporal resolution and can acquire an entire cardiac image in one heartbeat. This makes cardiac CT imaging useful for the assessment of coronary artery disease. Noncontrast cardiac CT is primarily used for the assessment of coronary artery calcium which is an indicator of atherosclerosis in the coronary arteries. A coronary calcium score helps in risk stratification of patients and identifies patients who benefit from cardiac preventive therapy.

Coronary CT angiography (CTA) uses intravenous iodinated contrast to increase vessel visualization. CTA uses cardiac ECG gating to acquire coronary images when cardiac movement is at its least. Sublingual nitroglycerin is used to enhance visualization of the coronary arteries. Two types of ECG gating are used for coronary CTA. Prospective ECG gating ideally requires the heart rate to be less than 65 bpm to reduce motion artifacts and acquires images during mid to end-diastolic phase which corresponds to around 70% of the R-R interval. β-Blockers or calcium channel blockers are used to reduce heart rate if it is more than 70 bpm and if there are no contraindications to their use. Retrospective ECG gating is used when the heart rate is high or in irregular heart rhythms like atrial fibrillation. In retrospective ECG-gated studies, images are acquired throughout the cardiac cycle and images from different phases of cardiac cycle are used to assess coronary anatomy. This technique can also be used to assess cardiac function with cine sequences. Compared to prospective CTA, retrospective CTA delivers a higher radiation dose. In addition, coronary CTA can provide an anatomical assessment of coronary artery disease such as plaque burden and plaque characteristics which may identify high-risk plaque. Coronary CTA can provide a noninvasive hemodynamic assessment of entire coronary tree from which fractional flow reserve can be calculated. This information helps in planning coronary interventions. With increases in spatial resolution, some CT scanners can assess coronary stent patency as well. Cardiac CTA has also shown great sensitivity in assessing coronary artery bypass graft patency and occlusion.

Other uses of cardiac CT include the assessment of pericardial disease such as calcification and cysts, although complex effusions and masses are better assessed by MRI. CT scanning is also very useful for detecting other potential causes of chest pain, including dissection of the aorta or a coronary artery and pulmonary embolism. With recent advances in structural heart interventions, cardiac CT has played a complimentary role along with other cardiac imaging modalities. With retrospective gating, cardiac function and valve excursion can be assessed. Cardiac CT with 3D imaging of the heart and surrounding structures provides valuable information for preprocedural planning, patient selection, and peripheral vascular access. Cardiac CT can also provide anatomic information regarding heart valves when poor acoustic windows or heavy calcification limit visualization of valve anatomy with echocardiography. Myocardial CT perfusion, Hybrid PET, or nuclear scanners plus CT scanners are now available and can provide anatomic, perfusion, and myocardial viability information.

C. MAGNETIC RESONANCE IMAGING—MRI has improved dramatically over the past two decades and is now increasingly used for cardiac imaging. Cardiac MRI (CMR) provides good spatial resolution, adequate temporal resolution, and has a unique ability to assess tissue characteristics such as edema, inflammation, fibrosis, and scar. Unlike cardiac CT or nuclear perfusion imaging, CMR does not use ionizing radiation for image acquisition. MRI uses a powerful superconducting electromagnet which creates a strong magnetic field. Hydrogen ions that are abundant in the body are used to generate signal for the image formation. The hydrogen nucleus has a single positively charged proton which spins along its own axis, causing a small electromagnetic field. When placed in a large magnetic field, these protons also spin about the axis of the external magnetic field which is called precession. When patient is placed in MRI machine, most of the protons precess aligning to the external magnetic field but some protons align opposite to the external magnetic field. The net magnetization which is aligned with the external magnetic field is called longitudinal magnetization. A radiofrequency (RF) pulse is used to excite the protons which flips them in the transverse plane causing net transverse magnetization. After the RF pulse is removed, the excited protons release energy and relax back to their resting state of longitudinal magnetization. This released signal is used to create the images in MRI. T1 is the time it takes for longitudinal magnetization to recover to 63% of its maximum value. Its value depends on the surrounding molecules and is specific for different tissues. T2 is the time it takes for transverse magnetization to decay to 37% of its maximum value. It depends on local magnetic field and is specific for different tissues. The differences in the T1 and T2 values of tissues are used to create the contrast for the T1- and T2-weighted imaging in MRI.

Different CMR techniques and sequences are used to assess anatomy, function, flow quantification, edema assessment, and tissue characterization. CMR is considered the gold standard for quantification of left and right ventricular volumetrics. It is widely used for anatomical assessment, functional assessment, and flow quantification in patients with congenital heart disease, cardiac shunts, and valvular heart disease. CMR is helpful for evaluating patients with poor-quality echocardiograms due to limited acoustic windows. Chamber volumes, wall function, blood flow quantification, and valve morphologies can be evaluated without the use of contrast agents.

Gadolinium is a noniodinated, paramagnetic contrast agent that is used intravenously in CMR for performing perfusion imaging, scar assessment, and magnetic resonance angiography. Gadolinium stays in the extracellular space and does not cross intact cell membranes. Late gadolinium enhancement (LGE) images are obtained 5–10 minutes after giving intravenous gadolinium contrast. Gadolinium persists in tissues with cellular injury, inflammation, necrosis, and washes out slowly in diseases with increased extracellular space like edema, infiltrative cardiomyopathy, and scar tissue. An inversion recovery sequence is used for LGE assessment which appears as a bright signal on a black/nulled myocardium. The major limitation of gadolinium-based contrast is the risk of nephrogenic systemic fibrosis (NSF) in chronic kidney disease patients with glomerular filtration rates less than 30 mL/kg/h. With the more recent use of macrocyclic gadolinium contrast, the incidence of NSF has been markedly reduced.

LGE patterns help in differentiating ischemic from nonischemic cardiomyopathy and can diagnose certain cardiomyopathies such as cardiac amyloidosis, hypereosinophilic endocarditis, sarcoidosis, and myocarditis. LGE in ischemic cardiomyopathy helps in risk stratification, the assessment of viability, and for predicting functional recovery post-revascularization. For arrhythmia patients, CMR with LGE helps with scar mapping in ventricular tachycardia and left atrial mapping in atrial fibrillation to plan ablation therapy. LGE also can risk stratify patients with hypertrophic cardiomyopathy by scar quantification and diagnose rare cardiomyopathies associated with arrhythmias. Apart from LGE sequences, myocardial parametric mapping sequences like T1 mapping, T2 mapping, and T^* mapping are used for tissue characterization and allows quantitative assessment of myocardial fibrosis, edema, and iron overload, respectively.

Stress CMR is performed with gadolinium-based contrast agents and vasodilators such as adenosine or regadenoson, or myocardial contractility stimulants such as dobutamine to evaluate perfusion reserve in coronary artery disease and assess for microvascular coronary disease. Magnetic resonance angiography with gadolinium-based contrast allows visualization of arterial and venous connections and can be used to assess structures such as the ascending and/or descending aorta, peripheral vasculature, and pulmonary veins. Vascular imaging can be performed with noncontrast CMR angiography sequences as well. CMR also plays an important role in assessment of cardiac masses, pericardial disease, and myopericarditis. Patients should be screened for metallic implants and cardiac implantable devices. Only patients with MRI conditional and MRI safe devices can get CMR. Some devices may require reprogramming into an MRI safe mode.

Some of the limitations of CMR at this time include the length of the studies, their cost, and the relative nonavailability of MRI systems in acute patient care areas compared to CT. CMR can last 45–60 minutes or more. This can be shortened by selecting focused imaging protocols that are specific for the indication of the study. CMR also needs patient cooperation for breath hold sequences to reduce respiratory and motion artifact. Unstable patients or patients with profound shortness of breath are not good candidates for the study. Patients with claustrophobia may need antianxiety medications or even sedation with anesthesia monitoring during image acquisition. Overall, CMR is a versatile tool for anatomic as well as functional assessment of the heart and has increasing indications in clinical practice.

5. Stress testing—Stress testing in various forms is most frequently applied in cases of suspected or overt ischemic heart disease (Table 5–3). Because ischemia represents an imbalance between myocardial oxygen supply and demand, exercise or pharmacologic stress increases myocardial oxygen demand and reveals an inadequate oxygen supply (hypoperfusion) in diseased coronary arteries. Stress testing can thus induce detectable ischemia in patients with no

Table 5–3. Some Indications for Stress Testing

Evaluation of exertional chest pain
Assess significance of known coronary artery disease
Risk stratification of ischemic heart disease
Determine exercise capacity
Evaluate other exercise symptoms
Detect exercise pulmonary hypertension
Evaluate the severity of valvular heart disease
Determine maximum oxygen consumption
Precipitate exercise-induced arrhythmias

evidence of ischemia at rest. It is also used to determine cardiac reserve in patients with valvular and myocardial disease. Deterioration of left ventricular performance during exercise or other stresses suggests a diminution in cardiac reserve that would have therapeutic and prognostic implications. In addition, exercise testing can be used to detect the development of pulmonary hypertension with exercise. Although most stress test studies use some technique (Table 5–4) for directly assessing the heart, it is important not to forget that the symptoms of angina pectoris, extreme dyspnea, lightheadedness, or syncope during stress testing can be equally important in evaluating patients. Physical findings such as the development of pulmonary crackles, ventricular gallops, murmurs, peripheral cyanosis, hypotension, excessive increases in heart rate, or inappropriate decreases in heart rate also have diagnostic and prognostic value. It is therefore important that a symptom assessment and physical examination always be done before, during, and after stress testing.

Electrocardiographic monitoring is the most common cardiac evaluation technique used during stress testing; it should be part of every stress test to assess heart rate and detect any arrhythmias. In patients with normal resting ECGs, diagnostic ST depression of myocardial ischemia has a fairly high sensitivity and specificity for detecting coronary artery disease in symptomatic patients if adequate stress is achieved (peak heart rate at least 85% of the patient's maximum predicted rate, based on age and sex). Exercise ECG testing is an excellent low-cost screening procedure for patients with chest pain consistent with coronary artery disease, normal resting ECGs, and the ability to exercise to maximal levels.

A **myocardial imaging** technique is usually added to the exercise evaluation in patients whose ECGs are abnormal or, for other reasons thought to be less accurate, for example, left bundle branch block. It is also used for determining the location and extent of myocardial ischemia in patients with known coronary artery disease. Imaging techniques, in general, enhance the sensitivity and specificity of the tests but are still not perfect, with false-positive and false-negative results occurring 5–10% of the time. Echocardiographic imaging in particular can assess the severity of valvular regurgitation and exercise-induced pulmonary hypertension, which can be helpful in evaluating patients with valvular heart disease. Finally, cardiopulmonary exercise testing is used to measure maximum oxygen uptake, which is of prognostic value in systolic heart failure patients.

Table 5–4. Methods of Detecting Myocardial Ischemia During Stress Testing

Electrocardiography
Echocardiography
Myocardial perfusion imaging
Positron emission tomography
Magnetic resonance imaging

Which adjunctive myocardial imaging technology to choose depends on the quality of the tests, their availability and cost, and the services provided by the laboratory. If these are all equal, the decision should be based on patient characteristics. For example, echocardiography might be appropriate when ischemia is suspected of developing during exercise and is profound enough to depress segmental left ventricular performance. On the other hand, perfusion scanning might be the best test to determine which coronary artery is producing the symptoms in a patient with known three-vessel coronary artery disease and recurrent angina after revascularization.

Choosing the appropriate form of stress is also important (Table 5–5). Exercise, the preferred stress for increasing myocardial oxygen demand, also simulates the patient's normal daily activities and is therefore highly relevant clinically. There are essentially only two reasons for not choosing exercise stress; however, the patient's inability to exercise adequately because of physical or psychological limitations, or the known superiority of pharmacologic stress in certain situations such as the presence of left bundle branch block.

6. Cardiac catheterization—Cardiac catheterization is now mainly used for the assessment of coronary artery anatomy by coronary angiography. In fact, the cardiac catheterization laboratory has become more of a therapeutic than a diagnostic arena. Once significant coronary artery disease is identified, a variety of catheter-based interventions

Table 5–5. Types of Stress Tests

Exercise
Treadmill
Bicycle
Pharmacologic
Adenosine
Dipyridamole
Dobutamine
Isoproterenol
Regadenoson
Other
Pacing

can be used to alleviate the obstruction to blood flow in the coronary arteries. At one time, hemodynamic measurements (pressure, flow, oxygen consumption) were necessary to accurately diagnose and quantitate the severity of valvular heart disease and intracardiac shunts. Currently, Doppler echocardiography has taken over this role almost completely, except in the few instances when Doppler studies are inadequate or believed to be inaccurate. Catheter-based hemodynamic assessments are still useful for differentiating cardiac constriction from restriction, despite advances in Doppler echocardiography. Currently, the catheterization laboratory is also more often used as a treatment arena for valvular and congenital heart disease. Certain stenotic valvular and arterial lesions can be treated successfully with catheter-delivered valve leaflet clips, the deployment of stents, or stent-mounted bioprosthetic valves. Congenital and acquired shunts can also be closed by catheter-delivered devices.

Myocardial biopsy is necessary to treat patients with heart transplants and is occasionally used to diagnose selected cases of suspected acute myocarditis. For this purpose, a bioptome is usually placed in the right heart, and several small pieces of myocardium are removed. Although this technique is relatively safe, myocardial perforation can occur.

7. Electrophysiologic testing and implantable devices—Electrophysiologic testing uses catheter-delivered electrodes in the heart to induce rhythm disorders, determine their mechanisms, and localize the abnormal circuits. Certain tachyarrhythmias and structural abnormalities that facilitate rhythm disturbances can be treated by heating (i.e., radiofrequency energy ablation) or freezing (i.e., cryoablation) the underlying tissue. Bradyarrhythmias (i.e., slow heart rates that cause symptoms) are treated by the placement of a pacemaker that monitors rhythm disturbances and treats them accordingly through pacing. On the other hand, patients who are at high risk of life-threatening tachyarrhythmias from the ventricles generally receive a defibrillator. A defibrillator can deliver defibrillation shocks internally and treat life-threatening rapid rhythms by resetting the heart. Electrophysiologic testing and treatment as well as implantable devices now dominate the management of arrhythmias; the test is more accurate than the surface ECG for diagnosing many arrhythmias and detecting their substrate, and catheter ablation and electronic devices have been more successful than pharmacologic approaches at treating many arrhythmias.

8. Test selection—In the current era of escalating health care costs, ordering multiple tests is rarely justifiable, and the physician must pick the one test that will best define the patient's problem. Unfortunately, cardiology offers multiple competing technologies that often address the same issues but in a different way. The following five principles should be followed when considering which test to order:

- What information is desired? If the test is not reasonably likely to provide the type of information needed to help the patient's problem, it should not be done, no matter how inexpensive and easy it is to obtain.
- What is the cost of the test? If two tests can provide the same information and one is much more expensive than the other, the less expensive test should be ordered.
- Is the test available? Sometimes the best test for the patient will not be available in the given facility. If it is available at a nearby facility and the patient can go there without undue cost, the test should be obtained. If expensive travel is required, the costs and benefits of that test versus local alternatives need to be carefully considered.
- What is the level of expertise of the laboratory and the physicians who interpret the tests? For many of the high-technology imaging tests, the level of expertise markedly affects the value of the test. Therefore, even though a given test may be available and inexpensive and could theoretically provide essential information, if the quality of the laboratory is not good, an alternative test should be sought.
- What quality of service is provided by the laboratory? Patients are customers, and they need to be satisfied. If a laboratory makes patients wait a long time, if it is tardy in getting the results to the physicians, or if great delays occur in accomplishing the test, choose an alternative laboratory or test.

Many other situations and considerations affect the choice of tests. Physicians are frequently solicited to use the latest emerging technologies, which often have not been proven to be superior to the standard techniques. It is generally unwise to begin using these usually more expensive methods until clinical trials have established their efficacy and cost-effectiveness.

Doherty JU, Kort S, Mehran R, et al. ACC/AATS/AHA/ASE/ASNC/HRS/SCAI/SCCT/SCMR/STS 2019 appropriate use criteria for multimodality imaging in the assessment of cardiac structure and function in nonvalvular heart disease. *J Am Coll Cardiol.* 2019;73:488–516. [PMID: 30630640]

Doherty JU, Kort S, Mehran R, Schoenhagen P, Soman P, et al. ACC/AATS/AHA/ASE/ASNC/HRS/SCAI/SCCT/SCMR/STS 2017 appropriate use criteria for multimodality imaging in valvular heart disease. *J Am Coll Cardiol.* 2017;70:1649–1667. [PMID: 28870679]

ACKNOWLEDGMENT

The expert assistance of Punita Kaveti, MD and Shadi Kalantarian, MD in editing the imaging and electrophysiology sections, respectively, is greatly appreciated.

6

Chronic Ischemic Heart Disease

Michael H. Crawford, MD

ESSENTIALS OF DIAGNOSIS

- Typical exertional angina pectoris or its equivalents.
- Objective evidence of myocardial ischemia by electrocardiography, myocardial imaging, or myocardial perfusion scanning.
- Likely occlusive coronary artery disease because of history and objective evidence of prior myocardial infarction.
- Known coronary artery disease shown by coronary angiography.

General Considerations

For clinical purposes, patients with chronic ischemic heart disease fall into two general categories: those with symptoms related to the disease and those who are asymptomatic. Although the latter are probably more common than the former, physicians typically see symptomatic patients more frequently. The issue of asymptomatic patients becomes important clinically when physicians are faced with estimating the risk to a particular patient who is undergoing some stressful intervention, such as major noncardiac surgery. Another issue is the patient with known coronary artery disease who is currently asymptomatic. Such individuals, especially if they have objective evidence of myocardial ischemia, are known to have a higher incidence of future cardiovascular morbidity and mortality. There is, understandably, a strong temptation to treat such patients, even though it is difficult to make an asymptomatic patient feel better, and some of the treatment modalities have their own risks. In such cases, strong evidence that longevity will be positively influenced by the treatment must be present for its benefits to outweigh its risks.

Pathophysiology & Etiology

In the industrialized nations, most patients with chronic ischemic heart disease have coronary atherosclerosis. Consequently, it is easy to become complacent and ignore the fact that other diseases can cause lesions in the coronary arteries (Table 6–1). In young people, coronary artery anomalies should be kept in mind; in older individuals, systemic vasculitites are not uncommon. Today, collagen vascular diseases are the most common vasculitis leading to coronary artery disease, but in the past, infections such as syphilis were a common cause of coronary vasculitis. Diseases of the ascending aorta, such as aortic dissection, can lead to coronary ostial occlusion. Isolated coronary artery dissection can also occur. Coronary artery emboli may occur as a result of infectious endocarditis or of atrial fibrillation with left atrial thrombus formation. Infiltrative diseases of the heart, such as tumor metastases, may also compromise coronary flow. Therefore, it is essential to keep in mind diagnostic possibilities other than atherosclerosis when managing chronic ischemic heart disease.

Myocardial ischemia is the result of an imbalance between myocardial oxygen supply and demand. Coronary atherosclerosis and other diseases reduce the supply of oxygenated blood by obstructing the coronary arteries. Although the obstructions may not be enough to produce myocardial ischemia at rest, increases in myocardial oxygen demand during activities can precipitate myocardial ischemia. This is the basis for using stress testing to detect ischemic heart disease. Transient increases in the degree of coronary artery obstruction may develop as a result of platelet and thrombus formation or through increased coronary vasomotor tone. Although it is rare in the United States, pure coronary vasospasm in the absence of atherosclerosis can occur and cause myocardial ischemia and even infarction. In addition, in the presence of other cardiac diseases, especially those that cause a pressure load on the left ventricle, myocardial oxygen

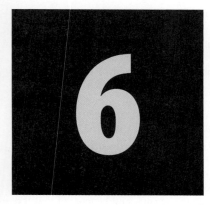

Table 6–1. Nonatherosclerotic Causes of Epicardial Coronary Artery Obstruction

Fixed	Congenital anomalies Myocardial bridges Vasculitites Aortic and coronary dissection Granulomas Tumors Scarring from trauma, radiation
Transient	Vasospasm Embolus Thrombus in situ

demand may outstrip the ability of normal coronary arteries to provide oxygenated blood, resulting in myocardial ischemia or infarction. A good example would be the patient with severe aortic stenosis, considerable left ventricular hypertrophy, and severely elevated left ventricular pressures who tries to exercise. The manifestations of chronic ischemic heart disease have their basis in a complex pathophysiology of multiple factors that affect myocardial oxygen supply and demand.

Clinical Findings

A. Risk Factors

Coronary atherosclerosis is more likely to occur in patients with certain risk factors for this disease (Table 6–2). These include advanced age, male gender or the postmenopausal state in females, a family history of coronary atherosclerosis, diabetes mellitus, systemic hypertension, high serum cholesterol and other associated lipoprotein abnormalities, and smoking and burning vegetable matter, for example, tobacco, marijuana. Additional minor risk factors include a sedentary lifestyle, obesity, high psychological stress levels, and such phenotypic characteristics as earlobe creases, auricular hirsutism, and a mesomorphic body type. The presence of other systemic diseases—hypothyroidism, pseudoxanthoma elasticum, and acromegaly, for example—can accelerate a propensity to coronary atherosclerosis. In the case of nonatherosclerotic coronary artery disease, evidence of systemic vasculitites such as lupus erythematosus and rheumatoid arthritis should be sought. Although none of these risk factors is diagnostic of coronary artery disease, the more of them that are present, the greater is the likelihood of the diagnosis. In this regard various structured formula have been developed to assess risk using clinical data in asymptomatic individuals. A popular one is the revised pooled cohort risk equation from the American Heart Association and the American College of Cardiology which estimates the 10 year and lifetime risk of developing atherosclerotic cardiovascular disease and can be found online. It is based on age, sex, race, cholesterol, blood pressure, smoking, and diabetes. (https://tools.acc.org/ldl/ascvd_risk_estimator/index.html#!/calulate/estimator/).

Table 6–2. Risk Factors for Coronary Heart Disease

Major independent risk factors
Advancing age
Tobacco smoking
Diabetes mellitus
Elevated total and low-density lipoprotein (LDL) cholesterol
Low high-density lipoprotein cholesterol
Hypertension
Conditional risk factors
Elevated serum homocysteine
Elevated serum lipoprotein(a)
Elevated apolipoprotein B
Elevated non–high-density cholesterol
Elevated serum triglycerides
Inflammatory markers (eg, C-reactive protein)
Prothrombotic factors (eg, plasminogen activator inhibitor-1)
Small, dense LDL particles
Predisposing risk factors
Abdominal obesity
Ethnic characteristics
Family history of premature coronary heart disease
Metabolic syndrome
Obesity
Physical inactivity
Psychosocial factors

Yadlowsky S, Hayward RA, Sussman JB, McClelland RL, Min YI, Basu S. Clinical implications of revised pooled cohort equations for estimating atherosclerotic cardiovascular disease risk. *Ann Intern Med.* 2018;169:20–29. [PMID: 29868850]

B. Symptoms & Signs

The major symptom of chronic ischemic heart disease is angina pectoris, with a clinical diagnosis based on five features:

- The character of the pain is a deep visceral pressure, tightness, squeezing or a heavy sensation, rather than sharp, stabbing, or pinprick-like pain. It may be accompanied by dyspnea, nausea or numbness, especially in women.
- The pain almost always has some substernal component, although some patients complain of pain only on the right or left side of the chest, upper back, or epigastrium.
- The pain may radiate from the thorax to the jaw, neck, or arm. Arm pain in angina pectoris typically involves the ulnar surface of the left arm. Occasionally, the radiated pain may be more noticeable to the patient than the origin of the pain, resulting in complaints of only jaw, arm, or upper back pain. These considerations have led some physicians to suggest that any pain between the umbilicus and the eyebrows, front and back, should be considered angina pectoris until proven otherwise.

- Angina is usually precipitated by exertion, emotional upset, or other events that obviously increase myocardial oxygen demand, such as rapid tachyarrhythmias or extreme elevations in blood pressure.
- Angina pectoris is transient, lasting between 2 and 30 minutes. It is relieved by cessation of the precipitating event, such as exercise, or by the administration of treatment, such as sublingual nitroglycerin. Chest pain that lasts longer than 30 minutes is more consistent with myocardial infarction; pain lasting less than 2 minutes is unlikely to be due to myocardial ischemia.

For reasons that are unclear, some patients with chronic ischemic heart disease do not manifest typical symptoms of angina pectoris but have other symptoms that are brought on by the same precipitating factors and are relieved in the same way as angina. Because myocardial ischemia can lead to transient left ventricular dysfunction, resulting in increased left ventricular end-diastolic pressure and consequent pulmonary capillary pressure, the sensation of dyspnea can occur during episodes of myocardial supply-and-demand imbalance. Dyspnea may be the patient's only symptom during myocardial ischemia, or it may overshadow the chest pain in the patient's mind. Therefore, dyspnea out of proportion to the degree of exercise or activity can be considered an angina equivalent. Severe myocardial ischemia may lead to ventricular tachyarrhythmias manifesting as palpitations, frank syncope, or sudden cardiac death. Severe episodes of myocardial ischemia may also lead to transient pulmonary edema, especially if the papillary muscles are involved in the ischemic myocardium and moderately severe mitral regurgitation is produced.

Patients with chronic myocardial ischemia can also have symptoms caused by the effects of repeated episodes of ischemia or infarction. Thus, patients may have manifestations of chronic cardiac rhythm disorders, especially ventricular arrhythmias, or chronic congestive heart failure. Patients may have symptoms related to atherosclerosis of other vascular systems. Patients with vascular disease in other organs are more likely to have coronary atherosclerosis. Those with prior cerebral vascular accidents or symptoms of peripheral vascular disease may be so disabled by these diseases that their ability to either perceive angina or generate enough myocardial oxygen demand to produce angina may be severely limited.

C. Physical Examination

The physical examination is often not helpful in the diagnosis of chronic ischemic heart disease. This is because many patients with chronic ischemic heart disease have no physical findings related to the disease, or if they do, the findings are not specific for coronary artery disease. For example, a fourth heart sound can be detected in patients with chronic ischemic heart disease, especially if they have had a prior myocardial infarction; however, fourth heart sounds are very common in hypertensive heart disease, valvular heart disease, and primary myocardial disease. Palpation of a systolic precordial bulge can occur in patients with prior myocardial infarction, but this sign is not specific and can occur in patients with left ventricular enlargement from any cause. Other signs can also be found in cases of chronic ischemic heart disease, such as those associated with congestive heart failure or mitral regurgitation. Again, these are nonspecific and can be caused by other disease processes. Because coronary atherosclerosis is the most common heart disease in industrialized nations, any physical findings suggestive of heart disease should raise the suspicion of chronic ischemic heart disease.

D. Laboratory Findings

A complete blood count is useful to detect anemia, which will aggravate angina. Thyroid function tests are also important because hyperthyroidism can aggravate angina and hypothyroidism can lead to atherosclerosis. Fasting blood glucose or hemoglobin A1c are indicated to detect diabetes as is a blood lipid panel to detect hypercholesterolemia. In addition, kidney function should be assessed. High-sensitivity C-reactive protein (CRP) has been used to detect the increased inflammation of active atherosclerosis. Values greater than 3 mg/L predict coronary events, but the additive value over standard risk factors is unclear. Mortality can be predicted by brain natriuretic peptide (BNP or NT-proBNP) or troponin levels in patients with coronary artery disease. Presumably, patients with high CRP, BNP, or troponin levels should be treated more aggressively to reduce risk factors.

Wong YK, Tse HF. Circulating biomarkers for cardiovascular disease risk prediction in patients with cardiovascular disease. *Front Cardiovasc Med.* 2021;8:713191. doi: 10.3389/fcvm.2021.713191. [PMID: 34660715]

E. Diagnostic Studies

1. Stress tests—Because angina pectoris or other manifestations of myocardial ischemia often occur during the patient's normal activities, it would be ideal to detect evidence of ischemia at that time. This can be done with ambulatory electrocardiography (ECG). Under unusual circumstances, a patient may have spontaneous angina or ischemia in a medical facility, where it is possible to perform an echocardiogram to assess wall motion abnormalities indicative of ischemia or to inject a radionuclide agent and immediately image the myocardium for perfusion defects. Detection of myocardial ischemia during a patient's normal activities, however, does not have as high a diagnostic yield as exercise stress testing does.

Of the various forms of exercise stress that can be used, the most popular is treadmill exercise, for several reasons. It involves walking, a familiar activity that often provokes symptoms. Because of the gravitational effects of being upright, walking requires higher levels of myocardial oxygen demand than do many other forms of exercise. In addition, walking can be performed on an inexpensive treadmill device, which makes evaluating the patient easy and cost-effective. Bicycling is an alternative form of exercise that is preferred by exercise physiologists because it is easier to quantitate the amount of work the person is performing on a bicycle than on a treadmill. Unfortunately, bicycle exercise does not produce as high a level of myocardial oxygen demand as does treadmill walking. Thus, a patient may become fatigued on the bicycle before myocardial ischemia is induced, resulting in lower diagnostic yields. On the other hand, bicycle exercise can be performed in the supine position, which facilitates some myocardial ischemia detection methods such as echocardiography. In patients with peripheral vascular disease or lower limb amputations, arm and upper trunk rowing or cranking exercises can be substituted for leg exercise. Arm exercise has a particularly low diagnostic yield because exercising with the small muscle mass of the arms does not increase myocardial oxygen demand by much. Rowing exercises that involve the arms and the trunk muscles produce higher levels of myocardial oxygen demand that can equal those achieved with bicycle exercise—but not quite the levels seen with treadmill exercise. For these reasons, patients who cannot perform leg exercises are usually evaluated using pharmacologic stress testing.

There are two basic kinds of pharmacologic stress tests. One uses drugs, such as the synthetic catecholamine dobutamine, that mimic exercise; the other uses vasodilator drugs, such as adenosine and regadenoson, that, by producing vasodilatation, increase the heart rate and stroke volume, thereby raising myocardial oxygen demand. In addition, vasodilators may dilate normal coronary arteries more than diseased coronary arteries, augmenting any differences in regional perfusion of the myocardium, which can be detected by perfusion scanning. In general, vasodilator stress is preferred for myocardial perfusion imaging, and synthetic catecholamine stress is preferred for wall motion imaging.

2. Electrocardiography—ECG is the most frequently used method for detecting myocardial ischemia because of its ready availability, low cost, and ease of application. If the resting ECG is abnormal, heart disease is more likely. ECG changes with stress testing are less specific for coronary artery disease. The usual criterion for diagnosing ischemia is horizontal or down-sloping ST-segment depression, achieving at least 0.1 mV at 80 milliseconds beyond the J point (junction of the QRS and the ST segment). This criterion provides the highest values of sensitivity and specificity. Sensitivity can be increased by using 0.5 mV, but at the expense of lower specificity; similarly, using 0.2 mV increases the specificity of the test at the expense of lower sensitivity. Furthermore, accuracy is highest when ECG changes are in the lateral precordial leads (V_4, V_5, V_6) instead of the inferior leads (II, III, aVF). In the usual middle-aged, predominantly male patients with chest pain syndromes, who have normal resting ECGs and can achieve more than 85% of their maximal predicted age-based heart rate during treadmill exercise, the preceding ECG criteria have a sensitivity and specificity of approximately 85%. If the resting ECG is abnormal, if the patient does not achieve 85% of maximum predicted heart rate, or if the patient is a woman, the sensitivity and specificity are lower and range from 70% to 80%. In an asymptomatic population with a low pretest probability of disease, sensitivity and specificity fall below 70%.

3. Myocardial perfusion scanning—This method detects differences in regional myocardial perfusion rather than ischemia per se; however, there is a high correlation between abnormal regional perfusion scans and the presence of significant coronary artery occlusive lesions. Thus, when coronary arteriography is used as the gold standard, the sensitivity and specificity of stress myocardial perfusion scanning in patients with symptoms are approximately 85–95%. Testing an asymptomatic population would result in lower values. Failure to achieve more than 85% of the maximal predicted heart rate during exercise also results in lower diagnostic accuracy. Although treadmill exercise is the preferred stress modality for myocardial perfusion imaging, pharmacologically induced stress produces nearly as good results and is an acceptable alternative in the patient who cannot exercise. **Positron emission tomography** with vasodilator stress also can be used to detect regional perfusion differences indicative of coronary artery disease and has the advantage of less radiation exposure.

4. Assessing wall motion abnormalities—Reduced myocardial oxygen supply results in diminishment and, if severe enough, failure of myocardial contraction. Using methods to visualize the left ventricular wall, a reduction in inward endocardial movement and systolic myocardial thickening is observed with ischemia. **Echocardiography** is an ideal detection system for wall motion abnormalities because it can examine the left ventricle from several imaging planes, maximizing the ability to detect subtle changes in wall motion. When images are suboptimal (< 5% of cases), intravenous contrast agents can be given to fill the left ventricular cavity and improve endocardial definition. The results with either exercise or pharmacologic stress are comparable to those of myocardial perfusion imaging and superior to the ECG stress test detection of ischemia. The preferred pharmacologic detection method with wall motion imaging is dobutamine because it directly stimulates the myocardium to increase contractility, as well as raising heart rate and blood pressure, all of which increase myocardial oxygen demand. Also, if the heart rate increase is not comparable to that usually achieved with exercise testing, atropine can be administered to increase heart rate and further increase myocardial oxygen demand. **Magnetic resonance imaging (MRI)** can also be used to assess left ventricular wall motion during pharmacologic stress testing, but there is less experience with this technique.

5. Evaluating coronary anatomy

A. Coronary angiography—Coronary angiography is the standard for evaluating the anatomy of the coronary artery tree. It is best at evaluating the large epicardial coronary vessels that are most frequently diseased in coronary atherosclerosis. Experimental studies suggest that lesions that reduce the lumen of the coronary artery by 70% or more in area (50% in diameter) significantly limit flow, especially during periods of increased myocardial oxygen demand. If such lesions are detected, they are considered compatible with symptoms or other signs of myocardial ischemia. This assessment is known to be imprecise for several reasons, however. First, the actual cross-sectional area of the coronary artery at the point of an atherosclerotic lesion must be estimated from two-dimensional diameter measurements in several planes. When compared with autopsy findings, stenosis severity is usually found to have been underestimated by coronary angiography. Second, the technique does not take into consideration that lesions in series in a coronary artery may incrementally reduce the flow to distal beds by more than is accounted for by any single lesion. Thus, a series of apparently insignificant lesions may reduce myocardial blood flow significantly. Third, the cross-sectional area is not actually measured routinely. It is instead referenced to a supposed normal segment of an artery in terms of a percentage of stenosis or percentage of reduction in the normal luminal diameter or cross-sectional area. The problem with this type of estimate is that it is often difficult to determine what a normal segment of artery is, especially in patients with diffuse coronary atherosclerosis.

Quantitative coronary angiogram measurements are an improvement over this visual inspection technique, but they are not commonly used. Epicardial coronary artery anatomy is a static representation at the time of the study. It does not take into consideration potential changes in coronary vasomotor tone that may occur under certain circumstances and further reduce coronary blood flow. Also, coronary angiography does not adequately evaluate disease in the intramyocardial blood vessels; this may be important in some patients, especially insulin-dependent diabetics. In addition, plaque characteristics are not well defined by angiography and can be better visualized by **optical coherence tomographic imaging** or **intravascular ultrasound**.

Even well-defined coronary anatomy does not always accurately determine the hemodynamic significance of a stenotic coronary lesion. The invasive **fractional flow reserve (FFR)** is the current standard for this assessment but requires the administration of adenosine to dilate the coronary artery and significantly prolongs the procedure time. Coronary CT angiography can also be used to determine FFR which may be useful for planning staged coronary procedures. More recently the **instantaneous wave-free ratio** has been employed to determine coronary flow above and below a lesion during coronary catheter pull-back and provides similar information as FFR in comparative studies.

In patients with vasospastic angina, the coronary arteries are usually normal or minimally diseased. To establish increased vasomotion as the cause of the angina, provocative tests have been used to induce coronary vasospasm in the cardiac catheterization laboratory. Traditionally an **ergonovine infusion,** which is reputed to produce focal vasospasm only in naturally susceptible arteries and not in normal coronary arteries, usually exhibits only a uniform reduction in vessel diameter. Ergonovine infusion has some risks, however, in that the resultant coronary vasospasm may be difficult to alleviate and can be quite profound. Consequently, it is no longer available in the United States but is widely available in Europe. In the United States an **acetylcholine infusion** is now used to induce coronary vasospasm. An alternative for some patients is ambulatory ECG monitoring during the patient's normal daily activities to detect transient ST elevation associated with coronary vasospasm.

B. Other techniques—ECG or imaging evidence of old myocardial infarction is often presumed to indicate that severe coronary artery stenoses are present in the involved vessel. Myocardial infarction, however, can occur as a result of thrombus on top of a minor plaque that has ruptured and occasionally from intense vasospasm or coronary emboli from the left heart. In these cases, coronary angiography would not detect significant (narrowing of > 50% of the diameter) coronary lesions despite the evidence of an old myocardial infarction. Therefore, coronary artery imaging is necessary because estimating the degree of stenosis from the presence of infarction is not accurate. The presence of inducible myocardial ischemia almost always correlates with significant coronary artery lesions. Under certain clinical circumstances, coronary angiography can be avoided if noninvasive stress testing produces myocardial ischemia. Coronary angiography could then be reserved for patients who have not responded to medical therapy and are being considered for revascularization, where visualizing the coronary anatomy is necessary.

Other imaging techniques have also had some success. Echocardiography, especially transesophageal, can often visualize the first few centimeters of the major epicardial coronary arteries, and MRI has also shown promise. At present, neither of these noninvasive imaging techniques has reached the degree of accuracy needed to replace contrast coronary angiography; however, technical improvements may change this in the future.

Cardiac computed tomography (CT) use is expanding. Noncontrast techniques can rapidly detect calcified coronary artery plaque. The amount of plaque can be quantitated, usually as the Agatston score, which is predictive of future coronary events in an incremental fashion beyond traditional risk factors. The major use of CT coronary calcium score may be to further stratify the risk of an event in intermediate-risk patients where the intensity of risk factor reduction could be altered accordingly. Contrast CT angiography can evaluate the lumen of the coronary arteries that are not heavily calcified and is a useful alternative to stress testing for low to intermediate pretest risk of coronary artery disease patients. More recently, hybrid CT and either single-photon emission CT or positron emission tomography scanners are being used to visualize coronary lesions and assess their physiologic significance at one setting.

F. Other Useful Tests

In selected patients a posteroanterior chest X-ray may be of value by detecting cardiac enlargement of pulmonary vascular congestion, which would increase the likelihood of significant cardiac disease. In patients with suspected carotid atherosclerosis, carotid ultrasound imaging can be done. Also, an ankle-brachial index test is useful in screening for peripheral vascular disease. The detection of atherosclerosis in these extra-cardiac vessels would increase the likelihood of coronary atherosclerosis. In addition, an echocardiogram is reasonable in patients suspected of having coronary artery disease to assess cardiac systolic and diastolic function and to detect any left ventricular wall motion abnormalities. These findings will also increase the likelihood of coronary artery disease.

G. Choosing a Diagnostic Approach

Normally, noninvasive testing is performed first in the evaluation of suspected coronary atherosclerosis in symptomatic patients with an intermediate pretest likelihood of disease. There are several reasons for this: There is less risk with stress testing than with invasive coronary angiography, and cardiac CT has almost no risks. Mortality rates for stress testing average about 1 per 10,000 patients, compared with 1 per 1000 for coronary angiography. The physiologic demonstration of myocardial ischemia and its extent forms the basis for the therapeutic approach irrespective of coronary anatomy. Mildly symptomatic patients who show small areas of ischemia at intense exercise levels have an excellent prognosis and are usually treated medically. Knowledge of the coronary anatomy is not necessary to make this therapeutic decision. In general, therefore, a noninvasive technique should be used to detect myocardial ischemia and its extent before considering invasive coronary angiography, which is both riskier and more costly. Asymptomatic patients with a low to intermediate pretest likelihood of coronary artery disease may be better served by a noninvasive coronary artery imaging technique, such as cardiac CT; symptomatic patients may be better served by undergoing the combination of cardiac CT and stress perfusion imaging.

Profound symptoms that occur with minimal exertion are almost certainly due to severe diffuse coronary atherosclerosis or left main obstruction, and it is prudent to proceed directly with coronary angiography. Patients with severe unstable angina should undergo coronary angiography because of the potential increased risk posed by stress testing. If this approach is not appropriate in a particular clinical setting, the clinician might medicate the patient and perform careful stress testing after demonstrating a lack of symptoms on medical therapy. If the clinical situation is such that it is likely that stress testing will be inaccurate or uninterpretable, CT or invasive coronary angiography should be performed. Left bundle branch block on the ECG, for example, not only renders the ECG useless for detecting myocardial ischemia but may also affect the results of myocardial perfusion imaging and wall motion studies. In general, patients whose medical conditions preclude accurate stress testing are candidates for direct coronary angiography.

Which type of noninvasive stress testing to select is based on several factors. First and most importantly is the type of information desired; second, certain characteristics of the patient may make one test more applicable than another; and third is the pretest likelihood of disease. For example, cardiac CT may be most useful in low-risk patients; stress imaging in intermediate-risk patients; and invasive angiography in high-risk patients. Stress perfusion scanning is more likely than echocardiographic imaging to provide adequate technical quality in obese individuals or those with chronic obstructive pulmonary disease. Cost is also an important consideration, and the ECG stress test is the least expensive. In most patients with a low-to-medium clinical pretest likelihood of disease, using the ECG stress test makes sense, especially because good exercise performance with a negative ECG response for ischemia indicates an excellent prognosis even if coronary artery disease is present. In the patient who is highly likely to have coronary artery disease, however, it is useful to not only confirm the presence of the disease but also document its extent. For this purpose, myocardial imaging techniques are better at determining the extent of coronary artery disease than is the ECG. It is also believed that myocardial perfusion scanning is somewhat better at identifying the coronary arteries involved in the production of ischemia than are techniques for detecting wall motion abnormalities. Finally, if revascularization is considered futile due to overwhelming comorbidities or frailty, no testing is necessary and you can proceed directly to symptom relieving medical therapy.

Baumann S, Chandra L, Skarga E, et al. Instantaneous wave-free ratio to determine hemodynamically significant coronary stenosis: A comprehensive review. *World J Cardiol.* 2018;10: 267–277. [PMID: 30622685]

Gulati M, Levy PD, Mukherjee D, et al. 2021 AHA/ACC/ASE/CHEST/SAEM/SCCT/SCMR guideline for the evaluation and diagnosis of chest pain: a report of the American College of Cardiology/American Heart Association Joint Committee on Clinical Practice Guidelines. *J Am Coll Cardiol.* 2021;78:e187–e285. [PMID: 34756653]

Treatment

A. General Approach

Because myocardial ischemia is produced by an imbalance between myocardial oxygen supply and demand, in general, treatment consists of increasing supply or reducing demand—or both. Heart rate is a major determinant of myocardial oxygen demand, and attention to its control is imperative. Any treatment that accelerates heart rate is generally not going to be efficacious in preventing myocardial ischemia. Therefore, care must be taken with potent vasodilator drugs, such as hydralazine, which may markedly lower blood pressure and induce reflex tachycardia. Furthermore, because most coronary blood flow occurs during diastole, the longer the diastole, the greater is the coronary blood flow; and the faster the heart rate, the shorter is diastole.

Blood pressure is another important factor. Increases in blood pressure raise myocardial oxygen demand by elevating left ventricular wall tension, but blood pressure is the driving pressure for coronary perfusion. A critical blood pressure is required that does not excessively increase demand yet keeps coronary perfusion pressure across stenotic lesions optimal. Unfortunately, determining what this level of blood pressure should be in any given patient is difficult, and a trial-and-error approach is often needed to achieve the right balance. Consequently, it is prudent to reduce blood pressure when it is very high, and it may be important to allow it to increase when it is very low. It is not uncommon to encounter patients whose myocardial ischemia has been so vigorously treated with a combination of pharmacologic agents that their blood pressure is too low to be compatible with adequate coronary perfusion. In such patients, withholding some of their medications may improve their symptoms. Although myocardial contractility and left ventricular volume also contribute to myocardial oxygen demand, they are less important than heart rate and blood pressure. Myocardial contractility usually parallels heart rate. Attention should be paid to reducing left ventricular volume in anyone with a dilated heart, but not at the expense of excessive hypotension or tachycardia because these factors are more important than volume for determining myocardial oxygen demand.

It is important to eliminate any aggravating factors that could increase myocardial oxygen demand or reduce coronary artery flow (Table 6–3). Hypertension and tachyarrhythmias are obvious factors that need to be controlled. Thyrotoxicosis leads to tachycardia and increases in myocardial oxygen demand. Anemia is a common problem that increases myocardial oxygen demand because of reflex tachycardia; it reduces oxygen supply by decreasing the oxygen-carrying capacity of the blood. Similarly, hypoxia from pulmonary disease reduces oxygen delivery to the heart. Heart failure increases angina because it often results in left ventricular dilatation, which increases wall stress, and in excess catecholamine tone, which increases contractility and produces tachycardia.

Table 6–3. Factors That Can Aggravate Myocardial Ischemia

Increased myocardial oxygen demand	Tachycardia Hypertension Thyrotoxicosis Heart failure Valvular heart disease Catecholamine analogues (eg, bronchodilators, tricyclic antidepressants, cocaine)
Reduced myocardial oxygen supply	Anemia Hypoxia Carbon monoxide poisoning Hypotension Tachycardia

The long-term outlook for patients with coronary atherosclerosis must be addressed by reducing their risk factors for the disease. Once a patient is known to have atherosclerosis, risk factor reduction should be vigorous. If diet has not reduced serum cholesterol, strong consideration should be given to pharmacologic therapy because it has been shown to reduce cardiac events. Patients should be encouraged to exercise, lose weight, quit smoking, and try to reduce stress levels. Daily low-dose aspirin is important for preventing coronary thrombosis. The use of megadoses of vitamin E, β-carotene, and vitamin C should be discouraged in the patient with known coronary atherosclerosis because clinical trials have not demonstrated efficacy, and some have shown harm.

B. Pharmacologic Therapy

Pharmacologic therapy has been shown to reduce or abrogate symptoms but, with the possible exception of β-blockers post myocardial infarction, not reduce mortality.

1. Nitrates—Nitrates, which work on both sides of the supply-and-demand equation, are the oldest drugs used to treat angina pectoris (Table 6–4). These agents are now available in several formulations to fit the patient's lifestyle and disease characteristics. Almost all patients with known coronary atherosclerosis should carry rapid-acting nitroglycerin to abort acute attacks of angina pectoris. Nitrates work principally by providing more nitrous oxide to the vascular endothelium and the arterial smooth muscle, resulting in vasodilation. This tends to ameliorate any increased coronary vasomotor tone and dilate coronary obstructions. If blood pressure does not fall excessively, nitrates increase coronary blood flow. Nitrates also cause venodilation, reducing preload and decreasing left ventricular end-diastolic volume. The reduced left ventricular volume decreases wall tension and myocardial oxygen demand.

Sublingual nitroglycerin takes 30–60 seconds to dissolve completely and begin to produce beneficial effects, which can last up to 30 minutes. Although most used to abort acute attacks of angina, the drug can be used prophylactically if the patient can anticipate its need 30 minutes prior to a precipitating event. Prophylactic therapy is best accomplished, however, with longer-acting nitrate preparations. Isosorbide dinitrate and mononitrate are available in oral formulations; each produces beneficial effects for several hours.

Table 6–4. Common Oral Antianginal Drugs

Drug	Available Doses	Comments/Adverse Effects
Nitrates		
Nitroglycerin	0.3–0.6 mg sublingual	Aborts acute attacks; headaches, hypotension
Nitroglycerin	0.4 mg spray	More convenient than pills
Nitroglycerin	0.5–2 in of 2% ointment	Prophylactic therapy; tolerance a problem
Nitroglycerin	0.1–0.6 mg/h patches	Prophylactic therapy; tolerance a problem
Isosorbide dinitrate	5–60 mg, ER 40–80 mg	Need 14 h off every 24 h to avoid tolerance
Isosorbide mononitrate	10–20 mg, ER 30–120 mg	Take immediate release form twice a day 7 h apart
Drug	**Daily Dosage (mg)**	**Comments; Adverse Effects**
β-Blockers		
Propranolol	10–80; ER 60–160	Central nervous system side effects—fatigue, impotence—common
Nadolol	20–80	Long half-life, noncardioselective
Timolol	5–20	Noncardioselective
Metoprolol	25–100 tartrate 25–200 succinate	Cardioselective; half-life succinate > tartrate Succinate has heart failure reduced EF indication
Atenolol	25–100	Cardioselective; once or twice daily
Bisoprolol	5–10	Cardioselective; heart failure reduced EF indication
Pindolol	5–20	Marked intrinsic sympathomimetic activity
Calcium Channel Blockers, Heart Rate Lowering		
Diltiazem	30–120; ER 60–420	Heart rate lowering; atrioventricular (AV) block, heart failure, edema
Verapamil	40–120; ER 100–360	Heart rate lowering; AV block, heart failure, constipation
Dihydropyridine Calcium Channel Blockers		
Amlodipine	5–10	Least myocardial depression
Nifedipine	10–20; ER 30–90	Hypotension, tachycardia
Nicardipine	20–30	Potent coronary vasodilator
Ranolazine	500–1000	May increase QT interval on electrocardiogram

Large doses of these agents must be taken orally to overcome nitrate reductases in the liver. Liver metabolism of the nitrates can also be avoided with cutaneous application. Nitroglycerin is available as a topical ointment that can be applied as a dressing; it is also available as a ready-made, self-adhesive patch that delivers accurate continuous dosing of the drug through a membrane. Although the paste and the patches produce similar effects, the patches are more convenient for patients to use.

Sublingual nitroglycerin tablets are extremely small and difficult for patients with arthritis to manipulate. A buccal preparation of nitroglycerin is available, which comes in a larger, more easily manipulable tablet that can be chewed and allowed to dissolve in the mouth, rather than being swallowed. This achieves nitrate effectiveness within 2–5 minutes and lasts about 30 minutes, as do the sublingual tablets. An oral nitroglycerin spray, which may be easier to manipulate and more convenient for some patients, is also available.

The major difficulty with all long-acting nitroglycerin preparations is the development of tolerance to their effects. The exact reason for tolerance development is not clearly understood, but it may involve liver enzyme induction or a lack of arterial responsiveness because of local adaptive factors. Regardless of the mechanism, round-the-clock nitrate administration will lead to progressively increasing tolerance to the drug after 24–48 hours. Because of this, nitroglycerin is usually taken over the 16-hour period each day that corresponds to the time period during which most of the ischemic episodes would be expected to occur. For most patients, this means not taking nitrate preparations before bed and allowing the ensuing 8 hours for the effects to wear off and responsiveness to the drug to be regained. This timing would have to be adjusted for patients with nocturnal angina. The difficulty with the 8-hour overnight hiatus in therapy, however, is that the patient has little protection during the critical early morning wakening period, when ischemic events are more likely to occur. Therefore, patients should take the nitrate preparation as soon as they arise in the morning. For this reason, the nitroglycerin patches have a small amount of paste on the outside of the membrane that delivers a bolus of drug through the skin, which quickly elevates the patient's blood level of the drug. It is important that the patient be careful not to wipe this paste off the patch before applying it.

Nitrates, which are effective in preventing the development of angina as well as aborting acute attacks, are helpful in both patients with fixed coronary artery occlusions and those with vasospastic angina. Their potency, compared with other agents, is limited, however, and patients with severe angina often must turn to other agents. In such patients, nitrates can be excellent adjunctive therapy.

2. β-Blockers—β-Adrenergic blocking agents are highly effective in the prophylactic therapy of angina pectoris. They have been shown to reduce or eliminate angina attacks and prolong exercise endurance time in double-blind, placebo-controlled studies. They can be used around the clock because no tachyphylaxis to their effects has been found. β-Blockers mainly work by lowering myocardial oxygen demand through decreasing heart rate, blood pressure, and myocardial contractility. As mentioned earlier, however, they also increase myocardial oxygen supply by increasing the duration of diastole through heart rate reduction. Currently, several β-blocker preparations are available, with one or more features that may make them more—or less—attractive for a particular patient.

Among these features is the agent's pharmacologic half-life, which ranges from 4 to 18 hours. Various delivery systems have been developed to slow down the delivery of short-acting agents and prolong the duration of drug activity through sustained-release or long-acting formulations. Note that the pharmacodynamic half-life of β-adrenergic blockers is often longer than their pharmacologic half-life, and drug effects can be detected for days after discontinuation of prolonged β-blocker therapy.

Ideally, β-blockers should be titrated against the heart rate response to exercise because blunting of the exercise heart rate response is the hallmark of their efficacy. Adverse effects of β-blockers include excessive bradycardia, heart block, and hypotension. Nonselective β-blockers can cause bronchospasm, but it occurs less often with the β_1-selective agents. Blocking β_2-peripheral vasodilatory actions may aggravate claudication in patients with severe peripheral vascular disease. β-Adrenergic stimulation is also important for the gluconeogenic response to hyperglycemia in severely insulin-dependent diabetic patients. Although β-blockers may impair this response, the major problem with their use in insulin-dependent diabetic patients is that the warning signals of hypoglycemia (sweating, tachycardia, piloerection) may be blocked. Because of their negative inotropic properties, β-blockers may also precipitate heart failure or cardiogenic shock in patients with markedly reduced left ventricular performance or acute heart failure.

Other side effects of β-blockers are less predictably related to their anti–β-adrenergic effects. Adverse central nervous system effects are especially troublesome and include fatigue, mental slowness, and impotence. These side effects are somewhat less common with agents that are less lipophilic, such as atenolol. Unfortunately, it is these side effects that make many patients unable to tolerate β-blockers.

3. Calcium channel antagonists—Calcium channel antagonists theoretically work on both sides of the supply-and-demand equation. By blocking calcium access to smooth muscle cells, they produce peripheral vasodilatation and are effective antihypertensive agents. In the myocardium, they block sinus node and atrioventricular node function and reduce the inotropic state. They dilate the coronary arteries and increase myocardial blood flow. The calcium channel blockers available today produce a variable spectrum of these basic pharmacologic effects. The biggest group is the dihydropyridine calcium channel blockers, which are potent arterial dilators and thereby cause reflex sympathetic activation, which may overshadow their negative chronotropic and inotropic effects.

A second major group of calcium channel blockers are those that lower the heart rate. The two most used drugs in this class are diltiazem and verapamil. Because these drugs have less peripheral vasodilatory action in individuals with normal blood pressure, they produce little reflex tachycardia. The average daily heart rate is usually reduced with these agents because their inherent negative chronotropic effects are not overridden. However, negative inotropic effects are also more common with these agents. Hypertensive and normotensive individuals seem to have a different vascular responsiveness to the rate-lowering calcium channel blockers. Interestingly, in hypertensive individuals, rate-lowering calcium channel blockers lower the blood pressure as well as the dihydropyridine agents. Diltiazem is more widely used because of its lower side effect profile. Verapamil has potent effects on the arteriovenous (AV) node; this can cause excessive bradycardia and heart block in patients with angina pectoris. Verapamil is also more likely than diltiazem to precipitate heart failure, and it often produces troublesome constipation, especially in elderly individuals. All the calcium channel blockers can produce peripheral edema. This is due not to their negative inotropic effects but rather to an imbalance between the efferent and afferent peripheral arteriolar tone, which increases capillary hydrostatic pressure. Other adverse effects of these drugs are idiosyncratic and include gastrointestinal and dermatologic effects.

Calcium channel blockers are titrated to the patient's symptoms because there is no physiologic marker of their effect, in contrast to the heart rate response to exercise with β-blockers. This makes choosing the appropriate dosage difficult, and many clinicians increase the dose until some side effect occurs and then they reduce it. The most common side effects are related to the pharmacologic effects of the drugs. With the dihydropyridines, vasodilatory side effects, such as orthostatic hypotension, flushing, and headache, occur. Hypotension is less common with the heart rate–lowering calcium channel blockers, and their side effects are more related to cardiac effects, such as excessive bradycardia. These drugs are very useful because they are excellent for preventing angina pectoris, lowering high blood pressure, and, in the case of the heart rate–lowering agents, controlling supraventricular arrhythmias.

4. Ranolazine—Ranolazine partially inhibits fatty acid oxidation and increases glucose oxidation, which generates more adenosine triphosphate for each molecule of oxygen consumed. This shift in substrate selection may reduce myocardial oxygen demand without altering hemodynamics. Because all other antianginal agents reduce blood pressure, this gives ranolazine an advantage. Studies have shown that ranolazine provides additive benefits to standard treatment described earlier and is useful as monotherapy. It has few adverse effects. However, it also selectively inhibits the inward sodium current which can prolong the QTc.

5. Combination therapy—Although monotherapy is desirable for patient convenience and cost considerations, many patients, especially those with severe coronary artery disease, require more than one antianginal agent to control their symptoms. Because all antianginal agents have a synergistic effect in preventing angina, the initial choices should be for agents with complementary pharmacologic effects. For example, nitrates can be added to β-blocker therapy. Nitrates dilate coronary arteries and increase coronary blood flow, and their peripheral effects may increase reflex sympathetic tone and counteract some of the negative inotropic and chronotropic effects of the β-blockers. This has proved to be a highly effective combination. Similarly, combining a β-blocker with dihydropyridine drugs, when the β-blockers suppress the reflex tachycardia produced by the dihydropyridine, has also proved to be highly effective. In addition, combinations of the heart rate-lowering calcium channel blockers and nitrates have proved efficacious. Extremely refractory patients may respond to the combination of a dihydropyridine calcium channel blocker and a heart rate-lowering calcium channel blocker.

Combining a dihydropyridine calcium channel blocker and nitrates makes little sense, however, because of the high likelihood of producing potent vasodilatory side effects. This combination may excessively lower blood pressure to the point that coronary perfusion pressure is compromised, and the patient's angina worsens. In fact, in as many as 10% of patients with moderately severe angina, both the nitrates and the dihydropyridine calcium channel blockers alone have been reported to aggravate angina. Although few corroborative data exist, this percentage is certainly higher with the combination of the two agents.

The most difficult cases often involve triple therapy, with a calcium channel blocker, a β-blocker, and a nitrate or even quadruple therapy with the addition of ranolazine. Although there are few objective data on the benefits of this approach, it has proven efficacious in selected patients. The major problem with triple therapy is that side effects, such as hypotension, are increased, which often limits therapy. Ranolazine has no hemodynamic effects and can be used for patients refractory to their current regimen or in patients whose heart rate or blood pressure levels are too low for the other agents.

6. Adjunctive therapy—All patients with coronary artery disease should take aspirin (81 mg/day) and selected high-risk patients should also take clopidogrel. These drugs reduce platelet aggregation and retard the growth of atherothrombosis. If patients are put on dual antiplatelet therapy and have a high bleeding risk, adjunctive proton pump inhibitor therapy should be considered. Also important is correction of dyslipidemia, smoking cessation, exercise, weight loss, control of hypertension, and management of stress. In patients with known coronary artery disease, it is important to decrease low-density lipoprotein (LDL) cholesterol. Angiotensin-converting enzyme inhibitors (ACEI) or angiotensin receptor blockers (ARB) may have a protective effect in patients with coronary artery disease, especially in those with reduced left ventricular ejection fraction, hypertension, or diabetes. β-Blockers are also indicated for patients after myocardial infarction, but their use in chronic coronary artery disease without infarct or angina is controversial. Finally, in patients with diabetes and ischemic heart disease treatment with a sodium-glucose cotransporter 2 inhibitors ("flozins") or a glucagon-like peptide-1 receptor agonist ("tides") for glucose reduction are recommended because of their beneficial effects on reducing cardiovascular events.

C. Revascularization

1. Catheter-based methods—The standard percutaneous coronary intervention (PCI) is balloon dilatation with placement of a stent. Such treatment is limited to the larger epicardial arteries and can be complicated by various types of acute vessel injury, which can result in myocardial infarction. Smaller arteries may be amenable to plain old balloon angioplasty (POBA), and large arteries with complicated lesions may be candidates for other forms of PCI. PCI requires intense antiplatelet therapy, usually with aspirin and a platelet P2Y12 receptor inhibitor such as clopidogrel, prasugrel, or ticagrelor to prevent stent thrombosis. After the stent has been covered with endothelium (1–3 months or more), this risk is much less and antiplatelet monotherapy is appropriate.

In the absence of acute complications, initial success rates for significantly dilating the coronary artery are greater than 90%, and the technique can be of tremendous benefit to patients—without their undergoing the risk of cardiac surgery. The principal disadvantage to PCI is restenosis, which occurs in about one-third of patients treated with a bare metal stent during the first 6 months. Drug-eluting stents have reduced restenosis to 10% or less but have been associated with a small incidence of late thrombosis. PCI is ideal for symptomatic patients with one or two discrete lesions in one or two arteries. In patients with more complex lesions or those with three or more vessels involved, bypass surgery is preferable for several reasons. First, the restenosis risk is the same for each lesion treated by PCI, so that if enough vessels are worked on the risk of restenosis in one of them will increase significantly. Second, the ability to completely revascularize patients with multivessel disease is less with PCI compared with bypass surgery. Finally, some clinical trials have shown that diabetic patients with multivessel disease have better outcomes after bypass surgery compared to PCI.

2. Coronary artery bypass graft surgery—Controlled clinical trials have shown that coronary artery bypass graft (CABG) surgery can successfully alleviate angina symptoms in up to 80% of patients. These results compare very favorably with pharmacologic therapy and catheter-based techniques and can be accomplished in selected patients with less than 2% operative mortality rates. Although the initial cost of surgery is high, studies have shown it can be competitive with repeated angioplasty and lifelong pharmacologic therapy in selected patients.

The standard surgical approach is to use the saphenous veins, which are sewn to the ascending aorta and then, distal to the obstruction, in the coronary artery, effectively bypassing the obstruction with blood from the aorta. Although single end-to-side saphenous-vein-to-coronary-artery grafts are preferred, occasionally surgeons will do side-to-side anastomoses in one coronary artery (or more) and then terminate the graft in an end-to-side anastomosis in the final coronary artery. There is some evidence that although these skip grafts are easier and quicker to place than multiple single saphenous grafts, they may not last as long. The major problems with saphenous vein grafts are recurrent atherosclerosis in the grafts, which is often quite bulky and friable, and ostial stenosis, probably from cicatrization at the anastomotic sites. Although these problems can be approached with PCI, the success rate of PCI to open obstructed saphenous vein grafts is not as high as that seen with native coronary artery obstructions, and many patients require repeat saphenous vein grafting after an average of about 8–10 years. It is believed that reducing LDL cholesterol, cessation of smoking, and the ingestion of one aspirin a day (81–100 mg) will retard the development of saphenous vein atherosclerosis; some patients do well for 20 years or more after CABG.

There is now considerable evidence that arterial conduits make better bypass graft materials. The difficulty is finding large enough arteries that are not essential to other parts of the body. The most popular arteries used today are the internal thoracic arteries. Their attachment to the subclavian artery is left intact, and the distal end is used as an end-to-side anastomosis into a single coronary artery. If a patient requires more than two grafts, some surgeons, rather than using a saphenous vein, have used the radial artery or abdominal vessels, such as the gastroepiploic. There are fewer data on these alternative conduits, but theoretically, they would have the same advantages as the internal thoracic arteries in terms of graft longevity. Efforts at preventing bypass graft failure are worthwhile because the risk of repeat surgery is usually higher than that of the initial surgery. There are several reasons for this, including the fact that the patient is older, the scar tissue from the first operation makes the second one more difficult, and finally, any progression of atherosclerosis in the coronary arteries makes finding good-quality insertion sites for the graft more difficult.

D. Selection of Therapy

Pharmacologic therapy is indicated when other conditions may be aggravating angina pectoris and can be successfully treated. For example, in the patient with coexistent hypertension and angina, it is often prudent to treat the hypertension and lower blood pressure to acceptable levels before pursuing revascularization for angina because lowering the blood pressure will often eliminate the angina. For this purpose, it is wise to use antihypertensive medications that are also antianginal (eg, β-blockers, calcium channel blockers) rather than other agents with no antianginal effects (eg, ACE inhibitors, centrally acting agents). The presence of heart failure can also produce or aggravate angina, and this should be treated. Care must be taken in choosing antianginal drugs that do not aggravate heart failure. For this reason, nitrates are frequently used in heart failure and angina because these drugs may benefit both conditions. Rate-lowering calcium channel blockers should be avoided if the left ventricular ejection fraction is below 35%, unless the heart failure is episodic and is being produced by ischemia. In this situation, however, revascularization may be a more effective strategy. β-Blockers can be effective for angina with heart failure, but they must be started at low doses and uptitrated carefully. Although β-blockers are now part of standard therapy for heart failure, there is little data on their use in patients with angina and reduced left ventricular performance. Finally, the presence of ventricular or supraventricular tachyarrhythmias may aggravate angina. Rhythm disorders also afford an opportunity for using dual-purpose drugs. The heart rate-lowering calcium channel blockers may effectively control supraventricular arrhythmias and benefit angina. β-Blockers can often be effective treatment for ventricular arrhythmias in patients with coronary artery disease and should be tried before other, more potent antiarrhythmics or devices are contemplated. Keep in mind that digoxin blood levels may be increased by concomitant treatment with calcium channel blockers. In addition, the combination of digoxin and either heart rate-lowering calcium channel blockers or β-blockers may cause synergistic effects on the atrioventricular node and lead to excessive bradycardia or heart block.

The major indication for revascularization of chronic ischemic heart disease is the failure of medications to control the patient's symptoms. Drug-refractory angina pectoris is the major indication for revascularization. Note that myocardial ischemia should be established as the source of the patient's symptoms before embarking on revascularization, since symptoms may be due to other conditions such as gastroesophageal reflux. Consequently, some form of stress testing that verifies the relationship between demonstrable ischemia and symptoms is advisable before performing any revascularization procedure in stable patients.

In some other instances—patient preference, for example—revascularization therapy might be considered before even trying pharmacologic therapy. Some patients do not like the prospect of lifelong drug therapy and would rather have open arteries. Although this is a valid reason to perform revascularization, the clinician must be careful that his or her own enthusiasm for revascularization as treatment does not pressure the patient into such a decision. Other candidates for direct revascularization are patients with high-risk occupations who cannot return to these occupations unless they are completely revascularized (eg, airline pilots).

Revascularization is preferred to medical therapy in managing certain types of coronary anatomy that are known (through clinical trials) to have a longer survival if treated with CABG rather than medically. Such lesions include left main obstructions of more than 50%, three-vessel disease, and two-vessel disease in which one of the vessels is the left anterior descending artery. Left main stenosis and two- and three-vessel coronary disease can be treated by PCI, and clinical trials have shown equivalent long-term outcomes between PCI and CABG in patients with left main and multivessel disease.

CABG is also recommended for patients with two- or three-vessel coronary artery disease and resultant heart failure from reduced left ventricular performance, especially if viable myocardium can be demonstrated. Because the tests for viable myocardium are not perfect, however, many clinicians believe that all these patients should be revascularized in the hope that some myocardial function will return. This seems a prudent approach, given that donor hearts for cardiac transplantation are difficult to obtain, and many patients with heart failure and coronary artery disease improve following bypass surgery. Surgery is also recommended when the patient has a concomitant disease that requires surgical therapy, such as significant valvular heart disease.

The risk of bypass surgery in each individual must also be considered because several factors can increase the risk significantly and might make catheter-based techniques or medical therapy more desirable. Age is always a risk factor for any major surgery, and CABG is no exception. Also, female sex tends to increase the risk of CABG, possibly because women are, on average, smaller and have smaller arteries than men. Some data indicate that if size is the only factor considered, sex disappears as a risk predictor with CABG. Other medical conditions that may complicate the perioperative period (eg, chronic kidney disease, obesity, lung disease, diabetes) also raise the risks of surgery. Another factor (discussed earlier) is whether this is a repeat bypass operation. The technical difficulties are especially troublesome when a prior internal thoracic artery graft has been placed because this artery lies right behind the sternum and can be easily compromised when reopening the chest.

The choice between catheter-based techniques and CABG surgery is based on several considerations: Is it technically feasible to perform either technique with a good result? What does the patient wish to do? The patient may have a strong preference for one technique over the other. Again, the clinician must be careful not to unduly influence the patient in this regard, lest it give the appearance of a conflict of interest. Consideration must also be given to factors that increase the risk of surgery. The most difficult decision involves the patient who is suitable for either surgery or a catheter-based technique. The few controlled, randomized clinical trials that have been done on such patients have shown equivalent clinical results with PCI and surgery in terms of mortality and symptom relief. Note that this is accomplished by PCI at the cost of repeated procedures in many patients. Despite the necessity for these repeated procedures, the overall cost of bypass surgery is higher over the short term. Unfortunately, the trials do not outline clear guidelines for choosing PCI or CABG in the patient who is a good candidate for either treatment; this continues to be a decision to be made by the clinician and the patient on a case-by-case basis. The availability of minimally invasive surgery has pushed the balance between CABG and PCI a little toward CABG, but not all patients are suitable for a minimally invasive approach.

Cosentino F, Grant PJ, Aboyans V, et al. 2019 ESC guidelines on diabetes, pre-diabetes, and cardiovascular diseases developed in collaboration with the EASD: The Task Force for diabetes, pre-diabetes, and cardiovascular diseases of the European Society of Cardiology (ESC) and the European Association for the Study of Diabetes (EASD). *Eur Heart J.* 2019;41:255–323. [PMID: 31497854]

Knuuti J, Wijns W, Saraste A, et al. 2019 ESC Guidelines for the diagnosis and management of chronic coronary syndromes. *Eur Heart J.* 2020;41:407. [PMID: 31504439]

Lawton JS, Tamis-Holland JE, Bangalore S, et al. 2021 ACC/AHA/SCAI guideline for coronary artery revascularization: a report of the American College of Cardiology/American Heart Association Joint Committee on Clinical Practice Guidelines. *J Am Coll Cardiol.* 2022;79:e21–e129. [PMID: 34895950]

Patel MR, Calhoon JH, Dehmer GJ, et al. ACC/AATS/AHA/ASE/ASNC/SCAI/SCCT/STS 2017 appropriate use criteria for coronary revascularization in patients with stable ischemic heart disease. *J Am Coll Cardiol.* 2017;69:2212–2241. [PMID: 28291663]

Prognosis

There are two major determinants of prognosis in patients with chronic ischemic heart disease. The first is the clinical status of the patient, which can be semi-quantitated by the Canadian Cardiovascular Society's angina functional class system. In this system, class I is asymptomatic, class II is angina with heavy exertion, class III is angina with mild-to-moderate exertion, and class IV comprises patients who cannot perform their daily activities without getting angina or who are experiencing angina decubitus. The higher the Canadian class, the worse is the prognosis. Clinical status can also be determined by exercise testing. If patients can exercise more than 9 minutes or into stage IV of the Bruce protocol, their prognosis is excellent. However, the presence of either angina or significant ischemic ST depression on the exercise test indicates a poorer prognosis. In addition, when using perfusion scanning, the more extensive the perfusion abnormalities with exercise, the worse is the prognosis. Left ventricular dysfunction with exercise, as evidenced by an increase in left ventricular volume or by a drop in left ventricular ejection fraction during stress perfusion imaging, also connotes a worse prognosis. Perhaps the most powerful predictor for future mortality is the resting left ventricular ejection fraction; values of less than 50% are associated with an exponential increase in mortality.

A second prognostic system is based solely on coronary anatomy. The more vessels involved and the more severely they are involved, the worse is the prognosis. This observation has formed the anatomic basis for revascularization in patients with coronary artery disease. Although this approach has some appeal, it has never been proven that revascularization in asymptomatic patients improves their prognosis. Even in patients with left main and severe three-vessel disease, proof is lacking that prophylactic revascularization is of any value if the patients are asymptomatic. Theoretical considerations suggest that ischemia—even in the absence of angina—that can be demonstrated by stress testing or ambulatory ECG recordings would support a decision to revascularize based on anatomy and the presence of ischemia. Although this seems like a much stronger case for revascularization in an asymptomatic patient, such treatment has not been proven efficacious in clinical trials.

The simplicity of the coronary anatomy approach to prognosis has resulted in considerable clinical data on the longevity of patients with chronic ischemic heart disease. Patients with one-vessel coronary artery disease have about a 3% per year mortality rate; this rate is less if the vessel is the right or circumflex coronary artery and somewhat more if it is the left anterior descending artery. Patients with two-vessel disease have a 5% or 6% mortality rate per year; in patients with three-vessel disease, this increases to 6–8% a year. Patients with left main disease, with or without other coronary occlusions, have about an 8–12% yearly mortality rate. Similar data do not exist for the clinical classification of patients because of the complexities of determining risk by this approach. A positive treadmill exercise test, at a low workload, for either angina or ischemic ST changes connotes a yearly mortality rate of 5%. This is less if the patient exercised a long time and had good left ventricular function and no previous myocardial infarction. It is worse if the patient exercised only a very short time on the treadmill and had evidence of left ventricular dysfunction or a prior myocardial infarction. Whether pharmacologic and revascularization therapy can influence these prognostic figures is unclear at present.

Unstable Angina/Non-ST Elevation Myocardial Infarction

7

Kuang-Yuh Chyu, MD, PhD
Prediman K. Shah, MD

ESSENTIALS OF DIAGNOSIS

- New or worsening symptoms (angina, pulmonary edema) or signs (electrocardiographic [ECG] changes) of myocardial ischemia.
- Absence or mild elevation of cardiac enzymes (troponin I or T) without prolonged ST-segment elevation on ECG.
- Unstable angina and non-ST elevation myocardial infarction (MI) (USA/NSTEMI) are closely related in pathogenesis and clinical presentation and are therefore discussed as one entity in this chapter.

General Considerations

A. Background

Unstable angina and non-ST elevation myocardial infarction (USA/NSTEMI) are a part of the wide spectrum of clinical manifestations of atherosclerotic coronary artery disease (Table 7–1). Compared with ST elevation myocardial infarction (STEMI), the incidence of USA/NSTEMI has been increasing. According to the Nationwide Inpatient Sample databases, from 2002 to 2011, the prevalence of NSTEMI increased from 52.8% to 68.6%. The risk-adjusted in-hospital mortality for NSTEMI patients has been gradually declining in the same period, likely due to advances in the treatment of acute coronary syndrome and increased utilization of early invasive strategy.

B. Pathophysiology

Angina pectoris is the symptomatic equivalent of transient myocardial ischemia that results from a temporary imbalance in the myocardial oxygen demand and supply. Most episodes of myocardial ischemia are generally believed to result from an absolute reduction in regional myocardial blood flow below basal levels, with the subendocardium carrying a greater burden of flow deficit relative to the epicardium, whether triggered by a primary reduction in coronary blood flow or an increase in oxygen demand. USA/NSTEMI shares a more or less common pathophysiologic substrate with STEMI, which is usually due to ruptured/eroded or unstable atherosclerotic plaques with overlying thrombus formation, leading to reduced coronary blood flow. The differences in clinical presentation result largely from the differences in the magnitude of coronary occlusion, the duration of the occlusion, the modifying influence of local and systemic blood flow, and the adequacy of coronary collaterals.

Clinical Findings

A. Symptoms

USA/NSTEMI is a clinical syndrome characterized by symptoms of ischemia, which may include classic retrosternal chest pain or such pain surrogates as a burning sensation, feeling of indigestion, or dyspnea (Table 7–2). Anginal symptoms may also be felt primarily or as radiation in the neck, jaw, teeth, arms, back, or epigastrium. The pain of unstable angina typically lasts 15–30 minutes; it can last longer in some patients. In some patients, particularly the elderly, dyspnea, fatigue, diaphoresis, light-headedness, a feeling of indigestion and the desire to burp or defecate, or nausea and emesis may accompany other symptoms or may be the only symptoms. It has been estimated that about 43.6% of patients with USA/NSTEMI presented without chest pain. The clinical presentation of unstable angina can take any one of several forms.

There may be an onset of ischemic symptoms in a patient who had been previously free of angina, with or without a history of coronary artery disease. If symptoms are effort induced, they are often rapidly progressive, with more frequent, easily provoked, and prolonged episodes. Rest pain may follow a period of crescendo effort angina or may exist from the beginning.

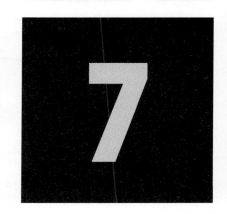

Table 7–1. Clinical Spectrum of Atherosclerotic Coronary Artery Disease

Subclinical or asymptomatic
Stable angina
Acute coronary syndrome
Unstable angina
NSTEMI
STEMI
Sudden death

Symptoms may intensify or change in a patient with antecedent angina. Pain may be provoked by less effort and be more frequent and prolonged than before. The response to nitrates may decrease and their consumption increase. The appearance of new pain at rest or with minimal exertion is particularly ominous. Ischemic symptoms may recur shortly after (usually within 4 weeks) an acute MI, coronary artery bypass surgery, or catheter-based coronary artery intervention. In some patients, an acute unstable coronary syndrome may manifest as acute pulmonary edema or sudden cardiac death.

B. Physical Examination

No physical finding is specific for USA/NSTEMI, and when the patient is free of pain, the examination may be entirely normal. During episodes of ischemia, a dyskinetic left ventricular apical impulse, a third or fourth heart sound, or a transient murmur of ischemic mitral regurgitation may be detected. Similarly, during episodes of prolonged or severe ischemia, there may be transient evidence of left ventricular failure, such as pulmonary congestion or edema, with dyspnea, diaphoresis, or hypotension. Arrhythmias and conduction disturbances may occur during episodes of myocardial ischemia.

The findings from physical examination, especially as they relate to signs of heart failure, provide important prognostic information. An analysis of data from four randomized clinical trials (GUSTO IIb, PURSUIT, and PARAGON A and B) revealed that Killip classification, a commonly used classification based on physical examination of patients at presentation of STEMI, is a strong independent predictor for short- and long-term mortality, with higher Killip class associated with higher mortality rate. This has also been confirmed using data from the Canadian Acute Coronary Syndrome Registries.

Table 7–2. Clinical Presentation of Unstable Angina

New onset of ischemic symptoms
At rest only
During exertion only
At rest and exertion
Intensification of previous ischemic symptoms
Increased frequency, severity, duration
Change in pattern (eg, symptoms at rest)
Recurrence of ischemic symptoms within 4–6 weeks after an acute myocardial infarction
Other
Recurrence of ischemia within 4–6 weeks following bypass surgery or coronary catheterization
Recurrent acute pulmonary edema
Prinzmetal (variant) angina

C. Diagnostic Studies

USA/NSTEMI is a common reason for admission to the hospital, and the diagnosis, in general, rests entirely on clinical grounds. In a patient with typical effort-induced chest discomfort that is new or rapidly progressive, the diagnosis is relatively straightforward, particularly (but not necessarily) when there are associated electrocardiogram (ECG) changes. Often, however, the symptoms are less clear-cut. The pain or discomfort may not be typical in terms of its location, radiation, character, and intensity, or the patient may have had a single, prolonged episode of pain, which may or may not have resolved by the time of presentation. The term "typical" or "atypical" to describe chest pain is now discouraged by the latest guideline. Instead the term "cardiac," "possible cardiac," and "non-cardiac" to describe chest pain (or discomfort) is recommended. The physician should strongly suspect unstable angina, particularly when coronary artery disease or its risk factors are present. When in doubt, it is safer to err on the side of caution and consider the diagnosis to be unstable angina until proven otherwise. Even though dynamic ST-T changes on the ECG make the diagnosis more certain, between 5% and 10% of patients with a compelling clinical history (especially middle-aged women) have no critical coronary stenosis on coronary angiography. In rare instances, especially in women, spontaneous coronary artery dissection, unrelated to coronary atherosclerosis, may be the basis for an acute coronary syndrome. In general, the more profound the ECG changes, the greater the likelihood of an ischemic origin for the pain and the worse the prognosis.

1. ECG and Holter monitoring—ECG abnormalities are common in patients with USA/NSTEMI and is recommended to obtain ECG within 10 minutes of patient's arrival to ER or at first medical contact with immediate transmission to qualified physicians for interpretation in prehospital setting. In view of the episodic nature of ischemia, however, the changes may not be present if the ECG is recorded during an ischemia-free period or the ischemia involves the myocardial territories (eg, the circumflex coronary artery territory) that are not well represented on the standard 12-lead ECG. Therefore, it is not surprising that 40–50% of patients admitted with a clinical diagnosis of unstable angina have no ECG abnormalities on initial presentation. The ECG abnormalities tend to be in the form of transient ST-segment depression or elevation and, less frequently, T-wave inversion, flattening, peaking, or pseudo-normalization (ie, the T wave becomes transiently upright from a baseline state of inversion or vice versa). It must be emphasized, however, that a normal or unremarkable ECG should never be used to disregard the diagnosis of unstable angina in a patient with a compelling clinical history and an appropriate risk-factor profile. Comparison with previous ECG, if possible, is always helpful, especially in patients with pre-existing ECG abnormalities such as left bundle branch block or left ventricular hypertrophy.

Continuous ambulatory ECG recording reveals a much higher prevalence of transient ST-T wave abnormalities, of which 70–80% are not accompanied by symptoms (silent ischemia). These episodes, which may be associated with transient ventricular dysfunction and reduced myocardial perfusion, are much more prevalent in patients with ST-T changes on their admission tracings (up to 80%) than in persons without such changes. Frequent and severe ECG changes on ECG monitoring, in general, indicate an increased risk of adverse clinical outcome.

2. Diagnostic coronary angiography—More than 90–95% of patients with a clinical syndrome of unstable angina have angiographically detectable atherosclerotic coronary artery disease of varying severity and extent. The prevalence of single-, two-, and three-vessel disease is roughly equal, especially in patients older than 55 and those with a past history of stable angina. In relatively younger patients and in those with no prior history of stable angina, the frequency of single-vessel disease is relatively higher (50–60%). Left main coronary disease is found in 10–15% of patients with unstable angina. A subset of patients (5–10%) with angiographically normal or near normal coronary arteries may have noncardiac symptoms masquerading as unstable angina, microvascular angina (syndrome X, ischemic symptoms with angiographically normal arteries and possible microvascular dysfunction), or the rare primary vasospastic syndrome of Prinzmetal (variant) angina. It should be recognized, however, that most patients (even those with Prinzmetal angina) tend to have a significant atherosclerotic lesion on which the spasm is superimposed. In general, the extent (number of vessels involved, location of lesions) and severity (the percentage of diameter narrowing, the minimal luminal diameter, or the length of the lesion) of coronary artery disease and the prevalence of collateral circulation, as judged by traditional angiographic criteria, do not differ between patients with unstable angina and those with stable coronary artery disease. The morphologic features of the culprit lesions do tend to differ, however. The culprit lesion in patients with unstable angina tends to be more eccentric and irregular, with overhanging margins and filling defects or lucencies. These findings (on autopsy or in vivo angioscopy) represent a fissured plaque, with or without a superimposed thrombus. Such unstable features in the culprit lesion are detected more frequently when angiography is performed early in the clinical course.

3. Noninvasive tests—Any form of provocative testing (exercise or pharmacologic stress) is contraindicated in the acute phase of the disease because of the inherent risk of provoking a serious complication. Several studies of patients who had been pain-free and clinically stable for more than 3–5 days, however, have shown that such testing, using ECG, scintigraphic, or echocardiographic evaluation, may be safe. Provocative testing is used primarily to stratify patients into low- and high-risk subsets. Aggressive diagnostic and therapeutic interventions can then be selectively applied to the high-risk patients; the low-risk patients are treated more conservatively. In general, these studies have shown that patients who have good exercise duration and ventricular function, without significant inducible ischemia or ECG changes on admission, are at a very low risk and can be managed conservatively. On the other hand, patients with ECG changes on admission, a history of prior MI, evidence of inducible ischemia, and ventricular dysfunction tend to be at a higher risk for adverse cardiac events and therefore in greater need of further and more invasive evaluation.

4. Biomarkers—Blood levels of specific myocardial biomarkers such as cardiac troponins are, by definition, not elevated in unstable angina; if they are high without ST-segment elevation on ECG, the diagnosis is generally an NSTEMI. This distinction is somewhat arbitrary, however. Cardiac troponin levels should be measured at presentation and 3–6 hours after symptom onset. Patients with negative biomarkers within 6 hours of symptom onset need to have them remeasured within 8–12 hours. A high sensitivity cardiac troponin test is available and widely used in Europe, and results in a 20% increase in the diagnosis of NSTEMI with a concomitant decrease in the diagnosis of unstable angina. High sensitivity troponin testing, using 0/1-hour, 0/2-hour, or 0/3-hour algorithm, allows early detection of biomarker changes in patients suspicious of having NSTEMI and substantially shortens the "rule-in" and "rule-out" protocol for NSTEMI.

Khers S, Kolte D, Aronow WS, et al. Non-ST-elevation myocardial infarction in the United States: contemporary trends in incidence, utilization of the early invasive strategy, and in-hospital outcomes. *J Am Heart Assoc.* 2014;28:e000995. [PMID: 25074695]

Gulati M, Levy PD, Mukherjee D, et al. 2021 AHA/ACC/ASE/CHEST/SAEM/SCCT/SCMR Guideline for the Evaluation and Diagnosis of Chest Pain: A Report of the American College of Cardiology/American Heart Association Joint Committee on Clinical Practice Guidelines. *Circulation.* 2021;144:e368–e454. [PMID: 34709879]

Differential Diagnosis

Conditions that simulate or masquerade as unstable angina include acute MI, acute aortic dissection, acute pericarditis, pulmonary embolism, esophageal spasm, hiatal hernia, and chest wall pain. Careful attention to the history, risk factors, and objective findings of ischemia (transient ST-T changes and mild elevations of troponins in particular) remain the cornerstones for the diagnosis.

A. Acute Myocardial Infarction

Although MI often produces more prolonged pain, the clinical presentation can be indistinguishable from that of unstable angina. As stated earlier, this distinction should be considered somewhat arbitrary because abnormal myocardial technetium-99m pyrophosphate uptake and mild increases in troponin T and I levels are observed in some patients with otherwise classic symptoms of unstable angina.

B. Acute Aortic Dissection

The pain of aortic dissection is usually prolonged and can be severe. It frequently begins in or radiates to the back and tends to be relatively unrelenting and often tearing in nature; transient ST-T changes are rare. An abnormal chest radiograph showing a widened mediastinum accompanied by asymmetry in arterial pulses and blood pressure can provide clues to the diagnosis of aortic dissection. However, the main and first-line diagnostic tests for aortic dissection are transesophageal echocardiography, CT aortography once aortic dissection is clinically suspected. Magnetic resonance imaging (MRI) is suitable for post-operative follow-up.

C. Acute Pericarditis or Myopericarditis

Acute pericarditis may be difficult to differentiate from unstable angina. A history of a febrile or respiratory illness suggests the former. The pain of pericarditis is classically pleuritic in nature and worsens with breathing, coughing, deglutition, truncal movement, and supine posture. A pericardial friction rub is diagnostic but is often evanescent and frequent auscultation may be needed. Prolonged, diffuse ST elevation that is not accompanied by reciprocal ST depression or myocardial necrosis is typical of pericarditis. Leukocytosis and an elevated erythrocyte sedimentation rate are common in pericarditis but not helpful to differentiate it from unstable angina. Echocardiography may detect pericardial effusion in patients with pericarditis; diffuse ventricular hypokinesis and troponin elevation may imply associated myocarditis. Regional dysfunction, especially if transient, is more likely to reflect myocardial ischemia.

D. Acute Pulmonary Embolism

Chest pain in acute pulmonary embolism is also pleuritic in nature and commonly accompanied by dyspnea. Arterial hypoxemia is common, and the ECG may show sinus tachycardia with a rightward axis shift. Precordial ST-T wave abnormalities may simulate patterns of anterior myocardial ischemia or infarction. A high index of suspicion, combined with a noninvasive assessment of pulmonary ventilation-perfusion mismatch, evidence of lower extremity deep venous thrombosis, CT angiography, and possibly pulmonary angiography, is necessary to exclude the diagnosis.

E. Gastrointestinal Causes of Pain

Various gastrointestinal pathologies can mimic unstable angina. These include esophageal spasm, peptic ulcer, hiatal hernia, cholecystitis, and acute pancreatitis. A history compatible with those conditions, the response to specific therapy, and appropriate biochemical tests and imaging procedures should help clarify the situation. It should be noted that these abdominal conditions may produce ECG changes that simulate acute myocardial ischemia.

F. Takotsubo Syndrome

Takotsubo syndrome is characterized by symptoms of myocardial ischemia with apical LV ballooning without significant obstructive coronary artery disease on coronary angiography. Clinically, in addition to myocardial ischemic symptoms, pateints with Takotsubo syndrome can present with positive troponin and ST-T changes on ECG mimicking classic acute coronary syndrome. Many attempts have been made to distinguish the ECG features between the two entities. ECGs from patients with Takotsubo syndrome are associated with absence of abnormal Q waves, absence of reciprocal ST-T changes, presence of ST-segment elevation in lead -aVR and absence of ST-segment elevation in lead V1 when compared to ECG changes in anterior STEMI; but such distinguishing features only have modest predictive accuracy. These ECG criteria were established retrospectively using ECGs from patients with confirmed diagnosis of Takotsubo syndrome. Prospective use of these criteria when evaluating patients has reduced accuracy in differentiating Takotsubo syndrome from anterior STEMI. Therefore coronary angiography still needs to be performed to exclude (or establish the diagnosis of and treat) anterior STEMI from obstructive CAD.

G. Other Causes of Chest Pain

Many patients present with noncardiac chest pain that mimics unstable angina, and sometimes no specific diagnosis can be reached. The pain may be musculoskeletal, or there may be nonspecific changes on the ECG that increase the diagnostic confusion. In these patients, a definite diagnosis sometimes cannot be reached despite careful clinical observation. When the pain has abated and the patient is stable, a provocative test for myocardial ischemia may help determine if chest pain is due to coronary artery disease. Although coronary angiography may provide evidence of atherosclerotic coronary artery disease, anatomic evidence does not necessarily prove an ischemic cause for the symptoms. In some patients, acute myocarditis may also produce chest pain syndromes or ECG changes simulating unstable angina and acute MI. Recreational drug use (eg, cocaine and methamphetamine) may also produce clinical syndromes of chest pain, sometimes related to drug-induced acute coronary syndrome precipitated by the vasoconstrictor and prothrombotic effects of these drugs.

Treatment

In treating unstable angina, the initial objective is to stratify patients for their short-term morbidity and mortality risks based on their clinical presentations. After risk stratification, management objectives include eliminating episodes of ischemia and preventing acute MI and death.

A. Initial Management

During this early in-hospital phase, therapy is primarily aimed at stabilizing the patient by stabilizing the culprit coronary lesion and thus preventing a recurrence of myocardial ischemia at rest and progression to MI.

1. General measures—Patients whose history is compatible with a diagnosis of unstable angina should be promptly hospitalized in an intensive or intermediate care unit. General supportive care includes bed rest with continuous monitoring of cardiac rate and rhythm and frequent evaluation of vital signs; relief of anxiety with appropriate reassurance and, if necessary, anxiolytic medication; and treatment of associated precipitating or aggravating factors such as hypoxia, hypertension, dysrhythmias, heart failure, acute blood loss, or thyrotoxicosis. A 12-lead ECG should be repeated if it is initially unrevealing or if any significant change has occurred in symptoms or clinical stability. Serial cardiac biomarker evaluation should be performed as a part of an NSTEMI rule-out protocol and to evaluate the extent of myocardial damage and used for outcome risk stratification.

2. Outcome risk stratification—The Global Registry of Acute Coronary Events (GRACE) and Thrombolysis in Myocardial Infarction (TIMI) risk scores are the two commonly used risk scores to predict short-term risk of events and are helpful for clinical decision-making. GRACE score is calculated based on the sum of the scores assigned to clinical parameters such as age, heart rate, systolic blood pressure, serum creatinine, Killip classification, presence of cardiac arrest, ST-segment deviation, and elevation of cardiac enzymes. The score predicts outcome events reasonably well both in test and validation cohorts, predicting greater than 3% in-hospital death with a score higher than 140. An online version of the GRACE risk score calculator is available at www.outcomes.org/grace. The TIMI score estimates risk of mortality, recurrent MI or ischemia requiring revascularization at 14 days. It contains less clinical variables hence, it is easier for clinical usage, but doesn't perform as well in predicting outcomes. The TIMI calculator is available at www.timi.org.

Table 7–3. Effects of Medical Therapy in USA/NSTEMI

Therapy	Recurrent Ischemia	Progression to Acute Myocardial Infarction	Mortality
Nitrates	↓↓	?	?
Calcium channel blockers	↓↓	?[1]	?[1]
β-Blockers	↓↓	↓?	↓?
Dual anti-platelets	↓?	↓↓	↓↓
UFH/LMWH	↓↓	↓↓↓	↓↓↓

↓, reduction in frequency; ?, benefit not clearly established.
[1]increased risk with nifedipine and decreased risk with diltiazem in non–Q wave infarction in two studies.
LMWH, low-molecular-weight heparin; UFH, unfractionated heparin.

3. Anti-ischemic medications

A. Nitrates—Nitrates are generally considered one of the cornerstones of therapy (Table 7–3); however, their use is largely based on clinical experience, not on randomized clinical trials. Reduction of left ventricular preload and afterload by peripheral vasodilator actions may contribute to the reduction of myocardial ischemia. Although nitrates may reduce the number of both symptomatic and asymptomatic episodes of myocardial ischemia in unstable angina, no effect has yet been demonstrated on the incidence of progression to MI or death.

In the very acute phase, it is preferable to use intravenous nitroglycerin to ensure adequate bioavailability, a rapid onset and cessation of action, and easy titration of doses. Oral, sublingual, transdermal, and transmucosal preparations are better suited for subacute and chronic use. To minimize the chances of abrupt hypotension, nitroglycerin infusion should be started at 10 mcg/min and the infusion rate titrated according to symptoms and blood pressure. The goal is to use the lowest dose that will relieve ischemic symptoms without incurring side effects. The side effects of nitrates include hypotension, reflex tachycardia associated with hypotension; occasional profound bradycardia, presumably related to vagal stimulation; headaches; and facial flushing. Rare side effects include methemoglobinemia, alcohol intoxication, and an increase in intraocular and intracranial pressure. Because the magnitude of reduced arterial pressure that a patient can tolerate without developing signs of organ hypoperfusion varies, it is difficult to define an absolute cut-off point. A reasonable approach in normotensive patients without heart failure is to maintain the arterial systolic blood pressure no lower than 100–110 mm Hg; in hypertensive patients, reduction below 120–130 mm Hg may be unwise.

Continuous and prolonged administration of intravenous nitroglycerin for more than 24 hours may lead to the development of tolerance in some patients with attenuation of both its peripheral and coronary dilator actions. At the present time, however, there is no easy and practical way to avoid or overcome this problem other than escalating the dose to maintain reduction in measurable end points (eg, the arterial blood pressure).

With the increasing use of phosphodiesterase-5 inhibitors (such as sildenafil) for erectile dysfunction among patients with coronary artery disease, it is important to obtain a history of whether the patient has taken such medication 24 hours prior to presentation of USA/NSTEMI. Nitrate-mediated vasodilation in the presence of phosphodiesterase-5 inhibition can lead to prolonged hypotension or even death.

B. β-BLOCKERS—The evidence for use of β-blockers in USA/NSTEMI extrapolates mostly from studies in STEMI or stable angina patients. Use of β-blockers has been shown to reduce the frequency of both symptomatic and asymptomatic ischemic episodes in stable as well as unstable angina. These protective effects are generally attributed to their negative chronotropic and inotropic effects, which reduce the imbalance of myocardial oxygen demand and supply. Their ability to reduce the risk of infarct development is less clear, but they do decrease reinfarction and mortality rates in postinfarction patients. The mechanism of their protective effect against reinfarction remains unexplained, although it has been speculated that they reduce the risk of plaque rupture by reducing mechanical stress on the vulnerable plaque. It is also unclear whether β-blockers offer any additional benefit in unstable angina patients who are already receiving nitrates and antiplatelet-anticoagulant therapy.

β-Blockers administered orally, not intravenously, can be started early (within 24 hours after admission) in the absence of contraindications such as congestive heart failure, hemodynamic instability, heart block, or active reactive airway disease. The choice of β-blockers depends on pharmacokinetic consideration as well as physician familiarity; however, β-blockers without intrinsic sympathomimetic activity, such as propranolol, atenolol, or metoprolol, are preferred.

C. CALCIUM CHANNEL BLOCKERS—Calcium channel blockers are also frequently used in managing ischemic heart disease due to their ability to improve myocardial blood flow by reducing coronary vascular tone and dilation of large epicardial vessels and coronary stenoses through an endothelium-independent action. They also reduce myocardial workload through their negative chronotropic (diltiazem and verapamil) and negative inotropic and peripheral vasodilator effects. Because exaggerated vasoconstriction may play a role in unstable angina, calcium channel blockers have been used in its management. In general, although calcium channel blockers have been shown to reduce the frequency of ischemic episodes in unstable angina, their protective effect against the development of acute MI has not been definitively demonstrated. In fact, the use of calcium channel blockers such as nifedipine tends to increase the risk of ischemic complications in unstable angina. Such adverse effects may well be due to reflex tachycardia or coronary steal caused by the arteriole-dilating actions of dihydropyridine calcium channel blockers. The protective effects of the heart rate-slowing calcium channel blocker diltiazem have been reported in patients with a non-Q wave MI and preserved ventricular function. The additive benefits of calcium channel blockers in patients with unstable angina who are receiving nitrates and antithrombotic therapy have not been defined, and their use should also be considered an adjunct to such drugs.

4. Antiplatelet therapy—Platelet activation and aggregation leading to coronary thrombosis is the hallmark feature underlying the pathophysiology of acute coronary syndrome. Hence, inhibition of platelet activation via pharmacologic blockade of signaling pathways such as cyclooxygenase-1 or $P2Y_{12}$ receptor plays a central role in managing acute coronary syndrome.

A. ASPIRIN—Aspirin irreversibly inhibits cyclooxygenase-1 and reduces thromboxane A_2 production; hence, it reduces platelet aggregation by this pathway. It has been shown to reduce the risk of developing MI by about 50% in at least four randomized trials. The protective effect of aspirin in unstable angina has been comparable, in the dosage range of 75–1200 mg/day. Because of the potential for gastrointestinal side effects, low doses of aspirin (75–81 mg/day) are preferable for daily maintenance. A higher loading dose of 160–325 mg on the first day is recommended to initiate the antiplatelet effect more rapidly.

B. $P2Y_{12}$ RECEPTOR INHIBITORS—Adenosine diphosphate (ADP) is one of the inducers of platelet activation by binding to a G-protein–coupled $P2Y_{12}$ receptor with subsequent activation of GP II_bIII_a receptor and stabilization of platelet aggregation. Currently available $P2Y_{12}$ receptor inhibitors include clopidogrel, prasugrel, and ticagrelor.

(1) Clopidogrel—Clopidogrel is a prodrug requiring hepatic metabolism via cytochrome P450 system to form active metabolite to irreversibly inhibit $P2Y_{12}$ receptor. Extrapolation based on the CURE trial suggested that the combination of aspirin and clopidogrel appears to modestly reduce the combined incidence of cardiovascular death, MI, or stroke in USA/NSTEMI patients who are not undergoing revascularization procedures. However, this small additional benefit is at the expense of increased major or minor bleeding and cost.

The majority of clinical trials (CREDO, PCI-CURE, CLARITY, and COMMIT) testing the efficacy of aspirin and clopidogrel focus on high-risk acute coronary syndrome patients undergoing percutaneous coronary intervention (PCI). Based on these trials, current guidelines recommend treatment with aspirin and clopidogrel for 12 months for acute coronary syndrome patients undergoing PCI.

The suggested loading and daily maintenance dose for clopidogrel are 300 mg and 75 mg, respectively. A higher loading dose (600 mg) and higher daily maintenance dose (150 mg) of clopidogrel for the first 7 days, using a dose of 75 mg/day thereafter, did not reduce the composite end point of cardiovascular death, MI, or stroke at 30 days when compared with the conventional dosing regimen but did result in a higher major bleeding rate, as demonstrated by the CURRENT-OASIS 7 trial. However in the subgroup of patients undergoing PCI, the high-dose clopidogrel approach reduced the risk of stent thrombosis and MI at the cost of excess bleeding risk.

Given that clopidogrel requires hepatic transformation into active metabolite, the gene polymorphism involving the key enzymes in the biotransformation has been detected, and such polymorphism may account for the variable platelet inhibition response in individual patients. It has been proposed that testing the degree of platelet inhibition after clopidogrel administration may identify patients with poor response to clopidogrel, and dosing of clopidogrel based on such results may improve clinical outcome. However, the results from the GRAVITAS trial failed to confirm this hypothesis. Hence, routine use of a platelet function test to dose clopidogrel in acute coronary syndrome patients is not recommended.

(2) Prasugrel—Prasugrel is a third-generation thienopyridine and a prodrug and, like clopidogrel, requires hepatic biotransformation to active metabolites. The biotransformation of prasugrel is more efficient compared to clopidogrel; hence, the onset of action is faster and the degree of platelet inhibition more potent.

The approved use of prasugrel is only for acute coronary syndrome patients undergoing PCI as tested in TRITON-TIMI 38 trial, with clinical benefit largely driven by reduction of non-fatal MI, not death or stroke, and at the expense of increasing life-threatening bleeding when compared to clopidogrel. The bleeding risk is increased in patients with history of stroke or transient ischemic attack, age greater than 75 years, or a body weight less than 60 kg; hence, the use of prasugrel in these patient populations should be avoided. The recommended dose in current guidelines is a loading dose of prasugrel 60 mg given promptly or no later than 1 hour after PCI with 10 mg daily as maintenance dose for at least 12 months. The benefit of prasugrel in medically managed patients with USA/NSTEMI has been evaluated in TRILOGY ACS trial. Compared to clopidogrel, medical management with Prasugrel did not reduce cardiovascular death, MI or stroke, hence Prasugrel is not recommended as an initial therapy in patients with NSTEMI especially if not undergoing PCI.

(3) Ticagrelor—Ticagrelor is a cyclopentyltriazolopyrimidine that directly and reversibly inhibits $P2Y_{12}$ receptors on platelets. It has several unique pharmacologic features including fast absorption and short half-life with rapid onset and offset. Based on the PLATO trial, its use in acute coronary syndrome patients, regardless of treatment strategy (medical management, revascularization via PCI or coronary artery bypass graft [CABG]), was approved by US Food and Drug Administration using a regimen with a loading dose of 180 mg followed by a maintenance dose of 90 mg twice daily. This approval is accompanied with a warning stating that use of ticagrelor with aspirin with a dose greater than 100 mg/day decreases its effectiveness. Its short half-life and twice-daily administration could potentially lead to adverse events in non-compliant patients after coronary stenting.

(4) Considerations when using $P2Y_{12}$ receptor inhibitors—For NSTEMI patients, pooled results from several clinical trials and registries including ACCOAST, ISAR-REACT 5, DUBIUS, ARIAM-Andalucia registry, and SCAAR do not support to routinely pretreat with $P2Y_{12}$ inhibitors in patients in whom coronary artery anatomy is not known and an early invasive management is planned. This approach decreases unnecessary bleeding risk in patients whose NSTEMI diagnosis is disproved or PCI is deemed not necessary by coronary angiogram, reduces the wait-time for CABG in patients with suitable coronary anatomy. Once coronary anatomy is defined and PCI deemed necessary, $P2Y_{12}$ inhibitor can be administered.

Current guidelines recommend to give aspirin and one of the $P2Y_{12}$ inhibitors for at least 12 months after PCI with stenting. Several trials have demonstrated it is feasible to discontinue aspirin after 1–3 months of DAPT with continued $P2Y_{12}$ monotherapy to reduce bleeding events without increasing ischemic risks. After 12 months of DAPT it is reasonable in patients who tolerate DAPT, do not have bleeding complications, and are not at high bleeding risk (such as prior bleeding on DAPT, coagulopathy, or oral anticoagulant use) to continue it indefinitely.

In patients who have indications to take oral anticoagulation therapy, 2021 ACC/AHA/SCAI guideline for coronary artery revascularization recommends to administer triple therapy (DAPT + anticoagulation) for 1–4 weeks followed by $P2Y_{12}$ inhibitor and oral anticoagulant. Direct-acting oral anticoagulants (DOAC) are preferred to vit-K antagonists as oral anticoagulants unless clinical condition prohibits the use of DOAC.

c. GP II_BIII_A Receptor inhibitor—Activation of GP II_bIII_a receptors leads to interaction of receptors with ligands such as fibrinogen followed by platelet aggregation. Currently available intravenous GP II_bIII_a receptor inhibitors are abciximab, a monoclonal antibody against the receptor; nonpeptidic inhibitors, lamifiban and tirofiban; and a peptidic inhibitor, eptifibatide.

Four major randomized clinical trials (PRISM, PRISM-PLUS, PURSUIT, and PARAGON) evaluated the efficacy of intravenous GP II_bIII_a receptor inhibitors in reducing clinical events (death, MI, or refractory angina) in patients with USA/NSTEMI. Different inhibitors were tested in the trials (tirofiban in PRISM and PRISM-PLUS, eptifibatide in PURSUIT, and lamifiban in PARAGON). These trials differed in tested patient population, experimental designs, angiographic strategies, and end point measurement, but showed consistent, although small, reductions in short-term composite event rates in the management of the acute phase of USA/NSTEMI when they were added to the background treatment of aspirin and heparin as a part of initial medical management. Meta-analysis of these trials indicated that patients with high-risk features would benefit more from the use of GP II_bIII_a inhibitors, especially when undergoing PCI.

The efficacy of intravenous abciximab on clinical outcome in patients with USA/NSTEMI **without early intervention** was tested in GUSTO-IV acute coronary syndrome trial. There was no survival benefit in patients receiving abciximab when compared with placebo at 30 days or at 1 year.

The efficacy of intravenous GP II_bIII_a inhibitors in reducing clinical events in patients with USA/NSTEMI **undergoing PCI** was also tested—abciximab in EPILOG and CAPTURE and tirofiban in RESTORE. These trials consistently showed a reduction of short-term clinical events (composite end point of death, MI, or urgent or repeat revascularization). The major benefit appears to be in nonfatal adverse events rather than mortality.

Thus, overall data suggest that intravenous GP II_bIII_a inhibitors used judiciously, along with aspirin and heparin, are beneficial in high-risk patients with USA/NSTEMI undergoing PCI.

In the modern era of frequent use of dual antiplatelet therapy (mostly aspirin and clopidogrel), routine addition of eptifibatide to aspirin and clopidogrel in managing USA/NSTEMI patients does not confer clinical benefit but increases bleeding risk as demonstrated by the EARLY-ACS trial. The efficacy and safety of GP II_bIII_a receptor inhibitors on top of Ticagrelor or Prasugrel have not been prospectively addressed. Current guidelines recommend to use intravenous GP II_bIII_a receptor inhibitors for high-risk patients with large thrombus burden, no-reflow or slow flow during PCI to improve procedural success.

5. Anticoagulant therapy

A. Unfractionated heparin and low-molecular-weight heparin—The protective effect of intravenous unfractionated heparin (UFH) in treating unstable angina has been demonstrated in randomized trials. During short-term use, the risk of MI in unstable angina is reduced by about 90%, and ischemic episodes are reduced by about 70%. Current US guideline recommends intravenous administration of a bolus of 60 U/kg (maximum 4000 IU) followed by infusion at 12 U/kg/h (maximum 1000 IU/h) titrated to an activated partial thromboplastin time of 1.5–2 times normal for 48 hours or until PCI is performed in patients with USA/NSTEMI. During PCI, UFH is given as an intravenous bolus under ACT guide in the range of 250–350 sec or 200–250 sec if a GP II_b/III_a inhibitor is given. UFH should be stopped after PCI unless other indications for UFH exist.

Low-molecular-weight heparin (LMWH) has been tested to examine its role as an alternative anticoagulation therapy to UFH in patients with USA/NSTEMI. LMWH has certain pharmacologically superior features to UFH: longer half-life, weaker binding to plasma protein, higher bioavailability with subcutaneous injection, more predictable dose response, and less incidence of heparin-induced thrombocytopenia. Dalteparin has been shown to be superior to placebo and equivalent to UFH for immediate, short-term treatment of USA/NSTEMI in reducing composite end points in the FRISC and FRIC trials, respectively. In the FRISC II trial, dalteparin also lowered the risk of death or MI in patients receiving invasive procedures, especially in high-risk patients. In the ESSENCE and TIMI 11B trials, enoxaparin (modestly but significantly) reduced the combined incidence of death, MI, or recurrent angina over UFH. This reduction is mainly due to a decrease in recurrent angina. But in the SYNERGY trial, enoxaparin was not superior to UFH in reducing mortality or nonfatal MI in high-risk patients undergoing early invasive therapy. Taken together, acute treatment with LMWH is likely as effective as UFH in USA/NSTEMI patients receiving aspirin. However, because LMWH is easier to use and does not require partial thromboplastin time monitoring, it is being increasingly preferred over UFH. Enoxaparin is the most studied LMWH, and its dose is 1 mg/kg subcutaneously twice daily with a treatment duration for the hospital stay or until PCI. In patients with creatinine clearance less than 30 mL/min the dose should be reduced to 1 mg/kg subcutaneously daily with consideration to use UFH as an alternative.

B. Direct thrombin inhibitors—Compared with heparin, direct thrombin inhibitors appear to offer a small reduction in death or MI in patients with USA/NSTEMI. Currently only bivalirudin is available for clinical use.

Bivalirudin was tested in the ACUITY trial in the setting of USA/NSTEMI. Bivalirudin was shown to be noninferior to heparin in composite ischemia end points (death, MI, or unplanned revascularization) in USA/NSTEMI patients with moderate- or high-risk features undergoing invasive therapy when it was used in conjunction with a GP II_bIII_a inhibitor. Taken together, direct thrombin inhibitors have not been routinely used in the medical management of USA/NSTEMI; however, they are alternative antithrombotics for patients with heparin-induced thrombocytopenia.

C. Fondaparinux—Fondaparinux is an indirect factor Xa inhibitor that works by reversible binding to antithrombin. When compared to enoxaparin in the OASIS-5 trial, fondaparinux was observed to have similar efficacy in reducing primary outcome of death, MI, or refractory ischemia with less major bleeding. However, catheter thrombus was noted to be more frequent than with enoxaparin, requiring additional bolus of UFH with empirically determined dose at the time of catheterization. Because of this disadvantage, fondaparinux is seldom used in USA/NSTEMI patients with planned early invasive approach. Fondaparinux is given at a dose of 2.5 mg/day subcutaneously and is contraindicated in patients with a creatinine clearance less than 30 mL/min because its excretion is predominantly by kidneys.

Figure 7–1 summarizes the use of various antiplatelet, antithrombotic, and GP II_bIII_a inhibitors in different USA/NSTEMI settings.

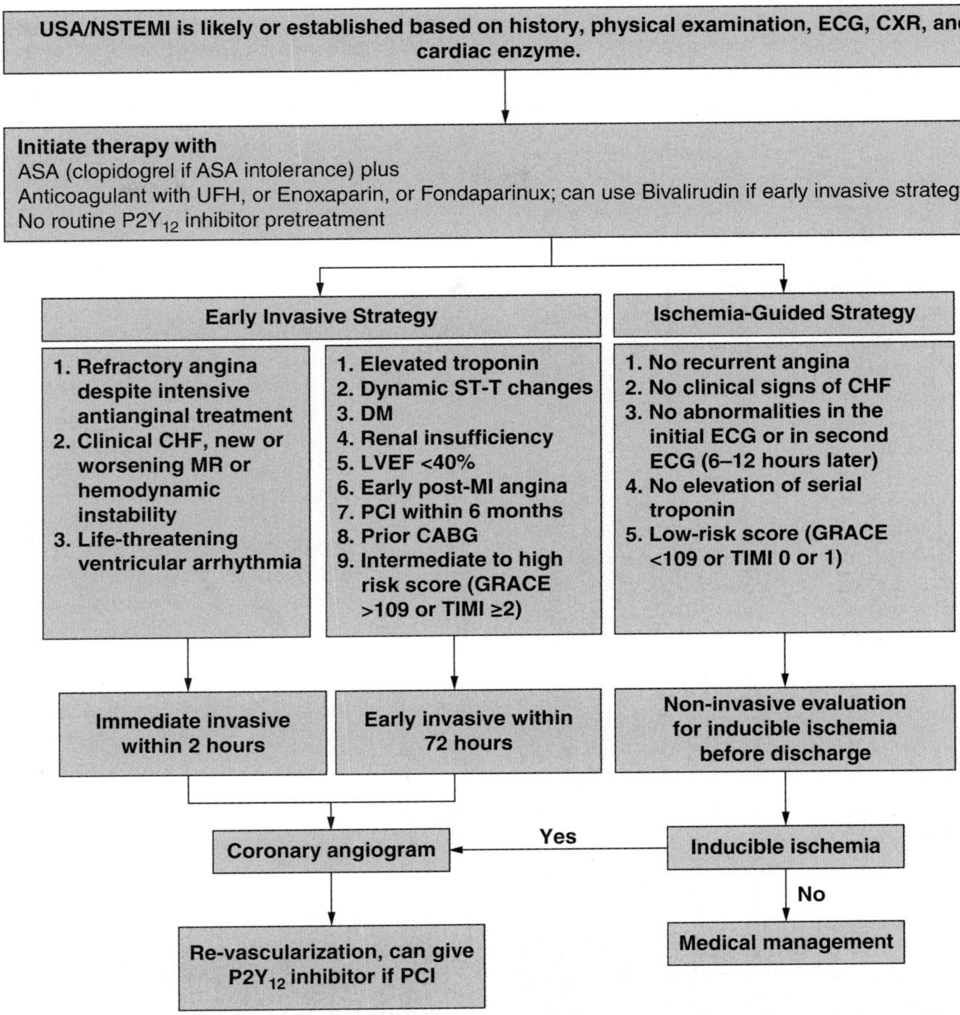

▲ **Figure 7–1.** Algorithm in risk stratification and management of unstable angina and non-ST elevation myocardial infarction (USA/NSTEMI). ASA, aspirin; CABG, coronary artery bypass graft; CHF, congestive heart failure; CXR, chest x-ray; d/c, discontinue; ECG, electrocardiogram; GP, glycoprotein; GRACE, Global Registry of Acute Coronary Events; LVEF, left ventricular ejection fraction; MI, myocardial infarction; MR, mitral regurgitation; PCI, percutaneous coronary intervention; UFH, unfractionated heparin.

Amsterdam EA, Wenger NK, Brindis RG, et al. 2014 ACC/AHA guideline for the management of patients with non-ST-elevation acute coronary syndromes: a report of the American College of Cardiology/American Heart Association Task Force on Practice Guidelines. *Circulation.* 2014;130:e344–e426. [PMID: 25249585]

Roffi M, Patrono C, Collet JP, et al. 2015 ESC Guidelines for the management of acute coronary syndromes in patients presenting without persistent ST-segment elevation: the task force for the management of acute coronary syndromes in patients presenting without persistent ST-segment elevation of the European Society of Cardiology (ESC). *Eur Heart J.* 2015 Aug 29. pii: ehv320. [PMID: 26320110]

B. Definitive Management

1. Percutaneous coronary revascularization—PCI with stenting are commonly performed in patients with unstable angina to reduce the critical stenosis in the culprit artery or in multiple coronary arteries. An important clinical decision in treating USA/NSTEMI patients is whether to choose a "conservative" versus "invasive" approach based on patients' clinical risk profile. Patients demonstrating highest risk for short-term morbidity or mortality from USA/NSTEMI are those with refractory angina despite intensive antianginal treatment, severe heart failure or unstable hemodynamics, and life-threatening ventricular arrhythmias, and these patients should undergo immediate angiography with intention for revascularization within 2 hours of presentation. Patients without the aforementioned high-risk features but with elevated troponin level, dynamic ST-T changes on ECG, diabetes mellitus, renal insufficiency, left ventricular ejection fraction less than 40%, early post-MI angina, PCI within 6 months, prior CABG, or intermediate to high GRACE score (> 109) should undergo invasive evaluation within 72 hours of admission. Other low-risk patients can undergo noninvasive evaluation for inducible ischemia before hospital discharge (conservative approach). If inducible ischemia is detected, patients should undergo coronary angiography (see Figure 7–1).

Although these interventions accomplish an acute reduction in the severity of stenosis in patients with unstable angina, they carry a somewhat higher risk of acute complications, including death (0–2%), abrupt closure (0–17%), acute MI (0–13%), and the need for urgent coronary artery bypass surgery (0–12%), than in patients with stable angina. The risk is especially great when the procedure is performed soon after the onset of symptoms, in the absence of prior treatment with heparin, or in the presence of an angiographically visible intracoronary thrombus. In the current era of stent placement for coronary intervention, the angiographic restenosis rate at 6- to 7-month follow-up with bare metal stents ranges from 22% to 32%, whereas it is less than 10% for drug-eluting stents even at longer follow-up, as demonstrated in clinical trials for uncomplicated lesions.

2. Surgical revascularization (Coronary artery bypass surgery)—In the current era of advanced percutaneous revascularization techniques, traditional surgical coronary diseases such as significant left main or triple vessel coronary disease can now be treated with PCI and stenting. In choosing surgical vs. percutaneous revascularization, it has been recommended to use the Heart Team approach with consideration of coronary anatomy complexity, comorbidity and patient factors to determine the best revascularization strategy for patients. Current guideline recommends surgical revascularization in patients with significant left main or multivessel coronary disease and complex coronary anatomy (eg, SYNTAX score > 33), especially in patients with DM or reduced left ventricular function. Patients who cannot tolerate or comply with dual antiplatelet therapy after PCI with stent, CABG is a reasonable option in preference to PCI even when patients coronary anatomy is suitable for CABG or PCI as premature interruption of dual antiplatelet therapy may result in catastrophic consequences such as early stent thrombosis leading to MI, congestive heart failure, or death. Surgical revascularization can be considered an appropriate option for patients with unstable angina who do not stabilize with aggressive medical therapy or for whom PCI is unsuccessful or is followed by acute complications not amenable to additional catheter-based intervention.

Many patients with USA/NSTEMI are on dual antiplatelet therapy when the decision of myocardial revascularization with CABG is made. CABG can be performed in patients on aspirin therapy with a small increase in bleeding risk. If possible, clopidogrel and ticagrelor should be discontinued for 5 days before CABG and prasugrel for 7 days before CABG to minimize bleeding risk from surgery. However the timing of CABG in patients on $P2Y_{12}$ inhibitors depends on the balance of benefit of revascularization from the urgent CABG and the risk of perioperative bleeding and increased need of blood transfusion.

3. Intra-aortic balloon counterpulsation (IABP)—IABP is a useful adjunct in managing selected cases of unstable angina. It helps maintain or improve coronary artery blood flow and myocardial perfusion by augmenting diastolic aortic pressure; at the same time, systolic unloading contributes to a reduction in ventricular wall tension and myocardial oxygen demand and an improvement in ventricular function. These beneficial effects on myocardial oxygen supply and demand help stabilize patients with recurrent myocardial ischemia and those with serious intermittent or persistent hemodynamic or electrical instability. Cardiac catheterization and revascularization can then be carried out with relative safety.

Intra-aortic balloon counterpulsation (and the percutaneous method of insertion) carries a significant risk of vascular complications involving the lower extremities, especially in women, in patients older than 70 years, and in the presence of diabetes or aortoiliac disease. It should be viewed as a temporary stabilizing measure, pending definitive revascularization.

Lawton JS, Holland JET, Bangalore S, et al. 2021 ACC/AHA/SCAI Guideline for Coronary Artery Revascularization: A Report of the American College of Cardiology/American Heart Association Joint Committee on Clinical Practice Guidelines. *J Am Coll Cardiol.* 2022 Jan,;79(2):e21–e129. [PMID: 34895950]

Prognosis

With the advances in treatment strategies, clinical event rates for refractory angina, MI, and death have been reduced substantially. For example, in patients who were not treated with aspirin and heparin, the rates of refractory angina, MI, and death were 23%, 12%, and 1.7%, respectively, within the first week of treatment, and the rates became 10.7%, 1.6%, and 0%, respectively, if the patients were treated with aspirin and heparin. With the addition of a GP II_bIII_a receptor inhibitor, the rates of refractory angina, MI, or death were 10.6%, 8.3%, and 6.9%, respectively, at 6 months in the PRISM-PLUS trial. With the combination of early invasive strategy, GP II_bIII_a inhibitor, heparin, and aspirin, the 6-month mortality rate decreased further to 3.3% in the TACTICS-TIMI 18 trial. Even with such decreases in the event rates, a substantial number of patients still continue to suffer from USA/NSTEMI and its complications due to the high prevalence of atherosclerosis. All patients should become acquainted with risk factor modification strategies, which include aggressive lipid lowering with high-intensity statin and PCSK9 antibody as an adjunct, smoking cessation, an exercise program, diabetes control, blood pressure control, dietary counseling, and weight control. Recently, the use of angiotensin-converting enzyme inhibitors has also been shown to reduce atherothrombotic events in patients with coronary artery disease especially in the presence of diabetes. With the advancement of therapies and risk factor modification, patients' short- and long-term outcomes can be further improved. The simple mnemonic ABCDE (Table 7–4) summarizes the long-term risk-reducing approach for patients with unstable coronary artery disease.

Table 7–4. ABCDE Approach for Long-Term Risk Reduction in Patients with USA/NSTEMI.

A:	Antiplatelet therapy, ACEI or ARB
B:	β-Blockers
	Blood pressure control
C:	Cholesterol-lowering medications (statins and others)
	Cessation of smoking
D:	Dietary management (Mediterranean, low-fat, or vegetarian diet)
	Diabetes control
E:	Exercise and weight control

8 Acute Myocardial Infarction

Andrew J. Boyle, MBBS, PhD

ESSENTIALS OF DIAGNOSIS

- Chest discomfort, usually described as "pressure," "dull," "squeezing," or "aching."
- Characteristic electrocardiographic changes.
- Elevated biomarkers, such as troponin.
- Imaging may show new regional wall motion abnormality with preserved wall thickness.
- The elderly, women, and diabetics may have atypical presentation.

General Considerations

Acute myocardial infarction (MI) is a clinical syndrome that results from the occlusion of a coronary artery, with resultant death of cardiac myocytes in the region supplied by that artery. Depending on the distribution of the affected coronary artery, acute MI can produce a wide range of clinical sequelae, varying from a small, clinically silent region of necrosis to a large overwhelming area of infarcted tissue resulting in cardiogenic shock and death. Over 1 million people experience MI in the United States each year; approximately one every 40 seconds.

The risk of having an acute MI increases with age, male gender, smoking, dyslipidemia, diabetes, hypertension, abdominal obesity, a lack of physical activity, low daily fruit and vegetable consumption, alcohol overconsumption, and psychosocial index. As much as 90% of the risk of acute MI has been attributed to the modifiable risk factors. The diagnostic criteria for acute MI are listed in Table 8–1.

Pathophysiology & Etiology

A prolonged imbalance between myocardial oxygen supply and demand leads to the death of myocardial tissue. Coronary atherosclerosis is an essential part of the process in most patients. Ischemic heart disease seems to progress through stages of fatty-streak deposition in coronary arteries to development of fibro-fatty plaque, which then increases in size until it causes luminal obstruction, leading to exertional angina (see Chapter 6). However, at any stage in this process, the atherosclerotic lesion may erode, ulcerate, fissure, or rupture, thereby exposing subendothelial vessel wall substances to the circulating blood. Procoagulant factors (such as tissue factor) reside within the plaque itself and, in the absence of counterbalancing antithrombotic factors (eg, heparin, tissue factor inhibitor) and fibrinolytic activities (tissue plasminogen activator [t-PA] and single-chain urokinase-type plasminogen activator) within the endothelial cells of the coronary artery, can cause thrombosis. This potent procoagulant stimulus results in thrombus development in this region. In general, larger transmural acute MI occurs when this thrombosis propagates and occludes flow within the artery, resulting in ischemia and necrosis of cardiomyocytes distal to the obstruction. This is often associated with ST-segment elevation on the electrocardiogram (ECG). Smaller nontransmural MI may occur when platelet thrombus on a plaque embolizes downstream and occludes very small branches. There is usually no ST elevation on the ECG in this situation. Recent work suggests that inflammation may play a pivotal role in the genesis of plaque rupture. Total thrombotic occlusion occurs most commonly in proximal coronary arteries; its presence has been documented during the first 4 hours after infarction in more than 85% of patients with ST-segment elevation.

A similar type of myocardial insult occurs occasionally despite angiographically normal coronary arteries and may be caused by emboli (eg, in patients with prosthetic valves or those with endocarditis), spontaneous dissection of the coronary artery (most commonly in pregnant women), or coronary vasospasm (on rare occasions). It can also be caused by thrombosis in situ, the probable mechanism by which patients who have variant angina or who abuse cocaine can suffer acute infarction. In these cases, vasoconstriction

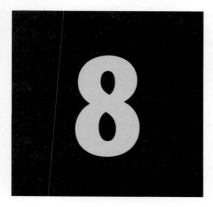

Table 8–1. ESC/ACC Definition of Myocardial Infarction

Criteria for acute MI

The term acute myocardial infarction (MI) should be used when there is evidence of *myocardial necrosis* in a clinical setting consistent with *acute myocardial ischemia*. Under these conditions, *any one of the following* criteria meets the diagnosis for MI:

1. Typical rise and fall of biochemical markers of myocardial necrosis (preferably cardiac troponin) with at least one of the following:
   a. Ischemic symptoms
   b. Development of pathologic Q waves on the ECG
   c. ECG changes indicative of ischemia (ST-segment/T-wave changes)
   d. Imaging evidence of new loss of viable myocardium or new regional wall motion abnormality.
   e. Identification of an intracoronary thrombus by angiography or autopsy
2. Cardiac death with symptoms suggestive of myocardial ischemia and presumed new ischemic ECG changes or new LBBB.
3. Percutaneous coronary intervention (PCI)–related MI is arbitrarily defined by elevation of cTn in patients with normal baseline values or a rise of cTn values > 20% if the baseline values are elevated and are stable or falling. In addition, either (i) symptoms suggestive of myocardial ischemia or (ii) new ischemic ECG changes or (iii) angiographic findings consistent with a procedural complication or (iv) imaging demonstrating new loss of viable myocardium or new regional wall motion abnormality are required.
4. Stent thrombosis associated with MI when detected by coronary angiography or autopsy in the setting of myocardial ischemia and with a rise and/or fall of cardiac biomarkers.
5. Coronary artery bypass grafting (CABG)–related MI is arbitrarily defined by elevation of cardiac biomarkers in patients with normal baseline values. In addition, either (i) new pathologic Q waves or new LBBB, or (ii) angiographic documented new graft or new native coronary artery occlusion, or (iii) imaging evidence of new loss of viable myocardium or new regional wall motion abnormality.

Criteria for prior MI

Any one of the following criteria satisfies the diagnosis for prior MI:

1. Development of new pathologic Q waves on serial ECGs. The patient may or may not remember previous symptoms. No other nonischemic cause.
2. Imaging evidence of a region of loss of viable myocardium that is thinned and fails to contract, in the absence of a nonischemic cause
3. Pathologic findings of a healed or healing MI.

cTn, cardiac troponin; CK-MB, myocardial muscle kinase isoenzyme; ECG, electrocardiogram; ESC/ACC, European Society of Cardiology/American College of Cardiology; LBBB, left bundle branch block; MI, myocardial infarction.

Adapted, from Thygesen K, et al. Fourth universal definition of myocardial infarction. *J Am Coll Cardiol.* 2018;72(18): 2231–2264.

secondary to endothelial dysfunction and a propensity to thrombosis are of sufficient magnitude and duration to cause thrombus formation. Oxygen consumption and possibly direct myocyte toxicity also increase with cocaine use. In addition, thrombosis in situ can apparently cause infarction among women who take estrogens (especially if they smoke). An increasingly recognized differential diagnosis of acute MI is stress cardiomyopathy (also known as apical ballooning syndrome or takotsubo cardiomyopathy). This entity can present with a variety of symptoms and ECG changes, including ST elevation, and there is akinesis of the anterior and inferior walls and apex of the left ventricle in the absence of coronary artery disease. It is more common in women and often is accompanied by severe emotional stress. The diagnosis is one of exclusion after angiography demonstrates patent coronary arteries. The treatment is supportive, and the prognosis is good; recovery of ventricular function is the norm.

In addition to blockage of coronary arteries (reduced "supply"), acute MI may be seen when myocardial oxygen requirements are elevated (increased "demand"). This often occurs when other medical illnesses coexist with ischemic heart disease. Pulmonary embolism, pneumonia, arrhythmia, septic shock, severe anemia, or great emotional distress can increase myocardial oxygen demand, reduce coronary perfusion pressure, or evoke paradoxical coronary artery responses and lead to MI. However, these tend to be smaller infarctions with no ECG ST elevation that are diagnosed by elevated biomarkers.

Tsao C, Aday AW, Almarzook ZI, et al. Heart disease and stroke statistics—2022 update. A report from the American Heart Association. *Circulation.* 2022;145:e153–e639. [PMID: 35078371]

Clinical Findings

A. Symptoms & Signs

Chest discomfort is the most common symptom; it is usually described as "pressure," "dull," "squeezing," or "aching," although it may be described differently because of individual variability, differences in articulation or verbal abilities, or concomitant disease processes. The discomfort is usually in the center of the chest and commonly radiates to the left arm or the neck. However, it may also radiate to the right arm, epigastrium, jaw, teeth, or back. The nature of the pain may lead patients to place a hand or fist over the sternum (Levine sign). These clinical signs and symptoms were originally defined in groups of males. It is now clear that women can have more atypical symptoms.

Associated symptoms may include dyspnea, nausea (particularly in inferior infarction), palpitations, and a sense of impending doom.

Patients, especially those with diabetes or hypertension, may have atypical presentations; for example, a diabetic person may have abdominal pain that mimics the discomfort commonly associated with gallstones. In elderly patients, heart failure is often the presenting symptom. Up to 42% of women and 30% of men present with MI without chest pain. The diagnosis of MI should be considered in patients in whom symptoms are atypical yet compatible with ischemia (eg, paroxysms of dyspnea) or in those with atypical chest discomfort. Patients can also have discomfort that is sharper or that radiates to the back. These patients can have pericarditis alone, pericarditis induced by infarction, or a dissecting aortic aneurysm—with or without concomitant infarction.

B. Physical Examination

The physical examination is a critical and underappreciated part of the initial assessment of patients with suspected acute MI. Findings may vary tremendously, from markedly abnormal, with signs of severe congestive heart failure (CHF), to totally normal.

On general inspection, most patients with a large MI appear pale or sweaty and may be agitated or restless. Heart rate should be measured for arrhythmia, heart block, or sinus tachycardia. This is crucial before administration of β-blockers. Assessment of blood pressure is important because severe hypertension (which may be due to the pain) is a contraindication to fibrinolytic treatment and must be treated emergently. Conversely, hypotension in the setting of acute MI may be due to cardiogenic shock, which alters treatment strategy. Fibrinolytic treatments are not effective in cardiogenic shock, and the patient should be considered for an urgent intra-aortic balloon pump (IABP) or percutaneous left ventricular assist device (eg, Impella) and primary percutaneous coronary intervention (PCI).

The jugular venous pulse should be carefully examined. Its elevation in the setting of inferior MI without left heart failure suggests right ventricular MI. Detection of right ventricular MI is vital because it portends a much worse prognosis than isolated inferior MI, and the management strategy is different than isolated inferior MI. Whereas elevated jugular venous pulse in left ventricular MI with left ventricular failure may respond to diuresis, right ventricular MI may require intravenous fluid therapy to maintain left ventricular filling.

Cardiac auscultation should be specifically targeted to complications of MI (see later discussion in this chapter) and detection of important comorbidities. Acute MI may result in ischemic mitral regurgitation with a soft S1 and a pansystolic murmur. Acquired ventricular septal defect (VSD) may also result in a pansystolic murmur, but it is usually loud and high-pitched and has a normal S1 and usually occurs later (see later Complications of Myocardial Infarction section). Both ischemic mitral regurgitation and acquired VSD may result in heart failure. The presence of a pericardial friction rub may indicate an established infarction that has happened days earlier. Heart failure due to large infarctions may result in a third heart sound. Signs of left heart failure, such as rales and pulmonary hypertension, should also be sought. Important comorbidities, such as concomitant severe aortic stenosis, should also be documented because they may change the initial reperfusion strategy from fibrinolysis or PCI to cardiac surgery with coronary artery bypass graft (CABG) and aortic valve replacement simultaneously.

Alternative diagnoses may also be suggested by clinical examination. The presence of atrial fibrillation or prosthetic valve may suggest that thromboembolism to the coronary artery is the cause of coronary occlusion. Furthermore, a brief assessment of pulse equality and blood pressure in both arms should be performed. Inequalities in perfusion between arms may indicate aortic dissection, causing compromised blood flow in the branch vessels of the aortic arch. Aortic dissection may also be responsible for occlusion of the ostium of the coronary artery causing the acute MI. This is a surgical emergency and should not be treated with anticoagulation or fibrinolysis. Therefore, a focused clinical examination is an essential part of the initial patient assessment and can be invaluable in guiding therapy.

C. Diagnostic Studies

1. Electrocardiography—The most rapid and helpful test in assessing patients with suspected acute MI is the 12-lead ECG. It should be performed as soon as possible, preferably within 10 minutes, after the patient's arrival in the emergency department or clinician's office, since the presence or absence of ST elevation determines the preferred management strategy. For a diagnosis of ST elevation MI (STEMI), greater than 0.1 mV of ST elevation must be present in at least two contiguous leads. For anterior MI, the precordial (V) leads demonstrate ST elevation (Figure 8–1), and if there is lateral wall involvement, leads I and aVL may also show ST elevation. In inferior MI, leads II, III, and aVF are affected.

In addition to standard ECG leads, right ventricular leads should be recorded in all patients with inferior MI. Inferior MI is usually caused by occlusion of the right coronary artery, which may also cause right ventricular infarction. Differentiating right ventricular infarction from left ventricular infarction is imperative because the management is different.

In posterior MI, usually due to circumflex artery occlusion, the only changes seen on a standard ECG may be reciprocal ST depression and R waves (reciprocal of Q waves) in the anterior leads. This ECG pattern should prompt the use of posterior ECG leads V7–9, which may show ST elevation. Even in the absence of ST elevation in posterior leads, true posterior infarction pattern on ECG in the presence of symptoms suggestive of MI should be treated like STEMI.

Non-ST elevation MI (NSTEMI) has a variable presentation on ECG. There may be no ECG changes, or patients may have ST depression, T-wave flattening, or T-wave inversion. Preexisting abnormalities like T-wave inversion may also "pseudo-normalize" in NSTEMI, making it even more difficult to diagnose on ECG. Because determining whether ECG changes are new or old may be difficult, serial ECGs are necessary to diagnose dynamic changes. In patients with symptoms suggestive of MI and no evidence of ST elevation

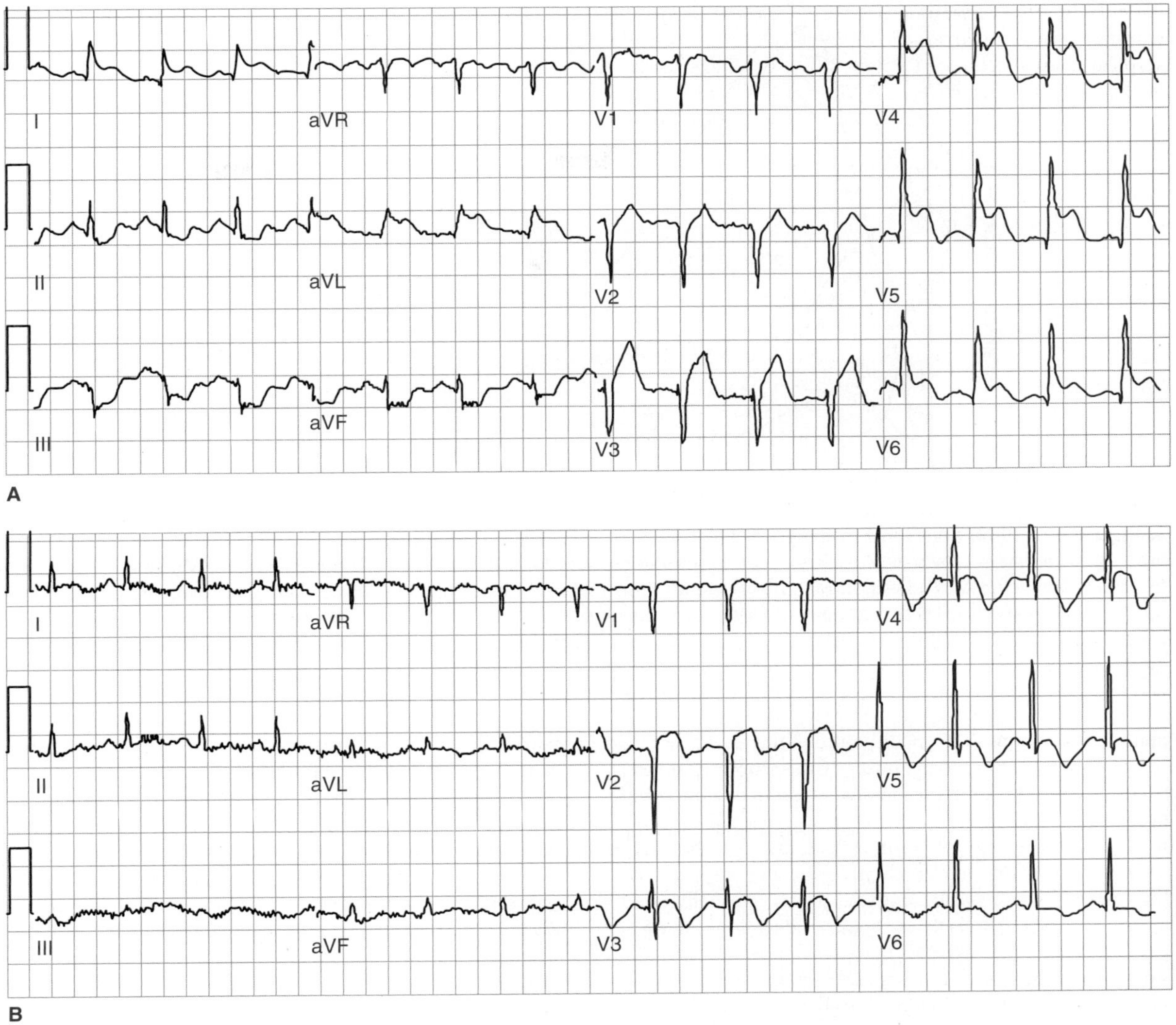

▲ **Figure 8–1.** Electrocardiogram (ECG) changes in anterolateral ST elevation myocardial infarction (STEMI). **A:** Initial ECG on presentation shows ST-segment elevation in the precordial leads, as well as I and aVL, indicative of acute anterolateral STEMI due to proximal left anterior descending (LAD) coronary artery occlusion. Note the reciprocal ST depression in the inferior leads. **B:** Following reperfusion, subsequent ECG 48 hours later demonstrates resolution of both the anterolateral ST elevation and the reciprocal changes. Note the Q wave in V2 and the development of T-wave inversion.

on ECG, the diagnosis of acute coronary syndrome is made. This encompasses unstable angina pectoris and NSTEMI. The distinction between these two entities is made on the presence or absence of elevated biomarkers of MI.

2. Cardiac biomarkers—The diagnosis of infarction requires increases in molecular markers of myocardial injury (Figure 8–2). Myoglobin release from injured myocardium occurs quite early and is very sensitive for detecting infarction. Unfortunately, it is not very specific because minor skeletal muscle trauma also releases myoglobin. Myoglobin is cleared renally, so even minor decreases in glomerular filtration rate lead to elevation. The other early markers advocated by some are isoforms of creatine kinase (CK). This marker has comparable early sensitivity and specificity to myoglobin. The marker of choice in past years was the MB isoenzyme of creatine kinase (CK-MB). A typical rising-and-falling pattern of CK and CK-MB (in the proper clinical setting) was sufficient for the diagnosis of acute infarction. In the typical pattern of CK release after infarction, the enzyme

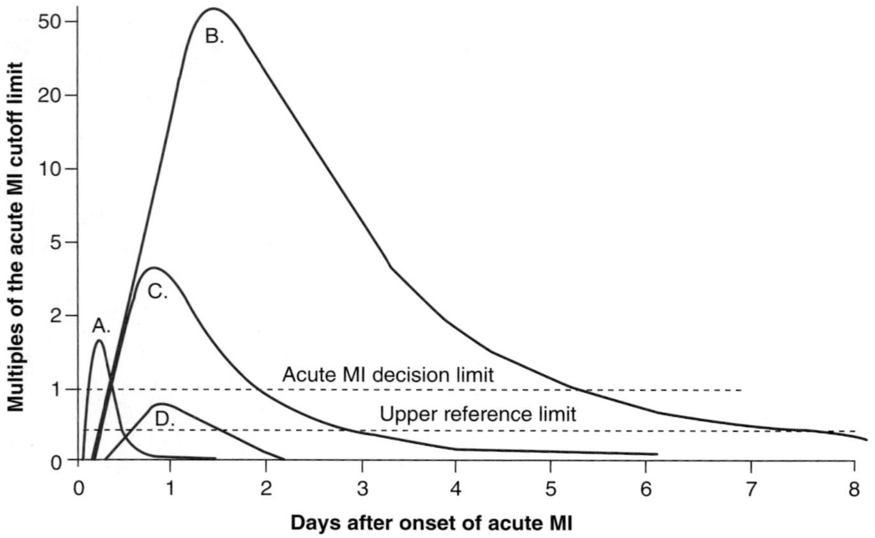

▲ **Figure 8–2.** Biomarkers in acute myocardial infarction (MI). Plot of the appearance of cardiac markers in blood versus time after the onset of symptoms. Peak A, early release of myoglobin or CK-MB isoforms after acute MI. Peak B, cardiac troponin after acute MI. Peak C, CK-MB after acute MI. Peak D, cardiac troponin after unstable angina. Data are plotted on a relative scale, where 1.0 is set at the acute MI cutoff concentration. (Reproduced with permission from Wu AH, Gibler WB, Jesse RL, Warshaw MM, Valdes R Jr. National Academy of Clinical Biochemistry Standards of Laboratory Practice: recommendations for the use of cardiac markers in coronary artery diseases. *Clin Chem*. 1999;45(7):1104–1121.)

marker level exceeds the upper bound of the reference range within 6–12 hours after the onset of infarction. Peak levels occur by 18–24 hours and generally return to baseline within no more than 48 hours. However, elevations can occur due to release of the enzyme from skeletal muscle. The lack of a rising-and-falling pattern should raise the suspicion that the release is from skeletal muscle, which is usually due to a chronic skeletal muscle myopathy. Elevations of CK in patients with hypothyroidism (where clearance of CK is slowed) and those with renal failure (where clearance is normal because CK is not cleared renally) are caused, in part, by myopathy.

Cardiac troponins I and T are proteins found in cardiac muscle cells and released into the circulation from damaged cardiac myocytes during acute MI. Troponin levels (either I or T) are significantly more sensitive and specific for myocardial damage than CK. Troponin becomes detectable in serum between 4 and 6 hours after onset of an acute MI, peaks and then falls to lower levels, and remains elevated at these low levels for 5–7 days (see Figure 8–2). Thus, the late or retrospective diagnosis of acute MI can be made with this marker, making the use of lactate dehydrogenase isoenzymes superfluous. Therefore, because of its sensitivity and specificity for cardiac muscle damage as well as its early rise and continued low-level detectability, troponin is the preferred biomarker for diagnosis of acute MI. Furthermore, it has been shown to correlate with prognosis even in the absence of CK or CK-MB elevation. Newer high-sensitivity troponin markers have the potential to detect myocardial necrosis at lower levels and more rapidly.

Coronary recanalization, whether spontaneous or induced pharmacologically or mechanically, alters the timing of all markers' appearance in the circulation. Because it increases the rapidity with which the marker is washed out from the heart, leading to rapid increases in plasma, the diagnosis of infarction can be made much earlier—generally within 2 hours of coronary recanalization. Although patency can be approximated from the marker rise, distinguishing between Thrombolysis in Myocardial Infarction (TIMI) II and TIMI III flow is not highly accurate. It should also be understood that peak elevations are accentuated, which must be taken into account if the clinician wants to use peak values as a surrogate for infarct size.

3. Imaging—In the emergency setting, most diagnoses of acute MI are made on history, ECG, and troponin level. However, when the history is atypical and the ECG is equivocal or uninterpretable, performance of a rapid bedside echocardiogram may demonstrate a new regional wall motion abnormality with preserved wall thickness, suggestive of acute MI. In most cases of STEMI, however, echocardiography is not warranted because it delays reperfusion therapy. Echocardiography is also helpful in diagnosing complications of MI, such as VSD, papillary muscle rupture or free wall rupture, and tamponade.

In NSTEMI that is diagnosed on elevated plasma levels of cardiac biomarkers, nuclear scintigraphy or echocardiography may help determine the region of the heart affected by the MI, but these are not standard diagnostic tools.

Gulati M, Levy P, Mukherjee D, et al. 2021 AHA/ACC/ASE/CHEST/SAEM/SCCT/SCMR Guideline for the Evaluation and Diagnosis of Chest Pain. *J Am Coll Cardiol.* 2021 Nov;78(22):e187–e285. [PMID: 34756653]

Jneid H, Addison D, Bhatt DL, et al. 2017 AHA/ACC Clinical Performance and Quality Measures for Adults With ST-Elevation and Non-ST-Elevation Myocardial Infarction. *J Am Coll Cardiol.* 2017;70(16):2048–2090. [PMID: 28943066]

Thygesen K, Alpert JS, Jaffe AS, et al. Fourth universal definition of myocardial infarction. *J Am Coll Cardiol.* 2018;72(18):2231–2264. [PMID: 30153967]

Treatment

The goals of treatment in acute MI are stabilization of the patient and salvage of as much myocardium as possible. A number of general measures should be performed in all patients. In patients with ST elevation—who are at highest risk for complications and have ongoing cardiomyocyte necrosis—immediate reperfusion of the infarct artery should be attempted. The management of acute MI is summarized in Table 8–2.

Table 8–2. Overview of Management of Acute Myocardial Infarction

Prehospital management
Aspirin
Call 911
Continuous cardiac monitoring
Consider prehospital 12-lead ECG
Emergency department treatment
Intravenous access
Continuous cardiac monitoring
12-lead ECG
Aspirin
Oxygen only to maintain normoxia
Nitroglycerin
Heparin
β-Blocker
Reperfusion strategies
Primary PCI vs fibrinolysis for STEMI
Antiplatelet therapy for NSTEMI, possibly followed by elective PCI
In-hospital management
Initial bedrest
Continuous cardiac monitoring
Oxygen for hypoxemia
Nitroglycerin for ongoing pain
ACE inhibitor, β-blocker, aspirin, thienopyridine, statin
Postdischarge
Prognostic indicators
Cardiac rehabilitation
Aggressive secondary prevention with smoking cessation, therapeutic lifestyle changes, and medications

ACE, angiotensin-converting enzyme; ECG, electrocardiogram; NSTEMI, non-ST elevation myocardial infarction; PCI, percutaneous coronary intervention; STEMI, ST-elevation myocardial infarction.

Early recognition of symptoms of myocardial ischemia may lead to faster treatment and salvage of myocardium. Therefore, it is recommended that patients at risk for MI be educated about the symptoms suggestive of acute MI and call for emergency help immediately if they have these symptoms.

A. Prehospital Management

Aspirin, 162–325 mg, should be given immediately. Continuous cardiac monitoring and sublingual nitroglycerin should be administered to all patients with suspected acute MI. Communities usually have organized protocols for ambulance personnel regarding (1) whether or not they should obtain a 12-lead ECG, (2) whether there are designated hospitals that receive patients in whom an acute MI is suspected, or (3) whether the patient should be taken to the nearest emergency department. In some regions of the world, fibrinolytic treatment is initiated in the ambulance, based on a 12-lead ECG.

B. Emergency Department Therapy

On arrival, all patients with suspected acute MI should have a 12-lead ECG performed immediately. If aspirin has not been given, then 162–325 mg of aspirin should be administered immediately. All patients with suspected MI should have continuous cardiac ECG monitoring, and intravenous access (two separate intravenous lines) should be gained in all patients. Sublingual nitroglycerin and intravenous morphine should be administered if patients have active chest pain. Oxygen saturations should be monitored noninvasively, rather than by arterial blood gas measurement. Supplemental oxygen, 2–4 L/min, should be given to all patients if they are hypoxemic, but routine administration of oxygen is not recommended if patients are not hypoxemic. A portable chest radiograph should be ordered but should not delay reperfusion, unless a diagnosis of aortic dissection is strongly considered. Echocardiography may be considered if the diagnosis of MI remains in doubt (eg, equivocal history, uninterpretable ECG). Oral β-blockers should be administered to all patients with acute MI, unless there is a contraindication, such as hypotension, bradycardia, or asthma. This has been shown to improve outcomes and limit the size of infarction. Intravenous β-blockers could be considered when there is hypertension or tachyarrhythmia, for example (Table 8–3). However, they should be avoided in patients with signs of heart failure, in those with contraindications to β-blockers, and in those at high risk for cardiogenic shock (age > 70 years, heart rate > 110/min or < 60/min, systolic blood pressure < 120 mm Hg, or prolonged time since the onset of symptoms).

An anticoagulant should be administered to all patients with acute MI, unless a contraindication exists. In patients with ST elevation who receive fibrinolytics, 48 hours of anticoagulant should be administered. Acceptable choices for anticoagulants include unfractionated heparin (UFH),

Table 8–3. Standard Doses of Commonly Used Agents in Patients with Acute Myocardial Infarction

Agents	Dosage	Comments
Antiarrhythmics		
Lidocaine	Initial bolus of 1 mg/kg and 2 mg/min infusion; additional bolus doses to 3 mg/kg may be necessary	For symptomatic arrhythmias and sustained ventricular tachycardia and ventricular fibrillation, not arrest
Procainamide	20 mg/min–1 g, then 2–4 mg/min drip	May cause hypotension, QRS or QT lengthening, or toxicity
Magnesium	1–2 g over 1–2 min or infusion of 8 g over 24 h	Observe for changes in heart rate, blood pressure
Amiodarone	15 mg/min × 10 min, then 1 mg/min × 6 h and 0.5 mg/min × 24 h	For refractory ventricular tachycardia, ventricular fibrillation and arrest
β-Blockers		
Esmolol	250 mcg/kg IV loading dose, then 25–50 mcg/kg/min to maximum dose of 300 mcg/kg/min	Very short half-life
Metoprolol	5 mg every 5 min IV × 3 then 25–50 mg every 12 h orally	Long duration of action; may exacerbate heart failure
Propranolol	0.1 mg/kg over 5 min IV, followed by 20–40 mg every 6 h orally	Long duration of action; may exacerbate heart failure
Calcium channel blockers		
Diltiazem	20–25 mg IV test dose, then 10–15 mg/h as needed; 90–120 mg three times daily orally	May exacerbate heart failure
Inotropes and pressors		
Dobutamine	Begin at 2.5 mcg/kg/min and titrate to effect	Increases in heart rate > 10% may exacerbate ischemia
Dopamine	Start at 2 mcg/kg/min, titrate to effect	May exacerbate pulmonary congestion and ischemia
Norepinephrine	Start at 2 mcg/min, titrate to effect	Temporizing treatment only
Vasodilators		
Nitroglycerin	Begin at 10 mcg/min IV, titrate to effect	Avoid reducing blood pressure by > 10% if normotensive, > 30% if hypertensive
Nitroprusside	Begin at 0.1 mcg/kg/min, titrate to effect	Mean dose 50–80 mcg/kg/min
Nesiritide	2 mcg/kg bolus followed by 0.01 mcg/kg/min infusion, can increase by 0.005 to maximum infusion 0.03 mcg/kg/min	Hold diuretics and other vasodilators. Keep systolic blood pressure > 100 mm Hg
Anticoagulants		
Unfractionated heparin	5000-unit bolus followed by 1000 units/h adjusted by aPTT	Less efficacious than LMWH
Enoxaparin	1 mg/kg SQ every 12 h, can give immediate 30-mg bolus intravenously if necessary	Hard to reverse effects; avoid in patients with renal failure
Fondaparinux	2.5 mg SQ daily	Contraindicated in patients with renal failure
Argatroban	2 mcg/kg/min	Titrate to aPTT; therefore, hepatic metabolism can be used in renal failure

(Continued)

Table 8–3. Standard Doses of Commonly Used Agents in Patients with Acute Myocardial Infarction (*Continued*)

Agents	Dosage	Comments
Eptifibatide	180 mcg/kg bolus × 2 (30 min later) followed by 2 mcg/kg/min for as long as 96 h for ACS, 24 h post PCI	Care necessary if renal failure
Tirofiban	0.4 mcg/kg/min × 30 min followed by 0.1 mcg/kg/min for up to 108 h for ACS, 12–19 h for PCI	Care necessary if renal failure
Clopidogrel	600 mg loading dose, then 75 mg/day × at least 1 month, preferably for 12 months	TTP possible
Prasugrel	60 mg loading dose, then 10 mg daily for 12 months	Contraindicated if prior stroke or TIA, weight < 60 kg, or age > 75 years
Ticagrelor	Ticagrelor 180-mg loading dose then 90 mg twice daily for 12 months	May cause bradycardia or shortness of breath Aspirin doses > 100 mg/day reduces efficacy

ACS, acute coronary syndromes; aPTT, activated partial thromboplastin time; IV, intravenous; LMWH, low-molecular-weight heparin; PCI, percutaneous coronary intervention; SQ, subcutaneous; TIA, transient ischemic attack; TTP, thrombotic thrombocytopenic purpura.

low-molecular-weight heparin (LMWH), and fondaparinux. For patients with ST elevation undergoing primary PCI, acceptable choices for anticoagulants include UFH, LMWH, and bivalirudin. UFH is preferred to LMWH in most institutions for primary PCI because it has a short half-life, it can be turned off rapidly if there is a complication during invasive therapy, and it can be monitored during procedures with a bedside activated clotting time test. In contrast, LMWHs have a long half-life, and there is no bedside test of their anticoagulant efficiency.

C. Reperfusion Therapy

1. Patients with STEMI—All patients with STEMI who seek medical care within the first 12 hours after symptom onset should be considered for urgent reperfusion of the infarct-related artery, but the earlier therapy is begun, the greater the benefit. In addition, patients who seek medical care within 12–24 hours of symptom onset may be considered for reperfusion, particularly if chest pain is ongoing or heart failure or shock has developed, but the benefit of reperfusion therapies after more than 12 hours is less well established. The definitive therapies for reperfusion in STEMI are fibrinolysis or PCI. Both of these strategies improve patency of the infarct-related artery, reduce infarct size, and lower mortality rates. Therefore, one or the other method should be performed as quickly as possible. The goal of reperfusion therapies in the United States is a door-to-needle time of 30 minutes (for fibrinolysis) and a door-to-balloon inflation time of less than 90 minutes (for PCI). PCI has been shown to be superior to fibrinolysis when it is performed without significant delay by experienced clinicians in experienced centers (Figure 8–3). However, significant delays in performing PCI reduce its benefit over fibrinolytic therapy. There are special cases where primary PCI is always preferred over fibrinolysis: cardiogenic shock, severe CHF, or pulmonary edema (Killip class III), or if there are contraindications to fibrinolysis (Table 8–4). These patients benefit from mechanical reperfusion with primary PCI. The different management of patients with these high-risk clinical features underscores the need for careful clinical examination of all patients with chest pain.

All patients with STEMI, whether they undergo primary PCI or fibrinolytic therapy, benefit from early administration of a thienopyridine in addition to aspirin. Acceptable alternatives include clopidogrel, prasugrel (only if undergoing primary PCI), or ticagrelor. However, thienopyridines may cause an increase in bleeding complications if the patient undergoes CABG surgery.

2. Patients with NSTEMI—These patients should not be treated with fibrinolytics. The definitive management of NSTEMI involves anticoagulation, platelet inhibition, and consideration for an early invasive strategy (ie, routine coronary angiography with or without PCI during the index hospitalization).

For detailed discussion of NSTEMI, see Chapter 7.

D. In-Hospital Management

All patients with acute MI should be admitted for continuous cardiac monitoring. Patients should have bed rest for the first 12–24 hours following MI and reperfusion, but in the absence of ongoing ischemia, they should be mobilized after this time. All patients should receive the appropriate cardiac diet, adhering to the dietary guidelines, as well as education regarding the necessary dietary changes they should make after discharge.

Within the first 24 hours of presentation, the long-term medical management of patients with both STEMI and NSTEMI should be commenced. Angiotensin-converting enzyme (ACE) inhibitors should be given on day 1, if the

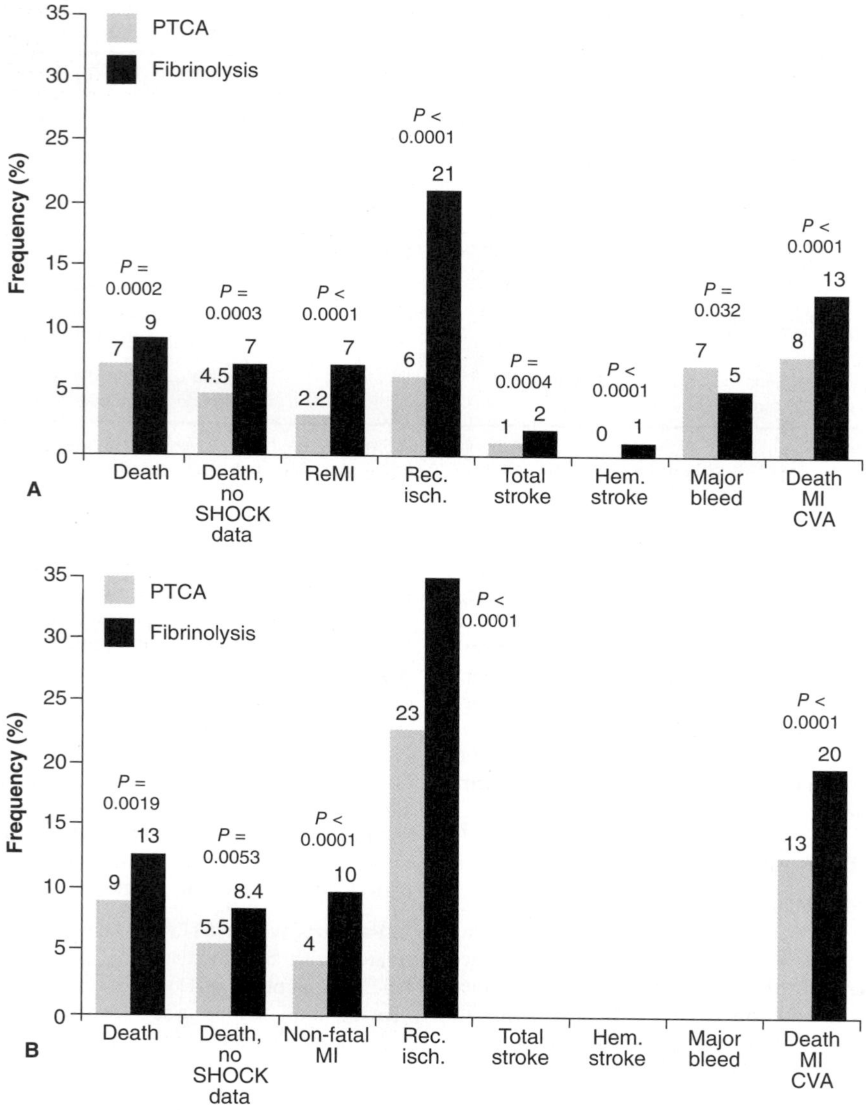

▲ **Figure 8–3.** Percutaneous coronary intervention (PCI) versus fibrinolysis for ST-elevation myocardial infarction (STEMI). Short-term (4–6 weeks; **A**) and long-term (**B**) outcomes for various end points shown are plotted for STEMI patients randomized to PCI or fibrinolysis for reperfusion in 23 trials (n = 7739). Primary angioplasty for acute STEMI improves both short- and long-term outcomes. CVA, cerebrovascular accident; Hem. stroke, hemorrhagic stroke; PTCA, percutaneous transluminal coronary angioplasty; Rec. isch., recurrent ischemia; ReMI, recurrent myocardial infarction. (Reproduced with permission from Keeley EC, Boura JA, Grines CL. Primary angioplasty versus intravenous thrombolytic therapy for acute myocardial infarction: a quantitative review of 23 randomised trials. *Lancet*. 2003;361(9351):13–20 and Antman EM, Anbe DT, Armstrong PW, et al. ACC/AHA guidelines for the management of patients with ST-elevation myocardial infarction—executive summary. A report of the American College of Cardiology/American Heart Association Task Force on Practice Guidelines (Writing Committee to revise the 1999 guidelines for the management of patients with acute myocardial infarction). *J Am Coll Cardiol*. 2004;44(3):671–719.)

Table 8–4. Contraindications for Fibrinolysis Use in STEMI

Absolute contraindications
Any prior ICH
Known structural cerebral vascular lesion (eg, AVM)
Known malignant intracranial neoplasm (primary or metastatic)
Ischemic stroke within previous 3 months
Suspected aortic dissection
Active bleeding or bleeding diathesis (excluding menses)
Significant closed head or facial trauma within 3 months
Severe uncontrolled hypertension (SBP > 180 mm Hg and/or DBP > 110 mm Hg)
Relative contraindications
History of prior ischemic stroke greater than 3 months, dementia, or known intracranial pathology not covered in contraindications
Traumatic or prolonged (> 10 minutes) CPR or major surgery in previous 3 weeks
Recent internal bleeding (within 4 weeks)
Noncompressible vascular punctures
For streptokinase/anistreplase: prior exposure (> 5 days ago) or prior allergic reaction to these agents
Pregnancy
Active peptic ulcer
Current use of anticoagulants: the higher the INR, the higher the risk of bleeding

AVM, arteriovenous malformation; CPR, cardiopulmonary resuscitation; DBP, diastolic blood pressure; ICH, intracranial hemorrhage; INR, international normalized ratio; SBP, systolic blood pressure; STEMI, ST-elevation myocardial infarction.

patient's blood pressure allows, particularly in those with anterior MI or impaired left ventricular function. ACE inhibitors reduce left ventricular remodeling and heart failure and should be continued long-term. β-Blockade should have already been started in the emergency department and should be continued orally in all patients, unless there are absolute contraindications, and should also be continued long-term. Aspirin, 162–325 mg daily, should be administered initially, then 81 mg daily for life. Thienopyridines (clopidogrel, prasugrel, or ticagrelor) should be continued for 12 months. Hydroxymethylglutaryl-coenzyme A (HMG-CoA) reductase inhibitors (statin therapy) should be given soon after MI and should be continued long-term at high doses.

During hospitalization, all patients should be educated about adhering to therapeutic lifestyle changes, including dietary and lifestyle measures, smoking cessation, and medication compliance. Patients should be referred to a cardiac rehabilitation program to consolidate these messages and develop an appropriate exercise regimen. This has been shown to reduce mortality after MI.

E. Primary Percutaneous Coronary Intervention Versus Fibrinolysis

The goal of reperfusion is to rapidly restore blood flow to the myocardium to prevent ongoing ischemic cell death. Therefore, whichever means can achieve reperfusion most quickly should be used. Primary PCI results in improved patency rates of the infarct-related artery, as well as improved TIMI flow grade, compared with fibrinolysis. In general, the patency rate with primary PCI is 90% or higher, whereas with thrombolysis, the rate is about 65% and recurrent events are more common. With modern advances, coronary stenting has further improved long-term outcomes over balloon angioplasty alone. Therefore, PCI has been widely accepted as the treatment of choice for STEMI in centers that can perform primary PCI rapidly and effectively (Figure 8–4). However, very early after the onset of symptoms, when the thrombus in the infarct-related artery is still soft, fibrinolysis may recanalize the artery as quickly as, if not more quickly

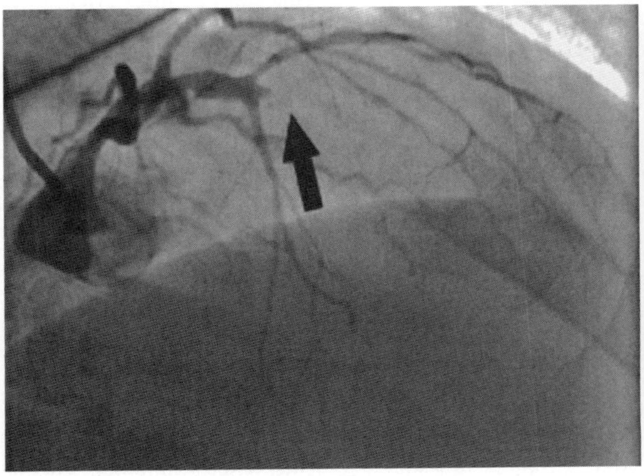

A

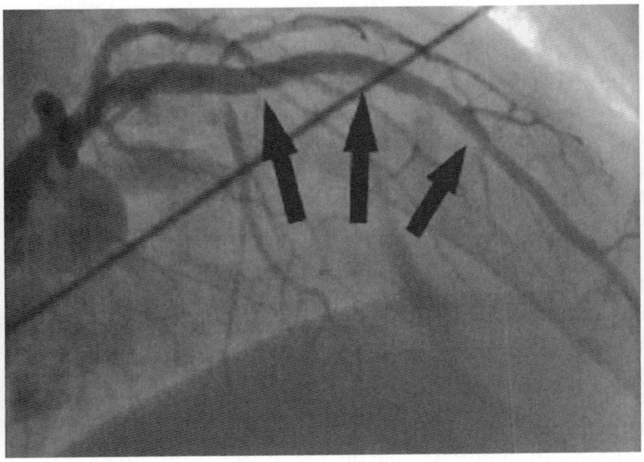

B

▲ **Figure 8–4.** Primary percutaneous coronary intervention (PCI) for acute myocardial infarction (MI). **A:** Initial angiography of a patient presenting with acute anterior ST-elevation myocardial infarction (STEMI) shows an occluded left anterior descending (LAD) coronary artery (*arrow*). **B:** Following angioplasty and stenting, patency of the LAD is restored.

than, primary PCI. This is true in the first hour and possibly the first 3 hours after symptom onset. Therefore, fibrinolysis is an acceptable treatment in these early time points. However, after 3 hours, primary PCI has a clear benefit over fibrinolysis and should be considered the preferred therapy. It bears restating that primary PCI should only be performed in centers skilled in the treatment of STEMI that can achieve rapid reperfusion, with a goal door-to-balloon inflation time of 90 minutes.

In deciding whether elderly patients with acute STEMI should undergo PCI or fibrinolytic therapy, the risks and benefits must be weighed carefully. Elderly patients with STEMI are at high risk for increased morbidity and mortality with thrombolytic agents. Indeed, some studies suggest that these agents have no benefit in this group. On the other hand, PCI is clearly beneficial. However, if PCI cannot be accomplished, individual decisions concerning the risk (which is substantial, especially in regard to intracranial bleeding) and the potential benefits must be balanced. Given the high (20–30%) mortality rate from STEMI in the elderly, some increased risk may be reasonable.

F. Fibrinolytic Agents

There are a number of fibrinolytic agents that have been successfully used in acute MI. Table 8–5 shows the currently approved agents for use in the United States. A brief discussion of each is warranted before deciding on the most appropriate agent. Plasmin, the key ingredient in the fibrinolytic system, degrades fibrin, fibrinogen, prothrombin, and a variety of other factors in the clotting and complement systems. This effect inhibits clot formation and can lead to bleeding. Patients with acute MI and ST-segment elevation have little evidence of spontaneous or intrinsic fibrinolysis, despite the intense thrombotic stimulus present. This may be due in part to increased levels of circulating plasminogen activator inhibitor-1 (PAI-1) in plasma or PAI-1 that is elaborated locally from platelets. The pharmacologic administration of fibrinolytic agents (see Table 8–5) to such patients seems reasonable. Plasminogen activators can be administered intravenously or directly into the coronary artery. Although more rapid patency occurs with local administration and lower doses can be used, given the need for early treatment, plasminogen activators are generally administered intravenously.

In addition to invoking fibrinolysis and inhibiting clotting by degrading clotting factors, all plasminogen activators enhance clot formation. These effects seem greater with nonspecific plasminogen activators such as streptokinase and urokinase and could partly explain why fibrin-specific activators such as t-PA open arteries more rapidly. The enhancement of coagulation by plasminogen activators suggests an important role for the concomitant use of antithrombotic agents.

All fibrinolytic agents increase the risk of bleeding, and therefore, patients at high risk for life-threatening bleeding should not be given fibrinolysis (see Table 8–4).

Table 8–5. Fibrinolytic Agents

Agent	Dosage	Adjunctive Treatments
Streptokinase	1,500,000 units over 1 h	Aspirin ± heparin
Tissue plasminogen activator		
Standard	15 mg bolus, then 50 mg over 30 min and 35 mg over next 60 min	Aspirin, heparin essential
Patients weighing less than 65 kg	1.25 mg/kg over 3 h, 10% of dose as initial bolus	
Urokinase	3,000,000 units over 1 h	Aspirin ± heparin
Reteplase	10 mg initial bolus, second 10-mg bolus after 30 min	Aspirin, heparin essential
Tenecteplase	< 60 kg: 30-mg bolus	Aspirin, heparin essential
	60–70 kg: 35-mg bolus	
	71–80 kg: 40-mg bolus	
	81–90 kg: 45-mg bolus	
	> 90 kg: 50-mg bolus	

1. Streptokinase—Streptokinase is derived from streptococcal bacteria and activates plasminogen indirectly, forming an activator complex with a slightly longer half-life than streptokinase alone (23 minutes versus 18 minutes after a bolus). Because it activates both circulating plasminogen and plasminogen bound to fibrin, both local and systemic effects occur; that is, circulating fibrinogen degrades substantially (both fibrinogenolysis and fibrinolysis occur).

Because antibodies to the streptococci exist in many patients, allergic reactions can occur; anaphylaxis is rare, however, and the use of corticosteroids to avoid allergic reactions is no longer recommended. When streptokinase is administered intravenously, a large dose is necessary to overcome antibody resistance. Because a dose of 250,000 units will suffice in 90% of patients, the recommended dose of 1.5 million units over a 1-hour period is generally more than adequate to overcome resistance. Patients who are known to have had a severe streptococcal infection or to have been treated with streptokinase within the preceding 5 or 6 months (or longer) should not receive the agent.

Rapid administration of streptokinase, even at the recommended dose, can cause a substantial reduction in blood pressure. Although this might be considered a potential benefit of the agent, it may also be detrimental. The rate of the infusion should therefore be reduced in response to significant hypotension, and the blood pressure should be monitored closely. Because streptokinase is more procoagulant than other thrombolytic agents, it should not be surprising that patients benefit to a greater extent from the concomitant use of potent antithrombins such as hirudin. However, in combination with glycoprotein (GP) II_bIII_a inhibitors, streptokinase seems to be associated with markedly increased bleeding rates.

2. Urokinase—Urokinase is a direct activator of plasminogen. It has a shorter half-life than streptokinase (14 ± 6 minutes) and is not antigenic. Its effects on both circulating and bound-to-fibrin plasminogen are similar to those from streptokinase. Therefore, it is difficult to understand why intravenous doses of urokinase (2.0 million units as bolus or 3 million units over 90 minutes) seem to induce coronary artery patency more rapidly than does streptokinase. There is substantial synergism between urokinase and t-PA.

3. Tissue plasminogen activator—The initial human t-PA was made by recombinant DNA technology. The half-life in plasma was short (4 minutes) as a bolus but longer (46 minutes) with prolonged infusions. Despite the short half-life, lytic activity persisted for many hours after clearance of the activator. Although t-PAs are considered "fibrin-specific," no activator is totally fibrin-specific, and fibrin specificity is lost at higher doses. At clinical doses, however, less fibrinogen degradation took place than with nonspecific activators. t-PA clearly opened coronary arteries more rapidly than nonspecific activators, and this is likely why its use improved mortality rates. Bleeding was not decreased, and there was a slight increase in the number of intracranial bleeds, which was in part due to the need for dosage adjustment for lighter-weight patients.

The original regimen for the use of t-PA was 100 mg over 3 hours: 10 mg as a bolus, followed by 50 mg over the first hour and 40 mg over the next 2 hours. Patients who weighed less than 65 kg received 1.25 mg/kg over 3 hours with 10% of the total dose given as a bolus. An alternative front-loaded regimen was found to be more effective and included an initial bolus of 15 mg, followed by 50 mg over 30 minutes and 35 mg over the next 60 minutes. Doses higher than 100 mg are associated with a higher incidence of intracranial bleeding.

4. Reteplase—Reteplase, a mutant form of t-PA, lacks several of the structural areas of the parent molecule (the finger domain, kringle 1, and the epidermal growth factor domain). It is less fibrin-specific (causes more systemic degradation of fibrinogen) than the parent molecule and has a longer half-life. Accordingly, it is used as a double bolus of 10 units initially followed by a second bolus 30 minutes later, and this requires no adjustment for patient weight. Although not shown to be superior to t-PA, many clinicians have elected to use reteplase because of the convenience of the double bolus administration.

5. Tenecteplase—Tenecteplase is also a mutant form of t-PA. It has substitutions in the kringle 1 and protease domains to increase its half-life, increase its fibrin specificity, and reduce its sensitivity to its native inhibitor (PAI-1). Although not shown to be superior to t-PA, tenecteplase is generally being used in preference to the parent molecule because of the convenience of a single bolus dose.

Regardless of the fibrinolytic agent used, all patients should receive aspirin and heparin (either UFH or LMWH) to counteract the procoagulant effect of the fibrinolytic agent.

Intravenous heparin, used with plasminogen activators, improves the rapidity with which patency is induced; it is essential for maintaining coronary patency, especially with t-PA–type agents. Its use is less necessary after treatment with streptokinase, probably because of the anticoagulant effects of fibrinogen depletion and degradation products.

The standard dose of UFH is usually a bolus of 5000 units, followed by a 1000-unit-per-hour infusion until the partial thromboplastin time can be used to titrate a dose between 1.5 and 2 times the normal range. It has become clear that optimal titration of UFH is problematic and that if the activated partial thromboplastin time is either too high or too low, some benefit is lost. For this reason, the use of LMWH has been recommended. With the exception of patients with renal failure, a dose of 1 mg/kg of enoxaparin and a dose of 120 units/kg of dalteparin provide consistent reduction in anti-Xa levels and thus consistent anticoagulation. This is probably the reason that recent studies suggest LMWH is more effective for the treatment of patients with acute MI. In addition, because LMWH inhibits Xa activity predominantly, there is some suggestion that discontinuing it may be less problematic than is the case for UFH, which has fewer effects on Xa and more direct effects (when combined with antithrombin 3) on thrombin itself. The ability to use LMWH intravenously in the catheterization laboratory has not been a problem in regions where this strategy has been embraced.

G. Adverse Effects of Fibrinolytic Therapy

The most serious complication of treatment with thrombolytic agents is bleeding, particularly intracranial hemorrhage; however, catheter-based interventions substantially reduce this complication. The mechanism of bleeding with thrombolytic agents is unclear but has been related to the efficacy of the agent; the concomitant use of antithrombotic agents, such as heparin and aspirin; and the degree of hemostatic perturbation induced by the plasminogen activators. In most studies, the incidence of stroke and intracranial bleeding has been slightly higher with t-PA–type activators. This may be in keeping with the greater efficacy and rapidity of their effects. Although most bleeding occurs early during treatment, bleeding can occur 24–48 hours later, and vigilance even after the first few hours is important.

Intracranial bleeding is by far the most dangerous bleeding complication because it is often fatal. For most plasminogen activators, the incidence of intracranial hemorrhage is less than 1%, but it may be as high as 2–3% in elderly patients. Risk factors for intracranial bleeding include a history of cerebrovascular disease, hypertension, and age. These factors must be taken into account when determining whether a thrombolytic agent has an appropriate benefit-to-risk relationship. Changes in mental status require an immediate evaluation—clinical and computed tomography or magnetic resonance imaging. If bleeding is strongly suspected, heparin should be discontinued or neutralized with protamine.

There also is a substantial incidence of nonhemorrhagic, probably thrombotic, stroke that may be partly due to dissolution of thrombus within the heart, followed by migration. The exact mechanisms of this phenomenon are unclear. In some studies, the excess of strokes with t-PA has been found to be related to this phenomenon, and in other studies, it has been due to an apparent increase in intracranial bleeding.

Bleeding outside the brain can occur in any organ bed and should be prevented whenever possible. The puncture of noncompressible arterial or venous vessels is relatively contraindicated in all cardiovascular patients: Those with unstable angina one day may be candidates for thrombolytic treatment on the next. Therefore, blood gas determinations should be avoided if possible and oximeters used instead in cardiovascular patients. It should be understood that central lines placed in cardiovascular patients pose a substantial risk should there be a subsequent need for a lytic agent. Foley catheters and endotracheal (especially nasotracheal) intubation can also predispose to significant hemorrhage. Bleeding should be watched for assiduously. If severe bleeding occurs while heparin is in use, it should be antagonized with protamine. In general, this and supportive measures are all that can be done. In some studies, there appears to be a slightly higher incidence of extracranial bleeding with nonspecific activators than with t-PA; this finding has not been consistent. In an occasional patient who begins to bleed shortly after receiving the plasminogen activator, aminocaproic acid, which changes the activation of plasminogen, may be useful. Otherwise, discontinuation of the drug and conservative local measures are all that can be done. If volume repletion is necessary, red blood cells are preferred to whole blood, and cryoprecipitate is preferred to fresh frozen plasma because it does not replenish plasminogen.

Allergic reactions related to the use of streptokinase are unusual but should be identified when they occur. Mild reactions, such as urticaria, can be treated with antihistamines; more severe reactions, such as bronchospasm, may require corticosteroids or epinephrine.

Bleeding after primary PCI can also be substantial, particularly if GP II_bIII_a agents are administered. The use of newer closure devices is touted by some clinicians, but close observation is the key to minimizing bleeding from the catheter site. On occasion, platelet transfusions may be necessary.

Ibanez B, James S, Agewall S, et al. 2017 ESC Guidelines for the management of acute myocardial infarction in patients presenting with ST-segment elevation: The Task Force for the management of acute myocardial infarction in patients presenting with ST-segment elevation of the European Society of Cardiology (ESC). *Eur Heart J.* 2018;39(2):119–177. [PMID: 28886621]

Jneid H, Addison D, Bhatt DL, et al. 2017 AHA/ACC Clinical Performance and Quality Measures for Adults With ST-Elevation and Non-ST-Elevation Myocardial Infarction. *J Am Coll Cardiol.* 2017;70(16):2048–2090. [PMID: 28943066]

Lichtenstein A, Appel LJ, Vadiveloo M, et al. 2021 Dietary Guidance to Improve Cardiovascular Health: A Scientific Statement From the American Heart Association. *Circulation.* 2021; 144(23): e472–e487. [PMID: 34724806]

Complications of Myocardial Infarction

The complications of acute MI are listed in Table 8–6.

A. Cardiogenic Shock

Cardiogenic shock is characterized by peripheral hypoperfusion and hypotension refractory to volume repletion. This occurs secondary to inadequate cardiac output resulting from severe left ventricular dysfunction.

Goals of therapy for cardiogenic shock include hemodynamic stabilization to ensure adequate oxygenation of perfused tissue and prompt assessment for reversible causes of the cardiogenic shock. If reversible causes are not found, immediate reperfusion, especially with PCI, is indicated (see Chapter 9).

B. Congestive Heart Failure

In general, there is greater urgency in treating patients with CHF during the early phases of acute MI because such patients often have multivessel disease and are at increased risk for recurrent infarction and increased infarct size. A high degree of suspicion and close monitoring are key to anticipating this complication of acute MI.

Echocardiography has been the technique of choice in evaluating such patients from a perspective of both valvular and myocardial function. Swan-Ganz pulmonary artery catheterization can also be used to aid diagnosis and to assess ongoing management in selected cases. Management strategies depend on the clinical history of the patient. Patients with new-onset acute CHF are typically euvolemic and benefit from nitrate therapy for ischemia. These patients in general should not receive diuretics initially because diuretic therapy often complicates the clinical course with the development of hypotension. In addition, reduced respiratory effort, reduced heart rate, and normalization of oxygen saturation are central to early clinical management.

Table 8–6. Complications of Acute Myocardial Infarction

Cardiogenic shock
Congestive heart failure
Ischemic mitral regurgitation
Ventricular septal defect
Free wall rupture
Recurrent ischemia
Pericarditis
Conduction disturbances
Arrhythmias
Mural thrombus
Aneurysm or pseudoaneurysm of the left ventricle
Right ventricular infarction

Nitroglycerin is often the best agent to use for ischemia in patients with CHF. In some instances, the hemodynamic profile provided by nitroprusside may be desirable. However, nitroprusside may exacerbate ischemia by inducing a coronary steal phenomenon; in this setting, nitroprusside would be a second-line therapy.

Continuous positive airway pressure can reduce the work of breathing in patients with pulmonary edema and should be considered early in these patients. Low-dose dobutamine, starting at 2.5 mcg/kg/min, can be used to achieve hemodynamic benefit. Also, phosphodiesterase inhibitors can be considered, although their vasodilating effects may limit their inotropic benefit in patients with significant hypotension.

The use of Swan-Ganz catheterization monitoring is controversial, and no randomized controlled data support their use as a first-line recommendation in the management of CHF with acute MI. However, Swan-Ganz monitoring can be beneficial in verifying diagnosis, and its use in the early phases of management may allow rapid titration of parenteral therapy.

Once hemodynamic stabilization has been achieved, which is generally within the first 6–12 hours, initiation of oral agents is appropriate. Drugs of choice in this setting are ACE inhibitors, which improve cardiac performance, have beneficial effects on ventricular remodeling, and have been demonstrated not only to reduce morbidity but also to reduce mortality rates in patients with CHF. Oral β-blocker therapy should also be initiated early in the treatment of these patients; however, this should be done in a stepwise fashion in relation to ACE inhibitor therapy to avoid hypotensive effects.

Aldosterone blockade with spironolactone or eplerenone should be given to patients with left ventricular impairment (left ventricular ejection fraction < 40%) or clinical heart failure or both following MI. Aldosterone blockade should be started, in addition to ACE inhibitors, in patients who do not have significant renal impairment or hyperkalemia. The serum potassium level should be monitored closely because both eplerenone and spironolactone can cause hyperkalemia.

C. Acute Mitral Valve Regurgitation

The development of acute severe mitral valve regurgitation occurs in approximately 1% of patients with acute MI and contributes to 5% of deaths. Acute mitral regurgitation occurs as a result of papillary muscle rupture most commonly involving the posterior medial papillary muscle because its singular blood vessel supply is derived from the posterior descending coronary artery. In contrast, the anterior lateral papillary muscle much less commonly ruptures because it has a dual blood supply derived from the left anterior descending and circumflex coronary arteries. Rupture of the papillary muscle may be complete or partial with the development of a flail mitral valve leaflet. Pulmonary edema usually ensues rapidly and occurs within 2–7 days after inferior infarction. The intensity of associated murmur varies depending on the extent of unobstructed flow back into the left atrium. If severe regurgitation is present, no murmur may be audible. As a result, a high degree of suspicion is needed to promptly diagnose acute mitral regurgitation. Two-dimensional echocardiography can be used to demonstrate the partial or completely ruptured papillary muscle head and the flail segment of the mitral valve. Typically, hyperdynamic left ventricular function is demonstrated, and its occurrence in severe CHF should prompt the diagnosis. The treatment of choice is to stabilize the patient hemodynamically with the use of intravenous vasodilators and possibly intra-aortic balloon counterpulsation. The basis of a successful outcome, however, is prompt emergency surgery. The operative mortality rate in this setting can be up to 10%, but this affords most opportunity for survival. Mitral valve repair with reimplantation of the severed papillary muscle is the preferred technique as an alternative to mitral valve replacement. The mortality rate is unacceptably high in the absence of prompt surgery.

Ischemic mitral regurgitation without papillary muscle rupture occurs in up to 50% of patients with acute inferior wall MI. In patients in whom severe CHF symptoms develop, hemodynamic compensation needs to be undertaken and could include the use of IABP for adequate afterload reduction. Treatment of ischemia in this setting may include reperfusion therapy with PCI, intravenous vasodilator therapy, and mechanical support. Once the acute phase of the infarction is passed, resolution of the severe mitral regurgitation may occur, which then avoids the need for surgery.

D. Acute Ventricular Septal Rupture

Rupture of the ventricular septum has been reported to occur in up to 3% of acute MIs and contributes to about 5% of deaths. Typically, half of VSDs occur in anterior wall MIs, often in patients with their first infarction, with peak incidence occurring 3–7 days after initial infarction. Findings associated with VSD can be confused with acute mitral regurgitation because both can result in hypotension, severe heart failure, and prominent murmur. However, the diagnosis of VSD should be suspected clinically when a new pansystolic murmur is noted. Generally, the murmur is most prominent along the left sternal border and may have an associated thrill. Prompt surgical intervention is recommended, which, if successful, can reduce the mortality rate from nearly 100% to below 50%.

Although percutaneous repair of postinfarction VSDs in the catheterization laboratory using septal occluding devices has been reported, surgical repair remains the gold standard.

E. Cardiac Rupture

Rupture of the free wall of the left ventricle occurs in approximately 1–3% of patients with acute infarction and accounts for up to 15% of peri-infarction deaths. Free wall rupture may occur as early as within the first 48 hours of infarction. Fifty percent of ruptures occur within the first 5 days of infarction and 90% within the first 2 weeks. Rupture may be due to expansion of the peri-infarct zone, with thinning of the infarcted wall occurring in response to increased stress. The paradoxical motion of the infarcted segment at the margin of the infarcted zone may also contribute stress, resulting in muscle rupture. Patients may complain of recurrence of chest pain, and an ECG may show persistent ST elevation with Q waves. Prompt intervention at that time may include echocardiography with pericardiocentesis, IABP placement, and urgent cardiac catheterization with anticipation of immediate surgery. Unfortunately, all too often, signs of cardiac rupture are not present until acute hemodynamic decompensation occurs with cardiac arrest due to electromechanical dissociation. The rate of cardiac rupture following MI is decreasing due to early reperfusion therapy. However, the mortality rate remains extremely high. Successful treatment of cardiac rupture requires the clinician to have a high index of suspicion and undertake immediate intervention if there is to be any possibility of preventing death.

F. Recurrent Ischemia

Episodes of chest pain recur in up to 60% of patients after infarction. When chest discomfort recurs early (within 24 hours of MI), the discomfort usually reflects the process of completing the infarction. However, chest discomfort may also reflect the effects of ongoing ischemia or recurrent infarction. In this situation, prompt reassessment and treatment are critical. Patients with hemodynamic compromise in association with new ECG changes in the distribution other than that of the infarct-related artery are at significant risk and require prompt attention, often including coronary angiography with catheter-based intervention.

In patients who were treated initially with reperfusion therapy and have recurrent chest pain, prompt evaluation is needed to assess the adequacy of anticoagulation and the possibility of reocclusion of the culprit coronary artery. Adequacy of adjunctive therapy in the setting of recurrent chest pain is necessary, and often adjustments in drug doses are required. Occasionally, short-term use of intravenous nitroglycerin and intravenous β-blockers is required to quiet the ischemic episode. In this setting, GP II_bIII_a inhibitors should be considered if no contraindications are present. In patients who have had coronary angiography and PCI, correlation between angiographic findings and the 12-lead ECG should be made. Acute stent thrombosis will usually be seen on the ECG as recurrence of ST elevation. This requires emergent repeat catheterization. Conversely, patients with diffuse coronary artery disease may have ischemia due to narrowing in the nonculprit coronary arteries, precipitated by stress or tachycardia, for example. The treatment of this is anticoagulation, GP II_bIII_a inhibitors, and β-blockers.

In patients with NSTEMI, recurrent chest pain is a marker of significant risk for reinfarction, especially if transient ST-segment and T-wave changes are noted or if persistent ST-segment depression is associated with the initial presentation. Prompt coronary angiography and PCI are often required in this setting.

G. Pericarditis

Pericarditis is common in patients with acute MI, particularly in the course of transmural infarctions. In general, the larger the area of infarction, the more likely pericarditis will develop. Pericarditis may be clinically silent or may be associated with a pericardial rub, pleuritic chest pain, or pericardial effusion as suggested by chest radiograph or two-dimensional echocardiography. The associated chest discomfort, classically described as being relieved by sitting up, may also be associated with a description of shortness of breath and epigastric discomfort with inflammation of the contiguous diaphragm. Pericardial rubs are most commonly heard when the patient is seated with held inspiration. Late pericardial inflammation occurring 2 weeks to 3 months after MI is termed Dressler syndrome and most likely reflects an autoimmune mechanism. Dressler syndrome is often associated with large serosanguinous pleural and pericardial effusions, and tamponade develops in persons who die of this syndrome. The treatment of choice for Dressler syndrome is aspirin or colchicine, and in some instances, corticosteroids may be necessary. The use of corticosteroids, however, is not generally advocated because of the high frequency of relapse when corticosteroid therapy is discontinued. Echocardiographic assessment is appropriate as a follow-up tool in these patients to determine the extent of effusion if present and to exclude tamponade or the possibility of partial myocardial rupture. Nonsteroidal anti-inflammatory drugs (NSAIDs) should be avoided in patients with ischemic heart disease, particularly those with evidence of acute infarction. Agents such as indomethacin inhibit new collagen deposition and, therefore, may impair the healing process necessary for stabilization of the infarcted region. This may, in a small number of patients, contribute to the development of myocardial rupture. When used in cases refractory to aspirin, NSAIDs should be used for the shortest time possible and tapered as rapidly as possible. In addition, recent data have linked the use of NSAIDs and cyclooxygenase-2 (COX-2) inhibitors to increased rates of cardiac events. Therefore, the use of NSAIDs and COX-2 inhibitors should be minimized or discouraged. Heparin use early in acute MI should not be stopped if pericarditis is present. However, the presence of Dressler syndrome is a contraindication to heparin use because of its high incidence of hemorrhage into the pericardial fluid with resulting tamponade.

H. Conduction Disturbances

The presence of a conduction disturbance is associated with increased in-hospital and long-term mortality rates. The prognostic significance and management of these disturbances may vary with the location of the infarction, the type of conduction disturbance, associated clinical findings, and the extent of hemodynamic compromise. Patients whose conduction disturbances result in bradycardias and produce hemodynamic compromise generally require transvenous pacing. Bradycardias, especially those associated with inferior infarction, can often be treated with atropine. Recurrent episodes, however, warrant insertion of a pacemaker. Often ventricular pacing to provide a backup rate is all that is required. A need for improved hemodynamics may be a reason to consider atrioventricular (AV) sequential pacing.

1. Anterior STEMI—The highest risk conduction disturbances occur in these patients. Abnormalities are present early after the onset of infarction and are usually the result of extensive infarction producing pump failure; treatment with a pacemaker may not improve the prognosis. Conduction disturbances in this circumstance are generally right bundle branch block (RBBB), with or without concomitant fascicular block. RBBB without fascicular block may have the same incidence of progression to complete heart block (20–40%) as does an RBBB with fascicular block. Patients with RBBB and a fascicular block with anterior MI should be considered for placement of temporary transvenous pacing and be observed for evidence of progression to complete heart block, warranting permanent transvenous pacing.

Left bundle branch block (LBBB) is most often a chronic manifestation of hypertension and myocardial dysfunction rather than an acute abnormality. In the setting of acute MI, however, it is often difficult to determine whether the LBBB is new. Recommendations have been to use pacemakers for patients with LBBB known to be new; this approach has also been advocated for patients with RBBB. Given the present availability of external pacemakers, these issues appear to be less critical.

In the absence of the signs and symptoms of hemodynamic instability or evidence of the progression to heart block, it is reasonable to observe patients with RBBBs or LBBBs and to use external pacing if conduction disturbances develop. Once such a disturbance develops, a transvenous pacemaker is indicated, and it is likely that AV sequential devices would be of benefit.

2. Inferior MI—Conduction disturbances with acute inferior MI are often less critical, but they do suggest a poorer prognosis. The conduction disturbances that commonly occur represent involvement of the AV node and usually include first-degree AV block, Mobitz I (Wenckebach) or Mobitz II second-degree AV block with narrow QRS complexes, and complete heart block with a junctional rhythm. Conduction disturbances are more common in patients with right ventricular infarction. If hemodynamic stability is maintained, patients with these conduction disturbances do not require pacemakers, and they often respond to the administration of atropine (0.5 mg intravenously). If hemodynamic compromise occurs in association with either Wenckebach block or a junctional rhythm, however, or if any arrhythmia requires treatment with more than one dose of atropine, a transvenous pacemaker is warranted. Large initial or total doses of atropine can lead to tachycardia with exacerbation of ischemia and, at times, ventricular tachycardia (VT) or ventricular fibrillation (VF). For patients with right ventricular infarction and hemodynamic compromise associated with the loss of atrial kick, an AV sequential pacemaker is recommended. In general, hemodynamically significant conduction disturbances occur in patients with inferior infarction early during the evolution of infarction; late conduction disturbances are usually well tolerated. Some of these conduction disturbances respond to an intravenous infusion of 250 mg of aminophylline.

3. Mobitz II second-degree AV block—Mobitz II second-degree AV block and complete heart block with a wide QRS complex are both absolute indications for transvenous pacemaker insertion. Such disturbances can occur from electrolyte abnormalities or conduction system disease, but they are most often associated with hemodynamic abnormalities caused by bradycardia. The use of temporary AV sequential pacing may benefit patients who have hemodynamic abnormalities; these patients are also likely to require permanent pacing (see the section Prognosis, Risk Stratification, & Management).

I. Other Arrhythmias

1. Sinus tachycardia—Sinus tachycardia occurs in up to 25% of patients with acute MI. It is a marker of physiologic stress (pain, anxiety, hypovolemia) and often indicates the presence of CHF. In some patients, such as those with right ventricular infarction, it may represent relative or absolute volume depletion. In general, although tachycardia increases myocardial oxygen consumption and can exacerbate ischemia, it should not be treated as a discrete entity. The proper approach is to treat the underlying physiologic drive. It may be unwise to block a tachycardia that is compensating for the increased cardiac work required, for example, by sepsis. Accordingly, β-blockers should only be used once it is clear that no underlying abnormality is inducing the tachycardia or that the underlying abnormality (eg, hyperthyroidism) is amenable to such treatment. Making this determination may require hemodynamic monitoring.

2. Supraventricular tachycardia—Paroxysmal supraventricular tachycardia (PSVT), atrial flutter, and atrial fibrillation can all occur with acute MI. Atrial fibrillation is by far the most common arrhythmia and is often associated with the presence of high atrial filling pressures. The presence of supraventricular tachycardia should lead to consideration of CHF as a cause. A complete differential diagnosis, including conditions such as hyperthyroidism, pulmonary embolism, pericarditis, and drug-induced arrhythmias, is appropriate. Paroxysmal supraventricular tachycardia should be treated immediately because of the high likelihood in this setting that the tachycardia will induce ischemia. Adenosine in bolus doses of 6–12 mg intravenously is the initial approach of choice and often terminates tachycardia. If it does not, cardioversion should be considered prior to other treatment, unless the PSVT terminates and restarts recurrently. Prolonged pharmacologic management before cardioversion may complicate the procedure, and the delay may induce toxicity if the heart rate is rapid, even in the absence of overt hemodynamic compromise. For recurrent or once-terminated PSVT (depending on the mechanisms of the tachycardia; see Chapter 11), small doses of digitalis, diltiazem, verapamil, or a class I antiarrhythmic agent are reasonable choices for maintenance, as long as the indications and contraindications for each of these agents are kept in mind.

Atrial flutter and atrial fibrillation are generally markers of CHF. Frequently the diagnosis of flutter or fibrillation is made after administration of adenosine; once diagnosed, control of the ventricular response is critical. This can generally be accomplished with digitalis, verapamil, or diltiazem in conventional doses (see Chapter 12) once the CHF is treated. Intravenous diltiazem is effective in an emergency situation, usually with an initial test dose of 20–25 mg. If the response is favorable, a titrated dose of 10–15 mg/h should be used. Intravenous diltiazem should be used cautiously in patients with acute MI and CHF. Cardioversion is indicated if a rapid ventricular response persists, the ventricular rate is difficult to control, or there are signs of hypotension, CHF, or recurrent ischemia. In general, PSVT and atrial flutter require 100 J as the initial shock energy; atrial fibrillation requires 200 J.

Arrhythmias that recur after transient reversion in response to pharmacologic maneuvers or cardioversion require additional treatment. Treatment of the underlying initiating stimulus is critical. β-Blockers can also be used to control the ventricular response acutely or for maintenance.

3. Ventricular arrhythmias—The incidence of postinfarct malignant ventricular arrhythmias in patients with acute MI appears to be diminishing, perhaps because of the use of reperfusion therapy. It also is conceivable that interventions such as intravenous β-blockers have also contributed to this decline. Because of the diminishing incidence of VT and fibrillation in patients with acute infarction, as well as an unfavorable benefit-risk ratio, the use of prophylactic lidocaine is not recommended. Although prophylactic lidocaine reduces the incidence of VF, it is associated in many series with an increase in cardiac death, possibly because it abolishes ventricular escape rhythms in patients who may also be prone to bradycardia. Because warning arrhythmias, once considered progenitors of VF, do not appear to be highly predictive, it is recommended that only symptomatic arrhythmias and VT be indications for treatment.

VT with hemodynamic compromise, angina, or pulmonary edema, and VF should be treated with immediate electric shock. Sustained monomorphic VT without hemodynamic compromise, angina, or pulmonary edema can be treated with amiodarone. Amiodarone should be administered as an initial bolus of 150 mg over 10 minutes. If arrhythmias persist, additional boluses of 150 mg every 10–15 minutes can be given; however, the total dose should never exceed 2.2 g in 24 hours. Hypotension and CHF can be induced during the acute administration of amiodarone as a result of its negative inotropic effects. If amiodarone does not relieve the symptoms or the arrhythmias, patients can be treated with intravenous procainamide. The initial loading dose is 1 g, at no more than 50 mg/min, followed by a 2–6 mg/min drip. The infusion rate should be reduced if hypotension occurs; this effect is due to procainamide's α-adrenergic effects. If successful, the drug is continued until the patient is hemodynamically stable; it can then be tapered after initiation of treatment with secondary prevention agents and an assessment made in terms of long-term risk stratification. On rare occasions, a pacemaker may need to be placed in the right ventricle to compete with or overdrive-suppress malignant ventricular arrhythmias. This is usually reserved for rhythms refractory to pharmacologic therapy and can, on occasion, be life-saving. The ventricular pacemaker is generally set at 90–110 bpm, or whatever rate is necessary to suppress the ventricular arrhythmias.

Accelerated idioventricular rhythm occurs in up to 40% of patients and can in some instances be a marker of reperfusion. This rhythm is generally thought to be benign and is usually not treated.

J. Mural Thrombi

Patients with acute MI are at risk for the development of endocardial thrombi for a variety of reasons. Left ventricular thrombus develops in up to 40% of patients with anterior wall infarction but this rate appears to be decreasing due to rapid reperfusion and early initiation of dual antiplatelet therapy. Left ventricular thrombus is uncommon in inferior infarcts. Large areas of dyskinesis with poor flow are prone to develop clots. Because there may be a return in contractility in the borders of the infarcted zone during the remodeling process, it could paradoxically be that clots develop more readily in patients with larger infarctions, but those with somewhat smaller infarctions tend to have their result in emboli more frequently. It has been recommended that all patients with an anterior wall MI be considered for anticoagulation during hospitalization and for 3–6 months thereafter. If anticoagulation is not used routinely, echocardiographic evaluation for the presence of mural thrombi is recommended. Because short-term anticoagulation until the ventricle is remodeled might well be adequate for most patients, the value of long-term (3 months or more) anticoagulation is unclear. In the absence of contraindications, it is probably worthwhile to use heparin during hospitalization and subsequently to use warfarin for 3 months for patients with anterior infarction. Because it has not been established whether low doses of warfarin are as effective as larger doses in inhibiting left ventricular mural thrombi, only a full dose (international normalized ratio [INR] 2.0–2.5) is recommended. Anticoagulation may be valuable for some patients for other reasons, such as atrial fibrillation. Patients with inferior or non–Q-wave infarctions do not require routine anticoagulation following MI but should receive warfarin if mural thrombi are detected by echocardiography. Some clinicians use echocardiographic criteria to select patients who should be treated; others would treat any thrombus detected.

In the current era of routine dual antiplatelet use after MI, there are few data on which patients should receive warfarin or non-vitamin K oral anticoagulants. It is prudent to fully anticoagulate patients with established mural thrombi and those with other reasons for oral anticoagulant therapy, such as atrial fibrillation or aspirin allergy. Other cases, including anterior MI, should be judged individually with the risk of thromboembolism from mural thrombus balanced against the risk of bleeding from warfarin.

Mural thrombi can form in the atrium as well as in the ventricle. Atrial fibrillation is common in patients with CHF; in the setting of atrial fibrillation, stagnation of blood in the atrial appendage leads to a high incidence of clots. This condition can be established only with transesophageal echocardiography, but it may explain the high incidence of emboli in patients with paroxysmal atrial fibrillation. Accordingly, patients with atrial fibrillation should receive anticoagulation, not only because of their increased incidence of thrombus but also because it appears that emboli can be prevented in this group with reasonably modest doses of anticoagulants (goal INR 2.0–2.5). Anticoagulation is discussed in depth in Chapter 4.

Patients with CHF and acute MI are at increased risk for pulmonary emboli because of deep venous thrombosis in the calf and thigh. This may be prevented by the use of warfarin. An argument can be made to consider the use of warfarin in any patient with acute infarction who has had no contraindications for several months. Because aspirin was withheld in some studies, it is unclear whether it offers similar benefits, which would allow it to be substituted for warfarin. In the current era of aspirin plus thienopyridine following MI, warfarin should be considered for MI with extensive wall motion abnormality, including anterior MI, and any MI with established mural thrombus on echocardiography. However, it is probably not necessary in other patients.

K. Aneurysms & Pseudo-Aneurysms

Large areas of infarction tend to thin and bulge paradoxically. These large dyskinetic areas eventually form discrete aneurysms with defined borders. In general, treatment involves the same principles as those for patients with heart failure: vasodilatation and adequate control of filling pressures to reduce pulmonary congestion. Often patients with large dyskinetic areas will have a component of heart failure.

Occasionally, while aneurysms are forming, a myocardial rupture will occur. A small amount of rupture can become tamponade by the pericardium, leading to what is known as a pseudo-aneurysm. Pseudo-aneurysms, which tend to have narrow necks and are not lined with endocardium, function like aneurysms in that they fill with blood during ejection, reducing systolic performance. In addition to reducing stroke volume and leading to increases in ventricular volume as a compensatory response with concomitant increases in pulmonary congestion, pseudo-aneurysms are prone to rupture. The larger the pseudo-aneurysm, the greater is the possibility of rupture. Accordingly, the diagnosis of pseudo-aneurysm usually leads to relatively prompt surgery. Although pseudo-aneurysms can occur with both anterior and inferior MIs, true aneurysms are unusual in the inferior-posterior distribution. A large aneurysmal dilatation is therefore more apt to be a pseudo-aneurysm in an inferior-posterior location.

L. Right Ventricular Infarction

Right ventricular involvement in acute inferior wall MI is common. Hemodynamically significant right ventricular dysfunction, however, is uncommon, occurring in relatively few patients with right ventricular infarction. Substantial right ventricular infarction contributing to hemodynamic compromise occurs in up to 20% of patients with inferior and posterior infarction. These patients often clinically demonstrate hypotension and elevated jugular venous pressure but clear lung fields in the setting of acute inferior wall infarction. ST-segment elevation in right-sided leads (V3R or V4R) and right ventricular wall motion abnormalities on echocardiography help confirm the diagnosis of right ventricular involvement. With right ventricular infarction, the right ventricle becomes noncontractile, and cardiac output is maintained by increased excursion of the septum into the right ventricle and by elevated right-sided filling pressures. The incidence of high-grade AV block is also increased in patients with right ventricular infarction.

If reperfusion is not possible, the stunned right ventricle tends to resolve its dysfunction. Support entails intravenous fluid administration if right ventricular filling pressures are reduced, and occasionally the use of positive inotropic therapy or AV sequential pacing, or both, is required. Early treatment with intravenous diuretics may lead to hypotension and confound patient presentation; therefore, focused clinical examination on presentation is paramount. Patients who display the development of shock despite supportive treatment may benefit from catheter-based intervention (angioplasty and stenting) of the occluded right coronary artery. The balance between the extent of right ventricular and left ventricular dysfunction, however, determines long-term outcome.

Prognosis, Risk Stratification, & Management

A. Risk Predictors

1. Infarct size—Infarct size is an important determinant of long-term risk: the larger the infarction, the poorer the long-term prognosis. This association is easy to demonstrate in patients with first infarctions. In patients with multiple infarctions, the cumulative amount of damage is predictive. Measures that estimate cumulative infarct size (eg, ejection fraction, sestamibi scanning) provide important prognostic information. Nonetheless, the presence of an adverse prognosis does not, in and of itself, mandate a more aggressive therapeutic approach. However, ACE inhibitors and β-blockers are important adjunctive therapies.

2. Infarct type—Patients with NSTEMI are more prone to recurrent episodes of chest discomfort and infarction than are patients with STEMI. Patients with STEMI have an adverse short-term prognosis and should be considered for immediate reperfusion therapy; they often manifest arrhythmias that, especially in association with a low left ventricular ejection fraction, are an important marker of an adverse prognosis. Often these are the patients who have CHF during hospitalization for acute infarction. Their prognosis is worse than that of patients without heart failure, even if the left ventricular ejection fraction appears reasonably well preserved.

3. Malignant arrhythmias—Many patients who suffer malignant arrhythmias during evolution of the infarction are also at increased risk. The one exception appears to be patients with primary VF (ie, VF with no complication of infarction).

B. Risk Assessment

Advanced age (> 65 years), prior MI, anterior location of infarction, multivessel disease involving non-culprit arteries, mechanical complications of infarction, CHF, reduced ejection fraction and the presence of diabetes all suggest higher risk for reinfarction or death in the 6 months following infarction. These patients require aggressive risk stratification prior to hospital discharge after infarction.

1. Myocardial ischemia—Patients with recurrent ischemia during hospitalization are generally considered unstable because of the adverse prognosis associated with recurrent angina following MI. For patients with multiple episodes of recurrent chest discomfort, or ischemia in a distribution distant from the current infarction, cardiac catheterization is recommended to permit consideration of PCI.

Patients who have received thrombolytics and/or PCI and have not had recurrent episodes of chest discomfort constitute a very low-risk group for which the ability of any stress testing method to predict events is significantly reduced. Patients who have been treated with thrombolytic agents should generally undergo invasive investigation with cardiac catheterization.

2. Ventricular function—Patients with complications of infarction or any findings of CHF should have a noninvasive evaluation of ventricular function during their acute hospitalization. Assuming the absence of intercurrent events, one evaluation of ventricular function generally suffices.

The evaluation of some patients with poor ventricular function may also require determining the presence of viable but dysfunctional myocardium (stunned or hibernating regions). Sophisticated metabolic studies using positron emission tomography seem to have the most promise for delineating the regions apt to improve with revascularization; however, they are not widely available for routine use. The response of dysfunctional regions may also be evaluated with dobutamine echocardiography (improved function is thought to be predictive of viable myocardium) or delayed thallium imaging (delayed uptake suggests viability). The absence of late gadolinium uptake by injured myocardium on magnetic resonance imaging also suggests viability.

3. Arrhythmias—Patients who have VT or recurrent episodes of VF after the first day require further evaluation. Evaluation is mandatory for patients who have recurrent arrhythmias without easily remediable causes, especially sustained VT, which generally requires invasive electrophysiologic studies. Although treadmill and ambulatory ECG-guided therapies are equivalent in some studies, the use of invasive electrophysiologic studies to select and titrate antiarrhythmic agents or choose a mechanical device provides one approach. Some data suggest that if the ejection fraction is less than 35% and VT is present then implantable cardioverter-defibrillators (ICDs) save lives.

At present, it is unclear how to manage less severe arrhythmias, which may include frequent ectopy or nonsustained VT. Signal-averaged ECG can be used in such patients; although a negative study is reassuring, the sensitivity of the procedure for detecting risk is inadequate. Recent data suggest that prophylactic external and ICDs in the 6 weeks following MI for ejection fraction less than 35% do not reduce mortality. Therefore, depressed ejection fraction alone, in the absence of life-threatening arrhythmias, following MI is not an indication for ICD therapy. Patients should have optimal medical therapy, and left ventricular ejection fraction should be reassessed after 6 weeks.

Patients who have had bradycardias often require pacemakers. Long-term pacemakers improve the prognosis for patients in whom complete heart block has developed via a mechanism involving bundle branch block. Some clinicians advocate pacing for patients who had transient complete heart block without the development of bundle branch blocks (those with inferior MI and narrow QRS complexes), but supportive data are not conclusive. There also is controversy concerning the use of pacemakers in patients with conduction disturbance such as RBBB and anterior fascicular block, who may (or may not) have had transient Mobitz II second-degree AV block; the benefits of pacing have yet to be established.

4. Multi-vessel disease—Multi-vessel disease detected during primary PCI is common. The culprit lesion should be treated during the initial procedure, as there is clear long-term benefit from this. There are multiple options for treating the other (non-culprit) lesions. Staged PCI is superior to medical therapy alone and is the recommended first choice. In more complex lesions, and particularly in diabetic patients, consideration could be given to coronary artery bypass graft surgery.

C. Risk Management

Patients with recurrent ischemia, severe ventricular arrhythmias, reduced ejection fraction (< 40%), or evidence of severe ischemia during stress testing require cardiac catheterization. Although, in general, treatment is guided by anatomic considerations and their relationship to a long-term prognosis, the ability to predict—from the anatomy—which vessels are apt to be involved in subsequent events is poor. Furthermore, it is unclear that mechanical interventions will reduce the incidence of infarction or death except in well-defined subsets of patients (eg, those with left main disease, proximal three-vessel disease, and a reduced ejection fraction).

1. Risk factor modification—Central to the patient's in-hospital treatment is the identification of factors that increase the risk for progression of coronary artery disease. These include the traditional risk factors for atherosclerosis: hypertension, diabetes, smoking, cholesterol abnormalities, family history, and a sedentary lifestyle. Attempts to modify the diet, stop smoking, and increase exercise should begin once the patient has left the intensive care unit. Although such efforts will vary with each patient, a structured program with active follow-up of patients to ensure some level of success may be helpful.

Recent statin therapy trials support aggressive reduction in cholesterol for the stabilization, and possibly regression, of atherosclerosis. Therefore, a very aggressive approach toward the reduction of low-density lipoprotein (LDL) cholesterol is justified early (within the first 24–48 hours) in postinfarction management. All post-MI patients should receive a statin and aim to achieve an LDL of less than 70 mg/dL.

2. Secondary prevention—β-Blockers should be given to all patients who have had acute STEMIs and NSTEMIs, with or without reperfusion therapy. Patients with CHF tend to benefit most with gradual titration of dose.

Although secondary prevention trials with aspirin have not indicated statistically significant benefits, most studies do show a trend toward improvement, and meta-analysis supports the concept that aspirin improves prognosis after acute infarction. Whether this benefit is synergistic with the effects of β-blockers is unclear. Nonetheless, it appears reasonable for patients to start taking low doses of aspirin (81–325 mg/day) after acute MI and to continue aspirin long-term. Patients treated with primary PCI should be treated with aspirin.

Long-term treatment with ACE inhibitors is recommended for patients at risk for ventricular remodeling and the sequelae associated with that process. In general, this includes patients with left ventricular ejection fractions of less than 45%. Given the results of recent trials, even patients with a low-normal ejection fraction after infarction should be considered for ACE inhibitor treatment, particularly with an anterior MI.

3. Rehabilitation—Studies of exercise rehabilitation have been confounded by the fact that individuals who participate in such programs generally have favorable risk factor and psychological profiles that lessen their risk of recurrent events. It has been argued that the improved prognosis of such patients is related to these initial characteristics—and not to the effects of exercise training. Nonetheless, exercise training clearly improves peripheral muscle efficiency, and intense long-term physical training (5 days a week for at least 9 months) has been shown to reduce the development of cardiac ischemia. Therefore, exercise rehabilitation programs are recommended whenever possible for postinfarction patients.

The amount of exercise prescribed must obviously be based on the patient's heart rate and blood pressure. These should be monitored as the patients start to walk during the convalescent phase in the hospital, and marked increases (eg, blood pressure > 140/90 mm Hg) should be avoided. The patient's rehabilitation activity schedule should be reduced if this level of hypertension occurs. This may also indicate the need for treatment with β-blockers or ACE inhibitors to reduce the labile hypertensive response. In any event, the response of blood pressure and heart rate to exercise must be monitored. Phase II of the program begins at hospital dismissal and generally continues for 8–12 weeks. Objectives should include further patient education, risk factor modification, and gradual resumption of normal work and recreational activities.

4. Psychological factors—It is now clear that as many as 20–25% of patients with acute MI meet formal clinical criteria for depression. It also appears that this is an adverse prognostic feature and that such patients have increased morbidity and mortality rates. Although there is some argument that this is so because these patients have more severe disease, this hypothesis has not been supported by recent studies. It may well be that whatever leads to depression is negatively synergistic with underlying coronary artery disease, as suggested by the increase in catecholamines in such patients. Regardless of the mechanism, however, careful consideration of the presence or absence of depression in patients is recommended. Psychological consultation should be sought for patients in whom depression is suspected, and treatment should be initiated to improve both the quality of the individual's life and—to the extent that there is an interaction with ischemic heart disease—the prognosis. Because tricyclic antidepressants initially liberate catecholamines and may thereby induce adverse effects, drug treatment has previously been thought to be problematic in cardiovascular patients. On the other hand, these agents have membrane-stabilizing effects that may reduce the propensity to arrhythmias, and it is believed that the potential for risk has been exaggerated. Newer agents that antagonize serotonin as their primary mode of action may be safer, but cognitive therapy has also been shown to be effective.

Lawton JS, Holland JET, Bangalore S, et al. 2021 ACC/AHA/SCAI Guideline for Coronary Artery Revascularization. *J Am Coll Cardiol.* 2022;79(2):e21–e129. [PMID: 34895950]

Olgin JE, Pletcher MJ, Vittinghoff E, et al. Wearable cardioverter-defibrillator after myocardial infarction. *N Engl J Med.* 2018; 379:1205–1215. [PMID: 30280654]

Thomas R, Balady G, Banka G, et al. 2018 ACC/AHA Clinical Performance and Quality Measures for Cardiac Rehabilitation. *J Am Coll Cardiol.* 2018;71(16):1814–1837. [PMID: 29606402]

Cardiogenic Shock

9

Richard Cheng, MD

ESSENTIALS OF DIAGNOSIS

- Hypotension: systolic blood pressure less than 90 mm Hg.
- Reduced cardiac output: cardiac index less than 2.2 L/min/m^2 in the absence of hypovolemia.
- Tissue hypoperfusion: depressed mental status, cool extremities, decreased urinary output.
- Laboratory abnormalities: elevated lactate, elevated creatinine, elevated liver enzyme tests, elevated b-type natriuretic peptide, decreased bicarbonate.

General Considerations

Cardiogenic shock results when the heart fails in its function as a pump resulting in inadequate cardiac output, systemic hypotension, and resultant tissue hypoperfusion. The acute insult leading to cardiogenic shock is often caused by acute myocardial infarction from an occluded artery, or from exacerbation of ischemic heart disease. Mechanical complications of delayed-presentation myocardial infarction, valve lesions, and arrhythmias can further complicate the clinical presentation. Cardiogenic shock remains an extremely morbid condition and despite advances in device-based treatment nearly 50% of patients with cardiogenic shock still do not survive hospital discharge in randomized control trials. However, recent advances in cardiogenic shock pathways and multidisciplinary shock teams have been associated with improved outcomes in acute myocardial infarction cardiogenic shock (AMI-CS) and acute decompensated heart failure cardiogenic shock (ADHF-CS).

Definition

Cardiogenic shock is defined by clinical and biochemical signs of reduced cardiac output, systemic hypotension, and tissue hypoperfusion. Clinical signs of reduced cardiac output include cool extremities, weak distal pulses, altered mental status, and diminished urinary output (< 30 mL/h). Hemodynamic findings in cardiogenic shock include a reduced cardiac output without evidence of hypovolemia. One commonly used set of hemodynamic criteria is as follows: (1) a systolic blood pressure of less than 90 mm Hg for at least 30 minutes (or the need for medications or devices to maintain a systolic blood pressure ≥ 90 mm Hg), (2) a pulmonary capillary wedge pressure (PCWP) of greater than 15 mm Hg, and (3) a cardiac index less than 2.2 L/min/m^2. A helpful hemodynamic measurement that summarizes some of the hemodynamic findings above is cardiac power output which is mean arterial pressure × cardiac output divided by 451, with cardiac power output less than 0.6 consistent with cardiogenic shock in the right clinical scenario. Supportive laboratory studies include elevated lactate, elevated b-type natriuretic peptide, increasing creatinine, elevated liver enzymes, and metabolic acidosis.

Etiology

Acute myocardial infarction accounts for many cases of cardiogenic shock and can occur due to an acutely occluded coronary artery, or due to active ischemia from increased demand in patients with a weakened heart from prior MIs. In patients with an acutely occluded coronary artery who present in a delayed fashion, cardiogenic shock can occur from mechanical complications including ventricular septal defect (VSD), acute mitral regurgitation as a result of papillary muscle rupture or dysfunction, and myocardial free wall rupture with tamponade. Right ventricular infarction in the absence of significant left ventricular infarction or dysfunction can lead to shock. Refractory tachyarrhythmias or bradyarrhythmias, usually in the setting of preexisting left ventricular dysfunction, are occasionally a cause of shock. Cardiogenic shock may also occur in patients with end-stage cardiomyopathies (ischemic, valvular, hypertrophic, restrictive, or idiopathic in origin). Cardiogenic shock may

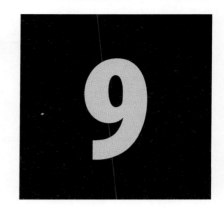

Table 9–1. Causes of Cardiogenic Shock

- I. Acute myocardial infarction (MI)
  - A. Pump failure
  - B. Mechanical complications of acute MI
    - 1. Acute mitral regurgitation
    - 2. Ventricular septal defect
    - 3. Free wall rupture/tamponade
  - C. Right ventricular MI
- II. End-stage, severe cardiomyopathies secondary to
  - A. Valvular disease
  - B. Chronic ischemic disease
  - C. Restrictive/infiltrative
  - D. Idiopathic
- III. Acute myocarditis: viral/infectious, toxic
- IV. Stress cardiomyopathy
- V. Endocrine disease (eg, hypothyroidism, pheochromocytoma)
  - A. Bradyarrhythmias
  - B. Tachyarrhythmias
- VI. Secondary to medications
- VII. Posttraumatic

also be the presenting manifestation of acute myocarditis (infectious, toxic, rheumatologic, or idiopathic). Stress cardiomyopathy (also known as apical ballooning syndrome or takotsubo cardiomyopathy) can also cause severe heart failure and sometimes cardiogenic shock from extreme emotional or physical distress. Finally, certain endocrine abnormalities may cause severe cardiac dysfunction and cardiogenic shock (Table 9–1).

Pathogenesis

The principal feature of shock is hypotension with end-organ hypoperfusion. In cardiogenic shock this occurs because of inadequate cardiac function. The usual response to low cardiac output is sympathetic stimulation to increase cardiac performance and maintain vascular tone. This results in tachycardia and increased myocardial contractility (β-adrenergic–mediated effects) and peripheral vasoconstriction (an α-adrenergic–mediated effect). The classic patient with cardiogenic shock has evidence of peripheral vasoconstriction (cool, moist skin) and tachycardia. Corresponding typical hemodynamics are a reduced cardiac output and increased systemic vascular resistance (SVR), defined as:

$$\text{SVR (in dynes} \times \text{s/cm}^5) = \text{(mean arterial pressure} - \text{right atrial pressure)/(cardiac output)}$$

However, not all patients with cardiogenic shock have this typical hemodynamic profile. Instead, in many patients a systemic inflammatory response-like syndrome may result in a low SVR. Crucially, the absence of cool and clammy extremities does not exclude cardiogenic shock.

A. Acute Myocardial Infarction Cardiogenic Shock

Cardiogenic shock from acute myocardial ischemia can occur in several broad clinical scenarios. A drop in cardiac output and blood pressure leads to decreased perfusion pressures in other coronary beds. (Coronary perfusion becomes compromised when the aortic diastolic pressure falls below 50–55 mm Hg.) This results in further ischemia.

1. In the setting of an ST-elevation myocardial infarction due to an acutely occluded coronary artery, whereby a substantial portion of left ventricular myocardial muscle mass is jeopardized (~40%) either acutely or as a result of prior damage, or in setting of malignant tachy- and bradyarrhythmias due to the myocardial infarction (Figure 9–1).
2. In patients with a delayed presentation acutely occluded coronary artery resulting in infarcted myocardium, and/or a mechanical complication.
3. Patients with prior myocardial infarction and resulting ischemic heart disease where additional ischemic insults are layered on due to increased myocardial oxygen demand (eg, volume overload, inadequate double product control, illicit substance use) resulting in further stunning and/or frank infarction of viable myocardium and pump failure.

The process of ischemia and infarction leading to myocardial dysfunction leading to further ischemia, and so on, has been appropriately termed "a vicious cycle." Evidence for this vicious cycle is found in autopsy studies that show infarct extension at the edges of an infarct in addition to discrete, remote infarctions throughout the ventricle. This also explains the finding that cardiogenic shock can occur immediately, provided sufficient myocardium is dysfunctional, or can occur hours after the initial infarct. Tissue hypoperfusion also leads to accumulation of lactic acid. Acidemia is detrimental to left ventricular contractility.

Mechanical complications of acute MI can occur if revascularization is not performed in a timely manner. The pathophysiology of cardiogenic shock due to mechanical complications of acute MI is somewhat different. The three main mechanical problems are (1) acute mitral regurgitation because of papillary muscle rupture or dysfunction, (2) VSD, and (3) myocardial free wall rupture leading to cardiac tamponade.

The papillary muscles anchor the mitral valve apparatus to the left ventricle. Proper papillary muscle function is vital in ensuring that the two mitral valve leaflets close completely to prevent the leakage or regurgitation of blood backward into the left atrium. In the setting of acute myocardial infarction, especially of multiple coronary distributions, papillary muscle rupture or dysfunction can lead to severe mitral regurgitation. As this process is acute, the left atrium is not able to remodel and compensate, leading to severely increased left

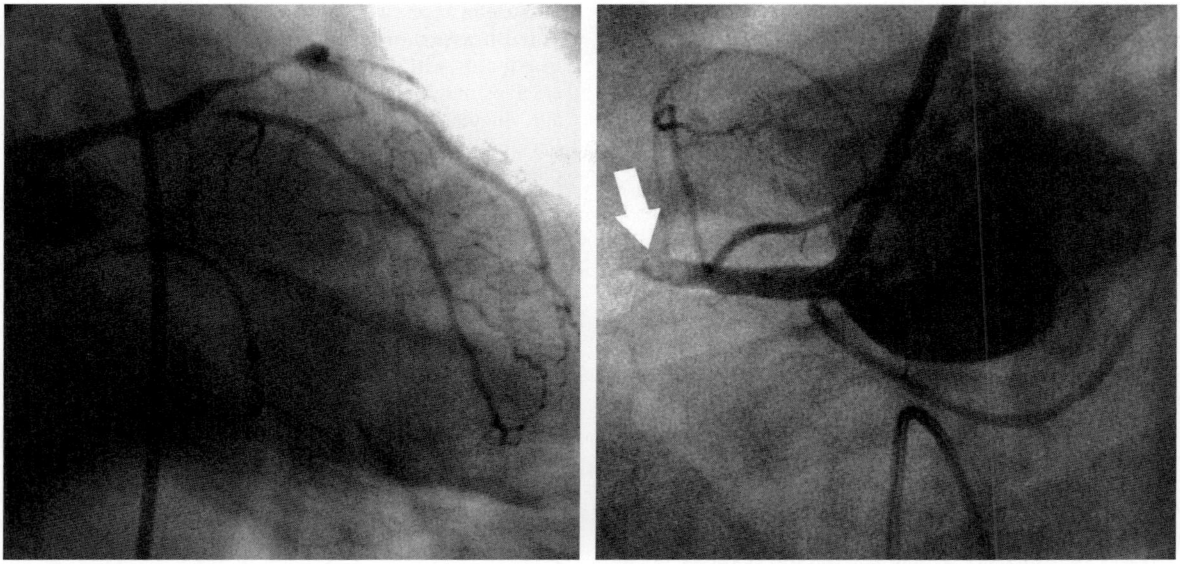

A B

▲ **Figure 9–1.** Coronary angiogram of patient with an acute myocardial infarction and cardiogenic shock. Severe disease in left coronary system (**A**) and acute occlusion with thrombus in the right coronary artery (**B**).

atrial pressures, pulmonary edema, and a reduced forward cardiac output. The sympathetic nervous system response to cardiac failure results in increased SVR (afterload) and a further increase in the regurgitant fraction, another example of a vicious cycle contributing to cardiogenic shock.

Rupture of the myocardial free wall results in bleeding into the relatively nondistendible pericardial space and leads rapidly to pericardial tamponade and cardiovascular collapse. Often this is immediately fatal.

Rupture of the intraventricular septum with the formation of a VSD can lead to significant shunting of blood from the left ventricle to the right ventricle and results in right ventricular volume and pressure overload (Figure 9–2) and decreased forward cardiac output. Also, the sympathetic nervous system response results in increased afterload, thereby shunting an even larger fraction of the cardiac output across the interventricular septum.

Patients with right ventricular infarction due to a proximally occluded right coronary artery may have resultant cardiogenic shock without significant left ventricular dysfunction. Failure of the right ventricle leads to diminished preload for the left ventricle, and the left ventricular function may appear abnormal due to inadequate filling. Since left ventricular filling pressures may not be elevated, pulmonary congestion will not be evident. The result is decreased systemic cardiac output. Bradyarrhythmias may occur leading to worsening cardiogenic shock in a heart

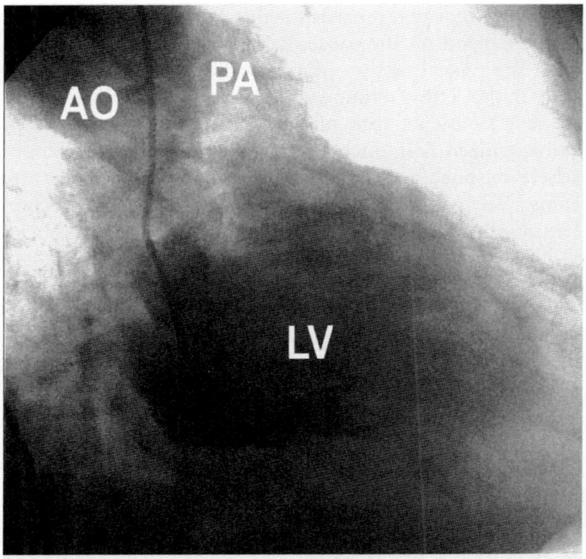

▲ **Figure 9–2.** Left ventriculogram of patient with ventricular septal defect. Note that contrast injected into the left ventricle (LV) opacifies both the aorta (AO) and the pulmonary artery (PA). (The right ventricle is superimposed on the left in this projection and therefore is not visualized.)

already compromised with inadequate stroke volume. While complete heart block resolves even without successful revascularization in right coronary artery occlusions, they can persist up to 2 weeks, and may require temporary pacing to support cardiac output and systemic perfusion.

B. Acute Decompensated Heart Failure Cardiogenic Shock

Cardiogenic shock can occur in the absence of coronary ischemia. Patients can be in an acutely decompensated state from heart failure exacerbation, and/or from progressive pump failure in end-stage cardiomyopathies. This population while large is not well studied in randomized control trials—the large majority of which enrolled patients in AMI-CS. In patients with recoverable heart failure, pharmacological and interventional device-based approaches to temporarily support the failing heart and interrupt the vicious cycle of cardiogenic shock can bridge the patient to recovery and the initiation of medications with acute and long-term hemodynamic/neurohormonal benefits. In patients with end-stage cardiomyopathies that are not recoverable, the same approaches can be used to support a patient to durable ventricular assist devices (VAD) and/or heart transplantation

Clinical Findings

A. History

The symptoms that precede the development of cardiogenic shock depend on the cause. Patients with acute MIs often have the typical history of acute onset of chest pain, possibly in the setting of known coronary artery disease. Often, however, patients seek medical care days later following unrecognized MIs once cardiogenic shock has developed where dyspnea and fatigue may be the presenting symptoms. For patients with nonischemic causes of decompensation that result in cardiogenic shock, the usual heart failure symptoms of dyspnea and orthopnea are often seen alongside forward symptoms like poor appetite and malaise. Mechanical complications of acute MI tend to occur several days to a week following the initial infarction. Patients may be obtunded and lethargic as a result of decreased central nervous system perfusion. Patients with end-stage heart disease with acute decompensated heart failure may slide into worsening cardiogenic shock even while in the acute care setting, unable to be rescued with usual inotropic and/or vasodilator therapies.

B. Physical Examination

The physical examination reveals signs consistent with hypoperfusion with systolic blood pressure less than 90 mm Hg. The heart rate is commonly elevated, and the respiratory rate is generally increased from pulmonary congestion. Patients may be confused, lethargic, or obtunded because of cerebral hypoperfusion. The chest examination in most cases shows diffuse crackles, often to the apices, but in patients with longstanding left-sided heart failure lung crackles may be absent due to increased lymphatic drainage. Jugular venous pulsations are commonly distended. Peripheral pulses may be weak. The apical impulse is displaced in patients with dilated cardiomyopathies, and the intensity of heart sounds is diminished, especially in patients with pericardial effusions. A third or fourth heart sound suggesting significant left ventricular dysfunction and/or elevated filling pressures may be present. A mitral regurgitation murmur (holosystolic, usually at the apex) or a VSD murmur (harsh, holosystolic at the sternal border) can help in diagnosing these causes. Patients with significant right heart failure may have signs on abdominal examination of liver enlargement with a pulsatile liver in the presence of significant tricuspid regurgitation. Peripheral edema may be present. Cyanosis and cool, moist extremities are indicative of diminished tissue perfusion, although vasodilation with warm extremities may herald a secondary distributive shock process or deteriorating cardiogenic shock with systemic inflammatory response.

C. Laboratory Findings

Patients with recent or acute MIs will have elevations in cardiac-specific enzymes (creatine phosphokinase-MB, troponin). Renal and hepatic hypoperfusion may result in elevations in serum creatinine and in transaminases (alanine transaminase [ALT] and aspartate transaminase [AST]). Coagulation abnormalities may be present in patients with hepatic congestion or hepatic hypoperfusion. An anion gap acidosis may be present, and the serum lactate level may be elevated. B-type natriuretic peptide may be elevated.

D. Diagnostic Studies

1. Electrocardiography—The electrocardiogram (ECG) may be helpful in distinguishing between causes of cardiogenic shock. Patients with coronary disease and acute MI may show evidence of both old (Q waves) and new infarctions (ST-segment changes). Right-sided chest leads in patients with inferior MIs can detect the presence of a right ventricular infarction (ST elevation in V_4R). Although ST elevations are often present on the ECGs of patients with cardiogenic shock, patients with non–ST-segment elevation MIs represent up to 50% of patients with cardiogenic shock. The ECG also readily aids in the diagnosis of arrhythmias contributing to cardiogenic shock.

2. Chest radiography—The chest radiograph may show an enlarged cardiac silhouette (cardiomegaly) and evidence of pulmonary congestion in patients with severe left ventricular failure. A VSD or severe mitral regurgitation associated with an acute infarction will lead to pulmonary congestion but not necessarily cardiomegaly. Findings of pulmonary congestion may be less prominent—or absent—in the case of predominantly right ventricular failure or in patients with longstanding left-sided heart failure due to increased lymphatic drainage.

3. Echocardiography—Echocardiography is extremely useful in the diagnosis of cardiogenic shock. Mechanical complications of an acute infarction can be readily diagnosed via echocardiography. Information obtained by echocardiography includes assessment of right and left ventricular size and function, valvular function (stenosis or regurgitation), right and left ventricular filling pressures, the presence of pericardial fluid with tamponade, and the absence or presence of left ventricular clot if a transaortic micro axial heart pump is being considered.

4. Hemodynamic monitoring—Routine use of invasive pulmonary artery catheters for patients in acute decompensated heart failure is not helpful but large randomized experiences in their use in cardiogenic shock is lacking. Their use however has been associated with lower in-hospital mortality in a large multicenter cardiogenic shock registry and right heart catheterization has become one of the centerpieces of many cardiogenic shock pathways. Catheters are usually placed from a central vein into the right heart and advanced into a pulmonary artery. By occluding flow temporarily in a branch of the pulmonary artery ("wedging" the catheter), an estimate of left atrial pressure can be obtained (the PCWP). A pulmonary artery catheter allows for right heart assessment, calculating right ventricular stroke work index, pulmonary artery pulsatility index, and right atrial pressure to PCWP ratio. It can be used to calculate pulmonary vascular resistance (PVR) to diagnose pulmonary hypertension and allows calculation of the SVR. Hemodynamic criteria for cardiogenic shock vary and include a cardiac index of less than 2.2 L/min/m^2, or a cardiac power output of less than 0.6 W.

5. Oxygen saturation—Invasive measurement of the mixed venous oxygen saturation can be obtained from pulmonary artery catheters and may be helpful in two ways. First, knowing the mixed venous oxygen saturation allows the arteriovenous difference in oxygen content to be calculated. The arteriovenous difference in oxygen content is inversely proportional to the cardiac output; it increases as more oxygen is extracted from the blood in the setting of low cardiac output. Serial determinations can be useful in monitoring a patient's course and response to therapy. Secondly, oxygen saturations obtained invasively with a pulmonary artery catheter may also be helpful in diagnosing a VSD. The shunting of oxygenated blood from the left ventricle to the right ventricle across the septal defect results in an abnormal "oxygen saturation step-up" when comparing oxygen saturations from the right atrium with those obtained from the right ventricle.

E. Left Heart (Cardiac) Catheterization & Pulmonary Artery Catheterization

Left heart catheterization and invasive coronary angiography should be performed without delay in patients with ST-segment elevation MI because survival and myocardial salvage depend on the time to reperfusion. This also applies to patients in cardiogenic shock with ST-segment elevation. In patients with cardiogenic shock without ST-segment elevation but with evidence of MI, cardiac catheterization should be expedited as well. In the cardiac catheterization laboratory, obstructions in coronary arteries or bypass grafts can be detected, appropriate treatments planned (either bypass surgery or percutaneous coronary intervention [PCI]), and an intra-aortic balloon pump (IABP) or other mechanical circulatory support device placed.

Classifications of Cardiogenic Shock

Newer classification systems have incorporated the "velocity" of cardiogenic shock. The Interagency Registry for Mechanically Assisted Circulatory Support (INTERMACS) created seven clinical profiles to classify patients with advanced heart failure being considered for VAD and assigned descriptions such as "stable on inotropes," "sliding on inotropes," and "crashing and burning." More recently, the Society for Cardiovascular Angiography and Interventions (SCAI) have also released new consensus classification for cardiogenic shock that incorporate "velocity" in addition to severity into its stages. SCAI Stage A for "at risk" for shock represents patients who are not experiencing cardiogenic shock but may have had a large AMI or are in decompensated heart failure. SCAI Stage B for "beginning" shock represents patients who may have hypotension, tachycardia, or abnormal systemic hemodynamics but do not yet have evidence of hypoperfusion. SCAI Stage C for "classic" shock represents patients who have clinical evidence of hypoperfusion that may require pharmacologic or mechanical support. Lactate, liver enzymes, creatinine, b-type natriuretic peptide may be elevated, and urine output might be less than 30 mL/h. SCAI Stage D for "deteriorating" shock represents patients who are worsening despite ongoing escalation of pharmacological and/or device-based therapies. SCAI Stage E for "extremis" shock represents patients with refractory shock or actual/impending circulatory collapse. Validation studies have subsequently been completed demonstrating increasing mortality with increasing stage of cardiogenic shock.

Treatment

Although some general therapeutic considerations are applicable to all patients in cardiogenic shock, treatment is most effective when the cause is identified (Table 9–2). In many situations, this identification allows rapid correction of the underlying problem. In fact, survival in most forms of shock requires a quick, accurate diagnosis, and avoidance

Table 9–2. Management of Cardiogenic Shock

I. Diagnosis[1]
   A. Electrocardiogram
   B. Chest radiography
   C. Laboratory tests (complete blood count, coagulation profile, CK-MB, cardiac troponin, electrolytes + blood urea nitrogen/creatinine, arterial blood gases)
   D. Echocardiography
   E. Pulmonary artery catheterization (if diagnosis is in question, patient receiving inotropes/vasopressors, or patient is not responding to treatment)
   F. Cardiac catheterization
   G. Classification of cardiogenic shock

II. Treatment
   A. Vasopressors/inotropes, arterial line and pulmonary artery catheter insertion to guide management; correct underlying causes of acidemia
   B. Intra-aortic balloon pump, microaxial pump, extracorporeal membrane oxygenation if needed
   C. For suspected acute MI: aspirin, heparin, urgent cardiac catheterization, revascularization (PCI, CABG)
   D. Durable ventricular assist device and/or heart transplantation
   E. Multidisciplinary discussions involving cardiac intensive care, interventional cardiology, cardiothoracic surgery, and advanced heart failure

[1]Patients with suspected acute MI should proceed directly to cardiac catheterization; this should generally not be delayed to facilitate additional diagnostic tests.
CABG, coronary artery bypass grafting; MI, myocardial infarction; PCI, percutaneous coronary intervention.

of any delays to treatment as the patient may already be in a downward spiral.

A. Inotropic/vasopressor Agents

A variety of drugs are available for intravenous administration to increase the contractility of the heart, the heart rate, and peripheral vascular tone. It is important to note that these agents also increase myocardial oxygen demand; improvements in hemodynamics and blood pressure therefore come at a cost, which can be deleterious in patients with ongoing ischemia. Furthermore, β-agonists can precipitate tachyarrhythmias, and α-agonists can lead to dangerous vasoconstriction and ischemia in vital organ beds. When using these agents, attention should be given to the whole patient rather than focusing solely on a desired arterial pressure. Moreover, their prolonged use before utilization of appropriate mechanical circulatory support has been associated with worse outcomes.

1. β-Adrenergic agonists—Dopamine is an endogenous catecholamine with qualitatively different effects at varying doses. At low doses (< 3 mcg/kg/min), it predominantly stimulates dopaminergic receptors that dilate various arterial beds, the most important being the renal vasculature. Although used frequently in low doses to improve renal perfusion, there is scant evidence to support the clinical usefulness of this strategy. Intermediate doses of 3–6 mcg/kg/min cause β_1-receptor stimulation and enhanced myocardial contractility. Further increases in dosage lead to predominant α-receptor stimulation (peripheral vasoconstriction) in addition to continued β_1 stimulation and tachycardia.

Dobutamine is a synthetic sympathomimetic agent that differs from dopamine in two important ways: It does not cause renal vasodilatation, and it has a much stronger β_2 (arteriolar vasodilatory) effect. The vasodilatory effect may be deleterious in hypotensive patients because a further drop in blood pressure may occur. On the other hand, many patients with cardiogenic shock experience excessive vasoconstriction with a resultant elevation in afterload (SVR) as a result of either the natural sympathetic discharge or the treatment with inotropic agents, such as dopamine, that also have prominent vasoconstrictor effects. In such patients, the combination of cardiac stimulation and decreased afterload with dobutamine may improve cardiac output without a loss of arterial pressure.

Norepinephrine has even stronger α and β_1 effects than dopamine and may be superior to dopamine in the treatment of cardiogenic shock. However, the potent vasoconstriction that can occur can exacerbate tissue hypoperfusion.

2. Vasodilators—Vasodilation (especially of the arterioles to reduce SVR) can be effective in increasing cardiac output of patients with heart failure by countering the peripheral vasoconstriction caused by endogenous catecholamines. Milrinone a phosphodiesterase 3 inhibitor with both inotropy and pulmonary and systemic vasodilatation properties can treat both low cardiac output and elevated SVR in cardiogenic shock with adequate systemic blood pressure. However, when studied against dobutamine in a randomized fashion no significant differences in clinical outcomes were found. Although these agents have a role in treating acute, decompensated heart failure, they are rarely used in patients with cardiogenic shock given the risk of worsening hypotension.

B. Mechanical Circulatory Support Devices

Mechanical devices developed to assist the left or right ventricle until myocardial recovery, or until more definitive therapy can be undertaken include the IABP, catheter-based micro axial pumps, and extracorporeal membrane oxygenation (ECMO) systems.

1. Intra-aortic balloon pump—The IABP is placed in the descending aorta, usually via the femoral artery. Its inflation and deflation are timed to the cardiac cycle (generally synchronized with the ECG). The balloon inflates in diastole immediately following aortic valve closure. The augmentation of diastolic pressure that occurs when the balloon inflates increases coronary perfusion as well as that of other organs. The balloon deflates at the end of diastole, immediately before left ventricular contraction, abruptly decreasing afterload and thereby enhancing left ventricular ejection. Unlike β-agonists, these benefits come without increases in myocardial demand.

IABP have been studied for routine use for AMI-CS in a randomized fashion, and a large IABP SHOCK II trial showed similar outcomes with or without IABP use following revascularization. They are therefore not used routinely in patients with AMI-CS. However, there are still several areas where their use is of value. In patients with cardiogenic shock caused by ventricular septal rupture and acute mitral regurgitation, the device decreases afterload without compromising blood pressure as the balloon deflates in systole; this results in a larger fraction of the left ventricular volume being ejected forward into the aorta rather than backward into the left atrium (mitral regurgitation) or into the right ventricle (ventricular septal rupture). Moreover, data from a large single center cohort of patients with chronic heart failure supported with IABP showed that mean CI increased by 0.26 on average, but demonstrated the benefit depends on the patient. Some patients had robust hemodynamic responses to IABP therapy. Factors associated with a robust hemodynamic response include older age, non-ischemic cardiomyopathy, elevated pulmonary artery pressures, and mitral regurgitation. In fact, patients with ADHF-CS, a cohort not studied in IABP SHOCK II, experienced roughly a five-fold greater cardiac output augmentation compared to patients with AMI-CS. Importantly, SVR was reduced among patients with ADHF-CS but not among AMI-CS.

Increasingly these pumps can be placed in the axillary position (Figure 9–3) to allow patient mobilization while awaiting recovery, durable VAD, or heart transplant. Outpatient ambulatory balloon pump systems and other IABPs designed specifically for the axillary position are being developed.

2. Catheter-based pumps—Micro-axial heart pumps are catheter-based temporary support VAD placed percutaneously from a femoral or axillary approach and positioned across the aortic valve (left-sided support devices) or across the tricuspid and pulmonic valves (for right-sided support). These devices offer improvement in left ventricular unloading when placed across the aortic valve by directly drawing blood from the ventricle and ejecting it into the ascending aorta. While early studies demonstrated more favorable hemodynamic profiles as compared with IABP, vascular complication rates and hemolysis are higher, and their routine use in AMI-CS was found not to be helpful following revascularization in randomized trials. However, large Impella 5.5 devices placed via a surgical vascular graft in the axillary position have been increasingly used to bridge patients to VAD or transplant and are associated with good outcomes. The Impella device is placed from a femoral venous approach and sits across the tricuspid and pulmonic valves and can be used for right ventricular infarction. Currently, Impella devices are the only micro axial catheter-based pumps in active clinical use, although other devices are being actively tested for cardiogenic shock and cardiorenal syndrome.

3. Extracorporeal pumps—Extracorporeal pumps with or without an oxygenation device can be used to support cardiogenic shock. The LifeSPARC extracorporeal disposable

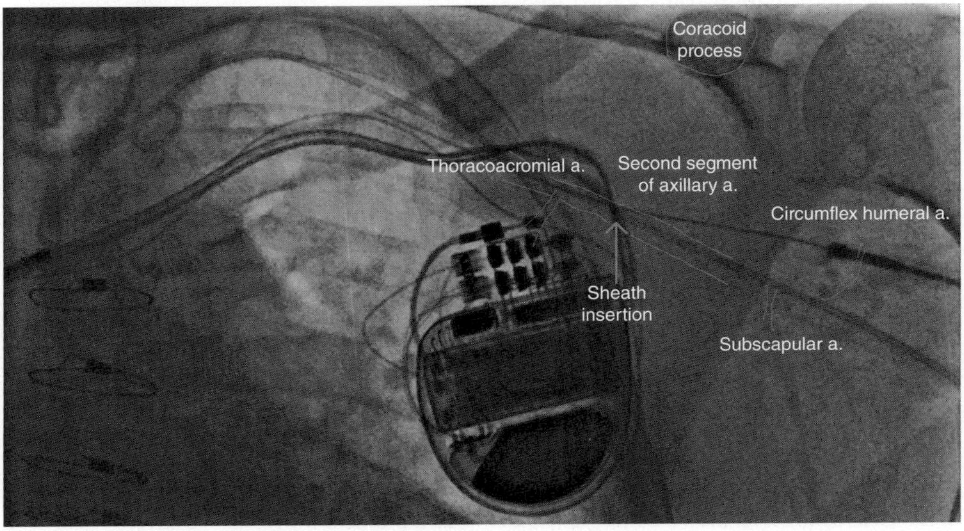

▲ **Figure 9–3.** Fluoroscopy in AP view of a microcatheter entering the left axillary artery between the thoracoacromial and subscapular arteries in the second segment, allowing for placement of an IABP or micro-axial pump. The device (and attached leads) is a dual chamber intracardiac defibrillator.

centrifugal pump can be attached to a TademHeart cannula kit to provide left atrial to femoral artery extracorporeal circulation, or to a ProTek cannula kit to provide right internal jugular to pulmonary artery right ventricular support. Both circuits can be connected to an oxygenator. Traditional ECMO with reusable pumps previously used primarily for postcardiotomy shock has been increasingly used to support cardiogenic shock and mostly support the right ventricle, but provide high flow rates, and can be quickly initiated at patient bedside in the catheterization laboratory or in a surgical suite. Therefore, it is the device of choice in patients with cardiopulmonary arrest refractory to resuscitation. A recent study randomized 30 patients to standard ACLS treatment or early ECMO-facilitated resuscitation in a cohort of patients undergoing active CPR without return of spontaneous circulation. Survival to hospital discharge was only observed in 1 patient of 15 in the standard ACLS group—the patient later died in follow-up—and observed in 6 of 14 in the ECMO-facilitated resuscitation group, resulting in the termination of the study early before target enrollment of 120 patients.

C. Revascularization

Revascularization, either by PCI or CABG surgery, decreases mortality in patients in whom cardiogenic shock develops following MI. The multicenter, randomized SHOCK (Should We Emergently Revascularize Occluded Coronaries for Cardiogenic Shock) trial showed a trend toward improved survival at 30 days in patients randomized to early revascularization (either PCI or CABG within 6 hours of enrollment). The survival benefit for early revascularization became significant at 6 months, a benefit that persisted to 6 years. Although the mortality of patients treated with a strategy of early revascularization was still high, the absolute reduction in mortality was substantial (13% at 1 year); stated alternatively, the "number needed to treat" with revascularization was approximately eight to prevent one death at 1 year. American College of Cardiology (ACC)/American Heart Association (AHA) guidelines recommend emergency revascularization for patients with cardiogenic shock complicating acute MI. This is supported by patients undergoing PCI in the SHOCK trial, who had a similar benefit to those having bypass surgery, and other studies from large populations showing that PCI use is associated with lower mortality in patients with cardiogenic shock. While revascularization of all lesions including non-culprit lesions was supported by the SHOCK trial, a more recent SHOCK-Culprit trial randomizing patients to culprit-lesion-only PCI versus multivessel PCI in the same setting (including PCI of chronic total occlusions) demonstrated increased risk of death and increased need for renal-replacement therapy in patients undergoing multivessel PCI, which has reversed guidelines previously recommending PCI of non-culprit lesions in cardiogenic shock.

D. Durable Mechanical Circulatory Support & Cardiac Transplantation

Patients with end-stage dilated cardiomyopathies without significant active coronary ischemia are presenting with cardiogenic shock and are increasingly supported with temporary mechanical circulatory support. While some patients can be bridged to recovery if their volume status and SVR can be optimized and guideline-directed medical therapy layered on, many have no realistic recovery options as revascularization would not help in the absence of acute myocardial ischemia. However, 1) the proliferation of VAD-capable centers and 2) the updated United Network of Organ Sharing (UNOS) heart allocation system in 2018 have resulted in the development of exit strategies for patients on temporary mechanical circulatory support without realistic myocardial recovery options.

Implant volumes for durable VAD have more than doubled between 2010 and 2019 corresponding with increasing experience, number of centers, and improving pump technologies. Most patients are implanted for "stable but inotrope dependent" or "sliding on inotropes" cardiogenic shock, accounting for 70% of patients. Patients supported on temporary mechanical circulatory support with critical "crashing and burning" cardiogenic shock make up 10–15% of implants (historically a cohort of patients with > 50% in-hospital mortality) and have worse outcomes after VAD implant than less sick patients. Nonetheless in this critically ill population, VAD implant resulted in much improved 3-month and 1-year survival, exceeding 80% and 70%, respectively. The availability of this exit strategy often then plays an important role in the upfront decision of offering temporary mechanical circulatory support in patients without a realistic path to myocardial recovery.

In 2018 the UNOS heart allocation system expanded to include six active statuses and prioritized patients with the highest waitlist mortality, separating patients supported on temporary mechanical circulatory support out into the highest statuses. This paved the path to directly transplanting patients off temporary mechanical circulatory support such as with a femoral or axillary IABP, or a surgical vascular graft micro-axial pump from the axillary artery. Previously, patients who needed temporary mechanical circulatory support often succumbed to their cardiogenic shock before they could be transplanted, waiting behind less sick patients in the newer listing statuses.

E. Cardiogenic Shock Pathways & Multidisciplinary Teams

Cardiogenic shock pathways that minimize variations in care have been associated with improved survival. The National Cardiogenic Shock Initiative includes a multicenter standardized protocol which standardizes care for AMI-CS. Patients who present with AMI-CS who meet hemodynamic criteria are first supported with temporary mechanical circulatory support prior to PCI. Post-PCI hemodynamics are mandated with the use of a right heart catheterization, and weaning of pressors and inotropes, and later the circulatory support is based on maintaining adequate cardiac power output and pulmonary artery pulsatility index. In the group's published early experience, 74% of patients had temporary support implanted prior to PCI. Right heart catheterization was performed in 92%. Survival to hospital discharge was 72%. One center that participated in the standardization protocol reported an improvement in survival from 50% to 58% prior to implantation of the protocol to 70–71% after initiation.

However, AMI-CS pathways do not fully capture the nuances of all cardiogenic shock, including that of ADHF-CS and the subset of patients with end-stage dilated cardiomyopathies. Growing experience and evidence in pharmacological and interventional device-based therapies targeted at different etiologies of pump failure have increasingly made cardiogenic shock a multiple subspecialty discipline and has led in part to fragmented care. In addition, as cardiogenic shock requires rapid diagnosis and early intervention, and ongoing hemodynamic assessment, this has led to the creation of shock pathways that rely on multidisciplinary teams to include cardiac intensivists, advanced heart failure cardiologists, and cardiothoracic surgeons in addition to interventional cardiologists. In addition to stabilization of shock around percutaneous or surgical revascularization, cardiogenic shock teams also consider different types of hemodynamic support, minimize complications from support devices, and consider treatment options and exit strategies including durable VAD and/or heart transplant. INOVA in Virginia has championed this approach, improving their 30-day survival from 47% to 57.9% and to 76.6% after the implementation of a multidisciplinary shock team. Notably, delays in care, including greater than 36 hours of vasopressor use at the time of team activation was associated with worse outcomes. In addition, the importance of initial and ongoing hemodynamic assessment with right heart catheterization has become a centerpiece of most published shock pathways and teams.

F. Special Considerations

Other presentations of cardiogenic shock such as right ventricular failure or arrythmias with targeted treatment options are summarized in Table 9–3.

Table 9–3. Special Considerations

	Presentation/Diagnosis	Treatment
Acute primary mitral regurgitation after myocardial infarction	Flash pulmonary edema from papillary muscle rupture	IABP Surgical repair/replacement TEER (off label indication)
Secondary mitral regurgitation after myocardial infarction	Due to left ventricular remodeling and/or scarring of left ventricle causing restriction of (usually) posterior leaflet	GDMT Consideration of TEER after maximally tolerated GDMT
Myocardial free-wall rupture	Refractory hypotension, pericardial effusion	Surgical repair/replacement Palliative care
Ventricular septal defect	Murmur on exam, left ventriculogram during left heart catheterization	IABP Surgical repair, operative mortality improves the longer patient survives from time of infarct and given time for myocardial tissue to demarcate Percutaneous closure
Right ventricular infarction	RHC showing decreased pulmonary artery pulsatility index, and increased RAP/PCWP ratio ST elevation in V1 and/or RV4 lead	Fluid resuscitation to target right atrial pressure of 10–15 mmHg Inotropes Treatment of bradyarrhythmia with pacemaker if needed (atrial-ventricular sequential pacing preferred) Right-sided temporary mechanical circulatory support
Arrythmias	ECG and telemetry monitoring	Tachyarrhythmias treated with electrical cardioversion in patients with hemodynamic compromise Antiarrhythmics
Bradyarrhythmias	Right coronary artery infarction, iatrogenic after aortic interventions, endocarditis	Due to right coronary artery infarction will improve with watchful waiting, up to 2 weeks Bradyarrhythmias may respond to atropine, isoproterenol, dopamine, epinephrine, or aminophylline

(*Continued*)

Table 9–3. Special Considerations (*Continued*)

	Presentation/Diagnosis	Treatment
Aortic regurgitation	Widened aortic pulse pressure	Dopamine, epinephrine, temporary pacing to minimize diastolic phase of cardiac cycle
Aortic stenosis	Syncope, global ischemia pattern on ECG	Fluid resuscitation Transcatheter aortic valve replacement
Mitral stenosis	Rheumatic mitral stenosis Calcific mitral stenosis	Phenylephrine and vasopressin Esmolol to increase filling time Preserve AV synchrony Percutaneous mitral balloon valvuloplasty for rheumatic mitral stenosis with low Wilkin's score, less than moderate mitral regurgitation No ideal transcatheter or surgical approach to calcific mitral stenosis
Left ventricular outflow tract obstruction	Hypertrophic cardiomyopathy Transcatheter mitral valve in mitral annular calcium	Phenylephrine and vasopressin Avoid inotropes Esmolol to increase filling time Preserve AV synchrony
Tamponade	Elevated jugular venous pressure, distended inferior vena cava, tachycardia, and pulsus paradoxus	Fluid resuscitation Pericardiocentesis
Giant cell myocarditis	Flu-like symptoms, elevated troponin without obstructive coronary disease, reduced left and/or right ventricular function, arrythmias	Endomyocardial biopsy Cardiac magnetic resonance imaging Steroids and immunosuppression ECMO with consideration of left ventricular venting
Multisystem inflammatory syndrome in adults associated with myocarditis	Flu-like symptoms, COVID-19 infection, elevated troponin	Steroids IVIG Interleukin-1 receptor antagonist
Toxins	History of drug overdose or toxin ingestion	Activated charcoal Targeted antidotes Poison control Inotropes and pressors to counteract drug effects ECMO
Post-cardiotomy cardiogenic shock	Inability to wean off pump	ECMO Consideration of other bridge options off bypass or ECMO such as an axillary graft percutaneous VAD
Heart allograft primary graft dysfunction	Decreased ejection fraction, persistent inotrope requirement, hemodynamic compromise on right-heart catheterization, need for IABP	Anti-thymocyte globulin and plasmapheresis if suspicious of acute rejection IABP ECMO
Heart allograft rejection	Decreased ejection fraction on echocardiogram, elevated cell-free DNA, molecular gene expression consistent with rejection, endomyocardial biopsy proven rejection	Steroids Anti-thymocyte globulin Plasmapheresis IVIG IABP ECMO

AV, atrioventricular; COVID-19, coronavirus disease of 2019; ECG, electrocardiogram; ECMO, extracorporeal membrane oxygenation; GDMT, guideline-directed medical therapy; IABP, intra-aortic balloon pump; IVIG, intravenous immune globulin; PCWP; pulmonary capillary wedge pressure; RHC, right-heart catheterization; RAP, right atrial pressure; TEER, transcatheter edge-to-edge repair; VAD, ventricular-assist device.

Prognosis

The prognosis of patients with cardiogenic shock has improved from 80% in-hospital mortality in the late 1970s to under 50% in recent years, with revascularization being a major contributor to improved outcomes. After the introduction of shock pathways, in-hospital mortality can now be seen under 30%. Delayed time to revascularization and delayed time to recognition of shock or activation of shock pathways remain reasons for worse outcomes. Several hemodynamic parameters are now used to prognosticate to allow decisions on treatment options for both left and right ventricles including cardiac power, pulmonary artery pulsatility index, and right atrial pressure to PCWP, among others. While VSD, acute myocardial infarction, primary mitral regurgitation, and other complications of acute myocardial infarction remain associated with worse outcomes, percutaneous structural interventions have emerged as additional options to halt the downward spiral of cardiogenic shock. In patients with end-stage heart failure without a chance of recovery in whom temporary mechanical support devices previously only delayed the inevitable, durable VAD and changes in the listing criteria for heart transplant to prioritize patients in cardiogenic shock have created attractive exit options, further improving outcomes.

Baran DA, Grines CL, Bailey S, et al. SCAI clinical expert consensus statement on the classification of cardiogenic shock. *Catheter Cardiovasc Interv*. 2019;94(1):29–37. [PMID: 31104355]

Basir MB, Kapur NK, Patel K, et al. Improved outcomes associated with the use of shock protocols: updates from the National Cardiogenic Shock Initiative. 2019;93(7):1173–1183. [PMID: 31025538]

Diepen, Katz JN, Albert NM, et al. Contemporary management of cardiogenic shock: a scientific statement from the American Heart Association. *Circulation*. 2017;136:e232–e268. [PMID: 28923988]

Fried JA. Clinical and hemodynamic effects of intra-aortic balloon pump therapy in chronic heart patients with cardiogenic shock. *J Heart Lung Transplant*. 2018;37(11):1313–1321. [PMID: 29678608]

Malick W, Fried JA, Masoumi A, et al. Comparison of the hemodynamic response to intra-aortic balloon pump counterpulsation in patients with cardiogenic shock resulting from acute myocardial infarction versus acute decompensated heart failure. *Am J Cardiol*. 2019;124(12):1947–1953. [PMID: 31648782]

Matthew R, Santo PD, Jung RG, et al. Milirnone as compared with dobutamine in the treatment of cardiogenic shock. *N Engl J Med*. 2021;385:516–525. [PMID: 34347952]

Ouweneel DM, Eriksen E, Sjauw KD, et al. Percutaneous mechanical circulatory support versus intra-aortic balloon pump in cardiogenic shock after acute myocardial infarction. *J Am Coll Cardiol*. 2017;69(3):278–287. [PMID: 27810347]

Tehrani BN, Truesdell AG, Sherwood MW, et al. Standardized team-based care for cardiogenic shock. *J Am Coll Cardiol*. 2019;73(13):1659–1669. [PMID: 30947919]

Thiele H, Akin I, Sandri M, et al. PCI strategies in patients with acute myocardial infarction and cardiogenic shock. *N Engl J Med*. 2017;377:2419–2432. [PMID: 29083953]

Yannopoulos D, Bartos J, Raveendran G, et al. Advanced reperfusion strategies for patients with out-of-hospital cardiac arrest and refractory ventricular fibrillation (ARREST). *Lancet*. 2020;396(10265):1807–1816. [PMID: 33197396]

10 Evaluation & Treatment of the Perioperative Patient

Michael H. Crawford, MD

The prevalence of cardiovascular disease and the death rate associated with it rise sharply after age 45, an age when the incidence of noncardiac surgeries is also increasing. Thus, about one-third of the surgical procedures done annually in the United States are performed in patients with cardiovascular diseases. Cardiac deaths and nonfatal myocardial infarction (MI) occur in about 0.2% of all cases of general anesthesia and surgery (about 500,000 events annually). Cardiac deaths account for approximately 40% of all perioperative mortality, the same proportion as sepsis, although in many cases, the cause of death is multisystem organ failure. These figures underestimate the total effect of cardiovascular diseases because another 500,000 persons a year suffer nonfatal MI, unstable angina, or congestive heart failure (CHF) perioperatively, prolonging both their time in the intensive care unit and the total hospital stay.

Although there is great potential to reduce perioperative cardiovascular risk, it is also impractical, unnecessary, and potentially harmful to perform cardiovascular testing in all patients prior to noncardiac surgery. Therefore, it is important to estimate perioperative risk, decide whether cardiac testing is appropriate, and provide prophylactic treatment to reduce risk when appropriate.

Preoperative Risk Assessment

An individual patient's preoperative risk profile depends on three main factors: the patient's age, current medical and functional status, and the type of surgery.

Table 10–1 lists cardiac risk based on type of noncardiac surgery. In the evaluation of perioperative patients, understanding the nature of the surgery is of prime importance. Is this an emergency surgery? If yes, the clinician should advise to proceed with the surgery and evaluate the patient's cardiac risk postoperatively. On the other hand, if the patient is young, without systemic disease, and undergoing a minor surgery or procedure, the clinician should advise to proceed with surgery without further cardiac workup. Also, in high-risk patients such as those with unstable angina, acute heart failure, symptomatic ventricular tachycardia, or recent MI, surgery should be postponed if possible until their risk is lowered. However, most patients are not so straightforward. In these patients, various algorithms can help identify perioperative risk and the need for further cardiac testing.

A. Algorithms

1. Revised Cardiac Risk Index (RCRI)—This algorithm is simple to use, and it helps identify patients who are at higher risk for major cardiac complications. *However, the RCRI may have less accuracy in patients undergoing major vascular surgery.* Use the RCRI as follows:

a. Assign 1 point to each of the following risk factors if present:

- High-risk surgery (see Table 10–1)
- Ischemic heart disease (history of MI or current angina, use of sublingual nitroglycerin, recent abnormal stress test, Q waves on electrocardiogram [ECG], or history of coronary revascularization with ongoing chest pain)
- History of heart failure or known left ventricular ejection fraction (EF) less than 30%
- History of cerebrovascular disease (stroke, transient ischemic attack)
- Diabetes mellitus requiring insulin
- Preoperative creatinine more than 2.0 mg/dL

b. Assign a risk class to determine the major cardiac complication rate to help counsel the patient:

- Class I: zero risk factors, 0.4%
- Class II: one risk factor, 0.9%
- Class III: two risk factors, 6.6%
- Class IV: three or more risk factors, 11.0%

c. Patients who are categorized as having risk Class III or IV may require additional cardiac testing for risk stratification and more aggressive perioperative medical management to reduce the risk of complications.

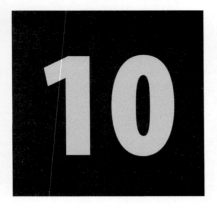

Table 10–1. Cardiac Risk Stratification for Noncardiac Surgical Procedures

High (reported cardiac risk often > 5%)
Emergent major operations, particularly in the elderly
Aortic and other major vascular surgery
Anticipated prolonged surgical procedures associated with large fluid shifts and/or blood loss (eg, liver or lung transplantation)
Pneumonectomy
Pancreatectomy
Esophagectomy
Intermediate (reported cardiac risk generally 1–5%)
Carotid endarterectomy surgery
Head and neck surgery
Intraperitoneal and intrathoracic non-major surgery
Orthopedic surgery
Peripheral vascular surgery
Prostatectomy
Low (reported cardiac risk generally < 1%)
Endoscopic procedures
Superficial procedure
Cataract or other eye surgery
Breast surgery
Minor urological surgery (eg, transurethral resection of the prostate)
Minor gynecological surgery
Minor orthopedic surgery

2. Online cardiac risk calculators—With the increased use of mobile computerized devices by physicians, access to interactive surgical databases is possible. This has been used successfully by cardiac surgeons to assess the risk of cardiac surgery using the Society of Thoracic Surgery (STS) database and the Euroscore from the European Society of Cardiology database. These societies collect data from their members about each surgery performed and its outcome. Then they use multiple regression analysis of the clinical variables in the database to compare with a specific patient's same variables entered in a Web-based calculator to determine the risk of a proposed surgery. The beauty of these databases is that they are frequently updated, so as surgical techniques and medical therapy improve these advances are reflected in the risk calculation. A similar schema has been proposed and tested for noncardiac surgery by the American College of Surgeons using data collected from over 1 million operations in 525 hospitals and has been shown to be superior to the RCRI. This index predicts MI and cardiac arrest based on the anatomic surgical site and other clinical variables. These online Web-based approaches are becoming the dominant approach to preoperative risk stratification for noncardiac surgery. One example from the American College of Surgeons can be found at https://riskcalculator.facs.org

3. Intermediate-risk patients—Although perioperative management of low-risk and high-risk patients is relatively straightforward, the management of patients who fall into the intermediate-risk group is more challenging. Low-risk patients can proceed to surgery without further cardiac evaluation. For high-risk patients, management should include one or more of the following: postpone or cancel surgery until high-risk features improve or resolve, start treatment of the underlying high-risk features, or proceed to invasive testing. In high-risk patients with a high pretest probability of disease, noninvasive tests are not helpful, because a negative result will most likely be a false negative. Intermediate-risk patients derive the most benefit from perioperative medical management or stress testing, or both.

A. Electrocardiography and echocardiography—Preoperative electrocardiography (ECG) can detect arrhythmias, left ventricular hypertrophy, conduction system disease and prior silent MI, but it rarely changes management. Therefore, preoperative ECG is only recommended in those with a history of cardiovascular disease, except for those undergoing low-risk surgery. Echocardiography can provide useful information, but the cost effectiveness of such testing has not been determined. Thus, it is only recommended for those with known or suspected heart failure or valvular heart disease undergoing intermediate to high-risk surgery.

B. Stress testing—The ACC/AHA guidelines recommend noninvasive cardiac stress testing in patients who are undergoing intermediate to high-risk surgery, have risk factors for coronary artery disease (CAD) and have poor functional capacity (less than four metabolic equivalents; cannot walk more than one or two blocks on level ground; cannot do light housework, such as washing dishes or dusting; cannot climb a flight of stairs or walk up a hill) or in whom functional capacity is unknown. However, cardiac stress testing is recommended only if the results would change perioperative management.

C. Exercise versus pharmacologic stress testing—The choice between exercise and pharmacologic stress testing follows the same guidelines as those for routine, nonperioperative stress testing. Exercise testing can provide valuable information on functional capacity, but patients may not be able to reach 85% of maximal predicted heart rate due to deconditioning or β-blocker use. Because β-blockers may be important in the perioperative period, withholding them is not ideal.

Dipyridamole, adenosine, or regadenoson is preferred in cases where arrhythmia (eg, rapid atrial fibrillation) or frequent premature atrial or ventricular beats are present. These agents are relatively contraindicated in patients with significant bronchospasm, in whom dobutamine is the agent of choice.

B. Type of Imaging Technique

When choosing either echocardiography or nuclear imaging (the two most commonly available stress imaging modalities), it is most important to determine which modality has better reliability and expertise at the clinician's hospital or clinic. In published studies, both imaging techniques have good negative predictive value (> 90%) but poor positive predictive value (< 25%). Echocardiography with contrast (to assist in endocardial border definition) may be more helpful in obese patients (who may have more attenuation defects on nuclear imaging). Nuclear imaging may be more useful in patients with left bundle branch block and when atrial fibrillation is present. Newer modalities include rubidium positron emission tomography (PET) scanning, which provides better resolution images. However, patients must be cooperative and must be able to hold still for longer periods of time. Cardiac computed tomography angiography provides an anatomic assessment of the coronary arteries but is not useful in those with coronary artery calcium and has not been adequately evaluated in the perioperative setting.

C. Biomarkers

Brain natriuretic peptide (BNP), troponin, and inflammatory markers such as high-sensitivity CRP have been studied as risk predictors, but suffer from low specificity, so are not recommended for routine preoperative testing. They can be useful in selected patients to confirm the presence of heart failure (BNP) or myocardial infarction (troponin). Also, some recommend obtaining a preoperative troponin level in those at high risk of MI to have a baseline comparative value.

D. Understanding Cardiac Complications

Despite the risks of general anesthesia, including myocardial depression, transient hypotension, and tachycardia, few cardiac events occur during the surgery itself. The incidence of perioperative cardiac complications peaks between 2 and 5 days postoperatively. These data imply that factors activated during or following surgery, not only the surgery itself, are crucial in determining adverse outcomes.

Pneumonitis and microatelectasis produce ventilation-perfusion mismatch, and sedation or analgesia may cause respiratory depression and interfere with coughing, all of which contribute to arterial hypoxemia. Thrombocytosis and a generalized hypercoagulable state, caused by increased fibrinogen and activators from the damaged tissue, favor thrombosis. At the same time, sympathetically mediated increases in heart rate, blood pressure, and contractility increase myocardial oxygen consumption, whereas thrombotic tendencies, anemia, and arterial desaturation impede oxygen delivery to the myocardium. In a patient with underlying CAD, this situation may lead to myocardial ischemia or infarction. The imbalance may be further exaggerated because antihypertensive or anginal medications are often withheld. Also, by the third or fourth postoperative day, the patient is hypermetabolic, with negative nitrogen and potassium balances. A natriuresis follows, which can produce hypovolemia and further activate the sympathetic nervous system.

All these factors provide the exact setting in which a perioperative myocardial ischemia or infarction may occur. The clinical manifestation may be that of ST elevation MI, non-ST elevation MI, or supply/demand myocardial blood flow imbalance ischemic injury. Perioperative MI carries a high mortality and often presents atypically (usually without chest pain) because of sedation and pain-relief medications. Clues such as hypotension, pulmonary edema, altered mental status, and arrhythmia may be the only signs alerting the clinician to the possibility of a perioperative MI. Therefore, those caring for perioperative patients must have a high level of suspicion to detect perioperative MI. Postoperative ECGs and troponin values help in making this determination.

Fleisher LA, Fleischmann KE, Auerbach AD, et al. 2014 ACC/AHA guideline on perioperative cardiovascular evaluation and management of patients undergoing noncardiac surgery: a report of the American College of Cardiology/American Heart Association Task Force on practice guidelines. *J Am Coll Cardiol.* 2014;64:e77–137. [PMID: 25091544]

Kristensen SD, Knuuti J, Saraste A, et al. 2022 ESC guidelines on cardiovascular assessment and management of patients undergoing non-cardiac surgery: Developed by the task force for cardiovascular assessment and management of patients undergoing non-cardiac surgery of the European Society of Cardiology (ESC) endorsed by the European Society of Anesthesiology and Intensive Care (ESAIC). *Eur Hear J.* 2022;43(39):3826–3924.

Ruetzler K, Smilowitz NR, Berger S, et al. Diagnosis and management of patients with myocardial injury after noncardiac surgery: a scientific statement from the American Heart Association. *Circulation.* 2021;144:e287–e305. [PMID: 34601955]

Smilowitz NR, Redel-Traub G, Hausvater A, et al. Myocardial injury after noncardiac surgery: a systematic review and meta-analysis. *Cardiol Rev.* 2019;27:267–273. [PMID: 34601955] doi:10.1097/CRD.0000000000000254

Treatment to Reduce Perioperative Risk

Knowledge of cardiac risk prediction has progressed rapidly in recent years. Risk management (through medicines such as β-blockers) has declined due to recent studies that have not shown compelling results in reducing perioperative major adverse cardiac events (MACE). However, the higher the patient's risk, the greater is the benefit derived from the use of therapies such as β-blockers. Therefore, healthcare providers should risk stratify patients, and then use this information to determine whether to treat the patient.

A. β-Blockers

These agents are first-line therapy to reduce perioperative morbidity and mortality in high-risk patients. Current guidelines consider β-blockers reasonable in almost all high-risk patients undergoing high-risk noncardiac surgery. However, they should not be given as a preoperative bolus, but rather be uptitrated days prior to surgery. Therefore, the decision to use β-blockers should be individualized. If the patient is already taking a β-blocker for other reasons (eg, CAD), usually β-blockers should be continued in the perioperative setting.

In patients deemed to benefit from β-blockers in the perioperative setting, oral atenolol, bisoprolol, or metoprolol is started on the day of the perioperative visit and the dose is titrated to a resting heart rate of 60–70 bpm. For patients who were taking β-blockers before the surgery, the dose the patient is taking is maintained. Oral β-blockers are then continued for 30 days postoperatively and indefinitely in patients who were previously taking these medications.

B. Statins

One small randomized controlled trial and several observational studies have found a benefit to statin use, with greater benefit in higher risk patients, especially major vascular surgery patients. Therefore, if there are no contraindications, high-risk patients should be taking a statin prior to high-risk noncardiac surgery. Also, patients already on statins should have them continued because there is evidence that stopping them is associated with a higher perioperative MI rate.

C. Angiotensin Converting Enzyme Inhibitors (ACEI) and Angiotensin Receptor Blockers (ARB)

These drugs should be continued in patients with heart failure or low EF but not given the day of surgery. They should be started in patients with heart failure or reduced EF who are not already on them well before surgery so the appropriate dose can be found. These drugs should be stopped preoperatively in patients taking them for hypertension and restarted soon after surgery.

D. Antiplatelet Drugs

Many patients are taking aspirin for known cardiovascular disease or for its prevention. Aspirin has been shown to mildly increase bleeding risk with surgery, but there are few data on how to manage aspirin perioperatively in patients without coronary stents. It seems reasonable to continue low-dose aspirin therapy if a small increase in bleeding risk is acceptable. This is often not the case for cerebral or eye surgery, but perfectly acceptable in orthopedic surgery, for example. If a patient is not on aspirin, it does not make sense to start it before surgery. If aspirin needs to be stopped, it should be stopped 7–10 days prior to surgery. $P2Y_{12}$ agents such as clopidogrel, should be stopped preoperatively and restarted once hemostasis is achieved.

Controversy exists regarding the optimal management of antiplatelet therapy in patients with coronary stents. The slower progression of endothelialization in drug-eluting stents predisposes these patients to stent thrombosis for quite some time after stent placement. Dual antiplatelet therapy is recommended for 6–12 months after stent placement depending on the type of stent, except for bare metal stents in which 30 days is recommended. During these time frames the risk of stent thrombosis greatly increases when aspirin and other antiplatelet drugs are stopped prematurely. If surgery cannot be deferred, aspirin should be continued and the $P2Y_{12}$ agents stopped 7 days prior to surgery and restarted once hemostasis is established.

E. Deep Venous Thrombosis Prophylaxis

Although not a routine part of perioperative cardiac risk assessment and treatment, it is important to check for appropriate perioperative deep venous thrombosis (DVT) prophylaxis since DVT (with resultant pulmonary embolism) can cause significant cardiac instability and death. Low-molecular-weight heparins are being used in place of unfractionated heparin, but the direct oral anticoagulants (OACs) are being used more frequently. Warfarin is rarely used. (See Chapter 29.)

F. Endocarditis Prophylaxis

Recommendations for management of endocarditis prophylaxis have changed dramatically with the publication of the new AHA guidelines. In general, the new AHA guidelines advocate less use of antibiotic prophylaxis because of the lack of evidence of benefit in humans and the fact that transient bacteremia occurs frequently, and there is no evidence that dental and other procedures increase rates of bacteremia more than activities of daily living alone. The AHA guidelines state that only patients at the highest risk for endocarditis should receive antibiotic prophylaxis. These high-risk patients include those with a prosthetic cardiac valve, previous infective endocarditis, unrepaired cyanotic congenital heart disease (including palliative shunts and conduits), completely repaired congenital heart defect with prosthetic material or device during the first 6 months after the procedure, repaired congenital heart defects with residual defects at site of prosthetic material that prevent endothelialization, and patients who have undergone heart transplantation in whom significant valvular heart disease develops.

Prophylaxis for dental procedures in the aforementioned patients is only recommended if the procedure involves manipulation of gingival tissue, manipulation of periapical region of teeth, or perforation of the oral mucosa.

Endocarditis prophylaxis is no longer recommended for genitourinary or gastrointestinal procedures.

G. Perioperative Medication Management

Management of outpatient medications in the perioperative period is underappreciated but extremely important for ensuring an optimal patient outcome. Often, essential medications are discontinued and not restarted before the patient is discharged from the hospital, leading to potentially disastrous outcomes.

1. Anticoagulation management—Nowhere is perioperative medication management more important than with anticoagulation, since the use of anticoagulants can cause increased bleeding intra- and postoperatively. Alternatively, too little anticoagulation can lead to severe morbidity (eg, stroke) and even death.

A. Oral anticoagulants—One of the most common reasons for cardiac consultation (besides assessing perioperative risk) is to manage oral anticoagulants (OACs) perioperatively. Although the risks of discontinuing OAC therapy 4 days prior to surgery are low, in the few patients with whom thromboembolism develops, the results (stroke, pulmonary embolism, or death) can be devastating. Therefore, in high-risk patients, bridging with unfractionated or intravenous heparin is important and can reduce the perioperative risk of thromboembolism. However, use of heparins can increase bleeding. Therefore, it is important to carefully select patients who will need bridging with heparin. The keys to optimal OAC management are to identify the indication for OAC and assess the patient's risk for thromboembolism. Bridging with heparin is advised in the following situations: atrial fibrillation associated with rheumatic mitral stenosis; history of thromboembolism; mechanical heart valve; hypercoagulable state; venous or arterial thromboembolism in the prior 3 months; or acute intracardiac thrombus visualized on echocardiogram. Bridging is not advised in patients with bioprosthetic valve in the aortic position, atrial fibrillation without multiple risk factors for cardiac embolism, or a history of one remote (> 6 months ago) venous thromboembolism.

Warfarin should be stopped 4 days prior to surgery if preoperative international normalized ratio (INR) is 2.0–3.0 (with modification of timing if INR is < 2.0 or > 3.0). Newer direct OACs can be held 48 hours prior to surgery. In patients who require bridging with a heparin, there is evidence that low-molecular-weight heparin (eg, enoxaparin) is just as effective and safe (if not more so) than unfractionated heparin. Enoxaparin (1 mg/kg twice daily), if not contraindicated, is started 36 hours after the last dose of warfarin and is discontinued 24 hours prior to surgery. On postoperative day 1, warfarin is restarted at the preoperative outpatient dose. At 24 hours postoperatively, the patient is evaluated, and enoxaparin is restarted if hemostasis has been achieved. Once INR is in the therapeutic range, enoxaparin can be discontinued. Consult manufacturer's guidelines for bridging with the newer OACs.

2. Antiarrhythmics—These medications should be continued up to the day of surgery and, if necessary, in the immediate postoperative period in intravenous form.

Amiodarone is a common oral antiarrhythmic that needs to be converted to an intravenous format in the perioperative period. Since an intravenous bolus of amiodarone can cause hypotension, it is ideal to add up the total daily oral dose of amiodarone and convert that dose to a prolonged or continuous infusion (eg, instead of giving 200 mg intravenously as a bolus once daily, give 0.15 mg/min intravenously continuously over 24 hours, or give the 200 mg intravenously over 4–6 hours).

Digoxin dose should generally be reduced slightly in the perioperative period, especially in elderly patients or those with whom worsening renal function is to be expected.

3. Nonsteroidal anti-inflammatory drugs (NSAIDs)—These medications can predispose elderly and other high-risk patients to perioperative renal failure, especially with perioperative dehydration and hypotension. Therefore, NSAIDs should be discontinued at least 3 days prior to surgery and restarted if necessary, on discharge from the hospital.

H. Prophylactic Coronary Revascularization

For patients who are intermediate or high risk and who eventually undergo coronary angiography, there are three possibilities: no significant CAD, left main or triple-vessel CAD, and single- or two-vessel CAD. In general, such patients should be treated the same as if no surgery was planned.

1. No significant coronary artery disease—Noncardiac surgery can proceed without further testing; aspirin can be stopped and β-blockers need not be initiated.

2. Left main or triple-vessel coronary artery disease—These patients, who are on the opposite extreme, are very high risk and should undergo prophylactic coronary artery bypass grafting or percutaneous coronary intervention and surgery should be postponed.

3. Single- or two-vessel coronary artery disease—In these patients, the decision for prophylactic revascularization is more difficult. However, there are no convincing data that revascularization, especially with surgery, is superior to maximal medical therapy for the prevention of short- and long-term cardiac events. Therefore, in patients found to have single- or two-vessel coronary disease, medical management in the perioperative period, even before high-risk vascular surgery, is just as safe as prophylactic revascularization and does not delay noncardiac surgery. If patients must undergo percutaneous coronary intervention preoperatively, balloon angioplasty alone avoids the necessity to continue dual antiplatelet therapy. If stents are placed, it is extremely important to follow recommendations for perioperative management of dual antiplatelet therapy (see earlier section, Perioperative Medication Management).

Special Populations

A. Liver Transplantation

Liver failure patients have a unique cardiovascular physiology characterized by high cardiac output and a reduced response to cardiac stress, which some have called cirrhotic cardiomyopathy. Often these patients have low peripheral vascular resistance, bradycardia, left ventricular hypertrophy, and prolonged QTc interval on ECG. Today, these patients are older, sicker, and have more comorbidities than before. The most common causes of perioperative death in these patients are arrhythmias, heart failure, and MI. Once the new liver is reperfused, there is an increase in preload, which will exacerbate cardiac stress. In addition, those with known CAD have worse outcomes. Thus, these are high-risk patients, and determining who has CAD is important because it may preclude liver transplantation.

Noninvasive stress testing has been less valuable in pre-liver transplant patients. Although preferred by many, dobutamine stress echo (DSE) has lower sensitivity in these patients. Nuclear perfusion testing has lower specificity. Given the enormous resources needed to transplant these patients successfully, many are assessed by coronary angiography, usually invasively. Coronary computed tomography angiography may be adequate, but there are few data on this technique in these patients. Certainly, patients with known CAD, diabetes, age older than 50 years, renal dysfunction, and two or more major risk factors are high risk for CAD and should be studied. Some centers study almost all patients. There are no data demonstrating improved outcomes with revascularization of significant coronary artery lesions but doing so may allow the patient to be transplanted.

Transthoracic echocardiography also is important in the evaluation of pre-liver transplant patients. Reduced left ventricular (LV) function may be detected but is not an absolute contraindication for transplant because it may improve afterward. However, it indicates that aggressive heart failure prophylactic measures should be taken. Some patients have LV outflow tract obstruction, which is also not a contraindication to surgery, but requires special management techniques during the perioperative period. Prolonged QTc on ECG is also not a contraindication to surgery, but should motivate a search for treatable causes, so the incidence of ventricular arrhythmias can be reduced. Some centers are employing cardiac magnetic resonance imaging to detect myocardial iron deposits, which indicate a higher risk of heart failure postoperatively but are not an absolute contraindication to surgery.

The most serious cardiovascular abnormality in pre-liver transplant patients is portopulmonary hypertension, which is caused by abnormal pulmonary vasoconstriction and, if not effectively treated, is a contraindication to transplantation. Echocardiographic screening that shows an elevated estimated systolic pulmonary artery pressure or right ventricular dysfunction indicates the need for right heart catheterization. A mean pulmonary artery pressure greater than 35 mm Hg, a pulmonary vascular resistance more than 3 Wood units, and a pulmonary artery wedge pressure less than 15 mm Hg contraindicate surgery unless treatment with pulmonary vasodilator drugs is successful in lowering the pulmonary pressure.

B. Severe Valvular Disease

In patients with severe or critical aortic stenosis, risks of a perioperative cardiac complication are high. The risk correlates with aortic valve mean gradient, as measured by echocardiography. Even moderate aortic stenosis (mean gradient of > 25 mm Hg) has been associated with an adjusted relative risk of 5.2% for perioperative cardiac complications.

Noninvasive stress testing is unnecessary and potentially dangerous in these patients. If the patient has symptomatic aortic stenosis, postpone the noncardiac surgery until after the patient undergoes coronary angiography, aortic valve replacement, and coronary intervention if the patient is found to have significant CAD. In asymptomatic patients with severe aortic stenosis, preoperative aortic valve replacement (prior to elective noncardiac surgery) is usually the best option because of the very high-risk nature of these patients. Also, the procedural risks must be weighed against the risk of canceling surgery or operating with significant aortic stenosis. Percutaneous aortic valve replacement is an attractive option but has not been tested extensively in this situation. Severe mitral stenosis is unusual today but should be handled similarly to severe aortic stenosis. Balloon mitral valvuloplasty prior to surgery is an attractive option.

Severe mitral and aortic regurgitation also increase the risk of MACE perioperatively. If these conditions cannot be corrected before surgery, then careful attention to the patient's fluid status during and after surgery is important and may require the use of a temporary right heart catheter monitoring.

C. Heart Failure

Patients with a history of hospitalization for heart failure, and especially those with current signs and symptoms of heart failure, are at high risk for perioperative cardiac events. In these patients, heart failure should be treated, and volume status optimized prior to surgery, since the risks of heart failure outweigh those associated with delaying surgery in most cases. As the number of patients with heart failure increases along with the aging population, more patients who undergo noncardiac surgery will have a history of heart failure. Even though heart failure indicates a greater risk of perioperative cardiac events than CAD, there are few studies on the optimal perioperative treatment of patients with heart failure, especially those with preserved EF. Selected patients may benefit from perioperative monitoring with a right heart catheter.

D. Pulmonary Hypertension

In patients with significant pulmonary hypertension, the risks of general anesthesia are extraordinarily high. Pulmonary hypertension can be thought of as a fixed obstruction to cardiopulmonary blood flow, and therefore, it prevents the increase in cardiac output necessary in the perioperative state. Therefore, it is very similar to critical aortic or mitral stenosis in this aspect. In these cases, a pulmonary hypertension specialist should be consulted. Elective surgeries should be postponed indefinitely until the patient is treated with pulmonary vasodilators to reduce the perioperative risk. If surgery is absolutely necessary, it is advisable that these patients undergo continuous monitoring with pulmonary artery catheter intraoperatively. Intraoperative inhaled nitric oxide can be used to decrease pulmonary artery pressures.

E. Pacemakers, Defibrillators, & Atrial Fibrillation

There is a small risk that prolonged electrocautery could trigger, reprogram, or inadvertently turn off an implantable cardioverter-defibrillator (ICD). Electrocautery may also interfere with pacemaker output, and anesthetic agents may interfere with pacing thresholds. Some manufacturers have recommended that these devices be inactivated during surgery. Supraventricular tachycardias, which are common in the postoperative period, may exceed the rate threshold of the ICD and can cause inappropriate shocks to be delivered. ICDs should be interrogated before surgery to assess underlying rhythm and frequency of discharges. In pacemaker-dependent patients, the rate response feature should be turned off. The ICD defibrillation capacity should be disengaged just prior to surgery and resumed immediately after surgery, and an external defibrillating device should be close to the patient at all times during the period that the ICD is off. Of note, an anteroposterior lead placement of the external paddles away from the device pocket is required in the event of external cardioversion or defibrillation. Preoperative atrial fibrillation is associated with a higher risk of perioperative adverse cardiovascular events, especially stroke. Anticoagulation should be restarted as soon as hemostasis is achieved postoperatively. The most common problem with atrial fibrillation patients is rapid rate after surgery. Optimization of rate control preoperatively should be accomplished if possible.

Duceppe E, Parlow J, MacDonald P, et al. Canadian Cardiovascular Society guidelines on perioperative cardiac risk assessment and management for patients who undergo noncardiac surgery. *Can J Cardiol.* 2017;33:17–32. [PMID: 27865641] doi: 10.1016/j.cjca.2016.09.008

Smilowitz NR, Gupta N, Guo Y, Beckman JA, Bangalore S, Berger JS. Trends in cardiovascular risk factor and disease prevalence in patients undergoing non-cardiac surgery. *Heart.* 2018;104:1180–1186. [PMID: 29305561] doi:10.1136/heartjnl-2017-312391

Supraventricular Tachycardias

11

Byron K. Lee, MD

ESSENTIALS OF DIAGNOSIS

- Heart rate greater than 100 bpm.
- Rhythm is supraventricular in origin.

General Considerations

Supraventricular tachycardias (SVTs) are rapid rhythm disturbances originating from the atria or the atrioventricular (AV) node. In the absence of a bundle branch block, there is intact conduction to the ventricles via the right and left bundles leading to a narrow and normal-appearing QRS. Therefore, these arrhythmias are also often called narrow complex tachycardias. Because many of the SVTs are episodic, many clinicians also refer to this group of arrhythmias as paroxysmal SVTs. Radiofrequency ablation has become an important therapeutic option in the management of SVTs because of its ability to cure these arrhythmias safely. Table 11–1 outlines the pharmacologic therapy for SVTs.

Pathophysiology & Etiology

Tachyarrhythmias occur as a result of three main mechanisms: reentry, which is most common; enhanced or abnormal automaticity; and triggered activity.

Reentrant arrhythmias sustain themselves by repetitively following a revolving pathway comprising two limbs, one that takes the impulse away from and one that carries it back to the site of origin. For reentry to exist, an area of slow conduction must occur, and each limb must have a different refractory period (see the discussion on AV nodal reentrant tachycardia). In this situation, ectopic beats or pacing (by inducing refractoriness in one limb of the circuit) can initiate a reentrant tachycardia. Once established, ectopic beats or pacing can also terminate the tachycardia by interfering with impulse propagation in one of the limbs.

The second mechanism, **automaticity**, refers to spontaneous and, often, repetitive firing from a single focus, which may either be ectopic or may originate in the sinus node. This mechanism comprises two subcategories. **Enhanced automaticity** is defined as a focus that fires spontaneously and may originate in the sinus node, subsidiary pacemakers in the atrium including the Eustachian ridge, Bachmann bundle, coronary sinus and AV valves, the AV node, His-Purkinje system, and the ventricles. **Abnormal automaticity** is usually secondary to a disease process causing alterations in ionic flow that produces a less negative resting diastolic membrane potential. Threshold potential is therefore more easily attained, thereby increasing the probability of a sustained arrhythmia.

The third mechanism, **triggered arrhythmias**, depends on oscillations in the membrane potential that closely follow an action potential. In the absence of a new external electrical stimulus, these oscillations, or **after-depolarizations**, cause new action potentials to develop. Thus, each new action potential results from the previous action potential. These arrhythmias can be produced by early or late after-depolarization, depending on the timing of the first after-depolarization relative to the preceding action potential (the one that spawned the triggered activity). In **early after-depolarizations**, membrane repolarization is incomplete, which allows an action potential to be initiated by a subthreshold stimulus. This type is often associated with electrolyte disturbance and may be the mechanism responsible for arrhythmogenesis related to the prolonged QT syndrome and torsades de pointes caused by quinidine. With **delayed after-depolarization**, membrane repolarization is complete, but an abnormal intracellular calcium load causes spontaneous depolarization. The high calcium levels can be related to the inhibition of the sodium pump by drugs such as digoxin. In either type of arrhythmia, the process may be repetitive and lead to a sustained tachycardia.

General Diagnostic Approach

A systematic approach to interpreting the 12-lead electrocardiogram (ECG) will allow accurate determination of the

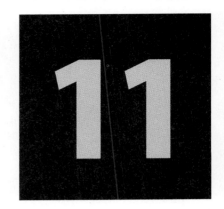

Table 11–1. Antiarrhythmic Drugs for Supraventricular Tachycardias

Agent	Indication	Intravenous Dose	Oral Dose	Adverse Effects	Drug Interactions
Class Ia					
Quinidine	AF, AFL, AVNRT, AVRT	6–10 mg/kg over 20–30 min	200–400 mg q4–6h; q8h with long-acting preparations	Hypotension (especially IV), ventricular proarrhythmia, GI disturbance, thrombocytopenia	↑ Digitalis level ↑ Warfarin effect ↑ Metoprolol, propranolol, propafenone levels
Procainamide	AF, AFL, AVNRT, AVRT	*Bolus:* 15 mg/kg given as 20 mg/min *Infusion:* 2–4 mg/min	50 mg/kg/day q3–4h; twice daily dosage with longacting preparation	GI disturbance, hypotension, SLE, agranulocytosis, FUO hemolytic anemia, myasthenia gravis aggravation, ventricular proarrhythmia	↑ Procainamide level with cimetidine, quinidine, and amiodarone
Class Ic					
Flecainide	AF, AFL, AT, AVNRT, AVRT	N/A	50–200 mg q12h	Ventricular proarrhythmia, CHF, GI disturbance, CNS (dizziness, tremor, light-headedness)	↑ Digitalis level ↑ Flecainide level with amiodarone, cimetidine, Norpace, propranolol ↓ Flecainide level with smoking
Propafenone	AF, AFL, AVNRT, AVRT	N/A	150–300 mg q8h or 225–425 mg bid (long-acting form)	GI disturbance, CNS (dizziness), metallic taste, CHF, first-degree AVB, IVCD, positive ANA	Synergism with β-blockers
Class II (IV)					
Esmolol	Ventricular rate control for AF, AFL, ST, AT	*Bolus:* 500 mcg/kg over 1–2 min *Infusion:* 50–200 mcg/kg/min	N/A	CHF, AVB, bradycardia, bronchospasm	
Propranolol	Ventricular rate control for AF, AFL, ST, AT	1–5 mg at 1 mg/min	20–320 mg/day q6h, q8h, q12h, or once daily, depending on preparation	CHF, AVB, bradycardia, bronchospasm	
Class III					
Sotalol	AF, AFL, AVNRT, AVRT, AT	N/A	80–160 mg q12h	Dyspnea, fatigue, dizziness, CHF, bradycardia, ventricular proarrhythmia, bronchospasm	Synergism with Ca^{2+} antagonists or β-blockers

Amiodarone	AF, AFL, AVNRT, AVRT, AT	*Bolus:* 150 mg over 10 min *Infusion:* 1 mg/min × 6 h, then 0.5 mg/min	100–400 mg once daily	Pulmonary toxicity, CHF, tremor, bradycardia, ↑ LFTs, corneal deposits, skin discoloration, GI intolerance, hyper-/hypothyroidism	↑ Digoxin levels ↑ Warfarin effect ↑ Quinidine, procainamide/NAPA, flecainide ↑ Phenytoin level
Ibutilide	AF, AFL	1 mg bolus over 10 min; second bolus, if needed, after 10-min wait	N/A	Ventricular proarrhythmia, hypotension, GI disturbance	
Dofetilide	AF, AFL	N/A	125–500 mcg twice daily modified by algorithm	Ventricular proarrhythmia, headache, chest pain, nausea, dizziness	Contraindicated with verapamil, cimetidine, ketoconazole, trimethoprim
Class IV					
Diltiazem	AF, AFL, AVNRT, AVRT, AT, MAT	*Bolus:* 0.25 mg/min over 2 min then 0.35 mg/kg in 15 min if needed *Infusion:* 5–15 mg/h	90–360 mg/day in 1–4 divided doses, depending on preparation	Hypotension, bradycardia, CHF, AVB	Synergism with β-blockers
Verapamil	AF, AFL, AVNRT, AVRT, AT, MAT	2.5–20 mg over 20 min in divided doses	40–120 mg q8h; 240–360 mg once daily of longacting preparation	Hypotension, bradycardia, CHF, AVB	Synergism with β-blockers
Class V					
Adenosine	SVT diagnosis, AVNRT, AVRT, AT termination	6 mg IV rapid bolus followed by 12 mg × 2 if needed; half dosage if administered in central line	N/A	Chest tightness, facial flushing, dyspnea, AVB	↑ Activity by dipyridamole ↓ Activity by theophylline
Digoxin	Ventricular rate control for AF, AFL, AT (generally not very effective in active patients)	Up to 1.0 mg bolus in divided doses followed by 0.125–0.375 mg/day	0.125–0.375 mg/day in single dose	GI disturbance, conduction defects, atrial/ventricular arrhythmias, headache, visual disturbances	↑ *Digoxin level:* amiodarone, quinidine, verapamil, indomethacin, spironolactone, alprazolam, erythromycin, tetracycline ↓ *Digoxin level:* antacids, cholestyramine, rifampin, neomycin ↑ Risk of digitalis toxicity with potassium-depleting diuretics

AF, atrial fibrillation; AFL, atrial flutter; ANA, antinuclear antigen; AT, atrial tachycardia; AVB, atrioventricular block; AVNRT, atrioventricular nodal reentrant tachycardia; AVRT, atrioventricular reciprocating tachycardia; CHF, congestive heart failure; CNS, central nervous system; FUO, fever of unknown origin; GI, gastrointestinal; IV, intravenous; IVCD, intraventricular conduction delay; LFT, liver function tests; MAT, multifocal atrial tachycardia; N/A, not applicable; NAPA, *N*-acetyl procainamide; SLE, systemic lupus erythematosus; ST, sinus tachycardia.

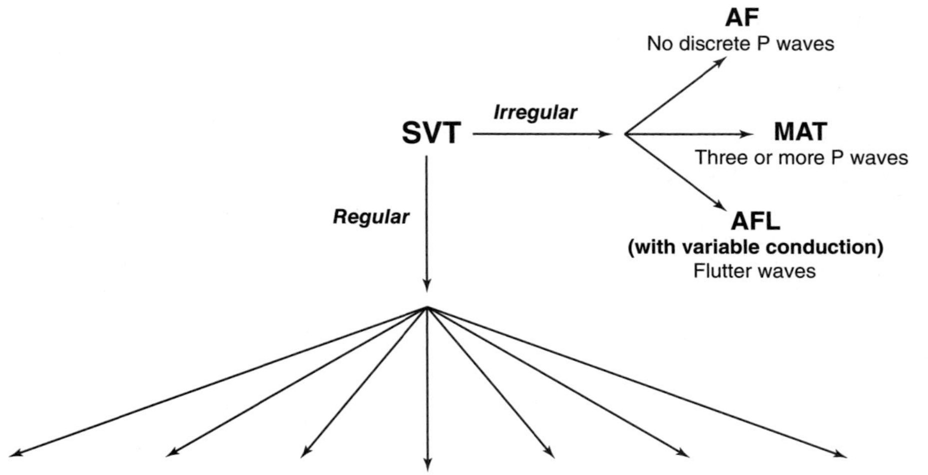

	ST	SN reentry	AFL	AT	AVNRT	JT (Accelerated AV junction rhythm)	AVRT
Onset and termination	Gradual	Sudden	Sudden	Sudden	Sudden	Gradual	Sudden
Heart rate (bpm)	100–(220 – age)	100–160	Multiple of 300	100–180	120–200	70–120	140–250
P wave	Sinus Ps	Sinus Ps	Flutter waves	Ectopic Ps	Retrograde Ps	Retrograde Ps	Ectopic Ps
R-P relationship	Long R-P	Long R-P	Undefined	Long R-P	Short R-P or no P	Short R-P or no P	Short R-P

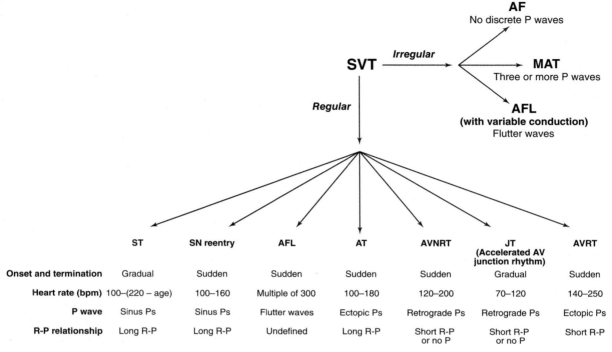

▲ **Figure 11–1.** Algorithm for distinguishing supraventricular tachycardias. AF, atrial fibrillation; AFL, atrial flutter; AT, atrial tachycardia; AVNRT, atrioventricular nodal reentrant tachycardia; AVRT, atrioventricular reciprocating tachycardia; JT, junctional tachycardia; MAT, multifocal atrial tachycardia; SN, sinus node; ST, sinus tachycardia; SVT, supraventricular tachycardia.

type of SVT in most cases (Figure 11–1). The first step is to determine whether the rhythm is regular or irregular. If it is irregular, the rhythm is likely either atrial fibrillation, atrial flutter with variable conduction, or multifocal atrial tachycardia (MAT). The appearance of the P waves or lack of P waves will usually distinguish between these three entities. In atrial fibrillation, there is chaotic atrial activity. In atrial flutter, P waves are seen at a rate of 240–320 bpm. In MAT, there are P waves preceding each QRS complex, and there are at least three different P-wave morphologies.

If the SVT is regular, there are several main types of SVT to consider. The SVT could be sinus tachycardia, sinus node reentry, atrial flutter, atrial tachycardia, AV nodal reentrant tachycardia (AVNRT), junctional tachycardia, or atrioventricular reciprocating tachycardia (AVRT). The type of regular SVT can be usually identified by examining four aspects of the 12-lead ECG: onset and termination, heart rate, P-wave morphology, and R-P relationship. Sinus tachycardia and junctional tachycardia typically have very gradual onset, whereas the other SVTs usually start and stop more suddenly. Rate can also be helpful since sinus tachycardia cannot typically go over 220 bpm minus age, and the heart rate in atrial flutter is often a multiple of 300. P-wave morphology can be helpful because retrograde P waves (negative in the inferior leads: II, III, and aVF) favor AVNRT and junctional tachycardia. Finally, R-P relationship refers to the distance from the R wave to the next P wave during tachycardia. If this distance is longer than the P-R interval, the SVT is termed "long R-P," whereas if this distance is short, it is termed "short R-P" (Figure 11–2).

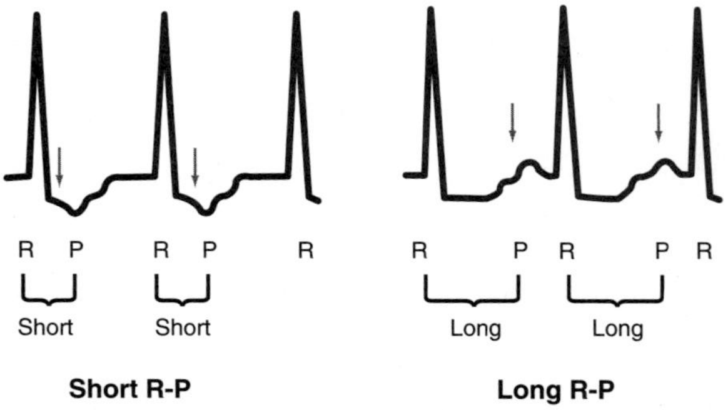

▲ **Figure 11–2.** *Short R-P* refers to a regular supraventricular tachycardia (SVT) where the R-P interval is shorter than the P-R interval. *Long R-P* refers to a regular SVT where the R-P interval is longer than the P-R interval.

SINUS TACHYCARDIA & SINUS NODE REENTRY

1. Sinus Tachycardia

ESSENTIALS OF DIAGNOSIS

- Onset and termination: gradual.
- Heart rate: over 100 to (220 – age) bpm.
- P wave: identical to normal sinus rhythm P wave.
- R-P relationship: long.

General Considerations

When the sinus node fires at a rate of more than 100 bpm, the rhythm is, with one exception, considered sinus tachycardia (see later section, Sinus Node Reentry). The onset and termination of sinus tachycardia are invariably gradual. The range for heart rate in sinus tachycardia is over 100 to (220 – age) bpm; faster rates usually imply a different cause. Confirming that the tachycardic P waves are identical in morphology and axis to the normal sinus rhythm P waves is essential to diagnosis. Like normal sinus rhythm, the R-P relationship in sinus tachycardia is typically long R-P, unless the patient has a very long P-R interval at baseline.

Sinus tachycardia is usually a normal physiologic response, activated when the body requires a higher heart rate to meet metabolic demands or maintain blood pressure. Common causes are exercise, hypotension, hypoxemia, heart failure, sepsis, fever, hyperthyroidism, fluid depletion, and blood loss.

The heart rate achieved is proportional to the intensity of the stimulus, but the rapidity with which the heart rate increases and decreases is a function of how quickly the stimulus is applied and withdrawn.

Treatment

Vagal maneuvers slow the tachycardia gradually but only while being performed; when the vagal stimulus is removed, the heart rate gradually returns to where it started.

Attempting to slow the heart rate pharmacologically can be detrimental because it counteracts the compensatory mechanism provided by tachycardia. Therefore, management is usually focused on treating the underlying cause of the sinus tachycardia.

2. Sinus Node Reentry

ESSENTIALS OF DIAGNOSIS

- Onset and termination: sudden.
- Heart rate: over 100–160 bpm.
- P wave: identical to normal sinus rhythm P wave.
- R-P relationship: long.

General Considerations

This uncommon reentrant rhythm accounts for less than 5% of SVTs. It uses the sinus node or perinodal tissue as a critical part of the reentrant circuit, producing P waves identical to those seen during normal sinus rhythm. The heart rate usually falls between 100 and 160 bpm. Like sinus tachycardia, the R-P relationship is typically long R-P. Unlike sinus tachycardia, sinus node reentry is initiated by an ectopic beat rather than a physiologic stimulus and possesses the characteristics typical of a reentrant circuit. Therefore, it begins and ends abruptly and responds to vagal maneuvers and pharmacologic interventions by terminating rather than slowing.

Treatment

The arrhythmia can be terminated quickly with intravenous adenosine, verapamil, or diltiazem, or via carotid massage. Long-term treatment uses β-blockers and calcium channel blockers. The largest reported series of patients treated with catheter ablation described success in all 10 patients. No complications were reported. Other smaller series found similar efficacy. Three-dimensional mapping can be helpful in ablation of sinus node reentry.

Yamabe H, Orita Y. Demonstration of the anatomical tachycardia circuit in sinoatrial node reentrant tachycardia: analysis using the entrainment method. *J Am Heart Assoc.* 2020 Jan 21;9(2):E014472. [PMID: 31928174]; PMCID: PMC7033835. doi: 10.1161/JAHA.119.014472.

ATRIAL FLUTTER

ESSENTIALS OF DIAGNOSIS

- Onset and termination: sudden.
- Heart rate: usually a multiple of 300.
- P waves: flutter waves at 250–340 bpm.
- R-P relationship: undefined due to flutter waves.
- Prominent neck vein pulsations of about 300/min.

General Considerations

Atrial flutter is usually associated with organic heart disease and is the second most common arrhythmia after atrial fibrillation in post–coronary artery bypass surgery patients, with an incidence of up to 33%. With a typical atrial rate of 300 bpm (range, 250–340 bpm), atrial flutter usually produces a "sawtooth" appearance (F waves). As is the case with atrial fibrillation (see Chapter 12), the ventricular rate depends on conduction through the AV node. Unlike atrial fibrillation, the ventricular impulses are transmitted at some integer fraction of the atrial rate. In rare circumstances, 1:1 conduction may occur. Fixed 2:1, 3:1, or 4:1 block is the usual scenario. However, variable block can also occur, leading to one of the three types of irregular SVTs (see Figure 11–1). If atrial flutter is suspected but F waves are not clearly visible, vagal maneuvers or pharmacologic agents, such as adenosine, can help unmask the flutter waves by enhancing the degree of AV block.

Pathophysiology

Atrial flutter occurs in a variety of forms; the most common is isthmus-dependent counterclockwise atrial flutter; followed by the isthmus-dependent clockwise atrial flutter; and then the atypical, non–isthmus-dependent variety. The counterclockwise flutter is recognized electrocardiographically by negative F waves in leads II, III, and aVF and positive F waves in lead V_1. The single reentrant wavefront proceeds up the interatrial septum, across the roof of the right atrium, down the lateral wall, and across the inferior wall. Clockwise flutter, on the other hand, has positive F waves in leads II, III, and aVF and negative F waves in lead V_1. The reentrant circuit in this case moves in the reverse direction. In both types of atrial flutter, the atrial rates usually range between 250 and 340 bpm.

Clinical Findings

Symptoms attributable to atrial flutter are secondary to the ventricular response in addition to any underlying cardiac diseases. Dizziness, palpitations, angina-type chest pain, dyspnea, weakness, fatigue, and, occasionally, syncope may be the presenting symptoms. In patients with poor left ventricular function, overt congestive heart failure may ensue.

Clinical evaluation is like that described for atrial fibrillation (see Chapter 12), but underlying heart disease is detected more often with atrial flutter than with atrial fibrillation.

Prevention

Several antiarrhythmic agents can prevent recurrences of atrial flutter. It appears that both class Ia and Ic agents are effective. Class III agents, such as sotalol and amiodarone, can also work very well. Dofetilide, a newer class III agent, which blocks the rapid form of the delayed rectifier current, Ik_r, has also been found effective in converting to sinus rhythm. Dofetilide administration requires initiation in the hospital and an ECG-monitored setting. Drugs that are contraindicated with its use include verapamil, ketoconazole, cimetidine, trimethoprim, prochlorperazine, megestrol, and hydrochlorothiazide. Regarding safety, dofetilide has an overall proarrhythmic event rate of approximately 0.9%, which is less than the 3.3% seen in patients with congestive heart failure or the 2.5% in patients with previous ventricular tachycardia.

It should be emphasized that an AV nodal blocking agent should be started before initiating a class I drug. If the AV node is unblocked, a type I agent could facilitate conduction of atrial flutter by improving nodal conduction or by slowing the flutter rate and paradoxically increasing the ventricular response.

Treatment

A. Conversion

Once the diagnosis of atrial flutter is made, assessment of the patient's status will dictate whether to perform cardioversion immediately. Immediate cardioversion can be accomplished with synchronized direct current (DC) cardioversion, rapid atrial pacing to interrupt the macroreentrant circuit, or intravenous infusion of an antiarrhythmic agent. For DC cardioversion, as little as 25 J may be all that is required; however, at least 50 J is recommended to avoid extra shocks, and 100 J will terminate almost all episodes of atrial flutter. The major drawback with DC cardioversion is the need to administer sedation.

Rapid atrial pacing is another method that may terminate this arrhythmia. Pacing is best performed in the right atrium at a rate faster than the atrial flutter rate, which allows the circuit to be entered by the pacing impulse. If the extrinsic pacing rate exceeds the rate that can be sustained through the zone of slow conduction, the flutter wavefront can be interrupted and will no longer be present when the pacing is stopped. If the patient has a pacemaker or implantable cardiac defibrillator with an atrial lead, pace termination can be done painlessly via the device. Of note, overdrive pacing may precipitate atrial fibrillation, which may terminate spontaneously. Should the atrial fibrillation persist, however, control of the ventricular response rate is typically easier when compared with atrial flutter.

Finally, rapid pharmacologic cardioversion can be considered with intravenous agents such as ibutilide. Ibutilide is a unique class III antiarrhythmic agent with a rate of conversion of approximately 60% in patients with atrial flutter of less than 45 days in duration. Cardioversion can be expected within 30 minutes of administration. The major complication with this agent is the development of torsades de pointes, which can occur in up to 12.5% of patients, with 1.7% requiring cardioversion for sustained polymorphic ventricular tachycardia. These occur primarily within the first hour after administration. For this reason, patients given ibutilide are typically kept on monitor for at least 4 hours after administration. Procainamide is another intravenous agent that can be given to pharmacologically convert atrial flutter.

B. Rate Control

In general, controlling the ventricular rate in atrial flutter is more difficult than in atrial fibrillation. β-Blockers and calcium channel blockers are moderately effective in controlling the rate. Digoxin is less helpful because it only weakly blocks AV node conduction. Intravenous amiodarone, which has some β-blocking effect, has been shown to be at least as efficacious as digoxin.

C. Catheter Ablation & Other Modalities

The reentrant circuit in typical atrial flutter includes an area of slow conduction called isthmus, which is bound by the tricuspid annulus, the inferior vena cava, and the os of the coronary sinus. Ablation in the isthmus region interrupts the reentrant circuit and has been shown to be highly successful (90–100%) in permanently eliminating atrial flutter. In cost-effective analysis, ablation appears to be the preferred approach over cardioversion and pharmacologic prevention. Recently, ablation for AFL in patients without prior AF was found to be associated with lower risks of all-cause mortality and CV events. Non–isthmus-dependent atypical atrial flutters can be more difficult to ablate. However, with current three-dimensional mapping systems, even these types of atrial flutter are being ablated with high success rates.

If attempts to ablate atrial flutter fail, the ventricular rate can be controlled by catheter ablation of the AV node or His bundle (AV junction) and pacemaker implantation. If the ejection fraction has been impaired by long-standing tachycardia, there may be a subsequent improvement in left ventricular function.

D. Stroke Prophylaxis

Atrial flutter is a recognized cause of peripheral embolization and stroke. The current recommendation is to treat patients with atrial flutter just as atrial fibrillation in terms of stroke prophylaxis. Many patients have bouts of atrial fibrillation even after successful atrial flutter ablation. Therefore, rigorous monitoring after atrial flutter ablation is recommended to determine which patients need long-term anticoagulant therapy.

January CT, Wann LS, Calkins H, et al. 2019 AHA/ACC/HRS Focused Update of the 2014 AHA/ACC/HRS Guideline for the Management of Patients With Atrial Fibrillation: A Report of the American College of Cardiology/American Heart Association Task Force on Clinical Practice Guidelines and the Heart Rhythm Society. *Heart Rhythm.* 2019 Aug;16(8):e66–e93. [PMID: 30703530]. doi: 10.1016/j.hrthm.2019.01.024. Epub 2019 JAN 28.

Yugo D, Chen YY, Linn YJ, et al. Long-term mortality and cardiovascular outcomes in patients with atrial flutter after catheter ablation. *Europace.* 2021 Dec 23:euab308. [PMID: 34939091]. doi: 10.1093/europace/euab308. epub ahead of print.

MULTIFOCAL ATRIAL TACHYCARDIA

ESSENTIALS OF DIAGNOSIS

- Heart rate: up to 150 bpm.
- P waves: three or more distinct P waves in a single lead.
- Variable P-P, P-R, and R-R intervals.

General Considerations

MAT is an irregular SVT that constitutes less than 1% of all arrhythmias. It is related to pulmonary disease in 60–85% of cases, with chronic obstructive pulmonary disease (COPD) exacerbation being the most common. In addition, MAT is precipitated by respiratory failure, acute decompensated cardiac function, and infection. It has also been reported to be associated with hypokalemia, hypomagnesemia, hyponatremia, pulmonary embolism, cancer, and valvular heart disease, and can also occur in the postoperative setting. It affects children and adults. Distention of the right atrium from elevated pulmonary pressures causes multiple ectopic foci to fire, with ventricular rates not usually exceeding 150 bpm. Whether this rhythm is due to abnormal automaticity or triggered activity is uncertain, but the ability of verapamil to suppress the ectopic atrial activity by virtue of its calcium channel–blocking properties supports the latter assumption.

Three ECG criteria must be met to diagnose MAT (Figure 11–3): (1) the presence of at least three distinct P-wave morphologies recorded in the same lead; (2) the absence of one dominant atrial pacemaker; and (3) varying P-P, P-R, and R-R intervals.

MAT is often misdiagnosed as atrial fibrillation. Although both are irregular, the former has clear P waves with an intervening isoelectric baseline. At times, MAT may progress to atrial fibrillation.

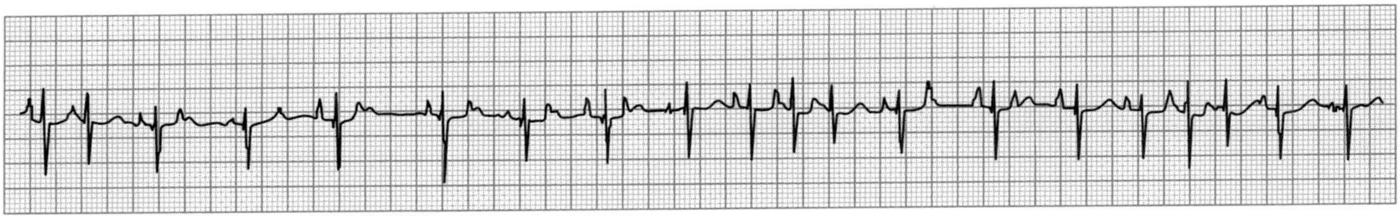

▲ **Figure 11–3.** Multifocal atrial tachycardia. The presence of at least three distinct P-wave morphologies, the absence of one dominant pacemaker focus, and varying P-P, R-R, and PR intervals establish the diagnosis.

Treatment

The primary treatment for MAT should be directed at the underlying disease state. Oral and intravenous verapamil and several formulations of intravenous β-blockers have been effective to varying degrees in either slowing the heart rate (without terminating the rhythm) or in converting the arrhythmia to sinus rhythm. Intravenous magnesium and potassium, even in patients with serum levels of these electrolytes within the normal range, convert a significant percentage of these patients to sinus rhythm. Ivabradine, a novel oral agent that blocks the I(f) cardiac channel, which is responsible for normal automaticity in pacemaker cells, may prove useful in MAT as one recent case report showed it decreased ectopy in an infant. Digoxin is not effective in treating MAT. Moreover, treatment with digoxin may precipitate digitalis intoxication. In addition, if the arrhythmia is secondary to delayed after-depolarizations, further aggravation may occur with digitalis because this drug increases delayed after-depolarizations. Medications that cause atrial irritability, such as theophylline and β-agonists, should be withdrawn whenever possible.

Application of radiofrequency energy for both AV node modification and AV node ablation with subsequent implantation of a pacemaker has been reported. The numbers of patients in the studies were very small. Nevertheless, ablation of the AV node has been shown to reduce symptomatic MAT, resulting in improved quality of life, reduced hospital admissions for recurrent symptomatic MAT, and improved left ventricular function.

Prognosis

Because of the severity of the precipitating underlying diseases, MAT portends a poor outcome. Mortality during the hospitalization when the arrhythmia is first diagnosed is between 30% and 60%, with death being attributed to the disease state rather than the tachycardia itself. In one study of patients with pulmonary disease who were admitted for acute respiratory failure, the in-hospital mortality rate for those with MAT was 87%, compared with 24% for those in a different rhythm.

Cohen MI, Cohen JA, Shope C, Stoller L, Collazo L. Ivabradine as a stabilising anti-arrhythmic agent for multifocal atrial tachycardia. *Cardiol Young*. 2020 Jun;30(6):899–902. [PMID: 32519627.] doi: 10.1017/S1047951120001195.

ATRIAL TACHYCARDIA

ESSENTIALS OF DIAGNOSIS

- Onset and termination: sudden.
- Heart rate: 100–180 bpm.
- P wave: distinct P waves that differ from sinus P waves.
- R-P relationship: long.

General Considerations

Atrial tachycardia originates from an ectopic site in the atrium, and therefore, the P waves are usually quite different than the sinus P waves. It has been demonstrated that these arrhythmias arise from well-defined anatomic regions, including the crista terminalis, the tricuspid and mitral annuli, the right and left atrial appendage, and the region within or surrounding the pulmonary veins. In situations where the P wave is identical to the sinus P wave, the SVT is usually designated to be sinus node reentry or sinus tachycardia. The onset of atrial tachycardia is typically sudden; however, there can be some acceleration at the very beginning, which is called the "warm-up" phase. Rates can range from 100 to 180 bpm and, rarely, over 200 bpm. The R-P relationship is usually long, unless there is a very long P-R interval, which can sometimes be appreciated on the baseline ECG. The episodes may either be brief and self-terminating or chronic and persistent, eventually leading to a tachycardia-induced cardiomyopathy if left untreated. Short nonsustained bursts of atrial tachycardia can be seen in 2–6% of young healthy adults on ambulatory ECG evaluations.

In patients with paroxysmal sustained atrial tachycardia, there is a higher likelihood of associated organic heart disease, including coronary artery disease, valvular heart disease, congenital heart disease, and other cardiomyopathies. Frequently, a transient automatic atrial tachycardia will be present, the cause of which can usually be determined from the associated clinical setting. Some of the most frequent causes include acute myocardial infarction (in which case, it is seen in 4–19% of patients), electrolyte disturbances (especially hypokalemia), chronic lung disease or pulmonary infection, acute alcohol ingestion, hypoxia, and use of cardiac stimulants (theophylline, cocaine).

The form that occurs almost exclusively, and not uncommonly, in children is a continuous tachycardia with heart rates of about 175 bpm. Symptoms can be severe, and congestive heart failure frequently develops as a result of a tachycardia-induced cardiomyopathy. The arrhythmia may be transient in younger children, but when it persists in older children, it should be treated. Fortunately, if the tachycardia can be terminated, cardiac function returns to normal. When it appears in adults, the continuous variety manifests milder symptoms.

Atrial tachycardias may have an automatic, triggered, or microreentrant mechanism. Although precisely defining the basic mechanism of a particular atrial tachycardia may be difficult, understanding their basic principles may help with choosing therapy.

Treatment

A. Pharmacologic Therapy

Although there are no large-scale trials in the medical treatment of atrial tachycardias, reported data show that β-blockers and calcium channel blockers are at least partially effective, particularly if the underlying mechanism of the tachycardia is abnormal automaticity or triggered activity. Because of their safety profile, these drugs are usually first-line medical therapy.

Other antiarrhythmic drugs may be effective in treating some patients with atrial tachycardias. However, there are no large-scale trials comparing the drugs or even trials comparing drugs to placebo. Therefore, drug therapy is largely empiric, and drug choice is determined more by side effect profile and risk of proarrhythmia than by suspected efficacy. The use of class Ic antiarrhythmic drugs may be successful. Flecainide and propafenone are often well tolerated in patients without structural heart disease and thus can be considered a reasonable first-line antiarrhythmic therapy. Class Ib agents are generally not effective for atrial tachycardias; however, there may be a small subset of lidocaine-sensitive atrial tachycardias in which mexiletine may be effective. Sotalol may also be effective, in part because of its inherent β-blocker (class II) properties and may provide rate control during recurrences. Nevertheless, because sotalol also has class III properties, it will prolong the QT interval and may predispose patients to torsades de pointes. Amiodarone may be effective, especially in resistant tachycardias. Since it is usually not proarrhythmic, amiodarone is generally used as first-line drug therapy in patients with depressed left ventricular function. Newer class III drugs, such as dofetilide, may be effective for atrial tachycardias, but there are few data about their use in atrial arrhythmias, except atrial fibrillation and atrial flutter. Recently, ivabradine has also been shown to be helpful, especially in incessant forms of atrial tachycardia.

B. Ablation

Ablation for atrial tachycardias has been proven safe and effective, with reported success rates between 77% and 100%. It also has been shown to improve patient quality of life. Therefore, ablation should be indicated for all symptomatic patients who have persistent symptoms despite medical therapy or intolerable side effects from medicines. Furthermore, patients who are not willing to undergo medical therapy should also be considered. Recently, the use of three-dimensional mapping systems has significantly improved ablation by decreasing fluoroscopic time, mapping time, and number of radiofrequency applications needed for success.

Banavalikar B, Shenthar J, Padmanabhan D, et al. Clinical and electrophysiological correlates of incessant ivabradine-sensitive atrial tachycardia. *Circ Arrhythm Electrophysiol.* 2019 Aug;12(8):e007387. [PMID: 31345093.] doi: 10.1161/CIRCEP.119.007387. Epub 2019 Jul 26.

ATRIOVENTRICULAR NODAL REENTRANT TACHYCARDIA

ESSENTIALS OF DIAGNOSIS

- Onset and termination: sudden.
- Heart rate: usually 120–200 bpm but can be faster; neck pulsations correspond to heart rate.
- P waves: retrograde P waves; P waves not visible in 50–60% of cases.
- R-P relationship: short, if P waves visible.

General Considerations

Atrioventricular nodal reentrant tachycardia (AVNRT) is more common in women than in men. Heart rates usually fall in the range of 120–200 bpm, although rates up to 250 bpm have been recorded. Palpitations are almost universally reported. Diuresis, noted with other supraventricular arrhythmias, is significantly more common in AVNRT and has been correlated with elevated right atrial pressures and elevated atrial natriuretic peptide. Neck pulsations are common (Brugada phenomenon) and are secondary to simultaneous contraction of the atria and ventricles against closed mitral and tricuspid valves. Dizziness and lightheadedness can occur, but frank syncope is very unusual. Sudden death has been reported but is extremely rare. Although symptoms may occur at any age, the distribution of when the tachycardia and symptoms commonly start appears to be bimodal. The initial episode may begin during the second decade of life, only to disappear and then reappear during the fourth and fifth decades of life.

Pathophysiology

Conduction from the right atrium to the ventricles is normally over a singular AV nodal pathway, with no route of reentry back into the atrium. In persons with dual AV nodal pathways, an atrial impulse may travel antegrade from the atrium over one limb of the AV node and then back to the atrium over another limb in a retrograde fashion. When only one cycle occurs, a single echo beat in the form of a retrograde P wave may be seen on the ECG. If this echo beat can again penetrate the AV node antegrade, the cycle can perpetuate itself, leading to AVNRT. It is estimated that dual AV nodal pathways exist in up to one-fourth of the population, but only a fraction of these people ever manifest this tachycardia.

If each limb of the circuit conducted impulses equally, echo beats and sustained AVNRT would not occur. An atrial impulse traveling down both limbs at the same speed would cause each limb to be refractory when that impulse reached the bottom of the node, preventing the impulse in each limb from going back up the other. Instead, the limbs have varying conduction speeds and refractory periods. The faster conducting limb, called the β or fast pathway, has a longer refractory period, whereas the reverse is true for the second limb, called the α or slow pathway. A premature atrial or ventricular depolarization is often the trigger of AVNRT. The typical AVNRT circuit occurs with a self-perpetuating impulse that travels down the slow pathway and up the fast pathway.

Conduction up the fast pathway is usually so rapid that retrograde atrial depolarization is simultaneous or almost simultaneous with antegrade ventricular activation. This causes the low-amplitude P wave to become obscured in the much higher amplitude QRS complex. Therefore, the P wave is not visible 50–60% of the time. In 20–30% of cases, the P wave distorts the terminal portion of the QRS causing a pseudo-S wave in the inferior leads and a pseudo-R′ in lead V_1, and in approximately 10% of cases, the P wave distorts the QRS complex (Figure 11–4). Since the P wave usually occurs simultaneous to or just after the QRS, the common variety of AVNRT is considered a short R-P tachycardia.

AVNRT, once initiated, can perpetuate itself without the participation of either the atria or ventricles. Therefore, on rare occasions, the tachycardia can occur with a 2:1 block in either direction, leading to two atrial depolarizations for every ventricular depolarization or two ventricular depolarizations for every atrial depolarization.

Prevention

Prevention of AVNRT is directed at slowing or blocking conduction in either the fast or slow pathway. Typical AV nodal blocking agents such as β-blockers, calcium channel blockers, and digoxin are most effective on the antegrade slow pathway. The more potent class Ia antiarrhythmic drugs may be necessary to inhibit conduction in the retrograde fast pathway. Class Ic drugs and amiodarone and sotalol (class III) affect both pathways.

Treatment

A. Vagal Maneuvers

Vagal maneuvers should be considered, barring any contraindications, before embarking on medical therapy. The Valsalva maneuver and carotid sinus massage can immediately terminate the tachycardia by increasing refractory time in the AV node. In patients older than 50 years, bruits should be ruled out before carotid sinus massage to avoid embolic stroke. Medications may render the arrhythmia more susceptible to termination with vagal maneuvers. Therefore, these can be attempted immediately after each round of drug therapy if the tachycardia persists.

B. Pharmacologic Therapy

Terminating an acute episode of AVNRT in the hospital setting has been made simpler with the availability of intravenous adenosine. Adenosine temporarily stops conduction in the AV node, thereby terminating the reentrant circuit in AVNRT. It is fast acting, typically reaching and acting on the AV node within seconds of administration. With a clinical half-life of 10 seconds, commonly reported sensations such as breathlessness, chest heaviness, and flushing disappear quickly. The routine dosage is 6 mg followed by up to two more boluses of 12 mg. If adenosine is ineffective, intravenous verapamil can be used, but it takes longer to act. Diltiazem, given as intravenous bolus, can also be effective in aborting the tachycardia. Hypotension occurs with about a 10% incidence and is usually rapidly reversed with fluid administration. Although intravenous β-blockers, procainamide, and digoxin are other second-line choices, they can be advantageous in recurrent cases because of their slower clearance from the body.

C. Catheter Ablation

Radiofrequency lesions delivered via an ablation catheter can be directed at either the fast or slow pathway; the latter is much preferred since it is associated with a lower risk of complete heart block.

The inferior origin of the slow pathway is variable within the triangle of Koch, but it is usually anterior and superior to (and sometimes within) the os of the coronary sinus. These anatomic landmarks and gross intracardiac electrogram patterns can be used to position the ablation catheter for successful ablation of the slow pathway. The fast pathway is left unaltered and can still be used for transmission of sinus impulses to the ventricles. Long-term freedom from recurrent AVNRT is about 95%, and the risk of complete heart block as a result of inadvertent fast pathway or nodal damage is 0–5%.

A relatively new form of ablation is cryoablation, using a supercooling catheter, which can reversibly or permanently damage endocardial tissue. This novel approach allows for testing the acceptability of a particular ablation site. Should heart block occur prior to irreversible tissue damage, then rewarming can be performed with no untoward effects.

Larroussi L, Badhwar N. Atrioventricular nodal reentrant tachycardia with 2:1 atrioventricular block. *Card Electrophysiol Clin.* 2016;8(1):51–55. [PMID: 26920169]

JUNCTIONAL TACHYCARDIA

ESSENTIALS OF DIAGNOSIS

- Onset and termination: gradual.
- Heart rate: 70–120 bpm.
- P waves: retrograde.
- R-P relationship: short, if P waves visible.

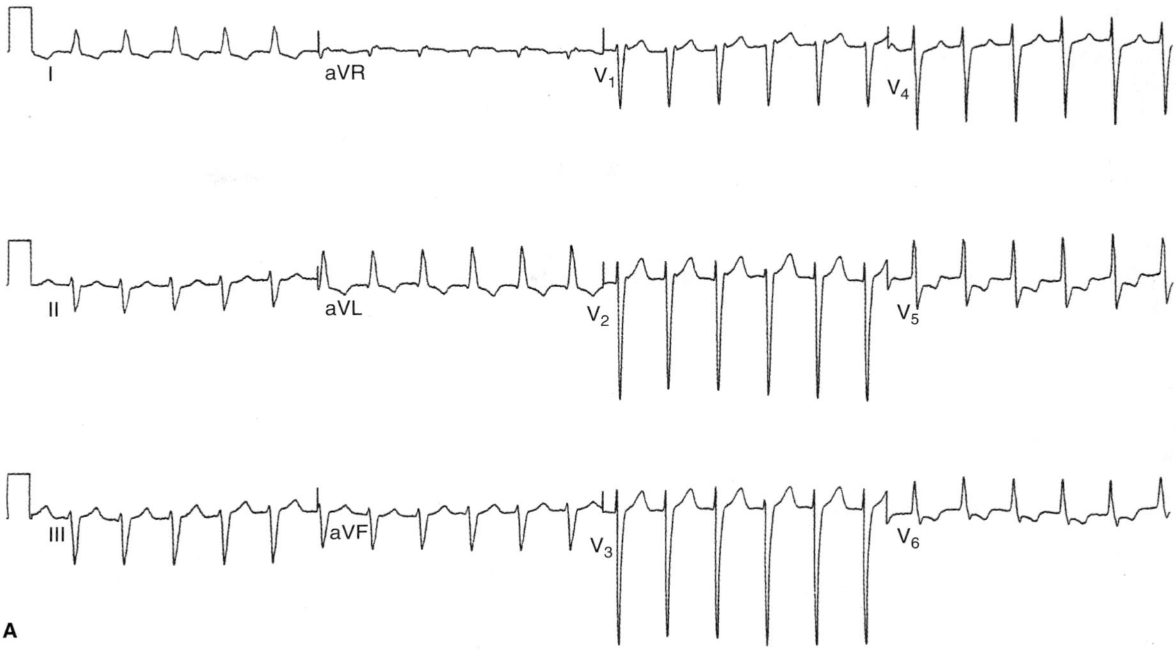

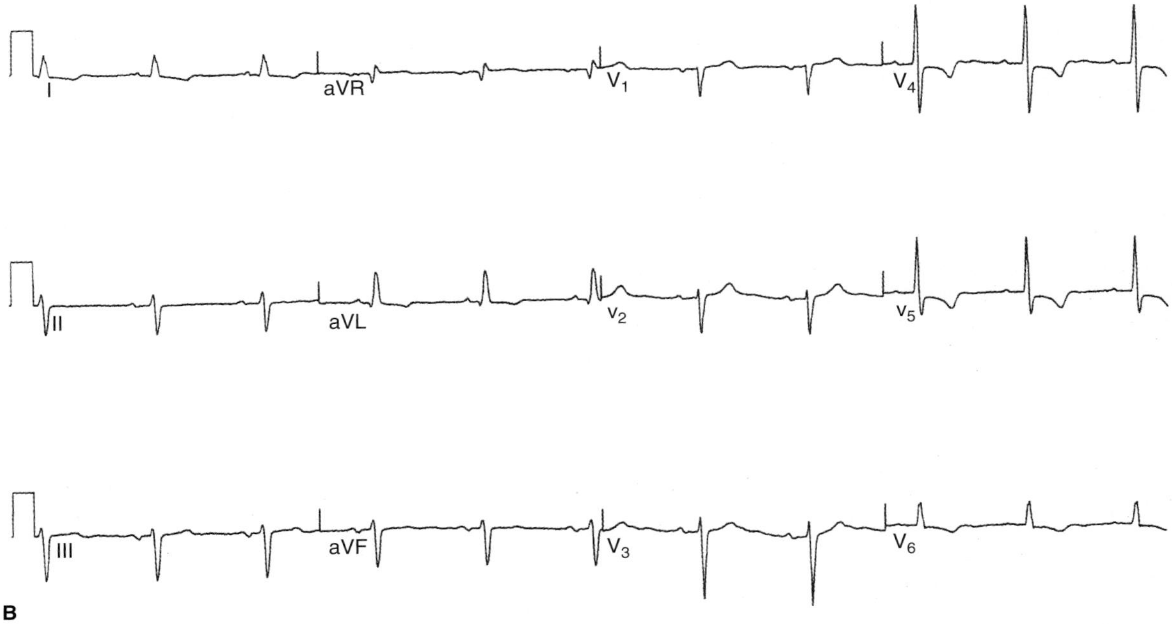

▲ **Figure 11–4.** **A:** Supraventricular tachycardia without easily identifiable P waves but with pseudo-R′ in lead V_1 compatible with atrioventricular nodal reentrant tachycardia. **B:** Post conversion tracing. Note normal QRS in lead V_1 when patient displays normal sinus rhythm.

General Considerations

Unlike AVNRT, which presents with recurrent tachycardia episodes of sudden onset, junctional tachycardia, which is sometimes also called nonparoxysmal junctional tachycardia (NPJT), usually starts gradually and sometimes almost imperceptibly. It is easily differentiated from AVNRT by a heart rate between 70 and 120 bpm, gradual onset and termination, and lack of termination with vagal maneuvers. Although heart rates of less than 100 bpm can be seen, it is considered a tachycardia because the rates are faster than the 40–60 bpm seen with a junctional escape rhythm.

Clinical Findings

The heart rate at onset is just slightly faster than that of the rhythm preceding it, with gradual acceleration until the final rate is achieved. AV dissociation is common, occurring in 85% of cases caused by digoxin (see following discussion). When the conduction to the atria is intact, retrograde P waves may appear immediately before or after the QRS complex, or they may be obscured within the QRS. Discharge from the AV node is regular, but if antegrade second-degree AV block (almost always the result of digoxin excess), exit block, or atrial capture beats coexist with junctional tachycardia, the rhythm will appear irregular. Enhanced vagal tone or vagolytic agents will either slow down or speed up the arrhythmia, respectively.

Usually seen in the setting of organic heart disease, the cause of this rhythm is almost always identifiable. At one time, digoxin excess accounted for up to 85% of cases of junctional tachycardia. With diminished use of digoxin, this arrhythmia has become less common. Nevertheless, in patients being treated with digoxin for atrial fibrillation, clinicians should suspect this arrhythmia when the ECG demonstrates a regularized ventricular response. Acute inferior infarction accounts for some junctional tachycardias outside of digoxin. This rhythm may be present in up to 10% of all infarcts in this location, with onset usually within the first 24 hours and disappearance in several days. Junctional tachycardia may follow open heart surgery (valve replacement more often than bypass surgery), or it can be caused by myocarditis (especially rheumatic) and, rarely, congenital heart disease. In all cases, the tachycardia resolves along with the acute underlying event or with digoxin withdrawal.

Treatment

Treatment is usually directed at the underlying causative factor. Because the rhythm rarely causes deleterious hemodynamic effects, treatment of the rhythm itself is usually not indicated. If digoxin toxicity is the cause, it should be withdrawn. If digoxin is not the cause, digoxin, β-blockers, or calcium channel blockers can be used to slow down the rate, if necessary. Catheter ablation can also be performed, but it carries a risk of complete heart block since the origin of the arrhythmia is near the AV node. Cryoablation has also been used in this setting and may be safer.

Di Biase L, Gianni C, Bagliani G, Padeletti L. Arrhythmias involving the atrioventricular junction. *Card Electrophysiol Clin.* 2017 Sep;9(3):435–452. [PMID: 28838549]. doi: 10.1016/j.ccep.2017.05.004.

ATRIOVENTRICULAR RECIPROCATING TACHYCARDIA

ESSENTIALS OF DIAGNOSIS

- Onset and termination: sudden.
- Heart rate: 140–250 bpm.
- P wave: ectopic.
- R-P relationship: short.
- Delta wave on baseline ECG if bypass tract conducts antegrade.

1. Bypass Tracts & Wolff-Parkinson-White Syndrome (WPW)

General Considerations

Congenital bands of tissue that can conduct impulses but lie outside the normal conduction system are called accessory pathways, or bypass tracts. These pathways are responsible for a variety of mechanistically distinct tachycardias by providing preferential conduction between different areas within the heart.

Epidemiology

Accessory pathways are quite prevalent in the general population, with a 2:1 male-to-female predominance. Evidence of an antegrade conducting accessory pathway on baseline ECG (WPW pattern), is seen in 0.1–0.3%. The presence of a bypass tract, however, does not mean that a tachyarrhythmia is a certainty because less than half of persons with documented bypass tracts ever sustain an arrhythmia. The actual number depends on the population studied and varies from 13% in a healthy outpatient population to 80% in the hospital setting.

Approximately 5–10% of patients with documented bypass tracts have concomitant structural heart disease. Ebstein anomaly is the most common, accounting for 25–50% of the anomalies in this group. Of patients with Ebstein anomaly, 8–10% have multiple bypass tracts, mostly on the right side. The association of right-sided accessory pathways with structural heart disease is strong: 45% of patients with right-sided (and only 5% of those with left-sided) pathways display some type of heart disease.

A familial tendency toward bypass tracts has been seen in some instances, with a fourfold to tenfold increase in incidence among first-degree family members.

Pathophysiology

A. Anatomy

Anatomically, the atria and ventricles are in apposition, separated by an invagination known as the AV groove. Paroxysmal tachycardias mediated by accessory pathways that cross this groove and electrically link the atria and ventricles, when combined with a short P-R interval (< 0.12 seconds), a wide QRS, and secondary repolarization abnormalities, define the Wolff-Parkinson-White syndrome. When this ECG pattern is seen without the tachycardia, it is called Wolff-Parkinson-White pattern or ventricular preexcitation.

Although the most common site of insertion is between the lateral aspect of the left atrium and left ventricular myocardium, pathways can cross the AV groove anywhere in its course (except the region between the aortic and mitral valves) to connect the left or right atrium to its respective ventricle (Figure 11–5). In noting the distribution of accessory pathways, 46–60% are in the left free wall, 25% within the posteroseptal space, 13–21% in the right free wall, and 2% in the anteroseptal space. Females have right-sided accessory pathways and Asians have right anterior accessory pathways more frequently than other groups, suggesting that pathogenesis of these pathways has a genetic component. Each location produces a distinct ECG pattern (Figure 11–6), but in the 13% of patients with two or more bypass tracts, the ECG tracing can be confounding and show multiple QRS morphologies.

B. Cardiac Electrical Conduction

Unlike the AV node, whose function is to delay atrial impulses en route to the ventricles, most bypass tracts conduct rapidly and without delay, which accounts for the short P-R interval often seen in sinus rhythm in these patients.

Impulses that reach the ventricles over a bypass tract spread through cell-to-cell conduction within the myocardium, activating the ventricles in series rather than in parallel. This relatively slow process is manifested as a wide QRS complex.

Sinus impulses are not restricted to using the AV node or the bypass tract only to reach the lower chambers. Instead, both may contribute to ventricular activation. This produces a QRS that is initially wide, reflecting conduction over the bypass tract, with the latter portion of the QRS appearing normal and narrow, indicating that the remainder of the ventricle has been depolarized via the normal conduction system (the AV node and His-Purkinje system). The initial slurred upstroke of the QRS, a delta wave, indicates ventricular preexcitation, which can be defined as ventricular

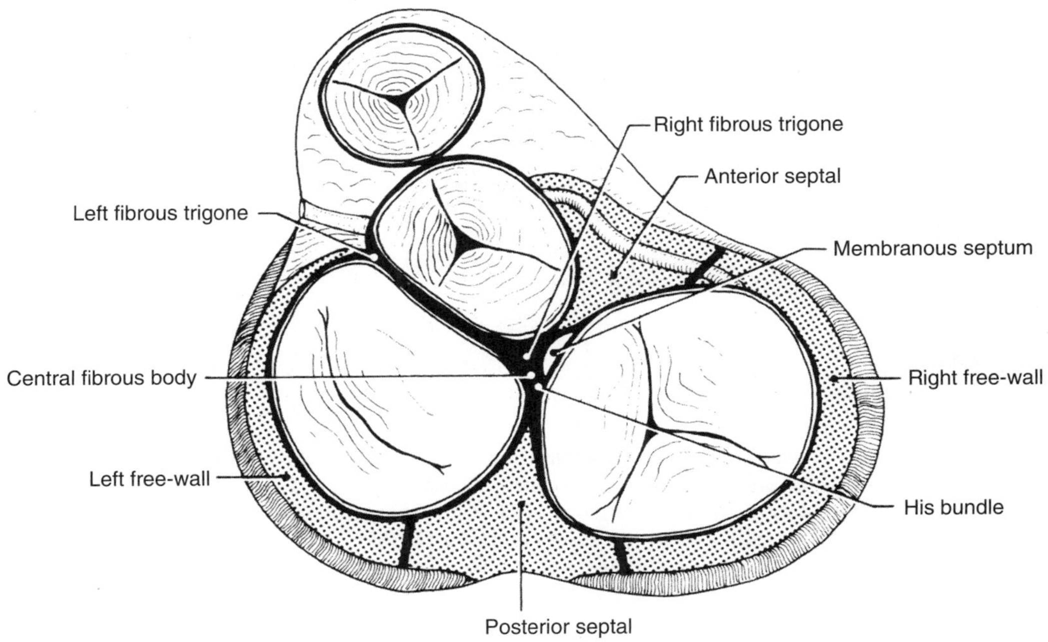

▲ **Figure 11–5.** Cross-sectional diagram of the atrioventricular groove. Atrioventricular bypass tracts may cross the groove anywhere in its course except in the region bounded by the left and right fibrous trigones. (Reproduced with permission from Cox JL, et al. Experience with 118 consecutive patients undergoing operation for the Wolff-Parkinson-White syndrome. *J Thorac Cardiovasc Surg.* 1985;90(4):490–501.)

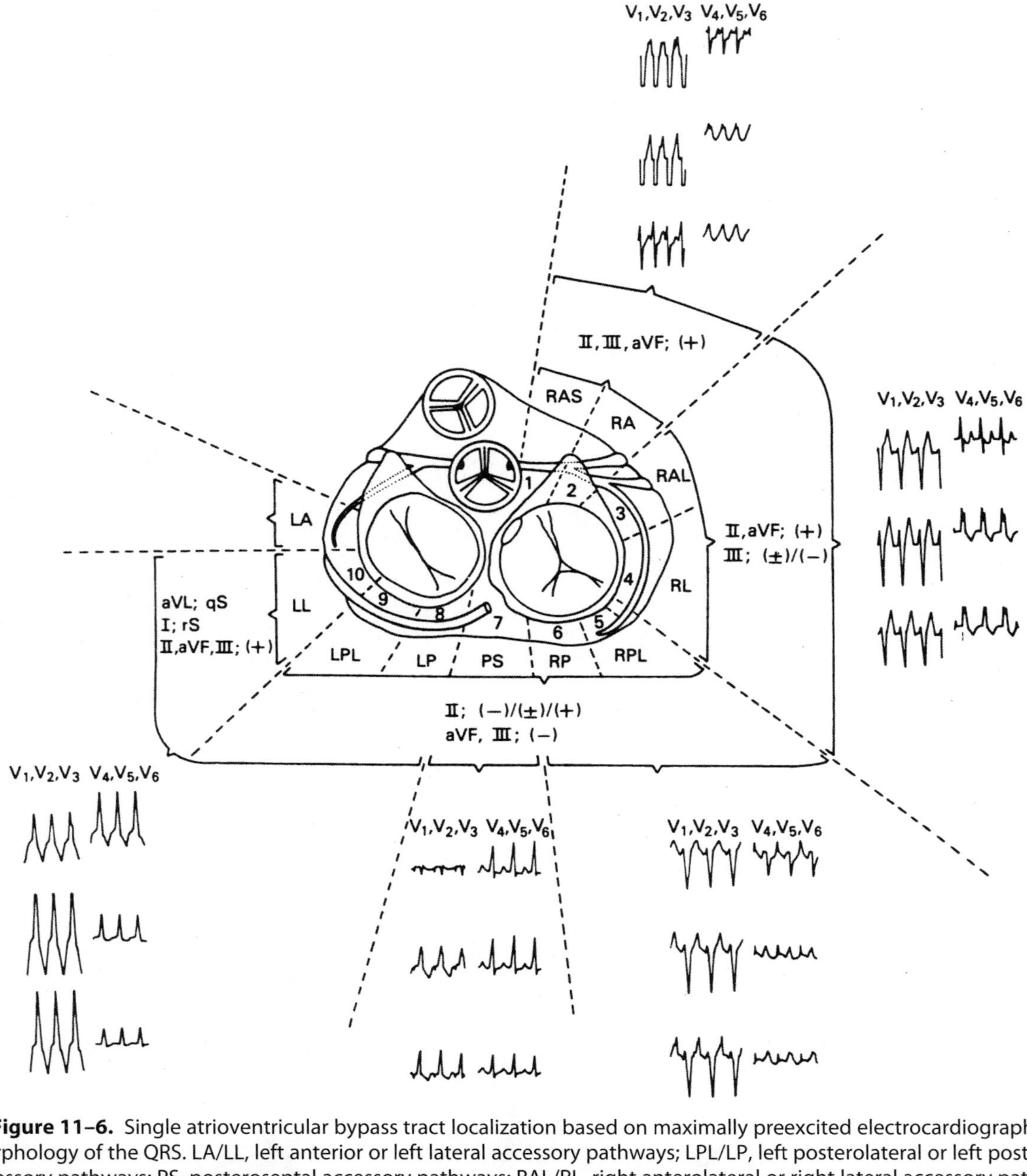

▲ **Figure 11–6.** Single atrioventricular bypass tract localization based on maximally preexcited electrocardiographic morphology of the QRS. LA/LL, left anterior or left lateral accessory pathways; LPL/LP, left posterolateral or left posterior accessory pathways; PS, posteroseptal accessory pathways; RAL/RL, right anterolateral or right lateral accessory pathways; RAS/RA, right anteroseptal or right anterior accessory pathways; RP/RPL, right posterior or right posterolateral accessory pathways; +, positive delta wave; –, negative delta wave; ±, isoelectric delta wave. (Reproduced with permission from Fananapazir L, et al. Importance of Preexcited QRS Morphology During Induced Atrial Fibrillation to the Diagnosis and Localization of Multiple Accessory Pathways. *Circulation*. 1990;81(2):578–585.)

depolarization that begins earlier than would be expected by conduction over the AV node alone. The degree of preexcitation and P-R shortening depends on the proportion of ventricular activation occurring over the AV node and the bypass tract. This, in turn, is related to two factors. The first is the conduction velocity of the bypass tract relative to the AV node. The faster the bypass tract can conduct impulses to the ventricles in relation to the AV node, the earlier the ventricle will preexcite, and vice versa. The second factor is the location of the tract, and more specifically, its proximity to the sinus node and AV node. A sinus impulse will encounter a right-sided free-wall bypass tract earlier than it will the AV node, and this favors a short P-R interval with a high degree of ventricular preexcitation (Figure 11–7A). On the other hand, a sinus beat will encounter the AV node early in its course while traveling to a pathway in the lateral left atrium, allowing ventricular activation to occur primarily by the normal conduction system. A narrow, minimally (if at all) preexcited QRS complex with a normal or near-normal P-R interval may be seen (Figure 11–7B). Changes in autonomic tone, by modifying the conduction velocity and refractoriness over both the pathway and the AV node, can produce varying degrees of preexcitation at different times in the same patient (Figure 11–7C).

If the delta wave axis of a maximally preexcited beat is discordant from the accompanying preexcited QRS axis, or if more than one preexcited QRS morphology is noted, there may be multiple bypass tracts.

C. Mechanism

1. Atrioventricular reciprocating tachycardia (AVRT)— An inherent property of accessory pathways is their ability to conduct in a retrograde direction more easily than antegrade. The AV node, on the other hand, conducts more efficiently antegrade. For this reason, reentrant rhythms in this setting most commonly use the AV node to go from atrium to ventricle and the bypass tract to return to the atrium. This mechanism is called orthodromic AVRT (antegrade conduction over the AV node) which accounts for 70–80% of arrhythmias in patients with AV bypass tracts, with heart rates of 140–250 bpm (Figure 11–8). Antidromic AVRT, in which the atrial impulse is carried to the ventricle over the bypass tract and reenters the atrium via

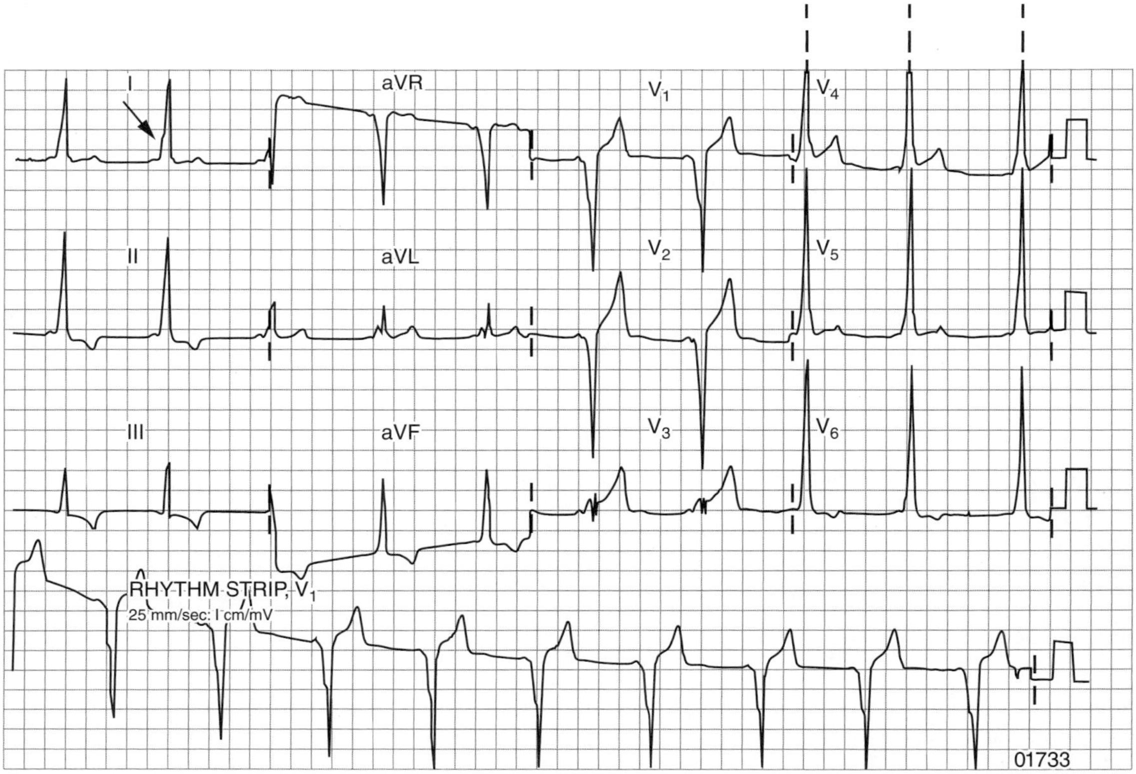

A

▲ **Figure 11–7.** Ventricular preexcitation over a bypass tract in sinus rhythm. Note the short P-R interval. **A:** Right anterior bypass tract. The delta wave is positive in most leads (*arrow*) and negative in a VR and V_1–V_3.

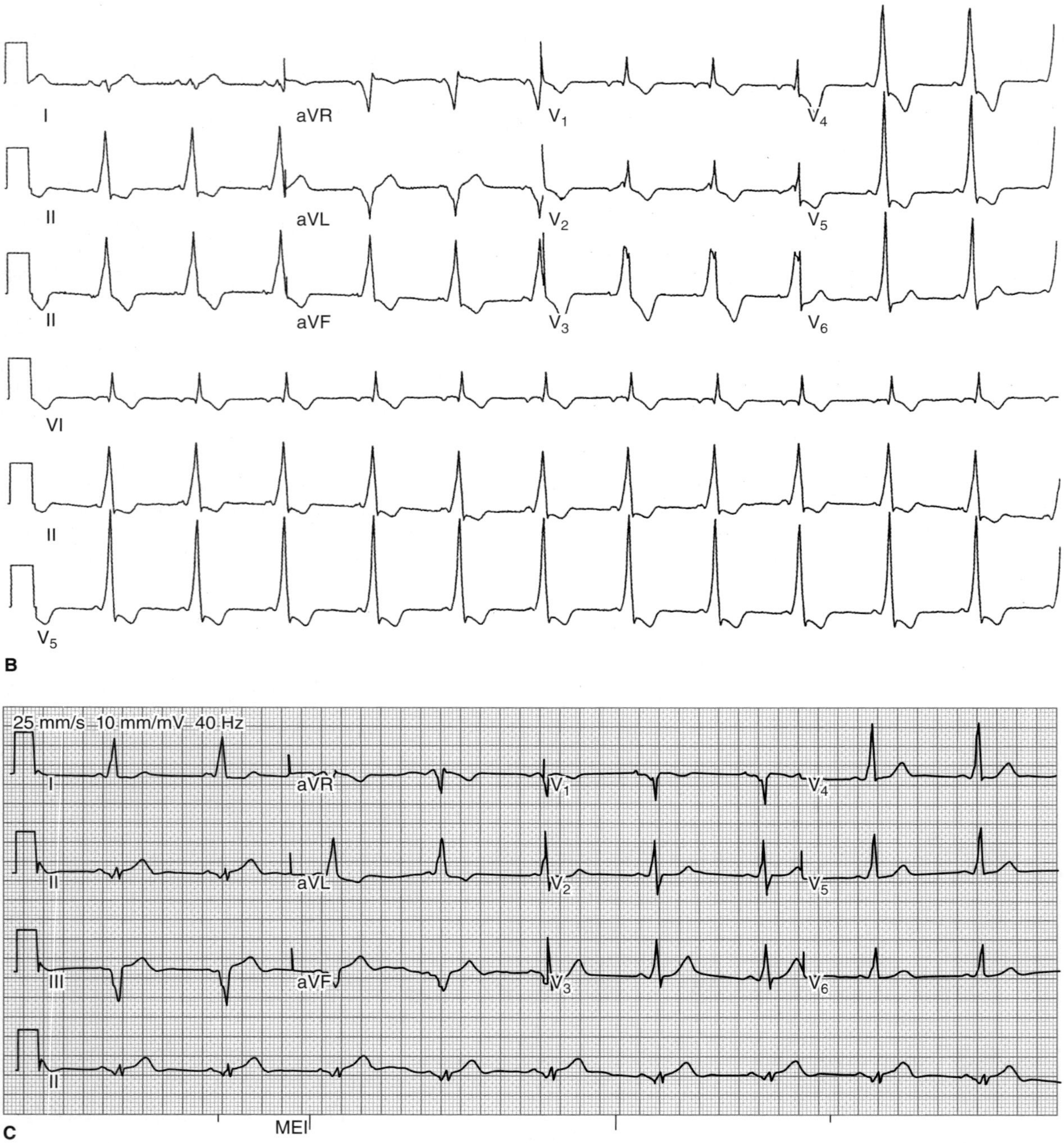

▲ **Figure 11–7.** (*Continued*) **B:** Left lateral bypass tract. The isoelectric delta wave in V_1 gives the appearance of a normal PR interval. Inspection of the simultaneously recorded rhythm strip leads (*lower three panels*) reveals delta wave onset to be at the end of the P wave in leads II and V_5. **C:** Posterior septal bypass tract. A short time after this tracing was obtained, the patient exhibited minimal to no preexcitation. This was due to fluctuations in autonomic tone causing enhanced conduction through the AV node.

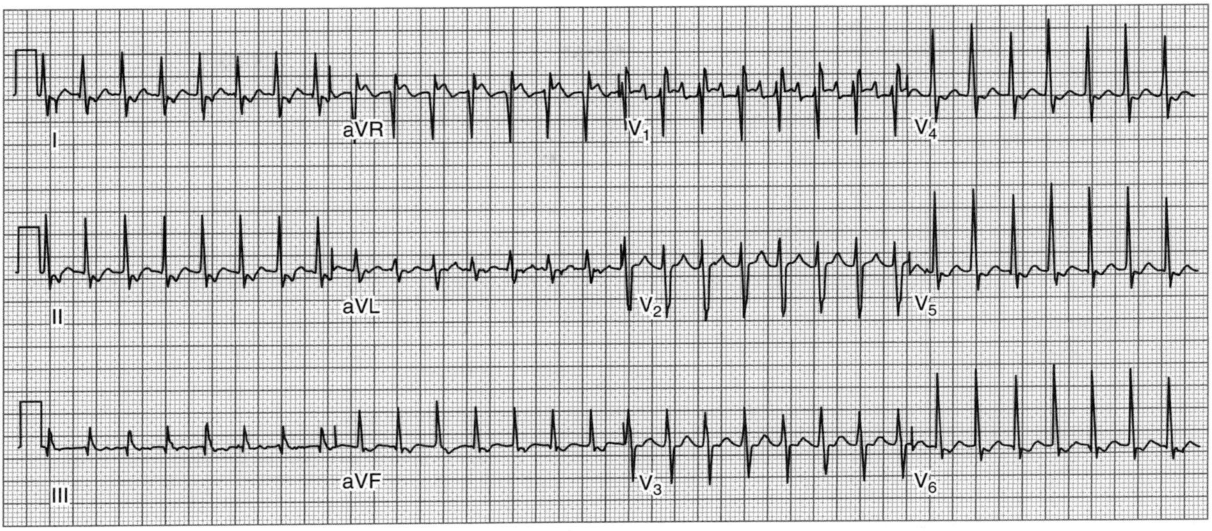

▲ **Figure 11–8.** Orthodromic atrioventricular reciprocating tachycardia (AVRT) in a patient with a left-sided bypass tract. The circuit conducts from atria to ventricles over the AV node and from ventricles to atria retrograde over the bypass tract. This mechanism accounts for the narrow QRS and the retrograde P waves inscribed in the early portion of the T waves. Although the electrocardiogram with atrioventricular nodal reentrant tachycardia (AVNRT) may appear similar, a ventriculoatrial conduction time of more than 100 ms, as measured from QRS onset to P-wave onset, greatly favors orthodromic AVRT. The time in this tracing is 110 ms.

retrograde conduction over the AV node, is rare, occurring in approximately 5–10% of cases. Because conduction to the ventricles during orthodromic AVRT occurs over the normal conduction system, the QRS is narrow, unless bundle branch aberrancy is present. During antidromic AVRT, the QRS is wide and maximally preexcited as a result of the complete lack of AV nodal contribution to ventricular depolarization. When two or more bypass tracts are present, each tract may act as the antegrade or retrograde limb (or both), especially with involvement of the AV node. There is a higher incidence of ventricular fibrillation in patients with multiple accessory pathways. In addition, multiple pathways are more common in patients with antidromic SVT and in patients with Ebstein anomaly.

Tachycardia is usually initiated by a premature atrial or ventricular beat. In orthodromic tachycardia, a premature atrial beat conducts down the AV node to depolarize the ventricle, and the bypass tract carries the impulse back to the atrium (Figure 11–9). A ventricular premature beat finding the AV node refractory might initiate an identical tachycardia by first conducting up the bypass tract to the atrium. Antidromic tachycardia initiates in an identical fashion but with a reversed direction of conduction.

Atrial fibrillation accounts for only 19–38% of arrhythmias in the population with accessory pathways, but it is potentially more lethal than the reciprocating tachycardias discussed earlier. It is more common in patients with antegrade conducting accessory pathways and in pathways with a short antegrade refractory period. By virtue of their short refractory periods, bypass tracts (unlike the AV node) have the potential to conduct very rapidly to the ventricles at ventricular rates of 250–350 bpm (Figure 11–10) with the possibility of degeneration to ventricular fibrillation. A reputed marker for sudden death in patients with atrial fibrillation is a shortest preexcited R-R interval of ≤ 250 ms (corresponding to a heart rate of ≥ 240 bpm) between two fully preexcited beats. The finding of a short R-R interval has a low positive predictive value, however, because sudden death in this syndrome is still rare.

During atrial fibrillation, the ECG reveals an irregularly irregular rhythm with QRS complexes of varying morphologies, representing conduction to the ventricles via the AV node (normally conducted narrow complexes), the bypass tract (wide, preexcited complexes), and both (fusion beats, harboring elements of both the normally conducted and preexcited beats). In this setting, the bypass tract may be called a bystander since it is not integral to the tachycardia. Patients with AV bypass tracts have a higher incidence of atrial fibrillation than the general population, possibly because of the degeneration of reentrant tachycardia or of microreentry within the atrial portion of the bypass tract. It has been shown that ablation of the bypass tract can frequently also eliminate atrial fibrillation.

2. Concealed bypass tracts—Between 15% and 50% of patients with no evidence of preexcitation during sinus rhythm are found to have bypass tracts that conduct only in

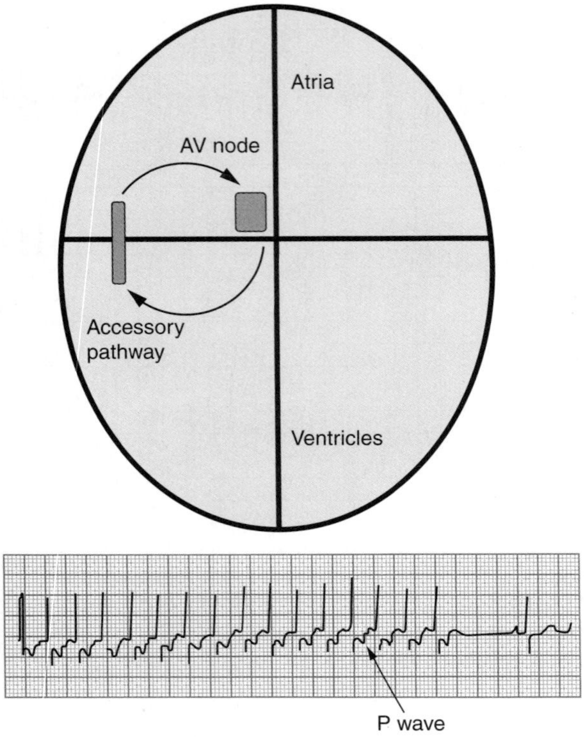

▲ **Figure 11–9.** The reentry circuit of orthodromic atrioventricular (reciprocating) tachycardia (AVRT). The atrioventricular (AV) node serves as the antegrade limb of the reentry circuit, and an accessory pathway serves as the retrograde limb. In this case, the accessory pathway is located in the free wall of the right ventricle. The wave of depolarization travels from the AV node to the accessory pathway through the ventricle and from the accessory pathway to the AV node through the atrium. Because the ventricles are depolarized by the normal conduction system, the QRS is narrow unless there is a bundle branch block. Also shown is an ECG example of orthodromic AVRT, at a rate of about 210 bpm. A P wave is present in the left half of the RR cycle (*arrow*) because retrograde conduction through the accessory pathway is more rapid than antegrade conduction through the AV node.

the retrograde direction. Concealed bypass tracts (their presence cannot be detected by standard ECG) do not display delta waves on the ECG during sinus rhythm, but they can still support an orthodromic AVRT and account for about 30% of orthodromic tachycardias.

Differentiating orthodromic AVRT from AVNRT on the ECG can be difficult. The incidence of both tachycardias being operative at different times in the same person is reported to be between 1.7% and 7%. Therefore, although the presence of a delta wave on the nontachycardic tracing makes it statistically unlikely that AVNRT was the documented tachycardia, it does not exclude the possibility completely.

Because of the simultaneous atrial and ventricular activation that occurs during AVNRT, the P waves formed as a result of retrograde conduction to the atrium are usually obscured by or merged with the QRS complex. Likewise, because of the short retrograde conduction time via the bypass tract, orthodromic AVRT usually is a short R-P tachycardia, albeit the R-P interval is typically longer than with AVNRT (see Figure 11–8). In AVRT, the P waves are usually located within the ST segment and are not obscured or merged with the QRS.

Treatment

A. Vagal Maneuvers

The management of orthodromic AVRT or antidromic AVRT is like that of AVNRT. Since the AV node is an integral part of the reentry circuit in AVRT, blocking the AV node terminates the tachycardia. Therefore, vagal maneuvers such as the Valsalva maneuver or carotid sinus massage can be tried first.

B. Pharmacologic Therapy

Intravenous adenosine almost always terminates these tachycardias. Other AV nodal blocking agents such as β-blockers, calcium channel blockers, and digoxin can also be helpful. Just as in AVNRT, vagal maneuvers can be retried after each dose of these longer-acting AV nodal blocking agents.

In contrast to orthodromic or antidromic AVRT, patients with atrial fibrillation or atrial flutter and a bystander bypass tract should **not** be given AV nodal blocking agents. This point is crucial since these types of medicines can precipitate ventricular fibrillation. Blocking the AV node promotes conduction down the bypass tract, making all the complexes wide. Furthermore, the bypass tract can often conduct faster than the AV node, increasing ventricular rates to sometimes over 200 bpm. The aberrant conduction and rapid rate can lead to disorganized ventricular conduction, resulting in ventricular fibrillation. The drug of choice for patients with atrial fibrillation or atrial flutter and a bystander bypass tract is intravenous procainamide or another drug that preferentially blocks the bypass tract. This shunts conduction through the AV node, which narrows the QRS complexes and often slows down the overall ventricular rate.

Asymptomatic patients showing delta waves on the ECG generally do not require treatment unless they are involved in a high-risk profession such as commercial pilots who may be restricted from flying if they have Wolff-Parkinson-White pattern on their ECG. Patients with occasional or rare bouts of minimal or mildly symptomatic palpitations from orthodromic or antidromic AVRT can often be safely treated with such agents as β-blockers or calcium channel blockers to prevent recurrent episodes. However, due to the

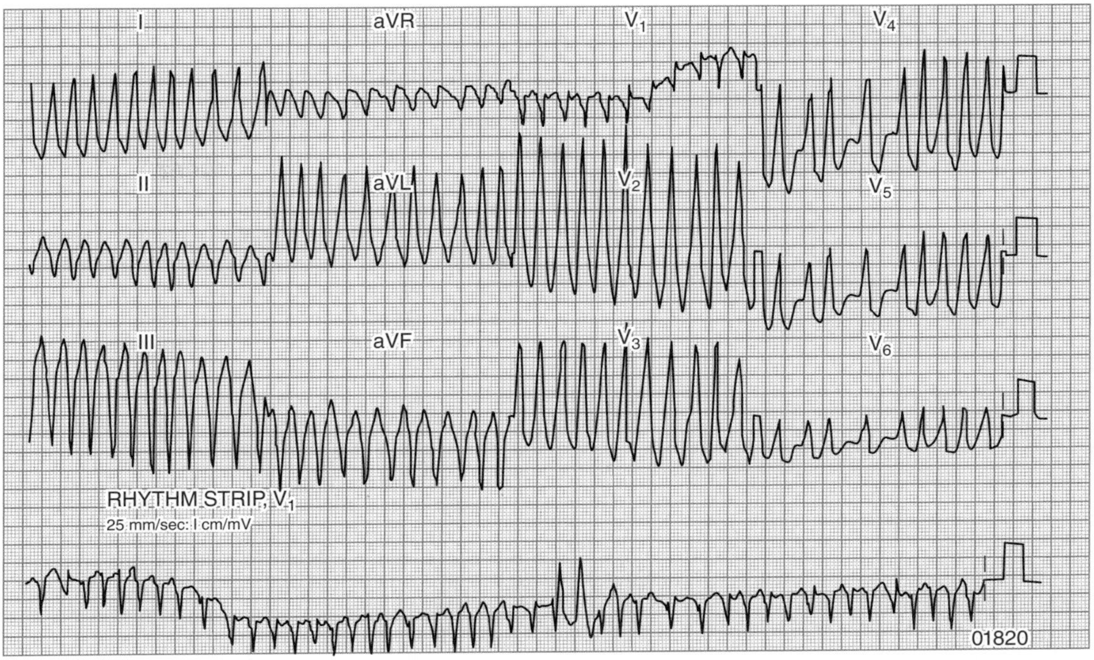

▲ **Figure 11–10.** Atrial fibrillation with antegrade conduction over a left posterolateral bypass tract. Although most beats are fully preexcited, several of the beats in the rhythm strip are narrower, indicating combined conduction over both the bypass tract and the atrioventricular node. Antidromic atrioventricular reciprocating tachycardia (AVRT) would have a similar appearance on 12-lead electrocardiogram, but the rhythm irregularity and the varying degrees of preexcitation nullify this possibility. (Reproduced with permission from Zipes DP. Specific arrhythmias: Diagnosis and treatment. In: Braunwald E, ed. *Heart Disease. A Textbook of Cardiovascular Medicine*. Philadelphia: WB Saunders; 1988.)

potential of ventricular fibrillation, these AV node blocking agents should be used with great caution or not at all in patients who have also demonstrated atrial fibrillation or atrial flutter.

C. Radiofrequency Catheter Ablation Therapy

Patients who experience significant symptoms such as dizziness, presyncope, or syncope should undergo an electrophysiologic study with concomitant radiofrequency ablation. In addition, patients with frequent palpitations who do not respond to or who wish to avoid drug therapy can also undergo ablative therapy. Recent guidelines indicate that ablation can be considered first-line therapy for patients with symptomatic Wolff-Parkinson-White syndrome.

In ablation, a steerable catheter is moved around the mitral or tricuspid annulus until the site of shortest impulse transit between the atrium and ventricle is found. This mapping process localizes the bypass tract. Frequently, an impulse can be recorded directly from the bypass tract, further confirming its localization. Once identified, radiofrequency energy delivered to the tract through the mapping catheter permanently eliminates the tract and prevents further transmission of electric impulses over it.

Given its curative potential, high success rate (95% in experienced hands, even with multiple bypass tracts), and low complication rate, radiofrequency catheter ablation is now a common treatment for accessory pathways (Table 11–2). As with other supraventricular arrhythmias, new three-dimensional mapping systems have been developed that decrease fluoroscopy and procedure time as well as allow the operator to return to specific locations if needed.

D. Surgical Ablation Therapy

In rare instances, patients will have multiple accessory pathways or pathways that are inaccessible to an ablation catheter. These patients may undergo surgical division of their tracts.

2. Other Bypass Tracts

A variety of bypass tracts other than AV tracts (Kent fibers) also exists. Atriohisian fibers connecting the atrium to the His bundle have been demonstrated. This led to the description of the Lown-Ganong-Levine (LGL) syndrome, which refers to patients with a short P-R interval, normal QRS, and recurrent SVT. However, current data suggest that LGL syndrome does

Table 11–2. Complications of Radiofrequency Ablation of Accessory Pathways[1]

Complication	Incidence (%)
Death	0.08
Nonfatal complications	
Cardiac tamponade	0.5
Atrioventricular block	0.5
Coronary artery spasm	0.2
Mild mitral regurgitation	0.2
Coronary artery thrombosis	0.1
Pericarditis	0.1
Mild aortic regurgitation	0.1
Transient neurologic deficit	0.1
Bacteremia	0.1
Femoral artery complications	
Thrombotic occlusion	0.2
Large hematoma	0.2
Atrioventricular fistula	0.1

[1]The incidence of death is based on unpublished data from the University of Oklahoma, the University of Alabama, the University of Michigan, Duke University, and the University of California, San Francisco. The incidence of nonfatal complications is based on pooled data from seven published studies.

not truly exist since atriohisian pathways have not been shown to support any type of reentry tachycardia.

Atriofascicular fibers, which are also known as Mahaim fibers, typically run from the lateral right atrium to the right bundle branch. The tract is capable of antegrade conduction only, and therefore, only antidromic AVRT is possible. Because the antegrade reentrant circuit engages the right bundle branch, the tachycardia QRS complex typically has a left bundle branch block pattern. Treatment considerations are the same as for Wolff-Parkinson-White syndrome.

Bunch TJ, May HT, Bair TL, et al. Long-term natural history of adult Wolff-Parkinson-White syndrome patients treated with and without catheter ablation. *Circ Arrhythm Electrophysiol.* 2015;8(6):1465–1471. [PMID: 26480930]

DIFFERENTIATION OF WIDE QRS COMPLEX TACHYCARDIAS

Except for the AV node, the refractory period of cardiac tissue for a given beat is directly related to the interval between that beat and the preceding beat; the slower the heart rate, the longer is the recovery period with each beat. Furthermore, because the stability of refractoriness depends on the stability of the heart rate, a beat-to-beat change in refractoriness accompanies variability in the heart rate.

When an early supraventricular beat occurs during a regular rhythm, the tissues do not have a chance to shorten (or reset) their refractory periods; the result may be aberrant conduction (a transient functional refractoriness, or block) in one of the bundle branches. The shorter the interval between the early beat and the preceding one, the greater is the probability that the early beat will be aberrant (Ashman phenomenon). Ashman phenomenon is also seen with the irregularity and frequent pauses of atrial fibrillation (Figure 11–11). Aberrancy may continue for a variable period before normal conduction resumes.

Aberrant conduction is often seen at the onset of any SVT that uses the AV node for antegrade conduction. (This excludes tachycardias that conduct antegrade over a bypass tract.) The right bundle branch, with its longer refractory period, is more subject to block than is the left, but occasionally, the left bundle becomes refractory earlier. Once the tachycardia has been established and refractory periods stabilized, this normal functional aberrancy may give way to normal conduction, with resumption of a narrow QRS.

Deciding whether a wide-complex tachycardia is supraventricular or ventricular in origin is often difficult. Only when AV dissociation or capture or fusion beats are present can a ventricular rhythm be diagnosed with near certainty. However, the low sensitivities of these findings (20% for AV dissociation) do not provide a firm diagnosis in a majority of wide-complex tachycardias.

Classic criteria that examine V_1 when a right bundle branch block pattern is present, the QRS width and axis, the presence of positive or negative concordance across the precordium, and various combinations of QRS patterns in different leads may support a diagnosis, but they have been found lacking in diagnostic power because of their low sensitivity, low specificity, or both. A proposed algorithm separates supraventricular from ventricular tachycardia

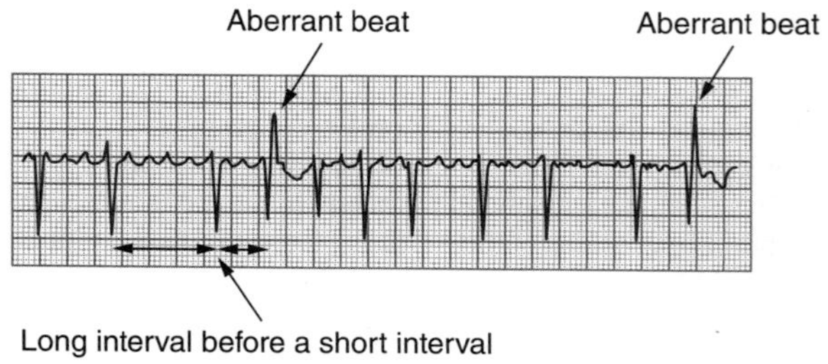

▲ **Figure 11–11.** Atrial fibrillation with ventricular aberration from Ashman phenomenon. The long interval before the short interval sets up the aberrant conduction in the ventricle.

with 99% sensitivity and 97% specificity. However, this algorithm, which is also known as the "Brugada Criteria," has demonstrated lower sensitivity and specificity in recent studies.

Kaiser E, Darrieux FCC, Barbosa SA, et al. Differential diagnosis of wide QRS tachycardias: comparison of two electrocardiographic algorithms. *Europace.* 2015;17(9):1422–1427. [PMID: 25600765]

OTHER SUPRAVENTRICULAR ARRHYTHMIAS

1. Sinus Arrhythmia

ESSENTIALS OF DIAGNOSIS

- Cyclic heart rate variation with respiration.
- P-P interval variability ≥ 160 ms or 10%.
- P-wave morphology identical to normal sinus rhythm P wave.

General Considerations

A cyclic increase and decrease in heart rate normally accompany inspiration and expiration, respectively, and this irregularity in rhythm (mediated by vagal tone) is often imperceptible. More marked degrees of rate excursion can occur, especially at slower heart rates, but these are not considered to be sinus arrhythmia unless the shortest and longest P-P interval varies by 0.16 seconds or more, or by 10% or more. This respiratory form of sinus arrhythmia is common in younger people and considered a normal finding. It becomes less prevalent with increasing age but can occur in conditions associated with autonomic dysfunction, such as diabetes mellitus. Enhancement of vagal tone with agents such as digoxin and morphine may also cause sinus arrhythmia.

Treatment

Because of its benign nature, no treatment is required for sinus arrhythmia.

2. Wandering Atrial Pacemaker

ESSENTIALS OF DIAGNOSIS

- Progressive cyclic alteration in P-wave morphology.
- Heart rate: 60–100 bpm.

General Considerations

The presence of more than one pacemaker within the atria (which may or may not include the sinus node) causes variation in the P-P interval, P-wave morphology, and P-R interval. The heart rate remains within the normal range.

There is controversy over the cause of this rhythm. Some authorities believe that wandering atrial pacemaker and MAT are the same rhythm artificially separated by heart rate and that both are attributable to underlying pulmonary disease. Others believe that wandering atrial pacemaker is an exaggerated form of a respiratory sinus arrhythmia, with the uncovering of latent atrial and sinus node pacemakers when the primary sinus node pacemaker cycles to a slow rate with expiration.

The significance ascribed to a wandering atrial pacemaker should probably be interpreted in the setting in which it is seen. In those with lung disease, it may be secondary to that process. In the elderly, it may suggest sinus node disease or sick sinus syndrome, and in the young and athletic heart, it may represent heightened vagal tone.

Treatment

The rhythm itself is usually benign and typically requires no intervention. If the rhythm is secondary, treating the underlying etiology may be warranted.

12 Atrial Fibrillation

Jonathan Hsu, MD, MAS
Melvin M. Scheinman, MD, MAS

ESSENTIALS OF DIAGNOSIS

- Absence of discrete P waves on the electrocardiogram.
- Irregularly irregular ventricular rhythm.

General Considerations

Atrial fibrillation, the most common sustained clinical arrhythmia, is diagnosed by the finding of an irregularly irregular ventricular rhythm without discrete P waves (Figure 12–1). The QRS complex is usually narrow, but it may be wide if aberrant conduction or bundle branch block is present. Atrial fibrillation associated with the Wolff-Parkinson-White syndrome may result in very rapid ventricular rates due to the conduction of atrial impulses over an accessory pathway and may be life-threatening. This arrhythmia is diagnosed by its very rapid, irregular rate associated with wide, preexcited QRS complexes, and requires emergency treatment.

Approximately 4% of the population older than 60 years have sustained an episode of atrial fibrillation, with a particularly steep increase in prevalence after the seventh decade of life. Other risk factors besides age for the development of atrial fibrillation include heart failure, hypertensive cardiovascular disease, coronary artery disease, valvular heart disease, chronic lung disease, thyroid disease, and alcohol consumption. Moreover, both sustained and paroxysmal atrial fibrillation can cause clot formation and embolism, most often clinically manifest by the development of a cerebrovascular accident (CVA) or other systemic emboli. It is estimated that 15–20% of CVAs in nonrheumatic patients are due to atrial fibrillation.

Clinical Findings

A. Symptoms & Signs

Symptoms associated with atrial fibrillation are often related to the irregularity of the rhythm and loss of atrial contraction. Common symptoms include palpitations, shortness of breath at rest or with exertion, and lightheadedness. Other nonspecific symptoms, including chest pain or generalized fatigue, can be manifestations of atrial fibrillation and add to the difficulty in diagnosing the abnormal cardiac rhythm based on symptoms alone.

When called on to manage new-onset atrial fibrillation, it is important to establish the precipitating factors, because the type of associated condition determines long-term prognosis. In some patients, episodes of atrial fibrillation may be initiated by alcohol or drug use. Atrial fibrillation may result from acute intercurrent ailments. For example, this arrhythmia may develop in patients with hyperthyroidism or lung disease or after either cardiac or pulmonary surgery, especially in older patients. Atrial fibrillation is also seen in patients with acute pulmonary embolism, myocarditis, or acute myocardial infarction, particularly when the last condition is complicated by either occlusion of the right coronary artery or heart failure. When atrial fibrillation occurs in these settings, it almost always abates spontaneously if the patient recovers from the underlying problem. Hence, management usually involves administration of drugs to control the heart rate, and long-term antiarrhythmic therapy is generally not needed. More recent observations, however, suggest that recurrent atrial fibrillation may occur after acute initiating events.

Alternatively, atrial fibrillation may occur in association with structural cardiac disease. Important associated conditions include rheumatic mitral stenosis, hypertension, hypertrophic cardiomyopathy, or chronic heart failure. In contrast to patients with acute intercurrent ailments, those with structural heart disease may expect (even with antiarrhythmic therapy) many recurrences, and chronic atrial fibrillation may supervene.

B. Initial Evaluation

The initial evaluation is mainly directed at diagnosing associated conditions (eg, valvular heart disease,

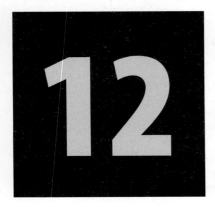

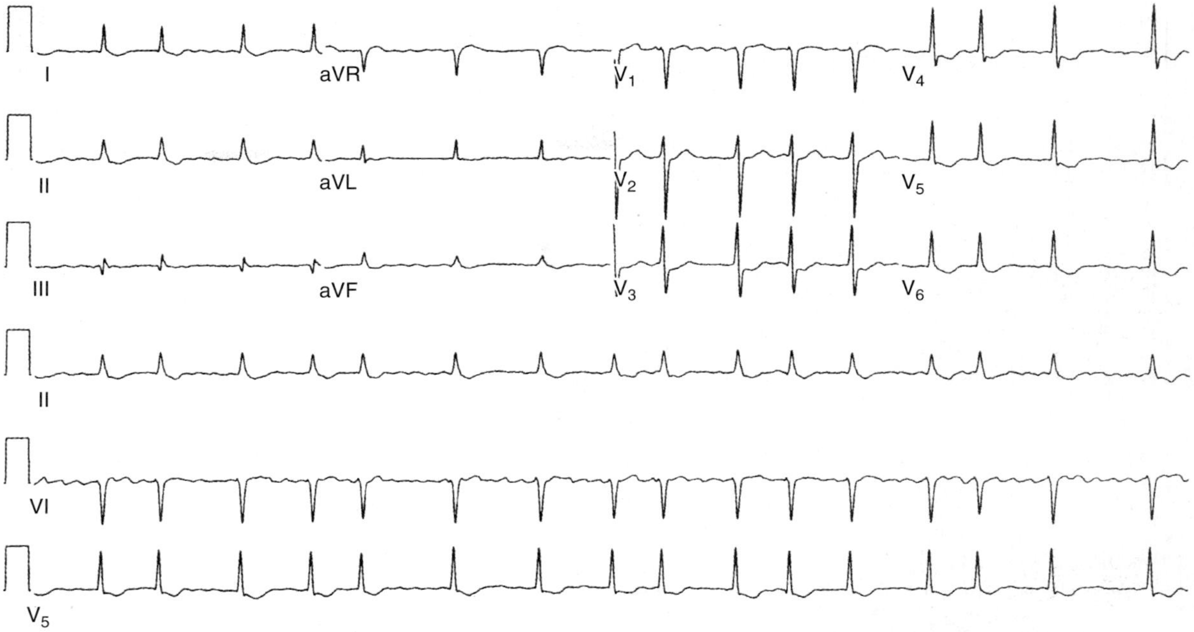

▲ **Figure 12–1.** The 12-lead electrocardiogram shows the typical rapid irregular rhythm seen with atrial fibrillation.

hypertension, evidence of heart failure). The cardiac examination during atrial fibrillation will show an irregularly irregular rhythm, variability of the first heart sound, and augmentation of a systolic ejection murmurs after long pauses. The initial evaluation of new-onset atrial fibrillation also includes a detailed history focusing on possible precipitating factors as well as the presence of organic cardiac disease. As such, the initial evaluation includes, at a minimum, a careful physical examination, 12-lead electrocardiogram (ECG), chest radiograph, echocardiogram, and tests of thyroid function. Further testing will depend on various aspects of the history or physical examination. Ambulatory ECG monitoring may be helpful in diagnosing the patient with paroxysmal atrial fibrillation. In the patient with frequent episodes of paroxysmal atrial fibrillation, a 24- to 48-hour ambulatory Holter ECG recording, or longer ambulatory ECG/mobile cardiac telemetry monitoring for 15–30 days may discern whether atrial fibrillation was triggered by another arrhythmia, such as a premature atrial complex alone, or whether the fibrillation was preceded by an episode of supraventricular tachycardia as well as to detail the burden of atrial fibrillation. Some patients have infrequent episodes and symptoms and require longer-term cardiac event monitoring to make the diagnosis. If atrial fibrillation is usually precipitated by exercise, then an exercise treadmill test is appropriate. In addition, patients with vagally mediated fibrillation will typically have episodes either after heavy meals or during sleep. These clues may help identify those patients who may respond to specific approaches (see later section, Treatment).

Differential Diagnosis

The ECG diagnosis of atrial fibrillation is usually straightforward and is characterized by an irregularly irregular ventricular rhythm with a narrow QRS complex unless there is associated bundle branch block, and no discrete P waves (signifying fibrillatory atrial activity). The chief diagnostic problem relates to patients showing short bursts of irregular atrial tachycardia (which are common on random ambulatory ECG recordings in the elderly) or frequent premature atrial contractions, which may result in an overall irregular rhythm but are characterized by distinct atrial depolarization as manifested by discrete P waves. In addition, patients with atrial flutter may have varying atrioventricular (AV) conduction, which may serve to mimic atrial fibrillation. Careful evaluation of all leads looking for the characteristic flutter pattern is important. Less commonly, patients presenting with multifocal atrial tachycardia may mimic the irregularity found in those with atrial fibrillation. Careful analysis in the latter group shows an irregular atrial tachycardia with at least three distinct P-wave morphologies. A very uncommon arrhythmia that may mimic atrial fibrillation is seen in patients with dual AV nodal physiology with dual conduction over the fast and slow AV nodal pathways. For this diagnosis, identify that a single sinus P wave is associated with two QRS complexes. These patients are readily cured with slow pathway ablation.

Treatment

The objectives of therapy for atrial fibrillation often include (1) achieving rate control of the ventricular response to atrial fibrillation, (2) restoring sinus rhythm (where feasible), and (3) decreasing the risk of CVA. The principles of treatment discussed in this chapter largely follow those promulgated in the most recent American College of Cardiology (ACC)/American Heart Association (AHA)/European Society of Cardiology (ESC) guidelines and updated guidelines.

January CT, Wann LS, Alpert JS, et al. 2014 AHA/ACC/HRS guideline for the management of patients with atrial fibrillation: a report of the American College of Cardiology/American Heart Association Task Force on Practice Guidelines and the Heart Rhythm Society. *J Am Coll Cardiol.* 2014;64(21):e1–e76. [PMID: 24685669]

January CT, Wann LS, Calkins H, et al. 2019 AHA/ACC/HRS focused update of the 2014 AHA/ACC/HRS guideline for he management of patients with atrial fibrillation. *J Am Coll Cardiol.* 2019;74:104–132. [PMID: 30703431]

Hindricks G, Potpara T, Dagres N, et al. 2020 ESC Guidelines for the diagnosis and management of atrial fibrillation developed in collaboration with the European Association for Cardio-thoracic Surgery (EACTS): the task force for the diagnosis and management of atrial fibrillation of the European Society of Cardiology (ESC) developed with the special contribution of the European Heart Rhythm Association (EHRA) of the ESC. *Eur Heart J.* 2020;42:373–498. [PMID: 32860505]

A. Rate Control

If the patient has atrial fibrillation and a rapid rate associated with hypotension, severe heart failure, or cardiogenic shock, emergency direct-current cardioversion is indicated. For patients with atrial fibrillation associated with rapid rate, but with stable hemodynamics, attempts to achieve acute rate control are indicated. Drugs to slow the ventricular rate in patients with atrial fibrillation (Table 12–1) include digitalis preparations, certain calcium channel blockers (verapamil or diltiazem), and β-blockers. If rapid rate control is desired, then calcium channel blockers and β-blockers are far more effective than digitalis. In addition, a common misconception is that digitalis therapy is associated with acute conversion to sinus rhythm, but carefully controlled studies have shown that conversion to sinus rhythm is no more likely with digoxin than with placebo. As emphasized later, digitalis, β-blockers, and calcium channel blockers are contraindicated in patients with Wolff-Parkinson-White syndrome and atrial fibrillation. Intravenous diltiazem has been shown to be safe and effective for patients with atrial fibrillation and a modest degree of heart failure. In patients refractory to these agents, intravenous amiodarone may be effective but requires many hours before rate control is achieved. In patients with a known history of congestive heart failure, use of intravenous β-blockers or calcium channel blockers may aggravate cardiac failure. In this subset, digitalis or intravenous amiodarone would be the preferred agent for rate control.

B. Long-Term Antiarrhythmic Therapy & Elective Cardioversion

For patients who have had a single, initial episode of atrial fibrillation with no significant hemodynamic problems, no specific therapy is required because repeat episodes may not occur for many years. In contrast, patients who manifest frequent recurrences may be candidates for long-term antiarrhythmic therapy with class Ia (quinidine, procainamide, and disopyramide), class Ic (propafenone and flecainide), or class III (sotalol, amiodarone, dronedarone, and dofetilide) agents, all of which are more effective than placebo in maintaining sinus rhythm (Table 12–2).

C. Antiarrhythmic Drug Therapy for Atrial Fibrillation

For patients with atrial fibrillation, use of any of the antiarrhythmic drugs listed is appropriate. In general, the class Ic agents (flecainide or propafenone) are the first choice in patients without ischemic heart disease in terms of efficacy

Table 12–1. Intravenous Pharmacologic Agents for Heart Rate Control in Atrial Fibrillation

Drug	Loading Dose	Onset	Maintenance Dose	Major Side Effects
Diltiazem	0.25 mg/kg IV over 2 min	2–7 min	5–15 mg/h infusion	Hypotension, heart block, HF
Esmolol	0.5 mg/kg over 1 min	5 min	0.05–0.2 mg kg^{-1} min^{-1}	Hypotension, heart block, bradycardia, asthma, HF
Metoprolol	2.5–5 mg IV bolus over 2 min; up to 3 doses	5 min	NA	Hypotension, heart block, bradycardia, asthma, HF
Propranolol	0.15 mg/kg IV	5 min	NA	Hypotension, heart block, bradycardia, asthma, HF
Verapamil	0.075–0.15 mg/kg IV over 2 min	3–5 min	NA	Hypotension, heart block, HF
Digoxin	0.25 mg IV each 2 h, up to 1.5 mg	2 h	0.125–0.25 mg daily	Digitalis toxicity, heart block, bradycardia

HF, heart failure; NA, not applicable.
Reproduced with permission from Fuster V, Rydén L, Asinger R, et al. ACC/AHA/ESC guidelines for the management of patients with atrial fibrillation. *J Am Coll Cardiol.* 2001;38(4):1266.

Table 12–2. Rhythm Control Strategies for Recurrent Paroxysmal or Persistent Atrial Fibrillation

Underlying Condition in Order of Increasing Seriousness	Therapy
No significant heart disease or hypertension without severe LVH: initial drug therapy	Dronedarone Flecainide Propafenone Sotalol
Failed initial drug therapy	Amiodarone Dofetilide Catheter ablation
Hypertension with severe LVH: initial drug therapy	Amiodarone
Failed initial drug therapy	Catheter ablation
Ischemic heart disease: initial drug therapy	Dofetilide Dronedarone Sotalol
Failed initial drug therapy	Amiodarone Catheter ablation
Heart failure: initial drug therapy	Amiodarone Dofetilide
Failed initial drug therapy	Catheter ablation

LVH, left ventricular hypertrophy. Drugs listed alphabetically, not in the order of suggested use. In patients with multiple conditions the selection of therapy depends on the most serious condition present.
Adapted from Wann SL, et al. *J Am Coll Cardiol.* 2011;57[2]:223–242.

and lowest incidence of side effects. It would be wise, for example, to withhold amiodarone as a first-line drug in view of the potential for adverse effects, particularly long-term. Only two drugs have been proven safe for patients with severe congestive heart failure: dofetilide and amiodarone.

For patients with atrial fibrillation associated with coronary artery disease, consider use of sotalol as initial drug therapy. This agent has class III antiarrhythmic effects and is a potent β-blocker. Class Ic drugs should not be used in patients with significant structural cardiac disease such as systolic heart failure or in those with ischemic heart disease. Sotalol or dronedarone may be safe and effective for patients with hypertension and atrial fibrillation without significant left ventricular hypotrophy. Similarly, class Ic drugs may be used in well-controlled hypertension, but without left ventricular hypertrophy.

In addition, extracardiac factors are important in the choice of antiarrhythmic drugs. For example, dose adjustments are mandatory for patients with renal insufficiency. This is especially true for sotalol and dofetilide. Dofetilide, for example, requires hospital admission, calculation of the creatinine clearance, and drug titration according to the QT corrected for heart rate as well as renal function. Antiarrhythmic drug usage is summarized in Table 12–2, and drug doses are listed in Table 12–3.

Even with drug therapy, recurrence rates for atrial fibrillation approach 50% per year (as opposed to recurrences with placebo therapy of 75% per year). In addition, these agents may be associated with significant side effects. For class Ia drugs, these include induction of torsades de pointes, especially for those with congestive heart failure. For example, a meta-analysis compared quinidine with placebo for patients with atrial fibrillation and found that death from all causes was higher in the groups

Table 12–3. Typical Doses of Drugs Used to Maintain Sinus Rhythm in Atrial Fibrillation, Listed Alphabetically

Drug	Daily Dosage	Potential Adverse Effects
Amiodarone	100–400 mg	Photosensitivity, pulmonary toxicity, polyneuropathy, GI upset, bradycardia, torsades de pointes (rare), hepatic toxicity, thyroid dysfunction
Disopyramide	400–750 mg	Torsades de pointes, HF, glaucoma, urinary retention, dry mouth
Dofetilide	500–1000 mcg	Torsades de pointes
Dronedarone	400–800 mg	Contraindicated for those with severe or worsening heart failure or in those with persistent AF and cardiovascular risk factors
Flecainide	200–300 mg	Ventricular tachycardia, congestive HF, increased rate with conversion to atrial flutter
Procainamide	1000–4000 mg	Torsades de pointes, lupus-like syndrome, GI symptoms
Propafenone	450–900 mg	Ventricular tachycardia, congestive HF, increased rate with conversion to atrial flutter
Quinidine	600–1500 mg	Torsades de pointes, GI upset, increased rate with conversion to atrial flutter
Sotalol	240–320 mg	Torsades de pointes, congestive HF, bradycardia, exacerbation of chronic obstructive or bronchospastic lung disease

AV, atrioventricular; GI, gastrointestinal; HF, heart failure.
Reproduced with permission from Fuster V, Rydén L, Asinger R, et al. ACC/AHA/ESC guidelines for the management of patients with atrial fibrillation. *J Am Coll Cardiol.* 2001;38(4):1266.

treated with quinidine. In addition, in the Stroke Prevention in Atrial Fibrillation (SPAF) trials, substantial numbers of patients were treated with antiarrhythmic agents; in patients with heart failure, those treated with class I drugs had significantly increased mortality rates compared with those not treated with antiarrhythmic drugs. Great care must be exercised in the use of these agents, balancing the benefits against the potential for adverse effects. General rules include avoidance of all class Ia drugs or sotalol for patients with congestive heart failure and avoidance of class Ic agents for patients with severe structural heart disease or ischemia. In addition, sotalol is contraindicated for patients with severe depression of the left ventricular ejection fraction and/or severe left ventricular hypertrophy. Patients with significant sinus node or AV conduction disease may require pacemaker therapy before use of antiarrhythmic drugs because these drugs may further depress sinus node or AV conduction. The only drugs that appear to be both effective and safe for patients with heart failure and atrial fibrillation are amiodarone and dofetilide. Amiodarone is associated with a host of both cardiac (eg, severe sinus bradycardia or arrest or AV block) and noncardiac (eg, liver abnormalities, thyroid abnormalities, pulmonary fibrosis) adverse effects, but low-dose amiodarone (ie, 200 mg/day) appears to be effective and well tolerated. Dofetilide has a narrow therapeutic window and can cause life-threatening arrhythmias; it can be used in patients with atrial fibrillation and congestive heart failure but requires a 2- to 3-day in-hospital stay for monitoring of the agent with regard to the QTc interval and for ventricular arrhythmias. Dronedarone is the newest agent approved for the treatment of atrial fibrillation. This drug is a derivative of amiodarone without the iodine moiety and has most of the physiologic effects of amiodarone. This drug may have less efficacy and should not be used in patients with severe or worsening heart failure or in those with persistent atrial fibrillation and cardiovascular risk factors (see later discussion of CHA_2DS_2-VASc score).

D. Chemical Cardioversion

Recent studies have emphasized the use of drugs for acute conversion of atrial fibrillation. It has been shown that intravenous ibutilide and intravenous dofetilide (not available in the United States) are effective for the conversion of approximately 50% of patients with recent-onset atrial fibrillation. It should be emphasized that ibutilide should be used only in a monitored hospital environment. The usual dose is 1 mg over 10 minutes, followed by a 10-minute interlude, followed by an additional 1 mg over 10 minutes if necessary. A defibrillator should be readily available because the incidence of sustained torsades de pointes is 1–2%. Ibutilide should be avoided in patients with severe heart failure, bradycardia, or a prolonged QT interval.

E. Other Drugs for Chemical Cardioversion

Other drug combinations have also been found effective. For example, it has been found that use of large oral doses of either flecainide (300 mg) or propafenone (600 mg) may terminate up to 80% of episodes of atrial fibrillation within 2 hours (pill-in-the-pocket). This approach should be used only in patients who are pretreated with β-blocking drugs and in the absence of significant cardiac disease or heart failure, to avoid accelerated conduction of atrial arrhythmias across the AV node. It is often best to assess first-time use of the "pill-in-the-pocket" approach in a hospital setting.

F. Anticoagulant Therapy & Left Atrial Appendage Occlusion

The risk of CVA in patients with nonrheumatic atrial fibrillation is 4–7% per year. Patients at particularly high risk include those older than 75 years or with hypertension, a history of heart failure, increased left atrial size, diabetes, or prior CVA. The risks of CVA are similar in patients with paroxysmal versus persistent atrial fibrillation. Risk of stroke was traditionally assessed by noting the $CHADS_2$ score: C (congestive heart failure), H (hypertension), A (age ≥ 75 years), D (diabetes), S (previous stroke or transient ischemic attack). According to previous AHA and ACC guidelines, aspirin therapy was acceptable for those with a $CHADS_2$ score of 0 or 1, whereas anticoagulants were advised for those with a $CHADS_2$ score ≥ 2 who had no contraindications for anticoagulant therapy. However, more recent risk criteria have been identified and include female sex, age 65 years or greater, and evidence of coronary or peripheral vascular disease (CHA_2DS_2-VASc score). When compared with $CHADS_2$, CHA_2DS_2-VASc performed better in predicting those at high risk or those at very low risk for stroke. Updated guidelines from the AHA and ACC advocate for the use of the CHA_2DS_2-VASc score as the preferred risk score for the estimation of thromboembolic risk in patients with atrial fibrillation. Warfarin or one of the non–vitamin K antagonist oral anticoagulants is recommended for those with a CHA_2DS_2-VASc score ≥ 2 (Table 12–4). Numerous studies have documented the remarkable efficacy of warfarin in decreasing the risk of emboli by 45–85% in patients with nonrheumatic atrial fibrillation with a low risk of significant hemorrhage, provided the international normalized ratio (INR) is in the range of 2.0–3.0. However, some patients have a considerable risk of bleeding, which can be estimated by scores such as the HAS-BLED (see Table 12–4).

Several direct oral anticoagulant drugs (dabigatran, rivaroxaban, apixaban, and edoxaban) have been approved to treat patients with nonvalvular atrial fibrillation and reduce the risk of thromboembolism. These drugs have proved to be either equivalent or superior in efficacy and safety compared with warfarin. The advantages of the newer agents include obviating the need for INR blood tests and fewer drug–drug or drug–food interactions compared with warfarin. All of the direct oral anticoagulant agents require careful monitoring of renal function by serial measurement of creatinine clearance (CrCl) because dose adjustment is required in the

Table 12–4. Risk Factor Scoring for Cerebrovascular Accident and Risk of Hemorrhage from Anticoagulant Therapy

	Risk Factor	Score
1. $CHADS_2$	Congestive heart failure	1
	Hypertension	1
	Age > 75	1
	Diabetes	1
	Stroke	2
2. CHA_2DS_2-VASc	Congestive heart failure or	1
	EF ≤ 35%	1
	Hypertension	1
	Age > 65	1
	Age > 75	2
	Diabetes	1
	Stroke (TIA or systemic emboli)	2
	Vascular disease (peripheral vascular disease, previous MI)	1
	Sex (female)	1
3. HAS-BLED	Hypertension (uncontrolled)	1
	Renal disease (Cr > 2.6 mg/dL)	1
	Liver disease (bilirubin 2× normal)	1
	Stroke history	1
	Prior major bleeding	1
	Labile INR	1
	Age ≥ 65	1
	Medications (NSAIDs)	1
	Alcohol usage	1

Cr, creatinine; EF, ejection fraction; INR, international normalized ratio; MI, myocardial infarction; NSAIDs, nonsteroidal anti-inflammatory drugs; TIA, transient ischemic attack.

face of reduced renal function (Table 12–5). In addition, specific antidotes (in the event of bleeding) are currently available for these agents. For the above reasons, the direct oral anticoagulant agents have become the preferred method for anticoagulation in patients with chronic atrial fibrillation.

The role of aspirin therapy for patients with atrial fibrillation remains controversial. In one study, 75 mg of aspirin failed to decrease the stroke risk compared with placebo (5.5% per year). In contrast, the SPAF I trial showed that a higher dose of aspirin, 325 mg, appeared to be of benefit in patients younger than 75 years. In a follow-up study (SPAF II), the incidence of stroke was higher with aspirin (4.8%) compared with warfarin (3.6%). The SPAF III trial demonstrated that aspirin (325 mg/day) and fixed low-dose warfarin (1, 2, or 3 mg) were ineffective for stroke prevention. Therefore, the weight of current data favors use of the direct oral anticoagulant agents or warfarin with an INR of 2.0–3.0 as the best strategy to prevent systemic embolization.

It is appreciated that 90% of clots emanate from the left atrial appendage. Left atrial appendage occlusion has been studied and approved for thromboembolic prophylaxis in patients with atrial fibrillation who are at risk for stroke but have an appropriate rationale for seeking a nonpharmacologic alternative for long-term stroke risk reduction. Approval of devices include the Watchman device by Boston Scientific and Amulet device by Abbott. These devices have been shown to be a viable alternative to long-term oral anticoagulation in patients with atrial fibrillation who cannot or will not take oral anticoagulant therapy and have been shown to be as effective as anticoagulant therapy for stroke prevention. The procedure involves percutaneous implantation of the device in the left atrial appendage, followed by antithrombotic therapy initially for 45 days to 6 months, followed by aspirin destination therapy thereafter.

G. Direct-Current Cardioversion

Direct-current cardioversion is an effective technique for restoration of sinus rhythm. Because of the benefits of sinus

Table 12–5. Anticoagulant Therapy

Drug	Dose	Side Effects or Precautions
Warfarin	Determined by INR measurement	Many drug–drug or drug–food (eg, green leafy vegetables) interactions
Dabigatran	150 mg bid for CrCl > 30 mL; 75 mg bid for CrCl 15–30 mL; contraindicated for CrCl < 15 mL	(1) When converting patients from warfarin to dabigatran, wait until INR > 2 (2) Gastrointestinal upset (3) Interactions with dronedarone, ketoconazole, etc.
Rivaroxaban	20 mg/day for CrCl > 50 mL/min; 15 mg/day for CrCl 15–50 mL/min	Interacts with drugs that inhibit (eg, ketoconazole) or induce CYP3A4 enzymes (eg, rifampin)
Apixaban	5 mg bid; 2.5 mg bid for patients with at least 2 of the following: age ≥ 80 years, weight < 60 kg, or Cr > 1.5	
Edoxaban	60 mg/day; 30 mg/day for CrCl 15–50 mL/min	Avoid use in patients with CrCl > 95 mL/min due to potential increased ischemic stroke risk in these patients

bid, twice a day; CrCl, creatinine clearance; INR, international normalized ratio.

rhythm in terms of improved cardiac output and decreased risk of embolic phenomena, in general, at least one attempt should be made to restore sinus rhythm in patients with atrial fibrillation. Several precautions are in order. If the patient has a history of recurrent episodes of atrial fibrillation, then the patient should be pretreated and continued with an antiarrhythmic agent because reversion to atrial fibrillation after shock therapy is high. Use of antiarrhythmic drugs before direct-current shock, however, is inappropriate for the patient with an initial episode of well-tolerated atrial fibrillation. Unless urgent cardioversion is required because of hemodynamic decompensation, severe ischemia, or congestive heart failure, it is imperative to follow one of several options for reducing the risk of systemic embolization after cardioversion:

a. For patients with atrial fibrillation of less than 48 hours in duration, it would appear to be safe to proceed with application of direct-current shock.

b. If atrial fibrillation persists for more than 48 hours prior to cardioversion, then the risk of embolization increases, and anticoagulants are required prior to conversion. One recommended option for patients with atrial fibrillation of more than 48 hours in duration is to perform transesophageal echocardiography (TEE), which is excellent for detecting clots in the left atrium or the left atrial appendage. Evidence from several studies indicates that the finding of either a clot or spontaneous echocardiographic contrast in the left atrium is associated with higher risks of systemic embolization. In the absence of such findings on TEE, systemic emboli are rare. Therefore, patients with recent-onset atrial fibrillation with no evidence of atrial clots or spontaneous contrast by TEE may undergo direct-current cardioversion after initiation of heparin or the new oral anticoagulants. A report from the ACUTE trial showed that patients with atrial fibrillation treated based on TEE-guided therapy versus a group treated with a 3-week course of anticoagulant therapy had similar rates of thromboembolism (< 1%). It must be appreciated that atrial function is depressed (atrial stunning) after cardioversion and that anticoagulant therapy is recommended for at least 1 month after cardioversion. This is true whether the duration of atrial fibrillation was either less than or greater than 48 hours. For patients with clot or dense spontaneous echocardiographic contrast with TEE, full anticoagulant therapy with direct oral anticoagulant therapy or warfarin therapy and an INR of 2.0–3.0 is recommended for at least 3 weeks before cardioversion.

c. An alternative approach is that patients with atrial fibrillation of greater than 48 hours be fully anticoagulated for at least 3 consecutive weeks before attempting direct-current cardioversion and for 4 weeks afterward to decrease the risk of an embolism after successful reversion to sinus rhythm. This approach tends to be less efficient than the TEE-guided approach for recent-onset atrial fibrillation but is an acceptable alternative treatment.

Direct-current external shock is usually performed in a monitored area under supervision of an anesthesiologist. Pads are placed in an anterior-posterior orientation to maximize current delivered to the atrium. It is wise to check the arterial oxygen saturation and serum potassium level before cardioversion. Direct-current shocks beginning with at least 150 J biphasic are used to achieve sinus rhythm. Multiple shocks of lesser energy are to be avoided. If the patient fails to revert after maximal external shocks (360 J biphasic), then successful cardioversion can almost always be achieved using supplemental doses of ibutilide. Ibutilide has been shown to lower the atrial defibrillation threshold. An attempt at internal cardioversion using small-energy shocks delivered between the coronary sinus and the right atrium is seldom necessary because the previously described treatments are almost always effective.

H. Long-Term Approach

Clinicians should be especially careful to identify patients whose atrial fibrillation might have a readily reversible cause. Examples include patients with hyperthyroidism as well as those in whom other cardiac arrhythmias appear to trigger atrial fibrillation. For example, patients with atrial flutter or paroxysmal supraventricular tachycardia may experience atrial premature impulses during tachycardia that trigger atrial fibrillation. In selected patients, it is possible to apply catheter ablation to cure the underlying supraventricular arrhythmia and, hence, prevent the trigger and modify the substrate for atrial fibrillation. Therefore, in the evaluation of patients with atrial fibrillation, initial testing should include obtaining a thyroid-stimulating hormone assay, an echocardiogram, and a 48-hour ambulatory ECG recording for those with paroxysmal atrial fibrillation. In analyses of these recordings, the clinician seeks evidence for triggering arrhythmias. In addition, the clinician looks for vagal triggers of atrial fibrillation, such as sinus bradycardia associated with sleep or heavy meals, that initially may be treated with vagolytic antiarrhythmic agents such as disopyramide. Alternatively, if atrial fibrillation appears only with enhanced sympathetic tone, such as with exercise, a trial of β-blocker therapy is appropriate.

One important special circumstance is that of atrial fibrillation in the patient with Wolff-Parkinson-White syndrome. These patients may have a very rapid irregular rate and wide complex tachycardia owing to conduction over the accessory pathway (Figure 12–2). After recognition of this entity, appropriate immediate therapy includes use of intravenous ibutilide or procainamide or direct-current cardioversion. It is important to remember that intravenous digoxin and calcium channel blockers are contraindicated. In addition, use of lidocaine, β-blockers, or adenosine is not effective and is contraindicated because they delay appropriate therapy. After the rhythm is stabilized, these patients should undergo catheter ablation of the accessory pathway.

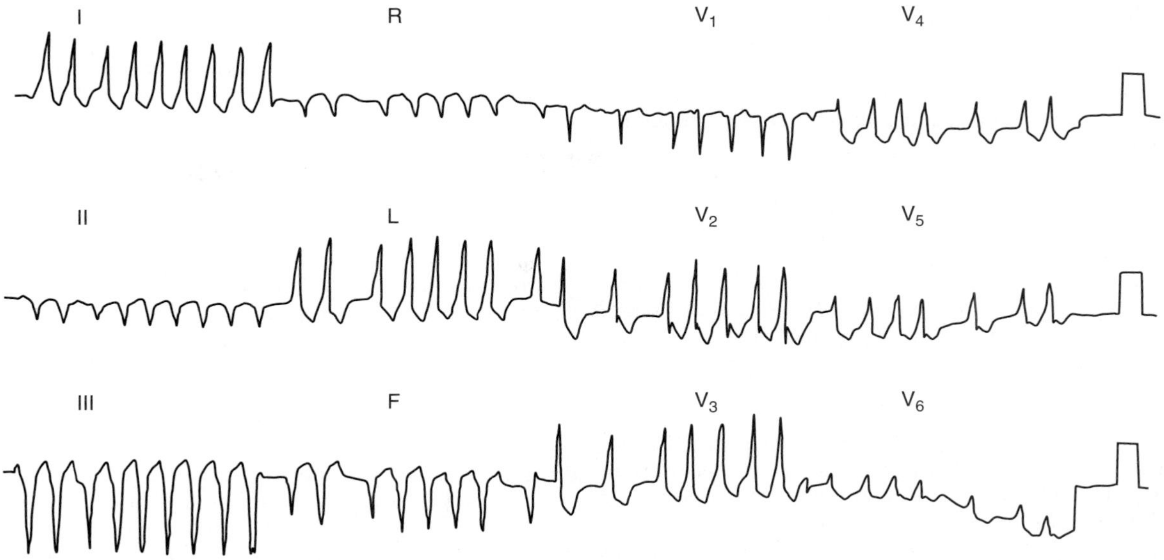

▲ **Figure 12–2.** The 12-lead electrocardiogram shows a rapid irregular rhythm with broad QRS complex. This is pathognomonic of atrial fibrillation in a patient with Wolff-Parkinson-White syndrome. This arrhythmia requires urgent treatment. Acceptable therapy includes use of intravenous ibutilide or procainamide or direct-current shock.

The natural history of atrial fibrillation associated with structural cardiac disease is spontaneous recurrence of the arrhythmia. Unfortunately, no drug is universally effective, and the decision of how many drugs to try before a judgment is made to terminate antiarrhythmic drugs and focus on rate control depends on how symptomatic the patient is during atrial fibrillation. If the episodes are poorly tolerated, then multiple drug trials or even various ablative procedures may be required (see later section, Nonpharmacologic Treatment of Atrial Fibrillation). On the other hand, if rate control can be readily achieved with drugs, such as digoxin, β-blockers, or calcium antagonists that block AV nodal conduction and the patient has a good symptomatic outcome, then an acceptable alternative is to use drugs that control the ventricular rate combined with long-term anticoagulant treatment. A large, randomized trial (AFFIRM) compared the strategy of rate control and anticoagulation versus maintaining sinus rhythm with antiarrhythmic drugs. The AFFIRM trial randomized over 4000 patients with atrial fibrillation to either rate or rhythm control. The patient cohort consisted in large measure of older (mean age 69 years) patients who were not very symptomatic. They found no difference in mortality or quality of life between groups. The rhythm control group had a higher incidence of hospitalizations and episodes of torsades de pointes. In addition, stroke risk was related to presence of no or inadequate anticoagulant treatment. This study showed that for most patients with atrial fibrillation, rate control was equally effective as rhythm control and that long-term anticoagulation therapy is required for both groups. More contemporary data from a multicenter randomized controlled trial (EAST-AFNET 4) showed that early rhythm control compared to usual care resulted in lower adverse cardiovascular outcomes in patients with early atrial fibrillation. These data suggest that earlier management with rhythm control strategy may improve long-term outcomes in patients with atrial fibrillation, by a strategy of antiarrhythmic drugs and/or ablation.

Kirchhof P, Camm AJ, Goette A, et al. Early rhythm-control therapy in patients with atrial fibrillation. *N Engl J Med.* 2020;383:1305–1316.

I. Nonpharmacologic Treatment of Atrial Fibrillation

Because pharmacologic therapy for atrial fibrillation may not be ideal, several nonpharmacologic treatment modalities have been introduced. Previous ACC/AHA/ESC guidelines allowed for catheter ablation for treatment of atrial fibrillation after one failed drug trial; however, Heart Rhythm Society guidelines allow for consideration of catheter ablation even prior to initiation of antiarrhythmic drug therapy. The mainstay of catheter ablation is pulmonary vein isolation aimed at pulmonary vein triggers that promote and sustain atrial fibrillation. Recent studies have used wide-area ablative lesions around the pulmonary veins to create entrance and exit block from those triggering foci. Other foci may emanate from the coronary sinus, vein of Marshall, or superior vena cava and may require ablation as well. In addition, some groups advocate ablation of complex fractionated potentials (CAFÉ), use of a roof line between the upper right and left superior pulmonary vein, full posterior wall ablation and isolation, or an ablation line from the mitral annulus to the left inferior pulmonary vein (mitral isthmus line). The initial success rate for ablation of paroxysmal atrial fibrillation is 70–90%, but the 5-year success rate is approximately 50%. Improvements in the risk of atrial fibrillation recurrence have been seen with additional ablative procedures in some, but not all, studies.

Patients with persistent tachycardia may suffer from a tachycardia-induced cardiomyopathy with left ventricular failure superimposed on their native cardiac disease. Hence, in the management of chronic atrial fibrillation, rate control is an important objective that must be achieved either via AV nodal blocking drugs or, failing these, with catheter ablative procedures. Catheter ablation of the AV junction involves insertion of an electrode catheter in the region of the His bundle with application of radiofrequency energy to destroy AV conduction. The chief benefit of this technique is the achievement of perfect rate control without need for rate control drugs. The drawbacks include the need for permanent pacing and a continued need for anticoagulant therapy.

For most of these patients, especially for those with left ventricular ejection fraction greater than 40%, single-chamber pacing appears to be sufficient. In some patients, left ventricular function may deteriorate, and biventricular pacing may be helpful (PAVE trial).

It has been shown that atrial-based pacing systems will decrease the incidence of atrial fibrillation in patients with the tachycardia-bradycardia syndrome. In addition, pacing may allow for safe use of antiarrhythmic drugs. In patients with vagally mediated atrial fibrillation, atrial pacing may be effective in decreasing episodes of atrial fibrillation.

Prognosis

Atrial fibrillation, particularly associated with rapid rates, carries significant negative prognostic implications for those with associated structural cardiac disease or heart failure. For example, loss of the atrial pump function for those with less compliant ventricles (ie, hypertrophic myopathy) may result in hemodynamic collapse. In addition, persistent, rapid rates may induce a tachycardia-mediated cardiomyopathy with similar negative prognostic implications. Therefore, depending on the clinical scenario, maintenance of sinus rhythm or rate control is such an important therapeutic concern.

Although anticoagulants, left atrial appendage occlusion, and perhaps aspirin can reduce the risk of stroke or other systemic emboli, the risk is never zero, regardless of whether the patient has paroxysmal, persistent, or permanent atrial fibrillation. Also, in patients with cardiovascular disease, the presence of atrial fibrillation always increases the risk of major adverse cardiac events. It is not clear whether various treatment approaches substantially alter this adverse prognosis.

Ventricular Tachycardia

13

Yaanik B. Desai, MD
Nitish Badhwar, MD

ESSENTIALS OF DIAGNOSIS

- Nonsustained: three or more consecutive QRS complexes of uniform configuration of ventricular origin at a rate of more than 100 bpm.
- Sustained: lasts more than 30 seconds; requires intervention for termination.
- Monomorphic ventricular tachycardia.
- Polymorphic ventricular tachycardia: beat-to-beat variation in QRS configuration.

The magnitude of ventricular tachycardia (VT), one of the most common health problems encountered in clinical practice, can best be appreciated in terms of its various clinical manifestations, which include ventricular fibrillation (sudden cardiac death [SCD]), syncope or near syncope, and wide QRS tachycardia.

The most serious is its degeneration into ventricular fibrillation, producing cardiac arrest and SCD that accounts for 200,000 deaths a year. The second most serious clinical presentation is syncope. Although the overall prevalence of VT-related syncope is unclear, it is estimated to be frequent because inducible VT (via electrical stimulation) is the most common arrhythmia detected in patients with unexplained syncope. A high prevalence of SCD (> 20% incidence within the ensuing 12 months) is noted in patients with syncope from cardiovascular causes, suggesting that undiagnosed VT may be an underlying cause of sudden death in patients with unexplained syncope. The third most significant clinical manifestation of VT is a wide QRS complex tachycardia that is often hemodynamically well tolerated.

DIAGNOSTIC ISSUES

1. Underdiagnosis

VT as a cause of morbidity and mortality is grossly underdiagnosed, potentially leading to mismanagement. This may be particularly true when the clinical presentation is unexplained syncope because no concomitant electrocardiographic (ECG) documentation is available. In the case of cardiac arrest or SCD, acute myocardial infarction rather than an arrhythmic problem is often assumed to be responsible. Most persons who have suffered sudden death have no evidence of acute myocardial necrosis, even though the episode often occurs in patients with underlying coronary artery disease. Managing the underlying coronary artery disease with no regard to treating the concomitant VT is inadequate.

2. Misdiagnosis

If a patient with a wide complex tachycardia is hemodynamically stable, it is often erroneously assumed that the rhythm must be a supraventricular tachycardia (SVT) with aberrant conduction rather than VT. In reality, the clinical presentation of VT can be quite variable, and the rate as well as the hemodynamic tolerance in a patient depends on many factors, including concomitant coronary artery disease, heart failure, the presence of cardioactive drugs, and even the patient's posture at the time of onset. Therefore, it is prudent not to exclude the diagnosis of VT on the basis of hemodynamic tolerance alone. Approximately 80% of the patients with sustained wide QRS tachycardia have VT. To avoid misdiagnosis, clinicians in emergency settings must become familiar with established ECG criteria (discussed in the next section) that distinguish VT from SVT with aberrant conduction. When there is uncertainty, it is best to

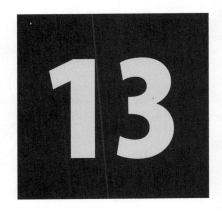

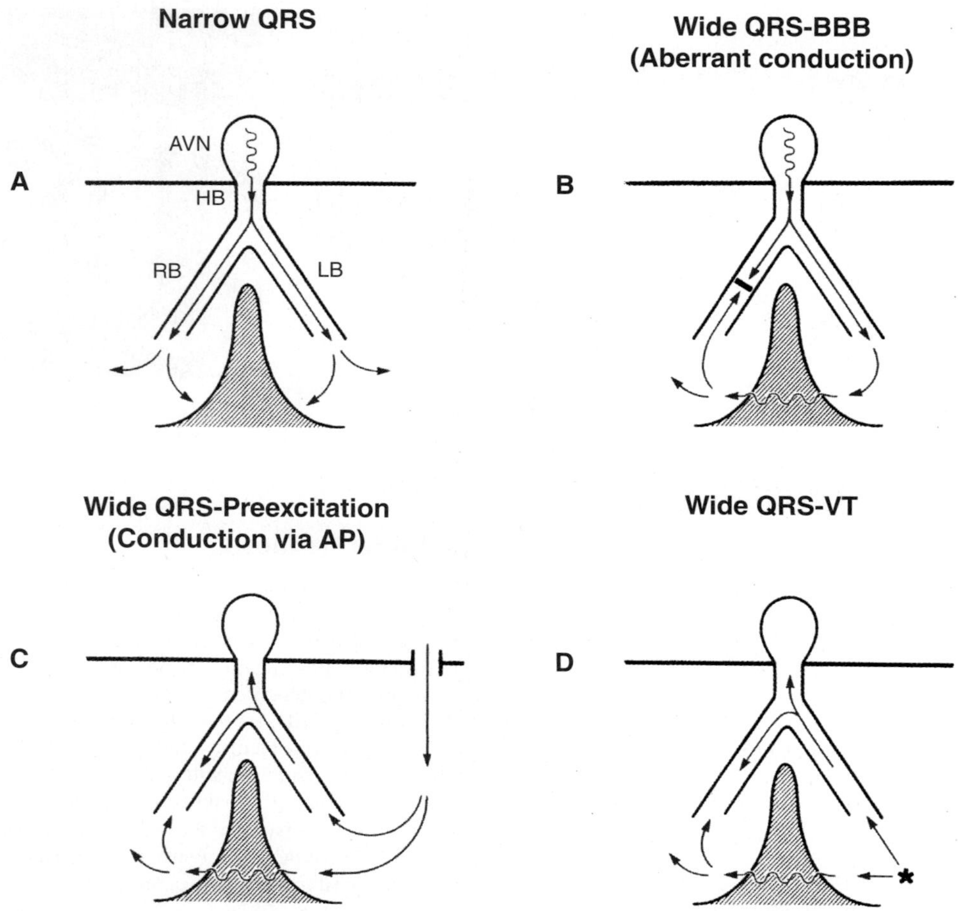

▲ **Figure 13–1.** Mechanism of wide QRS. **A:** Narrow QRS from simultaneous activation of the right and left ventricles. In the three types of wide QRS shown in **B–D,** there is sequential rather than simultaneous activation of the left and right ventricle and a variable amount of muscle-to-muscle conduction. AP, accessory pathway; AVN, atrioventricular node; BBB, bundle branch block; HB, His bundle; LB, left bundle; RB, right bundle. (Reproduced, with permission from Akhtar M, et al. Electrophysiological spectrum of wide QRS complex tachycardia. In: Zipes DP, et al., eds. *Cardiac Electrophysiology. From Cell to Bedside.* Philadelphia: WB Saunders; 1990.)

simply assume that the rhythm is VT—it is more often the correct assumption, and it is safer to treat SVT as VT than to leave VT untreated, given the risk of degeneration into sudden cardiac arrest.

3. Diagnostic Approach to the Patient with Wide QRS Complex Tachycardia

The diagnosis of wide QRS complex tachycardia by ECG analysis has always been a challenge for clinicians. The differential diagnosis includes VT, SVT with aberrant conduction, and preexcited tachycardia in patients with Wolff-Parkinson-White (WPW) syndrome. Figure 13–1 depicts, schematically, the reasons for normal and broad QRS complexes. Preexcited tachycardia results from antegrade activation of the ventricle via an accessory pathway in patients with WPW syndrome, which can present with atrial fibrillation, atrial flutter, atrial tachycardia, atrioventricular nodal reentry tachycardia (AVNRT), or antidromic tachycardia (Figure 13–2). Preexcited tachycardia is a rare cause of wide QRS complex tachycardia (5–8% of cases); however, the QRS pattern of preexcited QRS complex can be difficult to distinguish from VT because in both instances the QRS starts with myocyte-to-myocyte conduction. ECG artifact can also mimic wide QRS complex tachycardia and be misdiagnosed as VT, leading to expensive testing and even placement of implantable cardioverter-defibrillator (ICD). Clues to the diagnosis of artifact include: absence of hemodynamic

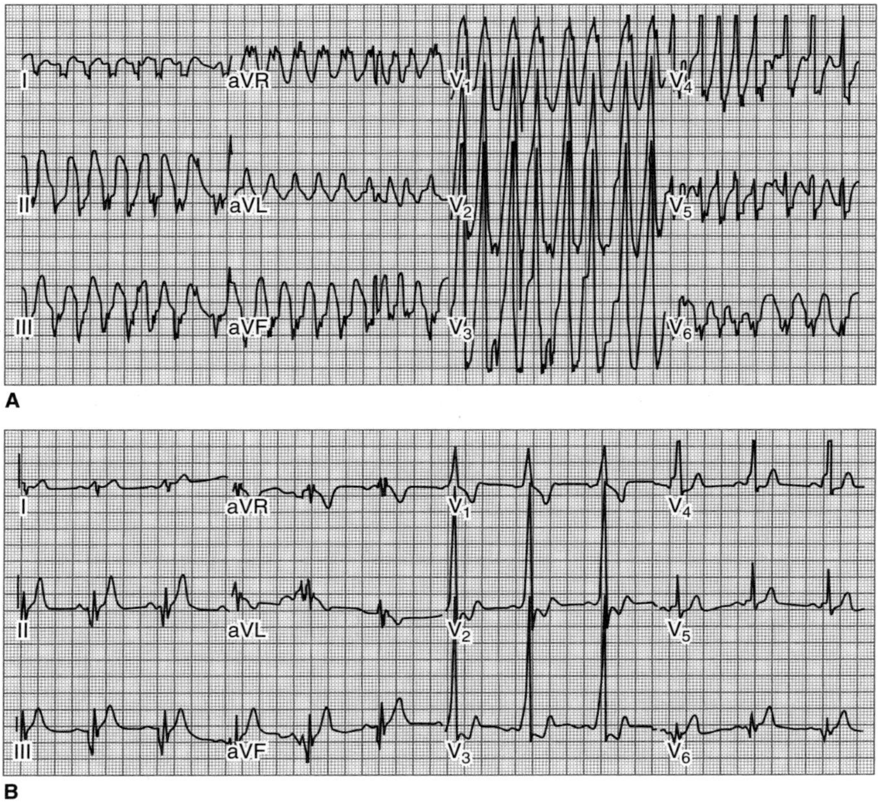

▲ **Figure 13–2. A:** Preexcited wide complex tachycardia in a patient with Wolff-Parkinson-White (WPW) and atrial fibrillation **B:** Sinus rhythm electrocardiogram showing short PR interval and delta wave consistent with left posterior WPW. (Reproduced, with permission from Turakhia MP, et al. Wolff-Parkinson-White syndrome: where is the pathway? *Indian Pacing Electrophysiol J.* 2009;9(2):130–133.)

deterioration, an unstable ECG baseline, association with body movement, and ability to march the normal QRS complexes through the artifact ("notches sign") at a sinus R-R interval (Figure 13–3). A number of surface ECG criteria, including the atrioventricular (AV) relationship, the QRS complex duration, specific QRS morphology, and the QRS complex axis, have been established to distinguish VT from SVT with aberrant conduction. These criteria are helpful in arriving at an accurate diagnosis if they are used in a systematic fashion.

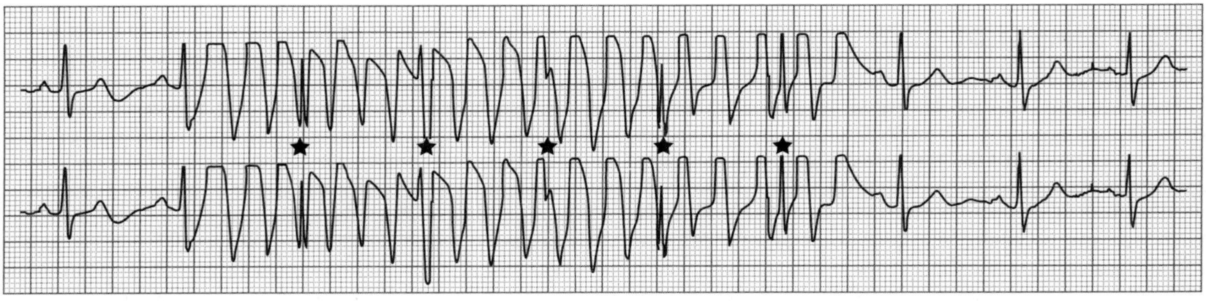

▲ **Figure 13–3.** Artifact mimicking ventricular tachycardia. The QRS complexes are seen as notches that are marching at the regular sinus interval (*). (Reproduced with permission from Badhwar N, Kusumoto F, Goldschlager N. Arrhythmias in the Coronary Care Unit. *Journal of Intensive Care Medicine.* 2012;27(5):267–289.)

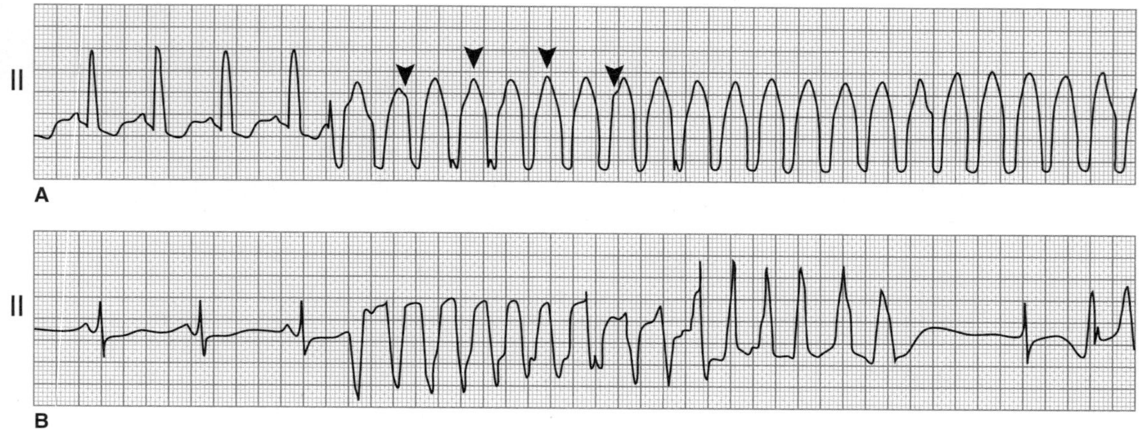

▲ **Figure 13–4. A:** Monomorphic ventricular tachycardia (VT), with a uniform QRS appearance for all complexes. Arrowheads indicate superimposed P waves. **B:** Polymorphic VT, with a beat-to-beat variation in the QRS morphology; QT-interval prolongation follows the termination of the VT episode. (Reproduced with permission from Akhtar M. Clinical spectrum of ventricular tachycardia. *Circulation*. 1990;82(5):1561–1573.)

Atrioventricular Relationship

In SVT, the arrhythmia arises in the atria or AV junction and reaches the ventricles through the AV node and His-Purkinje system. Because the atrial arrhythmia is the primary event, either a 1:1 AV response or a varying degree of AV block occurs, but in either case, the atrial rates equal or exceed ventricular rates. During VT, a retrograde block often leads to either AV dissociation or a varying degree of ventriculoatrial conduction ratios, but the ventricular rates equal or exceed the atrial rate. When AV dissociation can be recognized, it is the most reliable criterion for VT (Figures 13–4 and 13–5). This criterion lacks sensitivity, however, because the P waves can be identified on the surface ECG in only 25% of patients with VT. In patients with slower VT and AV dissociation, intermittent ventricular capture can result in fusion with narrow QRS complexes during wide QRS complex tachycardia. This useful but rarely observed finding is also 100% specific for the diagnosis of VT.

QRS Complex Duration

For the reasons listed earlier, the QRS complex duration is the widest in VT and narrowest in aberrant conduction. To distinguish VT from SVT with aberrant conduction on the basis of QRS duration alone, however, some specific aspects must be considered. In the absence of cardioactive drugs and extensive myocardial fibrosis, aberrancy rarely results in a QRS duration of more than 140 ms with a right bundle branch block (RBBB) pattern (see Figure 13–5) or more than 160 ms with a left bundle branch block (LBBB) configuration. However, in the presence of intramyocardial conduction delay from drugs (such as class I antiarrhythmic agents) or myocardial fibrosis, the QRS width may exceed these values in SVT with aberrant conduction. Conversely, on a rare occasion, VT can present as a narrow QRS tachycardia (< 120 ms that is narrower than the conducted QRS complex) when there is near-simultaneous activation of the two ventricles, perhaps from the septum.

Specific QRS Morphology

VT can have both LBBB or RBBB morphology, though because of the myocardial origin of most forms of VT, the QRS contrasts from typical RBBB and LBBB patterns. Many ECG criteria have therefore exploited these differences to distinguish VT from aberrant conduction. The typical RBBB (ie, in the case of aberrancy) is a triphasic complex best seen in V_1 as rsR′ or rSR′ pattern and in lead I as qRs, qRS pattern. Similarly, a typical LBBB has no initial q wave in lead I and a small r and a rapid S wave in V_1. One general principle that distinguishes the morphology of the QRS complex in SVT versus VT is that the initial portion of the complex in VT is slow, as it originates in myocardial tissue in contrast to the fast initial activation of SVT (which propagates initially down the native conduction system). A study that analyzed the morphology of premature ventricular complexes (PVC) and aberrantly conducted beats of RBBB morphology in V_1 found that the triphasic RsR′ pattern with R′ > R was predominant in aberrant conduction (70%) compared with PVC (6%). Monophasic pattern or R > R′ was seen in the PVC beats. The limitation of that study is that origin of the anomalous beats (SVT versus VT) was also based on the ECG (presence or absence of preceding P wave). A retrospective ECG analysis of 70 patients with SVT and 70 patients with VT in whom His bundle recordings were used to determine

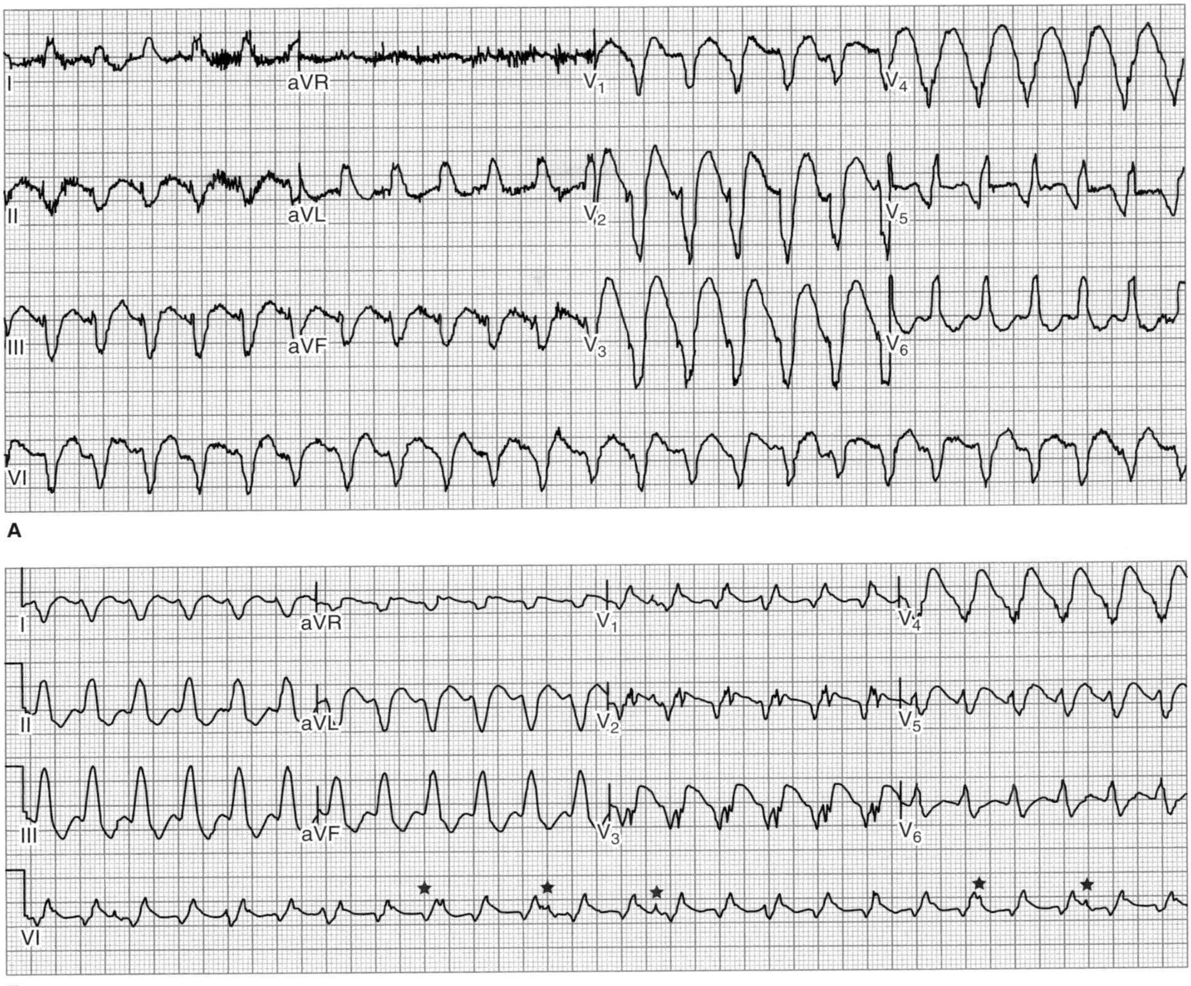

▲ **Figure 13–5. A:** Scar-related ventricular tachycardia (VT), with a left bundle branch block left axis morphology in a patient with ischemic cardiomyopathy and previous myocardial infarction. **B:** Right bundle branch block right axis morphology VT in the same patient at the same rate suggesting that both forms of VT have the same circuit (that revolves around the mitral annulus) with different exits causing the difference in morphology. Atrioventricular dissociation is noted in the rhythm strip on V_1 (*) that is 100% specific for VT.

the site of origin of the wide QRS complex tachycardia found that VT was favored by monophasic or biphasic R waves in V_1 and an R:S ratio less than 1 in V_6 in patients with RBBB morphology and any Q wave in V_6 in patients with LBBB morphology. A study of 150 consecutive wide QRS complex tachycardia cases found that 12-lead QRS morphology during wide QRS complex tachycardia was different from that during preexisting bundle branch block in sinus rhythm, favoring a diagnosis of VT. The investigators also noted that a positive QRS concordance (positive complexes V_1–V_6) is uncommon in aberrancy, but a negative QRS concordance can occur during aberrant conduction in a small percentage of cases. Another study that evaluated wide QRS complex tachycardia with LBBB morphology in V_1 found that an R wave of greater than 30 ms, notching in the down stroke of the S wave and an RS (beginning of QRS complex to nadir of S wave) interval greater than 60 ms in V_1 or V_2, and any Q wave in V_6 favored a diagnosis of VT. In a prospective analysis of wide QRS complex tachycardia (with RBBB and LBBB morphology), the following two criteria for a diagnosis of VT were proposed: (1) absence of R-S in all precordial leads and (2) R-S interval greater than 100 ms (measured from the beginning of the QRS complex to the nadir of the S wave) in any precordial lead. Finally, the presence of QR complex in any lead during wide QRS complex tachycardia also favors a diagnosis of VT.

QRS Complex Axis

The axis orientation on a 12-lead ECG ranging from normal (−30° to +90°), left (−31° to −90°), or right (+91° to +180°) has significant overlap across the causes of wide QRS complex tachycardia and is of little diagnostic value. The axis range of −91° to 180° (often referred to as a "northwest" axis), however, is usually not seen in aberrant conduction, unless there is a significant structural problem that predisposes the ECG vector to an abnormal axis (eg, severe R ventricular hypertrophy). Similarly, a combination of LBBB pattern with right axis deviation is almost always suggestive of VT over SVT. A previous history of myocardial infarction (MI) and an axis change of more than 40° between sinus rhythm and wide QRS complex tachycardia may independently favor VT over SVT.

History, Physical Examination, & 12-Lead ECG

A detailed history can provide clues to the diagnosis of wide QRS complex tachycardia. A history of prior MI strongly favors VT as the diagnosis in a patient with wide QRS complex tachycardia. The clinician must take note of drug and toxin ingestion to rule out secondary causes of VT. A detailed family history is also important, since it can reveal the presence of inherited arrhythmogenic cardiomyopathies.

There are also several salient features on physical examination that can be helpful. The presence of irregular cannon waves on jugular venous examination and variable intensity of S_1 on auscultation suggest AV dissociation and are indicative of VT in the setting of a wide QRS complex tachycardia. Carotid massage (performed carefully after ruling out a bruit) that leads to termination of wide QRS complex tachycardia typically suggests SVT as the mechanism of the arrhythmia (though an exception is idiopathic VT arising from the right ventricular outflow tract (RVOT), which can be responsive to vagal stimulation).

A prior ECG in sinus rhythm showing Q waves, indicative of infarcted tissue and scar, increases the likelihood that a subsequent wide QRS complex tachycardia is due to VT. SVT is the diagnosis if the old ECG shows bundle branch block pattern that matches the 12-lead ECG during wide QRS complex tachycardia. Preexcited tachycardia is inferred from the ECG showing WPW pattern that is similar to wide QRS complex tachycardia ECG pattern.

It is essential to obtain a 12-lead ECG during wide QRS complex tachycardia to compare it to the sinus rhythm ECG and look for subtle findings like AV dissociation and narrow beats (fusion and capture) that might not be evident in some leads. Table 13–1 outlines an approach to diagnosing wide QRS complex tachycardia by analyzing the ECG. The first step is to read the ECG with emphasis on rate, regularity (atrial fibrillation with preexcited tachycardia is irregular), axis (extreme northwest axis suggests VT), and morphology in V_1. The next step is to look for AV dissociation (V > A) by marching the sinus P waves at the onset and termination of the wide QRS complex tachycardia if available. Narrow QRS complexes in a wide QRS complex tachycardia (caused by capture and fusion of conducted beats through the AV node-His-Purkinje system) are 100% specific for VT. The next step is to use the Brugada criteria by evaluating the R-S complexes in precordial leads. Absence of R-S complex in all precordial leads or an R-S interval greater than 100 ms in one precordial lead favor a diagnosis of VT.

Table 13–1. Approach to the ECG with Wide QRS Complex Tachycardia

1. **Read the ECG:** rate, rhythm, axis, morphology in V_1 (predominantly upright, RBBB; downward, LBBB)
2. **AV dissociation**
3. **Narrow complex beat:** fusion or capture
4. **Brugada criteria:** RS (measured from beginning of QRS to the nadir of S wave) in precordial leads
   a. Absence of RS in all precordial leads favors VT
   b. RS > 100 ms in any precordial lead favors VT
5. **Morphology criteria:**
   a. RBBB (rsR′): R′ > r in lead V_1 favors SVT. Other morphologies favor VT
   b. LBBB: Kindwall criteria in leads V_1, V_2 favor VT
   R > 30 ms, notch in S wave, QRS onset to S > 60 ms Q wave in V_6
   c. Peak R-wave duration in lead II > 50 ms favors VT
   d. Lead aVR criteria that favor VT (any one of the following): Initial R wave, initial r or q wave > 40 ms, notch in initial downstroke of QRS complex, voltage change in initial 40 ms (v_i)/voltage change in terminal 40 ms (v_t) < 1

AV, atrioventricular; ECG, electrocardiogram; LBBB, left bundle branch block; RBBB, right bundle branch block; SVT, supraventricular tachycardia; VT, ventricular tachycardia.

The last step in the Brugada algorithm relies on QRS morphology criteria (discussed earlier) to differentiate VT from SVT. The onset of QRS complex to peak of the R wave or nadir of S wave in lead II greater than 50 ms favors a diagnosis of VT.

The morphology criteria have certain limitations. Idiopathic VTs (fascicular VT, outflow tract VT) and bundle branch reentrant VT can have a typical bundle branch block pattern on the ECG and can therefore be misdiagnosed as SVT with aberrancy. Furthermore, some antiarrhythmic medications can alter typical conduction and limit generalizability of the morphology criteria developed for the Brugada algorithm, that is, patients with an SVT with aberrancy may have an atypical bundle branch block pattern on the ECG, leading to a misdiagnosis of VT. In addition, patients with preexcited SVT may also have atypical bundle block patterns.

To address some of the limitations in morphology criteria, and to simplify detection, newer criteria have been developed that rely solely on aVR analysis. Criteria in aVR that favor VT include presence of initial R wave, initial r or q wave greater than 40 ms, notch in initial downstroke of QRS complex, and voltage change in initial 40 ms (v_i)/voltage change in terminal 40 ms (v_t) less than 1. Again, this criterion exploits the fact that the initial portion of the QRS in VT is slower than the terminal portion because the signal originates in slower myocardial tissue, before spreading across the ventricles and involving the faster native conduction tissue.

In clinical practice, traditional criteria and aVR criteria have generally similar sensitivity and specificity for distinguishing VT from SVT. Importantly, if the clinician is unsure of the diagnosis, it is safer to assume the signal is VT, and treat it as such.

Cerantola M, Arkles J, Frankel DS. Diagnostic approach to wide complex tachycardia. *JAMA Intern Med.* 2021 Sep 1;181(9):1231–1233. [PMID: 34279546]. doi: 10.1001/jamainternmed.2021.3189.

CLASSIFICATIONS OF VENTRICULAR TACHYCARDIA

The spectrum of VT in Table 13–2 lists the two most common varieties encountered in clinical practice and their underlying causes. This classification helps approach the diagnosis in a systematic fashion and directs the physician to specific therapeutic options.

Monomorphic VT is a form of VT in which the QRS complex configuration is uniform from beat to beat in all the surface ECG leads (see Figure 13–4A). In **polymorphic VT,** a beat-to-beat variation occurs in the QRS complex configuration in any of the ECG leads (see Figure 13–4B). These diagnoses may be difficult, however, when a single-surface ECG lead is recorded. As used in the literature, sustained VT is a tachycardia that lasts for 30 seconds or requires intervention for termination. Nonsustained VT is a term used to describe any three or more consecutive QRS complexes of ventricular origin with a rate of more than 100 bpm, that lasts less than 30 seconds. This time interval is, ultimately, an arbitrary cut point, and nonsustained VT can still be clinically significant, particularly if symptomatic and in the presence of structural heart disease. In this chapter, VT is considered sustained unless specifically stated otherwise.

VT is most commonly associated with structural heart disease, though up to 15–20% of VT is seen in patients with a structurally normal heart—referred to as idiopathic VT. This distinction is important because the therapeutic approach to VT is different in patients with structural heart disease compared with patients with idiopathic VT in which case catheter ablation can be curative.

Table 13–2. Classification and Causes of Common Ventricular Tachycardias

Monomorphic ventricular tachycardia
Chronic coronary artery disease
Idiopathic dilated cardiomyopathy
Arrhythmogenic right ventricular cardiomyopathy
No structural heart disease
Right bundle branch block configuration
Left bundle branch block configuration
Repetitive monomorphic ventricular tachycardia
Other forms
Polymorphic ventricular tachycardia
Prolonged QT interval (torsades de pointes)
Congenital
Acquired
Normal QT interval
Acute ischemia
Other

VENTRICULAR TACHYCARDIA ASSOCIATED WITH STRUCTURAL HEART DISEASE

1. Monomorphic Ventricular Tachycardia in Association with Chronic Coronary Artery Disease

This is the most common form encountered in clinical practice as well as the most extensively investigated in clinical and electrophysiology laboratories. The underlying substrate is usually an area of fibrosis that provides an anatomic obstacle around which the reentrant impulse can propagate. The extent and architecture of the scar may determine the propensity for VT in a given situation. For example, a homogeneous scar with no surviving conducting tissue is less likely to cause arrhythmias than is fibrosis interspersed with streaks of healthy myocardium. In some situations, acute myocardial ischemia or infarct can produce the conditions of slow conduction and block necessary for reentry. Although non-reentrant mechanisms (eg, abnormal automaticity, triggered activity) may cause VT in these settings, reentry is the most common mechanism.

As myocardial activation spreads from the reentrant circuit, the resultant QRS morphology is determined by the direction of the activation vector. Because of the myocardial origin of this type of VT, some characteristic features are expected: (1) The initial part of the QRS complex will generally be inscribed slowly because of muscle-to-muscle propagation. (2) The resultant QRS width is often markedly increased because of this intramyocardial conduction delay. (3) Because the impulse is not activating the ventricles via the bundle branches, the QRS pattern is not likely to be typical of either the RBBB or LBBB. (4) When there is no septal scar, VT originating in the left ventricle activates the surrounding left ventricular tissue, followed by the interventricular septum and then the right ventricle. This causes an atypical RBBB pattern. (5) Conversely, VT that originates in the right ventricle shows a LBBB pattern. (6) Because of the anterior position of the septum relative to the left ventricle, if the tachycardia originates close to a septal scar, it may show a LBBB pattern even if the reentrant circuit resides in the left ventricle. (7) ECG leads can be used to localize the site of origin of VT from the left ventricle as follows: (a) aVR and V_4 leads are nearly aligned along the apical-basal axis of the heart, such that a positive QRS complex in lead avR and negative in lead V_4 suggests apical site of origin and vice versa for basal sites. (b) Positive QRS complexes in leads II, III, and aVF suggest anterior site of origin, whereas negative QRS complex in these leads is seen in VT arising from inferior wall. (c) Positive QRS complex in leads I and aVL is seen in VT arising from the septum, whereas a negative QRS in these leads suggests origin from the lateral wall. Figure 13–5 shows scar-related VT in a patient with previous history of MI. The VT has one reentrant circuit in the left ventricle with two different morphologies based on different exit sites.

After an initial documentation on the surface ECG, or when VT is suspected by virtue of underlying coronary artery disease and symptoms such as syncope, a further workup is often critical for characterization of VT. Ambulatory monitoring is of limited value because sustained VT is not commonly seen on a daily basis. In most situations, invasive electrophysiologic studies are indicated for these patients for both diagnostic and therapeutic purposes.

2. Monomorphic Ventricular Tachycardia in Association with Idiopathic Dilated Cardiomyopathy

Monomorphic VT associated with idiopathic dilated cardiomyopathy and valvular disease is often difficult to distinguish from VT from chronic ischemic disease, because in both entities, the underlying substrate is fibrosis, providing both the anatomic obstacle and the pathway for reentry. Patients with idiopathic dilated cardiomyopathy, however, will often have conduction slowing in the His-Purkinje system as a part of the diffuse myocardial disease process, and the baseline ECG can show evidence of nonspecific intraventricular conduction defect. In this scenario, a special case of VT known as bundle branch reentry can occur. In this setting, the limbs of the reentry circuit are the two bundle branches themselves. The QRS pattern will either be a typical LBBB or RBBB pattern, depending on whether the signal travels antegrade via the RBBB or the LBBB, respectively (Figure 13–6). Although the prevalence of bundle branch reentry is particularly high in patients with idiopathic dilated cardiomyopathy, it can occur in the setting of advanced structural heart disease regardless of the underlying pathology.

Bundle branch reentry also occurs in the setting of aortic and mitral valve disease. Due to the close anatomic relationship between the proximal His-Purkinje system and annuli of these valves, His-Purkinje system conduction delays can occur in association with valvular disease. Frequently, sustained bundle branch reentry is observed soon after valve surgery, probably related to aggregation of local substrata.

3. Monomorphic Ventricular Tachycardia in Arrhythmogenic Cardiomyopathy

Arrhythmogenic cardiomyopathy is a broad classification of cardiac pathology that occurs in the setting of inflammation and/or genetic predisposition, where the predominant presentation is arrhythmia that is not explained by underlying ischemic, hypertensive, or valvular disease.

This classification includes infiltrative cardiomyopathies associated with systemic diseases like sarcoidosis, tuberculosis, and amyloidosis, which can manifest with conduction system disease and VT (reentrant VT or automatic VT). Cardiac sarcoidosis should be suspected in a patient with a new conduction block and a ventricular arrhythmia. Inflammatory processes resulting in myocarditis can also be associated with VT and SCD—and giant cell myocarditis is particularly malignant.

Arrhythmogenic cardiomyopathies also include diseases with infectious etiology which can cause ventricular arrhythmia. Chagas is a parasitic disease transmitted to humans by the *Reduvidaee* insect vector that is endemic in South and Central America. Infection can lead to dilated cardiomyopathy and fibrosis, and it is the most common cause of VT in South America. Risk factors for mortality in these patients include decreased ejection fraction, nonsustained VT on Holter monitoring, and advanced heart failure. There is a high incidence of epicardial VT in patients with Chagas disease, which requires a pericardial approach to VT ablation.

Of all the arrhythmogenic cardiomyopathies, the best characterized is arrhythmogenic right ventricular cardiomyopathy/dysplasia (ARVC/D). ARVC/D is classically described as a disease of fibrofatty infiltration in the right ventricular muscle, with a predilection for the development in athletes. These patients have inherited or de novo mutations in the desmosomal protein complex, which is responsible for cell-to-cell attachment. Functional problems in this complex disrupt the cell-to-cell connections and the mechanical integrity of the myocardium, leading to cell death and scar, which is the nidus for reentrant ventricular tachycardia.

Because scar and subsequent reentry occur in the right ventricle in the classic ARVC/D phenotype, the QRS morphology of the ventricular tachycardia has a LBBB pattern. The axis of the VT can be variable (and even normal), though consensus diagnostic criteria give more weight to a superiorly direct VT, which reflects an origin from the RV apex or body. Many patients with arrhythmogenic right ventricular cardiomyopathy have a VT circuit that arises from the epicardium rather than the endocardium and require a pericardial approach to VT ablation.

On the surface ECG in sinus rhythm, patients often have T-wave inversions in leads V_1–V_3, reflecting repolarization abnormalities within the RV (which is the most anterior chamber). Another finding while in sinus rhythm is the presence of an epsilon wave, which is a low-amplitude signal at the end of the QRS complex that reflects delayed depolarization of signal traveling through scar in the RV (Figure 13–7A).

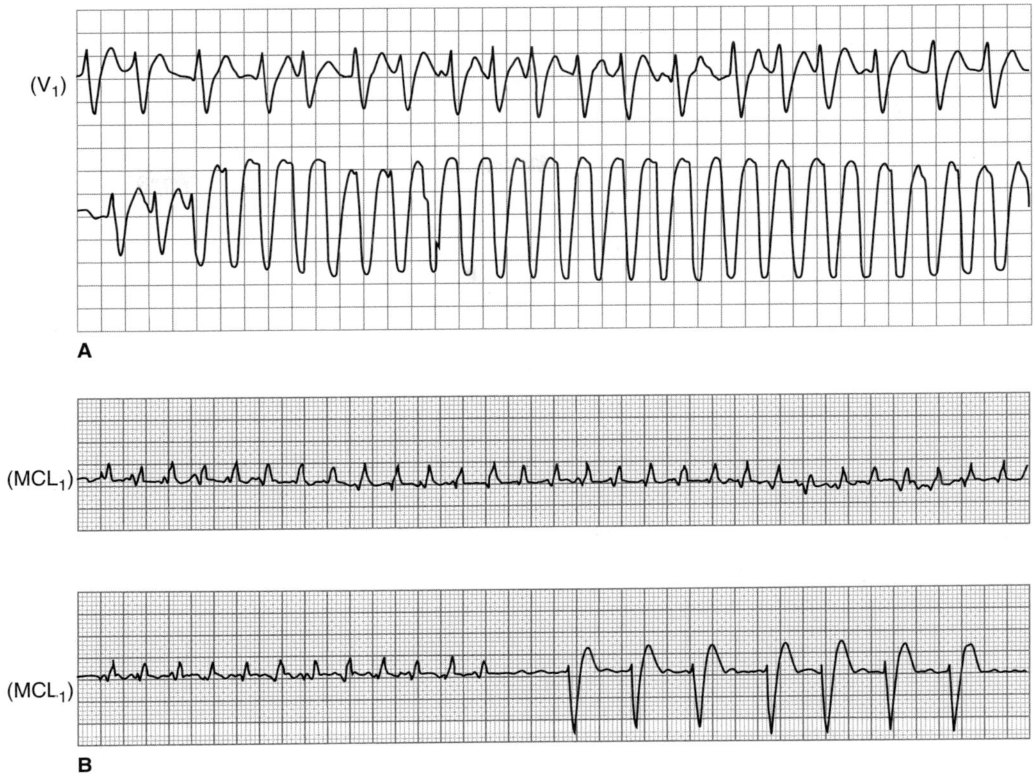

▲ **Figure 13–6.** Bundle branch reentrant ventricular tachycardia with typical left (**A**) and right (**B**) bundle branch morphologies, recorded at different times in a patient with idiopathic dilated cardiomyopathy. Note the underlying intraventricular conduction defect during baseline rhythm, before onset (**A**) and after termination (**B**). (Reproduced with permission from Tchou P, et al. Transcatheter electrical ablation of right bundle branch. A method of treating macroreentrant ventricular tachycardia attributed to bundle branch reentry. *Circulation*. 1988;78(2):246–257.)

The epsilon wave has limited sensitivity, as it is present in less than 25% of patients with ARVC/D. Another manifestation of delayed depolarization via diseased tissue is the presence of terminal activation delay, where the timing from the nadir of the S wave to the end of the QRS complex is greater than 55 ms. Of note, the resting ECG can also be normal in patients with ARVC/D. A signal averaged ECG can reveal low-amplitude late potentials that would otherwise not be visible, though it too is limited in sensitivity.

In addition to transthoracic echocardiography, cardiac magnetic resonance imaging (MRI) is an important diagnostic tool for the diagnosis of ARVC/D, because it allows for the assessment of RV function/ejection fraction, focal dyskinesia, and presence of scar (via deposition of gadolinium).

Diagnosis of ARVC/D can be difficult due to the limited sensitivity of consensus criteria, and the variable presentation and severity. Though the classic model of the disease describes primary right ventricular pathology, many of these patients also develop some degree of LV dysfunction (especially when queried by more sensitive imaging techniques like cMRI). The emerging use of rapid genetic testing is revealing new pathologic mutations and disease processes, which are broadening our understanding of arrhythmogenic cardiomyopathies that do not fit classically described phenotypes. Nevertheless, there must be high index of suspicion for ARVC/D in a young patient with LBBB pattern ventricular tachycardia and RV dysfunction.

4. Monomorphic Ventricular Tachycardia in Patients with Congenital Heart Disease

VT can present late in adult life in patients with congenital heart disease (eg, tetralogy of Fallot, aortic stenosis, pulmonary stenosis). The VT is usually due to reentrant circuits between fibrotic scars and healthy myocardium. Tetralogy of Fallot usually leads to enlargement of the right ventricle with VT arising from the RVOT. Severity of pulmonary valvular regurgitation, late surgical repair, and QRS duration greater than 180 ms are risk factors for VT and sudden death in patients with tetralogy of Fallot.

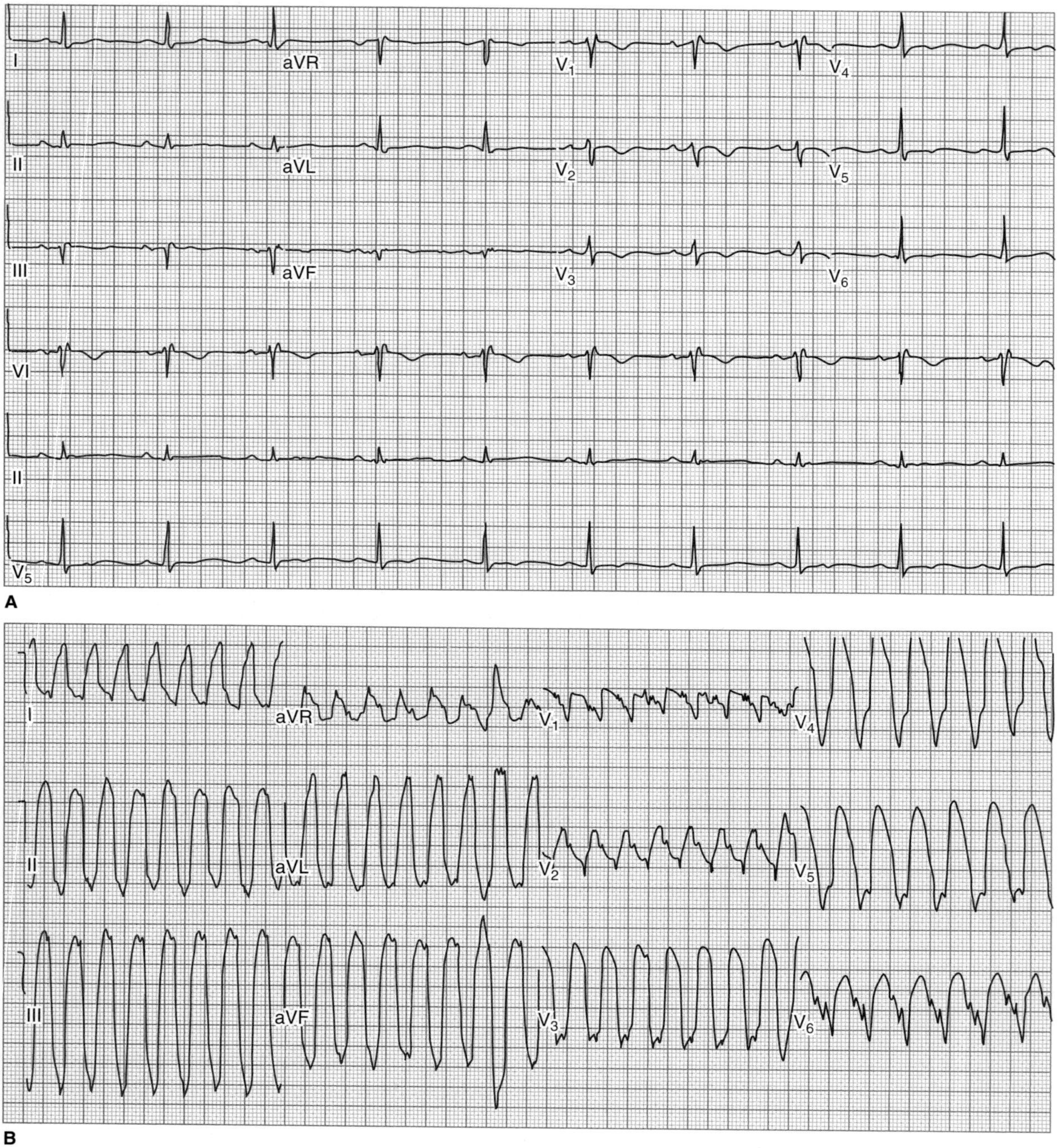

▲ **Figure 13–7. A:** Twelve-lead electrocardiogram in a patient with arrhythmogenic right ventricular cardiomyopathy (ARVC) showing T-wave inversions in V_1–V_3 and delayed depolarization in V_1. **B:** Ventricular tachycardia with a left bundle branch block left axis morphology in a patient with ARVC.

5. Monomorphic Ventricular Tachycardia in Other Forms of Structural Heart Disease

Hypertrophic cardiomyopathy is characterized by hypertrophy and enlargement of the left ventricle especially in the septum. There are fibrotic scars in the ventricle that give rise to VT. Although polymorphic VT is more common in these patients, they can also present with monomorphic VT. This is the most common cause of SCD in persons younger than 35 years (see Chapter 15). Skeletal muscle disorders like myotonic dystrophy and Kearns-Sayre syndrome are associated with degenerative changes in the myocardium and the conduction system that causes AV block and VT. Mitral valve prolapse can be associated with fibrotic and degenerative changes in the conduction system that forms the anatomic basis for VT and sudden death, though most patients with MVP do not manifest this, and the identification of arrhythmogenic variants of MVP is an active area of study.

VENTRICULAR TACHYCARDIA NOT ASSOCIATED WITH STRUCTURAL HEART DISEASE

Some patients have VT without any apparent structural heart disease and in this setting, the VT is characterized as "idiopathic." Idiopathic VTs are generally considered benign when compared to VT in the context of structural heart disease, and patients generally have good prognosis, with low risk of SCD. Importantly, the dilated and arrhythmogenic cardiomyopathies discussed earlier can be subtle and insidious in their presentation, and the clinician must thoroughly exclude other etiologies of VT before classifying a presentation as idiopathic.

Broadly, the idiopathic monomorphic VTs are classified by their site of origin (Table 13–3, left panel). In general, idiopathic VT is more likely to have a focal origin rather than reentrant mechanism (though fascicular ventricular tachycardia is an important exception, discussed later). The differing mechanisms also shed light on the differing responses to therapeutic agents—for example, focal VT due to cAMP-dependent triggered activity is more responsive to medications that decrease intracellular cAMP (eg, adenosine) compared to reentrant VT.

Table 13–3. Idiopathic Ventricular Tachycardia

Monomorphic Ventricular Tachycardia	Polymorphic Ventricular Tachycardia
Outflow Tract VT	Long QT syndrome
RVOT-VT	Brugada syndrome
LVOT-VT	Short coupled torsades
Aortic cusp VT	Short QT syndrome
Fascicular VT	Catecholaminergic polymorphic VT
LAF-VT	Idiopathic VF
LPF-VT	Early repolarization syndrome
Septal VT	
Papillary muscle VT	
VT arising from Cardiac Crux	
Annular VT	
Mitral annular	
Tricuspid annular	

LAF, left anterior fascicular; LPF, left posterior fascicular; LVOT, left ventricular outflow tract; RVOT, right ventricular outflow tract; VF, ventricular fibrillation; VT, ventricular tachycardia.
Reproduced with permission from Badhwar N, Scheinman MM. Idiopathic ventricular tachycardia: diagnosis and management. *Curr Probl Cardiol.* 2007;32(1):7–43.

1. Idiopathic Left Ventricular Tachycardia or Fascicular Ventricular Tachycardia

This form of VT arises from one of the three fascicles in the left ventricle: the posterior fascicle, the anterior fascicle, or the septal fascicle, The QRS morphology and axis help distinguish among the three. Fascicular VT involving the left posterior fascicle will have RBBB morphology (because it originates in the L ventricle) and will have a left axis deviation, as the vector escapes from the postero-inferiorly located fascicle and propagates through the remaining ventricle via myocyte-to-myocyte conduction. Conversely, left anterior fascicular VT has right axis deviation. Left upper septal VT (septal VT) is distinguished by a very narrow complex (which can have either RBBB or LBBB morphology since the septum is a more anterior structure. Because the reentrant circuit involves the native conduction system, the QRS duration in fascicular VT will tend to be shorter when compared to other VTs, and generally ranges between 140 and 150 ms (and even shorter in septal VT). The duration from the beginning of the QRS onset to the nadir of the S wave (RS interval) in the precordial leads is 60–80 ms, unlike VT associated with structural heart disease, which is usually associated with longer duration of QRS and RS intervals (Figure 13–8). The diagnosis of fascicular VT can be difficult, since the morphology criteria used to distinguish SVT with aberrancy from VT described earlier in the chapter will not apply. Rather, careful examination for capture/fusion beats and for AV dissociation are the most helpful clues.

Most of the affected patients are males (60–70%). The symptoms include palpitations, fatigue, dyspnea, dizziness, and presyncope. Syncope and sudden death are very rare. Most of the episodes occur at rest; however, this form of VT can be triggered by exercise and emotional stress. Because this VT responds to intravenous verapamil, it is often referred to as verapamil-sensitive VT. Radiofrequency catheter ablation is an appropriate management strategy for

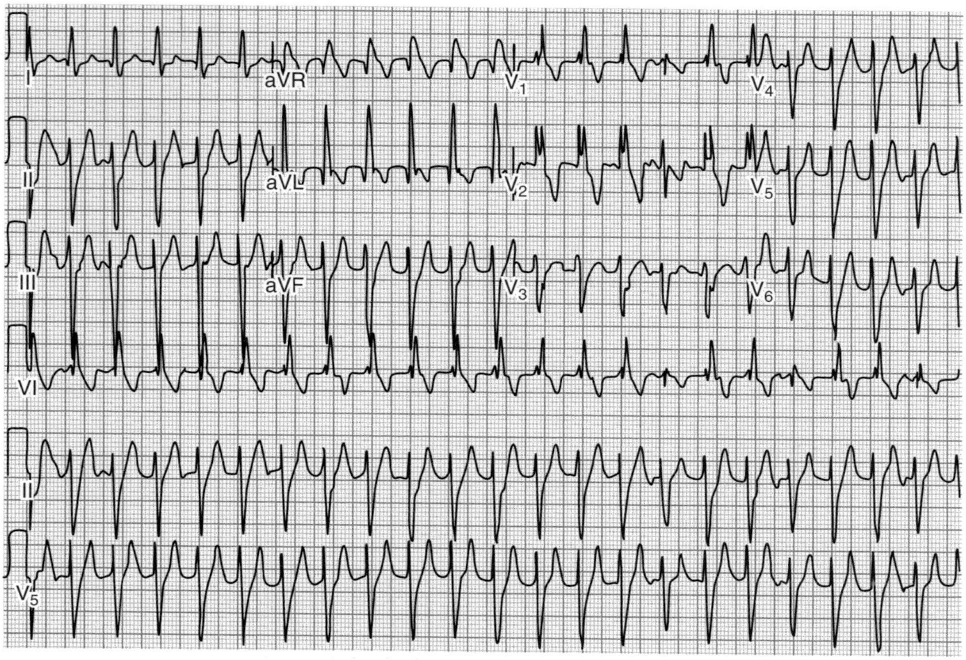

▲ **Figure 13–8.** Twelve-lead electrocardiogram of verapamil-sensitive idiopathic ventricular tachycardia (VT) arising from the left posterior fascicle with a right bundle branch block superior axis morphology. The duration of the QRS complex and the RS interval are narrower than that noted in VT associated with structural heart disease. However, the presence of atrioventricular dissociation and fusion beats (*arrows*) is diagnostic of VT. (Reproduced with permission from Badhwar N, Scheinman MM. Idiopathic ventricular tachycardia: diagnosis and management. *Curr Probl Cardiol*. 2007; 32(1):7–43.)

patients with severe symptoms or those intolerant or resistant to antiarrhythmic therapy with a success rate greater than 92%.

2. Outflow Tract Ventricular Tachycardia

This form of idiopathic VT arises from the outflow tract of the right or the left ventricle—because the outflow tracts are anterior and superior structures, the characteristic ECG morphology is LBBB pattern with inferior axis (Figure 13–9). Lead I has a QS or qR complex in anterior sites and dominant R wave in posterior sites, while aVL shows negative complex in septal sites and positive complex in lateral sites. Based on the site of origin, outflow tract VT can be classified as (1) VT that arises from the RVOT, (2) VT that arises from the left ventricular outflow tract (LVOT), or (3) VT that arises from the aortic cusps (cusp VT). Cusp VT shows earlier precordial transition (< V_2) and a broader R-wave duration in V_1 and V_2. It is important to differentiate RVOT VT from VT associated with arrhythmogenic right ventricular cardiomyopathy that also has an LBBB morphology.

Right ventricular outflow tract (RVOT) VTs are more common overall than left ventricular outflow tract (LVOT) VT. RVOT is more common in women is usually seen in third to fifth decade of life, whereas LVOT VT is equally distributed between men and women. Symptoms include palpitations, dizziness, atypical chest pain, and syncope. There are three predominant clinical forms of this syndrome: (1) nonsustained repetitive monomorphic VT alternating with periods of sinus rhythm, (2) paroxysmal exercise-induced sustained VT, and (3) frequent PVC that occasionally presents as bigeminal rhythm giving rise to tachycardia-induced cardiomyopathy. In some patients, the tachycardia is provoked by exercise and isoproterenol infusion, suggesting that the underlying mechanism is likely cAMP-dependent triggered activity from catecholamine, rather than reentry. As such, these VTs tend to terminate rapidly with the administration of adenosine, which reduces intracellular cAMP in myocytes. Immediate termination of RVOT VT can also be achieved with carotid sinus massage, verapamil, and lidocaine. Beta-blockers are especially effective for those with exercise-induced outflow tract VT, and a synergistic action is noted with calcium channel blockers. Antiarrhythmic agents, such as procainamide, flecainide, amiodarone, and sotalol, are also effective in these patients, though are generally reserved for patients who cannot tolerate beta or calcium channel blockade. Catheter ablation using radiofrequency

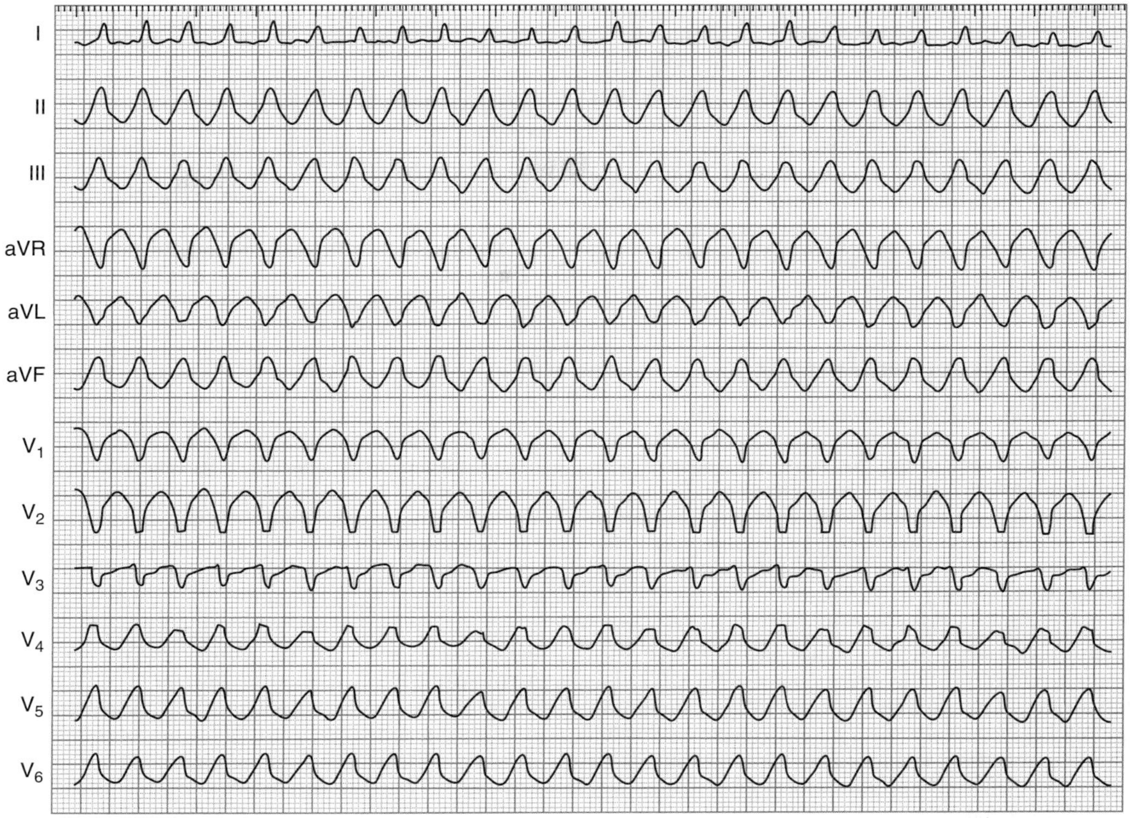

▲ **Figure 13–9.** Twelve-lead electrocardiogram that is typical of ventricular tachycardia (VT) in the absence of structural heart disease, originating in the right ventricular outflow tract. There is left bundle branch block morphology with late transition (V_4) in the precordial leads and an inferior axis in the limb leads. Negative QRS complex in lead avL suggest a septal origin. (Reproduced with permission from Badhwar N, Scheinman MM. Idiopathic ventricular tachycardia: diagnosis and management. *Curr Probl Cardiol.* 2007;32(1):7–43.)

energy is curative in most patients with outflow tract VT, due to the focal origin of the VT.

3. Annular Ventricular Tachycardia

Mitral annular VT arises from the mitral annulus in the left ventricle and is associated with RBBB morphology. Palpitations are the presenting manifestation in these patients due to repetitive monomorphic VT or frequent monomorphic PVC. The mechanism is thought to be triggered rhythm that terminates with the administration of intravenous adenosine and verapamil. The ECG in mitral annular VT shows a delta wave-like beginning of the QRS complex similar to that seen in patients with left-sided WPW syndrome. Catheter ablation is associated with a high success rate (> 90%), making it a suitable alternative to drug therapy in these patients.

VT arising from the tricuspid annulus has also been described which is associated with LBBB morphology. Tricuspid annulus VT originates more often in the septal region (74%) than in the free wall (26%). The septal VT has an early transition in precordial leads (V_3), narrower QRS complexes, and Qs in lead V_1 with absence of "notching" in the inferior leads, whereas the free wall VT has late precordial transition (> V_3), wider QRS complexes, absence of Q wave in lead V_1, and "notching" in the inferior leads. The success rate for catheter ablation of the free wall VT tends to be much higher when compared to septal origin, since the septal portion of the annulus is close to the AV node, and ablation in this region risks development of iatrogenic heart block.

4. Papillary Muscle VT

Following the advent of intracardiac echocardiography and improved visualization of endocardial structures, it became apparent that a subset of idiopathic VT arises from the papillary muscles. This form of VT is also seen in patients with mitral valve prolapse. Due to the proximity of the papillary muscles to the fascicular system, posteromedial and anterolateral papillary muscle VT closely resembles fascicular VT on ECG, though there are some notable differences. Papillary muscle VT tends to be wider and frequently exhibits a qR pattern in V1. Fascicular VTs classically have preserved septal q and r waves in leads I and aVL, while these are generally absent from papillary muscle VTs. Ablation of papillary muscle VT is more difficult compared to other forms of focal idiopathic VT, since it can be difficult to achieve continuous contact between the ablation catheter and papillary muscle during vigorous contractile activity. Further, the foci are frequently intramural instead of endocardial, which requires more advanced ablation strategies.

5. VT Arising From Cardiac Crux

The cardiac crux is a posteroseptal structure that lies at the intersection of the four chambers of the heart. Idiopathic epicardial VT arising from the crux has recently been described as a distinct entity with characteristic clinical and ECG findings. These patients present with very fast VT that can lead to syncope and cardiac arrest requiring resuscitation. Twelve-lead ECG shows morphology consistent with preexcited posteroseptal WPW pathway (Figure 13–10). They typically have a QS pattern in leads II and III, and a prolonged maximum deflection index (MDI) greater than 0.55, which is the ratio of the time of onset of the QRS complex to the maximum positive or negative deflection. A prolonged MDI reflects slower myocyte-to-myocyte conduction and has high sensitivity and specificity for an epicardial site of origin. Crux VT can be further subcategorized as arising from the more basal portion of the crux or the more apical portion. Basal crux VT predominantly has LBBB pattern, with R>S in V_6. Apical crux VT can have LBBB or RBBB pattern with R<S in V_6. Basal crux VT often can be successfully ablated in the proximal CS while apical crux VT requires percutaneous pericardial access for successful ablation.

DIAGNOSTIC STUDIES

Patients with either documented or suspected sustained VT should undergo additional workup to confirm the diagnosis, identify the underlying substrate, and determine the direction of therapy.

Noninvasive cardiovascular workup should start with a 12-lead ECG, though patients will often be in sinus rhythm at the time of evaluation, and baseline ECG may be normal. Ambulatory rhythm monitoring is useful to detect the presence of wide complex arrhythmia, to assess PVC burden, and to confirm whether a patient's symptoms are actually associated with ventricular ectopy. Exercise stress testing is indicated both to evaluate for coronary artery disease and to detect catecholamine-sensitive VTs, though typical exercise testing protocols unfortunately may not have high sensitivity for detecting exercise-induced ventricular arrhythmia (so the diagnosis should not be ruled out based on a negative stress test if suspicion is high). Transthoracic echocardiography is the essential initial imaging modality to uncover structural heart disease and should be performed in all patients with sustained VT. Cardiac MRI has emerged as a powerful adjunctive modality due to its ability to detect fibrosis (both in ischemic and nonischemic patterns). Coronary angiography (either via CT in suitable patients or via invasive catheterization) is recommended to evaluate for obstructive coronary artery disease in patients with VT.

When VT is suspected but not documented, its induction in the laboratory is critical to the decision to undertake any therapeutic approach. By inducing or replicating VT in the laboratory, its rate, morphology, origin, hemodynamic

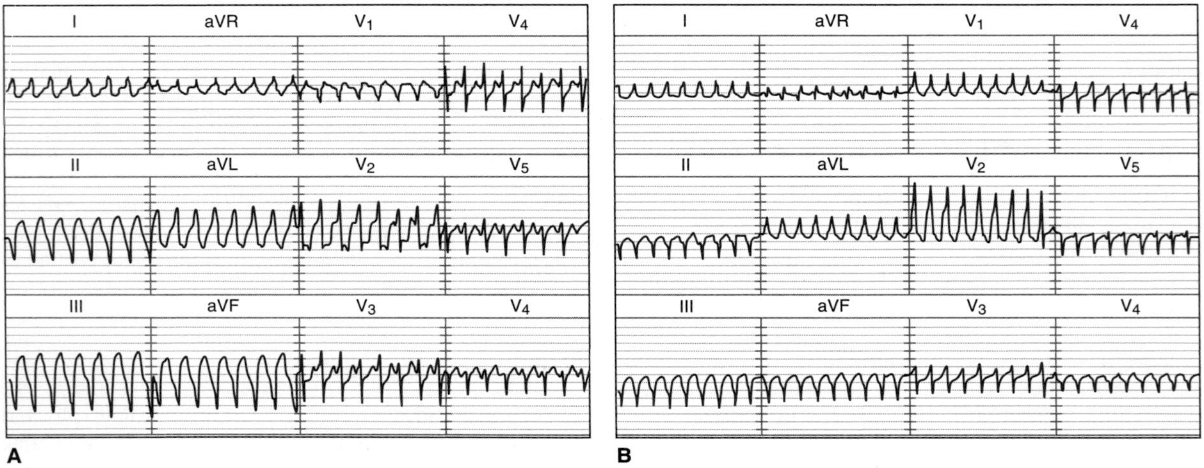

▲ **Figure 13–10.** Twelve-lead electrocardiogram that is typical of ventricular tachycardia (VT) arising from the crux of the heart. There is presence of Q waves in inferior leads, MDI > 0.55 in precordial leads and R<S in V_5 and V_6. Panel A shows LBBB morphology in V_1 with early transition while panel B shows RBBB morphology.

tolerance, and response to intravenous drugs can be evaluated.

Catheter ablation using radiofrequency or electrical energy is an effective form of treatment in patients with bundle branch reentry, idiopathic VT, and, in some cases, VT in association with prior MI. Thorough electrophysiologic testing is crucial for a successful outcome in these cases.

Many patients with VT have extensive cardiac pathology, including abnormalities of sinus node function and AV conduction. These abnormalities can be further aggravated with the administration of antiarrhythmic drugs. Electrophysiologic studies can frequently identify the nature and determine both the extent of these abnormalities and the need for additional therapeutic interventions (eg, permanent pacing for bradycardia).

There are, however, several important exceptions to routine electrophysiology testing identified in consensus guidelines. If a patient already meets criteria for ICD, direct implantation without an electrophysiology study is generally recommended. In addition, for patients with suspected channelopathies, exercise stress testing often provides more useful risk stratification than electrophysiologic testing.

Kobayashi Y. Idiopathic ventricular premature contraction and ventricular tachycardia: distribution of the origin, diagnostic algorithm, and catheter ablation. *J Nippon Med Sch*. 2018;85(2):87–94. [PMID: 29731502]. doi: 10.1272/jnms.2018_8514.

MANAGEMENT OF MONOMORPHIC VENTRICULAR TACHYCARDIA

Because monomorphic VT is most commonly due to underlying myocardial fibrosis, the pharmacologic treatment outlined here primarily relates to this substrate. The same approach can be used in other situations, but it may not be as applicable.

Immediate Termination

The method of VT termination in the acute settings depends on the hemodynamic tolerance of the tachycardia. When the patient has severe hypotension, loses consciousness, or has any other evidence of hemodynamic instability and hypoperfusion, a synchronized direct-current (DC) cardioversion should be attempted promptly. With hemodynamically well-tolerated VT, there is ample time to gather complete information, including a 12-lead ECG, before initiating therapy.

Regarding medications for acute treatment, intravenous amiodarone is the drug of choice. VT in association with acute MI may respond more readily to lidocaine (2–3 mg/kg). Intravenous procainamide (10–15 mg/kg) at a rate of 50–100 mg/min is also effective, but it can lead to hypotension, and is generally reserved for patients with VT refractory to amiodarone or lidocaine. For patients who have recurrent, incessant episodes of VT within a 24-hour period (known as "VT storm"), intubation and deep sedation with propofol may reduce burden.

Intravenous calcium channel blockers such as verapamil should not be administered unless there is a definitive diagnosis of SVT with aberrant conduction or verapamil-sensitive VT (though as discussed earlier, this diagnosis is uncommon). When VT is triggered or aggravated by exercise, intravenous beta-blockers may be tried as the initial therapy, if they can be tolerated. If there is any uncertainty regarding the safety of beta-blockers in patients with VT, it is reasonable to trial esmolol, which has a short half-life and can be rapidly downtitrated.

When pharmacologic intervention fails, overdrive termination via a pacing catheter can be attempted, though this should generally be done under consultation of an electrophysiologist. Cardioversion may also be necessary in hemodynamically stable patients with prolonged VT, since prolonged ventricular arrhythmia is undesirable, particularly in the setting of ischemic or structural heart disease. Careful attention should be paid to reversible factors contributing to ventricular arrhythmogenesis, such as acidosis, hypoxia, electrolyte abnormalities, and the use of pro-arrhythmic drugs (eg, beta agonists). If such factors are involved, pharmacologic treatment alone may fail to control the VT.

Prevention

Although acute termination of VT is relatively straightforward in most situations, the prevention of recurrences is often a challenge. The empiric use of antiarrhythmic drugs is not encouraged because of potential harm to the patient as well as their unproven efficacy. Because VT represents a potentially life-threatening arrhythmia, establishing an effective form of therapy is desirable before the patient is discharged, especially for patients with VT-related syncope or cardiac arrest. In most situations, the therapy must be individualized, which requires understanding the type of VT, any underlying heart disease, left ventricular function, and the clinical presentation.

A. Pharmacologic Therapy

For monomorphic VT in association with chronic coronary artery disease or any other type of fibrosis, a variety of therapeutic options are now available. These include antiarrhythmic drugs, ablative therapy, and ICDs. Among the antiarrhythmic drugs, the use of class I agents (Table 13–4) has progressively declined because of both excessive patient intolerance and availability. Class Ib drugs such as mexiletine are weak antiarrhythmic agents when used alone, but they seem more useful in combination with other antiarrhythmics. Class Ic drugs have moderate efficacy but a significant proarrhythmic potential, as well as an observed increase in mortality when used in patients with structural heart disease—they are therefore generally only used to treat ventricular arrhythmias in certain indications under expert management by an electrophysiologist.

Table 13–4. Antiarrhythmic Drugs

Class	Drug
Ia	Quinidine, procainamide, disopyramide
Ib	Mexiletine, lidocaine
Ic	Flecainide, propafenone, others (Ethmozine)
II	β-Blockers
III	Amiodarone, sotalol, bepridil
IV	Calcium channel blockers

Exercise-induced VT generally responds well to beta-blockers, and serial exercise stress tests can be used to monitor drug efficacy. Because other forms of VT in patients with coronary artery disease may respond to beta-blockers, they are frequently used alone or in combination with other antiarrhythmic drugs when the patient can tolerate them.

At present, class III agents (eg, amiodarone and sotalol) are the most promising antiarrhythmic agents for control of VT and ventricular fibrillation (VF). After a loading dose of 10 g over 1–2 weeks, amiodarone can be used in a maintenance dose of 200–400 mg/day. It is associated with long-term side effects that can affect the thyroid, lungs, gastrointestinal tract, eyes, skin, genitourinary system, and central nervous system. Baseline thyroid function test, liver function test, pulmonary function test, and ophthalmologic examination should be done in patients when amiodarone therapy is started, with repeat tests every 6 months. The usual daily dose of sotalol is 120–240 mg/day with monitoring of the ECG for QT prolongation during its administration or with any change in dosage.

It should be pointed out that in high-risk patients with coronary artery disease and reduced left ventricular function, none of the antiarrhythmics (apart from beta blockers), have been shown to decrease mortality compared with placebo. Failure of response to a drug or intolerance are indications for nonpharmacologic treatment, discussed in the following section.

Larson J, Rich L, Deshmukh A, Judge EC, Liang JJ. Pharmacologic management for ventricular arrhythmias: overview of antiarrhythmic drugs. *J Clin Med.* 2022 Jun 6;11(11):3233. [PMID: 35683620]. doi: 10.3390/jcm11113233.

B. Nonpharmacologic Therapy

1. Implantable cardioverter-defibrillators (ICD)—These devices are the mainstay of prevention of SCD in patients with VT. The highest quality of evidence for prevention of SCD with ICDs is in the secondary prevention of patients who have already experienced sudden cardiac arrest or sustained VT and in patients with LVEF lower than 35%. The main contraindications to placement are in VTs that have reversible causes (eg, acute ischemia, electrolyte abnormalities, antiarrhythmic drugs). ICDs do not prevent VT from occurring, but rather are designed to terminate the arrhythmia, which can be accomplished via anti-tachycardia pacing (ATP) or high energy shock

Most devices are programmed to first attempt ATP, which can frequently abolish VT (particularly if the mechanism is reentrant) without the need for a shock. ATP therapies have the advantage of being imperceptible to a patient and have been shown to reduce the need for shocks. ICDs have demonstrated a remarkable effectiveness in prevention of SCD, with an overall 1-year survival rate of 92% in patients with documented life-threatening ventricular tachyarrhythmias. A meta-analysis of ICD trials showed that the relative risk reduction of sudden death with ICDs in secondary prevention is 50% and that for primary prevention is 37% (see Chapter 15).

Identification of patients who are at highest risk for SCD—and therefore at greatest benefit from ICD implantation—remains an active area of investigation.

2. Catheter-based ablation—The development of radiofrequency catheter ablation as a therapeutic option for the treatment of arrhythmias has dramatically altered the approach to the tachycardic patient. Since its introduction in 1986, radiofrequency ablation has provided actual cure for thousands of patients with debilitating symptoms from paroxysmal SVTs and certain VTs. ICDs are the standard therapy for sustained VT in patients with structural heart disease. In patients who experience recurrent shocks from the ICD, radiofrequency catheter ablation may be used in an attempt to modify or eliminate the VT circuit and thereby reduce the number of shocks a patient may experience. Catheter ablation in this setting is usually palliative with elimination of all VT circuits achieved in 50–60% of patients by the most experienced operators.

It is almost always curative, however, for sustained VT from bundle branch reentry from any cause seen in patients with dilated cardiomyopathy. High success rates (85–100%) make radiofrequency catheter ablation a good alternative to drug therapy in patients with idiopathic VT. Radiofrequency catheter ablation is likely to play a greater role in management of VT in the future due to the development of advanced mapping systems, better catheter design, and incorporation of real-time anatomy using computed tomography scans and magnetic resonance imaging.

Recent consensus guidelines recommend catheter ablation for patients with structural heart disease in each of the following conditions: (1) symptomatic sustained monomorphic VT, including VT terminated by an ICD, that recurs despite antiarrhythmic drug therapy or when antiarrhythmic drugs are not tolerated or not desired; (2) incessant sustained monomorphic VT or VT storm that is not due to a transient reversible cause; (3) patients with frequent premature ventricular contractions, nonsustained VT, or VT that is presumed to cause ventricular dysfunction; (4) bundle branch reentrant or interfascicular VTs; and (5) recurrent sustained polymorphic VT and VF that is refractory to antiarrhythmic therapy when there is a suspected trigger that can be targeted for ablation.

3. Surgical ablation—Surgical ablation is rarely performed in the era of catheter ablation and is primarily reserved for cases when a patient already has an indication for cardiac surgery and has ventricular aneurysm, or when catheter ablation has failed.

Al-Khatib SM, Stevenson WG, Ackerman MJ, et al. 2017 AHA/ACC/HRS Guideline for management of patients with ventricular arrhythmias and prevention of sudden cardiac death. *J Am Coll Cardiol.* 2018 Oct 2;72(14):e91–e220. [PMID: 29097296]. Doi: 10.1016/j.jacc.2017.10.054. Epub 2018 Aug 16

Cronin EM, Bogun FM, Peichl P, et al. 2019 HRS/EHRA/APHRS/LAHRS expert consensus statement on catheter ablation of ventricular arrhythmias. *Heart Rhythm.* 2020;17:e2–e153. [PMID: 31085023].

Kanagaratnam A, Virk SA, Pham T, Anderson RD, et al. Catheter ablation for ventricular tachycardia in ischaemic versus non-ischaemic cardiomyopathy: a systematic review and meta-analysis. *Heart Lung Circ.* 2022 Aug;31(8):1064–1074. Doi: 10.1016/j.hlc.2022.02.014. Online ahead of print. [PMID: 35643798].

POLYMORPHIC VENTRICULAR TACHYCARDIA

Recognition of polymorphic VTs and their distinction from the monomorphic variety represent the crucial first step toward appropriate management. These tachycardias tend to be rapid; they generally produce symptoms of hypotension and can readily degenerate into VF. At least two types can be recognized that must be distinguished by the presence or absence of prolonged myocardial recovery.

1. Polymorphic Ventricular Tachycardia in the Setting of Prolonged QT Interval

This condition is often referred to as torsades de pointes. It can be congenital or acquired (ie, from QT-prolonging medications). In both cases, patients have a prolonged QT (QTc) interval and slow, prominent, or unusual-looking T waves.

Clinical Findings

Patients with congenital long QT syndrome have episodes of torsades de pointes that are often triggered by adrenergic stimulation, which can be brought about by physical exertion or mental or emotional stress. These patients can broadly be categorized in two distinct phenotypes, differentiated by the pattern of inheritance and by the presence or absence of deafness: "Jervell and Lange-Nielsen" syndrome is associated with deafness, and typically has an autosomal recessive pattern of inheritance, whereas patients with "Romano Ward" syndrome have intact hearing, and the inheritance is autosomal dominant (it is therefore more common). The QT interval prolongation in these patients may be subtle and can be unmasked by long pauses or adrenergic stimuli such as exercise. The electrophysiologic mechanism may be early after-depolarization for initiation and reentry for sustenance. The clinical presentation includes episodes of lightheadedness, near syncope, syncope, and, in some cases, cardiac arrest. There may not be any other obvious associated cardiac abnormalities. Generally, the age at diagnosis is between 9 and 12 years, though congenital LQTS has also been proposed as one of the causes of sudden infant death syndrome.

Genetic testing has revealed mutations in several ion channels that are culpable in congenital LQTS—the majority of phenotypes are accounted for by mutations in genes that encode KCNQ1 (potassium channel), KCNH2 (potassium channel), and SCN5A (sodium channel), and the syndrome is subclassified into LQT_1, LQT_2, and LQT_3 respectively, based on mutations in these genes (Figure 13–11). LQT_1 and LQT_2 account for the majority percentage of the cases of LQTS. LQT_3 is only seen in 10% of the cases, though it is the most morbid. Exercise and sudden auditory stimuli are triggers for LQT_1 and LQT_2, respectively, whereas LQT_3 patients have most of the events during sleep at slower heart rates. Female sex, congenital deafness, baseline QT interval greater than 500 ms, a prolonged interval from the peak of the T wave to the end of the T wave, and males with LQT_3 are associated with a high risk of sudden death.

Acquired LQTS can be caused by a variety of pharmacologic agents and metabolic factors (a partial list is given in Table 13–5). The main ECG abnormality is that of prolonged QT interval and often an unusual appearance of the T wave, frequently referred to as the slow wave (Figure 13–12). The QT interval prolongation may not always be striking at the normal rates but should show a measurable increase after a pause, for example, following a premature beat. Genetic testing in cohorts of patients with acquired long QT suggests that these patients likely have a "two-hit" mechanism that predisposes them to the syndrome: a mutation in ion channels (most commonly in the K^+ channel that drive I_{Kr} current) which results in a partial defect that only manifests in the presence of an offending medication (generally an agent which blocks the I_{Kr} current). Extreme caution must be exercised in such individuals because a recurrence is likely if challenged with the same triggers. The actual list of potentially offending agents may be quite long because many pharmacologic agents have not been tested for such adverse side effects as prolongation of the QT interval, and only the widely known culprits are listed in Table 13–5.

Management

The key to managing torsades de pointes related to acquired prolonged QT interval is recognizing it, promptly withdrawing the offending agent, and immediately replacing serum electrolytes magnesium infusion (even in the face of normal serum levels) reduces early after depolarizations

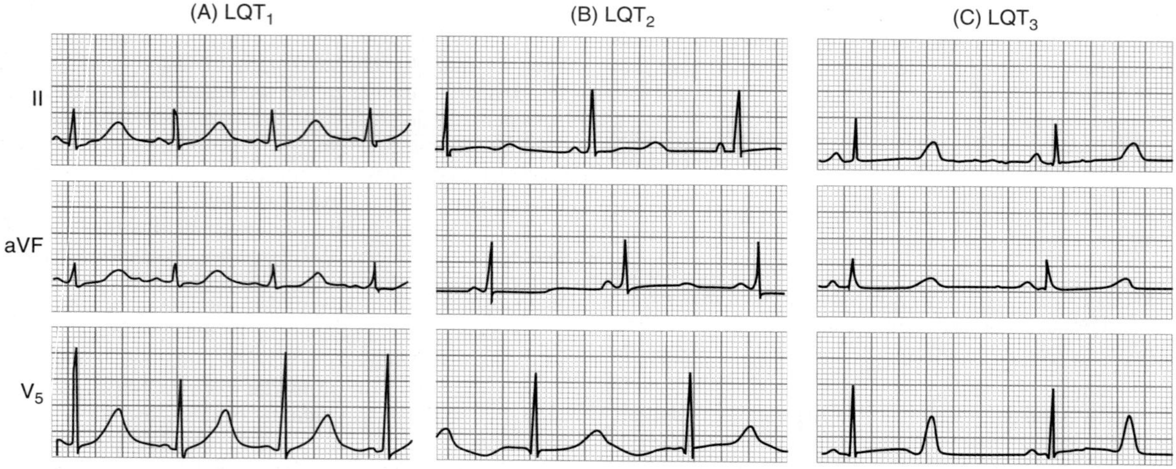

▲ **Figure 13–11.** Genotype-specific T-wave morphology on electrocardiogram (ECG) in long QT syndrome (LQTS) patients. **A:** ECG in LQT_1 showing broad-based T waves. **B:** ECG in LQT_2 showing low-amplitude T waves with notches. **C:** ECG in LQT_3 showing extended ST segment with relatively narrow peaked T waves. (Reproduced with permission from Moss AJ, Zareba W, Benhorin J, et al. ECG T-wave patterns in genetically distinct forms of the hereditary long QT syndrome. *Circulation*. 1995;92(10):2929–2934.)

by inhibiting inward calcium current. The prompt replacement of potassium and calcium is also critical. For patients with ongoing torsades despite magnesium infusion and electrolyte correction, often overdrive pacing (either via pacemaker wire or with isoproterenol infusion) is necessary to shorten the QT interval (particularly when the torsades is pause dependent). In patients with hemodynamic instability, standard emergency resuscitation algorithms should be employed.

Recognition of torsades can be particularly challenging in patients who have underlying monomorphic VT that is being treated with antiarrhythmic agents, which may themselves predispose a patient to prolonged QT and torsades de pointes. In this setting, offending antiarrhythmics should be discontinued.

The mainstay of treatment in congenital LQTS is beta-blockade—most commonly with nadolol or propranolol (often in high doses). Patients with LQT1 and LQT2 subtypes

Table 13–5. Causes of Acquired Long QT Syndrome

Antiarrhythmic drugs	**Psychiatry drugs**
Class Ia	Antidepressants (tetra/tricyclic), antipsychotic (phenothiazines, haloperidol, sertindole)
Quinidine (I_{Kr}, I_{To}, and I_{Ks}), disopyramide, procainamide	**Cholinergic antagonists**
Class III	Cisapride (I_{Kr}), organophosphates (insecticides)
Sotalol (I_{Kr}, I_{To}), d-sotalol, amiodarone (I_{Kr}, I_{Ks}), ibutilide, dofetilide (I_{Kr})	**Inotropic drugs**
Antibiotics	Amrinone, milrinone
Macrolides (erythromycin [I_{Kr}], clarithromycin, clindamycin), trimethoprim-sulfamethoxazole, pentamidine, imidazoles (ketoconazole)	**Poisons**
	Arsenic, organophosphates (insecticides, nerve gas)
Histamine receptor antagonists	**Metabolic abnormalities**
Terfenadine,[1] astemizole[1] (I_{Kr})	Hypokalemia (I_{Kr}), hypomagnesemia, hypocalcemia
Serotonin receptor antagonists	**Bradyarrhythmias**
Ketanserin (I_{Kr}, I_{To})[2]	Complete atrioventricular block, sick sinus syndrome
Serotonin receptor inhibitors	**Starvation**
Sertindole (I_{Kr}),[2] zimeldine[2]	Anorexia nervosa, "liquid protein" diets, gastroplasty, ileojejunal bypass
Diuretics	**Nervous system injury**
Indapamide (I_{Ks})	Subarachnoid hemorrhage, thalamic hematoma, right neck dissection or hematoma, pheochromocytoma

[1]Withdrawn from the U.S. market.
[2]Not available in the United States.

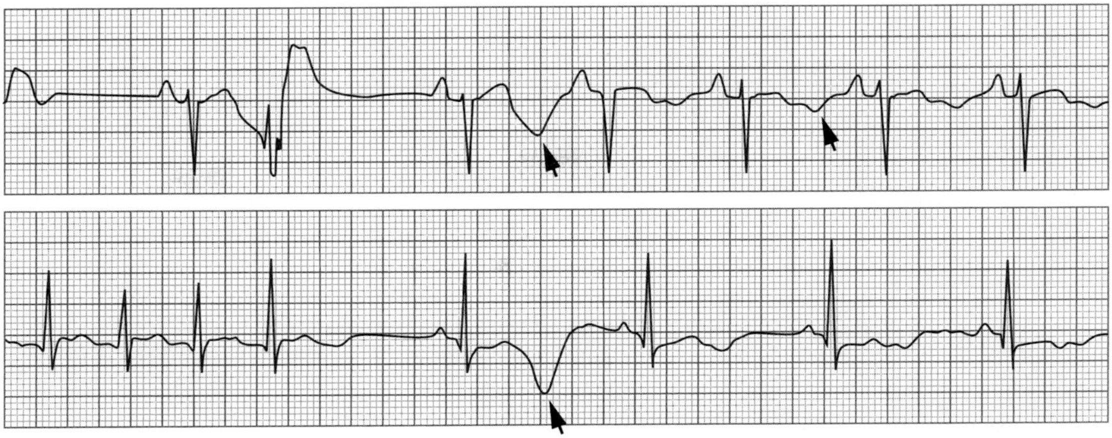

▲ **Figure 13–12. Prolonged QT interval with slow wave. The T wave has an unusual appearance, and both the QT-interval prolongation and T-wave morphologic abnormality are more pronounced after the pause. The slow wave is indicated by the *arrows*.** (Reproduced with permission from Jackman WM, Friday KJ, Anderson JL, Aliot EM, Clark M, Lazzara R. The long QT syndromes: a critical review, new clinical observations and a unifying hypothesis. *Prog Cardiovasc Dis.* 1988;31(2):115–172.)

appear to derive the greatest benefit from beta blockade, whereas patients with LQT3 tend to have arrhythmia triggered at lower heart rates—and may derive less benefit (particularly male patients with LQT3).

In patients who either do not tolerate beta blockade, or who have ongoing arrhythmia despite this medication, further treatment involves additional medications aimed at shortening the QT (eg, mexiletine, which is particularly useful in LQT3) or which prevent serum hypokalemia (eg, spironolactone, which is particularly helpful in LQT2). It is critical to avoid QT prolonging drugs in this patient population. Patients with refractory symptoms may also benefit from left stellate sympathectomy, which reduces catecholaminergic inputs to the ventricle, has been carried out with variable success in difficult cases. In individuals with recurrent syncope or sudden cardiac arrest, ICD placement is usually warranted to prevent SCD.

2. Polymorphic Ventricular Tachycardia with a Normal QT Interval

In the cases discussed earlier, the polymorphic VT is associated with a prolonged QT which is most readily appreciated in the QT interval prior to the onset of tachycardia or in the complex following termination of the tachycardia. However, polymorphic VT can also occur in the setting of a normal QT interval. In this case, acute ischemia—either from an acute coronary syndrome or coronary vasospasm—should be suspected as the etiology until proven otherwise. Ischemic polymorphic VT is rapid and has a tendency to degenerate into VF (Figure 13–13). Prompt diagnosis and therapy are critical for preventing VT-related SCD in these patients. The workup includes coronary arteriography and an assessment for coronary artery spasm. The traditional diagnostic criteria—history of chest pain or obvious ST abnormalities—may not be present prior to the episode. A high index of suspicion is likely to lead to a correct diagnosis. This type of VT can seldom be induced in the laboratory, and the electrophysiologic mechanism for it remains unclear. The treatment, in essence, is directed toward eliminating myocardial ischemia; it might include myocardial revascularization or anti-ischemic drugs such as beta-blockers or calcium channel blockers.

Polymorphic VT with normal QT interval can also occur in patients without substrates for myocardial ischemia but with chronic fibrosis or hypertrophy. Sometimes, it can occur with no obvious pathology. It is prudent to exclude all the previously mentioned correctable causes before a diagnosis of this idiopathic variety is made. In some cases, the polymorphic VT may be inducible, suggesting a reentrant nature. Although such an arrhythmia can occur in patients with healed MI, it is also sometimes seen in patients with hypertrophic and congestive cardiomyopathy. This type of polymorphic VT does not provide a reliable end point for drug testing or VT surgery. Antiarrhythmic drugs, particularly amiodarone, may be useful as are ICDs in preventing SCD in this population.

PROGNOSIS

The prognosis in a patient with VT depends considerably on the broader clinical context. The feared complication of VT is progression to sudden cardiac arrest and SCD. As discussed earlier, idiopathic VTs are less likely to degenerate into sudden cardiac arrest, and they can be treated with medications and ablation with excellent outcomes. On the other hand, VT in a patient with structural heart disease can

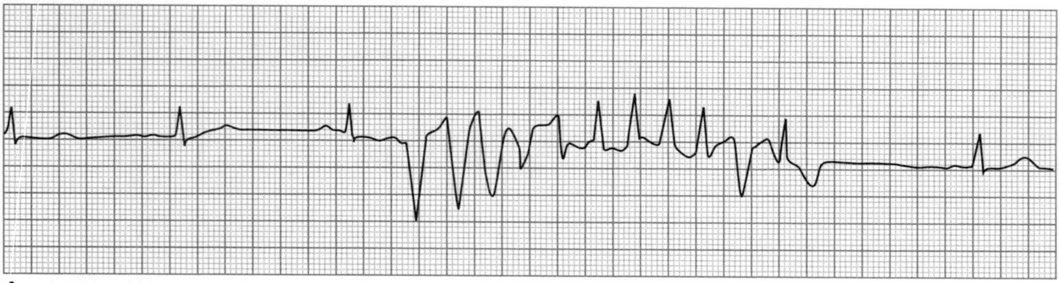

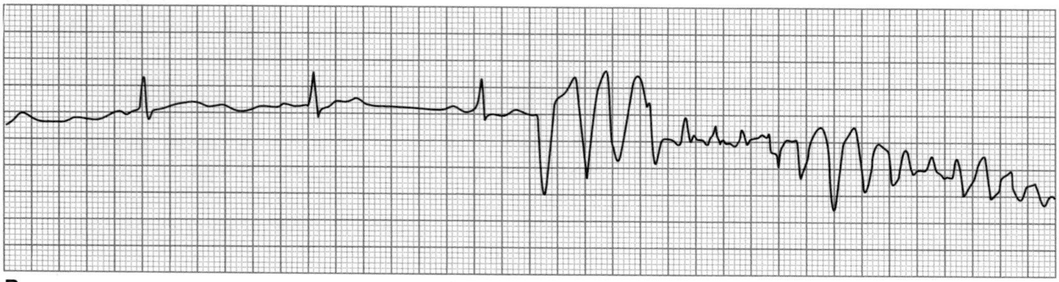

▲ **Figure 13–13.** Polymorphic ventricular tachycardia (VT) and normal QT interval in a patient with severe three-vessel disease. **A:** Several nonsustained polymorphic VT episodes. **B:** Degeneration to ventricular fibrillation, requiring direct-current cardioversion.

portend sudden cardiac arrest. Left ventricular dysfunction at initial presentation is perhaps the most important adverse predictor of a patient with VT. Patients with recurrent cardiac arrest, or recurrent syncope with VT also have poorer prognosis. Ultimately, it remains challenging to identify subpopulations that are at highest risk of sudden cardiac arrest, and further stratification remains an area of active study.

Conduction Disorders & Cardiac Pacing

14

Richard H. Hongo, MD
Nora F. Goldschlager, MD

ESSENTIALS OF DIAGNOSIS

Sinus node dysfunction ("sick sinus syndrome")

- Sinus bradycardia: sinus rate less than 50 bpm.
- Sinoatrial (SA) exit block.
  - Type I: P wave nonoccurrence preceded by decreasing P-P intervals.
  - Type II: abruptly longer P-P intervals that are multiples of sinus interval.
- Sinus pauses: P wave nonoccurrence more than 3 seconds.
- Sinus arrest: no evidence of P waves.

Atrioventricular (AV) block

- First degree: 1:1 AV conduction ratio and PR interval more than 200 ms.
- Second degree
  - Type I: failure of AV conduction and QRS complex nonoccurrence preceded by increasing PR intervals.
  - Type II: failure of AV conduction not preceded by increasing PR intervals.
  - "2:1": without consecutive PR intervals, unable to define as either type I or type II block.
  - Advanced ("high-grade" or "high-degree"): ≥ 3:1 AV conduction ratio.
- Third degree ("complete"): independent atrial and ventricular rhythms with failure of AV conduction despite temporal opportunity to occur

General Considerations

The clinical presentation of patients with conduction system disease is determined by two underlying abnormal conditions: the inability to increase or maintain the sinus rate in response to metabolic need and atrioventricular (AV) dyssynchrony (inappropriately timed atrial and ventricular depolarization and contraction sequences).

Pathophysiology & Etiology

A. Sinus Node Dysfunction

Sinus node dysfunction ("sick sinus syndrome") is usually due to age-dependent and progressive degenerative fibrosis of the sinus node and sinoatrial (SA) area (Table 14–1). Often, the degenerative process also involves the approaches to the AV node, the AV node itself, the His bundle, as well as the intraventricular conduction system; as many as 25–30% of patients with sinus node dysfunction have evidence of AV conduction disease.

Respiratory sinus arrhythmia, in which the sinus rate increases with inspiration and decreases with expiration, is not an abnormal rhythm and is mostly seen in young healthy persons. Nonrespiratory sinus arrhythmia, in which phasic changes in sinus rate are not due to respiration, may be accentuated by the use of vagotonic agents, such as digoxin and morphine, and is more likely to be observed in older patients who have underlying cardiac disease, although the arrhythmia itself is not a marker for structural heart disease; its mechanism is unknown. Ventriculophasic sinus arrhythmia is an unusual rhythm that occurs during advanced second-degree or complete AV block; it is characterized by shorter P-P intervals that enclose QRS complexes. The mechanism is not known with certainty but is thought to be related to the effects of mechanical ventricular systole. The ventricular contraction increases blood flow to the sinus node, thereby transiently increasing its firing rate; an increase in intra-atrial pressure causes subsequent reduction in sinus rate. Ventriculophasic sinus arrhythmia is not a pathologic arrhythmia and should not be confused with premature atrial depolarizations or SA block. None of the sinus arrhythmias indicate sinus node dysfunction.

Chronotropic incompetence is the inability to increase the heart rate to match the oxygen demand from

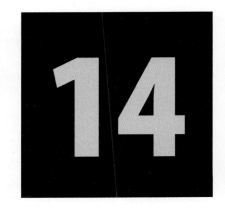

Table 14–1. Causes of Sinus Node Dysfunction

Degenerative
Ischemic (inferior wall MI, Bezold-Jarisch reflex)
Inflammatory (pericarditis, collagen vascular diseases)
Infiltrative (amyloidosis, sarcoidosis, hemochromatosis)
Hypothyroidism
Hypothermia
Hypoxemia
Medications
β-Blockers
Non-dihydropyridine calcium channel blockers (diltiazem, verapamil)
Digoxin (with high prevailing vagal tone)
Class I antiarrhythmic agents (flecainide, propafenone)
Class III antiarrhythmic agents (amiodarone, sotalol)
Other cellular ion channel blockers (ivabradine)
Acetylcholinesterase inhibitors (donepezil)
Sympatholytic drugs (clonidine, methyldopa)
Lithium

MI, myocardial infarction.

increased activity. Although the definition of chronotropic incompetence is not standardized and the underlying mechanism is still not fully understood, it is an important condition that is debilitating and has been reported to be an independent predictor of mortality. It appears to be related to dysfunction of autonomic regulation that can worsen with age and is frequently confounded by the effects of medications that cause sinus bradycardia (β-blockers, rate-limiting calcium channel–blocking agents diltiazem and verapamil, digoxin, and antiarrhythmic agents such as amiodarone and sotalol; Table 14–1 and Figure 14–2). If these medications are necessary treatments, permanent cardiac pacing is indicated.

Sinus node dysfunction can be present when sinus bradycardia, SA block, sinus pauses, sinus arrest, or a combination of these exist (Figures 14–1 through 14–5). Marked sinus bradycardia and prolonged sinus pauses, however, can be observed in clinically normal individuals without structural heart disease in the setting of increased vagal tone, such as during sleep. Hypoxemia from obstructive sleep apnea accentuates vagal tone, and both supplemental oxygen and continuous positive airway pressure can eliminate bradycardia and pauses. In some patients, coughing, swallowing, or vomiting can be identified as a trigger that causes sinus slowing or pause; in some cases, high acetylcholine levels may be responsible. Vagal stimulation, often from an identifiable trigger (Table 14–2), is commonly responsible for sinus bradyarrhythmias observed in patients in the intensive care setting. Vagally mediated sinus bradycardia or pauses should not prompt consideration for cardiac pacing, either temporary or permanent.

SA block occurs when the impulse generated by the sinus node fails to exit the sinus node through SA tissue, resulting in an absent P wave on the surface electrocardiogram (ECG). In second-degree type I (or Wenckebach) exit block, the P-P intervals progressively shortens prior to the absent P wave; this phenomenon is observed because there is less incremental delay with each successive impulse transmission (see Figures 14–1 and 14–4). In second-degree type II exit block, abruptly longer P-P intervals are seen without progressive shortening, and the longer P-P interval is a multiple of the underlying sinus interval (see Figure 14–1). SA exit block of 2:1 or higher degree cannot be distinguished from sinus bradycardia on the surface ECG.

Bradycardia-tachycardia syndrome is characterized by episodes of both bradycardias and supraventricular tachyarrhythmias (Figure 14–6). The bradycardia is due to sinus node dysfunction (sinus arrest or SA exit block); the supraventricular tachyarrhythmias may be atrial tachycardia, atrial flutter, atrial fibrillation, AV reciprocating tachycardia, or AV nodal reentry tachycardia (see Chapter 11); more than one type of tachycardia may occur in the same patient. Bradycardia-tachycardia syndrome often represents diffuse conduction system disease but is not necessarily associated with structural heart disease.

The natural history of sinus node dysfunction is one of variable progression to an absence of identifiable sinus activity, with the process taking from 10 to 30 years. The condition itself is not associated with a high risk of arrhythmic death, although the morbidity caused by sudden onset bradycardia can be considerable. The ultimate prognosis for the patient with sinus node dysfunction typically depends on the presence and severity of underlying heart disease or the involvement of other portions of the conduction system through diffuse fibrosis, rather than on the sinus bradyarrhythmia itself.

B. Atrioventricular Block

Delay or block can occur anywhere along the course of the AV conducting system, which is made up of the AV node, His bundle, bundle branches, and fascicles. Like sinus node dysfunction, AV nodal-His block and bundle branch block (BBB) are often the result of sclerodegenerative processes; these processes can also involve the approaches to the AV node. Acquired AV nodal block is often due to acute ischemia and infarction (especially involving the inferior wall and right ventricle), infection, medications, and trauma (Table 14–3).

The AV node (or junction) is made up of three regions: atrionodal, central compact, and nodal-His. Cells of the atrionodal region have a relatively fast depolarization rate (45–60 bpm) and are responsive to autonomic nervous system input, whereas cells of the nodal-His region have a slower depolarization rate (about 40 bpm) and are generally unresponsive to autonomic influences. The site of origin of a junctional rhythm will therefore determine its rate, responsiveness to vagal and adrenergic input, and consequently the presence and severity of clinical symptoms.

The natural history of patients with AV block depends on the prognosis of any underlying condition and on the site of AV block. When the site of block is at the level of the

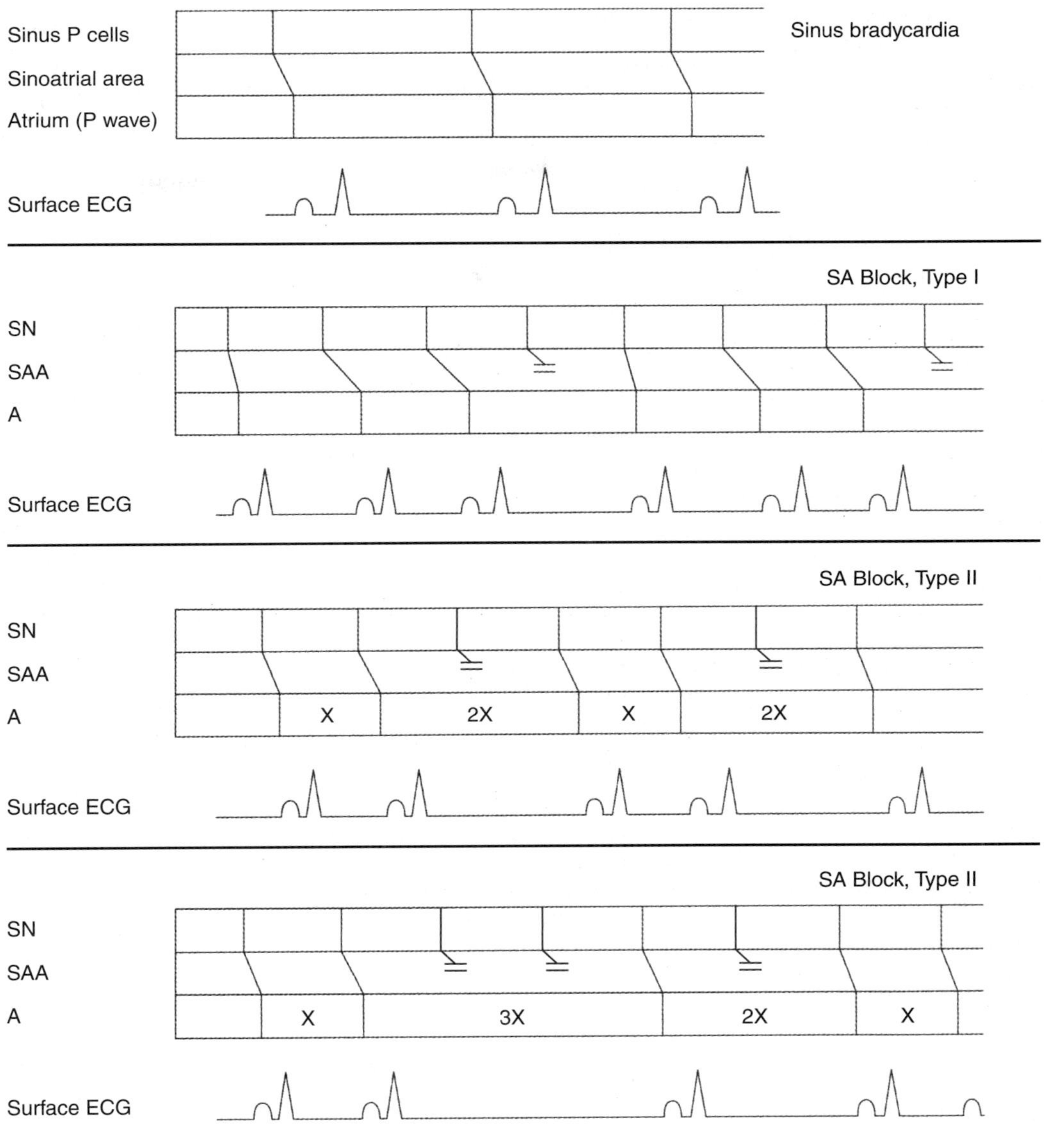

▲ **Figure 14–1.** Ladder diagrams illustrating sinus bradycardia and sinoatrial block, types I and II. ECG, electrocardiogram; SA, sinoatrial; SAA, sinoatrial area; SN, sinoatrial node.

AV node, there is a reliable escape rhythm that originates from AV node distal to the block; when the block is below the AV node, resulting ventricular escape rhythms can be slow and inconsistent and bradyasystolic arrests can ensue. First-degree AV block typically has little prognostic import. Marked PR prolongation, however, can physiologically resemble retrograde ventriculoatrial conduction with loss of optimal AV synchrony, thus causing debilitating symptoms. Persistent second-degree (type I, type II, 2:1, and advanced) and third-degree (or complete) AV block become increasingly symptomatic with higher degrees of block. Regardless of severity of block or symptoms, AV block below the level of the AV node can be associated with adverse outcomes including cardiac arrest and death.

Clinical Findings

A. Symptoms & Signs

The symptoms resulting from conduction disorders reflect cerebral hypoperfusion, low cardiac output at rest or during exercise, and rarely, hemodynamic collapse. Symptoms, which are often subtle, can be episodic or chronic

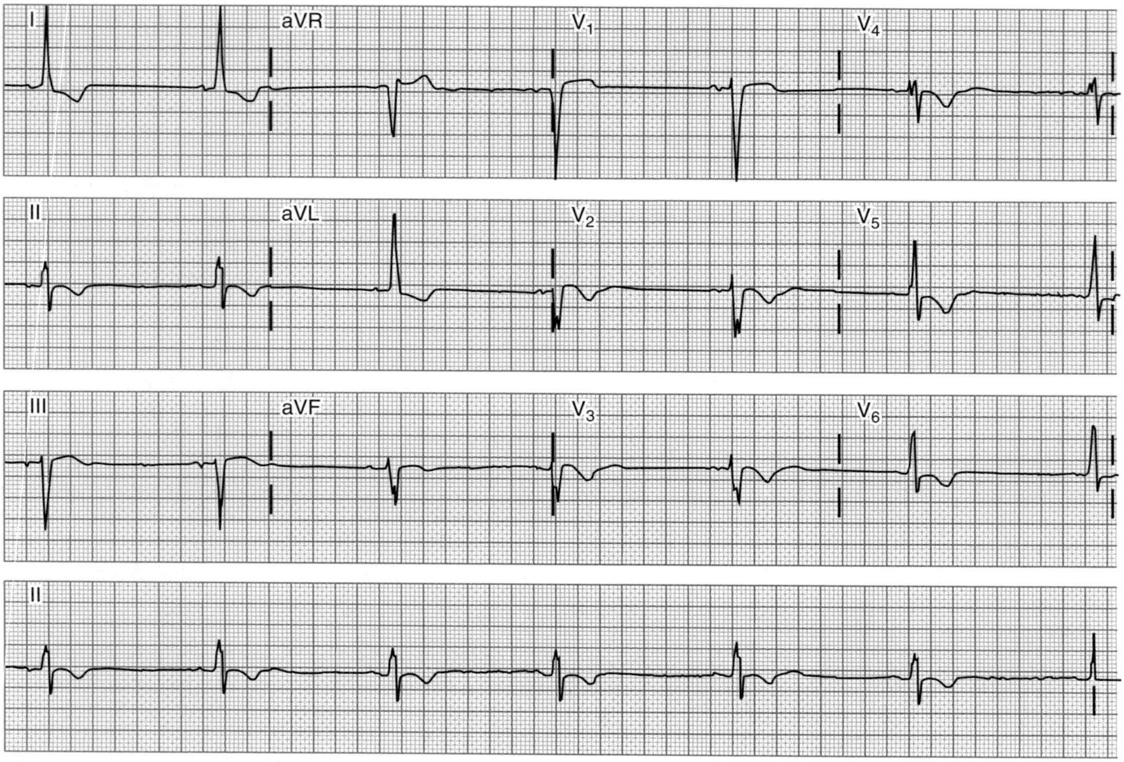

▲ **Figure 14–2.** This 83-year-old woman was being treated for heart failure with reduced ejection fraction and was receiving 200 mg/day of amiodarone for episodes of nonsustained ventricular tachycardia. She complained of profound effort fatigue but no symptoms of heart failure. Electrocardiogram reveals an atrial bradycardia at a rate of about 38 bpm. The P waves vary in morphology, suggesting some wandering of the atrial pacemaker. Left axis deviation and a left intraventricular conduction delay with ST- and T-wave abnormalities are present. The atrial bradycardia was presumed to be due to the amiodarone, which was discontinued, resulting in appreciable increase in a stable sinus rhythm, with amelioration of the patient's effort fatigue.

and can change over time. Because a patient often adapts activity levels to compensate for the impairment in heart rate response, significant symptoms may not be evident unless the patient is closely questioned about specific activities and effort tolerance, or the clinician actually observes the patient during performance of activities of daily living such as walking or during formal treadmill exercise tests.

Syncope is the classic symptom of cerebral hypoperfusion due to bradycardia; however, symptoms of presyncope such as dizziness, lightheadedness, and confusion can reflect the same pathophysiology and warrant the same aggressive approach to diagnosis and management. It should be emphasized that patients with cerebral hypoperfusion often have impairment of memory surrounding the syncopal or presyncopal episodes and may therefore be unable to provide an adequate or accurate history surrounding the events; witnesses, if present, can contribute significant information in these cases.

Patients with sinus node dysfunction, or AV block with an escape rhythm unresponsive to autonomic nervous system input, cannot increase their heart rate in response to increases in oxygen demand. These patients are, therefore, intolerant of effort and report symptoms of exercise-related breathlessness, weakness, and fatigue. These symptoms, which can be disabling, are often confused with other conditions such as hypothyroidism, medications, underlying heart disease, deconditioning, or simply older age.

During periods of AV block, the atria and ventricles often depolarize and contract asynchronously or with dyssynchronous timing. There are variable increases in atrial pressure and volume depending on the degree of AV valve opening at the onset of ventricular systole. The resulting atrial stretch and secretion of atrial natriuretic peptide produce reflex systemic hypotension and cerebral hypoperfusion. In addition, the increases in left atrial and pulmonary venous pressures can cause shortness of breath and pulmonary venous

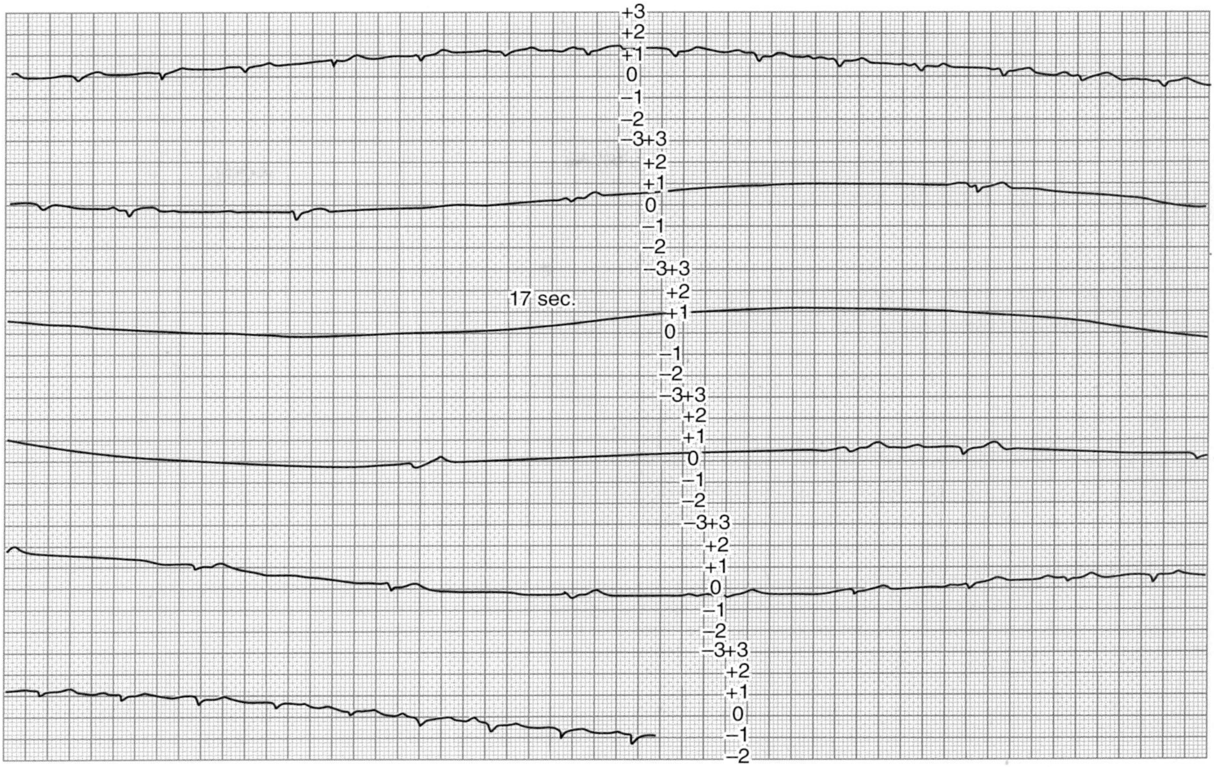

▲ **Figure 14–3.** Continuous modified lead II ambulatory electrocardiographic recording in a patient with recurrent presyncopal spells. Sinus rhythm is present in the top strip; the second strip shows marked sinus slowing, followed by a 17-second period of sinus arrest without the appearance of a QRS escape rhythm. Sinus rhythm reappears in the fourth strip, gradually increasing its rate until stable rhythm is restored in the bottom strip. The absence of an escape rhythm raises the possibility of diffuse disease of the conduction system and impulse-generating tissue.

congestion, including frank pulmonary edema. Misdiagnosis of refractory left ventricular dysfunction is not infrequently made in this situation.

Patients who have bradycardia-tachycardia syndrome (Figure 14–6) have symptoms attributable to both bradycardia and tachycardia. During tachyarrhythmias, the patient can experience uncomfortable palpitations, breathlessness, chest discomfort, and, at times, symptoms of cerebral hypoperfusion from excessively rapid heart rates.

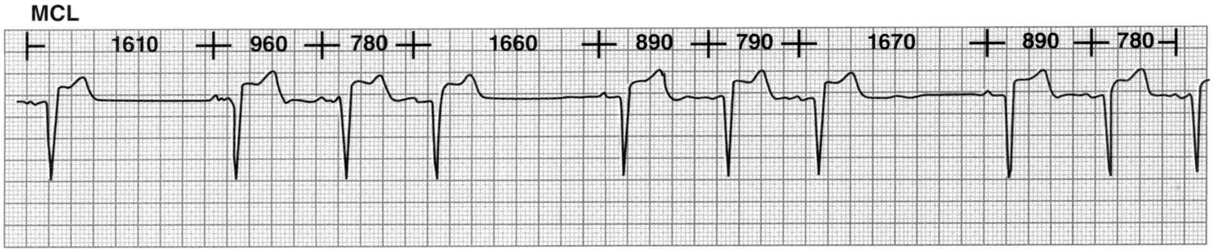

▲ **Figure 14–4.** Progressive decrease in P-wave cycle lengths followed by a pause in P-wave rate, indicating type I second-degree sinoatrial block. The pauses in sinus rate are less than twice the preceding sinus cycle lengths, satisfying the criteria for Wenckebach periodicity. MCL, modified chest lead.

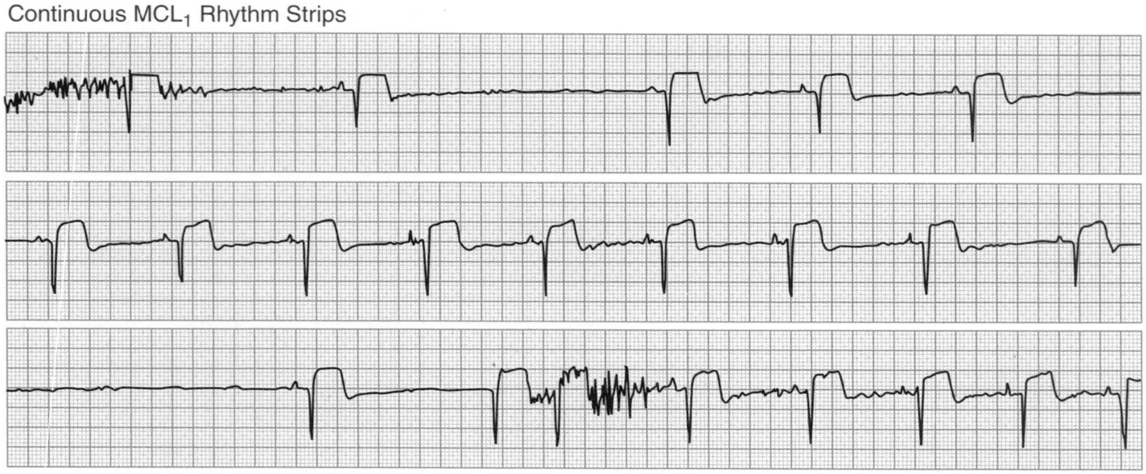

▲ **Figure 14–5.** Irregular pauses in sinus rate, which occur abruptly and are not multiples of a basic sinus-cycle length. Best characterized as sinus pauses rather than sinoatrial block or sinus arrest, this rhythm indicates the existence of sinus node dysfunction. MCL1, modified chest lead.

Distinct from bradycardia-tachycardia syndrome, bradycardias can, on occasion, lead to a potentially lethal form of polymorphic ventricular tachycardia known as bradycardia- or pause-dependent ventricular tachycardia (Figure 14–7). This is a manifestation of torsade de pointes as it occurs in the setting of QT interval prolongation brought on by the longer R-R intervals associated with either bradycardia or pauses. Symptoms in these patients can include not only palpitations, presyncope, and syncope, but also cardiac arrest.

B. Physical Examination

The physical examination of the patient with bradycardia reflects the origin of the QRS rhythm and the AV relationship more than the heart rate per se. Junctional or ventricular escape rhythms resulting from atrial bradycardia or AV block produce AV dyssynchrony. This dyssynchrony results in varying degrees of atrial contribution to ventricular filling, as well as varying stroke outputs and systolic blood pressures. Because AV dyssynchrony causes changes in the positions of the mitral and tricuspid valves relative to their fully closed or open positions, the intensity of the first heart sound will vary, as will the audibility of atrial gallop (S4) sounds and the intensity of semilunar valve systolic ejection murmurs and AV valve regurgitant murmurs.

Examination of the venous pulse contour in the neck can reveal cannon *a* waves (due to atrial systole occurring against closed AV valves) and prominent *cv* waves (due to ventricular contraction occurring with the AV valves partially or even completely open), and the diagnosis of AV block can be made by recognizing these findings. Central venous pressure elevation is a common physical finding that is independent of the venous pulse contour.

The carotid pulse may vary in volume and upstroke velocity in patients with AV dyssynchrony. Auscultation of the chest may disclose crackles, which reflect increased pulmonary venous pressure and valvular regurgitation rather than systolic or diastolic ventricular dysfunction. The liver may be enlarged and pulsatile because of transmitted *a* and *cv* waves. Peripheral edema may also be present if AV dyssynchrony is chronic.

These same physical findings can also occur in patients who have sinus rhythm but develop AV dyssynchrony from being paced by a single-chamber ventricular pacing system. In these patients, symptoms of weakness, fatigue, and congestive heart failure, together with physical findings indicating AV dyssynchrony, constitute "pacemaker syndrome." This syndrome is treated by upgrading the single-chamber

Table 14–2. Conditions Associated with Vagally-Mediated Bradyarrhythmias

Sleep
Highly conditioned state
Isotonic exercise conditioning
Coughing
Swallowing
Vomiting, retching
Suctioning
Nasal intubation
Gastric intubation
Urination
Defecation
Central nervous system trauma with high intracranial pressure

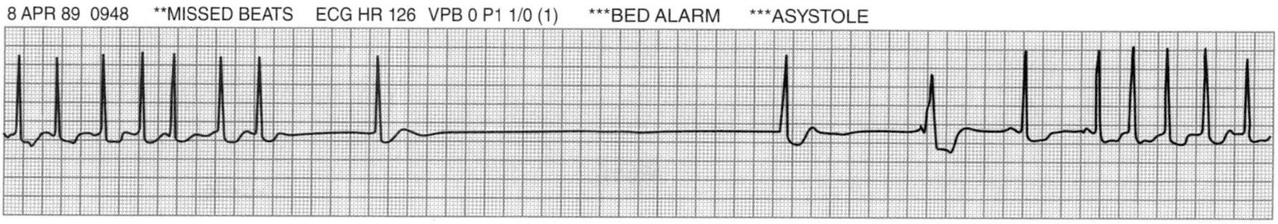

▲ **Figure 14–6.** Lead II rhythm strip characteristic of bradycardia-tachycardia syndrome, recorded from a patient with palpitations and intermittent dizzy spells.

ventricular pacing system to a dual-chamber system in which sensing of the atrial rhythm triggers a paced ventricular response that restores AV synchrony (see later section, Permanent Pacing).

In addition to the findings described earlier, significant bradycardia (<40 bpm) may result in ventricular dilation, and the Frank-Starling effect results in an increase in stroke volume and cardiac output despite the slow heart rate. This dilation may lead to left ventricular gallop sounds and regurgitant murmurs, which can disappear when normal heart rate is restored. The enlarged ventricles may be palpable.

C. Diagnostic Studies

1. Sinus node dysfunction

A. ELECTROCARDIOGRAPHY—The P waves inscribed on the surface ECG represent atrial depolarizations. Sinus node depolarization precedes atrial depolarization and is not seen on the surface ECG. The P waves that result from sinus-generated impulses must be inferred from their morphology and frontal plane axis.

The sinus P wave has a mean frontal plane axis of +15° to +75° and is upright in leads I, II, and aVF, inverted in lead aVR, and variable in leads III and aVL. In the horizontal plane, the sinus P wave can be inverted in lead V_1 but is upright in leads V_3–V_6. Respiratory variation in the sinus P-wave contour can be seen in the inferior leads and should not be confused with wandering atrial pacemaker, which is unrelated to breathing. Sinus arrhythmia is present when the P-wave morphology is normal and consistent, and the P-P intervals vary by more than 160 ms. SA block exists when some impulses generated by the sinus pacemaker cells do not exit the SA node to depolarize the atria; in the absence of atrial depolarization, a P wave will not be inscribed on the surface ECG. "Advanced" SA block, in which most of the sinus impulses fail to exit the SA node to the atrium, is inscribed on the surface ECG as pauses in sinus rhythm. These pauses often cannot be differentiated from sinus arrest caused by failure of impulse generation by the sinus node. If the pauses between sinus P waves are multiples of a basic P-wave rate, however, the diagnosis of type II second-degree or "advanced" SA block can be made.

Table 14–3. Causes of Atrioventricular Block

Congenital
Genetic (SCN5A mutations)
Degenerative (Lenègre and Lev's diseases)
Ischemic (inferior wall MI, anterior wall MI, ischemic cardiomyopathy)
Infectious (Lyme carditis, aortic valve endocarditis)
Inflammatory (myocarditis, collagen vascular diseases)
Infiltrative (amyloidosis, sarcoidosis, hemochromatosis, neoplasm)
Neuromuscular (myotonic muscular dystrophy, Kearns-Sayre syndrome, Erb dystrophy, peroneal muscular atrophy)
Calcific (aortic and mitral valve disease)
Iatrogenic
Medication (β-blockers, diltiazem, verapamil, digoxin, antiarrhythmic drugs, donepezil)
Valvular intervention (aortic valve surgery, TAVR)
Catheter ablation (AV nodal ablation)
Alcohol septal ablation

AV, atrioventricular; MI, myocardial infarction; TAVR, transcatheter aortic valve replacement.

B. ELECTROPHYSIOLOGIC STUDIES—Sinus node function can be evaluated in the electrophysiology laboratory by means of simultaneous surface and intracardiac electrographic recordings made during basal conditions, physiologic and pharmacologic interventions, and atrial pacing. This evaluation can be undertaken in patients with either symptomatic sinus bradycardia or bradycardia-tachycardia syndrome. It can also be used in patients with recurrent syncope of unclear etiology, although the diagnostic yield and predictive value for syncope is limited. Measurements include the intrinsic heart rate, the sinus node recovery time (SNRT), and the response to parasympathetic (vagal) stimulation as assessed by carotid sinus massage.

The intrinsic heart rate (ie, the rate independent of autonomic influences) is the sinus rate during pharmacologic denervation of the sinus node using a β-blocker and atropine. The intrinsic heart rate is sometimes used to distinguish healthy persons from those with sinus node dysfunction.

SNRT is the interval after sinus node suppression from overdrive atrial pacing to the first return of sinus node activity, manifested on the surface ECG by the postpacing sinus P-wave interval. The measured SNRT depends on several factors, among them the proximity of the pacing catheter to the sinus node, the presence or absence of SA entrance

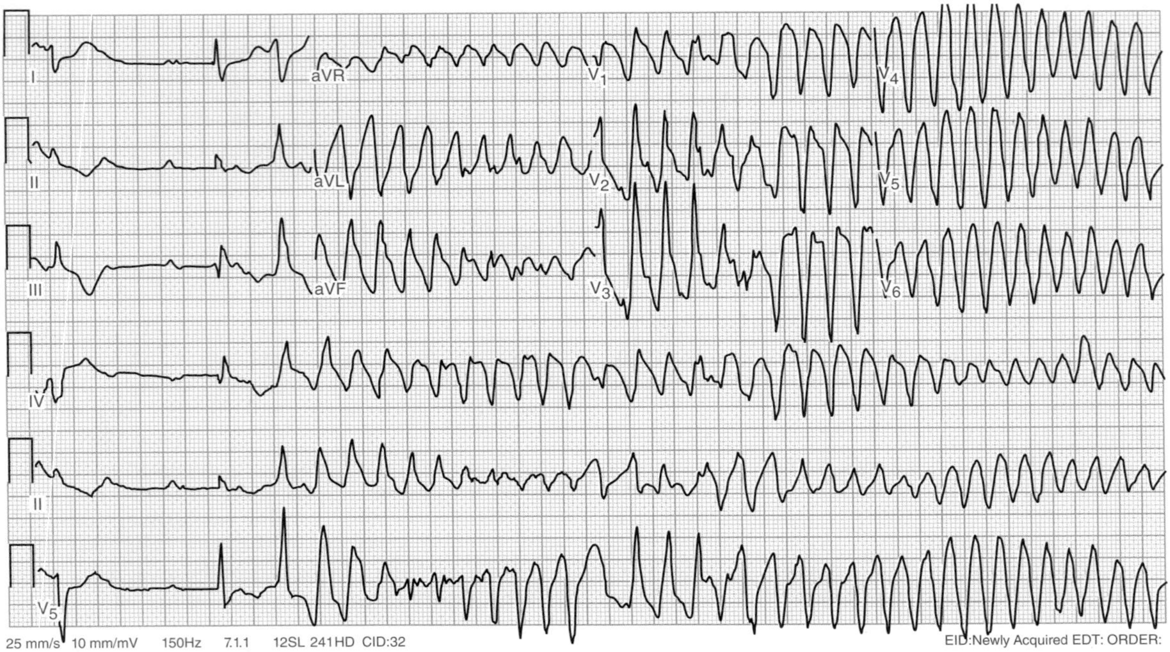

▲ **Figure 14–7.** Pause-dependent ventricular tachycardia. The initial seconds recorded on the 12-lead electrocardiogram and three-lead rhythm strips reveal complete heart block. The heart block results in a long RR cycle length and prolongation of the following QT interval. The QT prolongation results in polymorphic ventricular tachycardia (torsade de pointes).

block (in which atrial impulses fail to enter and depolarize the sinus node), and local neurohormonal influences. In normal persons, atrial pacing at rates of 120–130 bpm for 30 seconds or more is followed by a return of sinus node activity at a reproducible interval, with the basic sinus rate generally recovered within three postpacing beats. The usual SNRT is less than 1.5 seconds, although considerable variation may exist depending on the prevailing autonomic tone. A corrected SNRT can be calculated by subtracting the basic sinus rate from the SNRT; a normal value is usually between 350 and 550 ms. In patients with sinus node dysfunction, SNRT may not be reproducible and tend to be longer after more prolonged periods of pacing; return to the basic sinus rate within three postpacing beats is also inconstant and may be followed by additional (secondary) pauses in rate.

Electrophysiologic testing of sinus node function is neither specific nor sensitive; abnormal results can be seen in patients without sinus bradycardia and normal results in those with symptomatic sinus node disease. The diagnosis of sinus node dysfunction remains primarily a clinical one.

c. Ambulatory ECG monitoring—Establishing correlation between symptoms and documented bradycardia is necessary for the diagnosis of sinus node dysfunction, and essential when deciding if permanent pacing is indicated. Advances in ambulatory ECG monitoring have resulted in a wide range of modalities that allow for longer monitoring durations, and that are more accessible and convenient for patients.

Continuous ECG monitors have the advantage of uninterrupted recording over a period of time, but technology constraints have until recently limited the monitoring duration to 24–48 hours (eg, Holter monitors); the need for multiple electrodes and wires has also been a limitation that required application of the monitor by medical personnel and can be a cause of inconvenience for patients. Various patch monitors without wires have been designed that can be self-applied by the patient and can record continuously up to 2 weeks. If continuous monitoring is needed beyond 2 weeks, an implantable cardiac monitor with a battery longevity up to 4.5 years that is inserted subcutaneously overlying the chest wall can be considered.

Event monitors are able to be worn or carried for longer periods of time but have the limitation of recording only specific sequences. Wearable event monitors that utilize electrodes and wires can be worn up to 30 days. Portable ECG recorders have the advantage of longer observation durations but recording starts after the onset of symptoms and the patient must have the recorder on-hand. Personal portable ECG monitors have the advantage of being either wearable, as in the form of a smartwatch, or ultraportable, as being able to fit in a wallet, and are reliably available to record with the onset of symptoms; the ECG tracings from these portable monitors are increasingly being accepted by clinicians as achieving diagnostic quality.

D. EXERCISE TESTING—Treadmill exercise testing can be of substantial value in assessing chronotropic response ("chronotropic competence") to increases in metabolic needs in patients with sinus bradycardia in whom sinus node dysfunction is suspected. The definition of chronotropic incompetence is not agreed on, but it is reasonable to designate it as consisting of either an inability to achieve a heart rate exceeding 75% of age-predicted maximum (usually taken as 220 − age), or 100–120 bpm at maximum effort. Irregular (and nonreproducible) increases, and even decreases, in sinus rate during exercise can occur but are rare. Abrupt rate changes during the postexercise recovery period can also occur but are rare. Chronotropic incompetence can result from medications (Table 14–1) and should be distinguished from intrinsic sinus node dysfunction.

The Bruce treadmill exercise protocol, which is usually used to diagnose the presence and severity of coronary artery disease, is generally inappropriate for patients with sinus node dysfunction in whom the goal is to assess heart rate at lower workloads expected to be encountered during average daily activities. Specific protocols have been developed for this purpose. In addition to documenting chronotropic incompetence, treadmill exercise testing can be used to aid in optimal programming of rate-adaptive cardiac pacemakers that are usually required in these patients.

2. Atrioventricular block

A. ELECTROGRAPHY AND ELECTROCARDIOGRAPHY—His bundle electrography has provided important information regarding normal and abnormal AV conduction in humans. The technique involves positioning a multipolar electrode catheter across the tricuspid valve in proximity to the AV nodal-His bundle area to record electrical activity as it traverses these structures. Because of its location, the catheter records electrical activity at the level of the low right atrium, His bundle, proximal right bundle branch, and right ventricular septum. The sinus node pacemaker cells normally initiate the cardiac impulse, but they are not registered on the surface ECG; the onset of the P wave on the surface ECG signifies the beginning of atrial depolarization. Because the intracardiac electrode catheter lies at the level of the low right atrium, early atrial depolarization will not be detected by the catheter; as the atrial depolarization wavefront reaches the low right atrium, a deflection is registered (A). As the impulse traverses and depolarizes the His bundle, another deflection is registered (H). His bundle deflection is then followed by a ventricular deflection (V), which is registered at the time the wavefront of ventricular depolarization reaches the electrodes; ventricular deflection recorded by the catheter often occurs after the onset of QRS complex on the surface ECG.

His bundle electrography is useful in indicating the site of AV conduction delay or block. Normally, the conduction time through the AV node is 90–150 ms, and the conduction time through the His-Purkinje system is 35–55 ms. In a patient with a prolonged PR interval, a prolonged AH interval signifies delayed impulse conduction within the AV node, and a prolonged HV time represents delayed impulse conduction within the His bundle or the bundle branches. Conduction delay within the His bundle itself manifests as more than one His deflection ("split" His deflections).

In **first-degree AV block** (a delay in conduction between the atria and the ventricles), all atrial impulses are conducted to the ventricles; it is characterized by a prolonged PR interval that exceeds 200 ms (Figure 14–8). The components of a normal PR interval are interatrial conduction (10–50 ms), AV nodal conduction (90–150 ms), and intra-His and His-Purkinje conduction (35–55 ms). Conduction delay in first-degree AV block can thus represent prolonged intra-atrial, AV nodal, intra-His, or His-Purkinje conduction, and the His bundle electrographic recordings help clarify the location of the delay.

In patients with a QRS complex that is narrow and normal-appearing, first-degree AV block is AV nodal in more than 85% and is intra-His in less than 15%. In patients with a wide QRS complex due to BBB or nonspecific intraventricular conduction delay, first-degree AV block is AV nodal in less than 25%, infranodal in about 45%, and at more than one site in about 33%.

In **second-degree AV block,** not all atrial impulses are conducted to the ventricles. The ratio of P waves to QRS complexes is referred to as the *AV conduction ratio.* **Type I (Wenckebach) second-degree AV block** is present when the conduction of atrial impulses to the ventricles is progressively delayed because of AV (generally AV nodal) refractoriness, with eventual failure of conduction of an atrial impulse to the ventricles. The AV conduction ratio in type I second-degree AV block can be 3:2, 4:3, 5:4, and so on; this ratio is also referred to as a *Wenckebach period.* AV conduction ratios in type I second-degree AV block need not be constant, and therefore, the Wenckebach period may not be reproducible. Because type I second-degree AV block usually occurs within the AV node, the PR interval of the first conducted P wave of the Wenckebach period is often prolonged, and because this conduction disturbance does not involve the bundle branches, the QRS complexes are expected to be narrow and normal-appearing unless there is preexisting bundle branch disease.

In a typical, or classic, Wenckebach period, the PR intervals progressively lengthen, the R-R intervals progressively shorten, and the R-R interval encompassing the nonconducted P wave is less than twice the preceding R-R interval. Typical Wenckebach periods are usually seen with low AV conduction ratios (3:2, 4:3, and 5:4), but as the AV

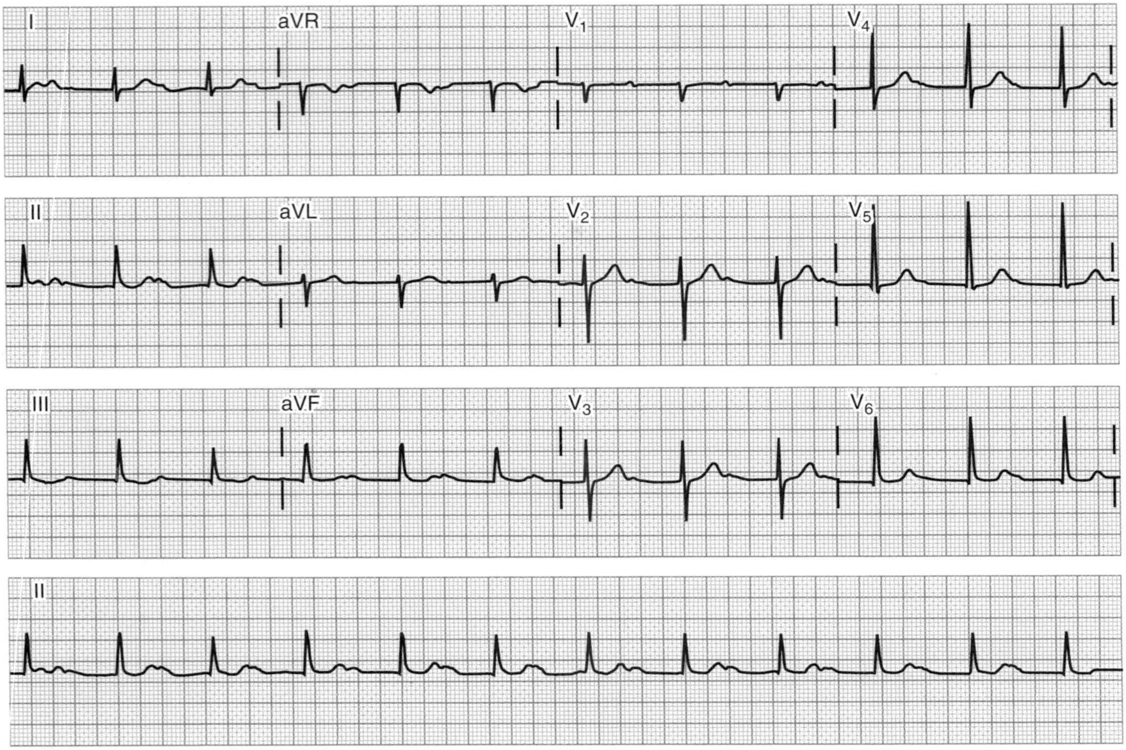

▲ **Figure 14–8.** Sinus rhythm with marked first-degree atrioventricular (AV) block. All P waves are conducted to the ventricles. The PR intervals are about 480 ms. The RP intervals are shorter than the PR intervals, which, in some patients, can cause symptoms due to suboptimally timed AV depolarization-contraction sequences. Despite the length of the PR intervals, this conduction disturbance is generally benign; evolution to second-degree AV block can take years.

conduction ratio increases (exceeding 6:5), more and more Wenckebach sequences are atypical. If the sinus rate is not constant, for example in vagally mediated bradyarrhythmias, sequences that resemble Wenckebach conduction often occur; they should not, however, be considered type I second-degree AV block, in which the sinus rate needs to be constant for the diagnosis to be made.

In **type II second-degree AV block,** atrial impulses intermittently fail to be transmitted to the ventricles, but progressive conduction delay prior to the AV conduction failure does not occur. Because prior conduction delay from the atria is not present, the failure of antegrade conduction is often abrupt and unpredictable (paroxysmal) and may be advanced. In contrast to type I second-degree AV block, in which the conduction delay is usually in the AV node, the conduction delay in type II second-degree AV block can be within the His bundle or, more commonly, distal to the His bundle in the bundle branches. If the block is within the His bundle, the QRS complexes will be narrow and normal-appearing, or only mildly aberrant, unless preexisting BBB is present. If the block is infra-His, the QRS complexes will show a BBB pattern. In contrast to type I second-degree AV block, the PR interval of the conducted P waves is constant and often (but not always) normal (Figure 14–9).

Second-degree AV block with 2:1 AV conduction ratio may represent either AV nodal or His-Purkinje block (Figures 14–10 and 14–11). Two consecutive PR intervals are not recorded in 2:1 AV conduction; therefore, the presence or absence of progressive PR prolongation cannot be ascertained and distinguishing the site of block may be difficult. If the PR interval of the conducted P waves is prolonged and the QRS complexes are narrow and normal-appearing, AV nodal block is probably present. If the PR interval of the conducted P waves is normal and the QRS complexes have a BBB pattern, His-Purkinje block is probably present. If the PR interval of the conducted P wave is prolonged and the QRS complexes have a BBB pattern, or if the PR interval of the conducted P wave is normal and the QRS complexes appear normal, it may not be possible to distinguish between the two types, and more than one site of AV block may also be present.

Altering the AV conduction ratio by means of carotid sinus massage or intravenous atropine will often allow identification of the nature of the AV block and thus its location

(Figure 14–9). If the site of block is in the AV node, the AV conduction ratio will increase due to the vagotonic effect of carotid sinus massage (eg, from 2:1 to 3:1 or 4:1) and improving with the vagolytic effect of intravenous atropine (eg, from 2:1 to 3:2 or 4:3). Conversely, His-Purkinje block is heart rate dependent, and AV conduction ratio improves (eg, from 2:1 to 3:2 or 4:3) due to the slower sinus rate caused by carotid sinus massage; with faster sinus rate due to the intravenous atropine, the AV conduction ratio will increase (eg, from 2:1 to 3:1 or 4:1).

In **advanced second-degree AV block,** the AV conduction ratio is 3:1 or greater, and atrial impulses are not consistently conducted to the ventricles. In contrast, in **third-degree ("complete") AV block,** no atrial impulses are conducted to the ventricles despite temporal opportunity for this to occur, and the atria and ventricles are depolarized by their respective pacemakers, which are independent of each other (Figure 14–12). The atrial rate in complete AV block is almost always faster than the ventricular rate. The QRS rhythm, or the escape rhythm, originates distal to the site of block and may be in the AV junction, His bundle, bundle branches, or distal Purkinje system. The morphology of the QRS complexes and their rate will depend on their site of origin. A narrow QRS complex escape rhythm originates from the AV junction. On the other hand, a wide QRS complex rhythm is not a reliable guide to the origin of the

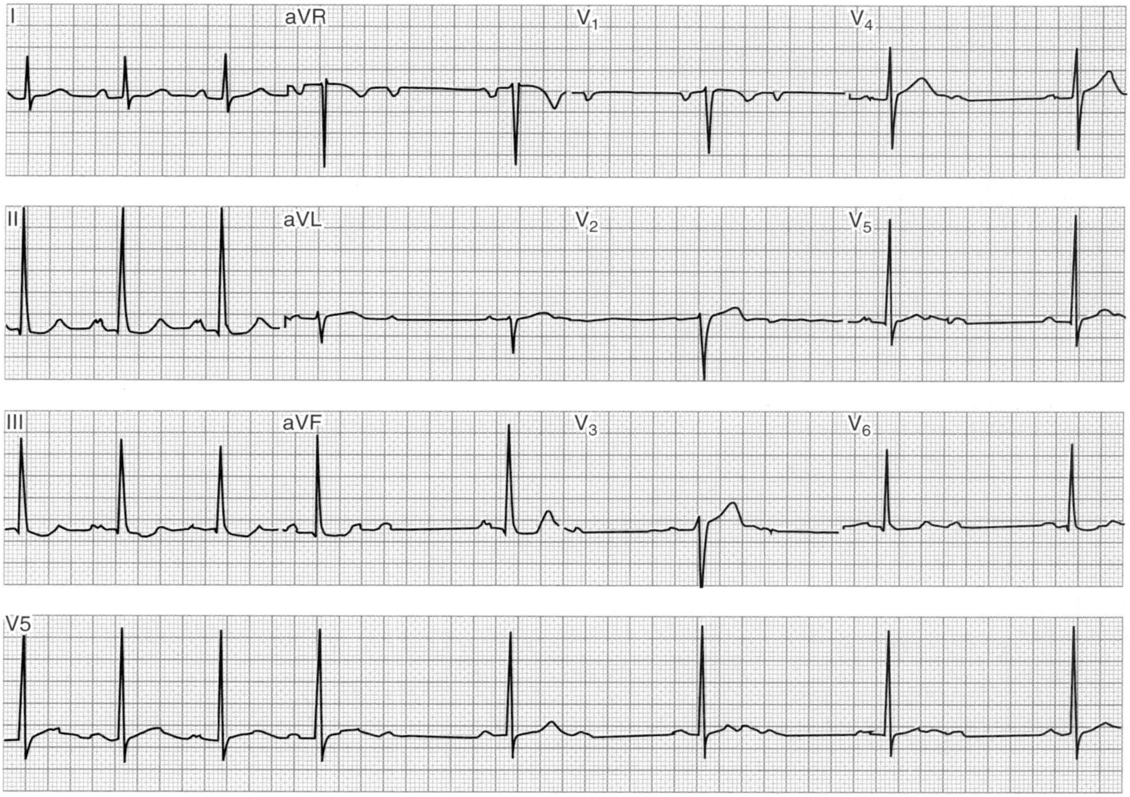

A

▲ **Figure 14–9. A:** This electrocardiogram was recorded in a patient with presyncopal spells who was about to undergo exercise treadmill testing. The atrial rhythm is sinus at a rate of about 68 bpm. The PR intervals of the conducted QRS complexes are all about 240 ms. The QRS complexes are narrow, and nondiagnostic ST- and T-wave abnormalities are present. A 2:1 atrioventricular (AV) conduction develops abruptly during the recording. The prolonged PR intervals of the conducted P waves, as well as the narrow morphology of the QRS complexes (indicating absence of bundle branch system disease), could suggest that the 2:1 AV conduction represents AV nodal block; intra-His block, however, is suggested by the absence of prolongation of the PR intervals prior to the nonconducted P waves. Changing of the AV conduction ratio from 2:1 to 3:2, 5:4, and so on, would help establish the presence of AV nodal block. This could be achieved by atropine or exercise testing, during which adrenergic drive would be expected to facilitate AV conduction.

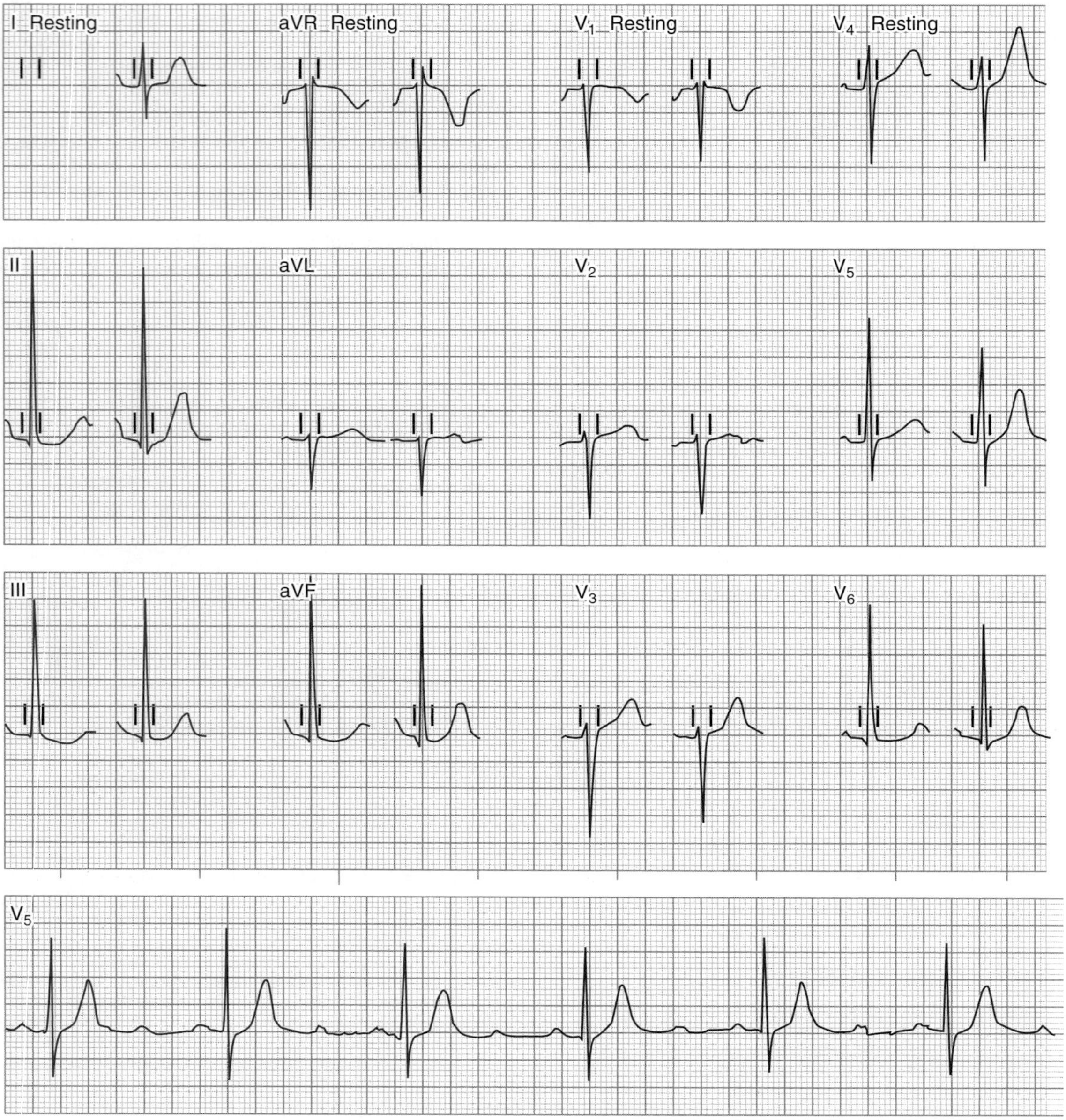

▲ **Figure 14–9.** (*Continued*) **B:** The patient achieved stage IV of the Bruce protocol during treadmill testing. The atrial rate was 150 bpm. At peak effort and for the first 2 minutes of the postexercise recovery period, 3:1 AV block developed abruptly and was associated with the patient's typical presyncopal symptoms. AV block developing during exercise, although rare, is always abnormal and, if the QRS complexes are narrow or normal appearing, indicates intra-His block. Permanent cardiac pacing is required.

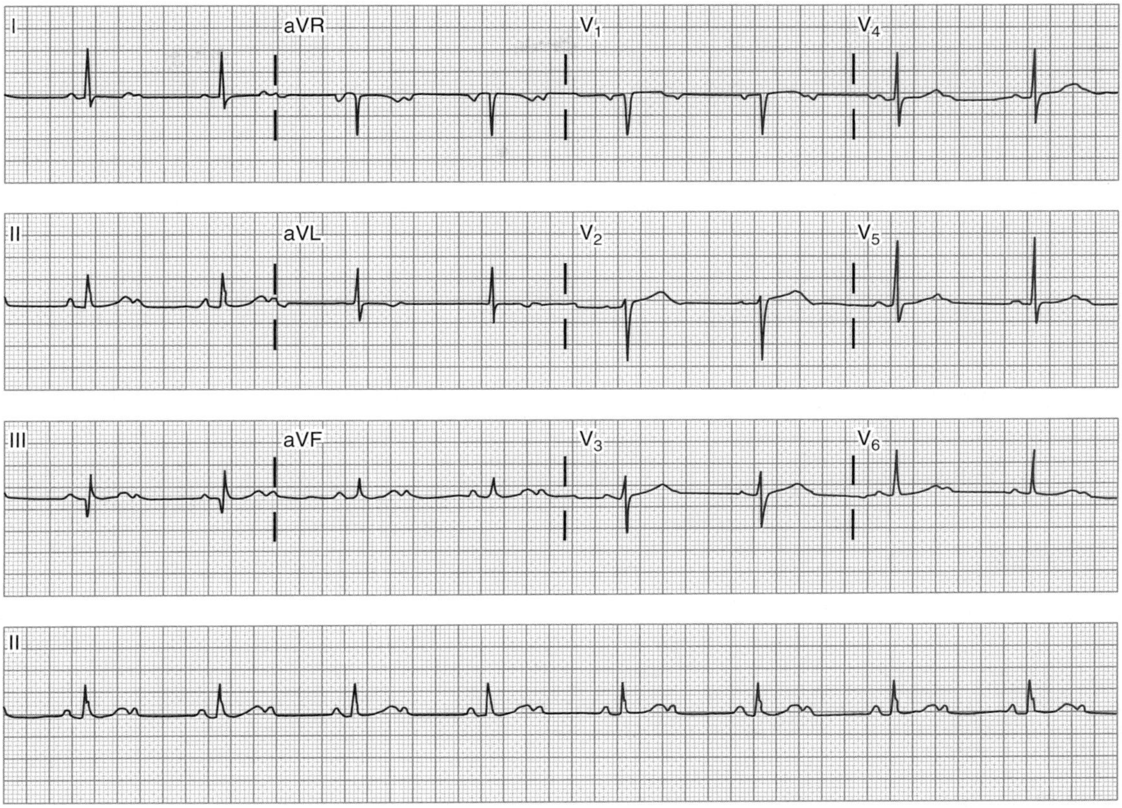

▲ **Figure 14–10.** The atrial rhythm is sinus, and 2:1 atrioventricular (AV) conduction is present. The PR intervals of the conducted beats are normal at about 190 ms. The QRS complexes are narrow and normal appearing. The 2:1 AV conduction could represent either AV nodal or His-Purkinje block. When AV nodal block is present, the PR intervals of the conducted complexes are often prolonged and the QRS complexes narrow and normal appearing, whereas in infra-Hisian block, the PR intervals of the conducted complexes are generally normal and the QRS complexes broad, indicating bundle branch disease. In this tracing, the PR intervals are normal. The site of block cannot be known with certainty from this tracing, and manipulation of the AV conduction ratio by atropine or exercise, which facilitates AV conduction, might be required. AV nodal block generally does not require cardiac pacing. If the block is within the His bundle, both the PR interval and QRS complex width are typically normal (electrophysiologic study may be needed to distinguish from AV nodal block), and permanent cardiac pacing is indicated.

rhythm because rhythms originating in the longitudinally separated predivisional region of the His bundle can have a wide QRS complex.

If the atrial rate is not sinus (eg, atrial fibrillation), the existence of advanced or complete AV block is diagnosed by the presence of a slow ventricular rate with varying intervals between the QRS complexes or by a slow and regular QRS rate (Figure 14–13), respectively. Atrial fibrillation and flutter are not uncommonly associated with advanced AV block and slow QRS rates. The rate of the ventricular rhythm, as well as the QRS-complex morphology, will depend on the site of origin of the rhythm. A regular rhythm in a patient with atrial fibrillation confirms the presence of complete AV block, with a QRS pacemaker originating below the level of conduction block that is independent of the atrial rhythm.

In **vagally mediated block,** a high degree of vagal tone, such as occurs with sympathetic withdrawal during sleep or in highly conditioned athletes, may be associated with slowing of the sinus rate, pauses in sinus rhythm, variable degrees of delay in AV conduction manifested by prolongation of PR intervals (often irregular), and failure of conduction of P waves resembling type I or II second-degree AV block (Table 14–4). It is important to recognize vagally mediated block because it often occurs in normal individuals as well as in patients with inferior or right ventricular myocardial infarction, or any other clinical condition in

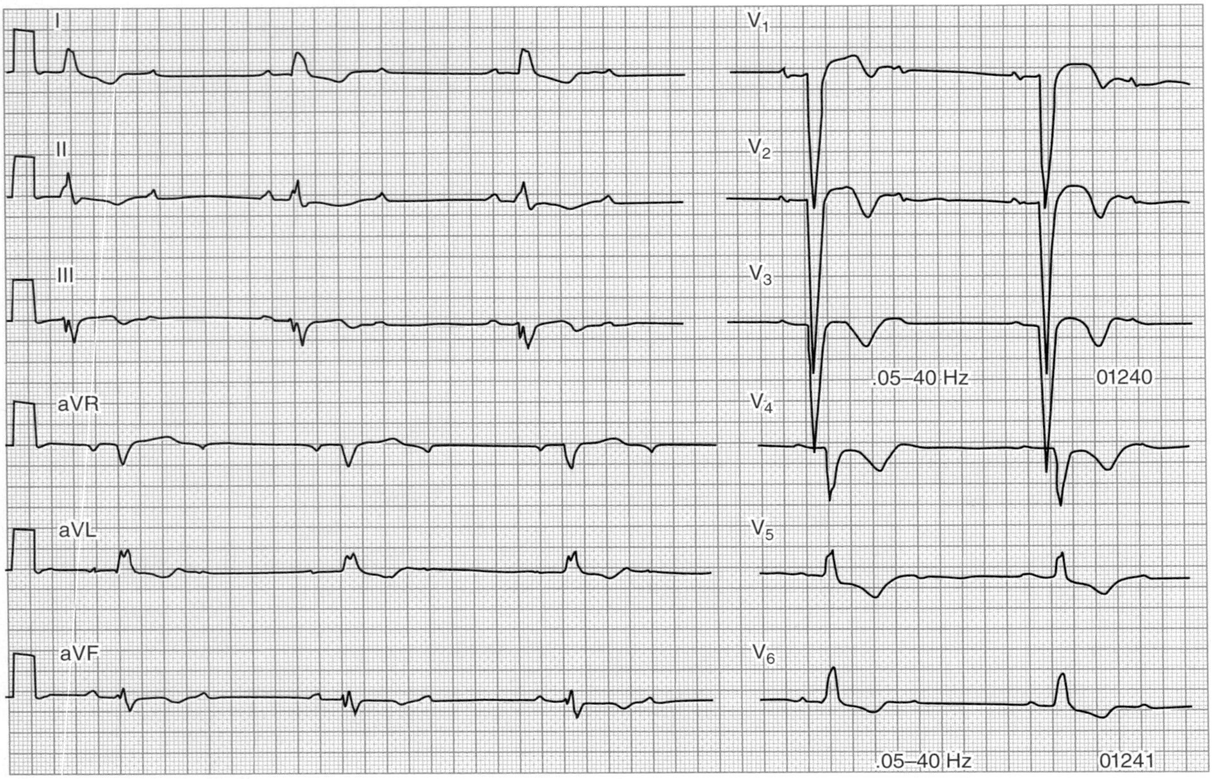

▲ **Figure 14–11.** Second-degree atrioventricular (AV) block, with 2:1 conduction ratio and evidence of bundle branch disease. The prolonged PR interval of the conducted P waves and the left bundle branch block pattern of the conducted QRS complexes make localization of the site of block difficult; the prolonged PR interval suggests AV nodal disease, whereas the wide QRS complexes support infra-Hisian disease; electrophysiologic study may be necessary to document the site of conduction delay and to decide whether permanent cardiac pacing is required.

which hypervagotonia is present (Table 14–2). It not uncommonly accompanies the use of certain medications, notably β-blocking agents, some antihypertensive drugs, and occasionally, digoxin. It can also be seen during coughing (tussive bradycardia), swallowing (deglutition bradycardia), and yawning. In the critical care setting, vagally mediated block (and significant bradycardia) can occur during endotracheal suctioning or esophagogastric intubation and in patients with elevated intracranial pressure.

B. Ambulatory ECG monitoring—In the diagnostic evaluation of AV block, ambulatory ECG monitoring takes on a different role from that in sinus node dysfunction. Because there is the potential for cardiac arrest with infranodal AV block, electrophysiologic studies will usually be considered to establish the location of the AV block prior to prolonged ECG monitoring. The transient nature of AV block, especially early in the course of disease, makes event monitoring less useful unless the monitor is capable of looping memory that retains data for a few minutes before it gets overwritten; this allows for capture of ECG tracings several minutes prior to onset of symptoms and activation of the event monitor. The intermittent nature of AV block, with sometimes months between symptoms, requires that monitoring be of prolonged duration. Implantable cardiac monitors can be useful if the diagnosis of AV block or the decision for permanent pacing therapy is not clear after electrophysiologic studies.

C. Exercise testing—Unlike the value of exercise testing in sinus node dysfunction for both diagnosis and evaluation of chronotropic competence, exercise testing in patients with AV block is generally less useful. AV node conduction is enhanced by the vagolysis and increased sympathetic drive that occurs with exercise. Thus, patients with first-degree AV block and type I second-degree AV block are expected to have shorter PR intervals during exercise; in patients with type I second-degree AV block, a longer Wenckebach period can develop (eg, 3:2 at rest becoming 6:5 during exercise). Patients with 2:1 AV conduction, in whom the

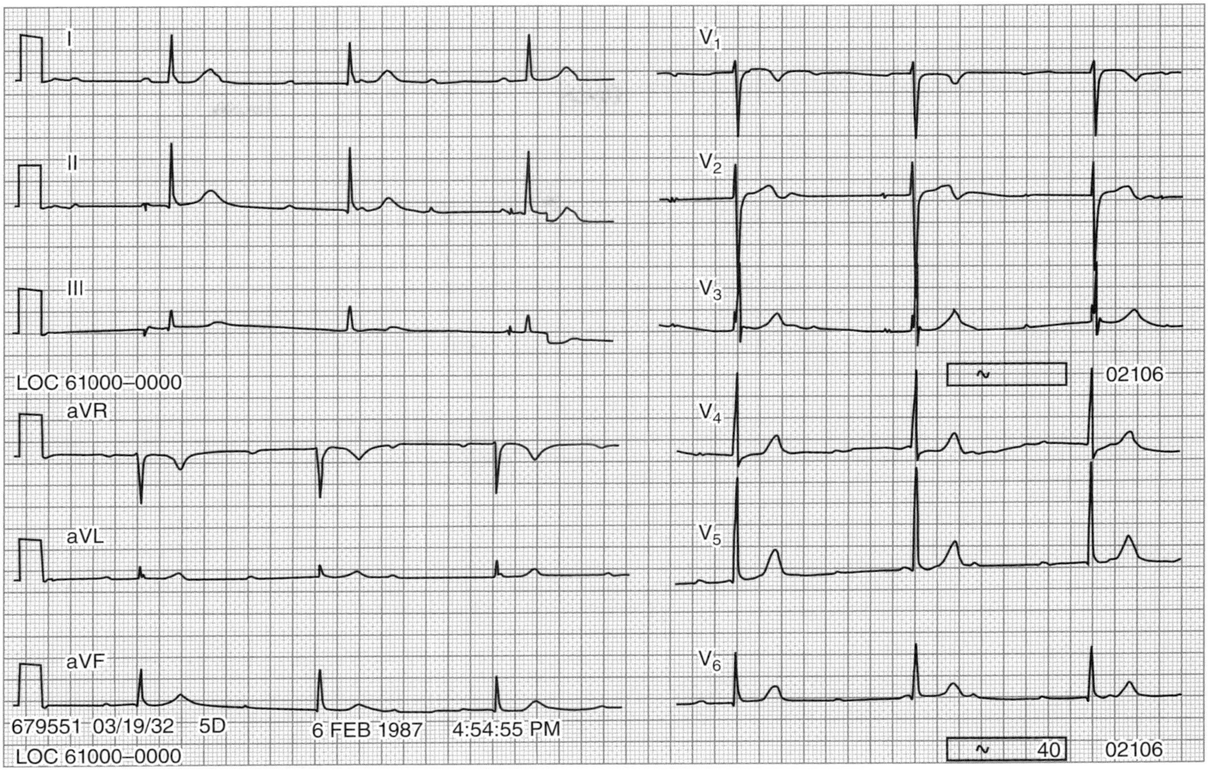

▲ **Figure 14–12.** Complete atrioventricular (AV) block. The atrial and ventricular rhythms are independent of each other. The narrow, normal-appearing QRS complexes establish that the AV block is within the AV node or the His bundle.

site of conduction block may be uncertain, can benefit from exercise testing by observing whether the AV conduction ratio increases in a Wenckebach-like manner (eg, to 3:2 or 4:3) or decreases (eg, to 3:1 or 4:1) (Figure 14–9). In the latter case, the increase in the sinus rate finds the His-Purkinje system refractory, causing the higher degrees of block. This response, when observed, is always abnormal because it indicates intra- or infra-His block, which will require permanent cardiac pacing.

Treatment

The major reversible causes of conduction system disturbances are high vagal tone and medications. High vagal tone, whether or not it is accompanied by withdrawal of sympathetic tone, can cause or contribute to both atrial and ventricular bradycardia. Vagally mediated bradycardias are usually transient and not accompanied by symptoms of presyncope or frank syncope, and no treatment is needed. Even when pauses are prolonged and symptomatic, permanent cardiac pacing is usually not indicated. If necessary, intravenous atropine can be used to facilitate AV nodal conduction to avoid ventricular bradycardia; however, the atropine-induced increase in atrial rate can lead to a paradoxical slowing of ventricular rate as a result of more rapid stimulation of, and encroachment on, the refractory period of the AV conduction system. Moreover, the effects of intravenous atropine are short-lived, and its long-term use is accompanied by significant side effects.

In contrast to the majority of vagally mediated bradycardias, "vasovagal" or vagally mediated syncope (hypotension with variable degrees of bradycardia or asystole) can be frequent, abrupt, unpredictable, and disabling. These highly symptomatic episodes, also referred to as "neurocardiogenic" or "neutrally mediated" syncopal syndromes, are generally not life-threatening but can have significant morbidity including serious injury. Predisposing factors such as volume depletion and prolonged standing should be avoided. Isometric contraction, such as by crossing legs, tensing the lower body, and vigorous handgripping, has been found to abort episodes, and patients should be instructed in these maneuvers.

Because left ventricular baroreceptor stimulation (from vigorous systolic ventricular contraction) and its consequent

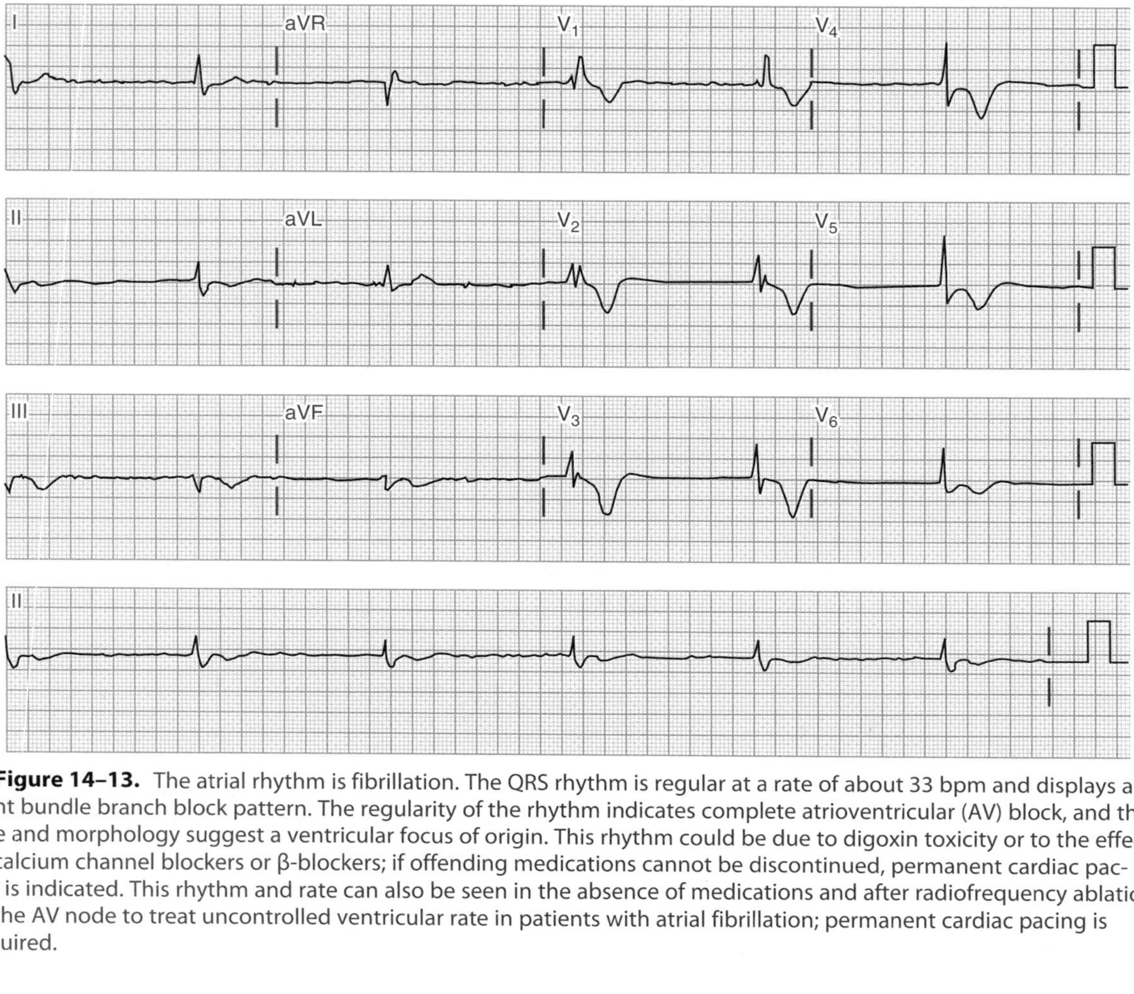

▲ **Figure 14–13.** The atrial rhythm is fibrillation. The QRS rhythm is regular at a rate of about 33 bpm and displays a right bundle branch block pattern. The regularity of the rhythm indicates complete atrioventricular (AV) block, and the rate and morphology suggest a ventricular focus of origin. This rhythm could be due to digoxin toxicity or to the effects of calcium channel blockers or β-blockers; if offending medications cannot be discontinued, permanent cardiac pacing is indicated. This rhythm and rate can also be seen in the absence of medications and after radiofrequency ablation of the AV node to treat uncontrolled ventricular rate in patients with atrial fibrillation; permanent cardiac pacing is required.

reflex peripheral vasodilation play a role in this syndrome, drugs having negative inotropic effects (eg, β-blockers) were postulated as potential medical therapies. Multiple studies have now shown β-blockers to be generally ineffective; there may be benefit among patients 42 years of age or older.

Table 14–4. Diagnostic Clues to Vagally Mediated Atrioventricular Block

Concomitant slowing of sinus rate
Changing PR intervals, often with irregularity of sinus rates
Atypical Wenckebach periods, often with inconstant PP intervals
Inconstant escape rates
Inconstant escape foci
Transient nature of episodes
Lack of reproducibility of episodes, duration
Reversed or abolished by intravenous atropine or an increase in sympathetic tone

α-Agonists, such as midodrine, have been used successfully with orthostatic hypotension, and to a lesser degree with vasovagal syncope. Fludrocortisone and selective serotonin reuptake inhibitors have been found to have variable degrees of effectiveness. The tendency for events to occur in clusters, sometimes separated by long periods of time, make daily use of medications typically unwarranted. In "malignant" vasovagal syncope (frequent attacks, severe events resulting in serious injury, prolonged asystole), permanent dual-chamber cardiac pacing can be considered, even though benefit of pacing has not been consistently shown. There is evidence that dual-chamber pacing reduces syncope in patients 40 years of age or older with spontaneous pauses ≥ 3 seconds documented with syncope or asymptomatic pauses ≥ 6 seconds. Special pacing algorithms can be used that detect abrupt falls in heart rate and respond with rapid pacing until the spontaneous heart rate increases.

Commonly used medications that cause or contribute to bradycardia do so by enhancing vagal tone (eg, digoxin), reducing the facilitation of AV conduction that results from sympathetic tone (eg, β-blockers and antiarrhythmic agents with β-blocking properties such as sotalol and propafenone), or acting directly on SA and AV conduction tissue (eg, verapamil and diltiazem). Simple withdrawal of these medications can reverse the bradycardia, although the process may require several days. If the offending medications are necessary to treat other conditions such as angina pectoris or heart failure and cannot be discontinued, permanent cardiac pacing will be required (Table 14–5).

It is important to exclude AV nodal blocking medications, such as digoxin, β-blockers, and rate-limiting calcium channel blockers, as a cause of, or contributor to, slow ventricular rates in atrial fibrillation and flutter; withdrawal of these drugs or reduction in dosage can result in reversal of the AV block, and permanent cardiac pacing can be avoided. If the ventricular rhythm is slow in the absence of these agents, intrinsic AV conduction system disease is likely to be present, and permanent cardiac pacing will usually be indicated. Electrical cardioversion of the atrial arrhythmia should be undertaken with caution in patients with slow ventricular rates in the absence of medication; because of diffuse underlying conduction disease, postcardioversion sinus bradycardia or even asystole can occur.

In bradycardia-tachycardia syndrome, prolonged pauses in sinus rhythm frequently occur following an abrupt termination of the tachycardia. These pauses are often associated with symptoms of cerebral insufficiency, and cardiac pacing can be required. Because catheter ablation is an effective treatment for most tachyarrhythmias (eg, atrial flutter, atrial fibrillation), elimination of the tachycardia should be considered as an alternative to permanent pacemaker implantation; severity of the underlying sinus node dysfunction, however, may still make cardiac pacing necessary even after ablation.

When treating bradycardia-tachycardia syndrome, current pacemakers use an algorithm to switch from a DDD or DDDR mode of operation to a VVI, VVIR, DDI, or DDIR mode on sensing an atrial tachyarrhythmia, and back again to DDD or DDDR mode when a normal atrial rate is sensed (see later section, Permanent Pacing); this helps maintain an even pulse rate, whether in or out of tachycardia, by avoiding rapid ventricular pacing in response to tracking of atrial tachyarrhythmias.

When tachycardia occurs despite antiarrhythmic drug therapy, or in the setting of permanent atrial fibrillation, more aggressive control of the ventricular rate becomes necessary. AV nodal blocking agents are often only partially effective in achieving this control; moreover, their use can be associated with significant side effects. AV node ablation, together with dual-chamber cardiac pacing, has been a useful and cost-effective technique in the management of drug-refractory supraventricular tachyarrhythmias.

Table 14–5. Common Indications for Permanent Cardiac Pacing

Sinus node dysfunction
With symptoms (including symptoms resulting from necessary medications)
Chronotropic incompetence
Atrioventricular block
Acute myocardial infarction
With persistent second-degree type II, advanced second-degree or third-degree AV block
With transient advanced second- or third-degree AV block, and bundle branch block
Second-degree
Type I, with symptoms
Type II
Third-degree (complete) and advanced second-degree
With symptoms (including symptoms resulting from necessary medications)
With asystole ≥3 seconds, escape rate <40 bpm, or escape rhythm below the AV node, in awake patients
With AF and ventricular pauses ≥5 seconds, in awake patients (including when resulting from necessary medications)
After AV node ablation
Bundle Branch Block
With syncope, HV interval ≥ 70 ms or infranodal block during EPS
With alternating bundle branch block
Carotid sinus hypersensitivity
With recurrent syncope caused by spontaneous carotid sinus stimulation
With cardioinhibitory response (asystole ≥ 3 seconds) during carotid sinus massage
Neurocardiogenic syncope
With symptomatic bradycardia documented spontaneously or during tilt-table testing

AV, atrioventricular; EPS, electrophysiology study; HV, His ventricular. Based on ACC/AHA/HRS 2008 guidelines for device-based therapy of cardiac rhythm abnormalities by Epstein AE, et al. *Circulation.* 2008;117:e350–e408, and 2018 ACC/AHA/HRS guideline on the evaluation and management of patients with bradycardia and cardiac conduction delay by Kusumoto FM, et al. *Circulation,* 2019;140: e282–e482.

A. Cardiac Pacing

Temporary or permanent cardiac pacing, in which an electrical stimulus depolarizes cardiac tissue, is indicated when bradycardia causes symptoms of cerebral hypoperfusion or hemodynamic decompensation (Tables 14–5 and 14–6). Occasionally, patients with bradycardia-dependent ventricular tachycardia require pacing to prevent the pauses in rhythm that lead to the tachyarrhythmia (Figure 14–7). Although emergency pacing can be accomplished temporarily by transcutaneous pacing systems, in all but the most critical situations, stable temporary pacing is best ensured by the transvenous insertion of electrodes into the right atrium, right ventricle, or both.

Permanent cardiac pacing is also usually performed by placement of leads through the transvenous route; in some circumstances, epicardial placement of electrodes via thoracotomy or a subxiphoid approach is still used

Table 14–6. Common Uses for Temporary Cardiac Pacing

Therapeutic
To provide adequate heart rate in patients with symptomatic sinus node dysfunction, advanced second- and third-degree AV block while awaiting resolution of reversible cause or awaiting permanent pacing
To terminate supraventricular and ventricular tachycardias by overdrive suppression or entrainment (eg, atrial flutter, monomorphic ventricular tachycardia)
Prophylactic
To prevent advanced second- and third-degree AV block in patients with acute myocardial infarction, after cardiac surgery (eg, aortic valve replacement), or after valve intervention (eg, TAVR)
To prevent bradycardia-dependent ventricular tachycardia (eg, torsade de pointes ventricular tachycardia)
Diagnostic
To determine the site of AV block (Wenckebach response during atrial pacing supports block at the AV node)
To determine the optimal type of permanent pacing system (AV block during atrial pacing supports use of dual-chamber device)

AV, atrioventricular; TAVR, transcatheter aortic valve replacement.

when necessary. Leadless pacemakers are miniaturized self-contained pulse generator and electrode systems that are directly implanted within the heart using a transcatheter approach from a femoral vein. While currently available systems are limited to right ventricular implants, the ability to sense mechanical atrial activity has enabled AV synchrony, and atrial devices in development today that communicate wirelessly with ventricular devices are expected to expand pacing indications in the near future.

Transcatheter aortic valve replacement (TAVR) has become an important alternative to aortic valve surgery for patients with aortic stenosis, and indications are expanding to include lower-risk patients. While periprocedural complications and death following TAVR have steadily decreased, the occurrence of conduction disturbances (high-degree and complete AV block, new-onset left bundle branch block [LBBB]) has not improved over time and is the most common complication of the procedure; post-TAVR patients represent an increasingly important group that requires conduction disorder management. The AV node, His bundle, and left bundle branch travel just below the aortic annulus and are susceptible to direct mechanical injury during TAVR prosthesis deployment. As such, the highest preprocedural features that predict the development of AV block requiring pacemaker implantation is preexisting right bundle branch block (RBBB) or first-degree AV block. High-degree or complete AV block that occur during the procedure but do not resolve by the end of the procedure, rarely improves with monitoring and usually requires permanent pacemaker implant. Temporary pacing is currently recommended for 24–48 hours in patients with preexisting RBBB, new-onset LBBB, or transient procedural AV block; permanent pacemaker implant is indicated

Table 14–7. Conditions Considered Risks for Advanced Second-Degree or Complete Atrioventricular Block During Acute Myocardial Infarction[1]

Inferior-wall MI, especially if it involves the interventricular septum, posterior wall, and right ventricle, with first-degree AV block; second-degree AV block, type I (usually intra-AV nodal); or second-degree AV block, type II (often intra-His)
Extensive anteroseptal MI, with new bifascicular block with a normal PR interval or with first-degree AV block; second-degree AV block, type II; first-degree AV block with bifascicular block (not known to be old); or alternating bundle branch block

[1]The incidence of AV block during acute MI has decreased considerably in the current era of percutaneous revascularization therapies.
AV, atrioventricular; MI, myocardial infarction.

if high-degree or complete AV block are observed during continuous telemetry monitoring.

1. Temporary pacing

A. Transcutaneous pacing—This method, in which electrical current is delivered to the heart through the skin via surface electrode patches, is usually reserved for standby prophylaxis in patients recognized to be at high risk for bradycardia, for example, during inferior and large anterior wall acute myocardial infarctions (Table 14–7), and in some patients with suspected sinus node dysfunction who are undergoing elective cardioversion.

The transcutaneous pacing system uses two large, low-impedance surface electrodes typically placed on the anterior and posterior chest walls. A long-duration pacing stimulus output of 20–40 ms (not programmable) and current output of more than 100 milliamperes (mA) (programmable) are often necessary to overcome the impedance offered by the chest wall, muscle and bone, and intrathoracic structures. The transcutaneous pacemaker paces the ventricle and inhibits its output when it senses spontaneous ventricular electrical activity, thus functioning in VVI (demand) mode (see later section, Permanent Pacing). Because the pacing pulses are 20–40 ms in duration and the current output is large, they create a deflection of high amplitude on the surface ECG recording that should not be confused with QRS complexes. If ventricular depolarization (capture) is occurring, the pacer output pulse will be followed by a QRS complex that is best seen on the pacemaker generator's oscilloscope and strip-chart recording. Significant distortion, or total obscuration, of the paced QRS complex can exist on the bedside rhythm monitor or surface ECG recording. Ventricular capture should always be verified by confirming the presence of a pulse, either through palpation or through visualizing a proper waveform with pulse oximetry or arterial pressure monitoring. Skeletal muscle twitching occurs at a stimulus output of 30 mA, but ventricular capture does not usually occur until 35–80 mA; sedation of the awake patient is usually required to mitigate the painful muscle contractions.

Transcutaneous cardiac pacing can be effective in up to 70% of patients and has its best use in an emergency situation when pacing of short duration is required or as a bridge to permanent cardiac pacemaker implantation. The majority of pacing failures (specifically, failure to capture) occur in patients during the advanced stages of cardiopulmonary arrest. The likelihood of successful transcutaneous pacing in patients with cardiac arrest of more than 15 minutes in duration is approximately 33–45%. Failure to capture can also occur after prolonged (hours to days) pacing and likely represents increases in impedance; repositioning of the electrodes can restore pacing capability.

B. Temporary transvenous pacing—Although transcutaneous pacing offers ease of use, rapid initiation of pacing therapy, and very low complication rates, transvenous pacing is far more stable and better tolerated if pacing is needed for longer than 20–30 minutes. Transvenous pacing is usually performed by positioning an electrode catheter in the right ventricle. In rare cases where temporary atrial pacing is also required, catheters can be positioned in the right atrium or in the proximal portion of the coronary sinus.

Venous access can be obtained by several approaches. The internal jugular, subclavian, and femoral veins are all potential sites for introduction of the pacing catheter into the right heart, although the femoral vein is the least desirable due to the potential for pacing lead dislodgement and infection. The median cubital and basilic veins can also be used, but these sites are also associated with a high incidence of lead dislodgement (because of arm motion) and are rarely, if ever, used today.

Prior to obtaining venous access, the existence of a bleeding diathesis or coagulopathy should be excluded or corrected if possible. If this is not possible, the femoral vein should be considered as the initial access site because it is easier to apply pressure and achieve hemostasis in this region if a complication occurs. Other factors, such as the patient's pulmonary status, location of dialysis shunts, previous neck surgery, or radiation therapy should be taken into account when considering the appropriate site for venous access. The presence of a prosthetic tricuspid valve can be a contraindication to right ventricular pacing because of the potential for disrupting valve function; in this circumstance, left ventricular pacing can be performed by positioning the pacing catheter in the left ventricular veins via the coronary sinus.

There are two main types of transvenous pacing catheters. The flexible balloon-tipped catheter is advanced into the heart in a similar way as a Swan-Ganz catheter, using blood flow to guide it into the right ventricle; it is important to note that during a cardiac arrest, the inflation of the balloon will be useless because of the lack of circulation. The position of the catheter tip within the heart is confirmed either through assessing the electrogram recorded from the pacing catheter tip (negative pole connected to any precordial lead on an ECG machine) or by observing capture of ventricular tissue. Once the catheter tip crosses the tricuspid valve, the balloon should be deflated to allow advancement into the ideal right ventricular apical position. Balloon-tipped pacing catheters can be inserted at the bedside if necessary. The non-floating, rigid, fixed-curve catheters are easier to manipulate and are more stable once positioned in the right ventricle; because of their rigid design, they are typically placed only under fluoroscopic guidance. In general, temporary transvenous pacing lead positioning should be accomplished using fluoroscopy.

Ventricular capture thresholds should be less than 2 mA (or < 2 volts [V] with some pulse generators) and ideally less than 1 mA (or <1 V) in stable lead positions and should not change with coughing or deep breathing. Atrial leads are typically less stable, and capture thresholds around 2 mA (or 1–2 V) are acceptable. The presence of myocardial infarction, ischemia, antiarrhythmic drug therapy, hyperkalemia, and other metabolic derangements can increase capture thresholds. Current or voltage output of the pulse generator should be programmed to at least twice capture threshold.

Sensing thresholds of the intracardiac electrical signal can also be affected by myocardial ischemia or infarction, hyperkalemia, and class I antiarrhythmic agents, leading to undersensing. Ectopic ventricular depolarizations are often undersensed because of poor intracardiac signal quality. These considerations need to be borne in mind when programming the sensitivity of the pacemaker; inappropriate pacing occurring due to an undersensed QRS complex can initiate ventricular tachyarrhythmias if the pacing stimulus falls on the middle to terminal portion of the T wave.

A daily chest radiograph and paced 12-lead ECG should be obtained and compared with prior studies to check for possible lead migration. Pacing and sensing thresholds should be checked at least daily, with any significant changes being investigated for possible lead migration, lead disconnection from the pulse generator, or change in the patient's clinical status. Pulse generator battery status should be monitored by the appropriate biomedical personnel, and batteries replaced as needed. Temporary leads and access sites should be changed at least every 3 or 4 days to decrease the risk of infection and venous thrombosis.

Although temporary transvenous pacing is relatively low risk, there are potentially serious complications. Complication rates range from 4% to 20% and include pneumothorax, hemothorax, arterial puncture, air embolism, serious bleeding, myocardial perforation, cardiac tamponade, nerve injury, thoracic duct injury, catheter-related arrhythmias, infection, and thromboembolism. The risk of complications is increased if pacing is initiated in emergent situations. To minimize risk, transvenous pacing should be accomplished when the patient is relatively hemodynamically stable. It is important to remember that if the patient has a preexisting LBBB, pacing catheter manipulation in the area of the right bundle branch can result in complete AV block; in these circumstances, transcutaneous pacing should be in place should rate support be required. To minimize, or avoid altogether, the risks associated with temporary pacing, permanent pacing should be accomplished as rapidly as possible in appropriate clinical circumstances.

2. Permanent pacing— Because of the complexity of pacing system design, an identification code has been developed that describes the function of currently available pacemaker generators. The "mode" code consists of three primary letters. The first letter stands for the chamber in which stimulus delivery is occurring: A for atrium, V for ventricle, and D for dual, or both. The second letter stands for the chamber in which sensing of the electrical signal occurs: A, V, D, or O for neither. The third letter refers to the type of response of the pulse generator to the sensed signal: I for inhibited output, D for both inhibited output within each chamber but triggered ventricular stimulus output in response to a sensed atrial signal (eg, a pacing stimulus delivered in response to a sensed P wave), and O for no response. Currently available pacing systems all have R as a potential fourth letter of the code, indicating incorporation of one or two sensors that when programmed "on" allow the pacing rate to increase and decrease with changes in metabolic need; sensor-based pacing systems thus adapt the pacing rate to the activities of daily living. Current pacemakers have numerous functions that can be altered noninvasively by a programmer (Table 14–8).

Table 14–8. Some Programmable Functions and Parameters of Cardiac Pacemakers

Lower rate limit, base rate: The rate at which the patient is paced unless the spontaneous rhythm is faster
Upper rate limit: The highest rate at which the ventricles are paced 1:1 in response to the atrial rate (atrial-based or sensor-based)
AV interval: The interval between the sensed or paced P wave and the delivery of the ventricular pacing stimulus
Atrial refractory period: The time after a sensed P wave or delivered atrial output during which the atrial channel is refractory to electrical signals; the refractory period that follows a paced QRS complex is referred to as the PVARP
Ventricular refractory period: The time after a sensed QRS or delivered ventricular output during which the ventricular channel is refractory to electrical signals
Sensitivity (atrial and ventricular channels): The amplitude of the intrinsic atrial and ventricular electrical signals that are to be sensed
Energy output (atrial and ventricular channels): Volts, current and pulse duration
Modes of function[1]: AAI, VVI, VDD, DDI, DDD, AOO, VOO, DOO
Sensor ("on" or "off"): Rate-adaptive programming either activated or deactivated (denoted by addition of R to the mode)
Sensor-based parameters: Time to achieve peak pacing rate; time to decline to standby rate; criteria for sensor activation
Mode switch ("on" or "off"): Upon sensing an atrial tachyarrhythmia, a DDD(R)[1] device will automatically switch to DDI(R)[1] or VVI(R)[1] mode of function, and will automatically switch back to DDD(R) mode upon sensing normal atrial rhythm

[1]Pacemaker codes: A, atrium; D, dual; I, inhibited; O, nonapplicable; R, rate-adaptive function; V, ventricle.
AV, atrioventricular; PVARP, postventricular atrial refractory period.

A. Modes of pacing

(1) Asynchronous pacing (VOO, AOO, DOO)—In the asynchronous mode of pacemaker function, no electrical signals are sensed, and the pulse generator delivers output pulses (nonprogrammable) without regard to any electrical activity occurring spontaneously within (or from outside) the heart (Figure 14–14). Because the native cardiac rhythm is not sensed, competitive rhythms (paced and native depolarizations) can result. Asynchronous pulse generators are no longer manufactured; however, the asynchronous pacing mode can be programmed. Asynchronous pacing also occurs whenever a magnet is placed over an implanted pulse generator to evaluate capture function. With a magnet in place, asynchronous pacing occurs at a manufacturer-specific rate; concomitant occurrence of the spontaneous rhythm result in iatrogenic parasystole (Figure 14–15). At the energy output of today's pulse generators (1.5–7.5 V), induction of repetitive ventricular or atrial rhythms is usually not observed, although this possibility exists, especially if myocardial ischemia or electrolyte imbalance is present. It is important to recognize that with implantable cardioverter-defibrillators, placement of a magnet over the pulse generator will suspend tachyarrhythmia therapies (eg, shocks) but will not affect pacing system function.

(2) Single-chamber demand pacing (VVI[R], AAI[R])—Both sensing and pacing circuits are present in these units. When a spontaneous intracardiac signal is sensed, VVI and AAI pulse generators will inhibit their output and no pacemaker stimulus artifact will appear. Electrical signals sensed by demand pacemaker pulse generators can originate not only from the heart but also from the environment (eg, electrocautery, some cell phones, electronic article surveillance systems, tasers), from the patient (muscle potentials), or from the pacing system itself (lead fracture or insulation breaks). Such sensed signals may cause inhibition of output, leading to pauses in paced rhythm; this phenomenon is termed *oversensing* (Tables 14–9 and 14–10), a problem that can generally be corrected by noninvasive programming or, in the case of lead fracture or insulation break, by replacement of the lead. Current pulse generator design and programming capability have not only helped to reduce problems of oversensing but have also simplified their correction.

The capture function of a demand pulse generator cannot be evaluated if the patient's spontaneous rhythm exceeds the programmed standby (base) rate of the generator. Applying a magnet over the pulse generator converts it to an asynchronous mode of function, and capture (stimulation) of the atria or ventricles by the pacemaker can be confirmed, provided that the pacing stimuli fall outside the refractory period of the cardiac tissue. Conversely, if the patient's rhythm is continually paced, the sensing function of the pulse generator cannot be evaluated. Programming the device to a lower rate may allow the emergence of a spontaneous cardiac rhythm, which should then be sensed, resulting in inhibition of pacemaker output.

Continuous single-chamber ventricular pacing will result in AV dyssynchrony (unless the atrial rhythm is fibrillation). Although the symptoms attributable to bradycardia are alleviated through ventricular rate support from the pacemaker, these may be replaced by symptoms due to AV dyssynchrony, or "pacemaker syndrome." Either single-chamber atrial pacing (with intact AV conduction) or dual-chamber pacing is a solution to avoid pacemaker syndrome.

(3) Single-lead P-synchronous pacing (VDD)—These are systems in which electrodes for both the atrium and the ventricle are located on a single lead. The lead is positioned in the right ventricle where the tip electrodes sense and pace the ventricle; atrial electrodes are located on the lead body, at the level of the atrium and are currently only capable of sensing. When the atrial electrode senses an electrical signal, a ventricular pacing stimulus is delivered after a programmable AV delay that corresponds to the PR interval. If a spontaneous QRS complex occurs, the ventricular output is inhibited. Tracking of the atrial rhythm in a 1:1 relationship allows the ventricular paced rate to change with the sinus rate. The programmed upper rate is the maximum ventricular paced rate that can occur in a 1:1 relationship to atrial activity and prevents rapid ventricular paced rates should the atrial rate become too fast. If the atrial rate exceeds the programmed upper rate limit, the paced ventricular rate can become irregular because of an electronic Wenckebach protection, can slow to one-half the programmed upper rate limit, or can fall back gradually until 1:1 tracking can resume. This last feature results in disengagement of the tracking function, which causes transient AV dyssynchrony (Figure 14–16).

If no atrial activity is sensed, as occurs in sinus bradycardia, most current VDD systems pace the ventricles on demand at the programmed base rate; atrial pacing does not occur. Thus, at slow atrial rates, the pacing system behaves as though it was a VVI system, and AV synchrony is lost (Figure 14–14). Although this pacing system seems ideal for patients with normal sinus rhythm and AV block, atrial bradycardia, which occurs commonly over ensuing years,

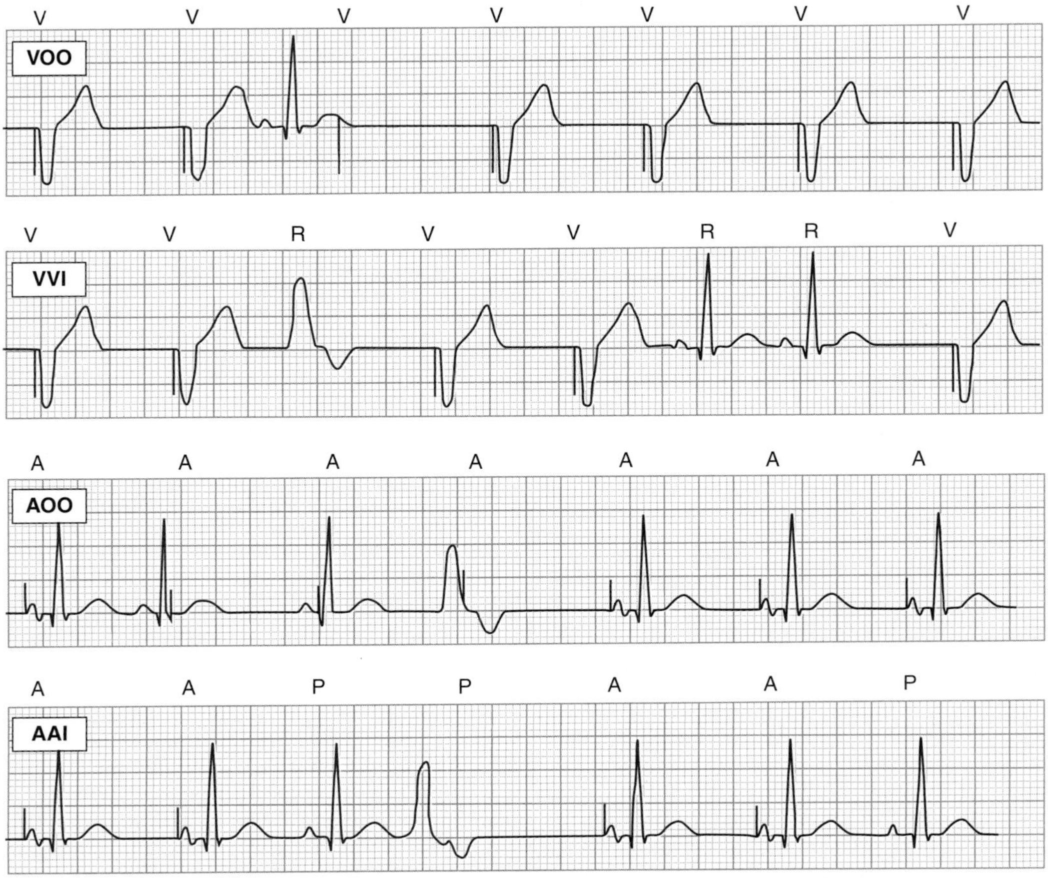

▲ **Figure 14–14.** Schematic illustrations of various pacing modes (see Permanent Pacing section for explanation of mode designations). A, atrial pacing stimulus; P, spontaneous P wave; R, spontaneous QRS; V, ventricular pacing stimulus.

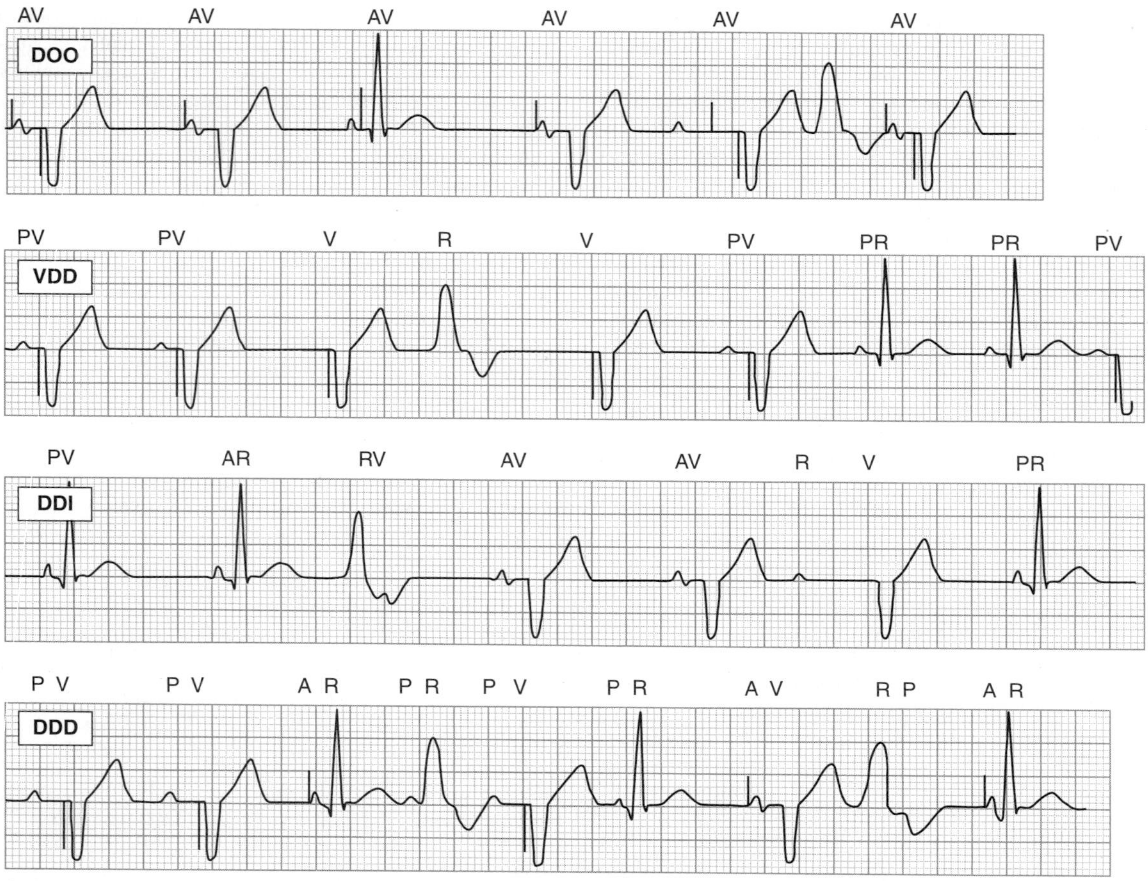

▲ **Figure 14–14.** *(Continued)*

either spontaneously or as a result of medications, makes VDD devices ultimately suboptimal for most patients, and they are rarely used today.

(4) Dual-chamber pacing (DDD[R])—These pacing systems are capable of sensing and pacing in both the atrium and the ventricle on demand (Figure 14–14). Therefore, they approach the physiology of normal AV conduction. The ability to sense retrograde atrial depolarizations can lead to ventricular stimulus delivery and ventricular pacing in response; if the paced ventricular depolarization travels retrograde to the atrium to depolarize it, the process can become repetitive. This event creates an artificial extra-AV-nodal bypass tract, causing a "pacemaker-mediated tachycardia." Specific algorithms have been designed to terminate these tachycardias and are automatic once they have been programmed "on."

Dual-chamber devices depend on a stable atrial rhythm for optimum function. Because of their potential for rapid paced ventricular rates, these systems should not be used with atrial arrhythmias such as permanent fibrillation or flutter, multifocal tachycardia, or refractory automatic tachycardia; unless catheter ablation can effectively treat the atrial arrhythmia (especially atrial flutter), single-chamber VVI(R) devices should be used instead.

If the atrial tachyarrhythmias are paroxysmal, however, a "mode switch" feature should be programmed "on" that automatically changes the mode from DDD(R) to either DDI(R) or VVI(R) modes when a rapid atrial rate is detected; this removes the ability to track the atrial rate as long as the atrial tachyarrhythmia persists (Figure 14–17). Some studies have shown that in patients with bradycardia, compared with ventricular pacing, atrial-based pacing reduces the incidence of atrial fibrillation.

Right ventricular pacing has been recognized as a cause of dyssynchrony-mediated cardiomyopathy. This process is similar to what has been observed in patients with spontaneous LBBB, where abnormal electrical activation can initiate electrical remodeling that then leads to myocardial remodeling. Dyssynchrony-mediated cardiomyopathy can

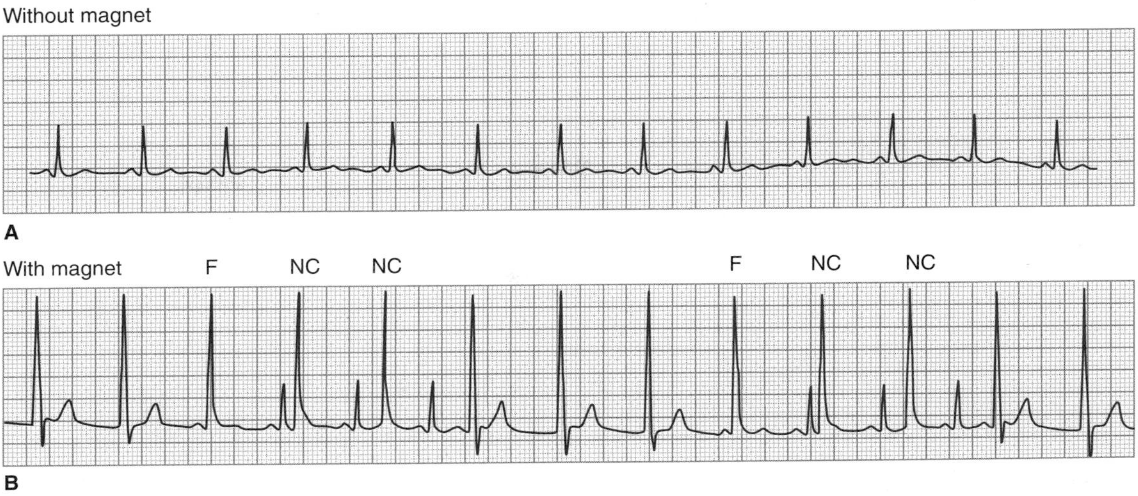

▲ **Figure 14–15.** VVI pacing system. **A:** Normal sinus rhythm is present. Sensing function is presumed to be normal because no ventricular pacing artifacts are occurring. **B:** With a magnet in place over the pulse generator, ventricular pacing stimuli are emitted asynchronously, resulting in a rhythm that competes with the sinus rhythm. The large magnitude of the pacing artifacts indicates that the lead configuration is unipolar. The large unipolar stimulus obscures the resulting QRS complex; however, because T waves are present following some of these pacing stimuli, capture is confirmed. Both sensing and pacing functions are normal. F, true fusion complexes, with ventricular depolarization resulting from both sinus and paced impulses. NC, noncapture because of pacing stimuli falling in the refractory period of ventricular muscle; this has been referred to as "functional" noncapture.

Table 14–9. Pacing System Malfunctions and Clues to Their Recognition

Undersensing
Single-chamber systems
ECG will show earlier-than-expected appearance of pacing-stimulus artifact
Dual-chamber systems
Atrial undersensing: Delivery of atrial pacing stimuli despite occurrence of spontaneous P waves; failure to track intrinsic atrial activity at the programmed AV interval
Ventricular undersensing: Delivery of ventricular pacing stimuli despite occurrence of spontaneous QRS complexes
Oversensing
ECG will show inappropriate inhibition of atrial or ventricular output stimuli; oversensing in the atrial channel results in earlier-than-expected ventricular pacing stimuli ("triggering," "tracking")
Noncapture
Pacing stimuli not followed by atrial or ventricular depolarization (assuming muscle tissue is not refractory)
Failure of output
Absence of pacing stimulus outputs, with oversensing excluded

AV, atrioventricular; ECG, electrocardiogram.

Table 14–10. Potential Causes of Pacemaker Oversensing

Electromagnetic interference
Power transformers, power lines; welding equipment; running motors and alternators; chainsaws; household appliances such as electric shavers and hair dryers (unusual with today's pulse generators); cell phones (some newer models); headphones and earbuds (if draped around neck); electric fences; metal-detector gates (older generation designs); electronic article surveillance systems; tasers; magnetic therapy products; transcutaneous nerve stimulators; therapeutic radiation; MRI; radiofrequency catheter ablation; cardioverting and defibrillating devices (external or implanted); electrocautery; electrocoagulation; diathermy; lithotripsy
Physiologic intracardiac signals
R-wave sensing (AAI[1] systems), T-wave sensing (VVI[1] systems), P-wave sensing (VVI systems) (unusual)
Physiologic extracardiac signals
Muscle potentials (myopotentials) (eg, diaphragm, pectoral)
Signals generated within the pacing system
Conductor-wire fracture causing a voltage transient
Lead insulation defect
Pulse generator component malfunction
Afterpotential sensing of late portions of the pacing stimulus itself (unusual)
Inappropriate programmed settings

[1]Pacemaker codes: A, atrium; I, inhibited; V, ventricle.
MRI, magnetic resonance imaging.

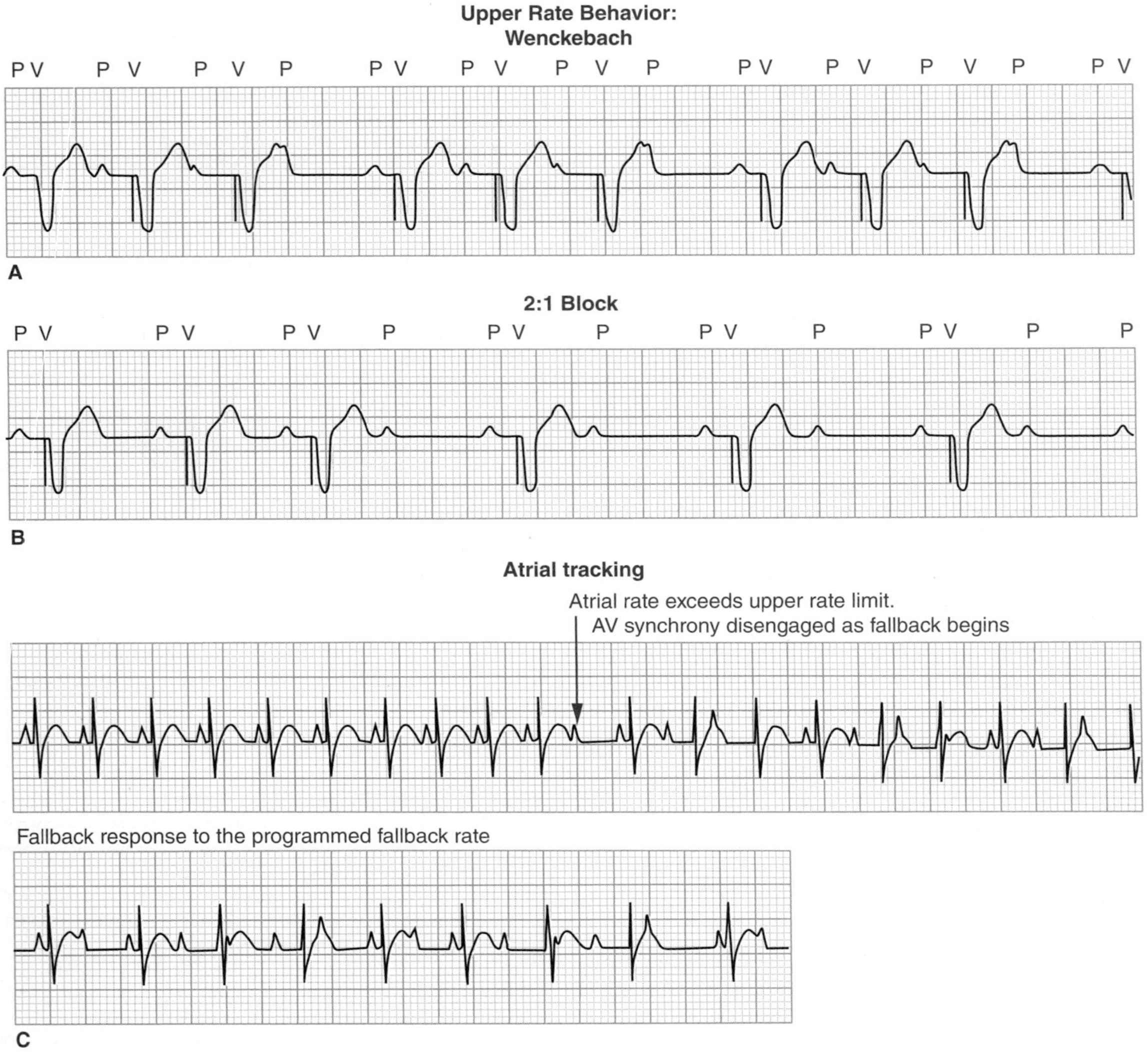

▲ **Figure 14–16.** Schematic illustration of responses from pulse generators at the atrial-driven programmed upper rate limit. The pacemaker will not allow the ventricular paced rate to exceed this upper rate (or "maximum tracking rate"). Atrial rhythms that can exceed the upper rate limit include sinus tachycardia, atrial tachycardia, atrial flutter and atrial fibrillation. The pacemaker-mediated tachycardia (see text) will also not exceed the programmed upper rate. **A:** Lengthening of the interval between the sensed P wave and the triggered ventricular-paced complex so as not to violate the upper rate limit (Wenckebach): the P wave that is not followed by a paced QRS complex falls in the refractory period of the atrial channel and is not sensed, resulting in absence (nondelivery) of the ventricular stimulus output. **B:** In 2:1 block, alternate P waves fall in the programmed atrial refractory period and are not sensed: they are not followed by a paced ventricular event. **C:** In "fallback," the ventricular paced rate gradually slows once the programmed upper rate has been achieved. During the fallback period, tracking of the atrial rate is disengaged, and atrioventricular synchrony is no longer present. The ventricular paced rate will again track the atrial rate once the latter falls below the programmed upper rate. The fallback response avoids abrupt decreases in paced ventricular rate. Pacemakers that function in a rate-adaptive mode can have their sensor-based upper rate limit exceed the previously described atrial-based upper tracking limit.

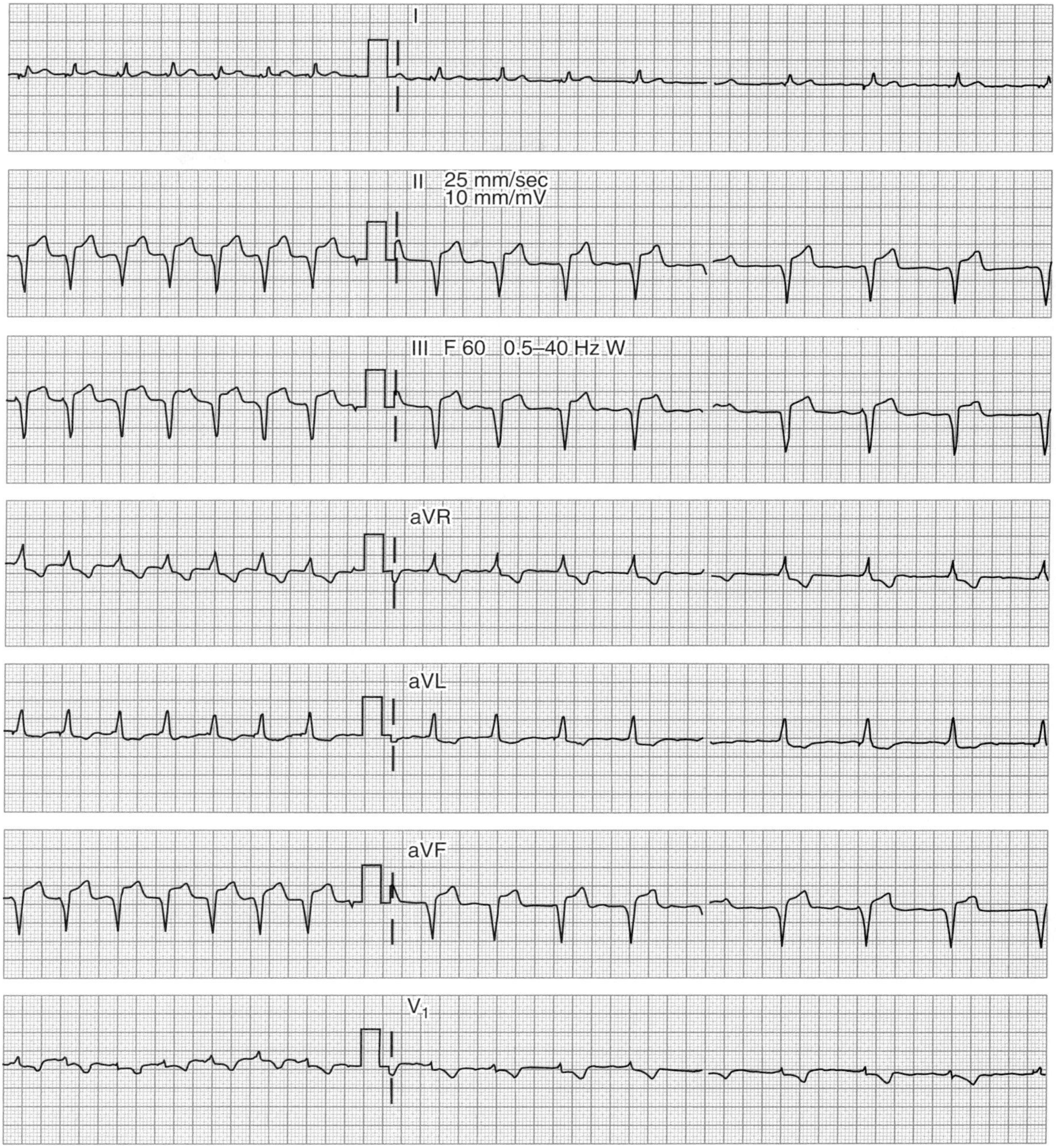

▲ **Figure 14–17.** Depiction of mode-switch operation of a dual-chamber pacemaker. In the initial portion of the rhythm strip, tracking of atrial fibrillation is occurring, resulting in a rapid paced ventricular rate. When the algorithm in the pacemaker recognizes the atrial tachyarrhythmia, automatic change of mode of function to VVIR takes place, terminating the rapid paced ventricular rate. On sensing restoration of a normal atrial rhythm, the device will automatically restore its dual-chamber mode of operation.

be reversed with cardiac resynchronization therapy (CRT) through biventricular pacing. In patients with preexisting cardiomyopathy, biventricular pacing can be considered at the time of pacemaker implant if ventricular pacing is deemed unavoidable. His bundle pacing is an alternative approach to right ventricular or biventricular pacing where the ventricular lead is affixed to the proximal intraventricular septum and the His bundle is directly activated; ventricular electrical activation then occurs in a more physiologic pattern via the His-Purkinje system. Ongoing clinical trial are evaluating the potential clinical benefit of His bundle pacing over right ventricular or biventricular pacing in both preventing and reversing dyssynchrony-mediated cardiomyopathy.

In patients who do not need continuous ventricular pacing, various parameters can be programmed to minimize unnecessary ventricular pacing. The AV delay can be programmed in most current pacemakers to automatically extend, allowing native AV conduction to occur as much as possible. There are also manufacturer-specific modes that maintain AAI(R) mode until AV block is detected, at which time they automatically switch to DDD(R) mode; AAI(R) mode is restored when the pacemaker detects resumption of native AV conduction.

The type of pacing system implanted is indicated on an identification card supplied to the patient by the manufacturer. It is important to note, however, that such information does not guarantee the operation of a particular mode of function, rate, or any parameter that can be programmed by the patient's pacemaker physician. As pulse-generator design and function increase in complexity, it is best to assume that the pacemaker is performing normally until proved otherwise (there are, of course, malfunctions and "pseudo" malfunctions; these are addressed in the following sections). Similarly, ECGs in paced patients should be considered to reflect normal device function unless they are interpreted otherwise by personnel experienced in pacemaker ECG.

Rate-adaptive pacing systems are appropriate for patients with permanent atrial arrhythmias with slow ventricular response and for patients whose sinus node dysfunction prevents rate acceleration, but who would benefit from an increase in paced ventricular or atrial rates, respectively, in response to increases in metabolic demand. Current sensors measure body motion and acceleration, minute ventilation, QT interval, or intracardiac impedance. Leadless pacemakers also have rate-adaptive capability utilizing a multiaxis accelerometer that detects activity in the presence of cardiac motion. Changes within the sensor's established parameters, designed to reflect physiologic needs, result in changes in paced rates. Sensor-based pacing rate depends on the individual sensor used, however; for example, if an activity sensor is being used, the paced rate can increase in response to body vibrations that are unrelated to actual physical activity, such as shivering or tremor. This can cause problems in hospitalized patients, especially those in intensive care units. Several manufacturers, therefore, currently incorporate two sensors into their pacemakers to confirm the need for appropriate changes in pacing rate. For example, the activity sensor input can be confirmed by a more physiologic sensor such as minute ventilation, resulting in a more specific and accurate response to the change in pacing rate for the change in metabolic need. Recognition of sensor-based pacing and changing pacing rates is necessary to avoid erroneous diagnoses of pacemaker malfunction.

B. Unipolar and bipolar pacing—Unipolar pacing systems have the cathode (stimulating electrode) in the heart and the anode at the pulse generator. The distance between the cathode and anode in these systems results in the inscription of large pacing artifacts whose direction (pacing-artifact axis) in the frontal plane points toward the anode in older analog ECG recorders, but not in contemporary digital recorders in which stimulus artifact amplitudes and axes vary due to digital sampling of the pacing stimulus.

Bipolar pacing systems have both lead electrodes within the heart, usually less than 1 cm apart, in either or both atrium and ventricle. Either the distal (tip) electrode or the proximal (ring) electrode of the lead can serve as the cathode. Because of the small interelectrode distance, the pacing artifacts are small and their direction in the frontal plane reflects the direction of current flow (Figure 14–18). It is common for the small pacing artifacts to be difficult to discern on ECGs and ECG monitoring strips; even computer-interpreted ECGs may fail to indicate that a pacemaker is present. Identification of paced (as opposed to spontaneous) P waves and QRS complexes must therefore be intentionally undertaken; often, magnet application with comparison of paced P and QRS morphologies with the initially recorded complexes is necessary to accomplish this.

In sum, ECGs recorded on digital rather than analog machines can show marked variations in both amplitude and polarity of pacing artifacts. Because the digital equipment samples the pacing stimuli at specific time intervals and then recreates them on paper, the inscribed stimulus artifacts are not seen in real time. In some ECG leads, the pacing stimuli may not be visible at all, raising the questions of spontaneous wide QRS complex rhythms or even failure of pulse generator output. It is important to recognize this recording artifact in patients with pacemakers to avoid an erroneous diagnosis of pacemaker malfunction. It is equally important to document the morphology of paced complexes so that when the pacing stimuli cannot be seen, normal pacemaker function can be assumed until an accurate evaluation can be made.

Some permanent bipolar pacing systems offer lead polarity that can be programmed to unipolar; therefore, the presence of a bipolar lead on chest radiograph does not ensure bipolar lead function, and the ECG appearance of the pacing artifacts may differ from what is expected. That being said, most pacing systems today use bipolar leads and are

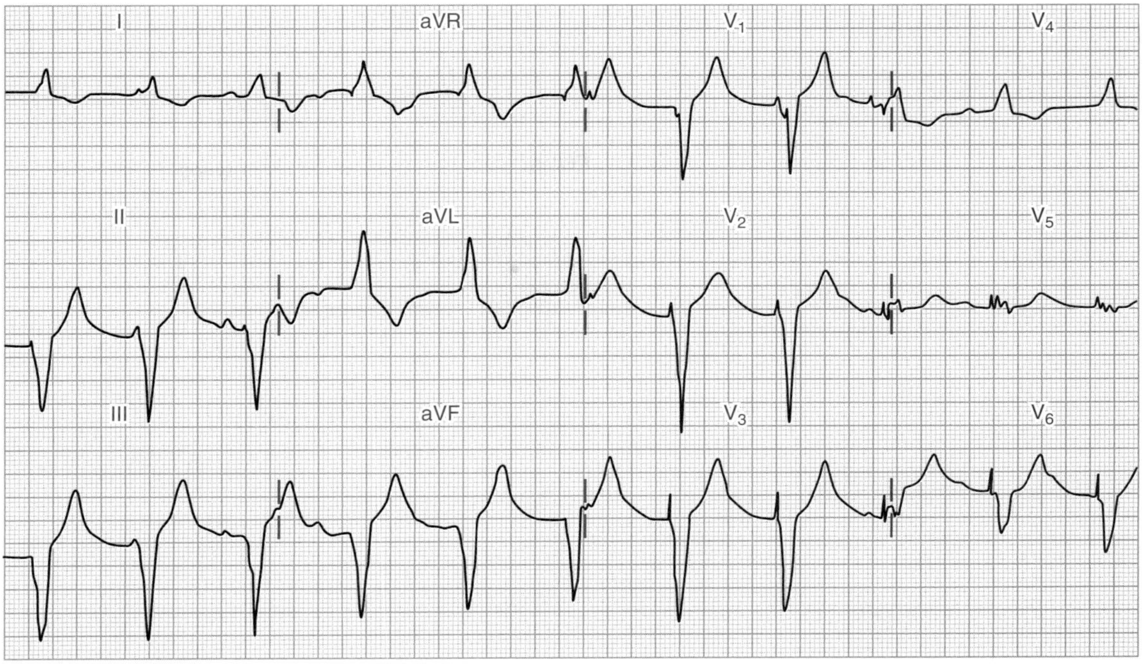

RHYTHM STRIP: II
25 mm/sec; 1 cm/mV

▲ **Figure 14–18.** Bipolar VVI pacing system. All QRS complexes are paced. Note the small magnitude of the pacing artifacts. The simultaneous recordings indicate that in some leads the pacing stimuli are virtually invisible.

programmed to function as bipolar leads unless there has been a revision undertaken for a specific reason.

C. Electrocardiographic patterns of paced complexes—These patterns depend on how the myocardium is depolarized. Paced atrial complexes reflect the sequence of atrial activation initiated by the pacing impulse and thus, in part, the site of the pacing electrode(s). Because the atrial electrodes can be located in the atrial appendage or affixed to any portion of atrial tissue, paced P-wave morphologies and axes will vary.

Pacing from the right ventricular apex produces paced QRS complexes that have a LBBB configuration (reflecting right ventricular myocardial depolarization occurring before left ventricular depolarization) and a superior mean frontal plane axis (the apex of the heart is depolarized before the base; Figure 14–19). Paced QRS complexes usually have a duration of 120–180 ms; if they are substantially longer, intrinsic myocardial disease, hyperkalemia, or antiarrhythmic drug therapy (eg, flecainide, amiodarone) should be suspected.

Pacing from the right ventricular outflow tract also results in QRS complexes that have a LBBB pattern, but the mean frontal plane axis is inferiorly directed (the base of the heart is depolarized before the apex). Occasionally, pacing from the interventricular septum can result in paced QRS complexes that show an indeterminate conduction delay pattern; they can even be narrow and relatively normal-appearing. This reflects almost simultaneous activation of both the right and left sides of the interventricular septum. Pacing from the His-bundle region can result in either normal-appearing narrow QRS complexes that reflect selective capture of the His bundle, or fusion complexes that are a combination of His bundle and right ventricular septal pacing.

Pacing from the left ventricular epicardium from electrodes positioned via the coronary sinus or placed directly at the time of cardiac surgery, produces paced QRS complexes having a RBBB pattern, reflecting left ventricular myocardial activation in advance of right ventricular activation. The mean frontal-plane QRS axis will depend on the location of the epicardial electrodes relative to each other (bipolar system) or to the pulse generator serving as anode (unipolar system).

Biventricular pacing can be recognized by tightly coupled double-pacing artifacts (Figure 14–20); biventricular pacing devices, however, can be programmed to deliver pacing in the left ventricle only, usually timed to coincide with native right ventricular activation, and the lack of double-pacing artifact does not exclude CRT. The resulting paced QRS complexes typically have a RBBB-like pattern since left

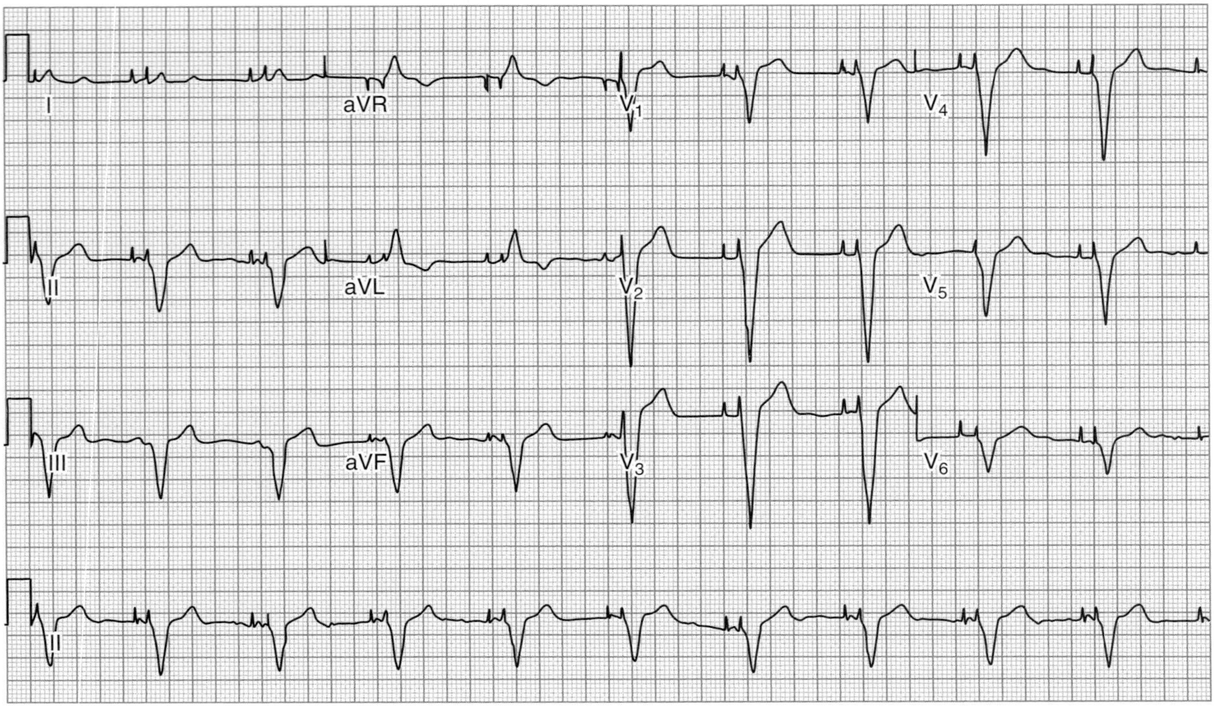

▲ **Figure 14–19.** Atrioventricular pacing at AV interval of 120 ms, with ventricular pacing from the area of the right ventricular apex, yielding superiorly directed paced QRS complexes with a left bundle branch block pattern. The paced P-wave morphology and axis are similarly determined by the location of the pacing lead tip.

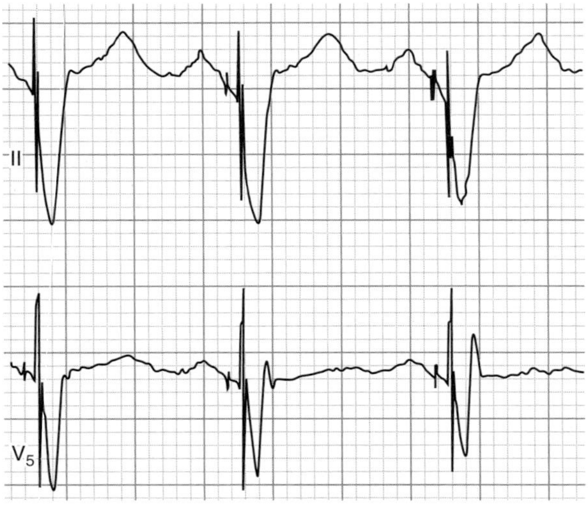

▲ **Figure 14–20.** Leads II and V5 in patient with a biventricular pacing system, programmed with a VV timing set to LV first by 60 ms. Two distinct ventricular stimulus output artifacts are seen tightly coupled at the onset of the paced QRS complex, following a sensed P wave.

ventricular pacing is usually programmed first, up to 80 ms earlier than right ventricular activation. The mean frontal plane axis will vary primarily with the location of the left ventricular electrode. Biventricular paced QRS complexes can be narrower than spontaneous QRS complexes, reflecting synchronized activation of left ventricular septum and free wall; electrical synchrony, however, does not necessarily correlate with mechanical synchrony, and a persistently wide biventricularly paced QRS complex does not predict failure of therapy. Because there are various programmable algorithms that trigger left ventricular or biventricular pacing when intrinsic ventricular activation is sensed, seemingly unusual responses to native conduction, rapidly conducted atrial fibrillation, and ventricular ectopy can be observed that require detailed knowledge of manufacturer-specific programming to properly decipher.

Spontaneous QRS complexes occurring in patients with pacemakers often show marked T-wave inversion (Figure 14–21). This phenomenon has been explained as "T-wave memory" or the persistence of abnormal repolarization "learned" by the myocardium during pacing. The ECG abnormality should not be interpreted as acute or chronic myocardial disease (including ischemia and infarction) in the absence of clinical correlations.

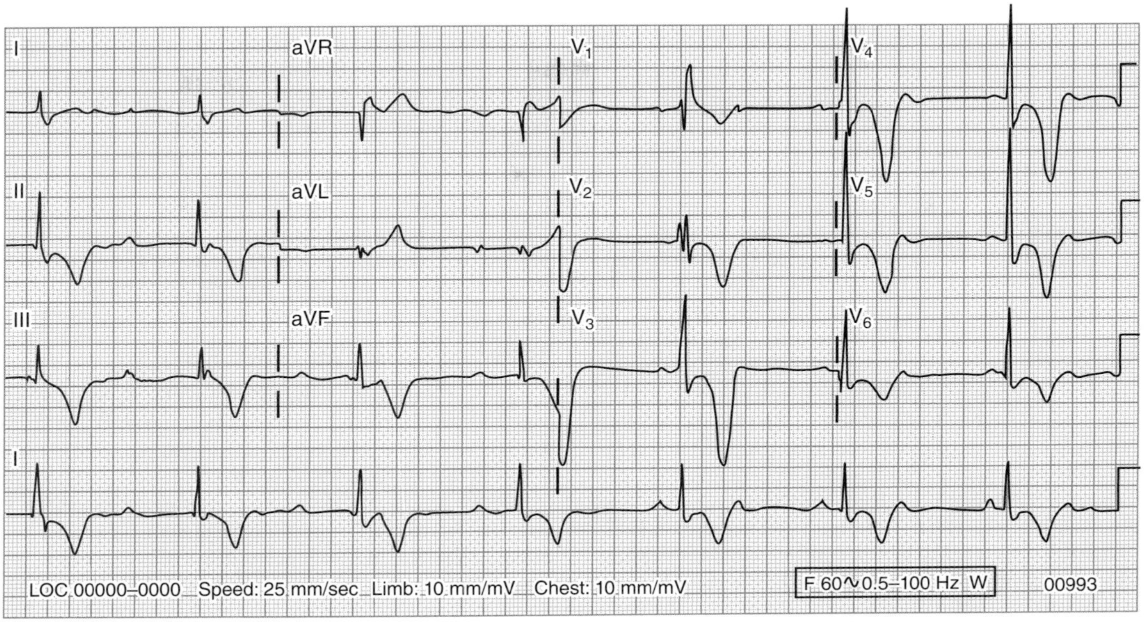

▲ **Figure 14–21.** Twelve-lead electrocardiogram in patient with a DDD pacing system, temporarily programmed to a rate of 30 bpm to permit emergence of the native rhythm. The intrinsic rhythm is sinus with complete atrioventricular block and right bundle branch block. Because no pacing artifacts are occurring, sensing function is normal in both atrium and ventricle. The deeply inverted T waves in the inferior and precordial leads represent a nonspecific abnormality (T-wave memory) commonly observed when pacing is suddenly suspended; they do not represent myocardial injury.

D. Pacemakers and Electromagnetic Interference—Electromagnetic interference (EMI) occurs when electrical or magnetic energy interferes with the normal function of a pacemaker. In general, EMI of pacemaker function is currently less of a problem than in previous years because of changes in the design of pacemakers, such as the use of titanium cases that are nonferromagnetic, the implementation of special filters or algorithms that distinguish EMI from intracardiac signals, and bipolar leads that have reduced the field of sensing to a few millimeters within the heart. Nonetheless, EMI can still occur, and understanding the potential effects of EMI on a pacemaker, as well as the potential sources of EMI, is important in the management of patients with pacemakers.

The most common effect of EMI is oversensing, or the sensing of unwanted electrical signal (Table 14–10). When oversensing occurs due to EMI, the environmental signal is sensed as intrinsic cardiac activity, and either inappropriate inhibition of pacing or unnecessary and unwanted triggered pacing occurs, depending on the pacemaker type and programmed mode of function. In patients who are pacemaker dependent (no intrinsic heart rate > 30 bpm or symptoms at lower-than-programmed rates), inhibition of pacing can result in dizziness, weakness, or syncope. With a dual-chamber pacemaker programmed in a synchronized mode such as DDD(R), patients can experience palpitations as triggered ventricular pacing occurs from electrical signals detected by the atrial lead. Rarely, EMI can also affect certain types of rate-adaptive algorithms, induce the device into reverting to a "reset mode" (a safety mode in some devices that paces at high output at a specific rate), or result in pulse generator damage.

In general, it is uncommon for EMI to cause serious harm, but it should be avoided in patients who are pacemaker dependent. Patients should be made aware of whether or not they are pacemaker dependent and of the potential causes of EMI. Sources of EMI in the typical surrounding environment are usually of low intensity, and EMI occurs only when the source is within inches of the pacemaker system. Although actual interference with cell phones is increasingly rare, certain phones that employ magnets have been found to cause interference and are advised to be kept at least 6 inches from the pacemaker generator. Interactions at airport screening are usually too transient to interfere with normal pacemaker function. Patients with pacemakers should know not to linger in the vicinity of any electronic surveillance equipment.

EMI can occur in a variety of medical settings (Table 14–10). The effect of unipolar electrocautery during surgery is the most common medical source of EMI. All patients with pacemakers undergoing surgery should have preoperative assessment of pacemaker dependency and pacemaker function, including the function and rate with magnet application. Reprogramming of the pacemaker to an asynchronous nonadaptive mode at rates higher than the patient's spontaneous rate can be recommended if the site of surgery is close enough to the pacing system. Other sources of EMI in the hospital include ionizing radiation (which can reset or damage the system), transcutaneous electrical nerve stimulation, radiofrequency ablation, external cardioversion or defibrillation, and lithotripsy, and therapy-specific precautions are necessary.

E. Pacemakers and magnetic resonance imaging—In past years, magnetic resonance imaging (MRI) has been contraindicated in patients with pacemakers. This is based on observed deleterious effects that strong magnetic fields can have on pacemakers, and on a handful of reported deaths not definitively associated with MRI scanning. Potential effects range from activation of rate-adaptive sensors causing rapid pacing rates, to reversion of pulse generators to default mode and settings. There is also the concern for electromagnetic current induction within leads that can give rise to heating at the lead tip-tissue interface and result in acute capture threshold increase; in a pacemaker-dependent patient, critical loss of capture could then ensue.

Pacemakers and leads that are approved by the U.S. Food and Drug Administration for use with MRI are now available from all major manufacturers, and should be used if there are underlying conditions that will likely require future MRI scans (eg, history of cancer, orthopedic problems, neurologic abnormalities). MRI compatibility is currently conditional only under specific pacing system and MRI scanning settings. When performing an MRI scan in a patient with an MRI-conditional pacing system, a specific protocol should be followed to ensure patient safety. Capture thresholds and lead impedances must be verified prior to scanning. The presence of a non-MRI-conditional lead, a lead adapter or extender, or any abandoned lead precludes the use of MRI scanning. After scanning, pacing system function must be reevaluated and reprogramed as necessary.

There are instances where the benefits of MRI scanning (eg, early detection of cancer, imaging of the brain) need to be weighed against the potential risks to the patient with a non-MRI-conditional pacemaker system. Protocols have been established by several institutions that allow for non–pacemaker-dependent patients to undergo MRI scanning under close observation after making temporary programming changes that will minimize interaction with the magnetic field. Pacemakers implanted in the last 15 years have advanced EMI protection, even if not MRI conditional, that decreases the likelihood of encountering a problem.

B. Pacing System Malfunctions

Pacing system malfunctions fall into four general categories: (1) undersensing (mistakenly referred to as "failure" to sense); (2) oversensing; (3) noncapture (mistakenly referred to as "failure" to capture); and (4) failure of output.

Undersensing of cardiac electrical signals because of poor intrinsic signal quality does not represent sensing failure as such, but rather the inability to detect the suboptimal signal itself; undersensed P waves and QRS complexes are not rare. Premature ventricular complexes (Table 14–9; Figure 14–22) generate suboptimal signals because they originate from within the myocardium, away from the normal conduction apparatus; they can occur in patients without structural heart disease, during acute myocardial ischemia and infarction, or as a result of drug toxicity and electrolyte imbalance (Table 14–11). Undersensed P waves can be due to changes in atrial volume, ectopic atrial rhythms, retrograde atrial depolarizations, or inappropriate programmed settings. Undersensing of spontaneous complexes and consequent failure to inhibit output results in the delivery of an earlier-than-expected pacing stimulus, which can, on occasion, induce repetitive rhythms.

Ventricular pacing artifacts can sometimes occur after the onset of spontaneous QRS complexes that have a RBBB

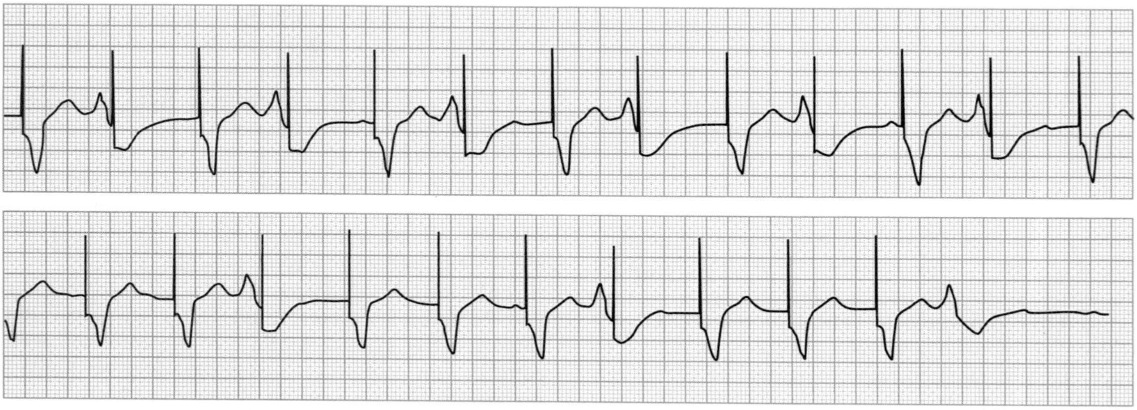

▲ **Figure 14–22.** Undersensing of spontaneous ventricular complexes in a patient with a VVI pacing system. Because the signal quality of depolarization originating in ventricular tissue is often poor, this is not uncommon. Repetitive ventricular beating induced by the stimulus-on-ST complex is, however, rare in stable patients.

Table 14–11. Potential Causes of Pacemaker Undersensing

Poor myocardial voltage signals
Change in conduction pattern (ectopy, new bundle branch block)
Electrolyte or metabolic abnormalities (hyperkalemia, acidosis)
Medications (flecainide, amiodarone)
Myocardial ischemia or infarction (scar)
Lead or pacing system problem
Poor lead positioning at the time of implant
Lead displacement
Lead tip-tissue fibrosis
Conductor-wire fracture causing non-transmission of signal
Lead insulation defect
Inappropriate programmed settings

configuration, raising concern of undersensing. This happens because of delay in conduction in the right bundle branch: the wavefront of ventricular depolarization does not reach the lead electrode in the right ventricle (especially the apex) in time to inhibit the output of the pacing stimulus. This phenomenon of stimulus delivery within a QRS complex, called "pseudofusion" (as opposed to true fusion), may also be observed in patients with inferior and right ventricular myocardial infarction and is probably due to the conduction delay resulting from ventricular scarring. The same principles apply to patients who have a left ventricular epicardial electrode and either underlying LBBB or ventricular scarring and to patients who have a right atrial electrode and an intra-atrial conduction delay. Undersensing in these cases is due to intrinsic conduction system disease rather than to a malfunctioning unit. The problem is managed by extending the programmed AV delay (in the case of ventricular pseudofusion), programming a higher sensitivity, or if necessary, increasing the pacing rate to overdrive the native rhythm.

Oversensing refers to sensing of unwanted electrical signals such as T waves, myopotentials, and environmental signals (eg, electrocautery; Table 14–10). Programming the pulse generator to sense only electrical signals of larger magnitude will often solve the problem. When a programmer is not immediately available, placing a magnet over the pulse generator will temporarily eliminate the oversensing by converting the generator to a non-sensing asynchronous mode of function. Because competitive rhythms with the magnet in place can induce ventricular tachyarrhythmias, these patients should be in a monitored unit.

Noncapture exists when pacing stimuli do not depolarize nonrefractory myocardium (Figure 14–23; Table 14–12). This condition may result from poor electrode position; a subthreshold programmed output; output reduction due to battery depletion; or an increase in myocardial stimulation threshold that can results from acute myocardial infarction, drug effect, electrolyte imbalance, cardiopulmonary resuscitation, or fibrosis at the electrode-tissue interface. Noncapture can be managed by noninvasive programming of the pulse generator's energy output (voltage and pulse duration), surgical repositioning of the lead, or generator exchange, depending on the underlying problem.

The difference between noncapture (stimulus artifact is present) and failure of output (lack of stimulus output when such output is expected and indicated) should be recognized. If the pacing stimulus has not been delivered (Table 14–13), capture cannot be ascertained. Applying a magnet will aid in determining the cause for the lack of stimulus output. Asynchronous pacing will result with magnet application if the lack of pacing stimulus output results from inhibition due to oversensing. If there is a true problem with delivery of a stimulus output, no stimulus output and therefore no paced complexes will be seen despite magnet application. The main causes of failure of output are battery depletion and pulse generator component failure. This is to be distinguished from the situation when pulse generator output is occurring normally but the current is not reaching body tissues to depolarize it, due to lead fracture or insulation break, and loose set screw (loss of connection between the lead connector pin and the pulse generator). Management of pacemaker failure of output will require replacement of the pulse generator, whereas lead problems usually require lead replacement, and loose set screws are addressed merely by restoring a good connection between the lead connector pin and the generator.

C. Assessment of Pacing System Function

All patients undergoing comprehensive pacing system assessment should have a 12-lead ECG, with and without a magnet applied, to allow identification of spontaneous (where present), purely paced, and fusion P waves and QRS

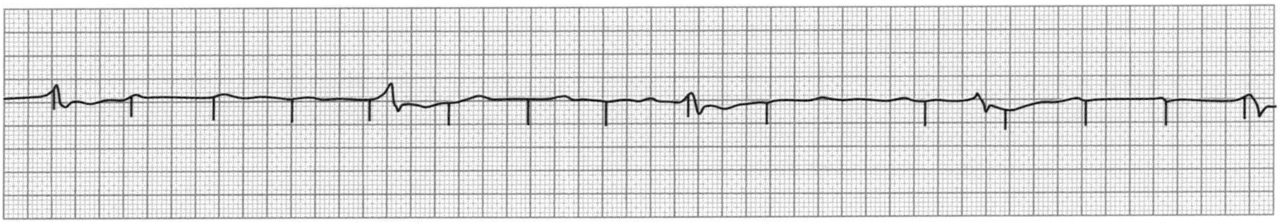

▲ **Figure 14–23.** Noncapture and undersensing in a patient following cardiac arrest; a temporary transvenous pacing system had been placed in the right ventricular apex. The QRS complexes are spontaneous and occur at a severely slow rate; they do not follow pacing stimuli.

Table 14–12. Causes and Management of Pacemaker Noncapture

Tissue refractoriness: Verify capture during temporal opportunity
Lead dislodgement: Reposition lead, or program lead polarity
Increase in myocardial stimulation threshold: Program higher energy output; treat underlying cause if possible
Lead-insulation break: Repair or replace lead; unipolarize lead
Conductor-wire fracture: Replace lead
Inappropriately low programmed output: Program higher output
Generator end of life: Replace generator

complexes, as well as sensing and pacing functions in both atria and ventricles. The (nonprogrammable) pacing rate with a magnet in place is not the same as the programmed rate, as indicated earlier, and the mode of function with the magnet in place may differ from the programmed mode (eg, a DDD system may have a magnet mode that is VOO, although this is currently a rare event; Figure 14–24). The magnet mode, rate, and AV interval for each device are manufacturer and model specific and may vary, sometimes with stimuli delivered at one rate and AV interval, followed by another rate and AV interval.

In addition, all patients should have highly penetrated posteroanterior and lateral chest radiographs to assess the

Table 14–13. Causes of Absence of Pacing Stimulus Output and Response to Magnet Application

Cause	Response to Magnet
Normal inhibition by P waves and QRS complexes	Pacing stimuli will be delivered asynchronously
Oversensing	Pacing stimuli will be delivered asynchronously
Lead fracture	Pacing stimuli may not be seen if the break in the wire is complete (current does not reach body tissues); may be seen as multiples of a basing pacing rate, or may be seen intermittently (make–break circuit); may have variable amplitude
Lead-generator disconnection or improper connection	Same as for lead fracture
Battery failure (end of life)	Pacing stimuli at slow rate, no visible pacing stimuli, noncapture, undersensing
Battery component failure	Variable response

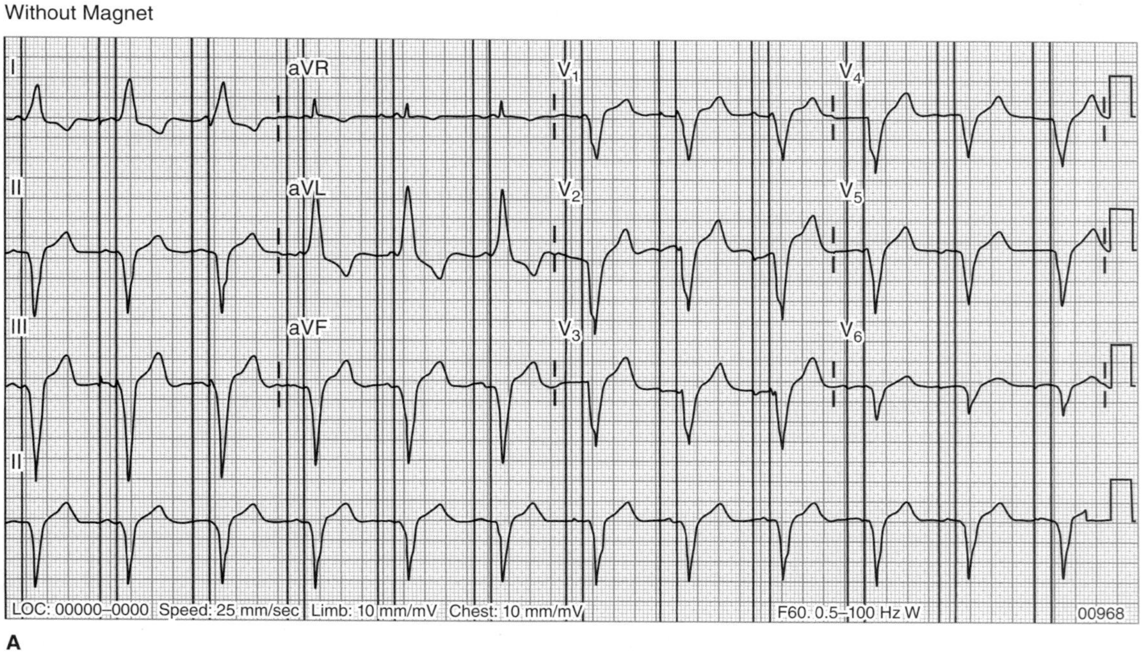

▲ **Figure 14–24. A:** Atrioventricular sequential pacing. The large magnitude of the pacing artifacts indicates unipolar pacing in both chambers. Because atrial pacing stimuli are followed by P waves, and ventricular stimuli are followed by QRS complexes, pacing function is normal in both chambers. Sensing function cannot be evaluated because spontaneous P waves and QRS complexes are not occurring.

With Magnet

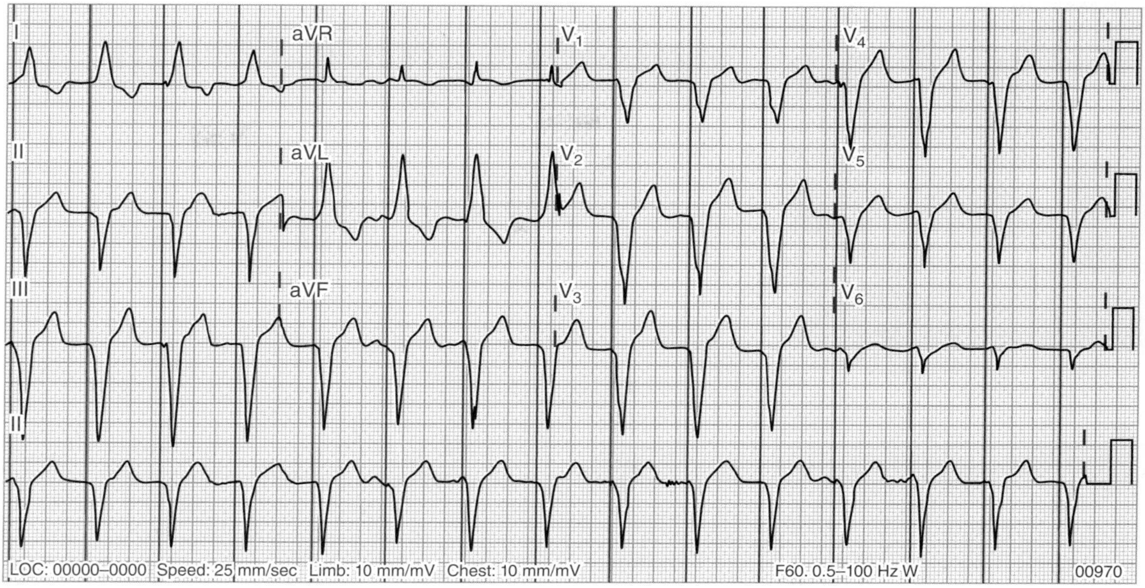

B

▲ **Figure 14–24.** (*Continued*) **B:** Twelve-lead electrocardiogram, recorded with magnet in place. The mode of function is VOO (asynchronous ventricular pacing) at 85 bpm.

leads and, when possible, to identify the pacemaker's manufacturer and model number. The number and type (unipolar, bipolar, MRI conditional) of leads can be ascertained, as well as the positions of the lead tips and pulse generator. Lead tips lying outside the cardiac silhouette suggest the possibility of myocardial perforation. Occasionally, lead insulation degradation, wire fracture, or improper connections between the lead and pulse generator can be seen. Smartphone applications are now available that can identify the manufacturer of the pulse generator by analyzing the chest radiograph.

More sophisticated evaluation techniques, such as interrogation of the programmed parameters of the pulse generator, sensing and pacing threshold determination, and recording of intracardiac electrograms, can be necessary to detect and then determine the cause of pacemaker malfunction; these evaluations should be performed by a pacemaker specialist.

Epstein AE, DiMarco JP, Ellenbogen KA, et al. ACC/AHA/HRS 2008 guidelines for device-based therapy of cardiac rhythm abnormalities. *Circulation.* 2008;117:e350–e408. [PMID: 18483207]

Gillis AM, Russo AM, Ellenbogen KA, et al. HRS/ACCF expert consensus statement on pacemaker device and mode selection. *Heart Rhythm.* 2012;9:1344–1365. [PMID: 22858114]

Kusumoto FM, Schoenfeld MH, Barrett C, et al. 2018 ACC/AHA/HRS guideline on the evaluation and management of patients with bradycardia and cardiac conduction delay. *Circulation.* 2019;140:e382–e482. [PMID: 30586772]

Nazarian S, Hansford R, Rahsepar AR, et al. Safety of magnetic resonance imaging in patients with cardiac devices. *N Engl J Med.* 2017;377:2555–2564. [PMID: 29281579]

15 Sudden Cardiac Death

James W. Salazar, MD, MAS
Zian H. Tseng, MD, MAS

ESSENTIALS OF DIAGNOSIS

- Sudden cardiac death is near instantaneous death due to underlying cardiac cause and may include arrhythmic and non-arrhythmic causes.
- Conventional definitions use death certificates, emergency medical systems records, or epidemiologic criteria to define sudden cardiac death, but these methods do not reliably exclude non-arrhythmic causes of sudden death.
- More recent studies use postmortem investigation to more accurately define sudden arrhythmic death.
- Sudden cardiac death is primarily intended to specify sudden deaths due to arrhythmic cause, that is, sudden arrhythmic death that is potentially rescuable with a defibrillator.
- Common underlying etiologies and risk factors for sudden arrhythmic death include coronary artery disease, nonischemic cardiomyopathy, and other structural heart diseases such as left ventricular hypertrophy; primary electrical diseases are a rare cause.
- Many noncardiac causes may underlie sudden cardiac arrest and sudden deaths, such as neurologic catastrophe, hemorrhage, occult overdose, and pulmonary embolism.

General Considerations

The effective study and prevention of **sudden cardiac death** is foremost dependent on understanding the pathophysiology of the condition it is intended to represent. As Hinkle and Thaler originally delineated in their classification of cardiac deaths in 1982, the primary mechanism presumed to underlie sudden cardiac deaths is lethal arrhythmia, most commonly ventricular tachycardia or fibrillation but also including heart block and bradyarrhythmias. These lethal arrhythmias usually occur in the setting of underlying chronic cardiovascular disease (eg, ischemic heart disease, cardiomyopathy). Although sudden cardiac death may also result from sudden hemodynamic collapse due to non-arrhythmic cardiac causes such as acute pump failure or tamponade, it is the arrhythmic phenotype that is the focus of interventions that include emergency medical systems resuscitation protocols, automated external defibrillators, or in high-risk populations, implantable cardioverter-defibrillators (ICD).

Investigators and clinicians have long sought an accurate and pragmatic definition that specifies arrhythmic and cardiac causes of instantaneous death. Broad consensus exists that the event is a sudden, unexpected, out-of-hospital death, but given its inherent sudden and unexpected nature, often limited diagnostic data are available to robustly exclude noncardiac causes which may also cause instantaneous death (eg, occult overdose, intracranial hemorrhage, aortic dissection, pulmonary embolism). Most definitions presume cardiac etiology or infer cardiac cause of death from limited pre-mortem and/or resuscitation records because these data are often the only records accessible and autopsies to verify cardiac cause are rarely performed. Moreover, due to variable investigative perspectives (emergency medicine, cardiology/electrophysiology, clinical trials, and pathology), data sources, and definitions (Table 15–1)—from death certificates to emergency medical services records to epidemiologic and societal definitions, to clinical trial definitions, and finally those based on pathology—incidence estimates of sudden cardiac death vary widely and sudden death due to primary arrhythmic cause is often presumed.

In this chapter, we will outline the various definitions that are critical to understand cardiac arrest and sudden cardiac death and the importance of discerning cardiac from noncardiac causes of sudden death. We will then focus on the conditions leading to sudden cardiac arrest and sudden cardiac death due to primary arrhythmia.

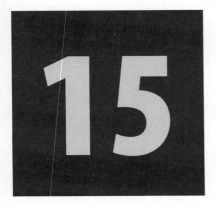

Table 15–1. Causes of Sudden Death

Sudden Arrhythmic Death	Non-Arrhythmic Sudden Cardiac Death	Noncardiac Sudden Death
Coronary artery disease	Mechanical complications of myocardial infarction	**H**ypoxia (eg, aspiration)
Atherosclerotic	Acute heart failure	**H**ypovolemia (eg, GI hemorrhage)
Acute ischemia or infarction (**T**hrombosis, coronary)	Acute valvular disease	**H**ypothermia
Prior infarction	**T**amponade	**H**yperkalemia/hypokalemia (eg, acute renal failure)
Other acute coronary syndromes	Pericarditis	**H**ydrogen ion (acidosis; eg, infection)
Coronary spasm		**T**oxins (eg, occult overdose)
Spontaneous dissection		**T**ension pneumothorax
Coronary embolism		**T**hrombosis, pulmonary
Congenital coronary anomalies		Other: aortic dissection, hypoglycemia
Myocardial diseases		
Hypertrophic cardiomyopathies		
Dilated cardiomyopathies		
Left ventricular noncompaction		
Valvular heart disease		
Arrhythmogenic right ventricular cardiomyopathy/ dysplasia		
Congenital heart disease		
Infiltrative cardiomyopathy (eg, sarcoidosis)		
Primary pulmonary hypertension		
Myocarditis		
Chagas disease		
Neuromuscular disorders with cardiac involvement		
Primary electrophysiologic disorders		
Long QT syndrome: acquired and congenital		
Brugada syndrome		
Catecholaminergic polymorphic ventricular tachycardia		
Preexcitation syndromes		
Congenital atrioventricular block		
Other		
Commotio cordis		
Diet related		

*Reversible causes of **Hs** and **Ts** of cardiac arrest are **bolded**.

Lastly, we will review the principles of prevention of sudden cardiac death—the identification, evaluation, and treatment of patients at elevated risk including strategies for primary and secondary prevention of SCD.

Definitions

Out-of-hospital cardiac arrest and sudden cardiac death are heterogeneous entities which are related and challenging to define. To develop an approach to cardiac arrest and sudden cardiac death it is important to know the most commonly accepted definitions for these entities (see Table 15–1) and how these vary in specificity for primary arrhythmic cause (Figure 15–1).

The most non-specific definition related to sudden cardiac death is **out-of-hospital cardiac arrest (OHCA)**. The American Heart Association Emergency Cardiovascular Care Committee proposed an OHCA as an event in which a person is evaluated by emergency medical services (EMS) and (1) receives defibrillation attempts or cardiopulmonary resuscitation (CPR) by EMS, or (2) is pulseless but does not receive defibrillation attempts or CPR from EMS personnel. Essential to the OHCA definition is that an EMS personnel responds to the patient, but notably this definition does not specify whether the event was unexpected (ie, existing severe illness) or sudden (ie, duration of symptoms prior to event), nor does it explicitly exclude noncardiac cause.

A **sudden cardiac arrest (SCA)** is generally defined as an OHCA that is sudden and unexpected. The most commonly adopted definition of suddenness is from the World Health Organization which classifies it as occurring within 1 hour of symptom onset in the case of a witnessed arrest or within 24 hours of having been observed alive and symptom free in the case of an unwitnessed arrest. Whether an arrest is unexpected is more variably defined, but generally sudden cardiac arrests exclude patients with (1) severe noncardiac chronic and terminal illness in which imminent death was anticipated or (2) identifiable noncardiac cause at presentation, including evidence of drug use at the scene, life-threatening trauma, homicide, or suicide. Definitions of sudden cardiac arrest do not exclude noncardiac causes of sudden arrest (eg, pulmonary embolism, intracranial hemorrhage, and aortic dissection), but it is more specific

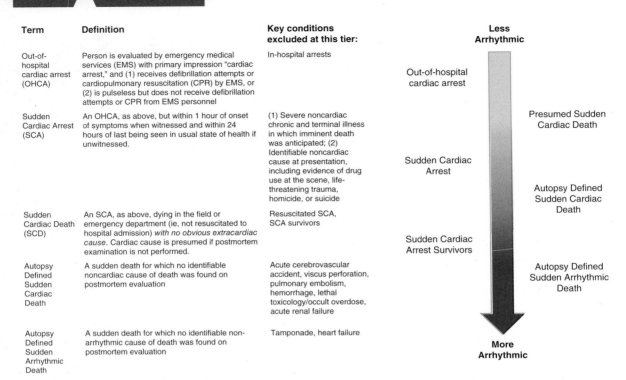

Term	Definition	Key conditions excluded at this tier:
Out-of-hospital cardiac arrest (OHCA)	Person is evaluated by emergency medical services (EMS) with primary impression "cardiac arrest," and (1) receives defibrillation attempts or cardiopulmonary resuscitation (CPR) by EMS, or (2) is pulseless but does not receive defibrillation attempts or CPR from EMS personnel	In-hospital arrests
Sudden Cardiac Arrest (SCA)	An OHCA, as above, but within 1 hour of onset of symptoms when witnessed and within 24 hours of last being seen in usual state of health if unwitnessed.	(1) Severe noncardiac chronic and terminal illness in which imminent death was anticipated; (2) Identifiable noncardiac cause at presentation, including evidence of drug use at the scene, life-threatening trauma, homicide, or suicide
Sudden Cardiac Death (SCD)	An SCA, as above, dying in the field or emergency department (ie, not resuscitated to hospital admission) *with no obvious extracardiac cause*. Cardiac cause is presumed if postmortem examination is not performed.	Resuscitated SCA, SCA survivors
Autopsy Defined Sudden Cardiac Death	A sudden death for which no identifiable noncardiac cause of death was found on postmortem evaluation	Acute cerebrovascular accident, viscus perforation, pulmonary embolism, hemorrhage, lethal toxicology/occult overdose, acute renal failure
Autopsy Defined Sudden Arrhythmic Death	A sudden death for which no identifiable non-arrhythmic cause of death was found on postmortem evaluation	Tamponade, heart failure

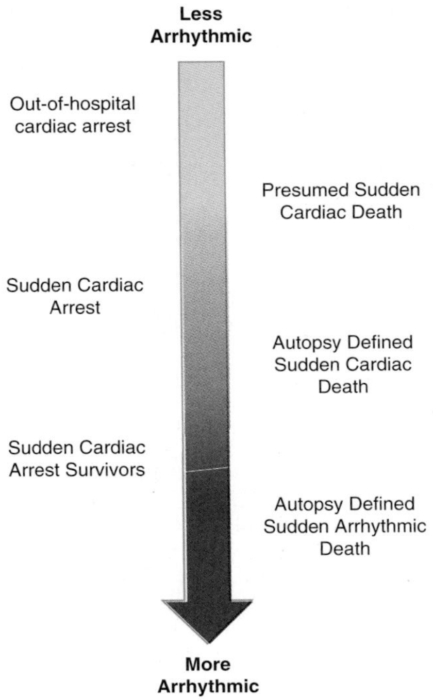

▲ Figure 15–1. Cardiac arrest and sudden cardiac death entities by specificity of underlying arrhythmic cause. Cardiac arrest and sudden cardiac death entities in order of specificity for primary arrhythmic cause. The least specific entity is the out-of-hospital cardiac arrest (OHCA) and the most specific entities are sudden cardiac arrest survivors and autopsy defined SAD. Definitions of sudden cardiac arrest do not exclude noncardiac causes of sudden arrest, but it is more specific for primary arrhythmic cause than the more generic OHCA definition, because sudden events are more likely arrhythmic. As sudden cardiac arrest victims survive further along the chain of survival, they are increasingly likely to have a primary cardiac and arrhythmic etiology for their arrest since resuscitation algorithms and treatments specifically target these etiologies. For sudden deaths, postmortem examination including a full autopsy, postmortem toxicology, postmortem vitreous chemistries, is an important tool to identify causes of death that would otherwise be indistinguishable (eg, occult overdose, pulmonary embolism, hemorrhage, stroke) and specify arrhythmic death.

for primary arrhythmic cause than the more generic OHCA definition.

A **sudden cardiac death (SCD)** is a sudden cardiac arrest that dies in the field or emergency department (ie, not resuscitated to hospital admission) *and is with no obvious extracardiac cause*. Notably, sudden cardiac arrests that are (1) resuscitated to hospitalization (ie, resuscitated SCAs) and (2) subsequently survive to discharge from hospitalization (ie, SCA survivors) are commonly equated but recent evidence demonstrates that these are distinct outcomes from sudden cardiac deaths. As sudden cardiac arrest victims survive further along the chain of survival, they are increasingly likely to have a primary cardiac and arrhythmic etiology for their arrest since resuscitation algorithms and treatments specifically target these etiologies. Patients resuscitated to hospitalization after cardiac arrest typically receive a broad workup to determine underlying causes. In contrast, the extent to which a possible extracardiac cause of sudden cardiac arrest for a victim dying in the field or emergency department (ie, sudden cardiac death) is evaluated is highly variable. The gold standard is a comprehensive postmortem examination, including a full autopsy, postmortem toxicology, postmortem vitreous chemistries, to identify causes of death that would otherwise be indistinguishable (eg, occult overdose, pulmonary embolism, hemorrhage, stroke). Cardiac cause is presumed if postmortem examination is not performed, therefore sudden cardiac deaths defined purely by epidemiologic or circumstantial criteria should be considered *presumed* sudden cardiac deaths.

Importantly an **autopsy defined sudden arrhythmic death (SAD)** provides the greatest level of specificity for deaths potentially rescuable with a defibrillator, and is distinct from **autopsy defined sudden cardiac deaths** which include cardiac, non-arrhythmic deaths that would not be rescuable with defibrillator (ie, acute heart failure, tamponade). SAD in this context should be distinguished from **sudden arrhythmic death syndrome (SADS)** as defined by the European Society of Cardiology in which by autopsy, histology, and toxicology the heart is structurally normal

Table 15–2. Notable Implantable Cardioverter-Defibrillator Trials

Trial	No. of Patients	Age (years)	LVEF	Follow-Up (months)	Mortality Control (%)	Mortality ICD (%)	Relative RR (%)	Absolute RR (%)	NNT (36 months)
Secondary Prevention									
AVID	1016	65	0.35	18	24	16	31	8.2	9
CIDS	659	64	0.34	36	30	25	23	4.3	23
CASH	228	58	0.45	57	44	36	23	8.1	20
Primary Prevention									
MADIT	196	63	0.26	27	39	16	54	22.8	3
MADIT II	1232	64	0.23	20	20	14	31	5.4	10
DEFINITE	458	58	0.21	29	14	8	35	5.2	24
SCD-HeFT	1676	60	0.25	46	28	22	23	6.8	23
CABG-Patch	900	64	0.27	32	21	23	7 (increase)	1.7 (increase)	
DINAMIT	674	62	0.31	30	17	19	8 (increase)	1.7 (increase)	
IRIS	898	63	0.35	37	26	26	4 (increase)	0	

AVID, antiarrhythmics versus implantable defibrillator; CABG-Patch, coronary artery bypass graft-patch trial; CASH, cardiac arrest study Hamburg; CIDS, Canadian Implantable Defibrillator Study; DEFINITE, defibrillators in nonischemic cardiomyopathy treatment evaluation; DINAMIT, The Defibrillator in Acute Myocardial Infarction Trial; ICD, implantable cardioverter-defibrillator; IRIS, immediate risk stratification improves survival; LVEF, left ventricular ejection fraction; MADIT I and II, Multicenter Automatic Implantable Defibrillator Trials I and II; NNT, number needed to treat; RR, risk reduction; SCD-HeFT, Sudden Cardiac Death in Heart Failure Trial.

and noncardiac etiologies are excluded. Some investigators have used "primary electrical disease" or "unexplained SCD" to define this normal heart condition at autopsy.

Al-Khatib SM, Stevenson WG, Ackerman MJ, et al. 2017 AHA/ACC/HRS Guideline for Management of Patients With Ventricular Arrhythmias and the Prevention of Sudden Cardiac Death. *Circulation*. 2018;138(13):e272–e391. [PMID: 29084733]

Priori SG, Blomström-Lundqvist C, Mazzanti A, et al. 2015 ESC Guidelines for the management of patients with ventricular arrhythmias and the prevention of sudden cardiac death: The Task Force for the Management of Patients with Ventricular Arrhythmias and the Prevention of Sudden Cardiac Death of the European Society of Cardiology (ESC). Endorsed by: Association for European Paediatric and Congenital Cardiology (AEPC). *Eur Heart J*. 2015;36(41):2793–2867. [PMID: 26320108]

Ricceri Santo, Salazar James W, Vu Andrew A, Vittinghoff Eric, Moffatt Ellen, Tseng Zian H. Factors predisposing to survival after resuscitation for sudden cardiac arrest. *J Am Coll Cardiol*. 2021;77(19):2353–2362. [PMID: 33985679]

Stiles MK, Wilde AAM, Abrams DJ, et al. 2020 APHRS/HRS expert consensus statement on the investigation of decedents with sudden unexplained death and patients with sudden cardiac arrest, and of their families. *Heart Rhythm*. 2021;18(1):e1–e50. [PMID: 33091602]

Tseng ZH, Salazar JW, Olgin JE, et al. Refining the World Health Organization Definition. *Circ Arrhythm Electrophysiol*. 2019;12(7):e007171. doi:10.1161/CIRCEP.119.007171. [PMID: 31248279]

Pathophysiology & Etiologies

A wide spectrum of cardiac and noncardiac causes may underlie sudden death (Table 15–2). Even when a death is sudden and unexpected, a recent prospective countywide postmortem study in the United States highlighted this diversity since 40% of presumed sudden cardiac deaths were found to have noncardiac causes, while a range of both arrhythmic and non-arrhythmic cardiac causes comprised the remaining 60% (Figure 15–2).

The focus of this chapter will be principally those sudden deaths for which an arrhythmia was the primary cause. Several different electrophysiologic mechanisms may be responsible for SAD. The prototypical sequence for a SAD is ventricular tachycardia which degenerates to ventricular fibrillation and ultimately, asystole. Ventricular tachycardia can either be monomorphic or polymorphic and can occur in the presence or absence of structural cardiac disease. Of approximately 300,000 persons with out-of-hospital cardiac arrests treated by emergency medical personnel in the United States, only 23% have an initial rhythm of ventricular tachycardia or ventricular fibrillation or are shockable by an automated external defibrillator. Autopsy studies of OHCA have demonstrated that while a presenting rhythm of VT/VF is widely regarded as synonymous with SAD and is fairly specific for arrhythmic

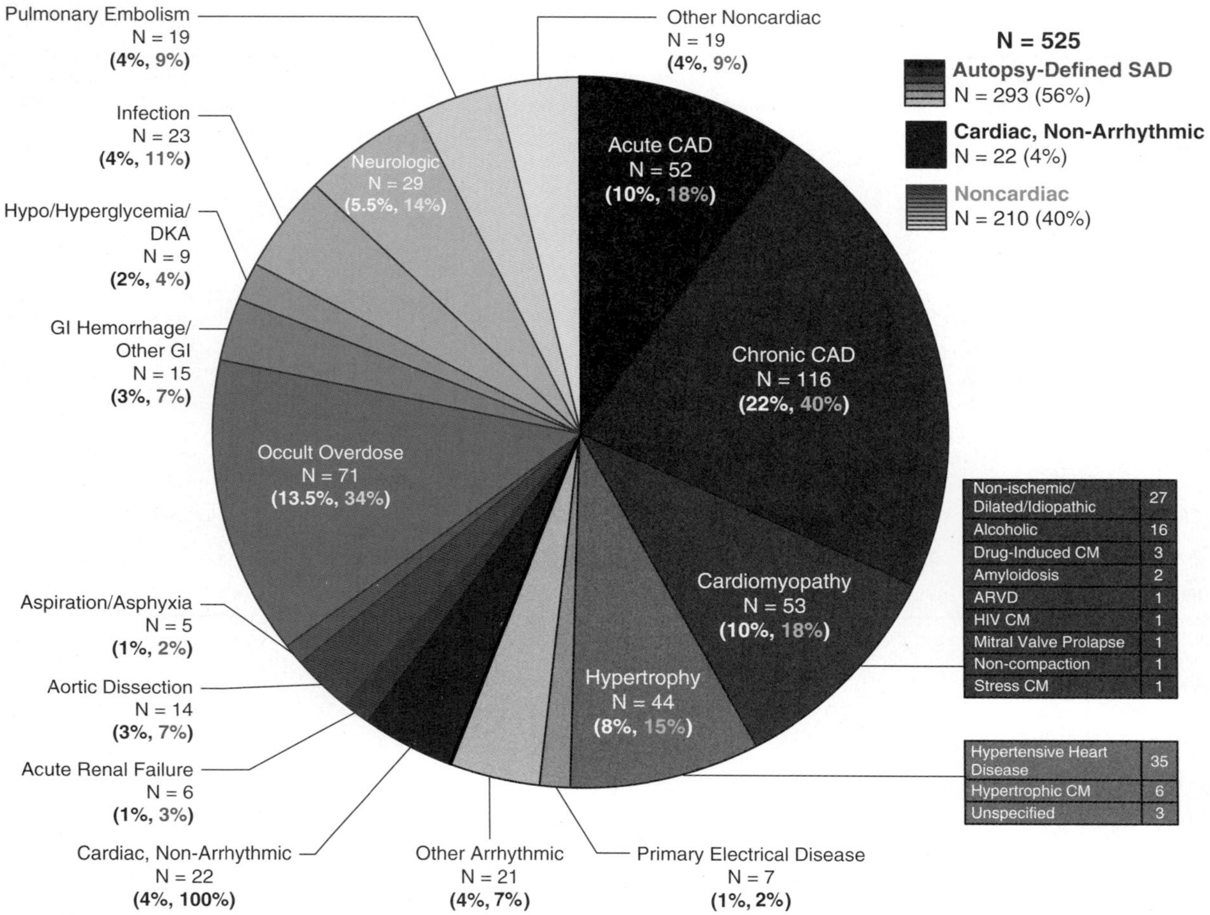

▲ **Figure 15–2. Adjudicated etiologies of autopsied WHO-defined SCDs from the POST SCD Study.**

The Postmortem Systematic Investigation of Sudden Cardiac Death (POST SCD) Study prospectively identified all incident deaths attributed to out-of-hospital cardiac arrest (emergency medical services primary impression, cardiac arrest) from February 1, 2011, and March 1, 2014 of persons between 18 and 90 years of age in San Francisco County for autopsy, toxicology, and histology via medical examiner surveillance of consecutive out-of-hospital deaths. This figure shows adjudicated etiologies of autopsied World Health Organization (WHO)-defined sudden cardiac deaths from this cohort after review of comprehensive medical records, emergency medical services runsheets, complete autopsy, toxicology, and postmortem chemistries. Autopsy-defined SAD required the absence of extracardiac (eg, pulmonary embolism, hemorrhage, lethal toxicology) or non-arrhythmic (tamponade, acute heart failure) cause of death. First % is of total WHO-defined SCDs, second % is of cause of death category. Overall autopsy-defined SAD accounted for 56% of all WHO-defined SCDs, 4% non-arrhythmic cardiac causes, and 40% noncardiac causes.

death, it may also be recorded as the perimortem rhythm for noncardiac causes of death such as overdose and neurologic catastrophe. Bradyarrhythmias including advanced atrioventricular block or electromechanical dissociation are also mechanisms of SAD.

Tseng ZH, Olgin JE, Vittinghoff E, et al. Prospective countywide surveillance and autopsy characterization of sudden cardiac death: POST SCD Study. *Circulation*. 2018;137(25):2689–2700. [PMID: 29915095]

Underlying Causes of Sudden Cardiac Arrest & Sudden Cardiac Death

A. Coronary Artery Disease

Postmortem studies in the 1980s–1990s remain the paradigm for our understanding of **coronary artery disease (CAD)**, acute and chronic, as the pathologic substrate of the majority of SADs, despite referral bias of the fraction of total sudden deaths autopsied. Advances in the treatment of ischemic heart disease and resuscitation science, and recent prospective postmortem studies of sudden cardiac death, have resulted in a contemporary trend of an increasing burden of nonischemic causes of SAD, but coronary artery disease remains the most common single etiology in SAD cohorts, accounting for approximately 60% of deaths adjudicated to be due to primary arrhythmia. Several mechanisms mediated by the coronary arteries can produce potentially lethal arrhythmias. Acute coronary syndromes refer to a sudden reduction in blood supply to the myocardium and primarily include phenomena related to atherosclerosis of the major coronary arteries (ie, plaque rupture and plaque erosion) but also include entities such as coronary spasm, spontaneous dissection, and embolism, which can be in the presence or absence of obstructive CAD. Acute coronary syndromes can lead to myocardial ischemia and infarction, which can rapidly give rise to fatal ventricular arrhythmia. On the chronic side of the spectrum, myocardial infarction, scar, and fibrosis mediated by a prior acute coronary syndrome or more indolent chronic ischemia may serve as a substrate for ventricular arrhythmia due to a triggering event such as ischemia, neurohormonal and autonomic nervous system alterations, or metabolic or hemodynamic imbalances, in conjunction with electrophysiologic substrate created by the prior infarction and myocardial fibrosis. Notably, acute myocardial infarction can also result in cardiac non-arrhythmic conditions not rescuable with an ICD such as wall rupture with tamponade (Figure 15–3, Panel B).

B. Nonischemic Dilated Cardiomyopathy

Nonischemic dilated cardiomyopathy (NICM) is a heterogeneous entity that is frequently categorized into primary cardiomyopathies characterized by myocardial dysfunction (eg, familial, idiopathic, or acquired causes such as alcohol or stimulant related) and secondary cardiomyopathies due to systemic diseases (eg, amyloid and sarcoid). Collectively, these account for the second leading cause of SAD. Although the pathophysiology is dependent on the subtype of NICM, SAD in this population is most often caused by ventricular tachyarrhythmias that are the result of micro/macroreentrant circuits and/or abnormalities of ventricular automaticity promoted by the characteristic structural, conduction, neurohormonal, and hemodynamic alterations comprising the substrate of NICM (Figure 15–3, Panel C).

As such, factors that have been associated with sudden cardiac death include reduced left ventricular ejection fraction, myocardial scar, biomarkers, and ECG markers.

As patients progress in severity of heart failure, specifically New York Heart Association classes III/IV, those with NICM are also presumed to have higher risk of death due to primary bradyarrhythmias or electromechanical dissociation leading to sudden death. In these severely ill patients with multiple comorbidities, cardiac arrests due to pulseless electrical activity that are truly sudden/unexpected and due to a primary cardiac process is hard to discern from those due to progressive hypoxemia as a result of chronic, indolent pulmonary edema, or a primary noncardiac process since these patients are also vulnerable to pneumonia, stroke, and other noncardiac causes of sudden death. However, progressively more sudden deaths observed in patients with severe left ventricular dysfunction are presumed due to pulseless electrical activity and the inability of cardiomyocytes to effectively contract despite existence of an action potential (ie, non-arrhythmic pump failure).

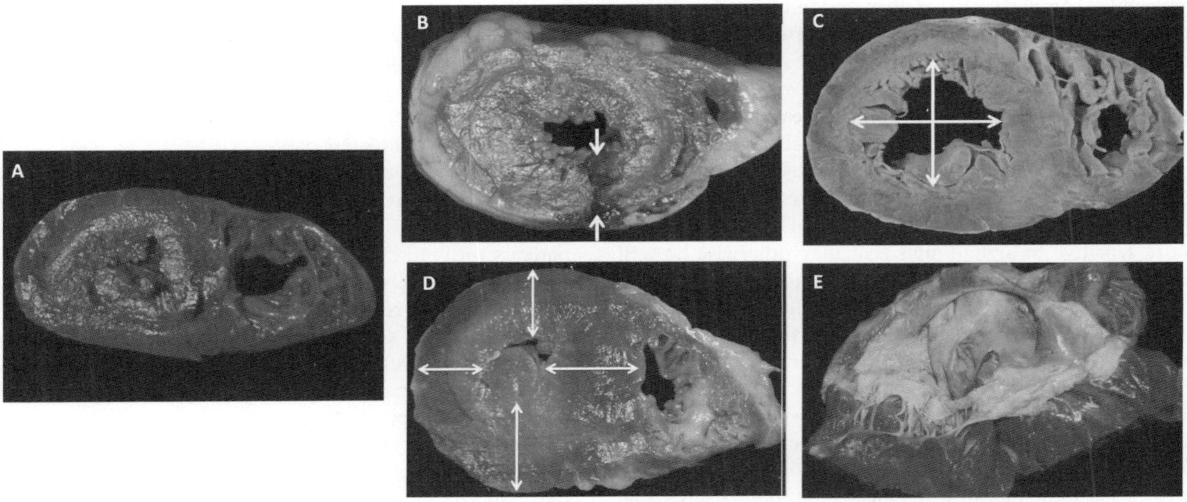

▲ Figure 15–3. Gross pathology examples of etiologies of sudden cardiac death from the POST SCD Study.

Representative examples of heart cross sections from autopsy. **A.** Normal heart. **B.** myocardial infarction with left ventricular rupture denoted by arrows. **C.** dilated cardiomyopathy with left ventricular chamber dimensions denoted by arrows. **D.** Hypertensive heart disease with LV wall thickness denoted by arrows. **E.** Mitral valve prolapse (opened longitudinally).

Steinberg BA, Mulpuru SK, Fang JC, Gersh BJ. Sudden death mechanisms in nonischemic cardiomyopathies: Insights gleaned from clinical implantable cardioverter-defibrillator trials. *Heart Rhythm*. 2017;14(12):1839–1848. [PMID: 28919378]

C. Hypertrophic Cardiomyopathy & Left Ventricular Hypertrophy

Hypertrophic cardiomyopathy (HCM) is an inherited condition defined by increased left ventricular wall thickness that is not explained solely by loading conditions. It is the most common inherited cardiovascular disorder with an estimated prevalence of 1 in 500 and primarily caused by cardiac sarcomere protein gene mutations. The annual rate of sudden death in patients with HCM is reported to be less than 1%; however, certain subpopulations have much higher incidence. Sudden death is often associated with vigorous exercise with the proposed mechanism being increased myocardial demand and ischemia and as such, may more commonly occur in young adults and account for the most sudden cardiac deaths among competitive athletes. Established clinical risk factors of SCD in HCM include history of syncope, cardiac arrest, family history of SCD or SCA, severe left ventricular hypertrophy (> 3.0 cm septal thickness), reduced left ventricular function, and history of nonsustained ventricular arrhythmias on ambulatory monitoring. Additional factors that may portend risk include myocardial fibrosis and scarring on cardiac magnetic resonance imaging.

Analyses of electrograms of patients with HCM and ICDs demonstrate that SAD in HCM is primarily mediated by polymorphic ventricular tachycardia or ventricular fibrillation commonly mediated by late-coupled premature ventricular complexes rather than monomorphic ventricular tachycardia. The underlying mechanisms of ventricular arrhythmia in HCM are an active area of study and include intraventricular dispersion of conduction due to cardiomyocyte fibrosis and disarray, and increased myofilament calcium sensitivity resulting in shorter effective refractory periods which collectively serve as the basis for ventricular arrhythmias, as well as an overall increased predilection for contributory ischemia. Patients with HCM may also be more sensitive to arrhythmias that may otherwise be well tolerated such as atrioventricular block and supraventricular arrhythmias. These arrhythmias may degenerate to fatal arrhythmias, however their overall contribution to SAD in patients with HCM remains poorly characterized.

Left ventricular hypertrophy (LVH) can be explained solely by loading conditions (ie, hypertension) is more common than HCM and shares much of the same proarrhythmic substrate of fibrosis, inflammation, and susceptibility to myocardial ischemia. In a prospective autopsy study of all sudden deaths in a United States county, hypertensive heart disease was found to be the primary cardiac substrate in ~12% of all SAD compared to hypertrophic cardiomyopathy which accounted for ~2% (Figure 15–3, Panel D). Numerous clinical studies have reported the association between left ventricular hypertrophy either ascertained by electrocardiogram or echocardiogram, however it is not currently used for routine prediction of SCD risk.

Ommen SR, Mital S, Burke MA, et al. 2020 AHA/ACC Guideline for the Diagnosis and Treatment of Patients With Hypertrophic Cardiomyopathy: Executive Summary: A Report of the American College of Cardiology/American Heart Association Joint Committee on Clinical Practice Guidelines. *Circulation*. 2020;142(25):e533–e557. [PMID 33215938]

D. Other Structural Cardiac Disease

Of the valvular disorders, **mitral valve prolapse (MVP)** is of the greatest relevance to SAD. MVP, characterized by systolic displacement of the anterior and/or posterior mitral leaflet into the left atrium, is a common condition with an estimated prevalence of 2–3% in the United States. Patients with MVP have varied clinical manifestations from a benign course to progressive heart failure necessitating mitral valve repair or replacement. It has long been established that MVP conveys some risk of SCD with estimates of 0.2–0.4% per year. However, more recently a subtype of MVP—malignant arrhythmic MVP—has been reported to have a multifold increased risk of SCD. Additional analysis of the same prospective autopsy study of sudden deaths found that lethal MVP accounted for 4% of all countywide SAD (Figure 15–3, Panel E). Morphologic characteristics of MVP that have been used to characterize this phenotype include mitral annular disjunction (an increased separation of the mitral leaflet and left atrial junction from the left ventricular posterior wall), increased leaflet thickness, and basal lateral left ventricular hypertrophy. These characteristics are hypothesized to cause papillary muscle traction, abnormal patterns of left ventricular strain, and fibrosis of the papillary muscles/inferobasal wall that may serve as arrhythmogenic substrate. Ongoing work involves the use of electrocardiographic, echocardiographic, and cardiac MRI findings to detect patients at greatest risk.

While sudden cardiac death is a feared complication of **aortic stenosis,** SCD is a rare consequence with a recent trial estimating a risk of 0.4%/patient-year in asymptomatic patients with mild to moderate AS and 0.6%/patient-year in severe AS, with the risk of SCD presumed primarily mediated through alternative risk factors. Hypothesized mechanisms of SCD in aortic stenosis include abnormal stimulation of LV baroreceptors leading to hypotension and bradycardia and ventricular tachyarrhythmia as the result of reduced, fixed cardiac output and subsequent demand ischemia.

Arrhythmogenic right ventricular cardiomyopathy (ARVC), also known as arrhythmogenic right ventricular dysplasia (ARVD), is a heritable condition with an estimated prevalence of ~1 in 5000 that affects primarily the right ventricle (but has recently been recognized to sometimes also affect the left ventricle) and can lead to heart failure and sudden cardiac death. ARVC is characterized by the replacement of myocytes by fibrous and fatty tissue predominantly in the right ventricular free wall and is mediated by genetic defects in the desmosomal proteins crucial to cell-to-cell adhesion, leading to myocyte cell death. This fibrofatty replacement serves as the substrate for ventricular arrhythmia either via scar mediated macro-reentry or irregularities in the coupling of myocytes on the cellular/molecular levels. ARVC is pleiotropic but often clinically manifests initially in young adulthood and in the form of arrhythmia ranging from palpitations, syncope, or SAD with heart failure usually being a late manifestation. Given the variable presentation of ARVC and similarities in presentations between other conditions that affect the right ventricle (eg, sarcoid, idiopathic right ventricular outflow tract tachycardia), ARVC remains a challenging diagnosis with consensus criteria using a host of electrocardiographic, echocardiographic, MRI features, along with family history. A mainstay in therapy of patients with ARVC is the cessation of intense exertion as this has been linked with arrhythmogenesis and SCD. Risk stratification in patients with ARVC is an ongoing area of research, but ICDs are recommended for the highest risk groups including secondary prevention and primary prevention for patients with severe ventricular dysfunction or multiple risk factors.

The rate of sudden cardiac death in **congenital heart disease (CHD)** is estimated to be 20–30 times the general population and account for up to 25% of deaths. The etiology of SCD in CHD is multifactorial and may be amenable to ICD therapy in only a minority of cases. Some risk factors for SCD in CHD are similar to the general population (ie, systemic ventricular function), others are specific to the CHD lesion and type of repair.

Delling FN, Aung S, Vittinghoff E, et al. Antemortem and post-mortem characteristics of lethal mitral valve prolapse among all countywide sudden deaths. *JACC Clin Electrophysiol.* 2021;7(8):1025–1034. [PMID: 33640349]

Ganatra S, Sharma A. Arrhythmogenic right ventricular cardiomyopathy. *N Engl J Med.* 2017;376(15):1489. [PMID: 28406281]

Khairy P, Silka MJ, Moore JP, et al. Sudden cardiac death in congenital heart disease. *Eur Heart J.* Published online March 18, 2022. [PMID: 35302168]

Minners J, Rossebo A, Chambers JB, et al. Sudden cardiac death in asymptomatic patients with aortic stenosis. *Heart.* 2020;106(21):1646–1650. [PMID: 32737125]

Muthukumar L, Jahangir A, Jan MF, Perez Moreno AC, Khandheria BK, Tajik AJ. Association between malignant mitral valve prolapse and sudden cardiac death: A review. *JAMA Cardiol.* 2020;5(9):1053–1061. [PMID: 32936277]

E. Primary Electrical Diseases—Inherited Arrhythmia Syndromes

Collectively, the inherited arrhythmia syndromes causing sudden cardiac death represent only a small fraction of the total burden of adult sudden cardiac death but are a more common cause of sudden death in children, adolescents, and young adults. For example, in the POST SCD study, primary electrical diseases accounted for 1% of all presumed sudden cardiac deaths, and 2% of autopsy defined SAD (see Figure 15–2).

The **congenital long QT syndrome (LQTS)** is a family of disorders characterized by prolongation of cardiac repolarization with a prolonged QT interval on the scalar ECG and a tendency to develop polymorphic ventricular tachycardia that may degenerate to ventricular fibrillation. It occurs with an estimated prevalence of 1 in 3000–5000 in the general population. The most common types of LQTS are caused by mutations in genes that encode ion channel proteins, causing a prolonged repolarization phase of the ventricular action potential. This promotes polymorphic ventricular tachycardia triggered by early after-depolarizations in the action potential. Electrolyte imbalance, bradycardia or pauses, sudden sympathetic stimulation, and drug effects all may further prolong repolarization in individuals with these mutations and trigger acute episodes. Factors significantly affecting outcome include QTc duration (ie, increased risk of ventricular arrhythmias with QTc > 500 ms), age–gender interactions (increased event rate in males during childhood and females after adolescence), LQTS genotype (LQT_3 responds less well to β-blocker therapy), and syncope despite treatment with a β-blocker. Notably, family history of sudden death does not seem to be a marker of life-threatening cardiac events in LQTS patients. It is important to recognize patients with LQTS because standard antiarrhythmic drugs may worsen their condition and other QT-prolonging agents must be avoided.

A **short QT syndrome** caused by a gain-of-function mutation in a repolarizing potassium current that is associated with sudden death has also been described. The syndrome is characterized by short QT intervals (< 350 ms) and high incidence of syncope, sudden death, and atrial fibrillation.

The **Brugada syndrome** is another familial condition associated with sudden death. These individuals have an incomplete or complete right bundle branch block with ST-segment elevation in V_1 and V_2 on ECG. These patients can manifest spontaneous episodes of polymorphic ventricular tachycardia and ventricular fibrillation, often during sleep. Some patients with Brugada syndrome have a mutation in the sodium channel gene (SCN5A) causing a decrease in the inward sodium current during the plateau phase of the action potential. The unusual ECG manifestations are postulated to be due to more pronounced ion channel dysfunction in the right ventricular epicardium.

Catecholaminergic polymorphic ventricular tachycardia (CPVT) is a rare syndrome in which bursts of rapid ventricular tachycardia occur during sympathetic stimulation or exercise. This syndrome is genetically heterogenous, with mutations in the genes encoding the cardiac ryanodine receptor type II and calsequestrin. These genetic mutations result in abnormal calcium homeostasis with increased intracellular calcium, thereby predisposing to an increased risk of ventricular arrhythmias. β-Blockers are indicated for symptomatic patients. An ICD may be indicated for CPVT patients with syncope or sustained ventricular tachycardia despite treatment with β-blockers.

Advancements in genetic testing have facilitated the diagnosis and risk stratification of patients with inherited arrhythmia syndromes. Most of these diseases are caused by single gene mutations that are often inherited in an autosomal dominant fashion. However, the genetic cause has been identified for only a portion of these life-threatening disorders (up to 50% of LQTS cases; 50% of hypertrophic cardiomyopathy; < 50% of ARVC and CPVT; and 25–30% of dilated cardiomyopathy and Brugada syndrome).

Notably, after thorough evaluation including comprehensive cardiovascular genetic testing 5–10% of resuscitated sudden cardiac arrest survivors remain unexplained and are termed idiopathic ventricular fibrillation (IVF).

F. Drug-Induced Sudden Death & Arrhythmias

Drug toxicity can also result in sudden death, directly in the form of occult (unrecognized) overdose causes of presumed sudden cardiac death, and by increasing risk of lethal arrhythmias by affecting cardiac electrophysiology, notably the QT prolonging medications. Even when prescribed for atrial fibrillation or supraventricular tachycardia, all antiarrhythmic drugs may be associated with pro-arrhythmic effects in the ventricle. Other cardiac and noncardiac drugs can also cause arrhythmias. The most common mechanism is I_{Kr} channel blockade leading to QT prolongation. A comprehensive, regularly updated list of QT prolonging medications and their associated risk is available for clinicians online. Multiple factors are often required for drug-induced arrhythmia, also termed acquired long QT syndrome. Risk factors include electrolyte disturbances, age, female gender, genetic polymorphisms or mutations, left ventricular hypertrophy, and bradycardia. Some patients with acquired long QT syndrome have been discovered to carry variants in channelopathy genes, therefore making them more susceptible to QT prolongation in the presence of an additional electrophysiologic stressor in the form of exposure to QT prolonging drugs. It is important to note, however, that even with high-risk QT prolonging medications the risk of sudden death also includes *non-arrhythmic* causes.

Patients with severe electrolyte disturbances and abnormal dietary histories (eg, anorexia nervosa and liquid protein diets) are also susceptible to potentially lethal ventricular arrhythmias even in the absence of significant heart disease.

Simpson TF, Salazar JW, Vittinghoff E, et al. Association of QT-prolonging medications with risk of autopsy-defined causes of sudden death. *JAMA Intern Med.* 2020;180(5):698–706. [PMID: 32119028]

Woosley RL, Heise CW, Gallo T, et al. CredibleMeds.org, QTdrugs List. Oro Valley, AZ: AZCERT, Inc. https://www.crediblemeds.org/.

G. Other Arrhythmias & Conditions

Several electrophysiologic abnormalities can result in sudden death without associated major structural heart disease. **Supraventricular arrhythmias,** if associated with very rapid ventricular rates, can cause hemodynamic collapse and degenerate to ventricular fibrillation, classically in the setting of **Wolff-Parkinson-White syndrome** whereby atrial fibrillation with rapid conduction over an accessory pathway is the supraventricular arrhythmia most frequently associated with sudden death, but other supraventricular arrhythmias have also been rarely implicated. Although sudden death due to a ventricular preexcitation syndrome is rare, it may be the first clinical manifestation of the condition.

Bradyarrhythmias may also be associated with sudden death. In **congenital complete heart block,** the escape pacemaker may deteriorate over time, with ventricular arrhythmias appearing as the patient's bradycardia becomes increasingly severe. Most previously healthy adults in whom bradycardia develops because of sinus node dysfunction or heart block will have some functioning escape pacemaker that can, at least briefly, support cardiac output. Therefore, sudden death is uncommon with these arrhythmias in the absence of severe ventricular dysfunction, other complicating disease, electrolyte imbalance, drug toxicity, or a prolonged delay in treatment of the bradycardia.

Commotio cordis can also cause sudden death in young individuals with structurally normal hearts. Ventricular fibrillation develops after the patient receives a sharp blow to the chest, often while engaged in sports. Animal models demonstrate that a critically timed and placed chest impact during the vulnerable portion of the T wave can initiate ventricular fibrillation. It is assumed that a similar mechanism is responsible in humans.

Prevention of SCD

Strategies for the prevention of sudden cardiac death are categorized as primary prevention or secondary prevention. Primary prevention is the use of lifestyle changes, medical, and device therapies to prevent SCD in patients prior to their first event, who have not had sustained VT or SCA but are at elevated risk. Secondary prevention is the use of similar efforts to prevent a second SCA in patients who have had prior event, sustained VT, or syncope caused by ventricular arrhythmia. Overall prevention strategies are dependent on (1) identification of the patient at risk, (2) the evaluation and treatment of the conditions conveying the risk, and (3) the consideration of ICD.

Identification of the Patient at Elevated Risk for SCD

A. Patients with Sudden Cardiac Arrest & Sustained Ventricular Arrhythmia

The patients at highest risk of sudden cardiac death are those who have already suffered a sudden cardiac arrest due to a primary arrhythmia or have experienced a sustained ventricular arrhythmia. As mentioned, the out-of-hospital cardiac arrest population is heterogeneous and noncardiac causes of sudden cardiac arrest (eg, pulmonary embolism, stroke, acute gastrointestinal hemorrhage, overdose) account for ~30% OHCAs resuscitated to hospitalization. These noncardiac conditions would not necessarily convey increased risk of sudden *cardiac* death and are important to exclude on initial in-hospital evaluation. Unfortunately, for multiple reasons (eg, high mortality of neurologic catastrophes, resuscitative strategies targeted toward cardiac causes), survival of SCA patients resuscitated to hospitalization with noncardiac etiology is poor. Thus, arrhythmic sudden cardiac arrest accounts for more than 90% of sudden cardiac arrest survivors.

B. Risk Assessment in Other Populations

An accurate tool for risk stratification of SCA and SCD for individual patients in the general population has remained elusive. Improving risk prediction at the level of individual patients is challenged by heterogeneity of both the underlying population—the individuals at highest risk of SCA/SCD may be easiest to identify yet contribute fewer overall cases than lower risk individuals who are more prevalent—and heterogeneity of the outcome of interest because definitions of sudden cardiac arrest and death often fail to exclude arrests/deaths due to noncardiac causes. To narrow the scope of this issue, efforts have often focused on the study of particular risk factors (eg, cardiac function, electrophysiologic properties, autonomic factors, genetic) and risk prediction in specific populations or disease states (eg, heart failure with reduced ejection fraction, hypertrophic cardiomyopathy). Important populations that have emerged as harboring sufficiently elevated risk for consideration of primary prevention ICD by consensus guidelines include those with moderately to severely reduced LV ejection fraction (based on evidence from randomized control trials), selected patients with hypertrophic cardiomyopathy and high-risk features (based on retrospective data), and other familial or inherited conditions with a high risk of life-threatening ventricular arrhythmias.

Narayan SM, Wang PJ, Daubert JP. New concepts in sudden cardiac arrest to address an intractable epidemic: JACC State-of-the-Art Review. *J Am Coll Cardiol.* 2019;73(1):70–88. [PMID: 30621954]

Evaluation of the Patient at Elevated Risk for SCD

Since the majority of SCDs are caused by ventricular arrhythmia, we will focus this section on evaluation of patients with sudden cardiac arrest or syncope due to documented or suspected ventricular arrhythmia. Although an unstable ventricular arrhythmia leading to sudden cardiac arrest requires expedited evaluation and may have a distinct differential diagnosis affecting prioritization of specific studies (eg, coronary angiography in acute coronary syndrome), the diagnostic tools employed to evaluate stable and lethal ventricular arrhythmia are shared and will be discussed together.

A. Noninvasive Evaluation

The evaluation of a patient with a suspected or documented ventricular arrhythmia begins with a thorough medical history and physical examination. The history of present illness should evaluate symptoms of ventricular arrhythmia including palpitations, chest pain, light-headedness, presyncope, or syncope with careful attention to factors including exercise, ingested substances/caffeine, or emotional. As most ventricular arrhythmias are caused by structural cardiac disease, past medical history should focus on cardiovascular disease and potential proarrhythmic medications should be elucidated. As many ventricular arrhythmias may be due to inherited conditions, a careful family history should be ascertained including any history of frequent miscarriages and unexpected deaths or unexplained drowning which may not have been initially attributed to ventricular arrhythmia. The physical examination should focus on identifying the structural cardiac conditions that underlie ventricular arrhythmias, including evidence of heart failure and valvular disease. Frequent premature ventricular contractions may manifest as an irregular rhythm on auscultation.

The standard 12-lead electrocardiogram may be a useful tool in many scenarios. In the patient with history concerning for prior ventricular arrhythmia, it should be evaluated for any electrocardiographic evidence of structural cardiac disease (eg, left ventricular hypertrophy, prior myocardial infarction, or conduction abnormalities) or specific evidence of inherited arrhythmia disorders as discussed previously (eg, Brugada pattern, prolonged QT interval). In ARVC, a characteristic epsilon wave, a small deflection at the end of the QRS complex in the right precordial leads, may be observed and is caused by post-excitation of right ventricular myocytes. A high-resolution signal-averaged electrocardiogram may be pursued to detect the subtle localized abnormalities of delayed depolarization if not detected on the standard electrocardiogram and there is suspicion for ARVC. In the patient with a stable ventricular tachycardia, the standard electrocardiogram is not only useful to differentiate ventricular tachycardia from supraventricular tachycardias with aberrancy, but also to localize the potential site of exit of the ventricular tachycardia. Some of the features suggestive of ventricular tachycardia include AV dissociation, fusion beats, capture beats, negative or positive concordance throughout the precordial leads, extreme axis deviation (QRS positive in lead aVR and negative in leads 1 + aVF), and several other morphologic criteria as covered in Chapter 13. In the patient who has recently been resuscitated from an episode of VT/VF, the electrocardiogram is critical to identify patients with a ST elevation myocardial infarction who should emergently be considered for catheterization and percutaneous coronary intervention. Lastly, stress testing with an electrocardiogram may be useful for patients with symptoms related to exertion such as CPVT.

Arrhythmias are rarely documented on first examination of a patient with suspected ventricular arrhythmia. In these cases, ambulatory rhythm monitoring may be useful. A variety of ambulatory rhythm monitoring tools ranging from 24-hour Holter monitors, adhesive patch electrocardiographic monitors which often record 1–2 weeks of data, and implantable loop recorders which can monitor over several years are available and can be selected based on the frequency of symptoms.

The two-dimensional echocardiogram can be used to ascertain structural cardiac abnormalities that may serve as the substrate for ventricular tachycardia, including chamber size, wall thickness, valvular abnormalities, coronary artery anomalies, and ventricular function. Cardiac MRI is increasingly used for the evaluation of ventricular arrhythmia. In addition to providing higher resolution of the structural and functional details assessed by the transthoracic echocardiogram, which can be useful in identifying specific cardiomyopathies such as ARVC. Cardiac MRI with late gadolinium enhancement can further characterize myocardial tissue composition, which can be critical in assessing inflammation, fibrosis, scar, and infiltrative diseases which may serve as the substrate for ventricular tachycardia. Coronary CT angiography may be useful to detect anomalous coronary arteries if invasive coronary angiography is not pursued.

Genetic testing should be employed on a case-by-case basis. Consideration of genetic testing should be performed in young patients without structural heart disease and unexplained ventricular arrhythmias or patients with a family history of sudden death. The yield of genetic testing is variable based on the suspected condition. For individuals with high suspicion of inherited cause but negative results, genetic testing may be repeated at regular intervals if the testing platform does not automatically update results of variant calls in tested genes, or to incorporate new genes as research advances.

B. Invasive Evaluation

Invasive coronary angiography may be employed in the evaluation of ventricular arrhythmias. In the context of a resuscitated out-of-hospital cardiac arrest with initial shockable rhythm and ST-segment elevation on ECG after return of spontaneous circulation, cardiac catheterization should be considered immediately with the decision dependent on the patient's neurologic status and other factors that denote a favorable or unfavorable outcome. In comatose patients with OHCA and concern for a **non-ST segment elevation MI,** irrespective of initial rhythm, recent trials suggest no significant difference in survival between early versus delayed cardiac catheterization. Unless a clear nonischemic culprit is found, most patients with cardiac arrest due to ventricular arrhythmia that are stabilized with neurologic recovery should be considered for cardiac catheterization to evaluate for coronary artery disease and potential revascularization. In patients with stable ventricular arrhythmias, ischemia should be considered as an etiology. Noninvasive strategies may be employed for evaluation of alternative etiologies, including CT coronary angiography in patients with low risk for CAD. However, in patients with high risk, or high concern for ischemia (eg, polymorphic VT) invasive coronary angiography should be considered for definitive evaluation.

In select patients in which the aforementioned diagnostic studies do not identify an etiology, an electrophysiologic study may be performed. Evaluation for ventricular arrhythmia by electrophysiologic study employs several maneuvers to induce VT/VF (ie, ventricular overdrive and extrastimulus pacing) to (1) confirm the presence of a ventricular arrhythmia causing symptoms, (2) localize the source of ventricular arrhythmia, and (3) guide further therapy. If VT/VF is successfully induced, catheter ablation of the substrate may be performed or this substrate information can be used to inform alternative antiarrhythmic strategies.

Desch S, Freund A, Akin I, et al. Angiography after out-of-hospital cardiac arrest without ST-segment elevation. *N Engl J Med.* 2021;385(27):2544–2553. [PMID: 34459570]

Lemkes JS, Janssens GN, van der Hoeven NW, et al. Coronary angiography after cardiac arrest without ST-segment elevation. *N Engl J Med.* 2019;380(15):1397–1407. [PMID: 3088305]

Lotfi, A, Klein, LW, Hira, RS, et al. SCAI expert consensus statement on out of hospital cardiac arrest. *Catheter Cardiovasc Interv.* 2020; 96: 844–861. [PMID: 32406999]

Treatment of the Patient at Elevated Risk for SCD

The treatment of patients with elevated risk of SCD can be divided into disease specific treatments (eg, guideline directed medical treatment of heart failure and ischemia), lifestyle changes and medical antiarrhythmic therapies, and consideration of ICD in high-risk populations. Disease specific treatments and non-device based antiarrhythmic strategies may be highly useful in mitigating SCA/SCD risk and mortality and are covered in other chapters. Here we will focus on ICD as it applies to secondary and primary prevention.

A. Implantable Cardioverter-Defibrillators

An **implantable cardioverter-defibrillator (ICD)** has two basic components: the ICD generator and a lead system for pacing and shock delivery. An ICD generator contains sensing circuits, memory storage, capacitors, voltage enhancers, a telemetry module, and a control microprocessor. Current devices have extensive programming options including, antitachycardia pacing (ATP), single- and dual-chamber rate-responsive pacing for bradycardia, biphasic defibrillation waveforms, enhanced arrhythmia detection features, and cardiac resynchronization.

The most important function of an ICD is to detect and terminate life-threatening ventricular arrhythmias. To accomplish this, the device is set to monitor heart rate, and various zones are set to detect ventricular tachycardia or ventricular fibrillation. When a heart rate in these zones is detected, programmable algorithms may be used to exclude supraventricular arrhythmias (eg, waveform matching to the patient's QRS waveform during sinus rhythm). Antitachycardia pacing is often attempted first to terminate ventricular tachycardia, but if this fails, the device will charge and deliver a high-energy shock.

The original systems required a thoracotomy to place epicardial patches, as a result, the implant procedure itself was associated with substantial morbidity and mortality rates. After transvenous leads were developed and the generator size was reduced, transvenous ICDs, typically implanted in the left pectoral region near the clavicle, became standard due to reduced implant morbidity. Recently, subcutaneous ICDs have been developed which feature a generator implanted outside of the left chest cavity with the lead for sensing and defibrillation implanted near the sternum in the subcutaneous tissue plane. While S-ICD systems have notable limitations such as the inability to pace, early evidence suggests that they may have similar efficacy in prevention of SCD as transvenous ICD systems and may be an attractive alternative for those in which transvenous access may present challenges (eg, patients with congenital anomalies, history of prior device infection). Current ICD systems are typically implanted by electrophysiologists using local or monitored anesthesia in a cardiac laboratory.

Initially ICDs were implanted chiefly in patients who did not respond to antiarrhythmic drug therapy. As the limitations of antiarrhythmic drugs became more apparent, ICDs became the primary treatment option. Three large randomized secondary prevention trials compared ICD therapy with antiarrhythmic therapy in survivors of cardiac arrest or hemodynamically unstable ventricular tachycardia (Table 15–2), each demonstrating a significant mortality benefit of ICDs over medical therapy and serving as the basis for guideline recommendations for ICDs as first-line therapy in cardiac arrest survivors due to documented ventricular arrhythmia.

ICD therapy has several notable limitations. Strategies to distinguish between supraventricular and ventricular arrhythmias are not always successful, and inappropriate shocks for supraventricular arrhythmias are not uncommon. An ICD shock results in significant discomfort, and patients who receive multiple shocks often report negative effects on their quality of life. Although several ICD programming strategies (eg, ATP, overdrive pacing, longer VT/VF detection parameters) may decrease shock frequency, antiarrhythmic drugs are often required as adjunctive therapy. Moreover, device issues such as under-sensing of ventricular arrhythmias and hardware failures such as lead fracture or rapid battery depletion remain problems that may lead to multiple invasive procedures to replace faulty components, or in the worst-case scenario directly contribute to death. Though these device complications are presumed to be rare, they are underestimated by the current passive device safety surveillance system by the Food and Drug Administration. Finally, ICD therapy is very costly—estimates of added cost over drug therapy per quality of life-year saved in the secondary prevention trials exceeded $100,000.

Knops RE, Olde Nordkamp LRA, Delnoy PPHM, et al. Subcutaneous or Transvenous Defibrillator Therapy. *N Engl J Med*. 2020;383(6):526–536. [PMID: 32757521]

Rordorf R, Casula M, Pezza L, et al. Subcutaneous versus transvenous implantable defibrillator: An updated meta-analysis. *Heart Rhythm*. 2021;18(3):382–391. [PMID: 33212250]

Tseng ZH, Hayward RM, Clark NM, et al. Sudden death in patients with cardiac implantable electronic devices. *JAMA Intern Med*. 2015;175(8):1342–1350. [PMID: 26098676]

Secondary Prevention for SCD

SCA survivors with a primary ventricular arrhythmic cause that is not transient or reversible (eg, acute myocardial infarction, electrolyte disturbance, or medication effects) and in whom survival greater than 1 year is expected are recommended for secondary prevention ICD, supported by a Class I recommendation by consensus guidelines (or pacemaker in the case of malignant heart block). Notably, secondary prevention does not only apply to cardiac arrest survivors but also patients with sustained spontaneous monomorphic VT or syncope attributed to ventricular arrhythmia. In patients with sustained hemodynamically stable VT related to ischemic heart disease, often revascularization is pursued before ICD consideration.

Primary Prevention for SCD

The sum total of evidence demonstrates the significant mortality benefit of guideline-directed treatment of underlying high-risk cardiac conditions (eg, heart failure, post-myocardial infarction) but not the use of specific antiarrhythmic medications for primary prevention of SCD. β-Adrenergic blocking agents, cholesterol-lowering drugs, and angiotensin-converting enzyme (ACE) inhibitors have been demonstrated to decrease both sudden and nonsudden deaths in patients with heart failure or after myocardial infarction, but these agents do not specifically treat arrhythmias. Also, clinical trials have shown that class I antiarrhythmic drugs did not decrease sudden mortality rates. The most definitive study—the Cardiac Arrhythmia Suppression Trial (CAST)—showed a higher mortality in patients who were randomized to drug therapy targeting suppression of spontaneous ventricular ectopy after myocardial infarction. Notably, in the larger context the CAST trial also serves as an exemplar in clinical medicine of the risks of equating surrogate outcomes (ventricular arrhythmias) with primary outcomes (sudden deaths). Several other large

Table 15–3. Indications and Contraindications for Implantable Cardioverter-Defibrillator Therapy

I. Indications for Secondary Prevention
   A. Documented episode of cardiac arrest due to ventricular fibrillation (VF), not due to a transient or reversible cause
   B. Documented sustained ventricular tachyarrhythmia (VT), either spontaneous or induced by an electrophysiology (EP) study (patients with syncope), not associated with an acute myocardial infarction (MI) and not due to a transient or reversible cause

II. Indications for Primary Prevention
   A. Documented familial or inherited conditions with a high risk of life-threatening VT, such as long QT syndrome or hypertrophic cardiomyopathy
   B. Coronary artery disease with a documented prior MI, a measured left ventricular ejection fraction (LVEF) < 35%, and inducible, sustained VT or VF at EP study. (The EP test must be performed more than 4 weeks after the qualifying MI.)
   C. Documented prior MI and a measured LVEF < 30%
   D. Patients with ischemic dilated cardiomyopathy, documented prior MI, New York Heart Association (NYHA) class II and III heart failure, and measured LVEF < 35%
   E. Patients with nonischemic dilated cardiomyopathy, NYHA class II and III heart failure, and measured LVEF < 35%, on optimal medical therapy > 3 months
   F. Require a patient shared decision-making interaction prior to ICD implantation

III. Exclusions
   A. NYHA classification IV without CRT
   B. Cardiogenic shock or symptomatic hypotension while in a stable baseline rhythm
   C. Had a coronary artery bypass graft or percutaneous transluminal coronary angioplasty within past 3 months
   D. Had an enzyme positive MI within past 40 days
   E. Clinical symptoms or findings that would make them a candidate for coronary revascularization
   F. Any disease, other than cardiac disease (eg, cancer, uremia, liver failure), associated with a likelihood of survival less than 1 year
   G. Patients must not have irreversible brain damage from preexisting cerebral disease

Modified from Medicare National Coverage Determinations Decision memo 02/15/2018: https://www.cms.gov/medicare-coverage-database/view/ncacal-decision-memo.aspx?proposed=N&NCAId=288

placebo-controlled studies—the European and Canadian Amiodarone Myocardial Infarction Trials (EMIAT and CAMIAT) and the Sudden Cardiac Death–Heart Failure Trial (SCD-HeFT)—also did not show any benefit for empiric amiodarone in high-risk populations. Cardiac resynchronization therapy in patients with advanced heart failure and a wide QRS has been shown to improve NYHA functional class, decrease hospitalizations, and reduce sudden and non-sudden cardiac deaths.

Randomized trials have indicated that ICD therapy for primary prevention of sudden death is effective in high-risk populations. The most definitive primary prevention trials used entry criteria based primarily on left ventricular ejection fraction (< 30% or 35%) and NYHA functional class with relative risk reductions in a range similar to those observed in the secondary prevention trials (20–30%). Summary data from notable clinical trials are shown in Table 15–2, and the current indications for ICD implantation accepted by the Centers for Medicare and Medicaid Services (CMS) are shown in Table 15–3. Individuals considered for primary prevention ICD should be on optimal guideline-directed medical therapy for their underlying cardiac conditions and have a reasonable expectation of survival at least 1 year after implant. Several studies failed to show benefit in patients who received an ICD either at the time of surgical coronary revascularization or within 40 days of an acute myocardial infarction. Therefore, current CMS guidelines (see Table 15–3) exclude implantation of ICDs within 40 days of myocardial infarction if no revascularization was performed, and within 3 months of stenting or surgical bypass.

The recent VEST (Vest Prevention of Early Sudden Death) Trial addressed the paradox of a high sudden death rate early after myocardial infarction among patients with a low ejection fraction but lack of benefit of ICDs in this setting, by randomizing patients to a wearable cardioverter–defibrillator in this vulnerable early period after infarction versus guideline-based medical therapy alone. The trial did not show a benefit with the device (relative risk, 0.67; 95% confidence interval, 0.37 to 1.21; P = 0.18) for the primary outcome of arrhythmic death (a composite of sudden death or death from ventricular arrhythmia). However, several factors likely contributed to the negative result—the trial was likely underpowered and the wear time of the device was low in the intervention arm. In an as-treated analysis, significantly fewer deaths occurred when patients were wearing the device than when they were not, therefore some experts still offer the wearable cardioverter–defibrillator in motivated high-risk patients.

Olgin JE, Pletcher MJ, Vittinghoff E, et al. Wearable cardioverter-defibrillator after myocardial infarction. *N Engl J Med.* 2018; 379(13):1205–1215. [PMID: 30280654]

16 Syncope

Bert Vandenberk, MD, PhD
Carlos A. Morillo, MD

ESSENTIALS OF DIAGNOSIS

- Sudden, unexpected, and transient loss of consciousness.
- Spontaneous and full recovery.
- Most common cause is neurally mediated reflex response (vasovagal).
- Cardiac syncope has high-risk morbidity and mortality.

General Considerations

Syncope is defined as a transient loss of consciousness (TLOC) with a common pathophysiologic mechanism associated with the reduction in cerebral blood flow leading to cerebral hypoperfusion. Syncope is common, with a similar incidence in men and women. The lifetime cumulative incidence of syncope is ≥ 35%, with peak prevalence of the first episode between ages 10 and 35. Incidence increases with age, especially after 70 years, and is bimodal with peaks at 20 and 80 years. It is estimated to account for 1–3% of emergency department (ED) annual visits and up to 6% of hospital admissions in North America and around the world.

Although most potential causes of syncope are benign and self-limited with a low rate of adverse events, some are associated with significant morbidity and mortality including cardiac arrhythmias and structural heart disease. Although many patients never experience a recurrence, a significant proportion do, and such recurrences can be extremely unpredictable. Management strategies are variable and often inefficient and costly.

Pathophysiology & Etiology

Syncope may be classified as reflex-mediated, orthostatic hypotension, and cardiac. Nonsyncopal causes of TLOC are always in the differential diagnosis because of obvious similarity in clinical presentation (Table 16–1). The most common cause, irrespective of age, sex, or comorbidity, is vasovagal syncope. The second most common cause is cardiac syncope. Carotid sinus hypersensitivity–associated syncope, adenosine-sensitive syncope, and orthostatic hypotension are rare causes of syncope in those under the age of 40.

A. Neurally Mediated Reflex Syncope

A heterogeneous group of disorders consisting of vasovagal syncope, situational syncope, carotid sinus hypersensitivity, and others is generally classified as reflex or neurally mediated syncope (NMS). Although the provoking stimuli may differ, they share a common final pathway characterized by hypotension and vasodilatation with relative or absolute bradycardia. This is likely related to an abrupt withdrawal of sympathetic tone and an increase in parasympathetic tone. Orthostatic stress is often the main trigger for NMS; however, NMS can occur in the absence of orthostatic stress in a supine position. The precise mechanism remains elusive, and a combination of central and peripheral mechanisms involving baroreceptor response and peripheral control of vasoconstriction is the most likely explanation. Strong or unexpected emotions or physical pain can also trigger NMS by poorly understood mechanisms. Some situational syncope appears to be triggered by distension of hollow viscera, including the esophagus, rectum, and bladder, which in turn activates sensory-proprioceptive or specialized afferent nerves resulting in syncope. NMS is primarily a benign form of syncope that can often be treated with patient education and avoidance of the precipitant factors. Approximately 30%, however, have recurrent episodes that may result in injuries and significantly impaired quality of life. Several therapies (discussed later) are available for patients who require intervention.

Adenosine-sensitive syncope is a rare subtype of reflex syncope that manifests typically in patients with older age (> 60 years) and otherwise negative work-up, including normal ECG and head-up tilt testing. Clinical diagnosis is suspected in elderly patients with abrupt sudden onset syncope not

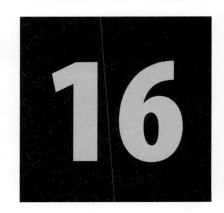

Table 16–1. The Causes of Loss of Consciousness and Their Prevalence

Syncope	Causes	Prevalence (%)
Reflex-mediated	• Vasovagal syncope • Situational syncope (cough, micturating, etc) • Adenosine-sensitive syncope • Carotid sinus syndrome	14 3 3 1
Orthostatic hypotension	• Primary autonomic dysfunction • Secondary autonomic dysfunction (drugs/diabetes/amyloid) • Acute massive hemorrhage • Addison disease	11
Cardiac	• Tachyarrhythmia and bradyarrhythmia • Hemodynamic/valvular (eg, hypertrophic obstructive cardiomyopathy, aortic stenosis, pulmonary hypertension, or massive pulmonary embolism)	14 3
Nonsyncope		
Seizures		7
Drop attacks		
Fall		
Vertebrobasilar transient ischemic attack	Left subclavian steal syndrome	
Metabolic	Medication/drug overdose Hypoglycemia Hypo-/hypernatremia Hypoxia/hypercapnia	7
Pseudosyncope		1

preceded by any prodromal symptoms and without history of prior typical vasovagal syncope, often presenting with trauma.

Finally, carotid sinus hypersensitivity–associated syncope typically occurs in the elderly, classically with neck stretching, but most often without obvious triggers, frequently presenting clinically as abrupt syncope with no prodrome. Clinical diagnosis is often one of exclusion or triggered by the reproduction of syncope associated with significant bradycardia and asystole by carotid sinus massage both in the supine and upright postures.

B. Orthostatic Hypotension

The common denominator in orthostatic hypotension is insufficient peripheral vasoconstriction (physiologic or pathologic) in response to orthostatic stress. Amongst patients with orthostatic hypotension, three different variants have been described. Initial orthostatic hypotension: defined as an immediate and transient drop in blood pressure within 15 seconds of standing of more than 40 mm Hg in systolic blood pressure and/or more than 20 mm Hg in diastolic blood pressure, which recovers within 30 seconds to 1 minute. Classical orthostatic hypotension is arbitrarily defined as a drop in systolic blood pressure of more than 20 mm Hg or diastolic blood pressure of more than 10 mm Hg within 3 minutes of standing. Delayed orthostatic hypotension is defined as symptomatic orthostatic hypotension occurring beyond 3 minutes of standing; however, its clinical significance remains uncertain and may reflect early forms of sympathetic adrenergic failure. Acute hemorrhage or excessive diuresis and rarely, Addison disease can lead to orthostatic hypotension. Autonomic insufficiency is frequently related to or aggravated by medication use, advancing age, or diabetes mellitus. Primary autonomic dysfunction is observed in Parkinson disease, Lewy body dementia, multisystem atrophy, or pure autonomic failure. Orthostatic hypotension may also trigger reflex-mediated syncope.

C. Cardiac Syncope

1. Tachycardia and bradycardia—Cardiac syncope is most often arrhythmic. Syncope during tachycardia is related to heart rate but modulated by the specific arrhythmia (supraventricular/ventricular), preload conditions, posture, integrity of cardiac autonomic reflexes, left ventricular function, and adequacy of vascular adaptation. Transient decreased cardiac output during ventricular or supraventricular tachycardias results when the ventricular rate is fast enough to decrease diastole significantly and thus decrease ventricular filling (preload). Simultaneous peripheral vasodepressor response leads to hypotension, and it frequently plays a role in precipitating syncope in subjects with supraventricular arrhythmias. Ventricular tachycardia (VT) occurs most frequently in patients with structural heart disease, particularly coronary artery disease with previous myocardial infarction or acute coronary syndrome. However, younger patients without evidence of structural heart disease may present with exercise-induced syncope and VT that is usually associated with right ventricular outflow tract VT. In the presence of ischemic heart disease or congenital channelopathies, VT is frequently a precursor of ventricular fibrillation, manifesting as sudden cardiac death. Symptoms and prognosis depend on the degree of underlying myocardial dysfunction and the rate and duration of the arrhythmia. Torsade de Pointes is a specific subtype of polymorphic VT classically known to cause syncope that can also present as sudden cardiac death. It is important to understand the reversible conditions that can precipitate these rhythm disorders. The congenital long QT syndrome can manifest with Torsade de Pointes triggered by exercise or pronounced bradycardia. An important proportion of Torsade de Pointes cases are due to acquired long QT syndromes triggered by drugs or drug-drug interactions (class Ia and III antiarrhythmics, macrolides, certain antihistamines, and tricyclic antidepressants), electrolyte abnormalities (hypomagnesemia, hypokalemia, and hypocalcemia), myocardial ischemia, and central nervous system disorders. Torsade de Pointes is typically initiated by a short-long-short sequence due to short-coupled premature beats and compensatory pauses during bradycardia that increase repolarization heterogeneity and trigger Torsade de pointes.

Supraventricular arrhythmias are more likely to cause palpitations and presyncope than true syncope. Supraventricular tachycardias rarely manifest initially as syncope. All atrial arrhythmias (fibrillation, flutter, and atrial tachycardia) and reentrant supraventricular tachycardias (atrioventricular [AV] nodal reentrant tachycardia and AV reentrant tachycardias associated with accessory pathways) have the potential to manifest with syncope; however, in the event of presenting with syncope, this is generally triggered by activation of neurally mediated reflexes during tachycardia. Elimination of the tachycardia usually prevents recurrence of syncope.

Bradycardia leads to symptoms when the heart rate is slow enough to prevent a compensatory increase in stroke volume, failing to maintain blood pressure and cerebral perfusion. Sinus node dysfunction (sinus exit block, sick sinus syndrome, extreme sinus bradycardia, or sinus arrest) or AV block (second- or third-degree block) may cause bradycardia directly or after tachycardia termination (tachy-brady). Periods of ventricular asystole as short as 5 seconds can cause syncope. Mobitz II second-degree AV block with paroxysms of several consecutive P waves that fail to conduct to the ventricle, known as Stokes-Adams syndrome, can manifest clinically with abrupt syncope frequently not associated with any triggers or warning symptoms. Medications, such as calcium channel blockers, digoxin, β-blockers (including optical formulations), sympatholytics, and antiarrhythmic drugs, can also cause syncope related to bradycardia. Finally, pacemaker malfunction, including a system problem, battery failure, or lead fracture, can lead to syncope.

2. Cardiac output abnormalities—Structural obstructive lesions of the heart can critically reduce cerebral blood flow. Exertional symptoms are common with obstructive lesions because cardiac output does not rise normally with exercise and cerebral perfusion is not maintained. Obstruction of the left ventricular outflow may occur with severe aortic valve stenosis, mitral valve stenosis, left atrial myxoma, prosthetic aortic or mitral valve dysfunction, and hypertrophic obstructive cardiomyopathy. Lesions that obstruct flow through the right side of the heart include right atrial myxoma, pulmonary stenosis, tricuspid stenosis, pulmonary hypertension, and pulmonary emboli. Non-exertional syncope can be the result of pulmonary emboli (hypoxia and obstruction of right ventricular outflow) and aortic dissection with pericardial tamponade, which impedes right ventricular filling and decreases cardiac output. Of note, these are all rare causes of syncope, and usually the diagnosis is one of exclusion, with the hallmark being syncope that is either abrupt with no warning or triggered during exercise.

Other possible causes of cardiogenic syncope include low-output states (ie, with either ischemic or dilated cardiomyopathy), which can sometimes be further exacerbated if the patient is taking vasoactive medications, as is common in those who have these disorders.

Saklani P, Krahn A, Klein G. Syncope. *Circulation*. 2013; 127(12):1330–1339. [PMID: 23529534]

Task Force for the Diagnosis and Management of Syncope, et al. Guidelines for the diagnosis and management of syncope (version 2018). *Eur Heart J*. 2018;39(21):1883–1948. [PMID: 29562304]

Clinical Findings

The history and physical examination remain the pillar for the diagnosis of syncope. The initial clinical evaluation establishes the cause of syncope or suggests the necessary diagnostic pathway in up to 85% of the patients in whom a diagnosis will eventually be reached. An account by a witness is often extremely helpful and worthy of pursuit. Witnesses may be able to provide information regarding the patient's complaints just prior to the event and observations during both the event (ie, pulse rate and rhythm, color, presence of spontaneous breathing, seizures, or seizure-like activity) and recovery.

The main challenge in assessing syncope patients is defining the risk of recurrence and promptly identifying subjects at risk of serious adverse cardiovascular outcomes, primarily sudden cardiac death.

A. Symptoms & Signs

- The circumstance: NMS is classically triggered by pain, medical procedures, prolonged standing, and hot or crowded environments. Syncope during cough, micturition, defecation, or swallowing suggests situational syncope, whereas syncope with shaving or neck extension suggests carotid sinus hypersensitivity syndrome. Syncope during exertion is generally worrisome and considered a marker of high risk. In contrast, syncope shortly after exertion is primarily related to NMS.
- The prodrome: NMS is classically associated with a prodrome of warmth, diaphoresis, nausea, ringing in the ears, tunnel vision, or abdominal pain. A thorough history is essential because, not infrequently, these warning symptoms are brief and often dismissed by the patient. Of note, NMS in the elderly often lacks significant warning, in part because retrograde amnesia is common, and patients may present with falls and injuries instead of syncope. An abrupt or very brief or absent prodrome is more typical of cardiac syncope. Syncope preceded by palpitations usually suggests tachyarrhythmia but is often

nonspecific. For clinicians in the ED, overlap between seizures and syncope is common, and TLOC associated with déjá vu, jamais vu, sensory aura, olfactory hallucinations, preoccupation, or behavior changes and lack of typical prodrome suggests seizure.

- During TLOC: Syncope involves brief TLOC, generally less than 5 minutes and typically less than 30 seconds. Pallor or diaphoresis suggests NMS. Cyanosis suggests cardiac syncope. Unusual posturing, head turning, tongue biting, and rhythmic limb jerking are more consistent with seizures. Syncope can cause seizure-like motor activity, and seizures may cause arrhythmia. Psychogenic syncope (pseudosyncope) may result in atypical features such as resistance to attempts to open the eyes or bizarre movements or inconsistencies.
- The postdrome: Syncope attributable to transient bradycardia or tachycardia is generally associated with relatively rapid recovery of mentation, whereas NMS frequently results in more protracted symptoms of fatigue, nausea, and somnolence from minutes to hours. Prolonged fatigue after the episode, often hours in duration, is more typical of NMS. TLOC involving postictal confusion and transient neurologic deficit suggests seizure.
- Associated cardiac disease including prior myocardial infarction, history of arrhythmias, valvular disease, and heart failure may be present.
- Family history of syncope, unexplained "seizures," or untimely sudden cardiac death may also be present.
- Medications (prescription or over-the-counter) that can affect blood pressure and heart rhythm should be noted and frequently de-escalated.
- Systematic assessment of clinical and electrocardiographic (ECG) features may be implemented in the ED to identify high-risk individuals and rule out cardiac arrhythmias. The Calgary Syncope Score may be a useful initial approach in patients who are under 60 years with no clinical evidence of structural heart disease (Table 16–2).

Table 16–2. Calgary Syncope Score

Points score for vasovagal syncope in healthy people < 60 years old	
	Points
For cardiac syncope	
Bifascicular block, asystole, supraventricular tachycardia, or diabetes	−5
Cyanosis noted by bystander	−4
Age of first syncope > 35 years	−3
Remembers something about the spell	−2
For vasovagal syncope	
Presyncope or syncope with prolong sitting or standing	+1
Sweating or warm feeling before the spell	+2
Presyncope or syncope with pain or medical procedure	+3

Vasovagal syncope is defined by total score > −3.

B. Physical Examination

Patients need a complete focused cardiac, peripheral vascular, and neurologic examination. The physical examination, although less useful, should be focused on the following:

- Heart rate (< 50 bpm) and pulse regularity
- Blood pressure—orthostatic hypotension: Assessed in the supine position followed by active standing for 3 minutes, preferably using a manual sphygmomanometer (fall in systolic blood pressure of ≥ 20 mm Hg or diastolic blood pressure of ≥ 10 mm Hg, or systolic blood pressure of < 90 mm Hg)
- Heart failure signs
- Valvular heart disease
- Focal neurologic deficit
- Carotid sinus massage is reasonable in patients older than 40 years presenting with syncope of unknown etiology after initial evaluation. Contraindications include myocardial infarction or stroke within 3 months and the presence of carotid bruits. Continuous ECG monitoring and ideally beat-to-beat blood pressure monitoring is necessary. A positive response associated with syncope or severe presyncope is characterized by an asystolic pause of ≥ 3 seconds or fall in systolic blood pressure of ≥ 50 mm Hg. This maneuver should be performed both in the supine and upright positions.
- Arm flexion and extension may be used to provoke symptoms of subclavian steal syndrome.
- Neck flexion and extension may elicit the symptoms of vertebrobasilar insufficiency.
- Open-mouthed hyperventilation for 1–3 minutes may elicit symptoms described in the history.

C. Risk Stratification

Risk stratification is mandatory at the initial evaluation to avoid unnecessary testing and admission. Risk stratification identifies subjects with repeated syncopal events and identifies subjects at risk of adverse cardiovascular outcomes, especially sudden cardiac death. This is particularly important because the peak of cardiovascular deaths is observed during the first month after presentation, whereas late adverse events are caused by associated cardiovascular diseases rather than by mechanisms of syncope.

The Canadian Syncope Risk Score showed excellent risk differentiation for 30-day serious adverse events after disposition of the emergency department. The risk score was derived from a prospective study including more than 4000 patients aged 16 or older presenting with syncope at the emergency department and is based on clinical evaluation, troponin levels, ECG, and the diagnosis in the emergency department. The risk of serious adverse events for the minimal score was 0.4%, whereas the maximal score was associated with 84% risk. A risk-based approach to the syncopal patient is shown in Figure 16–1. This approach focuses on first determining the safety of the patient and then establishing a diagnosis.

Hatoum T, Sheldon R. A practical approach to investigation of syncope. *Can J Cardiol.* 2014;30(6):671–674. [PMID: 24882540]

Thiruganasambandamoorthy V, Kwong K, Wells GA. Development of the Canadian Syncope Risk Score to predict serious adverse events after emergency department assessment of syncope. *CMAJ.* 2016;188(12):E289–E298. [PMID: 27378464]

Zimmermann T, de Lavallaz JF, Nestelberger T, et al. International validation of the Canadian syncope risk score. *Ann Int Med.* 2022;175(6):783–794. [PMID: 35467933] https://doi.org/10.7326/M21-2313

Diagnostic Studies

A. Noninvasive Diagnostic Investigations

1. Electrocardiography—A 12-lead ECG should always be part of the routine clinical evaluation of syncope. A normal 12-lead ECG generally indicates a good prognosis, with very low incidence of cardiac adverse events. Given the fact that syncope has an episodic nature that is unpredictable, it is rare that the ECG provides a diagnosis. A systematic approach to ECG interpretation in the context of syncope should always focus on rhythm, evidence of preexcitation, QRS complex morphology (bundle branch block), QT interval, and ST-T–wave changes. However, certain findings will suggest the possibility of a specific diagnosis, for example, Q waves suggestive of previous myocardial infarction correlate with the degree of ventricular dysfunction and likelihood of VT and sudden cardiac death. The ECG or rhythm strips recorded by paramedics, the ED, or hospital ward led to a specific diagnosis in about 10% of patients.

2. Echocardiography—Echocardiography is useful for assessing the severity of the underlying cardiac disease and for risk stratification in patients with unexplained syncope with a positive cardiac history or an abnormal ECG.

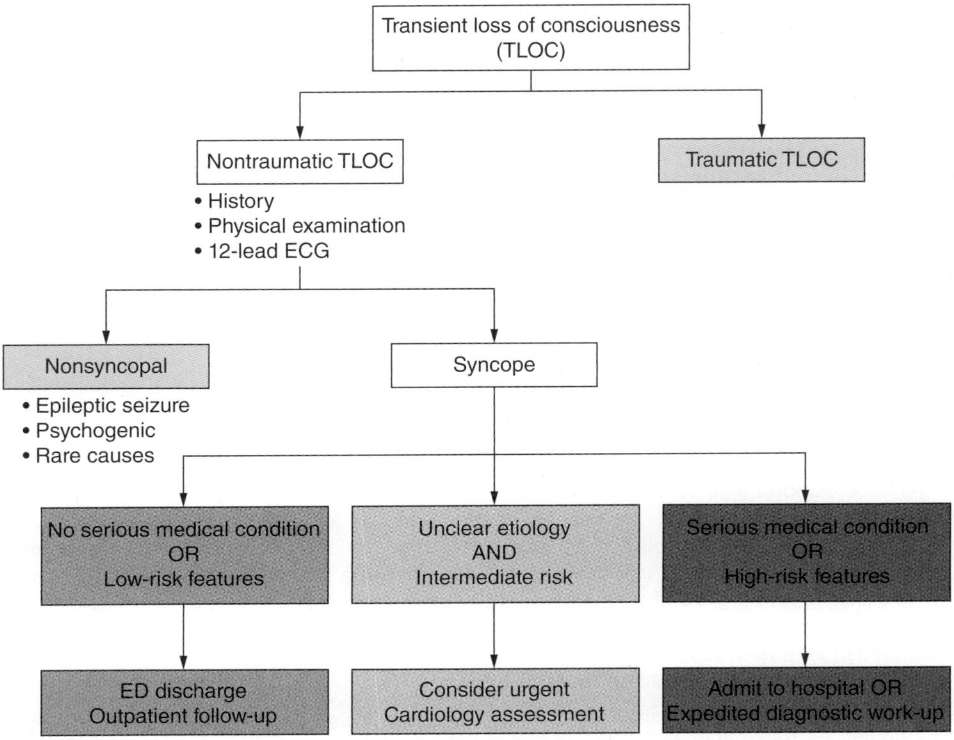

▲ **Figure 16–1.** A risk-based approach to the syncopal patient. (Reproduced with permission from Hatoum T, Sheldon R. A practical approach to investigation of syncope. *Can J Cardiol.* 2014;30(6):671–674.)

Echocardiographic findings that may be related with syncope include aortic stenosis, hypertrophic obstructive cardiomyopathy, global or localized contractility abnormalities, right ventricular dysfunction or enlargement suggestive of right ventricular arrhythmogenic cardiomyopathy, and pulmonary hypertension. Echocardiography plays an important role in risk stratification based on left ventricular dysfunction, helping the physician in assessing the patient's prognosis and the necessity for further invasive evaluation or implantable cardioverter-defibrillator management. Unsuspected findings on echocardiography are reported in 5–10% of unselected patients with syncope.

3. Exercise stress testing—Exercise-induced syncope is infrequent. Exercise testing should be performed in patients who have experienced episodes of syncope during or shortly after exertion, suggesting long QT syndrome, catecholaminergic polymorphic VT, ischemia, and other disorders. Careful ECG and blood pressure monitoring should be performed during both the testing and recovery phase because syncope can occur during or immediately after exercise. Exertional hypotension may occur because of underlying structural heart disease, chronotropic incompetence, or severe conduction disease resulting in AV block with increased atrial rates. Ventricular arrhythmias may be provoked with exercise, usually originate in the right ventricular outflow tract, and are easily approachable by invasive treatment. Hypotension and bradycardia at the termination of exercise can be diagnostic of reflex vasomotor instability. In addition, other forms of stress testing in those who cannot exercise may detect myocardial ischemia—a potential substrate for ventricular arrhythmias. In general, exercise-induced syncope is a high-risk feature and should be approached promptly.

4. Ambulatory monitoring and invasive long-term implantable cardiac monitoring—ECG monitoring of varying durations and types is one of the main diagnostic strategies in the assessment of syncope in the hope of obtaining symptom–rhythm correlation during the syncopal episode. Available technologies include ambulatory ECG (AECG) monitors, external loop recorders, event recorders, and implantable cardiac monitors. Overall, the diagnostic yield of each of these technologies is highly dependent on the frequency of syncope. AECG has a low diagnostic yield of around 5%, but it is important to remember that *only* rhythm alterations correlated with severe presyncope or syncope should be considered when ascribing an etiologic cause. External and event loop recorders have reportedly improved diagnostic yield to about 35% and are indicated in patients with a frequency of syncope of at least one episode a month due to the limited long-term capabilities and patient tolerability of these devices. Finally, implantable cardiac monitors are available and have the advantage of long-term recordings and should be indicated in patients with sporadic episodes (one episode every 6 months) or in those in whom exhaustive investigations remain undiagnostic. Some have proposed early use of these devices with the argument of having a higher diagnostic yield and promptly ruling out a cardiac arrhythmia. However, the cost of a first-line implantable monitor strategy may be untenable in some healthcare systems.

From the practical perspective, requesting one of the previously mentioned external ambulatory monitoring devices is reasonable in patients with a frequency of syncope of at least once a month, keeping in mind the low diagnostic yield of most of these devices. In our practice, a patient presenting with unexplained syncope under the age of 50 years with no ECG changes or evidence of structural heart disease is more likely to have a reflex-mediated cause than an arrhythmic cause of syncope. Those with either abrupt or no prodrome, some ECG features that can be as nonspecific as bradycardia, intraventricular conduction disorders, or Q waves should undergo one of the monitoring modalities described earlier.

5. Head-up tilt test—In the past decade, the routine use of head-up tilt testing for the assessment of unexplained syncope has markedly decreased. This is mostly due to our improved ability to identify vasovagal and other reflex-mediated causes of syncope which are the most frequent cause of syncope. The diagnostic yield of head-up tilt testing after appropriate application of the guidelines is approximately 80% in patients with unexplained syncope. Therefore, tilt testing may be most useful in patients with intermediate risk of NMS in whom clinical presentation is not typical, for example, elderly patients with limited or no prodromes. The response to tilt testing is classified according to the modified Vasovagal Syncope International Study (VASIS) classification as a cardio-inhibitory response with or without asystole, a vasodepressor response, or a mixed response. Further, tilt testing is a useful tool to characterize patients with orthostatic hypotension, particularly if beat-to-beat blood pressure and heart rate measurements are available. Additional provocative testing may unmask adenosine-sensitive syncope.

6. Other testing—Routine laboratory tests (blood counts and chemistries) rarely reveal useful diagnostic information. Unless specifically suggested by the history and physical examination, routine lab tests are not recommended in the evaluation of syncope. Likewise, electroencephalogram, computed tomography, and magnetic resonance imaging studies are of little use in patients whose history is not suggestive of a neurologic cause of TLOC. These tests may be considered only in patients whose neurologic history and physical examination are suggestive of seizure or other neurologic conditions.

B. Invasive Electrophysiologic Study

Today, electrophysiologic studies (EPS) have few indications in the overall assessment of the patient with recurrent syncope. In brief, according to the most recent guidelines an EPS is indicated in a setting of asymptomatic sinus bradycardia for suspected sinus arrest to assess the sinus node recovery time, bifascicular bundle branch block to assess the His-Ventricular interval for impending AV block, and suspected tachycardia. An EPS is only indicated in cases of intermediate risk in which either a bradyarrhythmia or tachyarrhythmia is suspected after routine thorough investigation. In these settings, the diagnostic yield of EPS is low, approximately 10%. In the case of tachyarrhythmia as a potential cause of syncope, reentrant supraventricular tachycardias and ventricular outflow tract tachycardia can be mapped and ablated with a high success rate and low complication rates. For conduction disorders, the negative predictive value based on older studies with intermittent ECG monitoring was approximately 93%. However, a recent meta-analysis including studies with continuous monitoring using implantable devices estimated a negative predictive value of 71%. Therefore, EPS should only be recommended in specific cases with the understanding that the diagnostic yield is low.

Barón-Esquivias G, Martín AJD, Castillo AMD, Quintanilla M, Solís CB, Morillo CA. Head-up tilt test diagnostic yield in syncope diagnosis. *J Electrocardiol.* 2020;63:46–50. [PMID: 33075618]

Brignole M, Menozzi C, Rosso AD, et al. New classification of haemodynamics of vasovagal syncope: beyond the VASIS classification. Analysis of the pre-syncopal phase of the tilt test without and with nitroglycerin challenge. Vasovagal Syncope International Study. *Europace.* 2000;2(1):66–76. [PMID: 11225598]

Giada F, Bartoletti A. Value of ambulatory electrocardiographic monitoring in syncope. *Cardiol Clin.* 2015;33(3):361–366. [PMID: 26115822]

Sheldon R, Lei LY, Solbiati M, et al. Electrophysiology studies for predicting atrioventricular block in patients with syncope: A systematic review and meta-analysis. *Heart Rhythm.* 2021;18(8):1310–1317. [PMID: 33887450]

Differential Diagnosis

A. Seizures

Seizures are rarely a cause of syncope, although they are frequently considered in the differential diagnosis. Epilepsy and seizures can cause TLOC; patients are nonresponsive, fall, and later have amnesia. This only occurs in tonic, clonic, tonic-clonic, and atonic generalized seizures. In absence epilepsy in children and partial complex epilepsy in adults, consciousness is altered, not lost; these patients remain upright during attacks, in contrast to TLOC. History of loss of bowel or bladder tone, witnessed tonic-clonic movements, a preceding aura, and slow recovery with prolonged postictal state strongly suggest seizure. Interestingly, myoclonic movements may occur with syncope due to cerebral hypoxia (from cerebral anoxia or ischemia), and this can be misinterpreted as syncope by eyewitnesses. A practical score to discriminate between syncope and seizure has been reported in the literature (Table 16–3).

Table 16–3. Diagnostic Questions to Determine Whether Loss of Consciousness Is a Result of Seizures or Syncope

Question	Points (if yes)
At times, do you wake with a cut tongue after your spells?	2
At times, do you have a sense of déjá vu or jamais vu before your spells?	1
At times, is emotional stress associated with losing consciousness?	
Has anyone ever noted your head turning during a spell?	1
Has anyone ever noted that you are unresponsive, have unusual posturing, or have jerking limbs during your spells or have no memory of your spells afterward?	1
Has anyone ever noted that you are confused after a spell?	1
Have you ever had lightheaded spells?	−2
At times, do you sweat before your spells?	−2
Is prolonged sitting or standing associated with your spells?	−2

The patient has seizures if the point score is ≥ 1 and syncope if the point score is < 1.

B. Psychiatric Disorders & Pseudosyncope

Syncope and psychiatry interact in two ways. Various psychiatric drugs can contribute to syncope through orthostatic hypotension and by prolonging the QT interval, increasing the risk of Torsade de Pointes. The second interaction concerns "functional" attacks. The term *functional* is used for conditions that resemble known somatic conditions without a somatic explanation being found and with a presumed psychological mechanism. Two types of patients must be included in the differential diagnosis of TLOC. In both, patients are nonresponsive and do not show normal motor control, implying that falls are common. In one type, gross movements resemble epileptic seizures; these attacks have been described as pseudoepilepsy, nonepileptic seizures, psychogenic nonepileptic seizures, and nonepileptic attack disorder. In the other type, there are no gross movements, so the attacks resemble syncope or longer lasting loss of consciousness. These attacks have been described as psychogenic syncope, pseudosyncope, syncope of psychiatric origin, and medically unexplained syncope. Note that the latter two terms are inconsistent with the definition of syncope because there is no cerebral hypoperfusion in functional TLOC. The frequency of such attacks is unknown and varies with the setting. Functional TLOC mimicking epilepsy occurs in 15–20% of cases in specialized epilepsy clinics and in up to 6% in syncope clinics.

C. Metabolic Disorders & Hypoxia

Any condition that starves the brain of essential nutrients (eg, electrolytes, oxygen, glucose) or markedly changes pH can cause somnolence or coma. These conditions are not usually associated with spontaneous recovery (ie, without intervention); they tend to be longer lasting, and treatment is directed at the underlying abnormality. Hypoglycemia in outpatient diabetics, resulting from excessive insulin injection, can cause somnolence with a normal pulse and blood pressure; it is rapidly correctable with glucose.

D. Cerebrovascular Insufficiency & Extracranial Vascular Disease

Although altered states of consciousness are known to occur with cerebral vascular events, true syncope is an uncommon presentation. Diseases of the intracranial and extracranial vessels can cause strokes and transient ischemic attacks, but rarely syncope. Focal neurologic defects found during the physical examination are clues to the presence of cerebrovascular insufficiency, and differential peripheral arterial pressures or bruits suggest extracranial arterial disease. The most involved extracranial arteries are the vertebrobasilar (occlusion), carotids (occlusion, emboli), aortic arch (dissection), and subclavian artery.

Treatment

Syncope treatment goals are focused on first reducing recurrence, followed by diminishing the risk of injury and improving quality of life. Identifying patients at risk of sudden death is always the challenge and goal when managing patients with recurrent syncope. Treatment should be directed at correction of the underlying cause when possible. However, preventive or curative treatment may be incomplete or not possible in some cases. Thus, risk stratification plays a key role in managing syncope since it allows the clinician to select populations at high risk of adverse cardiovascular outcomes and sudden cardiac death who will benefit from effective therapies such as permanent pacemakers, ICDs, and cardiovascular interventions that decrease mortality and prevent comorbid associated diseases.

A specific mechanistic preventive measure remains elusive in most cases of reflex-mediated syncope or orthostatic hypotension. Accordingly, treatment necessitates multiple measures that may, together, reduce frequency and associated morbidity. Finally, elderly patients have multiple causes of syncope and competing comorbidities that warrant treatment, making treatment of this population particularly challenging.

A. Neurally Mediated Reflex Syncope

1. Lifestyle changes—Lifestyle modification constitutes the foundation of NMS management. Patients should avoid triggers where possible, including severe dehydration, prolonged standing, pain, and emotional stress. Where feasible, increased fluid and salt intake are useful in decreasing the frequency and severity of events. Minimal alcohol intake is recommended, as well as avoiding medications with diuretic or vasodilator properties when possible. Finally, enhancing fitness and moderate exercise training may be beneficial.

2. Physical counterpressure maneuvers—When clear prodromal symptoms are present, the primary objective is usually to sit or lie down to avoid injury. One randomized controlled trial showed that counterpressure maneuvers including leg crossing, squatting, and tensing of legs and buttocks reduced the recurrence of syncope by 39% compared with conventional treatment. From the practical perspective, these maneuvers are recommended in younger patients but not older patients because older patients may have gait and other stability problems.

3. Pharmacologic treatment—Many agents have been prescribed for NMS, but results are disappointing. Conflicting data from small, short-term, nonrandomized, or uncontrolled trials abound, with a paucity of high-quality, randomized, placebo-controlled trial data.

A. β-BLOCKERS—Small, randomized trials of β-blockers have mostly been negative. The Prevention of Syncope Trial (POST I) was a relatively large multicenter, randomized, double blind, placebo-controlled study of β-blocker use in NMS that showed no benefit in reducing the frequency of syncopal events. However, a subgroup that was older than 42 years seemed to benefit, and a recent pooled analysis has shown that metoprolol may reduce syncope recurrence in those age $\geq$ 42 years by 48%. We use β-blockers, primarily metoprolol at a maximum dose of 100 mg twice a day, in patients older than 50 years with typical features of vasovagal syncope.

B. FLUDROCORTISONE—Fludrocortisone is a mineralocorticoid analogue that expands plasma volume and sensitizes peripheral α-adrenergic receptors, augmenting vasoconstriction. A small randomized, placebo-controlled trial of fludrocortisone and salt in pediatric NMS found it to be ineffective. However, the Second Prevention of Syncope Trial (POST II) trial showed that after 1 year of fludrocortisone therapy, the syncope rate was lower in the fludrocortisone group in both the intent-to-treat and on-treatment analyses, and a significant risk reduction was achieved when patients received the full dose of 0.1 mg twice a day. We use fludrocortisone in patients with recurrent episodes (ie, more than three episodes in past 2 years) or who have had injuries with syncope and are under 50 years because the risk of hypertension is lower.

C. α-AGONISTS—Currently, only midodrine, an α_1-agonist agent, seems to result in significant reductions in recurrent episodes, based on small trials and a meta-analysis. Recently, these findings were confirmed in the Fourth Prevention of

Syncope Trial (POST 4) study where midodrine was associated with a significantly lower risk of syncope recurrence after 1-year follow-up. Midodrine has a profile of few adverse events and, in clinical practice, seems to be highly effective in all age groups. In our practice, midodrine is the agent of choice due to the previously mentioned reasons and perceived efficacy. Practical prescribing tips include taking the first dose after waking up 30 minutes before getting out of bed and taking the last dose of the day before 4:00 p.m. or 5:00 p.m. to avoid, particularly in older patients, the risk of supine hypertension.

D. OTHER MEDICATIONS—A long list of alternative treatments, including serotonin reuptake inhibitors, angiotensin-converting enzyme inhibitors, vagolytics, and other central-acting agents, such as methylphenidate, have been tested but are rarely used. Theophylline, a nonselective adenosine receptor antagonist, has been shown to reduce syncope recurrence in adenosine-sensitive syncope in retrospective studies. In our practice, we occasionally use serotonin inhibitors if some of the personality traits are observed to respond to this therapy and syncope is refractory.

4. Device therapy—Cardiac pacing in NMS should be considered in several specific scenarios. First, pacing in reflex syncope is not indicated in the absence of any documented cardioinhibitory reflex. However, cardiac pacing may be considered in patients older than 40 years in the following settings:

- Symptomatic pauses more than 3 seconds or asymptomatic pauses more than 6 seconds due to sinus arrest or AV block (Class IIa)
- Presence of asystolic response during tilt-testing in patients with frequent unpredictable syncope (Class IIb)
- Cardioinhibitory carotid sinus syndrome with unpredictable syncope (Class IIa)
- Clinical features of adenosine-sensitive syncope as described earlier (Class IIb)

The indication for pacing in vasovagal syncope was recently established in two well-designed, randomized clinical trials. In the SPAIN Study, patients aged 40 years or older with a high burden of syncopal events were randomized to a crossover protocol including dual-chamber pacing for 12 months and sham pacing for 12 months. In this study, dual-chamber pacing significantly reduced syncope by sevenfold and prolonged the time to first recurrence. Similarly, the BioSync CLS trial showed a 77% relative risk reduction in patients implanted with a dual-chamber pacemaker when compared with an inactivated dual-chamber pacemaker, resulting in a number-needed-to-treat of 2.2. Both these studies were performed with closed loop stimulation (CLS), a feature only available in Biotronik pacemakers. Therefore, pacemakers play a limited, but significant role in a selected subgroup of patients with reflex syncope.

5. Cardioneuroablation—Ganglionic plexus ablation or cardioneuroablation aims to abolish the vagal innervation of the heart by targeting the epicardial ganglionated plexi. There is increasing data from observational nonrandomized studies, that cardioneuroablation may reduce vasovagal syncope recurrence in up to 90% of patients with therapy-refractory, recurrent vasovagal syncope. Similar success rates have been reported in vagal-mediated paroxysmal AV block. However, the current evidence originates from observational cohort studies with a wide variety in methods. There are no placebo-controlled randomized trials available, therefore this treatment should still be considered experimental.

B. Cardiac Implantable Electronic Devices & Electrophysiologic Therapies

Implantable devices, such as ICDs and pacemakers, and catheter ablation have all been used to treat syncope in appropriate patients. In patients presenting with syncope and structural heart disease with left ventricular function less than 35%, an ICD is the therapy of choice. In patients with evidence of conduction disorders or paroxysmal AV block, cardiac pacing is usually indicated. As discussed earlier, selected patients with reflex syncope might also benefit from pacemaker implantation. The SPRITELY trial randomized patients aged 50 years or older with bifascicular block between empiric pacing versus an implantable cardiac monitor. The composite primary outcome, defined as cardiovascular death, syncope, bradycardia resulting in pacemaker implant, and device complications, was observed in 76% of patients with an implantable monitor and in 35% of patients with empiric pacing. While empiric pacemaker implants reduced the risk of major adverse events, there was no difference in the prevalence of syncope. This indicates that the competing risk of fainting from other causes, such as vasodepressor syncope, remains relevant.

Catheter ablation techniques using radiofrequency energy are indicated when the cause of syncope is related to tachyarrhythmias, mostly paroxysmal supraventricular tachycardias and some VTs not associated with structural heart disease.

Baron-Esquivias G, Morillo CA, Mitjans AM, et al. Dual-chamber pacing with closed loop stimulation in recurrent reflex vasovagal syncope: The SPAIN Study. *J Am Coll Cardiol.* 2017;70(14):1720–1728. [PMID: 28958328]

Brignole M, Russo V, Arabia F, et al. Cardiac pacing in severe recurrent reflex syncope and tilt-induced asystole. *Eur Heart J.* 2021;42(5):508–516. [PMID: 33279955]

Sheldon R, Connolly S, Rose S, et al. Prevention of Syncope Trial (POST): a randomized, placebo-controlled study of metoprolol in the prevention of vasovagal syncope. *Circulation.* 2006;113(9):1164–1170. [PMID: 16505178]

Sheldon R, Faris P, Tang A, et al. Midodrine for the Prevention of Vasovagal Syncope: A Randomized Clinical Trial. *Ann Intern Med.* 2021;174(10):1349–1356. [PMID: 34339231]

Sheldon R, Talajic M, Tang A, et al. Randomized pragmatic trial of pacemaker versus implantable cardiac monitor in syncope and bifascicular block. *J Am Coll Cardiol EP.* Epublished Nov 24, 2021. [PMID: NA DOI: 10.1016/j.jacep.2021.10.003]

Task Force for the Diagnosis and Management of Syncope, et al. Guidelines for the diagnosis and management of syncope (version 2018). *Eur Heart J.* 2018;39(21):1883–1948. [PMID: 29562304]

Prognosis

The prognosis is determined by the underlying etiology, specifically the presence and severity of cardiac disease. Untreated, cardiac syncope mortality can be more than 10% (18–33%) at 6 months, whereas NMS has a generally favorable prognosis. Cardiac syncope has the highest risk of recurrence, usually within the first year of diagnosis. Long-term follow-up of patients with noncardiac syncope showed a recurrence rate of 37% over more than 4 years. Over a similar follow-up, mortality was 6.6% per year and was lowest in patients with vasovagal syncope. Recurrence of vasovagal syncope is best predicted by the frequency of events in the preceding year with rates of 7%, 22%, and 69% in those with no, less than two, or greater than six syncopal events, respectively, in the preceding year. Recurrences do not predict an increase in mortality, although they are associated with increased morbidity (ie, fractures, soft tissue injury) and impaired quality of life. Morbidity is particularly high in the elderly and ranges from loss of confidence, depressive illness, and fear of falling, to fractures and subsequent institutionalization.

An estimate of the composite mortality between 7 and 30 days after presentation for syncope according to a recent review of the literature is 0.7%. The risk increases to approximately 10% at 1 year. An average 7.5% of patients with syncope referred to the ED will have a severe nonfatal outcome (defined as a new diagnosis, clinical deterioration, syncope recurrence with injury, or a significant therapeutic intervention) while in the ED. A further 4.5% will have a severe nonfatal outcome in the subsequent 7–30 days. Only half of these events are attributable to cardiovascular causes.

A meta-analysis of prospective observational studies showed that the chance of being asymptomatic linearly progressively decreased over time after the first syncope. Short-term (10–30 days) mortality after syncope was less than 2%, and the overall 10-day rate of the composite endpoint of death and major events was approximately 9%. The knowledge of syncope prognosis could help clinicians to understand the prognosis of syncope patients and help researchers to design future studies.

Barón-Esquivias G, Quintanilla M, Martin AJD, et al. Long-term recurrences and mortality in patients with noncardiac syncope. *Rev Esp Cardiol (Engl Ed).* 2021. Epublished Dec 27, 2021. [PMID: 34969644]

Solbiati M, Cassaza G, Dipaola F, et al. Syncope recurrence and mortality: a systematic review. *Europace.* 2015;17(2):300–308. [PMID: 25476868]

Clinical Perspective

Syncope remains a challenging diagnostic and management encounter for clinicians. Simple principles such as a thorough history taking with particular attention to the circumstances surrounding the event and interrogation of any witnesses pave the way to a clear diagnosis. Overall, vasovagal syncope remains the most frequent cause of recurrent episodes in all ages. Features that should always alert the clinician include syncope during exercise, abrupt syncope without warning or prodrome, age greater than 60 years, history of structural heart disease (myocardial infarction, cardiomyopathy), and a family history of sudden death, recurrent syncope, or unexplained seizures; these features may suggest high risk and usually warrant in-hospital investigations. Detailed interpretation of ECG findings is also critical to identify high-risk patients and direct appropriate investigations and management.

Aortic Stenosis

17

Vishal Birk, MD
Amir E. Abbas, MD

ESSENTIALS OF DIAGNOSIS

- History
  - Angina, dyspnea, syncope
- Physical examination
  - Mid-systolic ejection murmur
  - Small and slow-rising carotid pulse contour (parvus et tardus)
- Echocardiography
  - Thickened immobile aortic valve leaflets
  - Increased peak transaortic jet velocity and mean gradient, reduced valve area

General Considerations & Etiology

Over the past century, there has been a linear climb in record life expectancy and an overall aging of the human race. Therefore, we are faced with an epidemic of aging and age-associated disease, not the least of which is valvular heart disease. Aortic stenosis, the narrowing of the aortic valve orifice caused by failure of the leaflets to open normally, is now the most common indication for valve replacement in North America and Europe.

The pathogenesis of aortic stenosis is most commonly progressive calcification and degeneration of a trileaflet or congenitally bicuspid valve. Although once thought to be a degenerative process, it is now recognized that calcific aortic stenosis is in fact an active disease process that shares similarities to atherosclerosis and involves inflammation, lipid accumulation, and calcification of the leaflets. The mechanisms by which some valves degenerate and become stenotic while others remain relatively normal are unknown but are probably related to genetic polymorphisms. Those with end-stage renal disease, Paget disease, or severe familial hypercholesterolemia may present with calcific aortic stenosis at a younger age and are susceptible to more rapid progression of stenosis severity.

Rheumatic valve disease is a rare cause of aortic stenosis in industrialized nations. However, for indigenous populations within these countries as well as in developing countries, there remains a significant prevalence of rheumatic valve disease. In contrast to calcific aortic valve stenosis, the rheumatic valve shows adhesion, leaflet retraction, and commissural fusion. Along or just a few millimeters away from the free margins of the valve leaflets, small sessile nodules develop that also contribute to leaflet malcoaptation. Therefore, the rheumatic aortic valve invariably will leak. Rheumatic aortic valve disease is almost never present in isolation, and there is invariably concomitant mitral valve disease. A patient with aortic stenosis and a perfectly normal mitral valve should be considered as having another cause for his or her disease. Other rare causes of aortic stenosis include connective tissues diseases such as systemic lupus erythematosus and ochronosis.

Clinical Findings

A. History

Those with acquired aortic stenosis generally have a long latent period before the onset of the salient clinical manifestations of the disease: effort-related dyspnea (heart failure), angina, and syncope. The most common initial clinical manifestations are a gradual decline in functional capacity and effort-related dyspnea. Regardless of the initial presenting symptom(s), it is imperative to ensure that the pathophysiologic mechanism of the symptoms is attributed to valve disease and not a manifestation of another mechanism such as concomitant coronary artery or lung disease because the onset of even mild symptoms attributed to aortic stenosis heralds a dramatic increase in the mortality rate for these patients if the valve is not replaced. Symptoms are therefore the guidepost for intervention, and understanding them is the key to understanding and managing the disease.

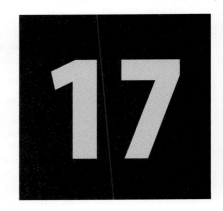

The primary determinants of left ventricular systolic function are contractility and afterload. The load on individual myocardial fibers can best be described as left ventricular wall stress and defined by the Laplace equation:

$$\text{Wall Stress} = \frac{\text{Pressure} \times \text{Radius}}{2 \times \text{Thickness}}$$

With acquired aortic stenosis, the obstruction will commonly progress gradually over time. Left ventricular adaptation to increases in systolic pressure is the parallel replication of sarcomeres to increase its thickness (concentric hypertrophy) in an effort to normalize wall stress and maintain systolic performance. As the severity of stenosis progresses, the increase in wall thickness may become insufficient to offset the rise in pressure ("afterload mismatch"), resulting in a rise in wall stress and a decline in ventricular function. The presence of aortic stenosis may also result in true depression of myocardial contractility, the exact mechanism of which is unclear but likely related to a loss of contractile elements secondary to reduced coronary blood flow. Thus, a decline in ejection fraction results from the interplay of varying degrees between excessive afterload and true myocardial depression. Those in whom the decline in function is largely attributed to afterload mismatch are more likely to experience restored ventricular function following aortic valve replacement. The evaluation of left ventricular ejection phase indices should be related to the global wall tension; however, clinically, it is difficult to tease out the extent to which wall stress (afterload) and contractility are contributing to a noted decline in ejection fraction.

1. Dyspnea and exercise intolerance—The increase in left ventricular wall thickness, although imposed in an effort to maintain wall stress and systolic performance, does have maladaptive physiologic consequences. The increase in wall thickness makes it harder to fill the ventricle, and therefore, higher filling pressures are required to achieve any given volume and end-diastolic volume will be required to increase to allow the maintenance of a normal ejection fraction (a rightward shift in the ventricular diastolic pressure-volume relationship) (Figure 17–1). In alignment with the concept of hemodynamic continuity, when the mitral valve opens, the left atrium is now exposed to the hemodynamic milieu of the left ventricle. The increased ventricular diastolic pressure is transmitted to atrium and further back into the pulmonary veins and lungs, resulting in pulmonary congestion and an increased work of breathing. In addition, with outflow obstruction, there is a prolongation of the ejection phase; this, in conjunction with an exercise-induced increase in heart rate, will result in a reduction of the diastolic filling time, and the ventricle will reach its limit of "preload reserve." Once limits of preload reserve are met, stroke volume becomes directly related to ventricular pressure (see Figure 17–1), resulting in an inability to increase cardiac

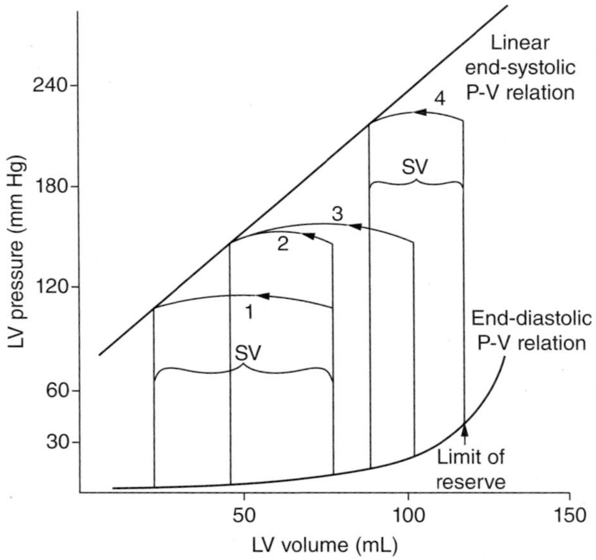

▲ **Figure 17–1.** Left ventricular (LV) pressure-volume (P-V) loops. As LV pressure increases, stroke volume (SV) would decrease if the end-diastolic volume were fixed (loop 2). The ventricle, however, adapts by increasing end-diastolic volume to maintain a normal SV (loop 3). Eventually, the limits of preload reserve are met whereby increases in LV pressure result in a decline in SV (SV is now directly related to LV pressure; loop 4). (Reproduced with permission from Ross J. Afterload mismatch in aortic and mitral valve disease: Implications for surgical therapy. *J Am Coll Cardiol*. 1985;5(4):811–826.)

output and further contributing to the presence of dyspnea and exercise intolerance.

2. Angina—Angina results from myocardial ischemia, which occurs when there is an imbalance between myocardial oxygen requirements/demand and myocardial oxygen supply. Although epicardial coronary artery disease often coexists with aortic stenosis, symptoms of angina frequently occur in those without epicardial coronary artery disease. Oxygen demand is best estimated clinically by the product of heart rate and wall stress, and as noted earlier, eventually the extent of hypertrophy cannot keep up with pressure demands of the ventricle and wall stress increases. In the absence of epicardial coronary artery disease, myocardial oxygen supply may also be decreased secondary to the rise in left ventricular end-diastolic pressure and a delayed rate of ventricular relaxation, with impaired coronary "diastolic suction" contributing to both reduced coronary perfusion and a decline in coronary flow reserve needed to offset increased oxygen demands during stress or exercise. In addition, with exercise and increased heart rates, there is reduced diastolic coronary perfusion time. Recently, coronary microvascular dysfunction has also been proposed as a mechanism of angina in patients with severe aortic stenosis as determined by adenosine-stress cardiac magnetic resonance.

3. Syncope—Syncope is a transient loss of consciousness due to cerebral hypoperfusion. Syncope in those with aortic stenosis usually occurs during exercise. There are two primary mechanisms, not mutually exclusive, that have been theorized to cause syncope. First, the narrowed aortic valve does not permit the appropriate increase in cardiac output necessary to offset the associated reduction in total peripheral resistance associated with exercise, resulting in a drop in blood pressure. Second, the very high ventricular pressure that develops with exercise when sensed by ventricular mechanoreceptors triggers a reflexive vasodepressor response, also leading to a decline in blood pressure. Less commonly, exercise can result in either ventricular or supraventricular arrhythmias, which can lead to a reduction in cardiac output and, consequently, a drop in blood pressure.

B. Physical Examination

1. Murmur—The character of a murmur can be described by its timing and shape, intensity and pitch, and location and radiation, along with changes in these characteristics imposed by transient changes in intracardiac hemodynamics.

A. TIMING AND SHAPE—The murmur of valvular aortic stenosis is a midsystolic murmur, which begins after the first heart sound and ends before the aortic (A_2) component of the second heart sound. During systole, as blood flow velocity accelerates across the valve, the intensity of the murmur increases, and as blood flow velocity decelerates, the intensity diminishes. Therefore, there is a classic "crescendo-decrescendo" configuration or shape to the murmur of valvular aortic stenosis. Further insights into the configuration of the murmur may help to discern the severity of disease; the later in systole the peak intensity occurs, generally the more severe is the stenosis.

B. INTENSITY AND PITCH—The intensity of the aortic stenosis murmur relates to the quantity and velocity of transaortic blood flow along with the ability to transmit sound through the chest. The pitch of the murmur relates to the pressure gradient and size of the "aperture" with which the blood flows through. In general, as the stenosis severity increases, the intensity and pitch of the murmur will increase. However, in those with a thick ventricle and low end-diastolic volume or in the presence of a decline in cardiac function, both of which may result in a low stroke volume, the intensity and pitch of the murmur may be lower than expected for the given severity of stenosis. In addition, the ability to transmit the sound through the chest is impaired in those with a pericardial effusion, emphysema, or obesity. Therefore, one should be cautious of excluding significant aortic stenosis solely based on murmur intensity/pitch.

C. LOCATION/RADIATION—The murmur of aortic stenosis typically is heard loudest in the "aortic area," the right second interspace at the sternal border, and will often radiate into the carotids and along a line from the aortic area toward the left ventricular apex. At the apex, the intensity and pitch of the murmur may change to more resemble that of the murmur of mitral regurgitation; however, the shape/configuration of the murmur does not change. This is known as the Gallavardin phenomenon.

D. RESPONSE TO MANEUVERS—A transient alteration in intracardiac hemodynamics may influence the characteristics of a murmur helping to further specify its etiology.

- Isometric handgrip: Increases systemic vascular resistance, decreasing the intensity of the murmur of aortic stenosis.
- Standing/Valsalva maneuver (phase II): Decreases ventricular filling, reducing the intensity of the murmur of aortic stenosis and most other valve murmurs, except that of hypertrophic cardiomyopathy and the duration of the murmur of mitral valve prolapse.
- Squatting: Increases ventricular filling but also increases systemic vascular resistance. Its effect on the murmur of aortic stenosis is therefore generally neutral; however, it will reduce the intensity of the murmur of hypertrophic cardiomyopathy.
- Cycle length: The intensity of the murmur of aortic stenosis may vary from beat to beat in those with atrial fibrillation or premature contractions, increasing in intensity in the beats following a longer R-R interval where diastolic filling time is increased.

2. Carotid pulse—The carotid artery pulse wave contour in those with aortic stenosis is characterized as small and slow rising (parvus et tardus). One may also appreciate a carotid shudder.

3. Heart sounds

A. SECOND HEART SOUND (S_2)—The presence of significant aortic stenosis may result in *paradoxical splitting* of the second heart sound where the A_2 component of S_2 is delayed, resulting in S_2 being more split during expiration than inspiration. Reduced movement of the aortic valve may render A_2 inaudible where only a *single* second heart sound can be appreciated.

B. FOURTH HEART SOUND (S_4)—As noted earlier, left ventricular hypertrophy imposed by the increase in wall stress reduces ventricular wall compliance. The fourth heart sound is a low-pitch sound heard coincident with late diastolic filling, due to atrial contraction, of a ventricle with reduced wall compliance and increased end-diastolic pressure.

4. Apical impulse—The apical impulse, which in aortic stenosis is generally the point of maximal impulse, remains in its normal position but is sustained due to prolongation of the ejection time. The atrial component of ventricular filling may also be palpable. With simultaneous palpation of the apical and carotid impulses, normally one will appreciate little delay in their peaks; however, they become separated in time proportional to the severity of stenosis.

C. Diagnostic Studies

The clinical severity of aortic stenosis is largely an operational classification based on the presence or absence of symptoms as discussed earlier. However, the indications for consideration of either a surgical or percutaneous aortic valve replacement rely on an estimate of stenosis severity.

1. Electrocardiogram—Left ventricular hypertrophy is the primary finding noted in those with aortic stenosis. Other common findings include left atrial abnormality along with ST- and T-wave abnormalities. There are, however, no electrocardiogram findings that are either sensitive or specific for aortic stenosis.

2. Chest radiography—With isolated aortic stenosis, the cardiac silhouette is generally normal in size with possible rounding of the left heart border consistent with concentric left ventricular hypertrophy. There may be signs of left atrial enlargement and pulmonary venous hypertension. The aortic shadow may become enlarged, and valve calcification may be appreciated.

3. Echocardiography—Echocardiography is the principal clinical tool used for the evaluation of aortic stenosis, and currently still remains the gold standard imaging modality for the assessment of aortic stenosis despite the advances in other cardiac imaging modalities. Appropriate use criteria deem transthoracic echocardiography appropriate on the initial evaluation of a patient when clinical evaluation provides "unexplained murmur or abnormal heart sounds, reasonable suspicion of valvular or structural heart disease, history of rheumatic heart disease, known systemic or acquired heart disease associated with valvular heart disease, first-degree family history of bicuspid aortic valve, or exposure to medications that could result in the development of valvular heart disease, syncope without other symptoms or signs of cardiovascular disease, hypotension or hemodynamic instability with suspected cardiac etiology, respiratory failure, or initial heart failure evaluation to exclude valvular cause." Re-evaluation of known valvular heart disease with echocardiography is appropriate "with a change in clinical status or cardiac exam or to guide therapy." Routine surveillance in the absence of a change in clinical status or cardiac examination is deemed appropriate at intervals of 6 months to 1 year when the aortic velocity is ≥ 4.0 m/s, 1–2 years when the aortic velocity is between 3.0 and 3.9 m/s, and 3–5 years when the aortic velocity is between 2.0 and 2.9 m/s. The echocardiogram should include not only anatomic and hemodynamic measures of stenosis severity, but also an assessment of the left ventricular response to the pressure load, insights into whether there is dilation of the ascending aorta, and assessment for the presence of coexisting valve regurgitation and other cardiac abnormalities. Myocardial imaging and a measure of global longitudinal peak systolic strain may detect adverse ventricular consequences to the hemodynamic load despite a preserved left ventricular ejection fraction.

A. ANATOMIC EVALUATION—Although most outcome data in those with aortic stenosis are based on the measures of the hemodynamic severity and physiologic orifice area, the anatomic evaluation of the valve is gaining increased importance in the evolving era of percutaneous valve replacement in guiding patient selection and procedural planning. From primarily the transthoracic parasternal views, or transesophageal imaging if the transthoracic images are suboptimal, the number of leaflets, extent of calcification, leaflet thickening, and mobility should be evaluated. An anatomic measure of the geometric valve area can be obtained by planimetry, either from echocardiography or cardiac CT. The fundamental limitations to accurate and reproducible measurements of the geometric orifice area are image attenuation secondary to leaflet calcification and the spatial integration of images required to ensure planimetry of the minimal opening area at the leaflet tips (Figure 17–2). It is for these reasons that the measure of geometric orifice area is reserved clinically primarily for those circumstances where Doppler measurements are unreliable. This holds true for classification of disease severity, however as we will discuss planimetry for procedural planning by cardiac CT has now become routine.

B. HEMODYNAMIC EVALUATION—The principal measures of the hemodynamic severity include peak transaortic jet velocity, peak instantaneous and mean pressure gradients, and valve area (effective orifice area by the continuity equation).

(1) Transaortic velocity and gradient calculations—The principle of conservation of energy states that the total

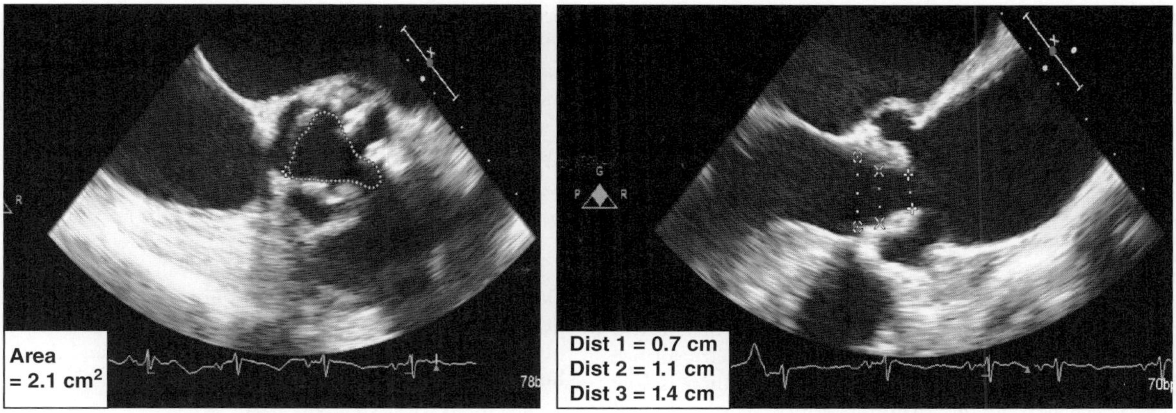

▲ **Figure 17–2.** Planimetry of the aortic valve. **A:** Short-axis image of the aortic valve and a calculated anatomic valve area by planimetry. Leaflet calcification and image attenuation limit accurate delineation of the leaflet borders. **B:** Long-axis image of the aortic valve noting that slight alteration in the tomographic slice obtained through the aortic valve will result in marked variation in the valve area calculated by planimetry. (AV VTI, aortic valve velocity time integral)

amount of energy in a closed system remains constant. Energy can change its location and form, but can be neither created nor destroyed. With respect to flow, as the flow stream approaches a narrowed orifice, its kinetic energy increases and potential energy decreases. Distal to the narrowed orifice, pressure is lost in part due to the dissipation of kinetic energy as heat. This creates a pressure gradient across the valve orifice. Continuous wave Doppler is used to determine the maximum jet velocity through the stenotic valve. Meticulous imaging from multiple acoustic windows is required to ensure that flow velocities are acquired with a parallel intercept angle to the direction of flow, limiting the error of underestimation of the peak velocity. The Bernoulli equation is then applied to the highest jet velocity obtained to calculate the peak instantaneous gradient (Figure 17–3).

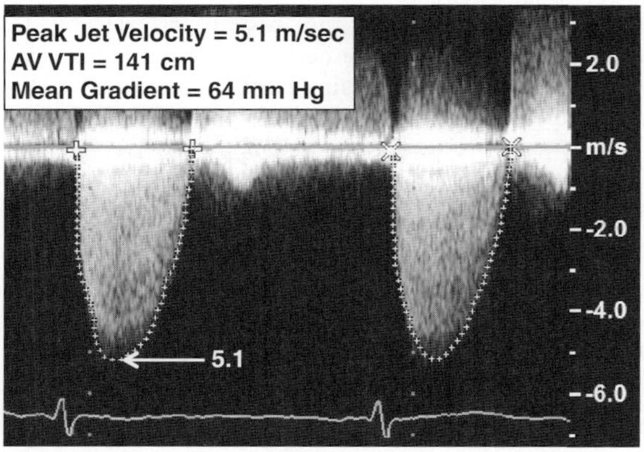

▲ **Figure 17–3.** Continuous wave Doppler of aortic stenosis.

Bernoulli equation:

$$\Delta P = 1/2\rho(V_2^2 - V_1^2) \quad \text{(Convective acceleration)}$$
$$+ \rho\int(dv/dt) * ds \quad \text{(Flow acceleration)}$$
$$+ R(\mu) \quad \text{(Viscous friction)}$$

ΔP = pressure gradient, ρ = mass density of blood, V_1 and V_2 = velocity proximal and distal to obstruction respectively, R = viscous resistance, μ = viscosity

Under most physiologic conditions, the latter two terms (flow acceleration and viscous friction) are negligible and can be ignored and $V_2 >>> V_1$ and thus V_1 can be ignored. Therefore, under most physiologic conditions, a simplified Bernoulli equation can be applied to the peak velocity obtained to derive the peak instantaneous gradient.

Simplified Bernoulli equation: $\Delta P = 4(V_2)^2$

When either V_1 is more than 1.5 m/s or V_2 is less than 3.0 m/s, the proximal velocity should be included in the simplified Bernoulli equation: $\Delta P = 4(V_2^2 - V_1^2)$. The final term, $R(\mu)$, represents energy losses due to viscous friction. Failing to recall this component may result in an overestimation of gradient in those who are anemic.

The mean gradient is obtained by averaging the instantaneous gradients over the ejection period. Because it is not possible to match each point on the ejection curve between the proximal and distal velocity profiles, it is not possible to "correct" the mean gradient when V_1 is significant, and in these circumstances, the measure of mean gradient should not be used to grade stenosis severity.

(2) Aortic valve area—Valve area calculations are based on the continuity equation, which assumes the principle of conservation of mass where flow across the left ventricular outflow tract (LVOT) is assumed equal to flow across the aortic valve (AV). Stroke volume is calculated as the product of the cross-sectional area (CSA) and velocity time integral (VTI). Therefore aortic valve area (AVA) is calculated as:

$$AVA = (CSA_{LVOT} \times VTI_{LVOT})/VTI_{AV}$$

The calculation of flow across the LVOT assumes the outflow tract is cylindrical in shape with the area of the LVOT therefore equal to π multiplied by its radius squared (πr^2); thus, an error in the calculation of LVOT diameter will be exponentially amplified. Note that the calculation of AVA is essentially the estimation of the "flow or effective orifice area" and not the true anatomic/geometric orifice area. As blood flows toward a narrowed orifice, there is flow convergence beyond the anatomic orifice. The narrowest point of the flow stream, the vena contracta, is located just distal to the anatomic orifice, and its area is smaller than the anatomic orifice. The ratio between the anatomic and effective orifice areas is called the correction coefficient.

Based on the principal measures of hemodynamic severity, the American Heart Association/American College of Cardiology guidelines categorize aortic stenosis in those with a normal transaortic flow volume as mild, moderate, or severe (Table 17–1).

The AVA should be indexed for body surface area in smaller individuals so as not to overestimate the severity of stenosis based on the valve area calculation. The role of indexed AVA in the obese is unclear, and it is not our practice to use this because it is difficult to integrate the relationship of weight in association to body "size" versus "adiposity."

(3) Dimensionless index—As noted earlier, an error in the measure of the LVOT diameter will be exponentially amplified notwithstanding the assumption that the LVOT is cylindrical in shape. Therefore, a proposed LVOT independent measure of stenosis severity, the dimensionless index, can be helpful to either confirm or dispute stenosis severity classification based on the effective orifice area calculation. The dimensionless index is defined as the ratio of the LVOT velocity to that of the transaortic jet velocity, and a value of less than 0.25 indicates severe aortic stenosis.

(4) Energy loss coefficient (ELCo)—The coefficient increases as the extent of pressure recovery (discussed later) increases. The magnitude of pressure recovery is determined by the ratio between the effective orifice area and the cross-sectional area of the ascending aorta (measured at the sinotubular junction) and is most significant when the valve area is less than 1.2 cm^2 and the aorta cross-sectional area is less than 3.0 cm.

$$ELCo = (EOA \times Aa)/(Aa - EOA)$$

where EOA = effective orifice area derived by the continuity equation and Aa = cross-sectional area of the aorta measured 1 cm distal to the sinotubular junction.

The ELCo then provides a value of valve area derived by Doppler echocardiography more equivalent to the valve area derived by the Gorlin equation, which is more representative of the actual energy loss caused by the stenosis and thus the burden it imposes on the ventricle.

Table 17–1. Categories of Aortic Stenosis Based on the Principal Measures of Hemodynamic Severity

	Transaortic Jet Velocity	Mean Gradient (mm Hg)	AVA (cm^2)	Indexed AVA (cm^2/m^2)
Mild	2.0–2.9	< 20	1.51–2.0	
Moderate	3.0–3.9	20–39	1.0–1.5	
Severe	≥ 4.0	≥ 40	≤ 1.0	≤ 0.6

AVA, aortic valve area.

4. Cardiac catheterization—The fundamental role of cardiac catheterization in those with aortic stenosis is to evaluate for the presence of coexisting coronary artery disease in those with symptoms of angina pectoris, helping clarify its pathophysiologic mechanism, and in whom AV replacement is being considered. Cardiac catheterization should not be routinely performed for the evaluation of the hemodynamic severity of aortic stenosis except for cases where echocardiographic data are of poor quality or when there remains a discrepancy between the clinical and echocardiographic determinations of stenosis severity.

The principal measures of the hemodynamic severity of aortic stenosis as assessed by cardiac catheterization include peak-to-peak and mean pressure gradients and valve area (derived by the Gorlin equation).

A. Pressure gradients—The transvalvular pressure gradient is calculated by placing one catheter into the left ventricle and a second into the proximal aorta. The difference in the pressure from simultaneous recordings from each catheter represents the peak-to-peak pressure gradient. Single-catheter techniques may include a pullback gradient and the use of a dual-lumen catheter. Note that Doppler echocardiography derives a maximum instantaneous gradient at a single point in time and by principle assumes that the pressure drop across the valve is irretrievably lost while the invasive measure derives a peak-to-peak gradient with the upstream pressure partially recovered. Therefore, the invasively derived measure of the peak pressure gradient is always lower than the Doppler-derived measure, and this difference is accentuated as the extent of pressure recovery increases (Figure 17–4). Mean gradients obtained by both Doppler and cardiac catheterization correlate well.

B. Valve area—During cardiac catheterization cardiac output is measured using primarily either the Fick or thermodilution principal and the pressure gradient measured as discussed earlier with values obtained used to calculate valve area using the Gorlin equation:

$$AVA = \frac{CO/SEP \times HR}{44.3\sqrt{\Delta P_{mean}}}$$

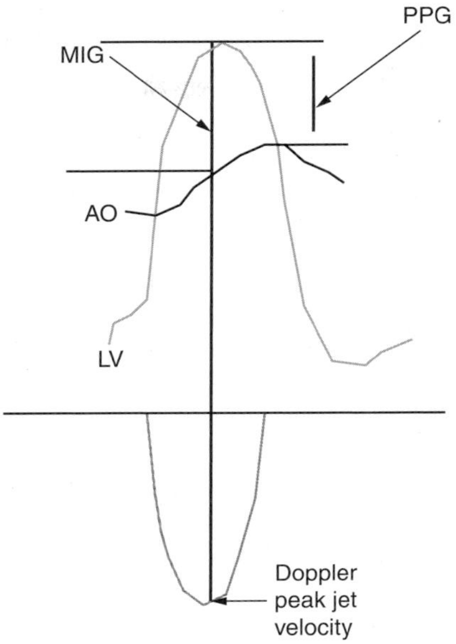

▲ **Figure 17–4.** *Top:* Simultaneous left ventricular and aortic pressure tracings. *Bottom:* Doppler echocardiography–derived transaortic velocity profile. AO, aortic pressure; LV, left ventricle; MIG, maximum instantaneous gradient (the gradient that is derived by applying the Bernoulli equation to the peak jet velocity obtained by Doppler echocardiography); PPG, peak-to-peak gradient (the gradient obtained with invasive catheterization).

where CO = cardiac output, SEP = systolic ejection period (in seconds), HR = heart rate, and ΔP = pressure gradient (mean). The presence of a measure of flow/cardiac output in the numerator of the Gorlin equation highlights the flow dependence on the derived values of AVA. Note that the valve area derived from the Gorlin equation is derived from recovered pressures, and as such, its value is higher than Doppler-derived valve areas by the continuity equation. The current guidelines, however, make no distinction between invasive and Doppler echocardiographic measurements in the characterization of stenosis severity by valve area and pressure gradients (see earlier discussion regarding the energy loss coefficient).

5. Cardiac computed tomography (CT)—Cardiac CT can be used to calculate the geometric valve area by planimetry and to quantify the extent and distribution of valve calcification, and although echocardiography remains the gold standard imaging modality, cardiac CT is becoming integral in the care of the patients with moderate to severe aortic stenosis (Figures 17–5 and 17–6). When echocardiography leaves the severity of the diagnosis inconclusive or is discordant between imaging and clinical suspicion, cardiac CT can be an invaluable tool to help classify severity, as it offers evaluation independent of hemodynamics of the patient. Cardiac CT quality continues to improve at an impressive rate. With upgrades in hardware, software, and scanning protocols which optimize gating and slice thickness, reconstruction image resolution continues to improve. These advances all aid in improving the accuracy of cardiac CT and limit the exposure of radiation to the patient. Quantification of AV calcification is strongly, but nonlinearly, associated with the hemodynamic severity of aortic stenosis, and the extent of calcification is predictive of event-free survival (survival without dyspnea, angina, syncope, heart failure, or need for valve replacement). Therefore, the measurement of AV calcium load should be considered for both diagnostic and prognostic purposes. Despite a similar degree of stenosis severity, women have lower valve calcium scores compared to men even after indexing for their smaller body size. For aortic stenosis severity purposes, the interpretation of the calcium load is thus different for men and women, where a score of more than 1300 AU for women and more than 2000 AU for men is considered severe.

In contemporary clinical practice, cardiac CT, in conjunction with two- and three-dimensional echocardiography, now has an essential role in the evaluation of patients being considered for a percutaneous valve replacement primarily for:

- The evaluation of the annular area and perimeter required for the appropriate selection of prosthetic valve size
- The assessment of the peripheral vasculature and suitability for arterial access
- The assessment of the geometric relationship/distance between the aortic annulus and the coronary ostia to ensure that the implanted valve, when in position, does not blanket the coronary ostia
- Characterizing the extent of valve, root, and LVOT calcification, which may impact the technical success, risk of implantation, and paravalvular regurgitation
- Allowing the prediction of post-implantation aortic regurgitation
- Determining the feasibility of transaortic transcatheter aortic valve replacement when the transfemoral route is not feasible

Doherty JU, Kort S, Mehran R, Schoenhagen P, Soman P. ACC/AATS/AHA/ASE/ASNC/HRS/SCAI/SCCT/SCMR/STS 2017 Appropriate Use Criteria for Multimodality Imaging in Valvular Heart Disease: A Report of the American College of Cardiology Appropriate Use Criteria Task Force, American Association for Thoracic Surgery, American Heart Association, American Society of Echocardiography, American Society of Nuclear Cardiology, Heart Rhythm Society, Society for Cardiovascular Angiography and Interventions, Society of Cardiovascular Computed Tomography, Society for Cardiovascular Magnetic Resonance, and Society of Thoracic Surgeons. *J Am Coll Cardiol.* 2017;70(13):1647–1672. [PMID: 28870679]

Pawade T, Sheth T, Guzzetti E, Dweck MR, Clavel MA. Why and how to measure aortic valve calcification in patients with aortic stenosis. *JACC Cardiovasc Img.* 2019;12:1835–1848. [PMID: 31488252]

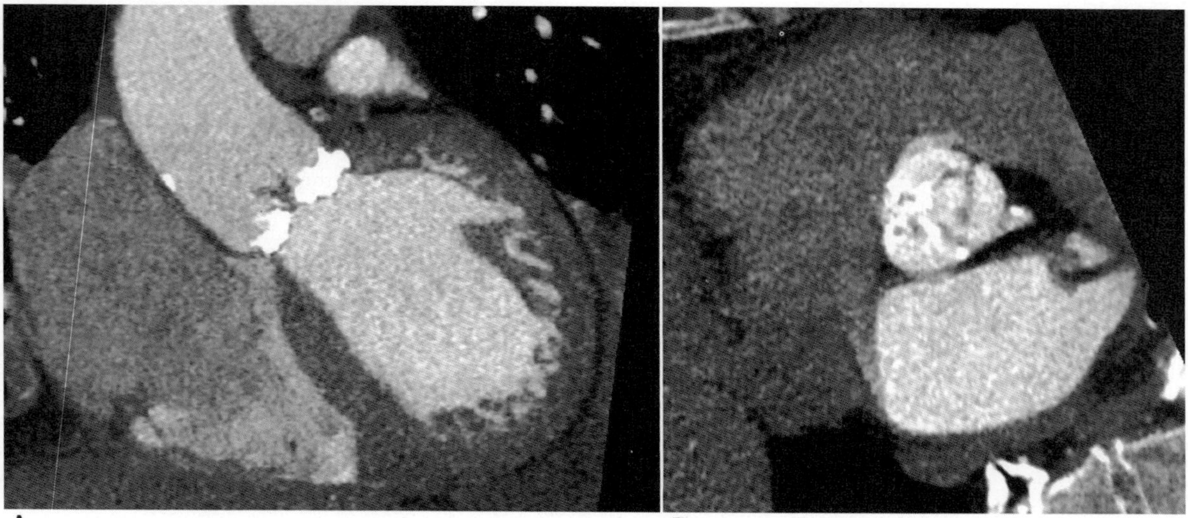

▲ **Figure 17–5.** **A:** Left; Cardiac CT showing the structures of the left ventricular outflow tract and aorta, along with the heavy calcifications (radio-opaque) on the aortic valve. **B:** right; Cross-sectional view of aortic valve on cardiac CT. Gating protocols allowing for the valve to be viewed at its opening during systole to allow for planimetry of the valve.

Diagnostic Dilemmas: Area-Gradient Mismatch

The principal parameters of stenosis severity, as discussed earlier, are directly related to transvalvular flow. As such, clinical scenarios where the AVA falls within the severe range, while the gradient remains nonsevere occur in clinical practice. This may occur in low-flow states (left ventricular stroke volume index < 35 mL/m^2) associated with either a low ejection fraction (EF) (low EF area-gradient mismatch) or a preserved EF (normal EF area-gradient mismatch). Less commonly, one notes the gradient in the severe range, while the AVA remains in the nonsevere range (reverse area-gradient mismatch). Deciphering the true severity of aortic stenosis in the presence of area-gradient mismatch is imperative to best understand patient prognosis and to guide the appropriate management of these patients.

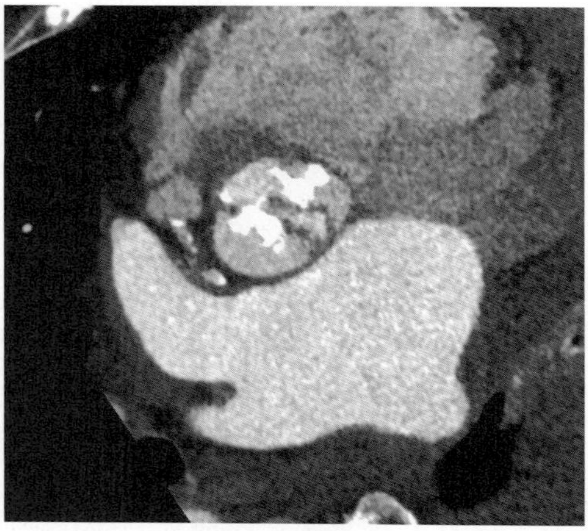

▲ **Figure 17–6.** Cross-sectional view of a bicuspid aortic valve on cardiac CT. Gating protocols allowing for the valve to be viewed at its opening during systole to allow for planimetry of the valve. Note the diminished AVA along with the heavy (radio-opaque) calcifications.

A. Low EF Area-Gradient Mismatch

This is also known as **low-flow, low-gradient (LF/LG) aortic stenosis with a depressed EF**.

- Effective orifice area less than 1.0 cm^2
- Left ventricular EF less than 40–50%
- Mean pressure gradient less than 30–40 mm Hg

Contemporary clinical protocol is to attempt to increase flow across the AV with a dobutamine infusion and to evaluate the ventricular response and transvalvular hemodynamics. One of three scenarios will evolve:

1. True or fixed severe aortic stenosis: Those in whom dobutamine can induce a greater than 20% increase in stroke volume with an associated increase in transvalvular gradient (peak velocity > 4.0 m/s, mean gradient > 40 mm Hg) and little or no change in AVA.
2. Pseudo or relative severe aortic stenosis: Those in whom dobutamine can induce a greater than 20% increase in stroke volume with an associated increase in

AVA (> 1 cm^2) and little or no change in transvalvular gradient (peak transvalvular velocity < 4.0 m/s).

3. Indeterminate aortic stenosis: Those in whom dobutamine is not able to increase stroke volume (no contractile reserve) with no change in AVA or transvalvular gradient.

The changes in valve area and gradient imposed during a dobutamine infusion are largely dependent on the extent of flow augmentation achieved, which can vary considerably between individuals. Recognizing the importance of flow rate in the determination of AS severity, the concept of standardizing flow rate has been proposed, allowing for the determination of a projected AVA (AVA_{proj}). The projected AVA is the estimated valve area at a normal flow rate (250 mL/min), and a value ≤ 1.0 cm^2 has been associated with true severe aortic stenosis, yet a value of ≤ 1.2 cm^2 (a value higher than proposed to identify true aortic stenosis) was noted to have a significant impact on survival. This highlights the fact that in the failing heart even moderate aortic stenosis may represent a detrimental hemodynamic burden to the ventricle.

$$AVA_{proj} = AVA_{rest} + VC\ (250 - Q_{rest})$$

$$\text{Where: VC (valve compliance)} = \frac{AVA_{peak} - AVA_{rest}}{Q_{peak} - Q_{rest}}$$

$$\text{and Q (mean flow)} = \frac{\text{Stroke Volume (mL)}}{\text{LV Ejection time (seconds)}}$$

Although at first glance the calculation of AVA_{proj} may seem complicated, in fact it really is not. One would use the same LVOT diameter for both the rest and stress calculation of AVA. You then must measure the VTI_{LVOT} and VTI_{AV} at rest and stress as we already do. Therefore, the only additional measurement required is the ejection time at rest and stress.

B. Normal EF Area-Gradient Mismatch

This is also known as **paradoxical low-flow, low-gradient (PLF/LG) aortic stenosis with preserved EF**.

- Effective orifice area less than 1.0 cm^2
- Left ventricular EF greater than 50% and left ventricular stroke volume index less than 35 mL/m^2
- Mean pressure gradient less than 30–40 mm Hg

This scenario is the result of the interaction of a *diastolic or preload component* whereby generally a thick ventricle with a small cavity is noted, a *myocardial or contractility component* whereby there is intrinsic myocardial dysfunction despite the persevered EF as noted with myocardial/strain imaging, and a *valvular-vascular or afterload component* imposing an increased global ventricular hemodynamic burden resulting from resistance in series between the valve stenosis and decreased systemic arterial compliance and increased vascular impedance. It has been proposed to characterize the valvular-vascular component through an index of valvuloarterial impedance (Zva). The Zva is defined as the ratio of the estimated left ventricular systolic pressure (systolic blood pressure + mean pressure gradient) to the stroke volume index. The Zva can be thought of as the cost in mm Hg for each mL of blood ejected. Other hemodynamic subgroups of aortic stenosis include those with normal flow (> 35 mL/m^2) and low-gradient (NF/LG) aortic stenosis, which carries a good prognosis and is considered an earlier form of the disease, and low-flow/high-gradient (LF/HG) aortic stenosis, which carries a worse prognosis intermediate between the NF/LG and the LF/LG subgroups.

C. Reverse Area-Gradient Mismatch

This may be noted when inappropriate assumptions or liberties are taken when applying the simplified Bernoulli equation to Doppler-derived blood flow velocities to estimate the transvalvular gradient, such as failure to include V_1 when significant or, as noted earlier, failing to recall the flow acceleration component and the viscous friction component in those with anemia. More commonly, this dilemma is secondary to the phenomenon of pressure recovery where downstream to the obstructed orifice as the blood flow velocity/kinetic energy decreases some of the kinetic energy will be converted to potential energy with associated increases in pressure. Pressure recovery is greatest in those in whom the ascending aorta diameter measures less than 3.0 cm. In this case, there will be a discrepancy between Doppler and catheter assessment of valve area and gradient, with the Doppler providing a more severe degree of stenosis. Finally, reverse area-gradient mismatch is noted in patients with eccentric jets. Due to jet eccentricity and collision with the aortic wall, the resultant pressure loss and diminished pressure recovery will lead to a disproportionately higher gradient by both Doppler and catheterization with respect to the geometric or anatomical valve area. The Doppler and catheter assessments of stenosis severity are, however, concordant.

Abbas AE, Pibarot P. Hemodynamic characterization of aortic stenosis states. *Catheter Cardiovasc Interv*. 2019;1;93(5):1002–1023. [PMID: 30790429]

Treatment

Aortic stenosis is a mechanical problem requiring a mechanical solution where the only effective treatment is valve replacement. The optimal time for valve replacement is therefore at the inflection point where the procedural risk and the long-term consequences of prosthetic heart valve disease become less then medical therapy.

A. Medical Therapy

There is no effective medical therapy for the treatment or cure of aortic stenosis. Because aortic stenosis is an active disease process that shares similarities and risk factors with atherosclerosis, there has been intellectual enthusiasm for aggressive atherosclerotic risk factor modification and the use of cholesterol-lowering drugs in an effort to slow stenosis progression and reduce the necessity for valve replacement. To date, studies evaluating the use of cholesterol-lowering therapies overall have not shown salutary effects with respect to disease progression or need for valve replacement.

In those with symptomatic aortic stenosis who are not candidates for valve replacement, medical therapy is directed at the relief of symptoms because there is no therapy that prolongs life. Treatment of the patient with heart failure may include the cautious use of diuretics and angiotensin-converting enzyme inhibitors. Initiation of such therapies should begin at low doses and be slowly increased. The concern is that diuretic-induced reduction in preload will lower cardiac output, resulting in a drop in systemic arterial pressure, adding to that imposed by angiotensin-converting enzyme inhibitors. β -Blockers should be used with great caution or avoided entirely as they may unmask the left ventricle's dependence on adrenergic support for pressure generation and thereby cause heart failure. Digoxin use is reserved primarily for those with left ventricular dysfunction and/or atrial fibrillation. Hypertension should be treated with careful titration of pharmacotherapy and frequent patient monitoring to avoid hypotension.

The latest guidelines have eliminated the need for antibiotic prophylaxis to prevent infective endocarditis in those with native valvular aortic stenosis. However, endocarditis prophylaxis remains essential in patients who have undergone aortic valve replacement.

B. Valve Replacement

1. Symptomatic patients—As noted earlier, survival in aortic stenosis abruptly declines once the classic symptoms of angina, effort syncope, or congestive heart failure appear. Fifty percent of patients with aortic stenosis in whom angina pectoris develops are dead within 5 years of its onset if AV replacement is not undertaken. Half of patients with syncope will be dead within 3 years and 50% of patients with congestive heart failure will be dead within 2 years without valve replacement (Figure 17–7). The exact pathophysiologic changes that produce the onset of symptoms and begin this rapid downhill course are unknown. The development of symptoms is a class I indication for valve replacement, and following successful valve replacement, symptoms and quality of life improve and survival, in general, is similar to an age-matched population. However, patients who, prior to valve replacement, have severe left ventricular hypertrophy, poor functional capacity, or a large area of myocardial scar and who, after valve replacement, have untreated coexisting coronary artery disease or suboptimal prosthesis hemodynamics are at risk for a less than ideal post-valve replacement outcome. Valve replacement may be either surgical or via a transcatheter approach.

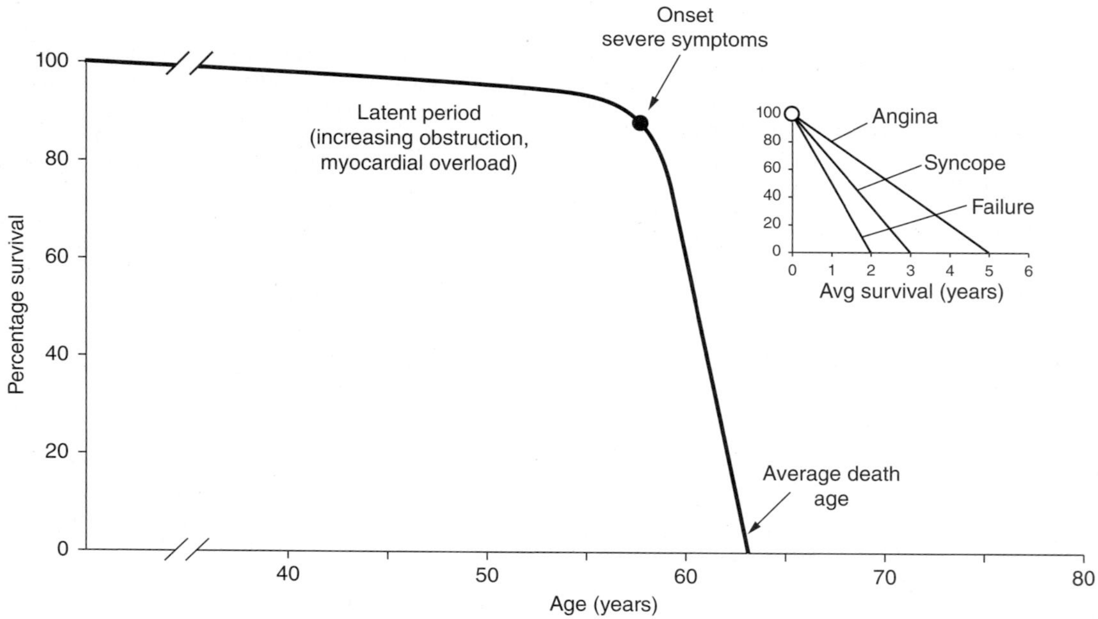

▲ **Figure 17–7.** The natural history of aortic stenosis. There is little change in survival until the symptoms of angina, syncope, or heart failure develop. (Reproduced with permission from Ross J Jr, Braunwald E. Aortic stenosis. *Circulation*. 1968;38[1 Suppl :61–67.)

A. Surgical aortic valve replacement—Surgical AV replacement is done primarily through a midline sternotomy, but in those without coexisting coronary artery disease requiring bypass or a chest wall deformity, valve replacement may be approached through a "mini-sternotomy"—minimally invasive valve surgery. The advantage of the minimally invasive approach is less blood loss, a faster recovery time, and a better cosmetic outcome at the expense of less surgical "exposure." There are a number of different types of valve prostheses including mechanical, stented, and stentless heterografts, xenografts, and homografts.

Mechanical valves used in the aortic position are primarily bileaflet valves, which are durable and provide a good hemodynamic profile particularly at the larger valve sizes. The primary drawback of mechanical valves is the need for lifelong anticoagulation and the associated risk of bleeding. However, new-generation heart valves may permit less aggressive anticoagulation regimens. The On-X bileaflet mechanical valve is the first and currently only heart valve that allows patients, beginning 3 months after their surgery, to be managed with an international normalized ratio of 1.5–2.0 along with low-dose aspirin. This regimen was associated with a 65% overall reduction in bleeding events with no increase in stroke rate.

Heterograft valves have the primary advantage of a low thromboembolism rate without anticoagulation. For any given prosthesis size, the stentless heterograft valves have a better hemodynamic profile when compared to the more commonly used stented bioprostheses. The primary drawback of heterograft valves is their reduced durability when compared to the mechanical valves. Homografts and pulmonary autografts (Ross procedure) are rarely used in the adult population because the operation is technically more challenging and the rate of structural valve failure appears to exceed that of the heterograft valves. The decision of which type of valve prosthesis is best suited for any given patient is based on a number of patient-related factors, such as the bleeding risk with anticoagulation or the need for anticoagulation in those already at high risk for thromboembolism (presence of atrial fibrillation, prior thromboembolism, or a hypercoagulable state). Age can be a factor as well, in a younger population for example, if medical co-morbidities and risk factors permit, a consideration of mechanical valve over bioprosthetic may be considered for durability. Those with renal failure, particularly if on dialysis, or hypercalcemia are at increased risk for structural valve failure with a bioprosthetic valve. The risk of a possible reoperation, if required, also must be considered along with the complex decision facing young women considering pregnancy.

B. Transcatheter aortic valve replacement (TAVR)—Despite the dismal prognosis, many symptomatic patients are either not referred, generally because of age and the perception of surgical risk, or are declined as candidates for surgical valve replacement. TAVR now provides an option for those with severe symptomatic aortic stenosis and a life expectancy in excess of 1 year who have been deemed to have a surgical risk that would preclude AV replacement. Initially, TAVR was an alternative to surgical valve replacement in those deemed surgical candidates but were stratified to have a high surgical risk. However, the FDA has expanded the indication now for patients who are not only high, but also intermediate and low surgical risk. The determination of surgical risk is based on a risk model from the Society of Thoracic Surgeons (STS) to estimate 30-day mortality. The score equals the predicted mortality expressed as a percentage. Patients deemed high surgical risk generally have an STS score greater than 8%. Increased operator experience and new-generation heart valves and delivery systems have resulted in lower TAVR-associated risk, making TAVR similar to surgical AV replacement with respect to death or disabling stroke in intermediate-risk patients. Intermediate-risk patient are generally those with an STS score between 4% and 8%. In the low-risk category, there have been trials to show that TAVR has been noninferior and occasionally shows lower rate of complications such as disabling stroke, complications due to bleeding, acute kidney injury, and atrial fibrillation as a result of transcatheter approach versus surgical approach. It should be noted however that there are higher rates of post-replacement aortic regurgitation and the need for permanent pacemakers after TAVR, especially with self-expanding valves.

TAVR is primarily performed through transfemoral arterial access. If delivery through the femoral artery is not possible, a transthoracic approach may be used (transapical or transaortic access route). Transsubclavian, transcaval, and transcarotid approaches have also been described. Although there are several transcatheter valves in development, at present, the Edwards SAPIEN 3 ultra (Edwards Lifesciences Inc., Irvine, CA) and EvolutPro/Pro Plus (Medtronic Inc., Minneapolis, MN) valves are the only valves approved for clinical use (Figure 17–8). In high-risk patients not deemed to be surgical candidates 1 year after TAVR, there was a 20% absolute reduction in mortality, significantly fewer cardiac symptoms, and lower New York Heart Association functional class with either the SAPIEN valve or the CoreValve when compared to those who received standard medical therapy. When high-risk patients were randomized to either surgical or transcatheter valve replacement, the 30-day mortality was lower with TAVR and the 1-year mortality was equivalent. The risks of TAVR include death, vascular complications, heart block requiring a pacemaker, neurologic events, and paravalvular regurgitation. Therefore, in high-risk patients who are still candidates for surgery, the European Society of Cardiology guidelines on valvular heart disease state that the decision "should be individualized and TAVR considered as an alternative to surgery in those patients for whom the heart team favors TAVR based on the individual's risk profile and anatomic suitability."

The concept of the multidisciplinary approach and the TAVR heart team has been one of the greatest collaborative successes in the field of cardiovascular diseases. The team

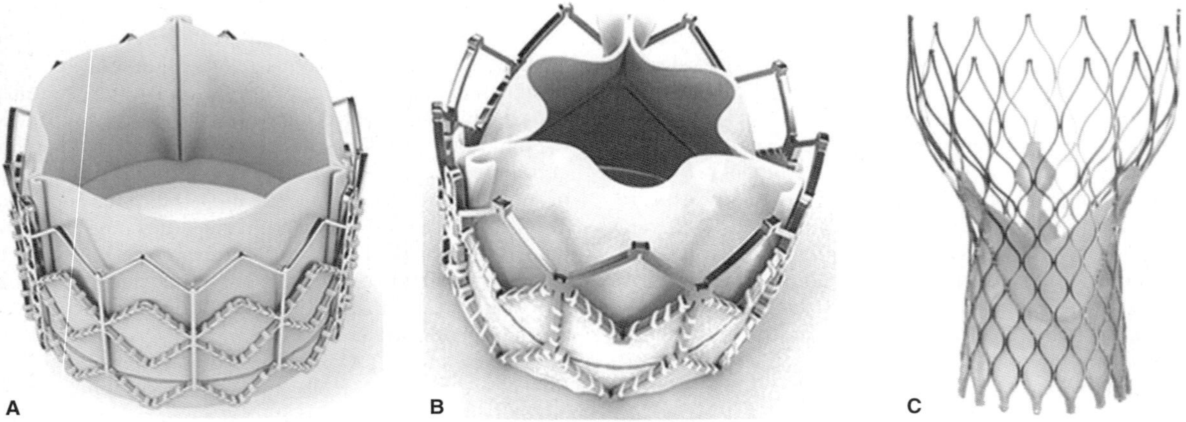

▲ **Figure 17–8. A:** The Edward SAPIEN balloon expandable valve (Edwards Lifesciences, Irvine, CA) incorporates a stainless-steel frame, bovine pericardial leaflets, and a fabric sealing cuff. **B:** The SAPIEN XT THV (Edwards Lifesciences) uses a cobalt chromium alloy frame and is compatible with lower profile delivery catheters. **C:** The Medtronic CoreValve (Medtronic, Minneapolis, MN) incorporates a self-expandable frame, porcine pericardial leaflets, and a pericardial seal. (Reproduced, with permission, from Webb J, Wood D. *J Am Coll Cardiol*. 2012;60:483–492. Copyright © American College of Cardiology Foundation.)

encompasses the patient at its center and involves the referring physician, imaging and interventional cardiologist, cardiac surgeon, valve clinic coordinator, anesthesiologist, and the cardiac and operating room staff. The patients are investigated clinically through assessing their frailty, STS score, imaging studies, cardiac catheterization, and assessment of social support. A plan is then conducted and conveyed to the patient and family.

Finally, there has been a shift from transesophageal echocardiography–guided/general anesthesia support for TAVR to a minimalist approach of local anesthesia with Perclose and transthoracic echocardiography. This has led to a decreased hospital stay, lesser morbidity, and lower cost at no penalty of increased mortality or morbidity.

c. Balloon aortic valvuloplasty (BAV)—Occasionally there will be circumstances in which patients with severe symptomatic aortic stenosis who would otherwise require TAVR or SAVR are unable to have valve replacements done. A possible alternative procedure to improve the stenotic lesion would be the balloon valvuloplasty. This is a nonsurgical, catheter-based technique in which balloon expansion at the stenotic aortic valve can fracture and force the calcified leaflets open. This of course comes with the obvious risk of causing aortic insufficiency which can be a contraindication to performing the procedure. Balloon aortic valvuloplasties can be useful procedures in a variety of clinical situations, for example, in patients who require urgent noncardiac surgery in whom their surgical risk otherwise would be too elevated due to their severe aortic stenosis. Other candidates to consider would be those who otherwise would have a contraindication or would be at elevated risk for SAVR or TAVR procedures. Occasionally a role for hemodynamic stabilization in those with decompensated heart disease due to obstruction of the aortic valve may find some relief from BAV procedure.

Debry N, Altes A, Vincent F, et al. Balloon aortic valvuloplasty for severe aortic stenosis before urgent non-cardiac surgery. *EuroIntervention*. 2021;17(8):e680–e687. [PMID: 34105511]

Kapadia SR, Leon MB, Makkar RR, et al. 5-year outcomes of transcatheter aortic valve replacement compared with standard treatment for patients with inoperable aortic stenosis (PARTNER 1): a randomised controlled trial. *Lancet*. 2015;385: 2485–2491. [PMID: 25788231]

Leon MB, Smith CR, Mack MJ, et al. Transcatheter or surgical aortic-valve replacement in intermediate-risk patients. *N Engl J Med*. 2016;374(17):1609–1620. [PMID: 27040324]

Mack MJ, Leon MB, Smith CR, et al. 5-year outcomes of transcatheter aortic valve replacement or surgical aortic valve replacement for high surgical risk patients with aortic stenosis (PARTNER 1): a randomised controlled trial. *Lancet*. 2015; 385:2477–2484. [PMID: 25788234]

Mack MJ, Leon MB, Thourani VH, et al. Transcatheter aortic-valve replacement with a balloon-expandable valve in low-risk patients. *N Engl J Med*. 2019;380(18):1695–1705. [PMID: 30883058]

Popma JJ, Deeb GM, Yakubov SJ, et al. Transcatheter aortic-valve replacement with a self-expanding valve in low-risk patients. *N Engl J Med*. 2019;380(18)1706–1715. [PMID: 30883053]

Reardon MJ, Mieghem NMV, Popma JJ, et al. Surgical or transcatheter aortic-valve replacement in intermediate-risk patients. *N Engl J Med*. 2017;376(14):1321–1331. [PMID: 28304219]

2. Asymptomatic patients—In distinct contrast to the universal recommendation for valve replacement in those with symptomatic severe aortic stenosis, the management of the asymptomatic patient remains controversial. As noted earlier, the decision to proceed with valve replacement occurs when the risk of native AV stenosis exceeds the procedural risk combined with the long-term risk of prosthetic heart valve disease. The primary concern in the strategy of watchful waiting is the risk of sudden death and the fact that symptoms are subjective and influenced by the patient's lifestyle and may be underreported.

The contemporary literature suggests that the risk of sudden death in the asymptomatic adult patient with severe aortic stenosis is approximately 1% per year. Conversely, in low-risk patients, there is an operative mortality of 1–3% and a 2–3% per year risk for a prosthesis-related complication such as thromboembolism, endocarditis, valve failure, bleeding (if anticoagulation is required), and death. Therefore, previous thought had been that surgical valve replacement risk exceeded any potential benefit to those with truly asymptomatic severe aortic stenosis and normal left ventricular systolic function. Patients may either not seek medical attention immediately following the onset of symptoms or truncate their lifestyle so as to negate symptoms. In addition, there is frequently some wait time until a valve replacement can be scheduled while the patient is symptomatic. These individuals are at increased risk, and the ideal situation is to better stratify risk in these "asymptomatic" patients and potentially offer valve replacement to those deemed at greatest risk. Features on the baseline echocardiogram including EF, left ventricular wall thickness, peak transaortic jet velocity, and the rate of hemodynamic progression are independent predictors of outcome. A noteworthy proportion of those who claim to be asymptomatic have an abnormal exercise test, defined as exercise-limiting symptoms and/or a fall in blood pressure below baseline, and these patients have a worse outcome. The added value of exercise-induced changes in echocardiographically derived valve hemodynamics is controversial, but reports state an incremental and independent prognostic value to an exercise-induced increase in mean gradient greater than 20 mm Hg, even in those with a normal exercise stress test—the "truly" asymptomatic. The extent of valve calcification, very severe stenosis, and plasma brain natriuretic peptide levels may also be helpful in refining risk. Both the North American and European valve disease guidelines primarily based on expert consensus (level of evidence C) make recommendations for valve replacement in those with asymptomatic severe aortic stenosis, but there is variability in the strength of the recommendation (Table 17–2).

Given the sharp decline in patient survival once symptomatic (angina, syncope, or congestive heart failure) aortic stenosis occurs, with a 50% mortality in 5 years, recent pushes to evaluate the potential benefit of early valve replacement have been sought. Specific populations have in fact shown benefit for early intervention prior to the onset of symptoms. In regard to surgical aortic valve replacement, the management of patient with asymptomatic very severe aortic stenosis has shown a lower incidence of operative mortality, acute MI, stroke, unplanned hospitalization, or cardiovascular death as compared to conservative care. Early surgical replacement has also been associated with an improved all-cause mortality in an asymptomatic patient with severe aortic stenosis. With the FDA approval for low- and intermediate-risk TAVR, there has been a shift now toward having a closer look on an individualized basis with a multidisciplinary Heart Team approach to determine if the risk of performing TAVR outweighs the risk of sudden cardiac death. There are ongoing clinical trials as well to assess the efficacy and safety of transcatheter aortic

Table 17–2. Asymptomatic Severe Aortic Stenosis: Indications for Isolated Aortic Valve Replacement

Class	ACC/AHA Guidelines	ESC Guidelines
I	Reduced LVEF < 50% not due to another cause	Reduced LVEF < 50% not due to another cause Abnormal exercise test showing symptoms on exercise clearly related to AS
IIa	Very severe AS (aortic velocity ≥ 5.0 m/s or mean gradient ≥ 60 mm Hg) and low surgical risk Decreased exercise tolerance or an exercise-related fall in blood pressure BNP 3× upper limit of normal and low surgical risk Rapid disease progression (increase in aortic velocity ≥ 0.3 m/s per year) and low surgical risk	Reduced LVEF < 55% not due to another cause Abnormal exercise test showing a fall in blood pressure > 20 mm Hg below baseline Low surgical risk with LVEF > 55% and one of the following: 1. Severe valve calcification by CCT and a rate of peak velocity progression ≥ 0.3 m/s per year 2. Very severe AS (peak transvalvular velocity > 5 m/s or mean gradient > 60 mm Hg) 3. BNP 3× upper limit of normal, age and sex corrected and confirmed on serial measures
IIb	Reduced LVEF < 60% not due to another cause on 3 serial studies	

ACC, American College of Cardiology; AHA, American Heart Association; AS, aortic stenosis; ESC, European Society of Cardiology; LV, left ventricular; LVEF, left ventricular ejection fraction.

valve replacement in the asymptotic severe aortic stenosis population.

Banovic M, Putnik S, Penicka M, et al. Aortic valve replacement versus conservative treatment in asymptomatic severe aortic stenosis: The AVATAR Trial [published correction appears in Circulation. 2022 Mar;145(9):e761]. *Circulation.* 2022;145(9):648–658. [PMID: 34779220]
Kang DH, Park SJ, Lee SA, et al. Early surgery or conservative care for asymptomatic aortic stenosis. *N Engl J Med.* 2020;382(2):111–119. [PMID:31733181]
Otto CM, Nishimura RA, Bonow RO, et al. 2020 ACC/AHA Guideline for the Management of Patients With Valvular Heart Disease: Executive Summary: A Report of the American College of Cardiology/American Heart Association Joint Committee on Clinical Practice Guidelines. [published correction appears in Circulation. 2021 Feb 2;143(5):e228] [published correction appears in Circulation. 2021 Mar 9;143(10):e784]. *Circulation.* 2021;143(5):e35–e71. [PMID: 33332149]
Vahanian A, Beyersdorf F, Praz F, et al. 2021 ESC/EACTS guidelines for the management of valvular heart disease: developed by the task force for the management of valvular heart disease of the European Society of Cardiology (ESC) and the European Association for Cardio-Thoracic Surgery (EACTS). *Eur Heart J.* 2022;43:561–632. [PMID: 34453165]

Special Circumstances

A. Low EF Area-Gradient Mismatch (LF/LG Aortic Stenosis)

Patients with LF/LG aortic stenosis have a poor prognosis with medical management. As noted earlier, deciphering the true severity of aortic stenosis in the presence of area-gradient mismatch is imperative in the evaluation of patient prognosis and to guide the appropriate management of patients. In those with LF/LG aortic stenosis, the contemporary clinical protocol is to attempt to increase flow across the AV with a dobutamine infusion and to evaluate the ventricular response and transvalvular hemodynamics. In general, those with true or fixed severe aortic stenosis should have valve replacement performed if it can be done with an acceptable risk. Those with indeterminate aortic stenosis because of the absence of contractile reserve (the inability to increase stroke volume ≥ 20% with a dobutamine infusion) have an abysmal prognosis with medical management but also a high operative risk (reported in some series to be up to 30%). However, those who survive surgery generally show an improvement in functional capacity, ventricular function, and overall survival. Thus, the management of those with LF/LG aortic stenosis and the absence of contractile reserve is controversial, but valve replacement has been given a class IIb recommendation in the European Society of Cardiology guidelines on valve disease. In those with significant valve calcification, a mean gradient greater than 20 mm Hg, and the absence of a large area of left ventricular scar, valve replacement should be considered. Note that the literature on risk and benefit of valve replacement in these patients is based on surgical valve replacement, and over time, we may find that TAVR offers a lower procedural risk alternative for these patients.

B. Normal EF Area-Gradient Mismatch (PLF/LG Aortic Stenosis)

These individuals present with a low valve area and low gradient despite a preserved left ventricular EF (LVEF). There is controversy about how best to manage these patients, and the mere presence of a low gradient cannot exclude severe aortic stenosis in some of these patients who would have a poor outcome if treated medically and would benefit from valve replacement. How best to characterize and select those with PLF/LG aortic stenosis who are most likely to benefit from valve replacement remains challenging. The American College of Cardiology/American Heart Association valvular heart disease guidelines state that AV replacement is "reasonable in symptomatic patients with low-flow/low-gradient severe AS who are normotensive (systolic blood pressure < 140 mm Hg) and have an LVEF ≥ 50% if clinical, hemodynamic and anatomic data support valve obstruction as the most likely cause of symptoms (class IIa recommendation)." Therefore, in patients with normal EF area-gradient mismatch, exercise testing is reasonable to help determine functional capacity and identify the presence of symptoms. If symptoms are noted, the first approach would be to ensure blood pressure is adequately controlled. If the patient is hypertensive (systolic blood pressure > 140 mm Hg), a repeat evaluation of stenosis severity should be performed once the blood pressure is controlled. The AVA should be indexed to body surface area, and an AVA index ≤ 0.6 cm^2/m^2 suggests severe aortic stenosis. If the patient is symptomatic but the blood pressure is well controlled, we will usually obtain a valve calcium score to help determine stenosis severity. A measure of AVA_{proj} ≤ 1.0 cm^2 is also predictive of true aortic stenosis, and its determination can help support clinical decision-making. As with those with low EF area-gradient mismatch, the literature on risk and benefit of valve replacement in these patients is based on surgical valve replacement; TAVR with its lower procedural risk may be an alternative for these patients.

C. Moderate Aortic Stenosis

The above discussions while often focusing on interventions for severe aortic stenosis, whether symptomatic or not, have all had the underlying theme of early intervention prior to poor survival and outcomes. It has been widely established that untreated severe aortic stenosis is associated with poor outcomes. Recent data have also suggested that those with known moderate aortic stenosis (mean trans-aortic gradient of 20–39 mm Hg or peak aortic blood velocity of 3.0–3.9 m/s), are also at an elevated risk of poor outcomes. These patients are not necessarily asymptomatic until reaching the severe grading as well; they are also at risk of, and often do develop symptoms related to their valvulopathy. Therefore, upcoming clinical trials aim to evaluate the utility in early intervention in a specific subset of patients known to have moderate aortic stenosis. The Medtronic Evolut (Medtronic, Minneapolis, MN) is currently being studied in symptomatic and asymptomatic patients with moderate aortic stenosis in the EXPAND TAVR I trial. The Edwards SAPIEN 3/SAPIEN 3 Ultra are currently being studied in patients with moderate calcific aortic stenosis in the PROGRESS trial. As well, patients with advanced heart failure with reduced ejection fraction will be studied to evaluate the safety and efficacy of TAVR using the Edward SAPIEN balloon expandable valve (Edwards Lifesciences, Irvine, CA), in the TAVR UNLOAD Trial.

Medtronic Evolut™ EXPAND TAVR I Feasibility Study. ClinicalTrials.gov identifier ***NCT04639258***

PROGRESS Trial: A Prospective, Randomized, Controlled Trial to Assess the Management of Moderate Aortic Stenosis by Clinical Surveillance or Transcatheter Aortic Valve Replacement. ClinicalTrials.gov identifier ***NCT04889872***

Spitzer E, Mieghem NMV, Pibarot P, et al. Rationale and design of the Transcatheter Aortic Valve Replacement to UNload the Left ventricle in patients with ADvanced heart failure (TAVR UNLOAD) trial. *Am Heart J*. 2016;182:80–88. [PMID: 27914503]

Strange G, Stewart S, Celermajer D, et al. Poor long-term survival in patients with moderate aortic stenosis. *J Am Coll Cardiol*. 2019;74(15):1851–1863. [PMID: 31491546]

Prognosis

As noted earlier, the prognosis of those with severe symptomatic and asymptomatic aortic stenosis, in the absence of valve replacement, is very poor. However, the age-adjusted survival following valve replacement is excellent, even in the elderly who are free of other cardiac or systemic diseases. Asymptomatic patients generally have a good prognosis, with the strongest predictor of clinical outcome (death or valve replacement) being stenosis severity. The likelihood of remaining alive without valve replacement at 2 years is approximately 20% in those with a peak jet velocity greater than 4.0 m/s, 66% if the jet velocity is between 3.0 and 4.0 m/s, and 84% for those with a jet velocity less than 3.0 m/s. Understanding the strong impact of stenosis severity along with other clinical predictors, such as functional capacity and the rate of hemodynamic progression, an outcome is useful when counseling patients about their prognosis and to help tailor the frequency of follow-up. As well, there are ongoing studies evaluating the prognosis without and with interventions in symptomatic and asymptomatic moderate aortic stenosis.

18 Aortic Regurgitation

Michael H. Crawford, MD

ESSENTIALS OF DIAGNOSIS

- Presentation dependent on the rapidity of onset of regurgitation: acute pulmonary edema or chronic dyspnea on exertion.
- Wide pulse pressure with associated peripheral signs.
- Diastolic decrescendo murmur at the left sternal border.
- Left ventricular dilation and hypertrophy with preserved function.
- Diagnosis confirmed and severity estimated by Doppler echocardiography, aortography, magnetic resonance imaging, or computed tomography angiography.

Etiology

Normally, the integrity of the aortic orifice during diastole is maintained by an intact aortic root and firm apposition of the free margins of the three aortic valve cusps. Aortic regurgitation (AR) may therefore be caused by a variety of disorders affecting the valve cusps, the aortic root, or the diastolic pressure in the proximal aorta (Table 18–1). With rheumatic heart disease becoming less common, nonrheumatic causes currently account for most of the underlying causes of AR, including congenitally malformed aortic valves, degenerative valve disease, and infective endocarditis. Disorders affecting the aortic root also account for many patients with AR. These conditions include Marfan syndrome, aortic dissection, and inflammatory diseases. Even in the absence of any obvious abnormality of the aortic valve or root, severe systemic hypertension has been reported to cause significant AR.

Pathophysiology

The presentation and findings in patients with AR depend on its severity and rapidity of onset. The hemodynamic effects of acute severe AR are entirely different from the chronic type, and the two will be discussed separately.

A. Chronic Aortic Regurgitation

In response to the left ventricular volume overload associated with AR, progressive left ventricular dilation occurs. This results in a higher wall stress, which stimulates ventricular hypertrophy and which, in turn, tends to normalize wall stress. Patients with severe AR may have the largest end-diastolic volumes produced by any other heart disease and yet their end-diastolic pressures are not uniformly elevated. In keeping with the Frank-Starling mechanism, the stroke volume is also increased. Thus, despite the presence of regurgitation, a normal effective forward cardiac output can be maintained. This state persists for several years. Gradually, left ventricular diastolic properties and contractile function start to decline. The adaptive dilation and hypertrophy can no longer match the loading conditions. The left ventricular end-diastolic pressure begins to rise, and the ejection fraction drops with a decline in effective forward output and development of heart failure.

B. Acute Aortic Regurgitation

In contrast to chronic AR, when sudden severe regurgitation occurs, the left ventricle has no time to adapt. The acute ventricular volume overload which results in a small increase in end-diastolic volume and severe elevation of end-diastolic pressure, which is transmitted to the left atrium and pulmonary veins, culminating in acute pulmonary edema. Because the ventricular end-diastolic volume is normal, the total stroke volume is not increased and the

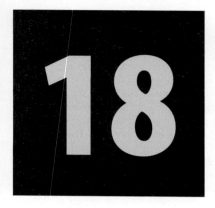

Table 18–1. Causes of Aortic Regurgitation

Aortic cusp abnormalities
Infectious: Bacterial endocarditis, rheumatic fever
Congenital: Bicuspid aortic valve
Inflammatory: Systemic lupus erythematosus, rheumatoid arthritis, Behçet syndrome
Degenerative: Myxomatous (floppy) valve, calcific aortic valve
Iatrogenic: Catheter
Postaortic valvuloplasty
Toxin-induced valvulopathy: Anorectics, carcinoid
Aortic root abnormalities
Aortic root dilatation: Marfan syndrome, syphilis, ankylosing spondylitis, relapsing polychondritis, idiopathic aortitis, annuloaortic ectasia, cystic medial necrosis, Ehlers-Danlos syndrome, syphilitic
Loss of commissural support: Aortic dissection, trauma, ventricular septal defect
Increased pressure
Systemic hypertension
Supravalvular aortic stenosis

effective forward cardiac output drops. To compensate for the low-output state, sympathetic stimulation occurs, which produces tachycardia and peripheral vasoconstriction, the latter further worsening AR.

Clinical Findings

A. Symptoms & Signs

1. Chronic aortic regurgitation—Patients with chronic AR remain asymptomatic for a long time. Palpitations are common and may be due to either awareness of forceful left ventricular contractions or the occurrence of premature atrial or ventricular beats. Angina may occur either from concomitant coronary disease or from a combination of low diastolic pressure and increased oxygen demand from ventricular hypertrophy. When left ventricular dysfunction supervenes, patients initially experience exertional dyspnea and fatigue. At a later stage, resting heart failure symptoms occur with orthopnea and paroxysmal nocturnal dyspnea.

On physical examination, visible cardiac pulsations are common. The area of the apical impulse is increased on palpation. The first heart sound is usually normal. The aortic component of the second heart sound may be decreased in conditions where cusp excursion is reduced, such as with valve calcification. An S_4 is often present due to underlying hypertrophy, and an S_3 is audible when ventricular failure occurs. On auscultation, the characteristic sound of AR is a soft, high-pitched diastolic decrescendo murmur best heard in the third intercostal space along the left sternal border at end expiration, with the patient sitting and leaning forward. In the presence of aortic root disease, the murmur may be best heard to the right of the sternum. A systolic ejection murmur may be present at the aortic area due to the high-flow state. Occasionally, a diastolic rumble may be heard at the apex, referred to as the Austin Flint murmur. The mechanism underlying this murmur remains unclear. Several different causes have been proposed, the most likely being the aortic jet encountering the mitral inflow resulting in turbulence.

The systolic arterial pressure is increased due to a large stroke volume, whereas the diastolic pressure is decreased due to runoff from the aorta into both the ventricle and peripheral arteries. This is the underlying reason for a wide pulse pressure and for a variety of associated eponymic peripheral signs in chronic significant AR (Table 18–2). However, it must be remembered that these signs are not specific for AR and may occur in any high-flow state such as occurs in anemia, thyrotoxicosis, and arteriovenous malformations. With the development of heart failure, the pulse pressure narrows and the peripheral signs of AR are attenuated.

2. Acute aortic regurgitation—In contrast to chronic AR, most patients with acute severe AR are symptomatic. Initial presentation may vary depending on the underlying cause, which most commonly is aortic dissection, infective endocarditis, or trauma. In the presence of associated acute AR, clinical manifestations of severe dyspnea, orthopnea, and weakness often develop. The onset of symptoms is sudden, with rapid progression to hemodynamic collapse if left untreated.

In acute AR, the left ventricle has had no time to adapt to the volume overload state. The peripheral signs associated with chronic AR are therefore absent. Pulse pressure is usually normal, and hypotension may be present in severe cases. Bilateral crackles are usually present on

Table 18–2. Peripheral Signs of Aortic Regurgitation

Name of Sign	Description
Corrigan pulse	Rapid and forceful distention of arterial pulse with quick collapse
De-Musset sign	To and fro head bobbing
Müller sign	Visible pulsation of uvula
Quincke sign	Capillary pulsations seen on light compression of nail bed
Traube sign	Systolic and diastolic sounds (pistol shots) over the femoral artery
Duroziez sign	Bruits heard over femoral artery on light compression by stethoscope
Hill sign	Popliteal cuff pressure exceeding brachial pressure by 60 mm Hg or greater

examination of the lungs and reflect underlying pulmonary edema. On precordial palpation, the apical impulse is not shifted. The rapid rise in left ventricular diastolic pressure causes premature closure of the mitral valve resulting in soft or absent first heart sound. An S_3 is often present, but an S_4 is usually absent because there is little or no atrial contribution to ventricular filling due to high left ventricular end-diastolic pressure. The typical diastolic murmur of AR is shortened in duration, often difficult to hear, and easily missed.

B. Laboratory Findings

Laboratory findings depend on the underlying cause of AR. Elevated white blood cell count and erythrocyte sedimentation rate are seen in inflammatory conditions, such as infection and aortitis. Abnormal antinuclear antigen and rheumatoid factor titers may be seen in patients with rheumatologic disorders. When syphilis is suspected, serologic tests may be indicated. Plasma brain natriuretic peptide (BNP and NT pro-BNP) levels are associated with prognosis in patients with AR and may contribute to the decision for surgery.

C. Diagnostic Studies

1. Electrocardiography—No specific electrocardiographic abnormalities are characteristic of AR. Signs of left atrial enlargement, left ventricular hypertrophy, and a "strain pattern" (ST depression with T-wave inversion in lateral leads) are often seen in chronic significant AR. Arrhythmias, including ventricular ectopy and ventricular tachycardia, may occur in advanced cases with left ventricular dysfunction. In acute AR, sinus tachycardia may be the only abnormality. In cases of infective endocarditis, inflammation or abscess formation may spread to the atrioventricular node, resulting in prolongation of the PR interval or development of atrioventricular block.

2. Chest radiography—Chest radiographic findings are not specific for AR and reflect an estimate of cardiac size and pulmonary vascular changes. In chronic significant AR, an increase in the size of the left heart chambers and the aorta is seen. In acute AR, the cardiac size is normal; the lung fields show increased markings due to pulmonary edema. When AR is due to aortic dissection, the chest film may show an enlarged ascending aorta. If calcification of the aortic knob is present, a helpful sign of dissection is increased separation between the outer margin of the aorta and the calcific density.

3. Echocardiography and Doppler techniques—Echocardiography is the method of choice for evaluating patients with AR. Two-dimensional echocardiography in combination with various Doppler modalities and, in selected cases, transesophageal imaging has provided a noninvasive means for not only diagnosing AR with a high sensitivity and specificity but also for assessing its etiology and severity. Furthermore, important information can be obtained on the hemodynamic impact of the regurgitant lesion, prognosis, and effectiveness of therapy.

A. DETECTION OF AORTIC REGURGITATION—Doppler techniques are extremely sensitive and specific in the detection of AR, manifested as a diastolic flow abnormality arising from the aortic valve, directed toward the left ventricle. Even trivial regurgitation can be detected, which commonly is not audible on physical examination. Although most cases of moderate-to-severe chronic AR have typical findings on physical examination, moderate lesions may occasionally be missed on examination because of the subtlety of auscultatory findings. Doppler echocardiography is also extremely valuable in patients with acute AR when the typical clinical findings of chronic AR are absent, and the brief murmur can often be missed. Color Doppler echocardiography has proven to be extremely helpful in the evaluation of AR (Figure 18–1). It provides a spatial orientation of the regurgitant jet arising from the aortic root. A completely negative color Doppler examination in multiple planes virtually excludes the presence of AR.

B. ASSESSMENT OF CAUSE—Because two-dimensional echocardiography can image cardiac structures, it provides valuable information on the cause of the AR. Structural abnormalities of the aortic valve, including calcifications or thickening, congenital deformities, vegetations, rupture, or prolapse, can be identified. Dilatation of the aortic root, calcifications, or dissection can also be evaluated. Although most of these conditions can be assessed with transthoracic echocardiography, transesophageal echocardiography has provided high-resolution images that allow for improved detection of such abnormalities, especially in technically difficult cases or in conditions such as infective endocarditis. In patients with AR due to aortic disease, precisely defining the morphology of the valve and involvement of the aortic root is important in determining the surgical approach and deciding whether the valve can be preserved or requires replacement.

C. ASSESSMENT OF SEVERITY—In addition to the detection of AR, Doppler echocardiography combined with two-dimensional echocardiographic imaging has recently allowed an assessment of the severity of the lesion. Several methods have been proposed, including color Doppler assessment of regurgitant jet size, continuous wave Doppler using the pressure half-time method, measurements of regurgitant volume and effective regurgitant orifice area derived from two-dimensional echocardiography and pulsed Doppler techniques, and three-dimensional echocardiography to directly visualize the size of the regurgitant orifice.

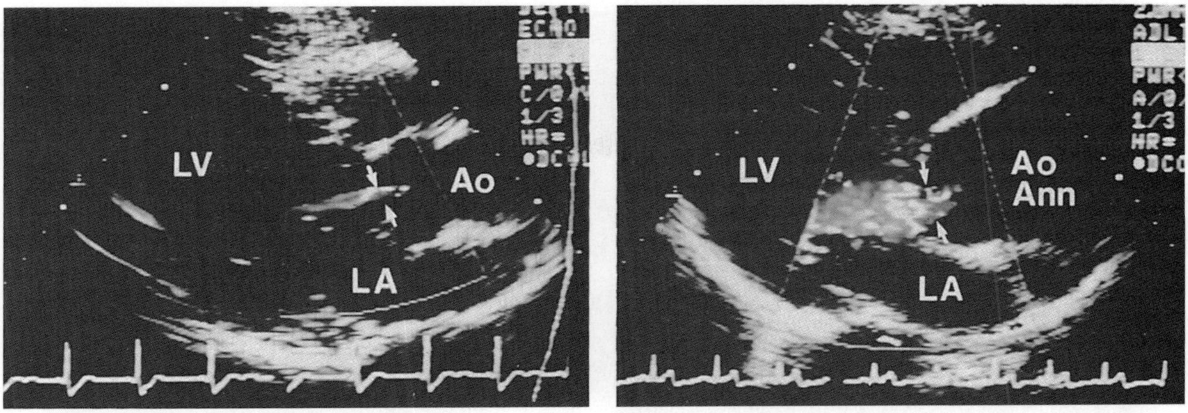

A B

▲ **Figure 18–1.** Color Doppler echocardiographic frames in diastole from the parasternal long-axis view in (**A**) a patient with mild aortic regurgitation and (**B**) another patient with severe regurgitation. The patient with severe aortic regurgitation (**B**) has a large ascending aortic aneurysm (Ao Ann). The width of the aortic regurgitation jet in the left ventricular outflow (*between arrows*) provides a good estimate of the severity of aortic regurgitation by color Doppler echocardiography. Ao, aorta; LA, left atrium; LV, left ventricle.

With color-flow Doppler, the AR jet can be spatially oriented in the two-dimensional plane arising from the aortic valve and directed toward the left ventricle. The measurement of the width of the AR jet at the level of the leaflets (vena contracta) has been used to quantitatively approximate AR severity. A vena contracta of greater than 0.6 cm is considered a sign of severe AR. On the other hand, it is important to note that the length of the AR jet does not correlate well with AR severity. This is in part because color Doppler flow mapping is also highly dependent on the velocity of regurgitation, or the driving pressure, in addition to the regurgitant volume. Also, ratio of the AR jet diameter just below the leaflets to that of the left ventricular outflow diameter has been shown to correlate well with the severity of regurgitation when compared with invasive angiography (Table 18–3; see Figure 18–1).

Another index of AR severity that has been useful clinically is the pressure half-time derived from continuous wave Doppler recordings of the AR jet velocity. The velocity of the regurgitant jet is related to the instantaneous pressure difference between the aorta and left ventricle in diastole by the modified Bernoulli equation: $\Delta P = 4V^2$, where ΔP is the pressure gradient in millimeters of mercury and V is the blood velocity in meters per second. The pressure half-time index is the time it takes for the initial maximal pressure gradient in diastole to fall by 50%. In patients with mild regurgitation, there is a gradual small drop in the pressure difference in diastole, whereas with severe AR, a more precipitous drop occurs (Figure 18–2). A pressure half-time greater than 500 ms is seen in mild AR, but more significant regurgitation is usually associated with a shorter pressure half-time (see Table 18–3 and Figure 18–2). The severity of AR using this index may be overestimated in patients who have elevated left ventricular end-diastolic pressure, especially those with reduced left ventricular compliance.

The severity of AR can also be assessed using regurgitant volume and regurgitant fraction derived from two-dimensional and pulsed Doppler echocardiography. This method is based on the continuity equation, which states

Table 18–3. Echocardiographic Parameter for Grading Aortic Regurgitation Severity

	Mild	Moderate	Severe
VC width, cm	< 0.3	0.3–0.6	> 0.6
Jet width/LVOT width, %	< 25	25–64	≥ 65
R Vol, mL/beat	< 30	30–59	≥ 60
RF, %	< 30	30–49	≥ 50
EROA, cm^2	< 0.10	0.10–0.29	≥ 0.30
Pressure half-time, ms	> 500	200–500	< 200
Diastolic flow reversal in descending aorta–PW	Brief, early diastolic reversal	Intermediate	Prominent holo-diastolic reversal

EROA, effective regurgitant orifice area; LVOT, left ventricular outflow tract; PW, pulsed wave Doppler; R Vol, regurgitant volume; RF, regurgitant fraction; VC, vena contracta.

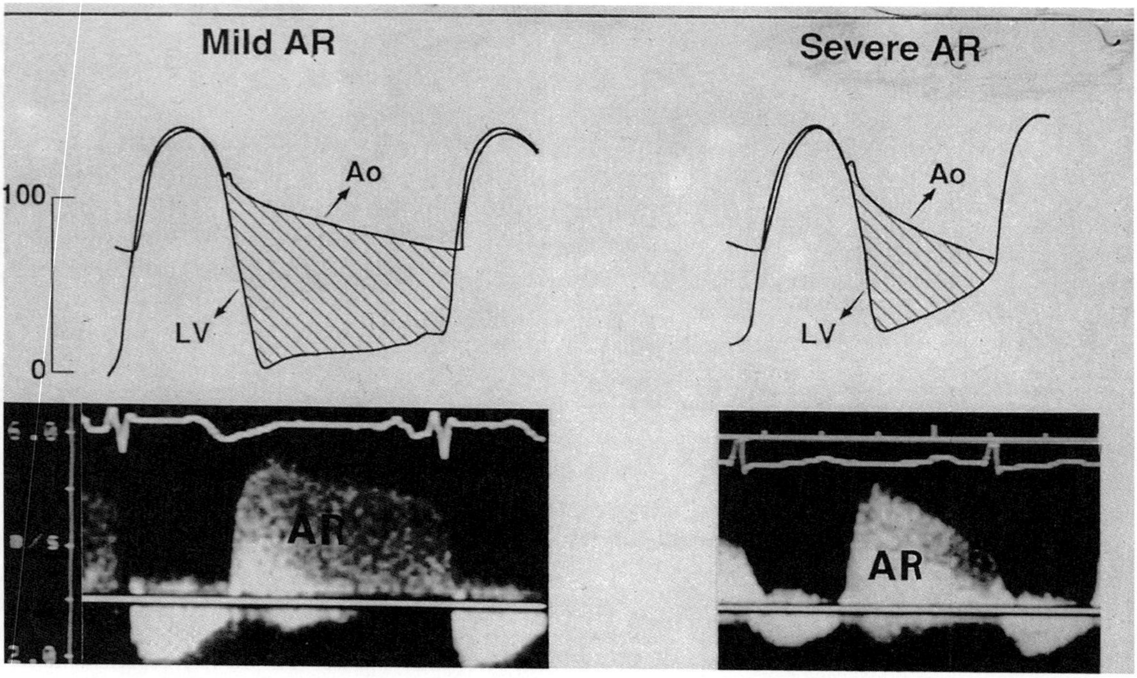

▲ **Figure 18–2.** Schematic of aortic and left ventricular pressure tracings in (*left*) a patient with mild and (*right*) another patient with severe aortic regurgitation and corresponding examples of continuous wave Doppler recording of aortic jet velocity in such patients. In mild aortic regurgitation, a gradual, small drop in the difference between aortic and ventricular pressures occurs in diastole, reflected by the small decrease in the velocity of the aortic regurgitation jet. In contrast, in severe aortic regurgitation, a more precipitous drop occurs in the pressure gradient and in the corresponding jet velocity. AR, aortic regurgitation; Ao, aorta; LV, left ventricle.

that, in the absence of regurgitation, blood flow is equal across all valves. Stroke volume at the level of a valve annulus is calculated as the product of the cross-sectional area obtained by two-dimensional echocardiography and the time velocity integral of flow recorded by pulsed Doppler. In the presence of AR, stroke volume at the left ventricular outflow tract is higher than that across another valve without regurgitation. Therefore, AR volume can be calculated as the difference between stroke volume at the left ventricular outflow and that derived at another valve site. Dividing the regurgitant volume by stroke volume across the aortic valve gives an estimate of regurgitant fraction. A regurgitant fraction of less than 30% is usually mild, whereas a regurgitant fraction greater than 50% denotes severe AR (see Table 18–3). A similar approach to estimating severity of AR can be achieved using pulsed Doppler echocardiography in the proximal descending aorta. In patients with significant AR, a large reversal of flow is observed in diastole toward the aortic arch and ascending aorta. This simple method should be used routinely to qualitatively grade the severity of regurgitation and can also be used quantitatively to derive a regurgitant fraction.

Proximal flow convergence is more difficult to identify in AR, but when it is present, the proximal isovelocity surface area (PISA) method can be used to determine the effective regurgitant orifice area (EROA). This method is less accurate in eccentric jets and aortic root dilatation. Also, shadowing from aortic valve and root calcium may obscure the flow convergence. Alternatively, dividing the regurgitant volume by the velocity time integral of the AR can provide an estimate of the EROA.

Although color-flow Doppler allows a good estimation of the severity of AR in most patients, its accuracy depends on optimization of the color Doppler examination, including gain settings, frame rate, and interrogation of multiple tomographic planes. The availability of other independent Doppler indices of AR severity further allows the corroboration of color Doppler findings. This is particularly helpful in patients with eccentric AR jets, for which severity may be difficult to assess by color-flow Doppler alone. A detailed transthoracic examination usually provides all the necessary information. When the transthoracic approach is inadequate or inconclusive, transesophageal echocardiography can be performed in this setting for the diagnosis and assessment of severity of the lesion.

Another important caveat in classifying the severity of AR is that it is in part dependent on hemodynamic status, including preload and, more importantly, afterload. Raising blood pressure may significantly increase AR severity.

D. Assessment of hemodynamic effects—The hemodynamic effects of AR are assessed with both echocardiographic imaging and Doppler echocardiography. Two-dimensional echocardiography provides quantitation of ventricular size and function, in addition to the degree of left ventricular hypertrophy and ventricular mass. End-diastolic and end-systolic left ventricular dimensions and volumes as well as left ventricular ejection fraction provide important measures of the hemodynamic effects of AR and help identify patients at higher risk. In patients with acute AR, premature closure of the mitral valve can be demonstrated by echocardiography. In these situations, diastolic mitral regurgitation can also be detected by Doppler echocardiography, reflecting the rapid rise of left ventricular pressure in diastole, exceeding that of left atrial pressure. These findings indicate severe AR. In patients with chronic AR, assessment of the ventricular and atrial filling dynamics at the mitral and pulmonary venous inflow, respectively, allows for noninvasive estimation of ventricular diastolic pressure, further adding to the overall evaluation of the hemodynamic effect of AR on ventricular function. Thus, in patients with chronic AR, two-dimensional echocardiography with Doppler provides serial assessment of left ventricular volumes, hypertrophy, and function and helps assess the progression of the disease and optimum timing of a valve intervention.

4. Cardiac catheterization and angiography—Cardiac catheterization is usually done to assess the patency of the coronary arteries in patients with AR who have angina or are being considered for valve replacement. Preoperative coronary angiography should be performed prior to elective surgery for AR in men older than 35 years, premenopausal women older than 35 years who have risk factors for coronary artery disease, postmenopausal women, and any patients with clinical suspicion of coronary artery disease.

At catheterization, the detection of AR can be achieved with the injection of radiopaque contrast into the aortic root and the appearance of dye in the left ventricle. In addition, aortography allows evaluation of the ascending aorta for dilatation or dissection. Some of the structural abnormalities of the aortic valve may also be identified. The severity of AR is quantitatively approximated using a grading system that considers the intensity of contrast dye in the left ventricle and its clearance. This grading system has been helpful clinically in the assessment of AR severity. However, it is important to emphasize that, like other diagnostic techniques, a number of technical factors may also affect interpretation. Positioning the catheter too close to the valve may itself cause regurgitation. The volume and rapidity of contrast injection, ventricular function, and type of catheter used are important factors that may affect the interpretation of AR severity.

At catheterization, the severity of AR can also be assessed by the determination of regurgitant volume and regurgitant fraction. In the absence of regurgitation or shunts, the left ventricular stroke volume derived from contrast ventriculography is equal to right ventricular stroke volume obtained by the Fick method or thermodilution. When isolated AR is present, subtracting left ventricular from right ventricular stroke volume gives the regurgitation volume. Regurgitant fraction is derived as the regurgitant volume divided by left ventricular stroke volume. In the presence of concomitant mitral regurgitation, a total regurgitant volume or fraction can only be assessed using this method. Because of inherent variability in the determination of stroke volume, a 10–15% error in these measurements is not infrequent and is like those obtained with Doppler echocardiography.

Cardiac catheterization provides an accurate assessment of the hemodynamic effect of AR. In compensated chronic AR, the only abnormality that may be observed is a widened pulse pressure on the aortic pressure tracing. As decompensation occurs, left ventricular end-diastolic pressure rises. In severe, particularly acute AR, aortic and left ventricular pressures may equalize at end-diastole.

With the improvement in noninvasive testing, routine cardiac catheterization is no longer necessary in most patients for the sole assessment of the lesion. Currently, cardiac catheterization is indicated in the assessment of AR severity when noninvasive testing is equivocal or discordant with the clinical presentation and, more commonly, in the assessment of coronary artery disease prior to aortic valve surgery.

5. Electrocardiographically gated multislice computed tomography angiography (CTA)—This test allows rapid diastolic frame rates from which the regurgitant orifice can be planimetered. Studies have shown excellent agreement with echo Doppler measures in the same patients. In addition, the size of the aorta and left ventricle can be determined as well as ejection fraction. CTA can also be used to detect significant coronary artery disease in patients with chest pain or who are being considered for surgery. Also, it provides excellent delineation of any abnormalities of the aorta such as dissection or dilatation.

6. Magnetic resonance imaging (MRI)—Currently, cardiac MRI is recommended for the evaluation of patients with AR in whom echocardiography is of poor quality or inconclusive. At present, three basic approaches are available: spin echo imaging, gradient echo imaging (cine-MRI), and phase velocity mapping. Spin echo imaging provides an excellent approach for depicting cardiac morphology and detecting aortic root disease. However, aortic valve visualization is poor. Using cine-MRI, AR is detected as a decrease in the signal intensity in the left ventricular outflow during diastole. The ratio of the area of low-intensity signal to the area of the left ventricular outflow has provided an accurate estimate of AR severity. Regurgitant fractions have been determined by comparing right and left ventricular volumes and stroke volumes. Furthermore, using phase velocity mapping, flow in a region of interest can be assessed. Regurgitant fraction with this method can be derived by comparing flows in the ascending aorta and pulmonary artery.

Cardiac MRI is particularly helpful in defining the severity and extent of AR. Imaging can be performed in any plane, without attenuation from lung or bone. Also, MRI is ideal for diagnosing and following abnormalities of the aorta. However, this modality cannot be used in many patients with certain metallic objects implanted in their bodies. Other current drawbacks are lack of widespread availability of cardiac MRI and high cost. It is an alternative to echocardiography for centers with expertise in cardiac MRI.

7. Exercise stress testing—Treadmill electrocardiogram (ECG) exercise stress testing can be used to evaluate patients with equivocal symptoms or to guide patients who wish to participate in athletic activities. Supine bicycle exercise echocardiography is useful for assessing the effect of exercise on estimated pulmonary artery systolic pressure (PASP), which can be helpful in evaluating equivocal symptoms. An excessive rise in PASP (to > 50 mm Hg) would suggest that the AR is producing the exercise-limiting symptoms.

Doherty JU, Kort S, Mehran R, Schoenhagen P, Soman P. ACC/AATS/AHA/ASE/ASNC/HRS/SCAI/SCCT/SCMR/STS 2017 appropriate use criteria for multimodality imaging in valvular heart disease. *J Am Coll Cardiol.* 2017;70:1648–1671. [PMID: 28870679]

Zoghbi WA, Adams D, Bonow RO, et al. Recommendations for noninvasive evaluation of native valvular regurgitation: a report from the American Society of Echocardiography developed in collaboration with the Society for Cardiovascular Magnetic Resonance. *J Am Soc Echocardiogr.* 2017;30:303–371. [PMID: 28314623]

Treatment

The treatment of AR depends on its underlying cause, severity, left ventricular function, hemodynamic perturbations, arrhythmias, and the presence or absence of symptoms. Mild-to-moderate AR may not require any specific treatment, whereas severe acute AR due to aortic dissection is a medical and surgical emergency.

A. Acute Aortic Regurgitation

Severe acute AR carries a high mortality rate if left untreated. It requires aggressive supportive measures, a rapid assessment of cause, and institution of definitive therapy. Because early death due to left ventricular failure and hemodynamic collapse is frequent in these patients despite intensive medical therapy, prompt surgical intervention is indicated. While the patient is being prepared for surgery, pharmacologic therapy can be initiated. Vasodilator therapy with intravenous sodium nitroprusside or nicardipine is the treatment of choice in acute AR because of its afterload and preload reduction. The dose is titrated to optimize forward cardiac output and pulmonary capillary wedge pressure. Positive inotropic agents such as dobutamine can be used if the patient remains hypotensive with a low systemic cardiac output. In cases of dissection of the aorta, β-blockers are useful to reduce left ventricular contractility and the rate of risk of aortic pressure. Unlike acute mitral regurgitation, intra-aortic balloon pumps are contraindicated in acute AR because the diastolic inflation of the balloon will worsen AR.

When acute AR is associated with hemodynamic instability, the only definitive therapy is surgical correction. The timing of surgery depends on the cause and degree of hemodynamic derangement. In infective endocarditis with severe AR, it is preferable to give several days of appropriate antibiotics prior to aortic valve replacement (AVR), provided the patient is hemodynamically stable. Indications for urgent surgery are New York Heart Association (NYHA) class III–IV congestive heart failure, systemic embolization, persistent bacteremia, fungal endocarditis, or abscess formation. When AR results from aortic dissection with disruption of commissural support, urgent surgical repair is indicated.

B. Chronic Aortic Regurgitation

1. Stage A: patients at risk of aortic regurgitation development—This category includes patients with a bicuspid aortic valve, degenerative aortic valve sclerosis, diseases producing ascending aorta dilatation such as Marfan syndrome, a history of rheumatic fever, connective tissue diseases, and infective endocarditis. For patients in whom a specific treatment for their predisposing condition exists, it should be administered. In patients with a history of rheumatic fever, prophylaxis using either penicillin or erythromycin is indicated until the age of 25 and 5 years after the last episode. If rheumatic carditis has already occurred, lifelong prophylaxis is recommended, even following valve replacement. Aortic sclerosis is common in older individuals and may be found on echocardiogram. The risk profile of these patients overlaps that of atherosclerotic vascular disease, and the risk factors present should be addressed. In addition, stage A patients should have periodic physical examinations and echocardiograms to detect the development of AR at a frequency consistent with the severity of the underlying disease.

2. Stage B: progressive but asymptomatic mild-to-moderate aortic regurgitation—Patients who have mild or moderate AR and are asymptomatic and who have normal or minimally increased cardiac size require no therapy for AR. They should be followed with clinical evaluation yearly and with echocardiography at 2- to 5-year intervals depending on the severity. Any occurrence of systemic hypertension (> 140/90 mm Hg) should be treated because it aggravates the degree of regurgitation. Ideally, antihypertensive therapy would avoid drugs that lower heart rate as this increases the time for regurgitation. Preferred agents include angiotensin-converting enzyme inhibitors, angiotensin receptor blockers, or dihydropyridine calcium antagonists. Patients with AR secondary to syphilis should receive a full course of penicillin therapy. Patients with moderate AR should avoid isometric exercise, competitive sports, and heavy physical exertion.

3. Stage C: severe asymptomatic aortic regurgitation— These patients should be followed every 6–12 months with echocardiograms at each visit. There are no data supporting long-term oral vasodilator therapy. However, hypertension or heart failure should be treated. AVR is recommended in patients with chronic severe AR and a left ventricular ejection fraction (LVEF) of less than 55% or a left ventricular end-systolic dimension (LVESD) by echocardiography that is greater than 5.0 cm or 2.5 cm/m^2 to prevent further left ventricular dysfunction and improve prognosis. However, once the ejection fraction is decreased, surgical risk is higher, and left ventricular dysfunction may become irreversible. Thus, the optimal timing of AVR in asymptomatic patients remains a challenging clinical decision. Some recommend considering AVR when the LV end-diastolic dimension exceeds 6.5 cm, but this criterion is less well supported. A consideration of LV volumes might be better but there are currently no supporting data on volumes, and measures of LV volume by different imaging techniques are somewhat discrepant. Also, a major limitation of end-diastolic indices is their dependence on preload, and thus, they may not reflect intrinsic myocardial contractile function. The use of BNP or other biomarkers to guide treatment lacks sufficient supportive data. Thus, when uncertain, it may be useful to assess exercise performance. AVR should be considered when serial testing shows decreased exercise tolerance, progressive left ventricular enlargement, worsening left ventricular function, or marked elevations in pulmonary artery pressure. Patients undergoing other cardiac operations should also be considered for AVR with moderate to severe AR. This is more controversial in those with strictly moderate AR because this condition can persist without symptoms or decompensation for years.

4. Stage D: severe symptomatic aortic regurgitation— Patients who have NYHA class III or IV symptoms or Canadian Cardiovascular Society class II–IV angina should undergo AVR. Patients with NYHA class II symptoms should be evaluated on a case-by-case basis. If the cause or severity of symptoms is unclear, an exercise test should be done. If exercise capacity is normal, treatment should be given as for asymptomatic patients, as outlined in the preceding section.

Table 18–4. Major Indications for Aortic Valve Replacement in Chronic Aortic Regurgitation

1. Symptomatic severe AR
2. Asymptomatic AR if LVEF < 55% or LVESD > 5.0 cm or > 2.5 cm/m^2
3. Moderate-severe AR if undergoing other cardiac surgery

AR, aortic regurgitation; LVEF, left ventricular ejection fraction; LVESD, left ventricular end-systolic dimension.

If new, even mild symptoms appear in a patient with chronic significant AR, particularly if left ventricular size is increased or the ejection fraction is 50–55%, then AVR should be considered (Table 18–4 and Figure 18–3).

Currently surgical AVR is the treatment of choice, especially if there is disease of the proximal aorta. In selected patients with aortic root disease, a loss of support of the aortic valve cusps can be surgically repaired. Also, some patients who are not candidates for surgical AVR may be candidates for transcatheter aortic valve replacement (TAVR) especially if there is calcium in the valve. However, at this time, experience with TAVR in AR is limited, but higher rates of valve migration and paravalvular leak have been observed.

C. Bicuspid Aortic Valve

Bicuspid aortic valves are often associated with an aortopathy that results in dilatation of the ascending aorta. Although less frequent than seen in Marfan syndrome, aortic dissection or rupture can occur. For this reason, ascending aortic size needs to be monitored in these patients. The bicuspid valve may become stenotic, regurgitant, or both independent of the aortopathy. Once the ascending aorta diameter exceeds 4.0 cm, imaging surveillance should begin. When the aorta exceeds 4.5 cm, yearly evaluations are recommended. If the ascending aorta can be well seen on echocardiography, this is a reasonable way to follow the patient. If not, MRI can be used. Aortic root replacement is recommended when the diameter exceeds 5.5 cm. In patients at higher risk of dissection, such as those with a family history of dissection or those in whom the aorta is increasing in size more than 0.5 cm/year, replacement is recommended at more than 5.0 cm. If a patient is undergoing aortic valve surgery, the aortic root should also be replaced if it is greater than 4.5 cm in diameter.

Otto CM, Nishimura RA, Bonow RO, et al. 2020 ACC/AHA guideline for the management of patients with valvular heart disease; a report of the American College of Cardiology/American Heart Association Joint Committee on Clinical Practice Guidelines; developed in collaboration with and endorsed by the American Association for Thoracic Surgery, American Society of Echocardiography, Society for Cardiovascular Angiography and Interventions, Society of Cardiovascular Anesthesiologists, and Society of Thoracic Surgeons. *J Am Coll Cardiol.* 2021;77:e25–e196. [PMID: 33342586]

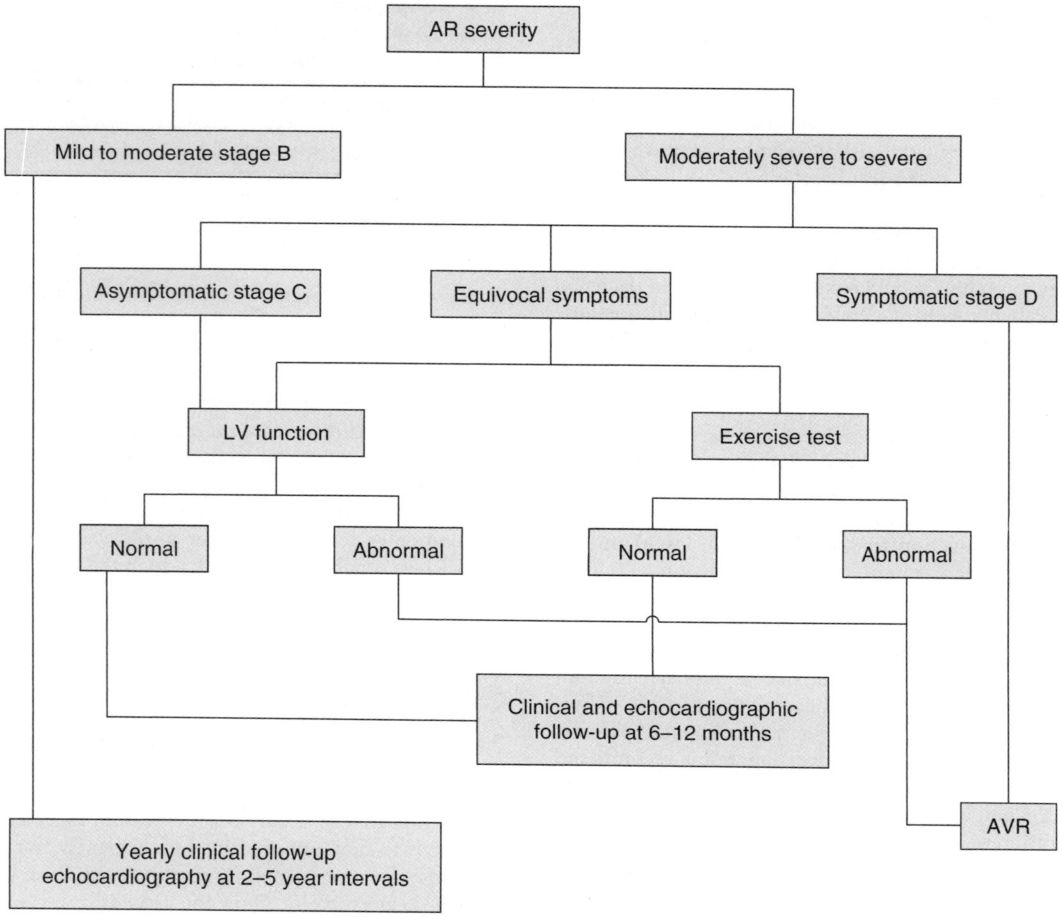

▲ **Figure 18–3.** Schematic of proposed treatment of patients with chronic significant aortic regurgitation. AR, aortic regurgitation; AVR, aortic valve replacement; LV, left ventricle.

Vahanian A, Byersdorf F, Praz F, et al. 2021 ESC/EACTS guidelines for the management of valvular heart disease: developed by the Task Force for the management of valvular heart disease of the European Society of Cardiology (ESC) and the European Association for Cardio-Thoracic Surgery (EACTS). *Eur Heart J.* 2022;43:561–632. [PMID: 34453165]

Prognosis

Asymptomatic patients with chronic AR have a stable course for many years. The mean rate of progression to surgery is approximately 4% per year. Symptoms are the major determinant of outcome in AR. The mortality rate for patients with NYHA class II–IV symptoms is more than 20% per year. Even for patients with class II symptoms, the mortality rate is 6% per year compared with 3% for patients with no symptoms. In general, good results have been observed with AVR with an average operative mortality rate of 3–4% and a 5-year survival rate of 85%. These results depend on several factors, including preoperative ventricular function, concomitant coronary artery disease, and the underlying cause of AR. AVR is necessary in most patients. In some cases of AR secondary to loss of commissural support, aortic valve repair can be performed. The feasibility of aortic valve repair often can be determined by a transesophageal echocardiogram. In patients with excessive aortic root dilatation or aneurysm, a composite aortic graft with reimplantation of the coronary arteries is performed more frequently.

Most patients show resolution of symptoms following surgery to correct AR. The end-diastolic volume is reduced immediately, with some further reduction occurring over several days after surgery. The LVEF continues to improve up to 1–2 years after surgery. There is also a gradual decline in left ventricular mass. About 20–30% of patients will have incomplete symptomatic relief and persistent left ventricular dysfunction. These findings are associated with the presence of preoperative left ventricular dysfunction, particularly if the duration of dysfunction is prolonged. Even though the outcome is less than optimal in patients with moderate left ventricular dysfunction, with recent surgical advances, many of them still do better with surgery than with medical management. Surgery should be considered in all symptomatic patients unless left ventricular dysfunction is very severe.

19 Mitral Stenosis

D. Elizabeth Le, MD

ESSENTIALS OF DIAGNOSIS

- Exertional dyspnea and fatigue.
- Opening snap, diastolic rumble murmur, loud S_1, presystolic accentuated murmur.
- Right ventricular heave and loud P_2 if pulmonary hypertension and right-heart failure are present.
- A2-OS interval ≤ 80 ms in severe mitral stenosis.
- Sinus rhythm or atrial fibrillation, notched P wave or P mitrale in leads II and III and/or biphasic P wave in V_1, right axis deviation, high amplitude of P wave in lead II, and large R wave in V_1 on electrocardiography.
- Flattening of left atrial border and/or double density, elevated left main bronchus, enlarged pulmonary arteries, and Kerley B lines on chest radiography.
- Thickened and/or calcified mitral leaflets and subvalvular apparatus resulting in "hockey-stick" motion of the anterior leaflet and fusion of commissures resulting in fish-mouth appearance of the rheumatic mitral valve on two- and three-dimensional echocardiography rheumatic valve disease.
- Calcification of the mitral annulus with extension to the basal mitral leaflets without commissural fusion resulting in tubular narrowing from the annulus to the leaflet tips on two- and three-dimensional echocardiography in degenerative calcific mitral stenosis.
- Mitral valve area ≤ 1.5 cm² by planimetry on two- or three-dimensional echocardiography and by pressure half-time, continuity equation, and proximal isovelocity surface area quantification methods on Doppler echocardiography and elevated mean transmitral valve gradient on Doppler echocardiography.

General Considerations

Mitral stenosis is a condition where the mitral valve area is reduced, causing obstruction of blood flow from the left atrium into the left ventricle during left ventricular diastole, which can lead to elevated left atrial pressure resulting in pulmonary hypertension, pulmonary edema, and right-heart failure. This valvular disease becomes clinically evident when the mitral valve area is reduced to approximately 1.5 cm².

Rheumatic mitral stenosis occurs predominantly in adults and is one of the sequelae of rheumatic fever in about 90% of cases. Approximately two-thirds of cases occur in women. Twenty-five percent of patients have isolated mitral stenosis, and 50% have mixed mitral valve disease or combined mitral and aortic valve involvement. Unlike mitral regurgitation, which can present during the initial acute rheumatic carditis episode, mitral stenosis often develops after recurrent attacks, follows an indolent course, and has a latent period up to 40 years after the index episode of rheumatic fever. Only about 50–70% patients recall having had antecedent group A β-hemolytic streptococcal tonsillopharyngitis.

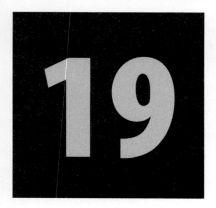

Rheumatic fever is a major public health problem in low-income countries in Oceania, South Asia, and sub-Saharan Africa. Approximately 60% of these patients will develop rheumatic heart disease. It is estimated that 40.5 million people worldwide have rheumatic heart disease in 2019 with an incidence of 2.8 million per year. The prevalence in high-income countries is 3.4 cases per 100,000 population and increases to more than 1000 case per 100,000 population in low-income countries. The prevalence in Western countries has not decreased substantially because of the increased rate of immigration from developing countries. Overall, the death rate from rheumatic heart disease is estimated to be 4.8 per 100,000 population. The pattern of valvular involvement is associated with the rate of recurrent or reactivation of streptococcal infection and thus varies geographically. Individuals in low-income countries are more likely to suffer from multiple episodes of rheumatic fever and thus become symptomatic at an earlier age compared to individuals in industrialized countries, who often do not present until they are ≥ 45 years old. Patients from low-income countries tend to have more severe stenosis, but less leaflet calcification and less atrial fibrillation. Due to the shorter latent period, younger patients tend to have more commissural thickening and pliable valves, whereas older patients with a longer latent period tend to have more calcified valves. A subgroup of patients, pregnant women, often present during the second trimester of pregnancy because increases in intravascular blood volume, cardiac output, and heart rate can make the impediment to flow more pronounced.

A. Anatomy

The mitral valve has two leaflets, anterior and posterior, which come together at the anterior and posterior commissures. The anterior leaflet occupies one-third of the saddle-shaped annular circumference, and the posterior occupies two-thirds of the circumference. Primary, secondary, and tertiary chordae tendineae originate from both the anterolateral and posteromedial papillary muscles of the left ventricle and insert into margin and base of both the anterior and posterior leaflets. A competent mitral valve requires precise and concerted motion of the leaflets, chordae, and left ventricular and atrial contraction. Alteration of any components of this complex geometry can result in stenosis, insufficiency, or both (Figure 19–1).

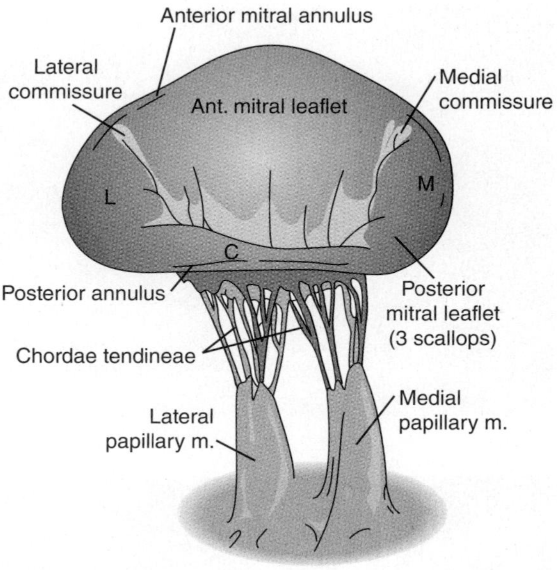

▲ **Figure 19–1.** The mitral valve apparatus. The anterior mitral leaflet attaches to a smaller portion of the circumference of the annulus than the posterior mitral leaflet, but the anterior leaflet is longer. The posterior leaflet consists of three segments designated the lateral (L or P1), central (C or P2), and medial (M or P3) scallops. Both leaflets attach to both the medial and lateral papillary muscles. (Reproduced with permission from Otto CM. *Textbook of Clinical Echocardiography*, 4th ed. Philadelphia: Elsevier; 2009.)

B. Etiology

Mitral stenosis is predominantly due to organic valve pathology and less commonly due to functional valve pathology where the mitral leaflets are anatomically normal, but their movement is altered. Approximately 90% of organic native valve mitral stenosis cases are associated with rheumatic fever or rheumatic heart disease, where the autoimmune response to group A streptococcal infection results in commissural thickening and fusion, valve and subvalvular apparatus thickening, calcification, and fusion, and consequently, restricted motion of the valve leaflets (Figure 19–2). Severe mitral annular calcification accounts for about 6–8% of cases and has steadily increased over the past decade in high-income countries. It is associated with advanced age, female gender, hypertension, hyperlipidemia, chronic kidney disease, and senile aortic stenosis. Other conditions associated with valve fibrosis are endocarditis, systemic lupus erythematous, rheumatoid arthritis, malignant carcinoid, and exposure to medications with direct serotonin receptors activation (ergotamine and methysergide for migraine headaches; fenfluramine, chlorphentermine, and benfluorex for weight reduction; and pergolide and cabergoline for Parkinson disease). In less than 1% of cases, mitral stenosis is due to congenital abnormalities and thus will present during infancy or childhood. These rare entities include supravalvar mitral ring, which is an abnormal connective tissue band located above the annulus or is adherent to the annulus and valve, hypoplasia of the mitral annulus, fusion of the commissures, a double orifice mitral valve, and a parachute mitral valve, where chordae from both the anterior and posterior leaflets insert into one papillary muscle. Another rare anomaly, cor triatriatum sinister, can result in stenotic physiology without valve involvement. In this condition, a membrane or a fibromuscular band separates the left atrium into two compartments. This abnormal tissue may vary in size and shape, may have fenestrations, or can be funnel-shaped, which restricts blood flow from the left atrium into the left ventricle.

Functional native mitral valve stenosis is rare and can result from a mass, such as a left atrial myxoma or a large left atrial thrombus, advancing across the mitral annulus and occupying a portion of the mitral orifice during left ventricular diastole. Acquired mitral stenosis can be iatrogenic where a portion of the mitral leaflet is inadvertently sutured to annular tissue during aortic or mitral valve surgery or a small annuloplasty ring is used during mitral valve repair, especially in a small left ventricle. Impingement of the anterior leaflet of the mitral valve with the bioprosthetic valve

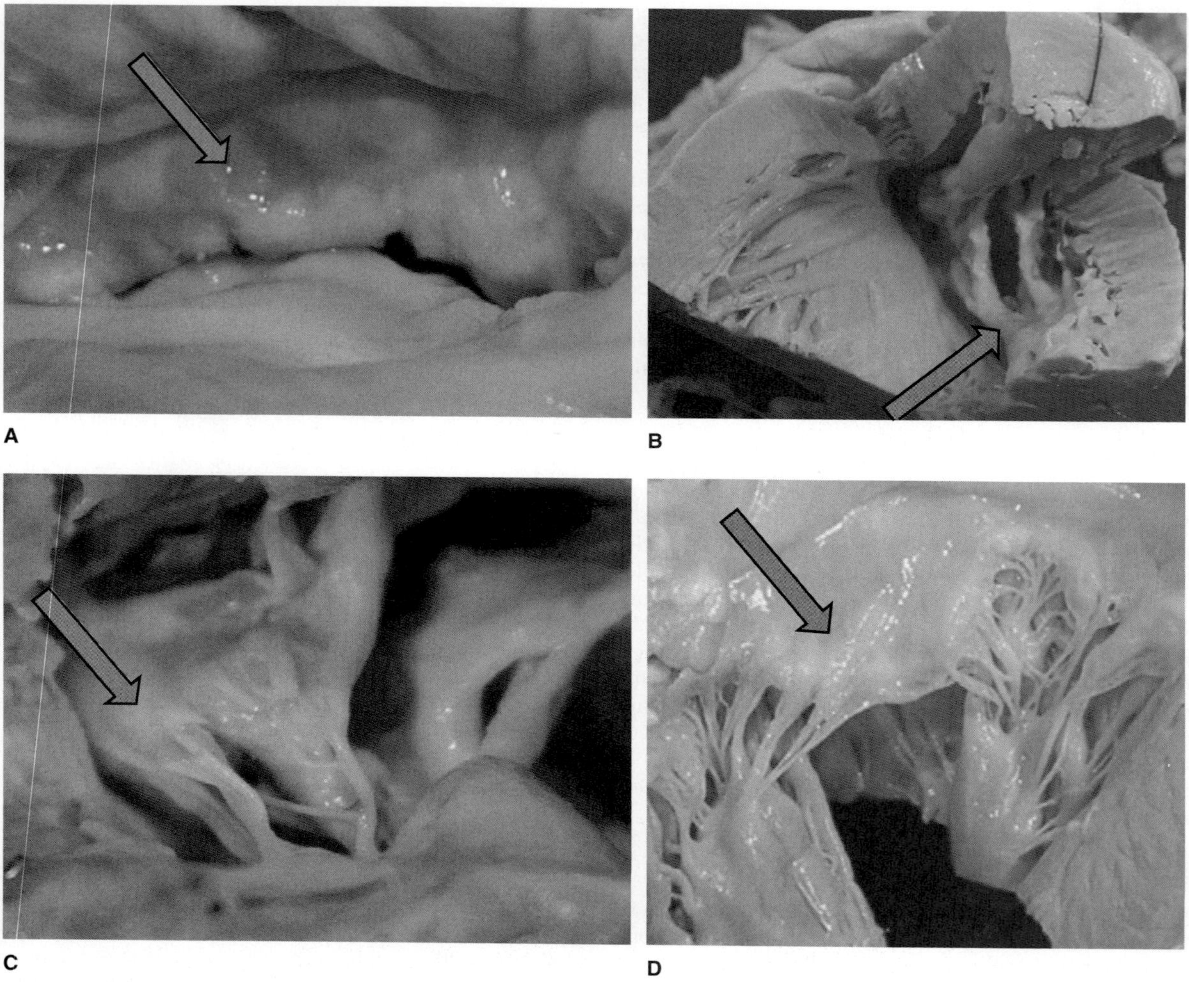

▲ **Figure 19–2.** Postmortem specimens of a rheumatic mitral valve and normal mitral valve. **A:** Thickened and nodular leaflet in rheumatic mitral valve. **B:** Calcified and fused commissure, fish-mouth shaped leaflets. **C:** Thickened, fused, and shortened subvalvular apparatus. **D:** Normal mitral leaflet and chordae tendineae. (Reproduced with permission from Chandrashekhar Y, et al. Mitral stenosis. *Lancet*. 2009;374(9697):1271–1283.)

deployed during percutaneous transcatheter aortic valve replacement to treat severe aortic stenosis can also result in mitral stenosis.

Mitral bioprosthetic valves can become stenotic when leaflets calcify over time with or without pannus overgrowth and cause similar pathophysiology seen in native valves. Mechanical mitral valves can also exhibit stenotic physiology when leaflet or poppet motion is impeded by thrombus, vegetation, or pannus.

C. Pathogenesis

The normal mitral valve area is 4–6 cm^2. Mild mitral stenosis occurs when the mitral valve area is reduced to 2 cm^2 and becomes severe when the area is $\leq$ 1.5 cm^2. In normal conditions, during early left ventricular diastole, blood flow from the left atrium into the left ventricle occurs from passive filling, is rapid, and peaks early, followed by diastasis, until active filling occurs from atrial contraction. Equalization of left atrial and left ventricular pressure occurs during mid-diastole. In the presence of mitral stenosis, the rate of passive filling is reduced and sustained throughout diastole, such that at end-diastole, left atrial pressure is higher than left ventricular pressure (Figure 19–3).

Within a cardiac cycle, the diastolic filling period (seconds per cycle) is the time between mitral valve opening

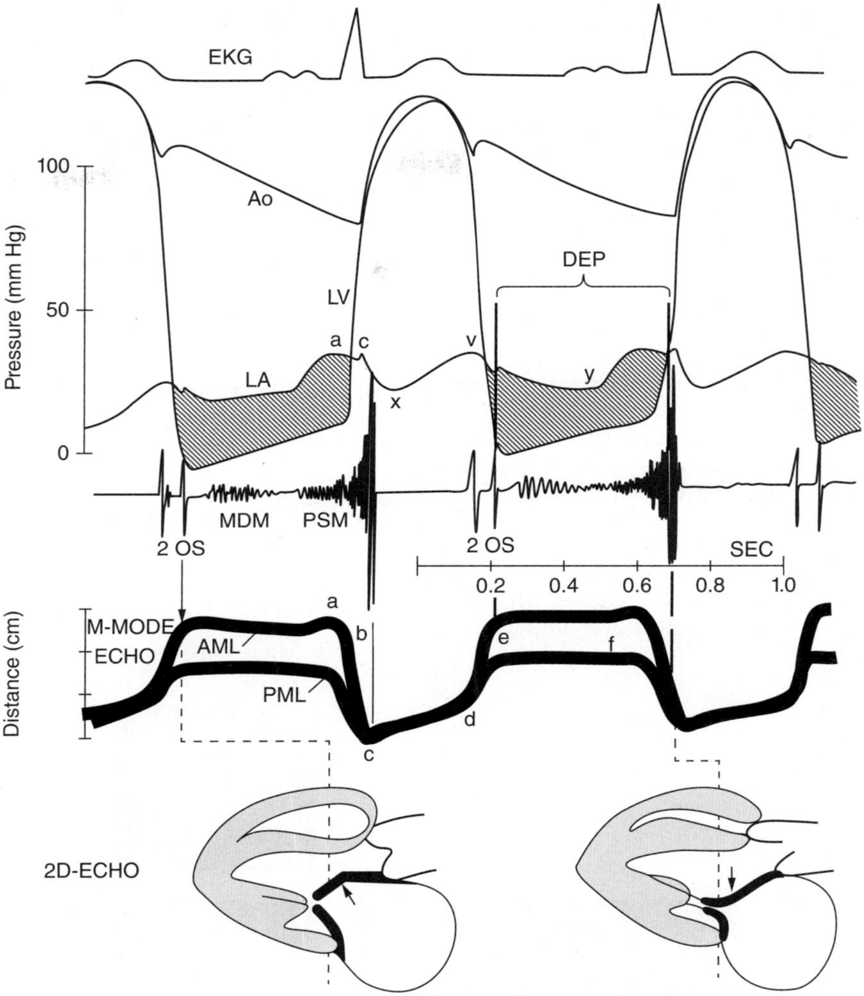

▲ **Figure 19–3.** Correlation of electrocardiogram (EKG), hemodynamic tracings, cardiac auscultation, M-mode, and two-dimensional (2D) echocardiography (ECHO) of mitral stenosis. The left atrium (LA) pressure tracing shows a prominent *a* wave and *v* wave. The atrioventricular pressure gradient (*shaded area*) is sustained throughout diastole with elevated LA pressure. The E-F slope is flat on M-mode recording of the mitral leaflets. AML, anterior mitral leaflet; AO, aorta; DFP, diastolic filling period; LV, left ventricle; MDM, mid-diastolic murmur; OS, opening snap; PML, posterior mitral leaflet; PSM, presystolic murmur. (Reproduced with permission from Heger JW, et al. *Cardiology*, 3rd ed. Baltimore: Williams & Wilkins; 1994.)

and closure. The diastolic filling time is determined using the following formula:

$$\text{Diastolic filling time (s/min)} = \text{Diastolic filling period (s/cycle)} \times \text{Heart rate (bpm)}$$

Mitral flow is a function of both the cardiac output and diastolic filling time and is calculated using the equation:

$$\text{Mitral flow (mL/s)} = \frac{\text{Cardiac output (mL/min)}}{\text{Diastolic filling time (s/min)}}$$

During each minute, the diastolic filling period averages about 30–32 seconds. As heart rate increases, more time of the 1 minute is devoted to systolic ejection and isovolumetric contraction and relaxation, thus leading to a reduction in the diastolic filling period (Table 19–1). At rest, the diastolic flow across the mitral valve is about 200 mL/s. During exercise, cardiac output can triple, and along with tachycardia and the compensatory reduction in diastolic filling, transmitral flow and gradient will increase. Assuming no change in left atrial and left ventricular compliance, as the mitral

Table 19–1. Relation Between Heart Rate, Diastolic Filling Time, and Mitral Valve Flow with a Constant Cardiac Output of 5 L/min

Heart Rate (bpm)	Diastolic Filling Time (s/min)	Mitral Valve Flow (mL/s)
50	38	132
75	30	167
100	26	192
150	18	278
175	12	417

valve area decreases, left atrial pressure and transmitral gradient will increase disproportionately with mitral flow (Figure 19–4). Chronically elevated left atrial pressure results in left atrial enlargement, which can lead to paroxysmal or permanent atrial fibrillation. Rapid atrial fibrillation reduces the diastolic filling time and cardiac output, which in turn, perpetuates the vicious circle by further increasing left atrial pressure. Chronic elevation of left atrial pressure causes a rise in pulmonary venous pressure and eventually pulmonary arterial pressure. When left atrial pressure exceeds 25 mm Hg, pulmonary edema develops. Consequently, chronic pulmonary arterial hypertension leads to right ventricular pressure overload and then volume overload when the right heart fails. Over time, the pulmonary vasculature becomes permanently damaged, leading to fixed pulmonary hypertension and elevation of pulmonary vascular resistance.

Mitral stenosis is associated with increased levels of prothrombotic metabolites. This hypercoagulable milieu poses a high risk of left atrial and left atrial appendage thrombus formation. Other factors that independently predict thrombosis in mitral stenosis are ≥ 1 year duration of atrial fibrillation, left atrial size ≥ 4.5 cm, left atrial spontaneous echo contrast on echocardiography, and a prior thromboembolic event.

Banovic M, DaCosta M. Degenerative mitral stenosis: from pathophysiology to challenging interventional treatment. *Curr Probl Cardiol.* 2019;44(1):10–35. [PMID: 29731112]

Coffey S, Thomson RR, Brown A, et al. Global epidemiology of valvular heart disease. *Nat Rev Cardiol.* 2021;18(12):853–864. [PMID: 34172950]

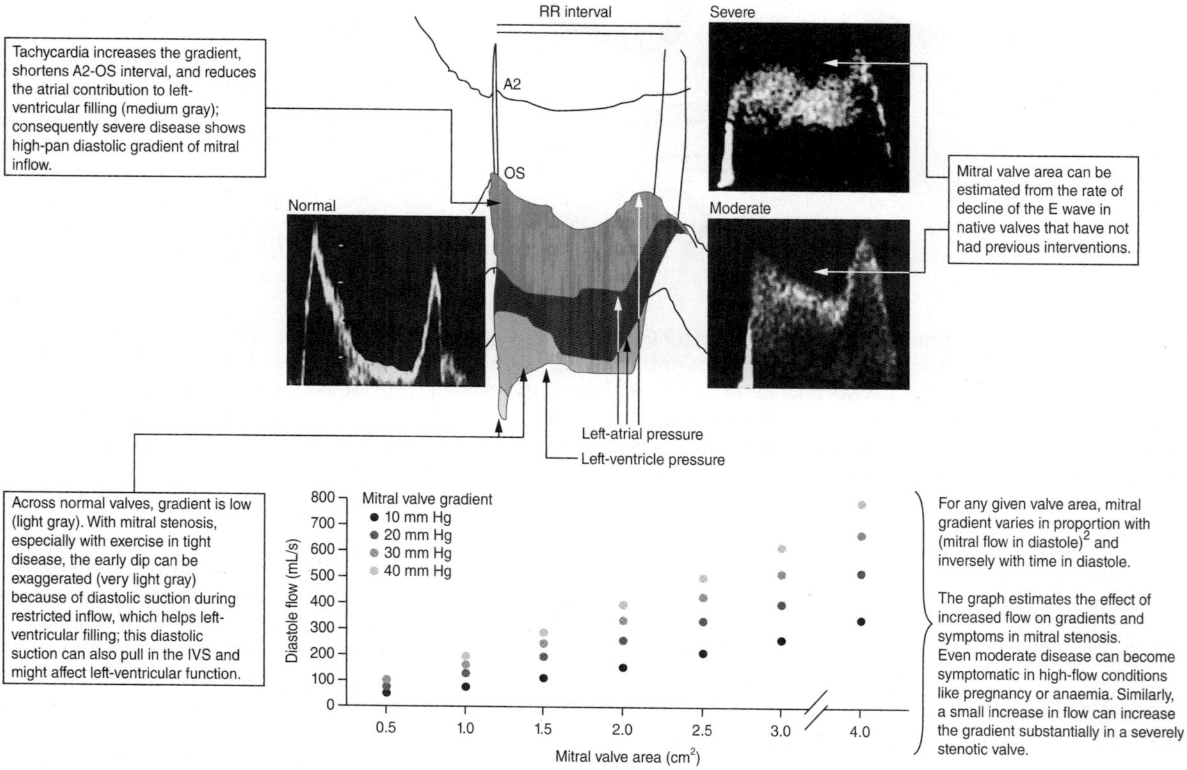

▲ **Figure 19–4. Pathophysiology of mitral stenosis.** (Reproduced with permission from Chandrashekhar Y, et al. Mitral stenosis. *Lancet.* 2009;374(9697):1271–1283.)

Kim JH, Lee SH, Joo HC, et al. Long-term clinical impacts of functional mitral stenosis after mitral valve repair. *Ann Thorac Surg.* 2021;111(4):1207–1215. [PMID: 32980324]

Roth GA, Mensah GA, Johnson CO, et al. Global burden of cardiovascular diseases and risk factors, 1990-2019: update from the GBD 2019 study. *J Am Coll Cardiol.* 2020;76:2982–3021. [PMID: 33309175]

Watkins DA, Johnson CO, Colquhoun SM, et al. Global, regional, and national burden of rheumatic heart disease, 1990-2015. *N Engl J Med.* 2017;377(8):713–722. [PMID: 28834488]

Prevention

Prompt diagnosis and treatment of group A β-hemolytic streptococcal infection can reduce the incidence of acute rheumatic fever. Secondary prevention of recurrent acute rheumatic fever with intramuscular benzathine penicillin G every four weeks to age 21, 40, or even lifelong, depending on the severity of rheumatic heart disease or social environment, can decrease progression of rheumatic heart disease.

Kumar R, Antunes, MJ, Beaton A, et al. Contemporary diagnosis and management of rheumatic heart disease: implications for closing the gap. *Circ.* 2020;142(20):e337–e357. [33073615]

Clinical Findings

A. Symptoms & Signs

1. Dyspnea and fatigue—The classic symptoms of mitral stenosis are dyspnea and fatigue during exercise or in the setting of any condition that results in sinus tachycardia such as hyperthyroidism, hypovolemia, anemia, fever/infection, emotional stress, pregnancy, or exposure to sympathomimetic agents. Those with more advanced disease can experience shortness of breath at rest. In addition, patients are predisposed to developing atrial fibrillation, and the loss of atrial contraction and synchronized contraction with the left ventricle during each cardiac cycle can exacerbate dyspnea on exertion or even produce shortness of breath at rest, especially in patients with left ventricular dysfunction. Chest pain is rare, but patients may have intermittent or sustained palpitations from paroxysmal or permanent atrial fibrillation. One of the most devastating morbidities associated with mitral stenosis is embolic cerebral vascular accident, which occasionally can be the presenting symptom.

2. Heart failure—As mitral stenosis becomes more severe, elevated left atrial pressure causes pulmonary vascular congestion. Pulmonary edema usually is manifested by dyspnea. In the early stages, pulmonary edema may occur only during exertion, and as the disease progresses, pulmonary edema occurs at rest. Occasionally, acute pulmonary edema can occur with exercise. Other signs of left-heart failure include weight gain, orthopnea, and paroxysmal nocturnal dyspnea. In patients with calcific mitral stenosis, long-standing left ventricular hypertrophy associated with chronic hypertension can lead to decompensated heart failure with preserved left ventricular function. In the late stages of mitral stenosis, there is irreversible adverse remodeling of the pulmonary vasculature, which results in elevated pulmonary artery pressure and pulmonary vascular resistance. Subsequently, right-heart failure ensues when right-heart hypertrophy can no longer adapt to the high pulmonary and right ventricular pressures. Symptoms of right-heart failure include exercise intolerance, dyspnea, abdominal fullness, and lower extremity edema.

3. Hemoptysis—When severe mitral stenosis leads to severe pulmonary hypertension, rarely the bronchial veins can rupture and cause hemoptysis.

B. Physical Examination

1. Arterial pulses—In severe stenosis, when stroke volume is reduced, pulses are diminished.

2. Rhythm—In the early stages of mitral stenosis, patients have normal sinus rhythm. In moderate to severe mitral stenosis, elevated left atrial pressure and atrial tissue fibrosis can lead to atrial arrhythmia, predominantly in the form of atrial fibrillation, where heart sounds will be rapid and irregularly irregular.

3. Opening snap—The opening snap (OS) is due to the abrupt opening of the mitral leaflets during left ventricular diastole, where the leaflets are still relatively mobile. It may not be detected if the valve is severely calcified and restricted. The OS is heard best at the base of the heart but can also be audible at the apex. The duration between aortic valve closure and OS, the A2-OS interval, can be used to determine stenosis severity. The astute clinician can estimate the duration of this interval on auscultation. An A2-OS duration of less than 80 ms is indicative of severe mitral stenosis with a corresponding left atrial pressure of at least 25 mm Hg. As left atrial pressure rises, the OS occurs earlier, leading to a shorter A2-OS interval (see Figure 19–3).

4. Diastolic rumble murmur—The diastolic murmur in mitral stenosis is due to turbulent flow across the mitral valve. This murmur is low-pitch and is heard best at the apex using the bell of the stethoscope when the patient lies in the left lateral decubitus position. The diastolic murmur can also be more prominent after exercise, although tachycardia results in a shorter diastolic filling time, which may make auscultation more challenging. Maneuvers that increase venous return accentuate the diastolic murmur and shorten the A2-OS interval, whereas maneuvers that decrease venous return decrease the murmur and lengthen the A2-OS interval. The duration of the murmur, and not the amplitude, correlates with stenosis severity. In mild stenosis, the diastolic murmur is audible during late ventricular diastole when atrial systole occurs and represents "presystolic accentuation." As the valve becomes more stenotic, the diastolic murmur is present throughout diastole. In very severe stenosis, the amplitude may be diminished significantly due to extremely low flow across the valve and may be inaudible.

5. Loud S_1—Closure of minimally calcified and pliable mitral leaflets transmits as a loud S_1. However, as calcification increases, the valve is less mobile and the S_1 is soft.

6. Findings with pulmonary hypertension—A loud pulmonic valve closure (P_2) can be audible in patients who have developed passive pulmonary hypertension. There may also be a systolic murmur from tricuspid regurgitation. If right ventricular hypertrophy is also present, a right ventricular heave may be palpable. Right-heart systolic dysfunction can present with elevated jugular venous pressure, hepatomegaly, ascites, and peripheral edema.

7. Other findings—If there is mixed valve disease, the holosystolic murmur of chronic mitral regurgitation is present. If there is concomitant aortic or pulmonary regurgitation, a high-pitch blowing diastolic murmur can be appreciated. In the presence of aortic stenosis, a systolic ejection murmur is audible. If a patient has left ventricular systolic or diastolic failure, pulmonary rales are heard.

C. Diagnostic Studies

1. Electrocardiography

The rhythm can be sinus or atrial fibrillation. A notched P wave or "P mitrale" in leads II and III and/or a biphasic P wave in lead V_1 can be present, which reflect left atrial enlargement. If there are right ventricular enlargement and failure, they manifest as right axis deviation, incomplete right bundle branch block, and tall R wave in V_2 or deep S wave in V_6. Right atrial enlargement is represented by high amplitude (≥ 2.5 mm) of the P wave in lead II (Figure 19–5).

2. Chest Radiography

Left atrial appendage enlargement on radiography results in straightening of the left superior cardiac border on the posteroanterior view, which is seen more commonly than the double density, where both the left and right atrial borders are seen when the left atrium enlarges to the right. Occasionally, the left main bronchus is also elevated due to left atrial enlargement. If there is enlargement of the pulmonary veins, an antler configuration is visible. In the frontal projection, when pulmonary hypertension coexists with mitral stenosis, the main pulmonary artery is enlarged and extends beyond the tangent line drawn from the aortic knob to the left

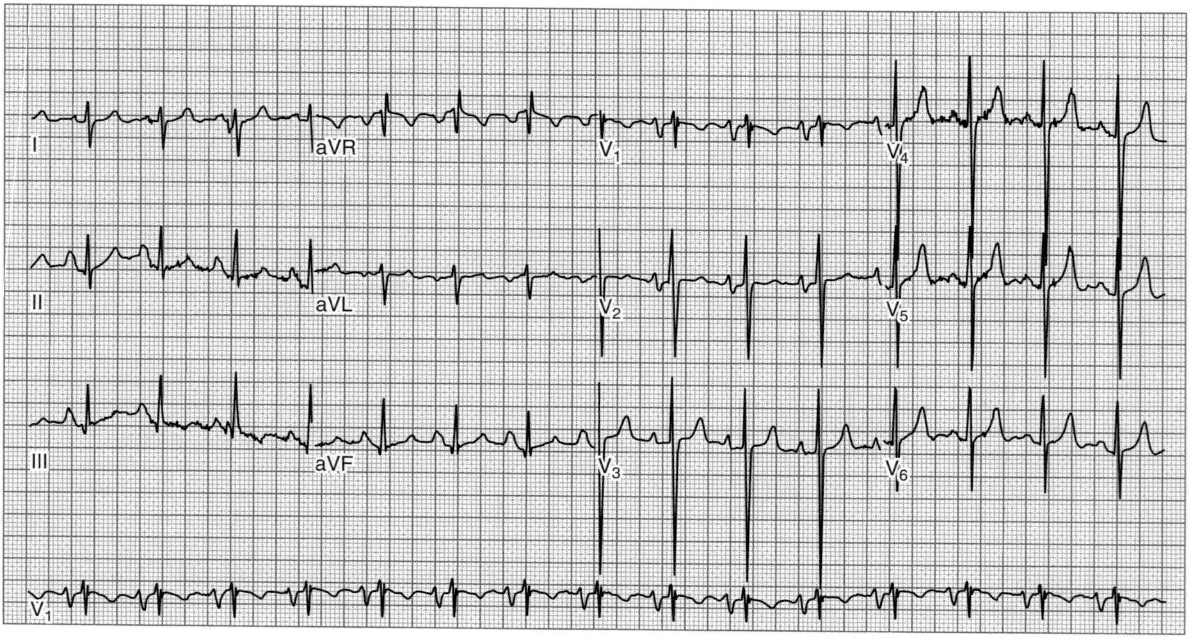

▲ Figure 19–5. Electrocardiogram demonstrating right axis deviation (+90° to +180°, negative amplitude in lead I, and positive amplitude in lead aVF), left atrial enlargement (notched P wave in lead II and biphasic P wave in leads V_1 and V_2), right atrial enlargement (P-wave amplitude of 4 mm in lead II), and right ventricular hypertrophy (right axis deviation > 90°, tall R in V_2, and prominent S wave in V_6) seen in mitral stenosis. (Reproduced with permission from American College of Cardiology ECG-SAPII. © 1997 American College of Cardiology Foundation.)

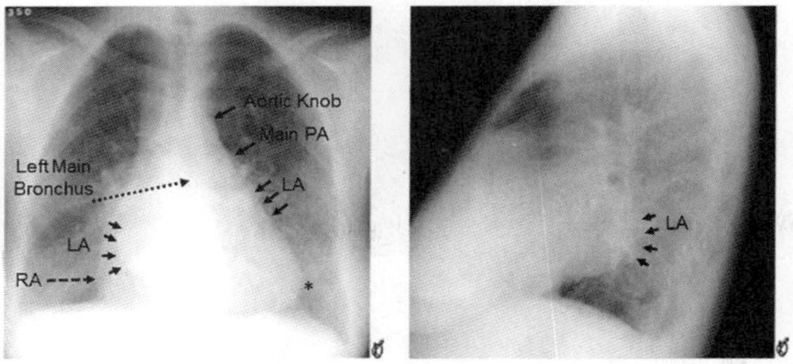

A B

▲ **Figure 19–6.** **A.** Posteroanterior view shows enlargement of the LA (arrows), double-density of the LA and RA borders (dashed arrow), elevation of the main stem bronchus (dotted arrow), and elevation of the cardiac apex suggestive of right ventricular enlargement (star). **B.** Lateral view shows left atrial enlargement (arrows) and filling of the retrosternal space by a dilated right ventricle. LA, left atrium; RA, right atrium. (Reproduced with permission from Patrick J. Lynch and C. Carl Jaffe, Yale University, 2006.)

ventricular apex (Figure 19–6). Chronically elevated pressure in the pulmonary veins can result in redistribution of blood flow to the upper lobes, seen as cephalization of the pulmonary vessels, and interlobular edema at the bases appearing as Kerley B lines. When pulmonary arterial hypertension ensues, pruning of the peripheral vessels is present. The left ventricular contour is usually normal, and if there is right-heart failure, the right ventricle fills the retrosternal space in the lateral projection.

3. Echocardiography

A. Descriptive anatomy—Echocardiography is the imaging modality of choice to investigate the severity of mitral stenosis because it offers both anatomic and functional information. Due to commissural fusion in rheumatic mitral stenosis, the anterior and posterior leaflets move anteriorly, and the E-F slope is reduced on M-mode images (Figure 19–7). Two-dimensional echo images show a funnel-shaped valve with fusion of the commissures and thickened and calcified leaflets and chordae tendineae. During diastole, the posterior leaflet is fixed, and the anterior leaflet opens and appears like a hockey stick in the parasternal long-axis view. In the parasternal short-axis view, the mitral valve has a "fish-mouth" appearance in the open position (Figure 19–8).

In degenerative calcific mitral stenosis, the posterior annulus is calcified, which over time, extends into the base of the leaflets resulting in displacement of the mitral valve hinge point into the left ventricle and formation of a tunnel-shaped valve. Patients with severe mitral annular calcification can exhibit circumferential calcification where the anterior mitral annulus is also involved (Figure 19–9). Mitral annular calcification is graded as mild when less than one-third of the annular circumference is calcified, moderate when one-third to one-half is calcified, and severe when more than one-half is calcified or the calcification thickness in the anteroposterior direction in the parasternal short axis view is more than 4 mm.

The left atrium is enlarged and could have visible thrombus on transesophageal echocardiography. The Wilkins

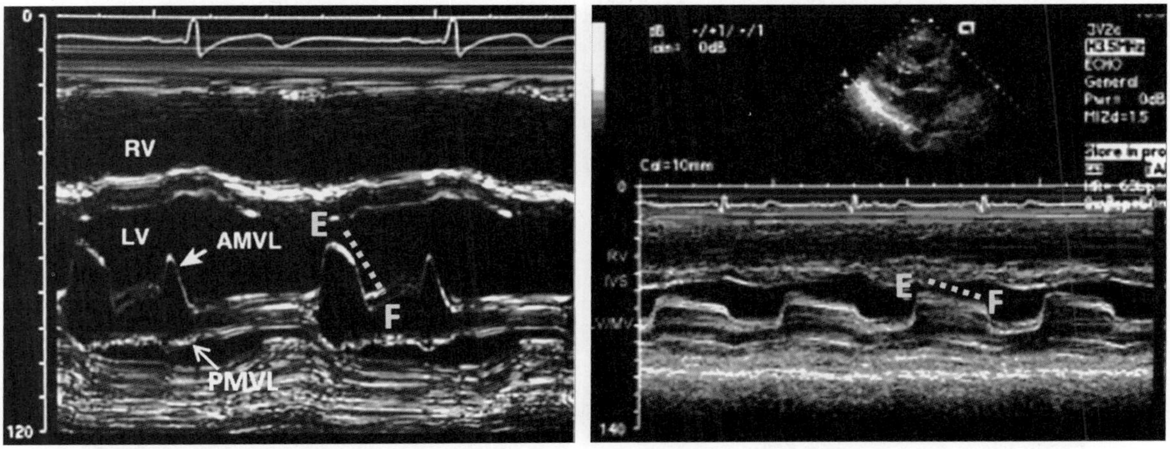

A B

▲ **Figure 19–7.** M-mode of a normal mitral valve (**A**) and of a rheumatic mitral valve (**B**). In the normal valve, the thin leaflets separate and the E-F slope is steep; whereas in the stenotic valve, the leaflets are thickened, the posterior leaflet moves anteriorly during diastole, and the E-F slope is flat. AMVL, anterior mitral valve leaflet; LV, left ventricle; PMVL, posterior mitral valve leaflet; RV, right ventricle. (A: Reproduced with permission from Otto CM. *Textbook of Clinical Echocardiography*, 4th ed. Philadelphia: Elsevier; 2009. Copyright © Elsevier. B: Reproduced, with permission, from Armstrong WF, Ryan T. *Feigenbaum's Echocardiography*, 7th ed. Philadelphia: Lippincott Williams & Wilkins; 2010.)

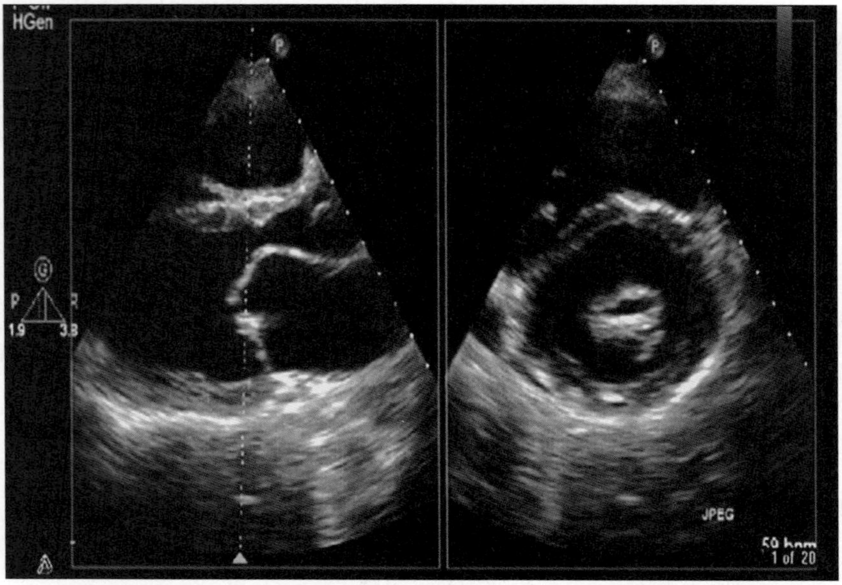

▲ **Figure 19–8.** Two-dimensional echocardiography orthogonal views of a rheumatic mitral valve confirm that measurement of the mitral orifice is at the tip of the leaflets and is the smallest area. **Left:** In the parasternal long axis view, hockey-stick appearance of anterior leaflet and fixed posterior leaflet is seen. **Right:** In the parasternal short axis view, the opened mitral valve has a fish-mouth configuration. (Reproduced, with permission, from de Augustin JA, et al. *Cardiol Clin*. 2007;25:311. Copyright © Elsevier.)

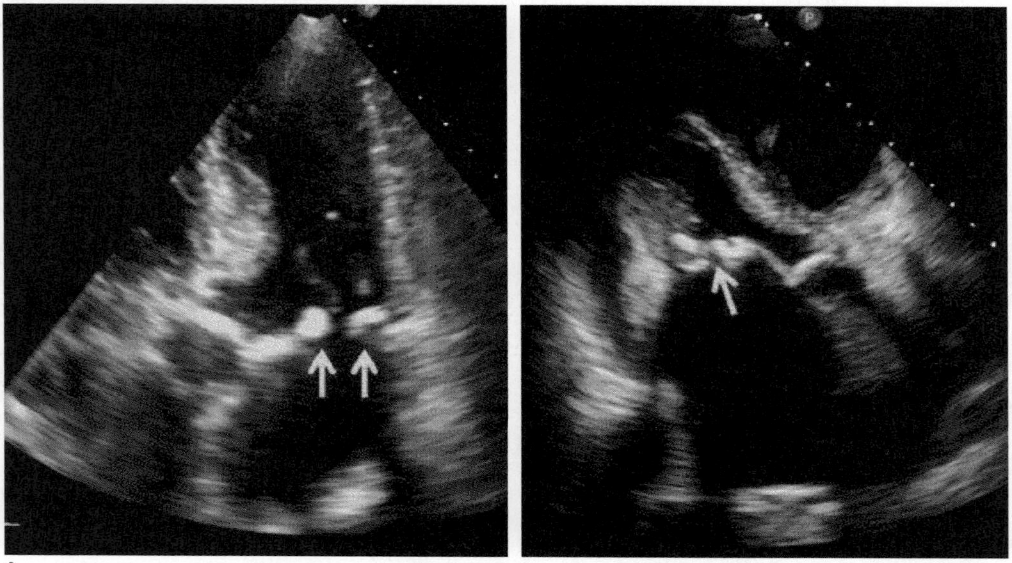

A B

▲ **Figure 19–9.** Main distinguishing characteristic between calcific versus rheumatic mitral stenosis (MS) is the location of the limiting orifice area. **A:** Calcific MS. Apical five-chamber view shows heavy calcification that extends from the level of mitral annulus to the base of the leaflet, resulting in a limiting orifice area at the base of the mitral leaflets (*arrow*) but lack of leaflet tip fusion. **B:** Rheumatic MS. Leaflet tip fusion (*arrow*) is shown in the apical long-axis view. Specifically, the decreased orifice area occurs at the leaflet tips, and the annular area is unaffected. (Reproduced from Zeng X, et al. *Prog Cardiovasc Dis*. 2014;57:55–73, with permission. Copyright © Elsevier.)

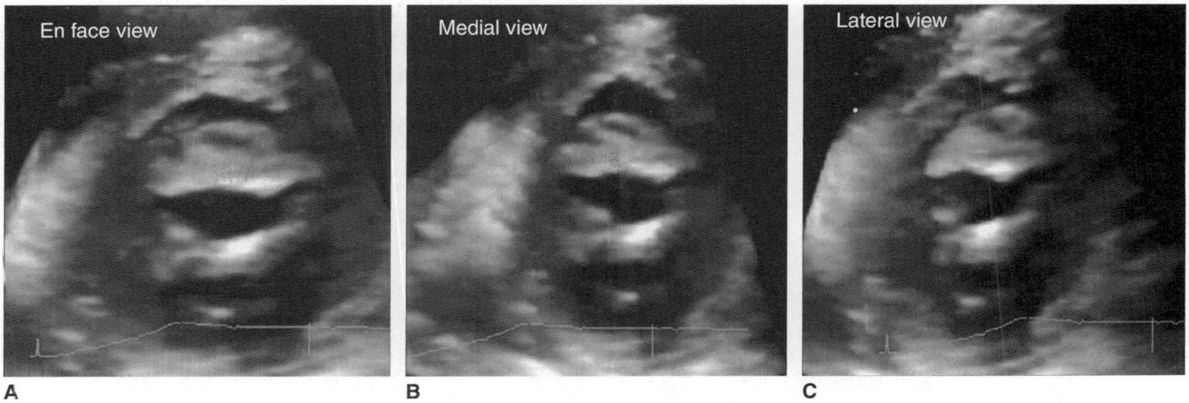

▲ **Figure 19–10.** Three-dimensional echo images of a stenotic rheumatic mitral valve in the parasternal short axis view after commissural opening. The (**A**) en face, (**B**) medial, and (**C**) lateral views showed opened commissures. (Reproduced with permission and was published in Messika-Zeitoun D, et al. *Arch Cardiovasc Dis*. 2008;101:653. Copyright © 2012 Published by Elsevier Masson SAS on behalf of the Éditions Françaises de Radiologie. All rights reserved.)

echocardiography score is commonly used to determine suitability for successful balloon valvotomy in rheumatic mitral stenosis, where 1 to 4 points are assigned in each of four categories: leaflet thickening, leaflet calcification, leaflet mobility, and subvalvular apparatus thickening. A score of ≤ 8 predicts a favorable outcome during balloon valvotomy.

Over the past three decades, the availability of real-time, three-dimensional (3D) echocardiographic imaging has allowed better visualization of the stenotic valve and commissural anatomy and has provided simultaneous acquisition of orthogonal views of the mitral valve, which has improved the accuracy of planimetry, especially when measured from the left ventricular side. 3D imaging also provides additional information on the orientation of the subvalvular apparatus, which permits detailed planning prior to interventional procedures (Figure 19–10).

B. Quantification—The parameters used to diagnose and quantify mitral stenosis are depicted in Table 19–2. Continuous wave Doppler flow is used to measure the mean mitral gradient based on the Bernoulli equation where velocities across the mitral valve are measured and the mean pressure gradient is the $\Sigma 4v^2/n$, where v is the velocity and n is the number of individual velocities measured. The mean gradient is determined by tracing the velocity time integral (VTI), which then is automatically calculated by ultrasound software packages. This measurement is straightforward to obtain but is dependent on heart rate, heart rhythm, and global left ventricular systolic function. The mean gradient can be low in bradycardia or in low cardiac output states (Figure 19–11). This parameter has not well validated in degenerative calcific mitral stenosis and appears to correlate with a larger mitral valve area (MVA) when compared to similar gradients in rheumatic mitral stenosis.

The MVA can be measured by planimetry of the mitral orifice in the parasternal short axis view. The area can be overestimated if the imaging plane is not at the level where the orifice is the smallest or underestimated when there is significant calcification. The availability of 3D echo images has improved the accuracy and reproducibility of this

Table 19–2. Quantification and Grading of Mitral Stenosis

Stage	Severity	MVA (cm²)	Mean Gradient (mm Hg)	PHT (ms)	PASP (mm Hg)	A2-OS Interval (ms)	Symptoms
A (At risk)	Normal	4–6	0	37–55	< 25	> 120	None
B (Progressive)	Mild/Moderate	> 1.5	1–4	< 150	25-29	> 120	None
C (Asymptomatic)	Severe	1.1–1.5	5–10	150–219	30–50	80–120	None
D (Symptomatic)	Very Severe	≤ 1.0	≥ 10	≥ 220	> 50	< 80	Decreased exercise tolerance Exertional dyspnea

Heart rate between 60 and 80 bpm, sinus rhythm
A2, aortic valve closure; MVA, mitral valve area; OS, opening snap; PASP, pulmonary artery systolic pressure; PHT, pressure half-time.

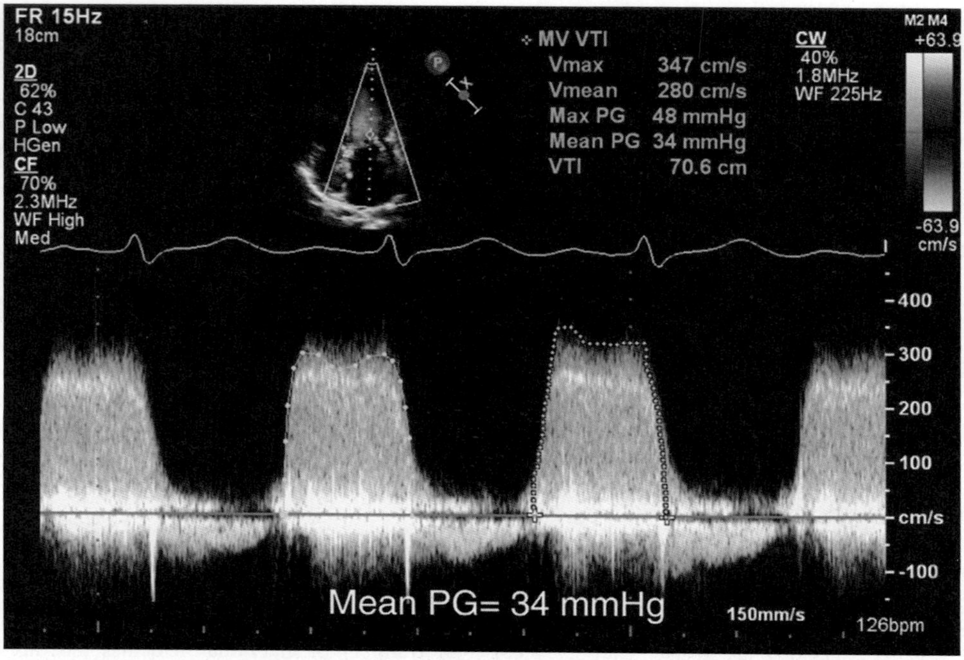

▲ **Figure 19–11.** **Doppler measurement of the mean mitral gradient.** (Reproduced with permission from Omran AS, et al. *J Saudi Heart Assoc*. 2011;23:51.)

technique. The advantage of this method is that it is easy to obtain if image quality is excellent (Figure 19–12A).

Using Doppler measurements, estimating the MVA by pressure half-time (PHT) is the simplest Doppler method. The PHT is the time during diastole when the transmitral gradient falls to 50% of the initial peak gradient.

$$\text{MVA (cm}^2\text{)} = \frac{220}{\text{PHT (ms)}}$$

This method is invalid immediately after balloon valvotomy and in patients with severe aortic regurgitation or in conditions with high-filling pressures or decreased left atrial and ventricular compliance. It also has not been well validated in degenerative mitral stenosis. In atrial fibrillation, at least five measurements should be recorded and averaged (Figure 19–12B).

The second Doppler method used to calculate MVA is based on the principle of energy conservation. The continuity equation used to calculate the cross-sectional area of the mitral valve is:

$$\text{MVA(cm}^2\text{)} = \frac{\text{LVOT D}^2 \times 0.785 \times \text{VTI}_{\text{LVOT}}}{\text{VTI}_{\text{MV}}}$$

where *LVOT D* is the diameter of the left ventricular outflow tract measured in the parasternal long axis view and *VTI* is the time velocity integral of the LVOT and mitral valve (MV), respectively. This method assumes that flow across the mitral valve is equivalent to flow across the aortic valve. It is inaccurate when there is significant concomitant mitral or aortic regurgitation. Mitral regurgitation can overestimate the severity of mitral stenosis, and aortic regurgitation can underestimate the severity of mitral stenosis. In addition, poor visualization of the LVOT on two-dimensional imaging can significantly affect the MVA (Figure 19–12C). This method is preferred for the measurement of MVA in calcific mitral stenosis.

The third Doppler method used in MVA calculation is the proximal isovelocity surface area (PISA) method, where

$$\text{MVA(cm}^2\text{)} = \frac{6.28 \times r^2 \times \text{Aliasing velocity}}{\text{Peak mitral stenosis velocity}} \times \frac{\alpha°}{180°}$$

This method is the most complex and technically challenging because it requires measuring the radius of PISA in the left atrium and the angle between the two mitral leaflets in the left atrium. However, since it is uses only velocity measurements, it is unaffected by factors that alter flow conditions (Figure 19–12D).

4. Exercise-Stress Echocardiography

When symptoms are discordant with two- or three-dimensional and Doppler findings, exercise-stress echocardiography can be used to assess mitral stenosis severity, since exercise increases cardiac output and gradient without

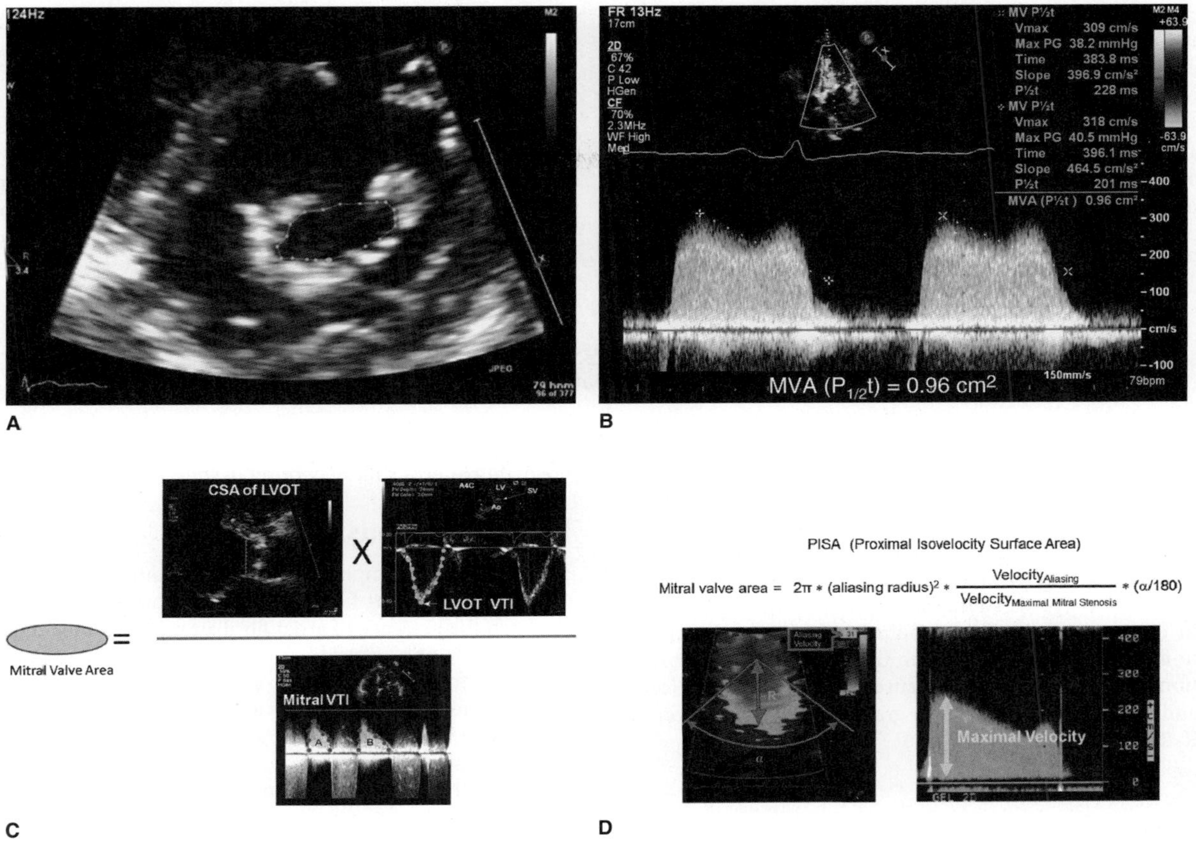

▲ **Figure 19–12.** Quantification of mitral stenosis using two-dimensional and Doppler echocardiography. **A:** Planimety of the mitral orifice. **B:** Calculation using the pressure half-time ($P_{1/2}t$) method. **C:** Calculation using the continuity equation. **D:** Calculation using the proximal isovelocity surface area (PISA) method. CSA, cross-sectional area; LVOT, left ventricular outflow tract; MVA, mitral valve area; $P_{1/2}t$, pressure half-time; PG, peak gradient; R, aliasing radius; Va, aliasing velocity; Vmax, maximum velocity; VTI, velocity time integral; α/180, corrected angle between the two mitral leaflets on the left atrial side. (Panels A and B were Reproduced with permission from Omran AS, et al. *J Saudi Heart Assoc.* 2011;23:51. Panel C was Reproduced with permission, from Baumgartner H, et al. J *Am Soc Echocardiogr.* 2009;22:1. Panel D was Reproduced, with permission, from Messika-Zeitoun D, et al. *Arch Cardiovasc Dis.* 2008;101:653. Copyright © 2012 Published by Elsevier Masson SAS on behalf of the Éditions Françaises de Radiologie. All rights reserved.)

changing the MVA. The mean mitral gradient and pulmonary artery systolic pressure (PASP) are measured during each stage of treadmill or bicycle exercise and are correlated with the perception of dyspnea. The recommended threshold for intervention consideration is a mean transmitral gradient more than 15 mm Hg or PASP more than 60 mm Hg during stress. Dobutamine stress can also be employed, and a dobutamine-induced mean transmitral gradient of ≥ 18 mm Hg has a 90% accuracy rate for predicting a high-risk subpopulation. The tricuspid annulus S-wave velocity reflects right ventricular function, and its response during exercise is an independent predictor of functional capacity. A reduced S-wave velocity is a marker of poor prognosis.

5. Cardiac Computed Tomography and Magnetic Resonance Imaging

Computed tomography can detect valve calcification and provide MVA by planimetry but lacks validation data in hemodynamic assessment. Cardiac magnetic resonance imaging overestimates the valve area by planimetry and PHT and is limited by artifact from calcification and atrial fibrillation. These two imaging modalities are not routinely used in rheumatic or degenerative mitral stenosis assessment.

6. Cardiac Catheterization

When echocardiographic data are ambiguous and/or suboptimal, often in situations when left atrial and left ventricular compliance are altered, cardiac catheterization is used to simultaneously and directly measure the left atrial and left ventricular pressures during diastole. On the left atrial pressure tracing, the "a" wave is accentuated, due to elevated pressure during atrial contraction. The left atrial pressure tracing also records an enlarged V wave, but it is not exclusively seen in mitral stenosis (Figure 19–13). If direct left atrial access is not performed, then the pulmonary capillary wedge (PCW) pressure is used as the surrogate for left atrial pressure. When PCW pressure is used, the operator must be absolutely certain that the balloon right-heart catheter is in the "wedged" position by evaluating the hemodynamic waveform and, ideally, by measuring the oxygen saturation distal to the catheter, which originates from the oxygenated blood of a pulmonary vein. The diagnostic finding of mitral stenosis is the presence of a diastolic gradient when the PCW pressure or left atrial pressure is measured simultaneously with the left ventricular pressure. The magnitude of difference in gradients at end-diastole reflects the severity of obstruction. Tachycardia will increase and bradycardia will decrease the transmitral gradients. The Gorlin formula is used to calculate the MVA, where

$$\text{MVA}(\text{cm}^2) = \frac{(\text{Cardiac output (mL/min)/Diastolic filling period(s)}) \times \text{Heart rate (bpm)}}{\text{Constant } 37.9 \times \sqrt{\text{Mean transmitral gradient (mm Hg)}}}$$

This formula accurately determines MVA only in patients with isolated mitral stenosis. In those who also have mitral regurgitation, the Gorlin formula overestimates the degree of mitral stenosis because it does not account for the increased regurgitant flow across the valve. Pulmonary arterial pressure is also measured and is usually elevated proportionally with left atrial hypertension in the absence of intrinsic pulmonary disease. Similar to noninvasive measurements, in the setting of atrial fibrillation, a minimum of five measurements should be collected and averaged since the mean gradient is dependent on the R-R interval.

Pressman GS, Ranjan R, Park DH, Shim CY, Hong GR. Degenerative mitral stenosis versus rheumatic mitral stenosis. *Am J Cardiol.* 2020;125(10):1536–1542. [PMID: 32241552]

Silbiger JJ. Advances in rheumatic mitral stenosis: echocardiographic, pathophysiologic, and hemodynamic considerations. *J Am Soc Echocardiogr.* 2021;34(7):709–722. [PMID: 33652082]

Silbiger JJ. Mitral annular calcification and calcific mitral stenosis: role of echocardiography in hemodynamic assessment and management. *J Am Soc Echocardiogr.* 2021;34(9):923–931. [PMID: 33857624]

Wunderlich NC, Dalvi B, Ho SY, Küx H, Siegel RJ. Rheumatic mitral valve stenosis: diagnosis and treatment options. *Curr Cardiol Rep.* 2019;21(3):14. [PMID: 30815750]

Differential Diagnosis

Dyspnea on exertion and exercise intolerance are nonspecific symptoms that can be present in many other cardiac and noncardiac conditions. It is important to consider left- and right-heart cardiomyopathy; valvular pathology such as aortic stenosis, aortic insufficiency, and mitral regurgitation; pericardial disease such as chronic constrictive pericarditis; intracardiac shunting; and bradyarrhythmias and tachyarrhythmias. Obviously, numerous pulmonary processes can lead to dyspnea, including obstructive and restrictive lung disease and interstitial lung disease. Other etiologies of dyspnea and fatigue to consider are chronic anemia, hypothyroidism, thyrotoxicosis, and obesity. The likelihood of mitral stenosis should always be considered when evaluating pregnant patients with new-onset dyspnea.

Complications

The three major complications of severe mitral stenosis are decompensated heart failure, atrial fibrillation, and embolic stroke in the presence of atrial fibrillation. The annual incidence of new-onset atrial fibrillation is 3.5% and increases to 6% if the left atrium is dilated to at least 47 mm. Endocarditis is uncommon, but if present, is associated with a high mortality rate. Untreated moderate and severe rheumatic mitral stenosis during pregnancy can result in significant maternal morbidity with 50% developing heart failure and 11% arrhythmia. The maternal mortality rate ranges between 1.9% and 50%, depending on geographic region. Fetal outcome can also be poor with 23% preterm delivery and 21% intrauterine growth retardation.

Cupido B, Zuhlke L, Osman A, van Dyk D, Sliwa K. Managing rheumatic heart disease in pregnancy: a practical evidence-based multidisciplinary approach. *Can J Cardiol.* 2021;37(12):2045–2055. [PMID: 34571164]

Lewey J, Andrade L, Levine LD. Valvular heart disease in pregnancy. *Cardiol Clinics.* 2021:39(1);151–161. [PMID: 33222810]

Treatment

Management is guided by symptoms, and in a subset of patients, symptoms are only elicited during rigorous exercise protocols. The 2020 American Heart Association/American College of Cardiology Valvular Heart Disease Guidelines classifies mitral stenosis in four stages according to symptoms. Stage A patients are at risk of stenosis and only have valve doming during diastole. Stage B patients have progressive stenosis with additional commissural fusion and mild to moderate left atrial enlargement, MVA more than 1.5 cm^2, PHT less than 150 ms, and normal PASP at rest. Stage C patients have asymptomatic severe stenosis with MVA $\leq$ 1.5 cm^2 and PHT $\geq$ 150 ms or very severe stenosis with MVA $\leq$ 1.0 cm^2 and PHT $\geq$ 220 ms with severe left

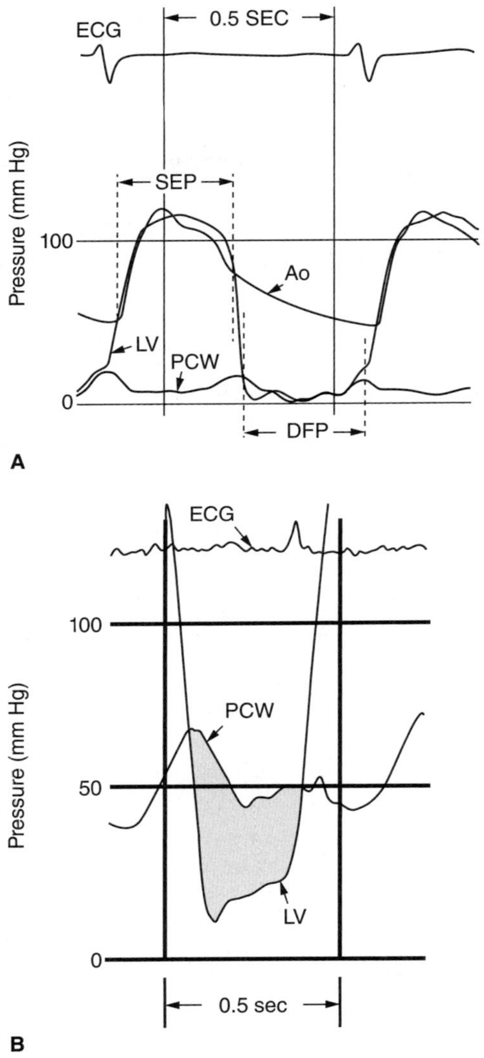

▲ **Figure 19–13.** Invasive simultaneous hemodynamic tracings of (**A**) normal left ventricular (LV), left atrial, and aortic (Ao) pressure and (**B**) pressure gradient between pulmonary capillary wedge (PCW) pressure and LV (*shaded in gray in mitral stenosis*). The LV end-diastolic pressure is atypically elevated with coincident mitral regurgitation. The PCW tracing has a large V wave. The PCW-LV pressure gradient is marked throughout diastole. DFP, diastolic filling period; SEP, systolic ejection period. (Reproduced, with permission, from Carabello BA, Grossman W. Calculation of stenotic valve orifice area. In: Baim DS, Grossman W, ed. *Grossman's Cardiac Catheterization, Angiography, and Intervention*, 5th ed. Philadelphia: Lippincott Williams & Wilkins; 1996.)

atrial enlargement and PASP more than 30 mm Hg. Stage D patients have the same findings as in stage C, except they are symptomatic with decreased exercise tolerance and exertional dyspnea. In general, the MVA in rheumatic mitral stenosis decreases by 0.1 cm^2 per year. However, the rate of progression can be variable and is more rapid in patients living in low-income countries due to recurrent episodes of symptomatic and asymptomatic rheumatic fever.

A. Lifestyle Modifications

Patients with moderate or severe mitral stenosis should be counseled to avoid strenuous activities and thereby reduce risk of tachycardia. They also benefit from consuming a low-sodium diet to avoid fluid retention and to prevent development of pulmonary edema.

B. Pharmacologic Therapy

1. Secondary prevention of rheumatic fever—Since recurrent rheumatic fever is associated with progression of mitral stenosis, secondary prevention with antimicrobial therapy is recommended and the duration of therapy is dependent on the individual's age, extent of initial cardiac involvement, and risk of recurrent infection. Intramuscular benzathine penicillin G (1.2 million units every 4 weeks) is recommended in most cases. In populations with a high incidence of rheumatic fever, a 3-week schedule is more effective. Patients with rheumatic fever with carditis and residual valvular disease should take antimicrobial therapy for 10 years or until age 40, whichever is longer. Those without residual cardiac disease should continue for 10 years or until age 21, whichever is longer. Individuals who had only rheumatic fever, without carditis, can take prophylactic therapy for 5 years or until age 21, whichever is longer. Alternatively, oral penicillin V 250 mg twice daily or sulfadiazine 0.5 g (< 27 kg) to 1.0 g (≥ 27 kg) daily can be used.

2. Atrial fibrillation—Since tachycardia decreases the diastolic filling time, the ventricular rate should be aggressively treated with negative chronotropic agents, including β-blockers, nondihydropyridine calcium channel blockers, digoxin, and ivrabadine. When tachycardia is refractory to medical therapy, pharmacologic cardioversion with antiarrhythmic medications or direct-current synchronized cardioversion is appropriate. In patients with atrial fibrillation, it is imperative that anticoagulation with warfarin be initiated with a therapeutic international normalized ratio goal of 2–3. The risk of systemic embolic events ranges from 1.5 to 4.7% per year without anticoagulation and decreases to about 0.7–0.8% per year on therapeutic vitamin K antagonist. Successful valvotomy does not reduce the thrombotic risk, and thus patients still require indefinite anticoagulation. While tempting, there are no data to support empiric vitamin K antagonist therapy in the absence of atrial fibrillation. Of note, the CHA_2DS_2-VASc score used to estimate stroke risk associated with atrial fibrillation is not applicable in valvular or rheumatic mitral stenosis. The INVICTUS-VKA trial demonstrated that vitamin K antagonist was superior to rivaroxaban in reducing a composite of stroke, systemic embolism, myocardial infarction, and death and did not increase major bleeding.

3. Heart failure—Diuretics and sodium restriction are used to treat pulmonary edema. In the setting of concomitant right ventricular failure, venodilators can be added.

C. Surveillance Imaging

Patients with stage B progressive rheumatic mitral stenosis, can undergo surveillance transthoracic echo every 3–5 years when the MVA is more than 1.5 cm^2. For those with stage C asymptomatic severe stenosis with MVA 1.0–1.5 cm^2 and compensated left and right ventricular function, imaging can be performed every 1–2 years. If there is left or right ventricular decompensation, imaging can be repeated sooner. Patients with very severe mitral stenosis where the MVA is less than 1.0 cm^2, echo is recommended every year. The frequency of echocardiograms in calcific mitral stenosis has not been established.

D. Interventional Therapy

Mechanical therapy should be considered in symptomatic patients when the MVA is less than 1.5 cm^2 or when the mitral valve index is less than 0.6 cm^2/m^2 and in asymptomatic patients with MVA $\leq$ 1.0 cm^2 and favorable valve morphology. Intervention can also be contemplated in asymptomatic patients with PASP more than 50 mm Hg at rest or more than 60 mm Hg during exercise, mean transmitral gradient more than 15 mm Hg during exercise, new-onset atrial fibrillation, or prior embolization or dense left atrial contrast. In New York Heart Association (NYHA) congestive heart failure class III/IV patients, invasive intervention should be pursued when symptoms become refractory to optimal medical therapy. Prior to conception, patients with symptomatic moderate or severe mitral stenosis or PASP more than 50 mm Hg at rest should be counseled to undergo intervention. Currently, percutaneous balloon valvotomy is the preferred method for enlarging the mitral orifice in patients with favorable anatomy. Finally, in patients undergoing other cardiac surgery, concomitant mitral valve surgery is indicated for those classified as stage C and D and may be considered in patients with MVA of 1.6–2.0 cm^2.

1. Percutaneous balloon valvotomy—Percutaneous balloon valvotomy is reserved for individuals with pliable valves with minimal calcification and mild or no mitral regurgitation and can be considered in those who are poor surgical candidates with the above valve morphology. It can also be performed safely in pregnant patients. All patients considered for valvotomy need to have an invasive assessment of mitral valve hemodynamic data prior to the procedure and immediately after completion of the procedure. Meticulous patient selection is absolutely essential for procedural success. The Wilkins echocardiographic score of $\leq$ 8 predicts a very favorable outcome. On average, the mitral gradient decreases by approximately 7–10 mm Hg, mitral orifice increases by approximately 0.7–1 cm^2, and cardiac output increases by about 0.6 L/min. The immediate, short-, and long-term results are excellent. For those with a score of $\leq$ 8, the survival rate at 12 years was 82% versus 57% in those with higher scores, and event-free survival was 38% versus 22%. At 19 years, restenosis-free survival ranges from 22 to 30%, and event-free survival ranges from 21 to 35%. Successful valvotomy can last for decades in flexible, noncalcified valves and is comparable to surgical commissurotomy. In some patients, the stenotic mitral valve can undergo repeat balloon valvotomy. In addition, successful valvotomy can result in normalization of PASP, regression of tricuspid regurgitation, and improvement of left ventricular systolic function if it is reduced prior to intervention (Figure 19–14).

Even though the success rate ranges from 85 to 99% in appropriately selected patients, the procedure is associated with a 0–0.5% mortality rate, up to a 12% incidence of hemopericardium, and a 1–2% rate of systemic embolization. The most catastrophic complication of balloon valvotomy is severe mitral regurgitation, which occurs in 2–10% of cases when the heavily calcified leaflets, and not the commissures, are split. In 1.6–3% of cases, surgical treatment of mitral regurgitation is necessary. Use of transesophageal and intracardiac echocardiography during valvotomy assists in balloon placement, septal puncture guidance, and detection of complications.

2. Surgical commissurotomy—Surgical commissurotomy can be performed either by the closed or open approach. The surgical mortality rate is 2–5% in isolated mitral valve repair or replacement. After surgical commissurotomy, the postoperation mean mitral gradient and MVA can be measured noninvasively. In countries where percutaneous balloon valvotomy is not available or is cost-prohibitive, surgical commissurotomy can be performed with similar results. In populations with a high Wilkins echocardiographic score or atrial fibrillation, compared with balloon valvotomy, surgical open mitral commissurotomy or mitral valve replacement is associated with a higher event-free survival rate of 94% versus 80% at 9 years. However, compared to the percutaneous approach, surgical commissurotomy is associated with greater morbidity, longer hospital stay, and longer recovery. Similar to the balloon valvotomy, a relatively larger mitral orifice does not reduce the risk of thrombosis.

3. Surgical mitral valve replacement—If the valve is heavily calcified or commissurotomy does not sufficiently increase the mitral orifice area, then mitral valve replacement is indicated. A Wilkins echocardiographic score $\geq$ 8 and at least moderate mitral regurgitation are independent risk factors for surgery after balloon valvotomy. The choice of a bioprosthetic valve versus a mechanical valve depends on the age of the

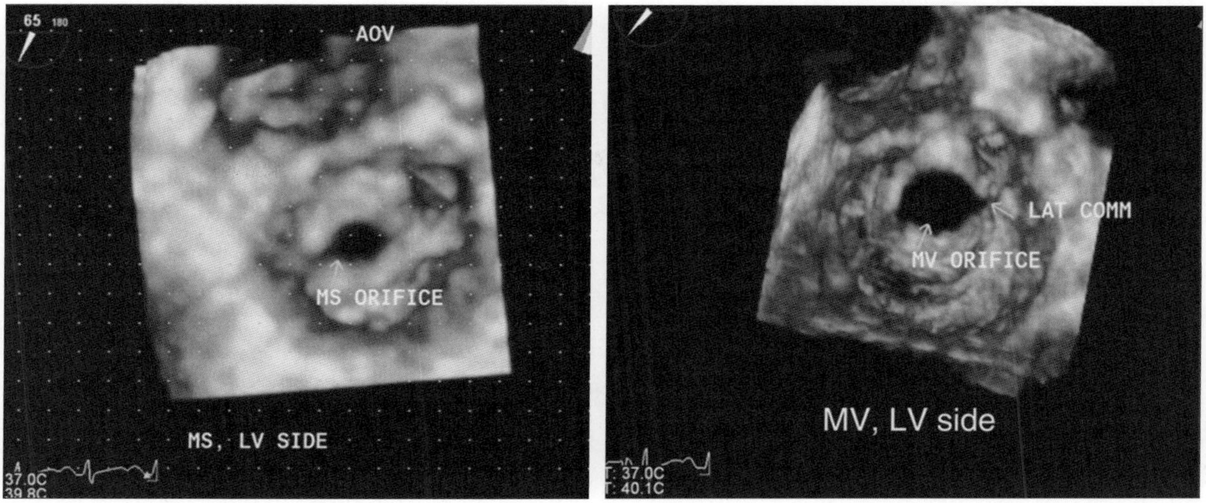

A B

▲ **Figure 19–14.** Three-dimensional echocardiography images of the mitral orifice before (**A**) and after (**B**) mitral valve balloon valvotomy. AOV, aortic valve; LV, left ventricle; MS, mitral stenosis; MV, mitral valve. (Reproduced from Omran AS, et al. *J Saudi Heart Assoc*. 2011;23:51, with permission.)

patient, existing comorbid conditions, and ability to comply with oral anticoagulant therapy. A mechanical valve is preferable in young patients to avoid accelerated bioprosthetic valve calcification, especially in those who are hemodialysis dependent. In individuals of childbearing age who are interested in future pregnancies, a bioprosthetic valve is often selected to avoid warfarin-induced embryopathy.

4. Surgical and transcatheter mitral valve implantation— Patients with degenerative calcific mitral stenosis are not candidates for balloon valvulotomy because they lack commissural fusion. They have both high anatomic risk and high surgical morbidity and mortality risk due to advanced age and concomitant comorbid conditions. In 2014 and 2015, two bioprosthetic mitral valves were implanted via the transapical approach after thoracotomy. Over the past few years, these valves have been implanted percutaneously in clinical investigations, which is a promising option for patients with degenerative calcific mitral stenosis with unfavorable valve morphology and unacceptable surgical morbidity and mortality risks.

Alexis SL, Malik AH, Eshmawi AE, et al. Surgical and transcatheter mitral valve replacement in mitral annular calcification: a systematic review. *J Am Heart Assoc*. 2021;10(7):e018514. [PMID: 33728929]

Connolly SJ, Karthikeyan G, Ntsekhe M, et al. Rivaroxaban in rheumatic heart disease-associated atrial fibrillation. *N Engl J Med*. 2022;387(11):978–988. [PIMD: 36036525]

Ghadimi N, Kaveh S, Shabaninejad H, Lijassi A, Mehr AZ. Comparative efficacy of ivabradine versus beta-blockers in patients with mitral stenosis in sinus rhythm: systemic review and meta-analysis. *Int J Clin Pharm*. 2019:41(1):22–29. [PMID: 30659493]

Karthikeyan G, Connolly SJ, Ntsekhe M, et al. The INVICTUS rheumatic heart disease research program: rationale, design and baseline characteristic of a randomized trial of rivaroxaban compared to vitamin K antagonists in rheumatic valvular disease and atrial fibrillation. *Am Heart J*. 2020;225:69–77. [PMID: 32474206]

Rmilah AAA, Tahboub MA, Alkurashi AK, et al. Efficacy and safety of percutaneous mitral balloon valvotomy in patients with mitral stenosis: a systematic review and meta-analysis. *Int J Cardiol Heart Vasc*. 2021;33:100765. [PMID: 33889711]

Russell EA, Walsh WF, Costello B, et al. Medical management of rheumatic heart disease: systematic review of the evidence. *Cardiol Rev*. 2018;26(4):187–195. [PMID: 29608495]

Prognosis

Prognosis of uncorrected rheumatic mitral stenosis is closely linked with NYHA congestive heart failure class at the time of diagnosis. The 10-year mortality rate for patients who are asymptomatic is less than 20%. NYHA class II and III patients have a mortality rate of 40%, and patients in class IV approach a rate of 80–85%. Sixty to 70% of patients with severe mitral stenosis die from congestive heart failure, 20–30% from systemic thromboembolism, and 1–5% from infection (Figure 19–15). Without intervention, the 5-year calculated mortality rate of patients with calcific mitral stenosis is approximately 53%, which is 3 times that of age- and gender-matched cohort.

Bertrand PB, Mihos CG, Yucel E. Mitral annular calcification and calcific mitral stenosis: therapeutic challenges and considerations. *Curr Treat Options Cardiovasc Med*. 2019;21(4):19. [PMID: 30929092]

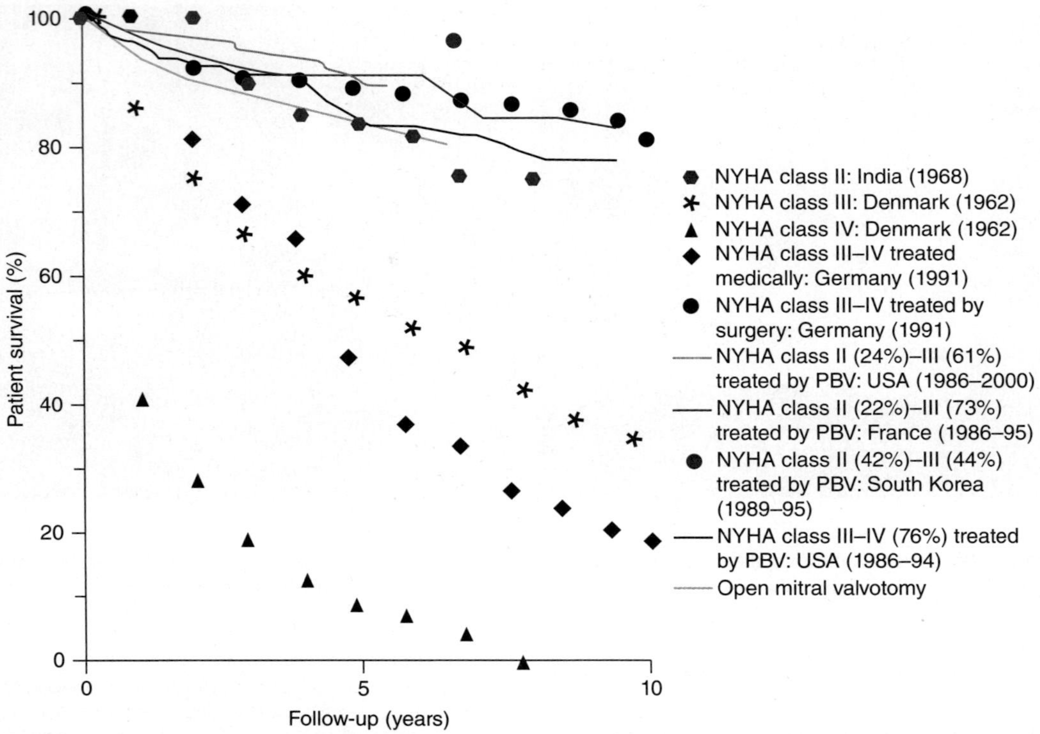

▲ **Figure 19–15.** **Natural history of mitral stenosis and the effect of intervention. NYHA, New York Heart Association; PBV, percutaneous balloon valvotomy.** (Reproduced with permission from Chandrashekhar Y, et al. Mitral stenosis. *Lancet.* 2009;374(9697):1271–1283.)

When to Refer or Admit

Referral to cardiology subspecialty care is warranted when patients have stage C or D severe mitral stenosis or when symptoms of dyspnea and fatigue are disproportionately greater than the severity of mitral stenosis determined by echocardiography imaging. In addition, the electrophysiologist can assist with sinus rhythm restoration using direct current cardioversion and maintenance of sinus rhythm using anti-arrhythmic medications in patients with new-onset atrial fibrillation to optimize hemodynamics.

Mitral Regurgitation

20

Michael H. Crawford, MD

ESSENTIALS OF DIAGNOSIS

- Dyspnea or orthopnea.
- Characteristic apical systolic murmur.
- Color-flow Doppler echocardiographic evidence of systolic regurgitation into the left atrium.

General Considerations

The mitral apparatus consists of the left ventricular walls that support the papillary muscles, the chordae tendineae, mitral leaflets, annulus, and adjacent left atrial walls. Because defects in any of these components can lead to systolic regurgitation, the list of diseases that can cause mitral regurgitation includes many types of heart disease. Anything that causes left ventricular dilatation may disrupt the alignment of the papillary muscles, impairing their function and dilating the annulus, resulting in mitral regurgitation. Myocardial infarction involving the papillary muscles or the left ventricular walls that support them can impair the function of the mitral apparatus. Mitral chordae can rupture, especially in patients with hypertension or mitral valve prolapse. The most common diseases affecting the mitral leaflets are systolic left ventricular dysfunction and the myxomatous changes of mitral valve prolapse. In addition, infective endocarditis can destroy the mitral leaflets, and mitral annular calcification can impair the normal systolic contraction of the annulus, leading to mitral regurgitation. Finally, left atrial dilatation from any cause, eg, atrial fibrillation, can dilate the mitral annulus and disrupt annular function leading to mitral regurgitation. Some patients have combinations of these defects, making mitral regurgitation both more likely and more severe.

For clinical purposes, mitral regurgitation can be divided into two broad categories: primary or degenerative and secondary or functional. The former refers to diseases that involve the valve leaflets and their immediate supporting apparatus (ie, chordae and annulus). The latter refers to diseases that affect the left ventricle and atrium, leaving the valve apparatus intact (Table 20–1).

Mitral valve prolapse is the most common cause of primary mitral regurgitation and is unique in many ways. An increase in the middle connective tissue layer of the mitral valve causes an increase in leaflet size and elongated chordae. The resultant systolic prolapse of the valve into the left atrium may or may not be accompanied by regurgitation. In some patients, regurgitation depends on left ventricular volume. Large volumes tend to reduce prolapse and hence regurgitation; small volumes have the opposite effect. Consequently, the presence or absence of regurgitation and its severity and timing in systole (the ventricle becomes progressively smaller during systole) are determined by a complex interplay of left ventricular volume, pressure, and contractile state.

Patients with mitral valve prolapse are also unique because the condition can be hereditary. A minority have mitral valve prolapse as part of a syndrome such as Marfan, Ehlers-Danlos, and Loeys-Dietzs. Also, it can be familial with an autosomal dominant pattern. Rarely in men it can be X-linked and present with a more severe phenotype. In most cases it is of polygenetic origin with at least 33 genes currently identified by genome-wide association studies. Some patients exhibit abnormalities of connective tissue in other organs (eg, thoracic skeleton) and have demonstrable abnormalities in the autonomic nervous system. In addition, there is a rare phenotype usually in women that is associated with repolarization abnormalities on ECG, premature ventricular contractions, mitral annular dysjunction, papillary muscle fibrosis, and sudden cardiac death. Thus, the clinical presentation of mitral valve prolapse varies from one that is similar to other forms of mitral regurgitation to a unique presentation in which extracardiac manifestations are prominent. Age is a factor as well. In younger patients severe myxomatous changes can result in extensive deformity of both valve

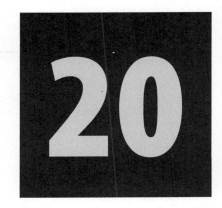

Table 20–1. Etiologic Classification of Mitral Regurgitation

Primary Mitral Regurgitation
Myxomatous changes (mitral valve prolapse)
Rheumatic heart disease
Infective endocarditis
Spontaneous chordal rupture
Collagen vascular disease
Radiation therapy
Secondary Mitral Regurgitation
Coronary artery disease
Hypertrophic cardiomyopathy
Dilated cardiomyopathy
Left atrial dilatation

leaflets with marked prolapse, the so-called Barlow valve. In older patients, fibroelastic deficiency may predominate, resulting in thin stiff leaflets and chordal rupture.

Primary mitral regurgitation can also be acquired from rheumatic heart disease, connective tissue diseases, infective endocarditis, or radiation therapy, especially to the left chest for breast cancer. Secondary or functional mitral regurgitation is usually due to left ventricular dilatation or ischemic wall motion abnormalities involving the papillary muscles or their supporting left ventricular wall. Common etiologies are ischemic heart disease and dilated cardiomyopathies.

Clinically mitral valve prolapse can present as acute or chronic mitral regurgitation. In **chronic mitral regurgitation**, the more common of the two clinical presentations, the mitral regurgitation progressively worsens as the underlying heart disease worsens. In this situation, the heart has time to adapt to the mitral leak. The increased pressure in the left atrium during systole causes left atrial dilatation. If this left atrial enlargement is not adequate to decompress the left atrial pressure, the pulmonary arterial tone increases to protect the pulmonary capillaries from increased hydrostatic pressure, resulting in pulmonary hypertension. Because the regurgitated blood returns to the left ventricle in diastole, along with the normal atrial stroke volume, the volume load on the left ventricle results in left ventricular dilatation and eccentric hypertrophy.

Initially, the loading conditions in mitral regurgitation enhance left ventricular performance because preload is increased, and afterload is normal. Preload is increased by the augmentation of left ventricular diastolic volume, which increases left ventricular systolic function via the Frank-Starling mechanism. Afterload, or the left ventricular wall tension after the aortic valve opens in systole, is not increased, despite increased left ventricular volume, because much of the increased volume is regurgitated into the left atrium in early systole before the aortic valve opens and because the continued regurgitation during systole reduces forward stroke volume and blood pressure. As the severity of mitral regurgitation increases over time, the ability of the dilated left ventricle to augment systolic function reaches its limits, left ventricular systolic function falls, and heart failure ensues.

Acute mitral regurgitation presents differently because there is insufficient time for these compensatory mechanisms to develop. Sudden rupture of the chordae tendineae, for example, may result in severe acute mitral regurgitation, which markedly increases left atrial pressure. Because the left atrium has no time to dilate, the pulmonary capillary pressure rises markedly, and pulmonary edema usually ensues. The left ventricle also does not dilate adequately to handle the tremendous volume load, and forward failure occurs because of an impaired left ventricular stroke volume. Acute mitral regurgitation (caused by the abrupt failure of a component of the mitral apparatus) can precipitate or aggravate symptoms in a patient with chronic mitral regurgitation.

Trenkwalker T, Krane M. Mitral valve prolapse: will genetics finally solve the puzzle? *Eur Heart J*. 2022;43:1681–1683. [PMID: 35265976]

Clinical Findings

A. Symptoms & Signs

1. Chronic mitral regurgitation—The medical history of patients with chronic mitral regurgitation may suggest its cause. Look for a possible history of acute rheumatic fever, coronary artery disease, or a cardiomyopathy. The most common symptom in patients with chronic mitral regurgitation is progressive dyspnea, beginning with dyspnea on exertion and progressing to paroxysmal nocturnal dyspnea, and finally orthopnea. Patients may also complain of fatigue and other symptoms associated with congestive heart failure, such as edema. Chronic mitral regurgitation can lead to atrial fibrillation, and palpitations or other symptoms related to this rhythm disturbance may present in patients. Some patients with mitral valve prolapse may have atypical chest pain or inappropriate autonomic nervous system activation (eg, inappropriate tachycardia, orthostatic hypotension).

2. Acute mitral regurgitation—The patient with acute mitral regurgitation is usually markedly symptomatic, with severe orthopnea or frank pulmonary edema. Although sudden pulmonary edema may suggest the diagnosis, other features of the history may point to the cause of mitral apparatus failure, such as a history of acute myocardial infarction, uncontrolled hypertension, or symptoms of infective endocarditis.

B. Physical Examination

1. Chronic mitral regurgitation—In chronic mitral regurgitation, the heart rate may be increased because of atrial fibrillation or heart failure. The carotid pulse is usually brief and of low amplitude, and blood pressure examination shows a narrow pulse pressure. These findings reflect the reduced forward stroke volume. In the presence of heart failure, the respiratory rate may be increased and lung crackles, pleural effusion, edema, increased jugular venous pressure, or ascites may be present. Left ventricular enlargement may result in an enlarged apical impulse, and right ventricular enlargement due to pulmonary hypertension may produce a right ventricular lift along the left sternal border. The first and second heart sounds are usually normal, but the pulmonic component of the second heart sound may be increased if pulmonary hypertension is evident. A third heart sound is common because of the left ventricular volume overload, but it does not necessarily indicate heart failure. A fourth heart sound is unusual unless associated coronary artery disease or hypertension is present. The characteristic murmur of chronic mitral regurgitation is usually holosystolic and heard best at the apex, with radiation to the axilla. Occasionally, in patients with posterior leaflet defects, the direction of the regurgitant jet may be anterior, and the murmur is heard in the aortic area. With anterior leaflet defects, the direction of the mitral jet may be posterior and transmitted to the back, where it can be heard up and down the spine. In patients with mitral valve prolapse, the murmur can be crescendo and late systolic. This type of murmur, in fact, almost always represents mitral regurgitation. Often, the late systolic crescendo murmur of mitral valve prolapse is preceded by a midsystolic click from the sudden tensing of the prolapsing leaflets when the end of chordal tethering is reached. Some patients may manifest only a midsystolic click. Occasionally, mitral murmurs will be honking or musical in quality, presumably from a prolapsing leaflet that vibrates in the regurgitant stream. Some patients occasionally have other murmur configurations, whereas others with echocardiographically documented mitral regurgitation have no audible murmur, especially if the regurgitation is mild.

Because murmur configuration and radiation vary in mitral regurgitation, dynamic auscultation is of a great deal of value at the bedside for differentiating this murmur from other heart murmurs (Table 20–2). Handgrip exercise is the favored bedside maneuver because it frequently increases the intensity of a mitral regurgitation murmur. The murmur of mitral valve prolapse behaves like that of mitral regurgitation from any cause, but it has a few unique features. Any maneuver that increases left ventricular volume will (as noted earlier) decrease the amount of mitral valve prolapse and decrease the amount of mitral regurgitation, thereby lessening the intensity of the murmur. Thus, rapid squatting will diminish the murmur of mitral valve prolapse and move the timing of the click-murmur complex later in systole (Figure 20–1). Conversely, maneuvers that decrease left ventricular volume increase the intensity and duration of the murmur of mitral valve prolapse. Thus, standing rapidly from a squatting position will make the murmur louder and move the click-murmur complex toward early systole. Extreme left ventricular volume increases can eliminate the click-murmur and mitral regurgitation, and extreme decrease can result in a pansystolic murmur without a click.

Table 20–2. Differentiation of Systolic Murmurs Based on Changes in Their Intensity from Physiologic Maneuvers

	Origin of Murmur					
Maneuver	**Flow**	**TR**	**AS**	**MR/VSD**	**MVP**	**HOCM**
Inspiration	– or ↑	↑	—	—	—	—
Stand	↓	—	—	—	↑	↑
Squat	↑	—	—	—	↓	↓
Valsalva maneuver	↓	↓	↓	↓	↑	↑
Handgrip/TAO	↓	—	—	↑	↑	↓
Post-PVC	↑	—	↑	—	—	↑

AS, aortic stenosis; Flow, benign flow murmur; HOCM, hypertrophic obstructive cardiomyopathy; MR, mitral regurgitation; MVP, mitral valve prolapse; PVC, premature ventricular contraction; TAO, transient arterial occlusion; TR, tricuspid regurgitation; VSD, ventricular septal defect; ↑, increase in murmur intensity; ↓, decrease in murmur intensity; —, no predictable change.

Consequently, the auscultatory findings in mitral valve prolapse vary greatly, which can make accurate clinical diagnosis difficult.

2. Acute mitral regurgitation—In acute mitral regurgitation, the physical findings are different. The marked increase in left atrial pressure, caused by regurgitation into a noncompliant left atrium, may raise left atrial pressure in late systole to the point that there is no longer any gradient for regurgitant flow. The murmur thus becomes an early systolic murmur rather than the holosystolic murmur characteristic of patients with chronic mitral regurgitation. In fact, when the acute

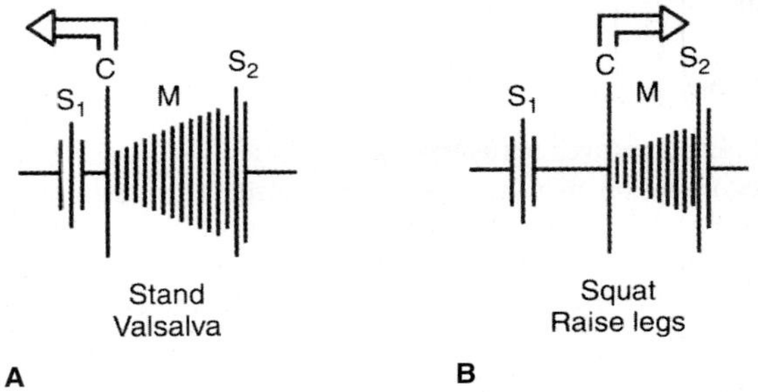

▲ **Figure 20–1.** Change in the position of the click (C)-murmur (M) complex during systole and the intensity of the murmur as a result of bedside maneuvers. **A:** Maneuvers that lengthen the murmur and increase intensity. **B:** Maneuvers that shorten the murmur and reduce its intensity. Note that the position of the midsystolic click also changes with these maneuvers.

mitral regurgitation is very severe, the murmur may not be audible. In mild-to-moderate acute mitral regurgitation, the murmur responds like the murmur of chronic mitral regurgitation with dynamic auscultation. More severe acute regurgitation is associated with high catecholamine tone and a lack of responsiveness to bedside maneuvers. Other characteristic features of acute mitral regurgitation include a fourth heart sound caused by vigorous atrial contraction following exaggerated expansion during ventricular systole (atrial diastole). In the presence of pulmonary hypertension, the pulmonary second sound increases, and murmurs of pulmonic and tricuspid regurgitation may be present. As mentioned earlier, acute mitral regurgitation invariably results in pulmonary edema. Consequently, the patient will have an increased respiratory rate, diffuse lung crackles, evidence of plural effusion, increased heart rate, a narrow pulse pressure with low systolic blood pressure, and signs of acute right-heart failure, such as increased jugular venous pressure.

3. Mixed valvular disease—Patients with rheumatic valvular disease often have mixed mitral disease, which is defined as at least moderate mitral regurgitation, with a mean mitral valve diastolic gradient of more than 10 mm Hg. The clinical course of mixed mitral valve disease is like that of mitral regurgitation, and such patients should be treated similarly. Aortic regurgitation frequently occurs with mitral regurgitation, either because of left ventricular dilatation or because the same disease process affects the aortic valve (eg, Marfan syndrome). This places an additional volume load on the left ventricle and usually accelerates the patient's clinical deterioration.

When aortic stenosis and mitral regurgitation occur together, it is sometimes difficult to ascertain whether the same disease process (eg, rheumatic disease) involved both valves or whether the pressure load of significant aortic stenosis altered left ventricular geometry, performance, or both, resulting in functional or secondary mitral regurgitation. Diagnostic imaging studies usually resolve this issue and help direct therapy.

C. Diagnostic Studies

1. Electrocardiography—Patients with chronic mitral regurgitation may have evidence of left ventricular hypertrophy, left atrial abnormality, and sometimes, right ventricular enlargement. Patients with coronary artery disease might have evidence of myocardial infarction or ischemia. Electrocardiographic (ECG) exercise testing is usually done only to confirm the patient's physical limitations, because ECG changes in the face of a left ventricular volume load are not likely to be accurate for the diagnosis of coronary artery disease. Ambulatory ECG monitoring can be helpful in patients with palpitations to document atrial fibrillation or other intermittent rhythm disorders.

2. Chest radiography—In cases of chronic mitral regurgitation, an enlarged left ventricle and left atrium would be expected. In severe regurgitation, right-heart enlargement and pulmonary hypertension may be evident. Patients in heart failure will show pulmonary congestion and pleural effusions. In acute mitral regurgitation, there are often signs of pulmonary congestion without enlargement of the heart.

3. Echocardiography—Doppler echocardiography is the technique of choice for the initial evaluation of mitral regurgitation and the color-flow Doppler identification of a systolic regurgitant jet across the mitral valve into the left atrium is diagnostic of mitral regurgitation (Figure 20–2). There are several ways of estimating the severity of mitral regurgitation by analyzing the characteristics of the regurgitant jet on color-flow Doppler. The first method is the depth of penetration of the jet into the left atrium. A penetration of 1 cm or less is considered mild; 2–3 cm, moderate; and 4 cm or more, severe. If the jet is very narrow, the actual volume of regurgitant flow may not be as great as occurs with a more voluminous flow disturbance that penetrates to the same depth. Some investigators have therefore suggested also taking the area of the jet into consideration. One problem with this assessment system, however, is that if the jet impinges on a wall of the left atrium, it appears to penetrate less and be of a smaller area than if it is free in the atrial cavity. There is thus a tendency to underestimate the severity of mitral regurgitation when the jet hits the atrial wall. Also, a regurgitant jet of any size occurring in a large left atrium will not appear as impressive as the same size jet in a small left atrium. In addition, a jet that only occurs in late systole will exaggerate the severity of regurgitation. The size of the leak

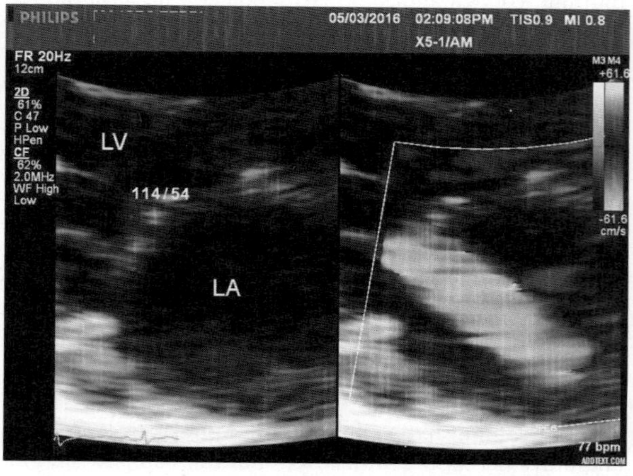

▲ **Figure 20–2.** *Left panel*: Two-dimensional echocardiographic still frame image from the parasternal long-axis view of the closed mitral valve in systole (patient's blood pressure value written over the valve). *Right panel*: The color-flow Doppler has been turned on, and the large regurgitant jet is visible emanating from the closed valve and striking the posterior wall of the left atrium. LA, left atrium; LV, left ventricle.

Table 20–3. Qualitative and Quantitative Parameters Useful in Grading Mitral Regurgitation Severity by Echocardiography

	Mild	Moderate	Severe
Structural parameters			
LA size	Normal	Normal to dilated	Usually dilated
LV size	Normal	Normal to dilated	Usually dilated
Mitral leaflets or support apparatus	Normal or mild thickening/prolapse	Normal or abnormal	Abnormal: loss of leaflet coaptation, flail leaflet, thickened leaflets, ruptured papillary muscle, prior IE
Doppler parameters			
Color-flow jet area	Small central jet (< 4 cm^2 or < 20% of LA area)	Variable central jet 20–40% of LA area or late systolic or eccentric	Large central jet (usually > 10 cm^2 or > 40% of LA area) or variable size wall-impinging jet swirling in LA
Mitral inflow-PW	E wave dominant but usually < 0.8 m/s	Variable	E wave dominant, but usually E > 1.2 m/s
Jet density-CW	Incomplete or faint	Dense	Dense
Jet contour-CW	Parabolic	Usually parabolic	Early peaking-triangular
Pulmonary vein flow	Systolic dominance	Systolic blunting	Systolic flow reversal
Quantitative parameters			
VC width (cm)	< 0.3	0.3–0.69	≥ 0.7
R Vol (mL/beat)	< 30	30–59	≥ 60
RF (%)	< 30	30–49	≥ 50
EROA (cm^2)	< 0.20	0.20–0.39	≥ 0.40

CW, continuous wave; EROA, effective regurgitation orifice area; IE, infective endocarditis; LA, left atrium; LV, left ventricle; PW, pulsed wave; RF, regurgitant fraction; R Vol, regurgitant volume; VC vena contracta.

in the mitral valve can be determined by evaluating the jet longitudinally or in a cross-sectional plane at the level of the mitral valve. This method gives an estimate of the size of the hole through which the jet is originating (vena contracta).

These qualitative criteria for mitral regurgitation severity can be highly subjective. Accordingly, there has been interest in more quantitative methods for estimating the severity of mitral regurgitation (Table 20–3). The proximal isovelocity surface area observed where flow acceleration and convergence occur on the left ventricular side of the mitral leaflets allows the estimate of regurgitant volume and effective regurgitant orifice area. Fluid dynamics theory states that flow through an isovelocity surface is equal to the velocity times the surface area, which yields instantaneous regurgitant flow. This technique uses the color-flow Doppler color change interfaces observed with accelerating velocity through the orifice to estimate isovelocity surface area. Also, pulsed wave Doppler echocardiography can be used to quantitate regurgitant volume. The principle used is that of flow continuity. Systolic flow through the left ventricular outflow tract represents the forward stroke volume. This can be determined by multiplying the outflow tract area (measured on the two-dimensional echocardiographic image) times the outflow tract Doppler systolic velocity–time integral. Flow across the mitral valve in diastole represents the total stroke volume (forward plus regurgitant flow) and can be determined by multiplying mitral annulus area times the diastolic velocity–time integral. Regurgitant volume is the difference between the total and forward stroke volume. Typically, the regurgitant volume is reported as the regurgitant fraction, which is the regurgitant stroke volume divided by the total stroke volume. Unfortunately, the calculation of regurgitant stroke volume has many possible sources of error, the largest of which is measuring the flow areas—mitral annular and outflow tract. Thus, individuals without valvular regurgitation can have regurgitant fractions of up to 20%. Also, the calculation of regurgitant flow is time-consuming and requires considerable skill. Effective regurgitant orifice area can be estimated as the ratio of regurgitant volume to the regurgitant jet velocity–time integral by pulsed Doppler.

Assessment of pulmonary venous flow velocity by pulsed Doppler echocardiography can also be of value in estimating the severity of mitral regurgitation. Normal pulmonary venous flow velocity is biphasic, with a predominant systolic forward velocity and a lesser diastolic forward velocity in older adults. Systolic forward velocity is reduced in patients with mitral regurgitation, and often the diastolic velocity predominates. In severe mitral regurgitation, the systolic flow in the pulmonary vein signal may reverse. Systolic flow reversal is highly specific for severe regurgitation, but sensitivity is low. Unfortunately, pulmonary venous flow velocity patterns vary considerably in patients with mitral regurgitation, and the predictive value for regurgitation severity is low. It is recommended that all these factors are integrated to produce a composite estimate of the severity of regurgitation.

Echocardiography can be used to evaluate the anatomy of the mitral apparatus to determine where the defect lies and what its cause may be. For example, patients with rheumatic mitral valve disease have thickening of the mitral leaflets, especially at the tips, with rolled edges and regurgitation along the commissural fissure lines. Patients with mitral valve prolapse have voluminous mitral leaflets that prolapse into the left atrium in the latter part of systole. Patients with coronary artery disease have wall motion abnormalities near the papillary muscle attachments. Ruptured and flail chordae tendineae are readily detected by echocardiography, as is mitral annular calcification.

The echocardiogram is also useful for assessing the compensatory changes in the cardiovascular system resulting from mitral regurgitation. The degree of left ventricular and left atrial enlargement is related to the severity of the mitral regurgitation and its chronicity. Left ventricular systolic performance is an important determinant of prognosis in mitral regurgitation. Doppler estimation of pulmonary artery pressures from pulmonic or tricuspid regurgitant jets is valuable for estimating the effect of mitral regurgitation on the pulmonary circulation. An assessment of right-heart chamber sizes and function is additional useful information. Echocardiography can be deployed during bicycle exercise to assess exercise-induced changes in mitral regurgitation severity and pulmonary artery systolic pressure (PASP). Increases in either suggest a worse prognosis. Exercise echocardiography is especially useful for detecting physical limitations in asymptomatic patients with severe mitral regurgitation. Color-flow Doppler echocardiography can detect trivial or mild mitral regurgitation in up to half of otherwise healthy adults. The incidence increases with age and with the rigor with which the operator interrogates the valve. In the absence of anatomic abnormalities, small degrees of regurgitation are probably benign effects of aging.

Transesophageal echocardiography (TEE) can provide the anatomic details of leaflet anatomy needed to plan surgical repair. The probe is rotated progressively to identify the scallops of the two mitral valve leaflets in midesophageal long axis views. The direction of the color-flow jet helps confirm the incompetent scallops. In addition, annular size can be determined and the subvalvular apparatus interrogated. TEE during surgery can be of value to the surgeon. Also, three-dimensional echocardiography is useful for identifying the culprit scallops especially with TEE because an *en face* or surgeons view (looking from the atrial side) of the valve can be obtained.

4. Magnetic resonance imaging—MRI is useful when the echocardiographic grading of the severity of regurgitation is inconsistent or not technically feasible. Although MRI can visualize the regurgitant flow, its main use is quantitating the stroke volume of the left and right ventricles since the difference between the two is the regurgitant volume. Also, MRI is the reference standard for measuring left ventricular and left atrial volume. In addition, late gadolinium enhancement can reveal fibrosis in the papillary muscles which has been associated with ventricular arrhythmias and sudden cardiac death.

5. Cardiac catheterization—Cardiac catheterization is rarely needed to diagnose mitral regurgitation, nor is it usually needed to assess the severity of the regurgitation, left ventricular size and function, or any resultant pulmonary hypertension. Coronary angiography is useful, however, for establishing coronary artery disease as the likely cause of mitral regurgitation as well as the risk from surgical correction of mitral regurgitation from any cause.

Hemodynamic evaluation at the time of cardiac catheterization in patients with moderate-to-severe mitral regurgitation will show an increase in pulmonary artery pressures, increases in the pulmonary capillary wedge pressure (PCWP), and possibly a reduction in forward cardiac output. The PCWP tracing often displays a large *v* wave, which is more than 50% greater than the height of the *a* wave. Although much has been made of the diagnostic value of large *v* waves in the PCWP tracing (especially in the intensive care unit setting), it must be remembered that any cause of left atrial pressure elevation will elevate the height of the *v* wave. It is only when the *v* wave is elevated out of proportion to the *a* wave that the diagnosis of mitral regurgitation is likely (> 150% of the *a* wave).

Left ventricular angiography is graded with a 1–4+ system, where 1+ is mild and 4+ is severe, indicating regurgitation of the angiographic dye into the pulmonary veins. This assessment method correlates well with the color-flow Doppler system. In addition, left ventricular angiography can be used to estimate left ventricular volume and ejection fraction.

6. Laboratory measures—Brain natriuretic peptides (BNP or NT-proBNP) serum levels have been associated with mortality in mitral regurgitation patients. Thus, they can be supportive of a decision to intervene on the valve in borderline cases or be used to follow patients on the verge of needing an intervention. However, the specificity of BNP or NT-proBNP for predicting death is low, so they are not considered a key element of interventional decision-making.

Doherty JU, Kort S, Mehran R, Schoenhagen P, Soman P. ACC/AATS/AHA/ASE/ASNC/HRS/SCAI/SCCT/SCMR/STS 2017 appropriate use criteria for multimodality imaging in valvular heart disease. *J Am Coll Cardiol.* 2017;70:1648–1671. [PMID: 28870679]

Zoghbi WA, Adams D, Bonow RO, et al. Recommendations for noninvasive evaluation of native valvular regurgitation: a report form the American Society of Echocardiography developed in collaboration with the Society for Cardiovascular Magnetic Resonance. J Am Soc Echocardiogr 2017;30:303-371. [PMID: 28314623]

Treatment

A. Medical Therapy

1. Vasodilators—Vasodilators are useful in acute mitral regurgitation to decrease aortic pressure and impedance, favoring forward over regurgitant flow during systole. This decreases left ventricular size and left ventricular and atrial pressures, improves forward cardiac output, and decreases the amount of regurgitation. Studies of acute regurgitation with vasodilators, such as nicardapine and nitroprusside, have demonstrated effectiveness for managing acute mitral regurgitation. Studies on the pharmacologic treatment of patients with chronic mitral regurgitation are scant, and the available data are not encouraging. Because afterload is not increased in patients with well-compensated chronic mitral regurgitation, lowering it further may not improve forward flow and would more likely reduce it. Many patients experience vasodilator side effects, and if forward cardiac output is not improved, the patient's overall hemodynamic status is worsened. Thus, there is no evidence to support vasodilator therapy for asymptomatic patients with chronic mitral regurgitation. However, patients with systemic hypertension and those with functional mitral regurgitation due to systolic dysfunction can be treated with vasodilators.

2. Antibiotic prophylaxis—Only valve disease patients with prosthetic heart valves or prior infective endocarditis now require antibiotics to prevent the development of bacterial endocarditis with dental procedures that involve trauma to gingival tissue, the periapical region of the tooth, or oral mucosa. Patients in whom rheumatic heart disease is the likely cause of mitral regurgitation should have rheumatic fever antibiotic prophylaxis.

B. Valve Repair or Replacement

Surgery to repair or replace the mitral valve is the primary intervention for symptomatic mitral regurgitation. Patients with acute, severe, or decompensated chronic severe mitral regurgitation will need urgent surgical therapy—if it is appropriate to their general medical condition. Such patients can usually be stabilized with intravenous vasodilators, such as nicardipine or nitroprusside, and other therapies for heart failure, such as diuretics. If there is no response to pharmacologic therapy, intra-aortic balloon pump insertion can be lifesaving. It will selectively decrease afterload in systole with balloon deflation and augment coronary artery flow in diastole with balloon inflation. There are few data on left ventricular assist devices or extracorporeal membrane oxygenation in such patients, but they may be helpful as a bridge to valve repair or replacement if pharmacologic therapy and a balloon pump are ineffective. Most patients will stabilize on this therapy, allowing for an appropriate evaluation (eg, coronary angiography) and thereby maximizing the benefits of any valve surgery.

Patients with primary chronic mitral regurgitation will eventually need surgery as this is usually a progressive disease. The issue is the appropriate timing of surgery. If the physician waits until marked symptoms develop because of left-heart failure with depressed left ventricular systolic function and severe pulmonary hypertension, not much symptomatic improvement is achieved after surgery, and left ventricular function often remains depressed. On the other hand, if surgery is performed earlier, the patient may become relatively asymptomatic, with normal left ventricular function. Considerable effort has been directed at determining prognostic indicators for avoiding a poor response to surgical therapy. Prospective studies have shown that the following are all markers of a poor prognosis following surgery: an ejection fraction of 60% or less, an end-systolic volume index of 50 mL/m^2 or more, an end-systolic dimension on echocardiography of 40 mm or more, significant pulmonary hypertension (PASP > 50 mm Hg or peak exercise PASP > 60 mm Hg), and atrial fibrillation. Although it seems logical that surgery should therefore be performed before these indicators are obtained in a patient, even one who is asymptomatic, this decision analysis has never been tested in clinical trials (Table 20–4).

In patients with aortic and mitral regurgitation, if the mitral valve is not obviously diseased and the mitral regurgitation is mild to moderate (1–2+), replacing the aortic valve will often diminish left ventricular size enough to reduce or eliminate the mitral regurgitation. Sometimes a mitral annular ring will be required to reduce mitral annular size. In cases where the mitral valve leaflets and chordae are diseased or the regurgitation is moderate to severe, valve repair or replacement will be necessary—at the cost of a higher likelihood of operative mortality or postoperative morbidity.

Table 20–4. General Indications for Considering Mitral Valve Surgery in Patients with Chronic Severe Primary Mitral Regurgitation

Symptoms such as dyspnea
Left ventricular ejection fraction ≤ 60%
Left ventricular end-systolic dimension ≥ 40 mm
Left ventricular end-systolic volume index ≥ 50 mL/m^2
Atrial fibrillation
Pulmonary artery systolic pressure > 50 mm Hg at rest or > 60 mm Hg with exercise

Severe aortic stenosis is often accompanied by mild-to-moderate mitral regurgitation. In this situation, the reduction in left ventricular pressure produced by aortic valve replacement usually reduces the mitral regurgitation, and additional mitral surgery can often be avoided.

The pulmonary hypertension that can accompany mitral regurgitation may lead to tricuspid and pulmonic regurgitation. The latter usually resolves when the pulmonary pressure is reduced by mitral valve surgery, and pulmonary valve replacement is rarely necessary. Tricuspid regurgitation, if mild-to-moderate and associated with moderately severe pulmonary hypertension, will usually resolve after successful mitral surgery. If the tricuspid regurgitation is moderate to severe, but the leaflets are not diseased, a tricuspid ring may be effective; if tricuspid valve disease is present, repair or replacement will be necessary. A clinical indicator for the need for tricuspid valve repair or replacement is a mean right atrial pressure of more than 15 mm Hg or the presence of severe tricuspid regurgitation. With the availability of catheter delivered valve clipping devices concomitant tricuspid valve surgery is being done less often (see later).

The onset of heart failure symptoms should prompt consideration of surgical treatment. Symptoms such as dyspnea, fatigue, and edema develop in some patients before the echocardiographic signs of severe mitral regurgitation develop. Other factors to be considered when deciding when to perform surgery are the type of operation—valve repair or replacement—and the type of prosthetic valve, should one be needed. It is now possible in many patients with mitral regurgitation to repair rather than replace the mitral valve. Patients with mitral valve prolapse, ruptured chordae tendineae, or marked annular dilatation are especially likely to respond to reparative surgery, whereas patients with markedly deformed valves and fused chordae from rheumatic heart disease or patients with infective endocarditis are less likely to be helped by mitral valve repair and often require valve replacement. Repair is preferable, especially for the patient with normal sinus rhythm because there is no need for long-term anticoagulation therapy following surgery. In addition, mitral valve repair is generally associated with better preservation of left ventricular systolic function following surgery and is therefore highly advantageous for patients with a low left ventricular ejection fraction and a repairable mitral valve. Thus, if it is highly likely that mitral valve repair can be done successfully, there is less reluctance about operating in asymptomatic patients that otherwise meet criteria for surgery.

If valve replacement is necessary, ventricular function can be preserved by leaving the chordae intact; chordal tethering of the papillary muscles is presumed to improve left ventricular performance. With valve replacement, the choice between a mechanical and a bioprosthetic valve may influence the timing of surgery.

In general, mechanical prosthetic valves have better long-term durability, but they require oral anticoagulant therapy. Bioprosthetic valves can be chosen when valve longevity is not an issue or when patients want to try to avoid anticoagulation therapy. These valves will need to be replaced in approximately 10–15 years, as a result of deterioration. However, now that percutaneous transcatheter bioprosthetic valves can be placed within a degenerated bioprosthesis, many surgeons are selecting bioprostheses for almost all mitral valve replacements. At present, there are no acceptable transcatheter valves for initial valve replacement, but several are in development. The incidence of systemic emboli is higher with mitral than with aortic prosthetic valves. Without anticoagulation, there is a 1–3% per year chance of systemic emboli with a bioprosthetic valve in the mitral position, so aspirin therapy is recommended for patients with bioprosthetic valves. The use of warfarin for 3 months after bioprosthetic mitral valve replacement is sometimes done until the endothelium grows over the sewing ring, reducing the risk of thrombus development. Patients with other risks for thrombus formation, such as atrial fibrillation, should also receive warfarin.

Percutaneous approaches to mitral valve repair and replacement are developing rapidly. One currently available approach is to put a clip at the tip of the mitral leaflets, creating a double orifice valve like the surgical Alfieri technique. It is FDA approved in the United States for patients with primary mitral regurgitation who are not candidates for or are at too high a risk for surgery. Initial studies suggest that it may be useful for patients with severe functional mitral regurgitation out of proportion to the severity of left ventricular dilatation. Another technique currently in development is to deliver an annuloplasty ring percutaneously, reducing the annulus size.

Otto CM, Nishimura RA, Bonow RO, et al. 2020 ACC/AHA guideline for the management of patients with valvular heart disease; a report of the American College of Cardiology/American Heart Association Joint Committee on Clinical Practice Guidelines; developed in collaboration with and endorsed by the American Association for Thoracic Surgery, American Society of Echocardiography, Society for Cardiovascular Angiography and Interventions, Society of Cardiovascular Anesthesiologists , and Society of Thoracic Surgeons. *J Am Coll Cardiol.* 2021;77:e25–e196. [PMID: 33342586]

Vahanian A, Byersdorf F, Praz F, et al. 2021 ESC/EACTS guidelines for the management of valvular heart disease: developed by the Task Force for the management of valvular heart disease of the European Society of Cardiology (ESC) and the European Association for Cardio-Thoracic Surgery (EACTS). *Eur Heart J.* 2022;43:561–632. [PMID: 34453165]

Prognosis

Chronic primary mitral regurgitation is often slowly progressive with a survival curve that dips below the population average. The cause of the chronic secondary mitral regurgitation in individual patients influences the prognosis. In general, patients with coronary artery disease and dilated cardiomyopathy have a poor prognosis. Also, the onset of infective endocarditis can markedly alter prognosis. In addition, any sudden deterioration of mitral valve function that leads to acute worsening of the mitral regurgitation lessens the prognosis.

The prognosis in acute mitral regurgitation, when it is associated with acute pulmonary edema and severe symptoms, is guarded; it also depends on the cause. For example, patients with acute severe mitral regurgitation from acute myocardial infarction have a much worse prognosis than do otherwise healthy individuals who rupture a chorda. In general, most patients with acute mitral regurgitation require immediate valve repair or replacement, and their prognosis is not as good as that for patients with chronic mitral regurgitation.

21 Tricuspid & Pulmonic Valve Disease

Brian D. Hoit, MD

TRICUSPID VALVE DISEASE

ESSENTIALS OF DIAGNOSIS

Tricuspid regurgitation

- Prominent *v* wave in jugular venous pulse.
- Systolic murmur at left lower sternal border that increases with inspiration.
- Characteristic Doppler echocardiographic findings, including right ventricular (RV) volume overload (RV enlargement, paradoxical septal motion, and diastolic flattening of the interventricular septum), right atrial enlargement, and systolic turbulence in the right atrium.

Tricuspid stenosis

- Prominent *a* wave and reduced *y* descent in jugular venous pulse.
- Diastolic murmur at left lower sternal border that increases with inspiration.
- Characteristic Doppler echocardiographic findings, including a thickened and domed valve with restricted motion, right atrial enlargement, and increased diastolic velocity across the tricuspid valve.

General Considerations

Clinical interest in tricuspid valve disorders has increased because of several distinct but interrelated events in clinical cardiology. First, high-resolution, noninvasive imaging techniques have been developed and validated, allowing clinicians to easily assess the morphology and function of the tricuspid valve. Second, the frequency of tricuspid valve endocarditis has increased significantly, owing largely to an increasing population of injection drug users, patients with implanted cardiac devices or long-term central venous catheters, and, to a lesser extent, a growing number of immunocompromised patients. Third, several reparative percutaneous and surgical techniques with acceptable morbidity and mortality rates now exist. In addition, investigations in both animals and humans have demonstrated the influence of right-heart disease on cardiovascular performance vis-á-vis series and parallel interactions with the left ventricle.

Staging Valvular Heart Disease

Valvular heart disease (VHD) progresses through stages A to D. Stage A is defined by the possession of risk factors for the development of VHD; stage B is defined as progressive VHD (asymptomatic mild to moderate severity); stage C is defined as asymptomatic severe disease, and is subcategorized into those with (C1) and without (C2) ventricular compensation; and stage D is defined by severe, symptomatic VHD.

Pathophysiology & Etiology

The tricuspid valve has three leaflets that are unequal in size (anterior > septal > posterior). The papillary muscles are not as well defined as those of the left ventricle and are subject to considerable variation in both their size and leaflet support. Like the mitral valve, the leaflets, annulus, chordae, papillary muscles, and contiguous myocardium contribute individually to normal valve function and can be altered by pathophysiologic processes (Table 21–1).

A. Tricuspid Regurgitation

Tricuspid regurgitation most frequently occurs with a structurally normal tricuspid valve (functional tricuspid regurgitation), which is the result of a dilated right ventricle and tricuspid annulus and papillary muscle dysfunction.

Functional (or secondary) tricuspid regurgitation is usually observed in patients with disease of the left heart (eg, left ventricular [LV] dysfunction, mitral valve disease), pulmonary vascular and parenchymal disease, right ventricular (RV)

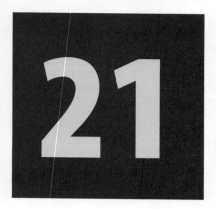

Table 21–1. Causes of Tricuspid Valve Disease

Tricuspid Regurgitation	Tricuspid Stenosis
Functional (structurally normal tricuspid valve)	Rheumatic
Rheumatic	Carcinoid heart disease
Infective endocarditis	Tumors
Congenital (eg, tricuspid valve prolapse, Ebstein anomaly)	Congenital (eg, Ebstein anomaly)
Carcinoid heart disease	Systemic lupus erythematosus
Systemic lupus erythematosus	Whipple disease
Catheter-induced	Fabry disease
Trauma	Infective endocarditis
Tumors	Endomyocardial fibrosis
Orthotopic heart transplantation	Endocardial fibroelastosis
Endomyocardial fibrosis	Methysergide therapy
Antiphospholipid syndrome	Antiphospholipid syndrome

infarction, arrhythmogenic RV dysplasia, and congenital heart disease. Underlying mechanisms include tricuspid annular dilatation, leaflet tethering, and RV remodeling. A recently recognized etiology, atrial functional tricuspid regurgitation, is characterized by atrial fibrillation, annular dilatation, and atrial remodeling in the absence of coexisting pulmonary hypertension and left-heart disease.

By contrast, **organic (or primary) tricuspid regurgitation** occurs when the intrinsic structure of the valve is anatomically abnormal.

Rheumatic tricuspid regurgitation almost always coexists with mitral valve involvement and is aggravated by associated pulmonary hypertension. Although two-thirds of patients with rheumatic mitral valve disease have pathologic evidence of tricuspid valve involvement, clinically significant tricuspid disease, which generally affects young and middle-aged women, is much less common. Rheumatic tricuspid involvement is usually mild and generally is manifested clinically as pure regurgitation or mixed regurgitation and stenosis, caused by the fibrosis of the valve leaflets and chordae tendineae. Contracture of the leaflets and commissural fusion, produce regurgitation and stenosis, respectively.

Tricuspid valve endocarditis occurs primarily in injection drug users and patients with chronic intravascular hardware, left-to-right shunts, burns, and immunocompromised states. Infective endocarditis is more common in injecting drug users who are human immunodeficiency virus (HIV) positive than in those who are HIV negative. Infective endocarditis is typically caused by virulent pathogens that infect structurally normal valves. *Staphylococcus aureus* is the most common organism; the next most common pathogens are streptococci and enterococci. *Pseudomonas* and *Candida* species also predominate, and polymicrobial infections are not uncommon. Geographic location should also be considered when attempting to identify the responsible pathogens. Fungal endocarditis should be considered when vegetations are large; they occasionally cause obstruction. Abscesses may involve the annulus and septum, and chordal rupture or valve perforations may cause tricuspid regurgitation.

Carcinoid tumors are a rare cause of both tricuspid and pulmonic valve disease. Cardiac involvement is about 50% by the time the carcinoid syndrome becomes clinically apparent. The vasoactive substances (principally serotonin) produced by these tumors are believed to be causal, and patients with carcinoid valvular disease have higher serum levels of serotonin and increased urinary excretion of its metabolite, 5-hydroxyindoleacetic acid (5-HIAA), than those without cardiac disease. Left-sided valve involvement is unusual due to the inactivation of these vasoactive molecules by monoamine oxidase in the lungs, but can be seen in patients with right-to-left shunts or bronchial tumors. The valve exhibits pathognomonic plaque-like deposits of fibrous tissue (which may also deposit on the endocardium); leaflet distortion leads to regurgitation, stenosis, or both. Tricuspid regurgitation is the most common lesion and is detected by echocardiography in virtually all patients with carcinoid tricuspid valve disease. Cardiac involvement is progressive and causes significant morbidity and mortality in such patients, but early detection and surgical management may prolong survival. Long-term survival has been reported after tricuspid valve replacement, but carcinoid plaques may deposit on the bioprosthetic leaflets. Somatostatin analogues used to treat symptoms of the carcinoid syndrome offer no survival benefit.

Tricuspid valve prolapse, owing to myxomatous degeneration, is seen almost exclusively in patients with mitral valve prolapse and occurs in as many as 50% of cases. Isolated involvement has been confirmed, however, by both echocardiography and necropsy. Anterior leaflet prolapse is most common, followed by septal and posterior leaflet prolapse. The associated tricuspid regurgitation is usually mild. Although tricuspid valve prolapse may be a marker of generalized connective tissue disease and a poor prognostic indicator in patients with mitral valve prolapse, its clinical significance remains undefined. Like mitral valve prolapse, the precise incidence of tricuspid valve prolapse is difficult to determine because of inconsistent clinical, echocardiographic, and angiographic definitions.

Tricuspid regurgitation is a frequent component of **Ebstein anomaly** of the tricuspid valve because of the apical displacement of septal and posterior tricuspid leaflets. This results in "atrialization" of a variable portion of the right ventricle and a range of abnormalities involving the anterior leaflet and atrial septum. The downward displacement of the tricuspid valve frequently causes a tricuspid regurgitant murmur (heard best in the apical area). This uncommon congenital abnormality is associated with right-to-left intra-atrial shunting, RV dysfunction, supraventricular arrhythmias, and sudden death.

Tricuspid regurgitation of at least moderate severity may complicate as many as 25% of cases of **systemic lupus erythematosus**; significant tricuspid regurgitation is usually due to the pulmonary hypertension produced by lupus pulmonary disease. Libman-Sacks endocarditis that involves the tricuspid valve is far less common. However, Libman-Sacks endocarditis has been associated with antiphospholipid antibodies, which has been shown to cause valvular thickening, isolated tricuspid involvement, and the development of nonbacterial vegetations. The cause of the valve disease is poorly understood, but intravalvular capillary thrombosis is believed to be a factor. Most patients present with combined tricuspid regurgitation and stenosis, and the regurgitation is typically moderate or severe. Pulmonary hypertension is usually present and contributes to the valvular dysfunction.

Although **catheter-induced** tricuspid regurgitation occurs in approximately 50% of cases with catheters across the valve, the regurgitation is quantitatively small, clinically unimportant, and usually disappears when the catheter is removed. In contrast, clinically significant TR may result from pacing wires and internal defibrillators. A clear association between implantable device lead position relative to the tricuspid valve leaflets and regurgitation due to leaflet adherence and impingement-induced malcoaptation has been demonstrated by three-dimensional echocardiography.

Tricuspid regurgitation can occur as a late complication of successful **mitral valve replacement** (MVR). In one series, Doppler-detected moderate-to-severe regurgitation occurred in two-thirds of patients at a mean of more than 11 years following MVR; over one-third of these patients had clinically evident tricuspid regurgitation. Other causes include blunt and penetrating trauma (rupture of papillary muscles, chordal disruption or detachment, leaflet rupture, complete valve destruction), primary or secondary cardiac tumors, right ventricular biopsy, and endomyocardial fibrosis.

B. Tricuspid Stenosis

Tricuspid stenosis is an uncommon lesion that is usually rheumatic in origin and almost exclusively accompanies mitral stenosis. Isolated rheumatic tricuspid stenosis is rare, and subvalvular disease is usually less severe in tricuspid than in mitral stenosis. Isolated carcinoid tricuspid stenosis is also rare; tricuspid regurgitation is more frequent and often occurs with pulmonic stenosis. Right atrial (RA) myxomas and obstructing metastatic tumors may produce hemodynamic changes that are indistinguishable from tricuspid stenosis. Tricuspid stenosis may be congenital and is infrequently predominant in Ebstein anomaly. Other unusual causes include systemic lupus erythematosus, Whipple disease, Fabry disease, antiphospholipid syndrome, infective endocarditis, endocardial fibroelastosis, and as a sequela to methysergide therapy. It should be noted that prosthetic tricuspid valves, like all prosthetic valves, are inherently stenotic.

Addetia K, Harb SC, Hahn RT, Kapadia S, Lang RM. Cardiac implantable electronic device lead-induced tricuspid regurgitation. *J Am Coll Cardiol Img.* 2019;12:622–636. [PMID: 30947905]

Baron T, Bergsten J, Albage A, et al. Cardiac imaging in carcinoid heart disease. *JACC Cardiovasc Imaging.* 2021;14:2240–2253. [PMID: 33865761]

Florescu DR, Muraru D, Volpato V, et al. Atrial functional tricuspid regurgitation as a distinct pathophysiological clinical entity: No idiopathic tricuspid regurgitation anymore. *J Clin Med.* 2022;11:382. [PMID: 33054074]

Clinical Findings

A. Symptoms & Signs

Tricuspid valve disease can be difficult to recognize clinically. The symptoms may be overshadowed by associated illness, such as systemic lupus erythematosus, infective endocarditis, trauma, or neoplasia. The dominant presenting features may be symptoms that are usually not considered cardiac in origin: abdominal discomfort, ascites, jaundice, wasting, and inanition. In addition, patients with associated cardiovascular disease may have nonspecific symptoms (exertional dyspnea and fatigue in mitral stenosis) that obfuscate the diagnosis and deflect the suspicion of tricuspid valve disease. In patients with mitral stenosis, for example, tricuspid valve disease protects the pulmonary circulation and exertional dyspnea, pulmonary edema, and hemoptysis are less commonly reported, although a history of excessive fatigue may be elicited. Most often, however, the history is insufficient to diagnose tricuspid valve disease, and only a careful physical examination provides the necessary clues.

B. Physical Examination

1. Jugular venous pulse—Because the internal jugular veins lack effective valves, they should be inspected for an estimate of RA pressure (Figure 21–1 shows a normal jugular venous pulse). There are three waves (*a, c,* and *v*) and two descents, *x* and *y* (which correspond to the *a* and *v* waves, respectively). The *a* wave and the initial descent are produced by atrial contraction and relaxation, respectively. The *x* descent is interrupted by a *c* wave that is caused by isovolumetric contraction of the right ventricle and resultant bowing of the tricuspid valve toward the right atrium. The continuation of the *x* descent (sometimes called *x′*) is caused by the descent of the arteriovenous (AV) ring toward the apex during RV ejection. The right atrium fills and, because the tricuspid valve is closed, RA pressure rises, causing the *v* wave. The rapid fall in volume and pressure when the valve opens produces the *y* descent. Except for a small but variable delay, the jugular venous pulse and RA pressure contours are similar.

When inspecting the jugular venous pulse, the examiner should pay careful attention to the magnitude of the central

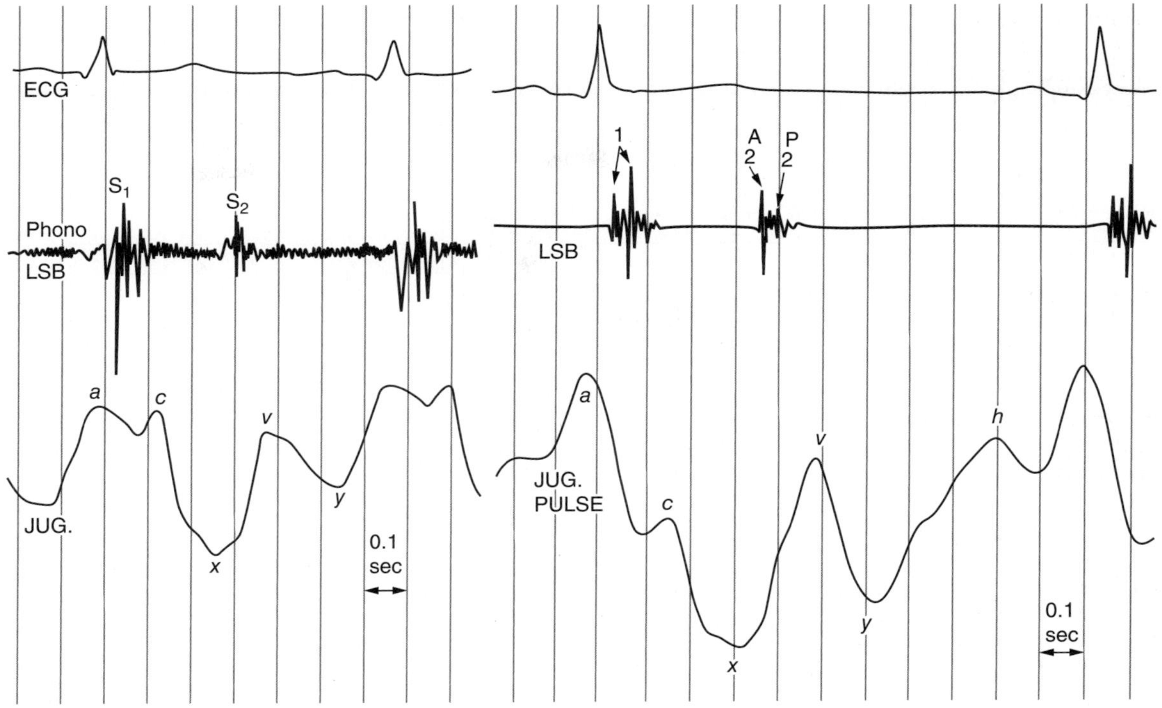

▲ **Figure 21–1.** Electrocardiogram, phonocardiogram, and normal jugular venous pulse tracings at fast (**A**) and slow (**B**) heart rates. The *a* wave is the dominant reflection. At slow heart rates, an *h* wave signifying the end of right ventricular filling can be seen. LSB, left sternal border. (Reproduced, with permission, from Tavel ME. *Clinical Phonocardiograpy and External Pulse Recording.* Yearbook Medical Publishers, 1978.)

venous (mean RA) pressure, the dominant wave (*a* or *v*), and changes in pulse contour with respiration. Tricuspid valve disease is typically associated with increased central venous pressure.

A. Tricuspid regurgitation—The *x* descent of the jugular venous pulse is interrupted by an early *v* wave (*c-v* wave) with a rapid *y* descent. These findings are characteristically augmented during inspiration. The neck veins are distended, and the earlobes may pulsate. Because venous distention may obscure the jugular pulse contour, it is important to elevate the patient's head. RV volume overload leads to prominent pulsations over the left lower sternal border.

B. Tricuspid stenosis—In tricuspid **stenosis** (Figure 21–2), inspection of the jugular veins reveals a dominant *a* wave (assuming sinus rhythm), which increases with inspiration, and a slow and shallow *y* descent due to resistance to early RV diastolic filling.

2. Cardiac auscultation

A. Tricuspid regurgitation—Tricuspid regurgitation is classically associated with a holosystolic murmur that is best heard at the right or left midsternal border, but when the right ventricle is markedly dilated, the location of the murmur may move toward the left and suggest mitral regurgitation. The auscultatory hallmark of tricuspid regurgitation is an inspiratory augmentation from increased systemic venous return and tricuspid valve flow. Under such circumstances as severe tricuspid regurgitation, markedly increased RA pressures, and RV systolic failure, the murmur may not increase with inspiration. Although usually described as holosystolic, the timing of the murmur may be early, mid, or late systolic. The murmur may be decrescendo when tricuspid regurgitation is severe and acute, and its character reflects the presence of a giant *c-v* wave; there may be a mid-diastolic flow rumble that resembles tricuspid stenosis. The murmur of tricuspid regurgitation is usually not accompanied by a thrill, and there is little radiation of the murmur. When the tricuspid valve is wide open in systole, there may be no murmur. An S_3, which can vary in intensity and with inspiration, is often associated with an extremely dilated right ventricle. An S_4 may also be heard if there is significant RV hypertrophy.

B. Tricuspid stenosis—The tricuspid opening snap is difficult to distinguish from the mitral opening snap, and

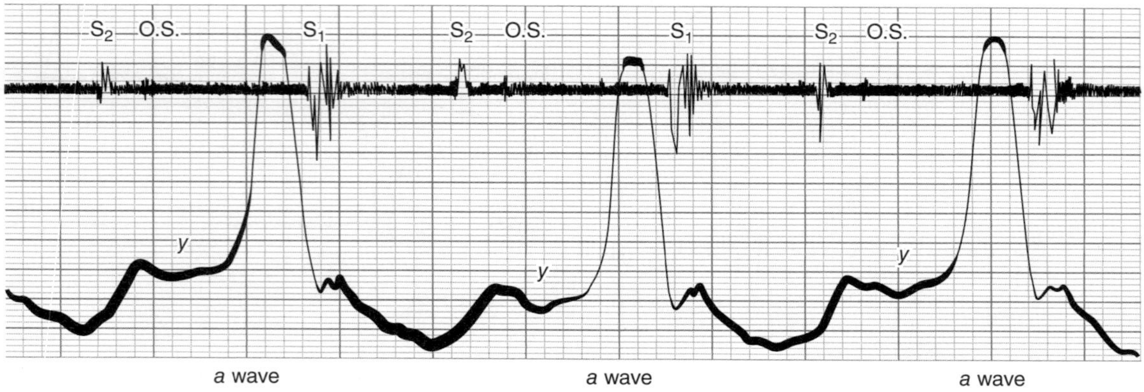

▲ **Figure 21–2.** Jugular venous pulse tracing and phonocardiogram from a patient with rheumatic tricuspid stenosis. Note the striking *a* waves and the shallow *y* descents. A loud S_1 and opening snap (O.S.) are evident on the accompanying phonocardiogram.

auscultatory findings may be difficult to distinguish from existing mitral stenosis. Unlike mitral stenosis, however, the diastolic rumble of tricuspid stenosis has a higher pitch, increases with inspiration, is usually loudest at the lower left sternal border, and follows the opening snap of mitral stenosis. The tricuspid stenosis murmur is often scratchy, ends before the first heart sound, and has no presystolic crescendo in patients with normal sinus rhythm. A diastolic murmur from relative tricuspid stenosis may be heard with large atrial septal defects and severe tricuspid regurgitation. In patients with normal sinus rhythm, a presystolic hepatic pulsation may be felt; this is due to reflux from atrial contraction against the stenotic valve. Both tricuspid stenosis and regurgitation can, if chronic, lead to ascites, peripheral edema, jaundice, wasting, and muscle loss. Tricuspid valve disease, which is often diagnosed or suspected at the bedside, can almost always be confirmed with echocardiography.

C. Diagnostic Studies

The diagnostic evaluation of suspected tricuspid valve disease includes electrocardiography (ECG), plain chest film, echocardiography, and cardiac catheterization. Experience with cine magnetic resonance imaging (MRI) and computed tomography (CT) suggests that, except in certain instances (such as the evaluation of carcinoid heart disease), these techniques offer no clear advantage over echocardiography.

1. Electrocardiography—P waves characteristic of RA enlargement with no evidence of RV hypertrophy suggest isolated tricuspid stenosis. Most often, however, the rhythm is atrial fibrillation. When pulmonary hypertension is the cause of tricuspid regurgitation, the ECG may show evidence of RV hypertrophy with right axis deviation and tall R waves in V_1 to V_2 and RA enlargement (Figure 21–3A). Atrial fibrillation is also common, and incomplete right bundle branch block and Q waves in V_1 are occasionally seen. Preexcitation frequently accompanies Ebstein anomaly (Figure 21–3B).

2. Chest radiography—In tricuspid stenosis, the chest film is characterized by cardiomegaly, with a prominent right-heart border caused by RA enlargement, and a dilated superior vena cava and azygos vein. Pulmonary vascular markings may be notably absent. The chest film in tricuspid regurgitation shows cardiomegaly from RA and RV enlargement; pleural effusions and elevated diaphragms from ascites may be seen. In general, a dilated heart in the absence of pulmonary congestion or pulmonary hypertension should suggest either tricuspid valve disease or pericardial effusion. Massive RA enlargement suggests Ebstein anomaly.

3. Echocardiography—Echocardiography is the most useful noninvasive diagnostic test for evaluating tricuspid valve disease. Two-dimensional and Doppler echocardiographic examinations can identify associated disease of the left ventricle and other cardiac valves (eg, mitral stenosis), show the anatomic sequelae of chronic tricuspid valve disease (eg, dilated right heart chambers), and detect structural abnormalities of the tricuspid valve (eg, a thickened tricuspid valve with decreased mobility, compression of the tricuspid annulus, or involvement by tumor or prolapsing or displaced leaflets and vegetations; Figure 21–4). Three-dimensional echocardiography can be helpful in defining the anatomy of the tricuspid valve.

A. TRICUSPID REGURGITATION—In tricuspid regurgitation, the echocardiographic findings usually show RV volume overload with a dilated right ventricle, paradoxical septal motion, and diastolic flattening of the interventricular septum. Color-flow Doppler echocardiography can visualize the tricuspid regurgitant jet. The tricuspid valve diastolic gradient can be quantified using continuous wave Doppler,

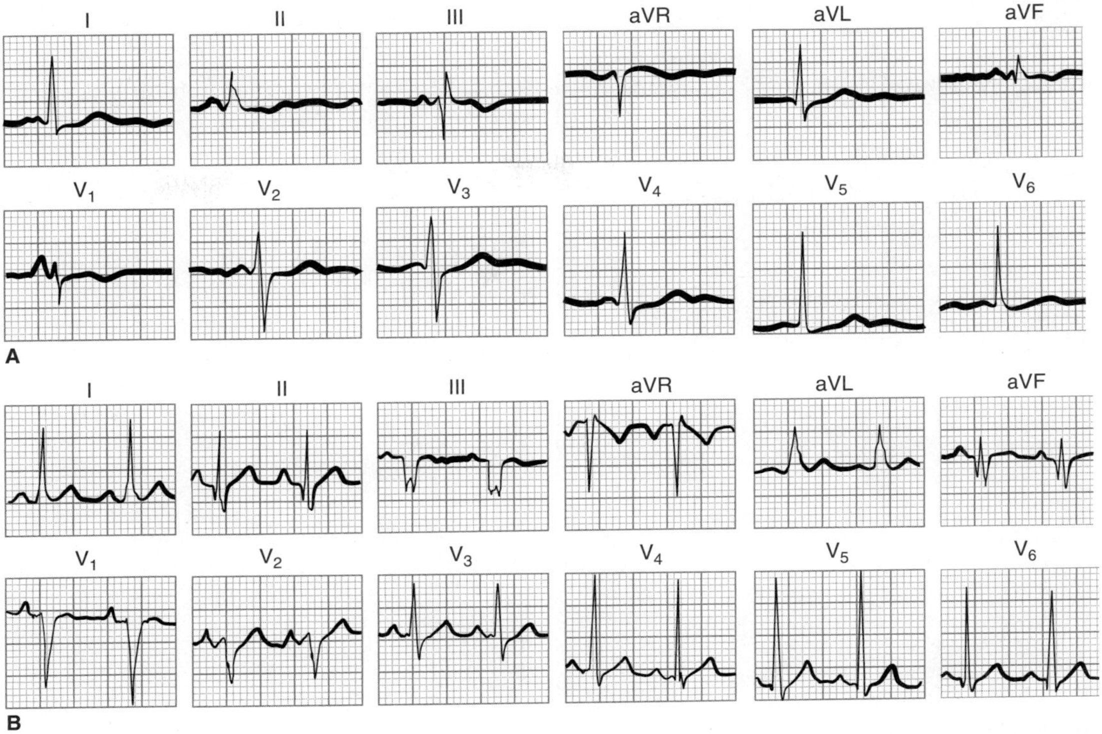

▲ **Figure 21–3.** Electrocardiograms from patients with tricuspid valve disease. **A:** Mitral stenosis and isolated tricuspid stenosis. The tall initial P-wave forces in lead V_1 indicate right atrial enlargement. There is no electrocardiographic evidence of right ventricular hypertrophy. **B:** Patient with Ebstein anomaly and preexcitation. Delta waves create a pseudoinfarct pattern in leads II, III and aVF. P-wave amplitude in leads II and V_2 is consistent with right atrial enlargement. (A: Reproduced with permission from Chou TE. *Electrocardiography in Clinical Practice*, 3rd ed. Philadelphia: WB Saunders; 1991.)

and pulmonary arterial pressure can be estimated from the pulmonary artery acceleration time or the peak velocity of the tricuspid regurgitant jet. Two-dimensional echocardiography distinguishes between primary disease of the left heart and RV disease, both of which cause functional tricuspid regurgitation, and organic disease of the tricuspid valve. Contrast found in the inferior vena cava and hepatic veins following injection of agitated saline into an arm vein implies significant tricuspid regurgitation. On the other hand, a tricuspid valve annulus less than 3.4 cm in diameter during diastole virtually excludes significant tricuspid regurgitation. The temporal and spatial distribution of systolic turbulence in the right atrium, using color-flow mapping, can be a means of estimating the severity of the regurgitation. Systolic reversal of the Doppler signal in the hepatic veins indicates significant tricuspid regurgitation. Doppler techniques that quantitatively estimate effective regurgitant orifice, regurgitant volume, and regurgitant fraction have been developed and validated but are not widely used. It should be recognized that Doppler-detected tricuspid regurgitation occurs commonly in normal individuals. In such cases, the Doppler signal tends not to be holosystolic, and systolic turbulence occupies only a small area of the right atrium.

B. Tricuspid stenosis—As shown in Figure 21–5, the stenotic tricuspid valve is thickened and domed and has restricted motion. The echocardiographic appearance alone may be misleading because many patients with two-dimensional echocardiographic findings that suggest tricuspid stenosis have normal tricuspid valve diastolic pressure gradients. Although the right atrium is usually dilated, the right ventricle is not enlarged in isolated tricuspid stenosis. The severity of the stenosis is determined with continuous wave Doppler. Accurate peak instantaneous and mean gradients across the stenotic tricuspid valve are readily calculated using the modified **Bernoulli equation,** which relates a pressure drop (dP) to the velocity (V) across a stenosis ($dP = 4V^2$). The pressure half-time method for calculating valve orifice area, used successfully for the mitral valve, has not been well validated for the tricuspid valve, but values greater than 190 ms are considered consistent with severe tricuspid stenosis. Also, a tricuspid valve area less than 1.0 cm^2 indicates severe tricuspid stenosis.

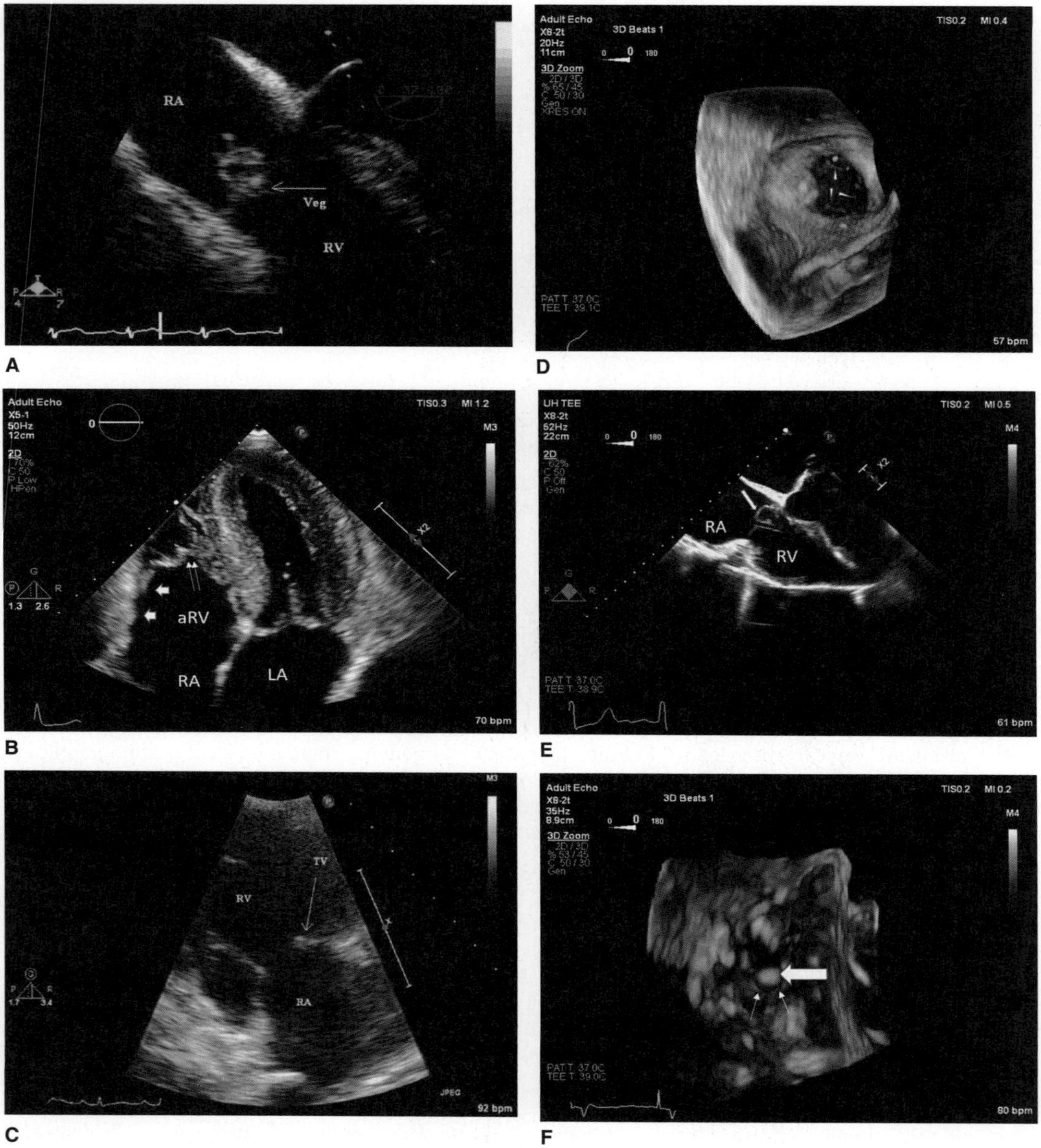

▲ **Figure 21–4.** Two- and three-dimensional echocardiograms illustrating abnormalities of the tricuspid valve leaflets. **A:** Infective endocarditis. RA, right atrium; RV, right ventricle; Veg, tricuspid valve vegetation. **B:** Ebstein anomaly. Note the apical displacement of the septal leaflet (double arrows) and the tricuspid valve orifice, resulting in atrialization of the RV (aRV). Note the tethering of the elongated anterior tricuspid leaflet (arrowheads). LV, left ventricle; RA, right atrium. **C:** Carcinoid syndrome. Note the thickened and rigid tricuspid leaflets (*arrows*). **D:** Three-dimensional echocardiogram of the tricuspid valve in carcinoid. Leaflets are thickened, fixed, and immobile resulting in severe tricuspid regurgitation. **E:** Tricuspid valve prolapse. As is usually the case, there is mitral valve prolapse. The anterior leaflet is most commonly involved; in this case it is the septal leaflet (arrow). **F:** Three-dimensional echocardiogram from the RV perspective. There is impingement of the septal leaflet (small arrows) by the pacing lead (large arrow).

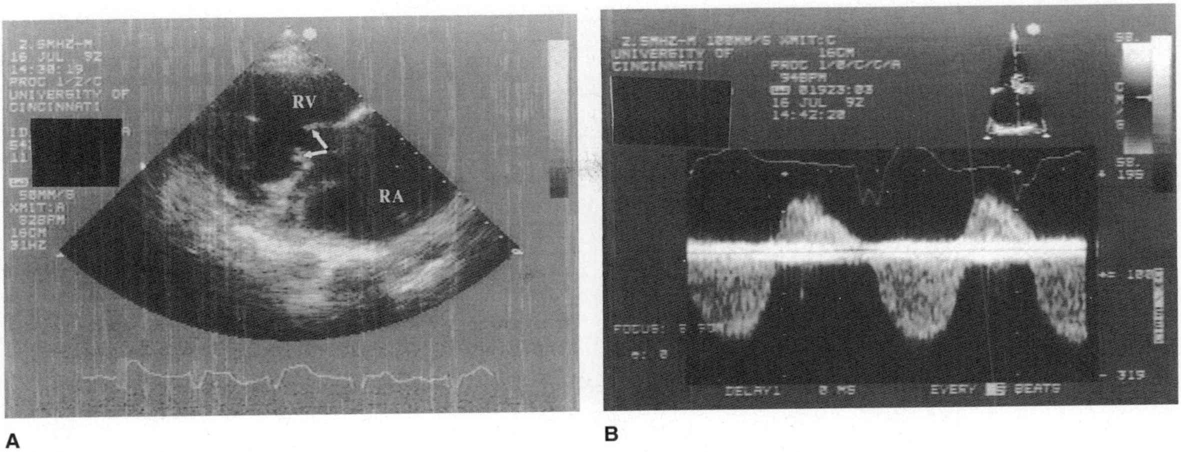

▲ **Figure 21–5. A:** Two-dimensional echocardiogram from a patient with rheumatic tricuspid valve disease, showing a thickened and domed tricuspid valve (*arrows*). The right atrium (RA) is considerably dilated, and the right ventricle (RV) is enlarged. **B:** Continuous wave Doppler study from the same patient confirms tricuspid stenosis and regurgitation. The high-velocity signal above the baseline during diastole represents right ventricular inflow; the signal below the baseline during systole represents tricuspid regurgitation.

4. Cardiac catheterization

A. Tricuspid regurgitation—Opacification of the right atrium following injection of radiographic contrast into the right ventricle detects and estimates the severity of the regurgitation. Although right ventriculography requires a catheter across the tricuspid valve, there is no significant contrast leak into the right atrium under normal circumstances. Right atrial and ventricular pressures are elevated, and the RA pressure may become "ventricularized" as a result of a large *c-v* wave and an absent *x* descent (Figure 21–6A). **Kussmaul sign** (increased RA pressure with inspiration or the absence of a normal fall in RA pressure) may be seen when the regurgitation is severe.

B. Tricuspid stenosis—In tricuspid stenosis, the mean RA pressure is increased; characteristically, the *a* wave is prominent and the *y* descent is slow. The hallmark of tricuspid stenosis is a diastolic gradient between the right atrium and right ventricle that increases with inspiration (Figure 21–6B). The gradients are frequently small; however, their detection is enhanced by recording RA and RV pressures simultaneously with two optimally damped catheters and equally sensitive transducers. Because of the low gradient, calculation of the valve area is unreliable. Rapid volume infusion or an injection of atropine to increase the heart rate can increase the diastolic gradient and facilitate the diagnosis.

Treatment

A. Medical

Tricuspid regurgitation is usually well tolerated in the absence of pulmonary hypertension but may require chronic diuretic therapy. When pulmonary arterial pressures increase, cardiac output falls, leading to symptoms of right-heart failure (edema, fatigue, dyspnea). Restriction of sodium and the use of potent loop diuretics to decrease RA pressure are indicated. Medical therapy is also aimed at the cause of pulmonary hypertension. Treatment of associated systemic diseases is a critically important aspect of the therapeutic paradigm; it is, however, beyond the scope of this discussion. Severe symptomatic tricuspid stenosis is usually treated surgically.

B. Surgical

Surgery on the tricuspid valve may involve repair, reconstruction, excision, or replacement with a prosthetic valve. The decision to operate on the stenotic tricuspid valve is a straightforward one; the decision to operate on a regurgitant valve is more challenging. The surgeon must determine whether the regurgitation is functional or organic (ie, associated with a structurally normal or abnormal tricuspid valve), and if it is functional, the response of the pulmonary arterial pressure to the primary procedure should be anticipated. For example, repair may be unnecessary for functional tricuspid regurgitation if there is a high likelihood of a postoperative fall in pulmonary arterial pressure. In addition, repair of the functionally regurgitant tricuspid valve in patients with severe right ventricular dysfunction is unlikely to improve their status. However, the response of tricuspid regurgitation to reduced pulmonary artery pressure can be difficult to predict, and, as mentioned previously, significant tricuspid regurgitation often complicates successful MVR despite reduced pulmonary artery pressures. Given the high morbidity and mortality associated with reoperation to correct

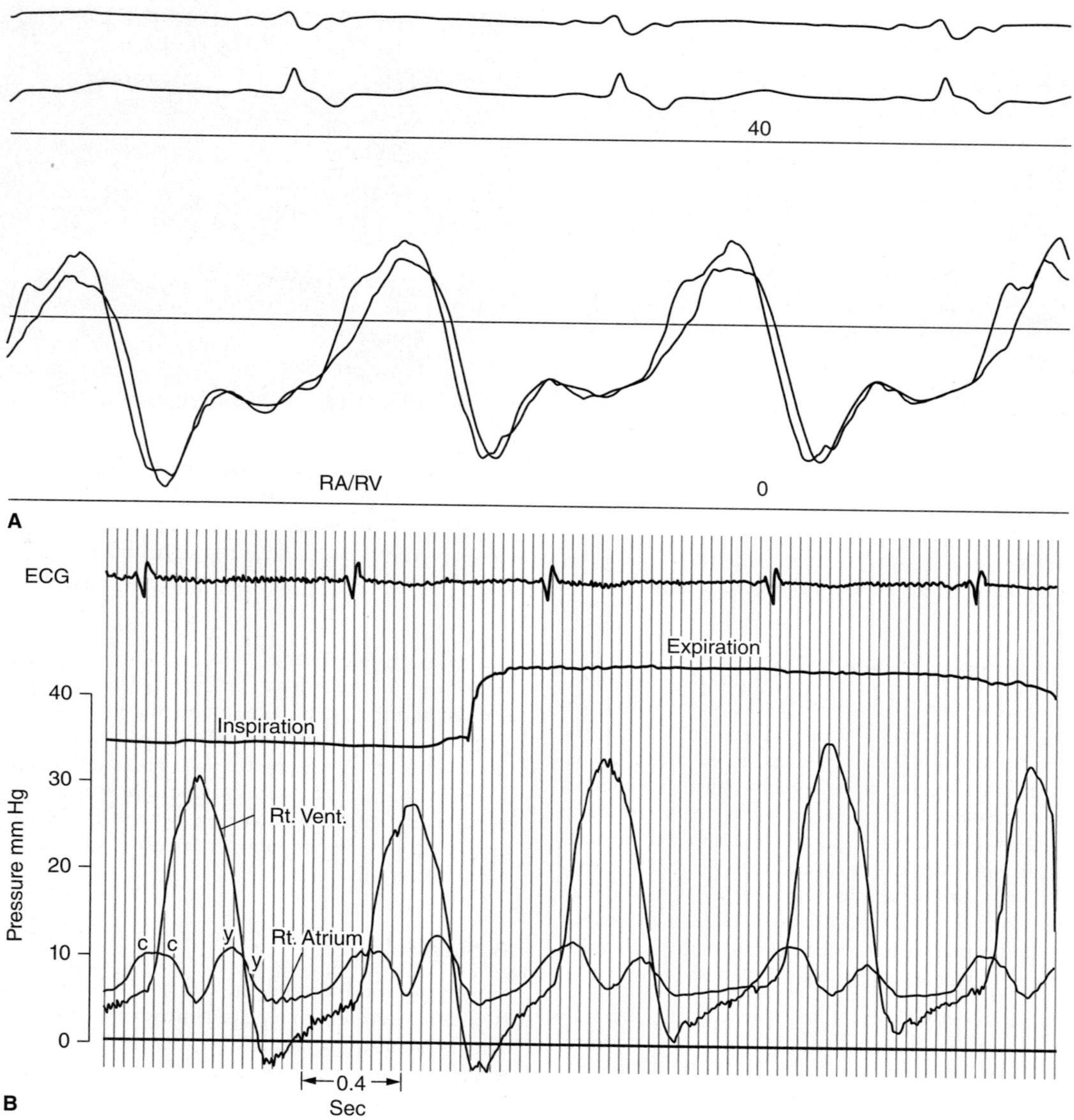

▲ **Figure 21–6.** Electrocardiogram and hemodynamic recordings from patients with tricuspid valve disease. **A:** Severe tricuspid regurgitation. There is "ventricularization" of the right atrial (RA) pressures, which are indistinguishable from the right ventricular (RV) pressures. **B:** Simultaneous and equally sensitive recordings of RA and RV pressures from a patient with rheumatic tricuspid stenosis. Note the RA-RV gradient throughout diastole, which increases with inspiration. (Reproduced, with permission, from Fowler N, et al. *Diagnosis of Heart Disease*. New York: Springer-Verlag; 1991.)

tricuspid regurgitation following MVR, the presence of any degree of preoperative tricuspid regurgitation, especially organic regurgitation, warrants consideration of concurrent tricuspid valve repair. Moreover, because "functional" tricuspid regurgitation may be due to unrecognized annular involvement and because annular dilation may be progressive, "prophylactic" tricuspid annuloplasty has been recommended when the annular diameter exceeds 21 mm/m^2. Interestingly, in patients with chronic pulmonary thromboembolic disease, pulmonary thromboendarterectomy dramatically reduces functional tricuspid regurgitation without a change in tricuspid annular diameter.

The decision whether to repair or replace the tricuspid valve with a prosthesis depends on the suitability of valve repair, the associated surgical procedures, and the underlying disease. Thrombosis is a more frequent problem with tricuspid than with mitral prostheses. Thus, primary valve repair, when possible, is the preferred procedure. Repair of the stenotic tricuspid valve involves identifying and separating the fan chordae (the chords that support the leaflets in the area of the commissure), leaflet decalcification, and chordal or papillary muscle division.

Annuloplasty procedures correct dilatation of the tricuspid valve annulus. The dilatation, which is not symmetric, typically involves the annulus around the anterior and posterior leaflets (posterior more than anterior). The procedure involves sizing and selectively plicating the anterior and posterior annuli. Although the routine use of an annuloplasty ring is considered superior to non-ring methods and is recommended by some groups, this position is not universally accepted.

When the tricuspid valve cannot be repaired and replacement is necessary, a bioprosthesis is often used because of the lower risk of thrombosis, although recent changes in valve design have significantly lowered the risk of thrombosis with mechanical prostheses. Bioprosthetic valves are also more prone to late failure than mechanical prostheses. If anticoagulation is necessary for other reasons, a St. Jude prosthesis is preferred by some surgeons—especially for younger patients. Also, there is a risk of complete heart block requiring permanent pacing with tricuspid valve replacement. Recent studies indicate that long-term outcomes (mortality, thrombosis, structural deterioration) for bioprosthetic and mechanical valves are similar.

The primary indications for surgery in patients with tricuspid valve endocarditis are uncontrollable infection, septic emboli, or refractory congestive heart failure. Because virulent organisms are the rule, they are not, per se, an indication for surgery. Total excision of the tricuspid valve is an attractive option in injection drug users, considering both recidivism and the threat of prosthetic valve endocarditis. As noted earlier, tricuspid regurgitation without pulmonary hypertension is well tolerated; however, 20% of these patients ultimately may require valve replacement for right-heart failure. Debridement and valve repair have been suggested as alternative procedures to valve excision.

Successful percutaneous balloon valvuloplasty has been reported for native valve tricuspid stenosis and stenotic bioprosthetic tricuspid valves, but experience is limited. There are no published studies to compare percutaneous balloon valvotomy with surgical valvuloplasty, and only limited long-term results have been published. In selected patients with failing bioprostheses, preliminary data suggest that percutaneous tricuspid valve-in-valve implantation is feasible and effective. Initial tricuspid valve replacement with percutaneously delivered stent-mounted bioprostheses is under development.

Percutaneous treatment of TR can be accomplished by edge-to-edge valve repair and vena cava valves; in addition, a number of annuloplasty systems are in clinical trials. Despite considerable evidence that more severe TR is associated with adverse outcomes, it is uncertain whether TR is a marker of increased risk if TR is causal, independent of mitral valve disease, pulmonary hypertension, arrhythmias or RV dysfunction. Randomized controlled trials of surgical and percutaneous techniques compared to optimal medical therapy are needed.

Asmarats L, Puri R, Latib A, Navia JL, Cabau JR. Transcatheter tricuspid valve interventions: landscape, challenges, and future directions. *J Am Coll Cardiol.* 2018;71:2935–2956. [PMID: 29929618]

Hamandi M, Smith RL, Ryan WH, et al. Outcomes of isolated tricuspid valve surgery have improved in the modern era. *Ann Thorac Surg.* 2019;108:11–15. [PMID: 30951698]

Otto CM, Nishimura RA, Bonow RO, et al. 2020 AHA/ACC guideline for the management of patients with valvular heart disease: A report of the American College of Cardiology/American Heart Association joint committee on clinical practice guidelines. *J Am Coll Cardiol.* 2021;77:e25–e197. [PMID: 33342586]

Prognosis

The natural history of tricuspid valve disease is a function of the associated valvular lesions and the underlying disease. Isolated tricuspid regurgitation is unusual, and its natural history is unknown.

Regardless of etiology, tricuspid regurgitation is associated with decreased survival, and mortality increases as severity of regurgitation increases. In general, the results of tricuspid valve surgery depend on the types of valve lesions, the corrective procedures, the degree and reversibility of LV and RV function, and the pulmonary vascular resistance. Residual tricuspid regurgitation usually occurs when the pulmonary vascular resistance remains elevated. Many patients have small-to-moderate tricuspid valve gradients after tricuspid valve replacement; like residual tricuspid valve leaks, these are usually not clinically important. Although most surgeons favor repair over replacement, the superiority of this approach is difficult to prove.

Raikhelkar J, Lin HM, Neckman D, Afonso A, Scurlock C. Isolated tricuspid valve surgery: predictors of adverse outcome and survival. *Heart Lung Circ.* 2013;22:211–220. [PMID: 23103071]

PULMONIC VALVE DISEASE

ESSENTIALS OF DIAGNOSIS

Pulmonic regurgitation

- Diastolic murmur at the left upper sternal border that increases with inspiration.
- Split S_2 with a loud P_2.
- Characteristic Doppler echocardiographic findings, including valvular abnormalities (depending on etiology), right ventricular enlargement, and diastolic turbulence in the right ventricular outflow tract.

Pulmonic stenosis

- Systolic murmur at the left second intercostal space preceded by a systolic click.
- Split S_2 with a soft P_2.
- Characteristic Doppler echocardiographic findings, including thickened and domed leaflets, and increased systolic velocities across the pulmonic valve.

General Considerations

The technologic advances made in the fields of noninvasive cardiac imaging, interventional cardiology, and cardiac surgery over the past few decades have had a noticeable effect on the diagnosis and management of pulmonic valve disease.

Pathophysiology & Etiology

The normal pulmonic valve is a semilunar valve with anterior, left, and right leaflets. The function and texture of the valve leaflets, as well as the size of the valve annulus, can be adversely affected in a variety of diseases.

A. Pulmonic Regurgitation

Trivial to mild pulmonic regurgitation occurs in almost everyone at any age, but more severe pulmonic regurgitation commonly occurs in the setting of pulmonary hypertension. The regurgitation is caused by dilatation of the pulmonic valve ring, and any cause of pulmonary hypertension can precipitate pulmonic regurgitation. **Idiopathic dilation** of the pulmonary trunk and **Marfan syndrome** also cause pulmonic regurgitation via a similar distortion of the valve ring. **Infective endocarditis** is unusual, but when present, often causes pulmonic regurgitation, with vegetations causing dysfunction of the leaflets themselves. Although the pulmonic valve is the least likely to be seeded in endocarditis, the rising number of injecting drug users, immunocompromised persons, and patients with subclinical pulmonic stenosis represent a growing population at risk. Pulmonic regurgitation can also occur as a consequence of surgical treatment for **tetralogy of Fallot** or balloon valvuloplasty of **congenital pulmonic stenosis**. The pulmonic regurgitation is generally mild and hemodynamically insignificant, but in rare cases, it can progress to RV dilation, necessitating pulmonic valve replacement. **Rheumatic heart disease** is an infrequent cause of pulmonic regurgitation, and it invariably occurs in the setting of multiple valve disease. Other rare causes of pulmonic regurgitation include chest trauma, carcinoid tumors, syphilis, and catheter-related valve dysfunction.

B. Pulmonic Stenosis

Pulmonic stenosis is a congenital disorder in more than 95% of cases. Congenital pulmonic stenosis is usually caused by a valvular lesion, although subvalvular (infundibular hypertrophy) and supravalvular (rare intracardiac tumors, congenital rubella syndrome) lesions do occur. Valvular pulmonic stenosis is most often due to fibrosis of the valve with thickening of the leaflets. The leaflets dome into the pulmonary trunk during systole, producing a narrow central aperture. Less commonly, the valve leaflets are dysplastic and rubbery with a small valve annulus. Bicuspid pulmonic valves also occur. The pathologic distinctions made earlier do have some clinical relevance, as dysplastic valves are less responsive to balloon dilatation than dome-shaped valves. **Isolated congenital pulmonic stenosis** is the most commonly encountered congenital pulmonic valve disease in adulthood, and it typically causes valvular pulmonic stenosis. **Tetralogy of Fallot** also causes pulmonic stenosis, and **Noonan syndrome** can be associated with dysplastic pulmonic stenosis. Other congenital syndromes associated with pulmonic stenosis include double-outlet right ventricle, atrioventricular canal defect, and univentricular atrioventricular connection.

The most common acquired form of pulmonic stenosis occurs with **carcinoid heart disease**. The proposed mechanism for carcinoid valve disease has been discussed earlier in this chapter. The whitish carcinoid plaques adhere to the valve leaflets and can cause both pulmonic stenosis and pulmonic regurgitation. Rheumatic heart disease is a rare cause of pulmonic stenosis and, when present, is generally seen with multiple valve disease. Large vegetations on an infected pulmonic valve can rarely cause pulmonic stenosis.

Clinical Findings

A. Symptoms & Signs

As with tricuspid disease, the symptoms of pulmonic valve disease can be subtle and overshadowed by coexisting illnesses. Patients with pulmonic regurgitation are often asymptomatic unless symptoms of pulmonary hypertension and RV failure eventuate. Patients with pulmonic stenosis are also frequently asymptomatic. Symptoms can appear gradually as the pulmonic valve pressure gradient increases and include exertional dyspnea, chest pain, and fatigue.

B. Physical Examination

1. Jugular venous waveform—The presence of pulmonic stenosis is suggested by a prominent jugular venous *a* wave in the setting of a relatively normal central venous pressure.

2. Cardiac auscultation

A. PULMONIC REGURGITATION—The pulmonic component of S_2 is usually loud because most patients have pulmonary hypertension, and the second heart sound is often widely split due to prolonged RV emptying. RV S_3 and S_4 gallops are sometimes heard in the left parasternal area. In the absence of pulmonary hypertension, the murmur of pulmonic regurgitation is a low-pitched, crescendo–decrescendo diastolic murmur that is best heard near the left second or third intercostal space. The murmur is augmented during inspiration.

However, in patients with significant pulmonary hypertension, the murmur assumes a different quality. The dilatation of the pulmonic valve annulus allows for a more forceful regurgitant jet, resulting in a high-pitched, decrescendo murmur that is best heard at the left parasternal border near the second or third intercostal space, otherwise known as the **Graham Steell murmur.**

B. Pulmonic stenosis—The second heart sound is also widely split with pulmonic stenosis, and this splitting is proportional to the degree of stenosis. Unlike in pulmonic regurgitation, the pulmonic component of S_2 is soft in pulmonic stenosis, and an S_4 can frequently be appreciated over the lower left sternal border. A high-frequency systolic click can be heard near the left upper sternal border that precedes the late-peaking crescendo–decrescendo systolic murmur that typifies pulmonic stenosis. Unlike the murmur, the click becomes softer during inspiration due to enhanced late diastolic pulmonic valve opening with the increased RV filling. The murmur can be associated with a thrill, and an RV impulse is frequently palpable.

C. Diagnostic Studies

The diagnostic evaluation of pulmonic valve disease should include an ECG, chest film, and a transthoracic echocardiogram. Cardiac catheterization is generally unnecessary given the high degree of agreement between echocardiographic and catheterization data in pulmonic valve disease.

1. Electrocardiography—Pulmonic regurgitation and pulmonic stenosis can both cause ECG evidence of RV enlargement. Typical findings include right bundle branch block, right axis deviation, and RV hypertrophy. Mild or moderate pulmonic stenosis frequently presents with a normal ECG.

2. Chest radiography—Nonspecific enlargement of the right ventricle and pulmonary arteries can be seen with pulmonic regurgitation. Characteristically, pulmonic stenosis is associated with dilatation of the main pulmonary artery.

3. Echocardiography—In pulmonic regurgitation, color-flow and pulsed Doppler techniques are used to accurately detect the presence and severity of pulmonic regurgitation. In addition, the presence of pulmonary hypertension, RV hypertrophy and dilation, and coexistent valve disease can be detected. Transesophageal echocardiography has a role in the evaluation of suspected pulmonic valve endocarditis.

Two-dimensional and Doppler echocardiography determine the nature, location, and severity of pulmonic stenosis. The severity of the stenosis can be quantitated by Doppler echocardiography; peak transvalvular velocities greater than 4 m/s (estimated pressure gradient > 64 mm Hg) are considered consistent with severe stenosis. As with pulmonic regurgitation, data regarding the status of the ventricles and other valves can also be obtained. Transesophageal studies may be useful when the location of the stenosis is unclear from the surface study.

4. Cardiac catheterization—Cardiac catheterization is recommended in adolescents and young adults with congenital pulmonic stenosis for evaluation of the valvular gradient if the Doppler peak jet velocity is greater than 3 m/s and balloon valvotomy is feasible.

5. Magnetic resonance imaging (MRI)—MRI provides excellent images of the pulmonary outflow tract and valve and is especially useful for planning percutaneous bioprosthetic valve placement. It can also visualize the main pulmonary artery anatomy to assess for branch stenosis. In addition, it provides for accurate assessment of RV size and function. Finally, it can assess both stenosis and regurgitation quantitatively.

Stout KK, Daniels CJ, Aboulhosn JA, et al. 2018 AHA/ACC Guideline for the management of adults with congenital heart disease: a report of the American College of Cardiology/American Heart Association Task Force on Clinical Practice Guidelines. *J Am Coll Cardiol.* 2019;73:e81–e192. [PMID: 30121239]

Treatment

Pulmonic regurgitation rarely requires specific treatment. Treatment of predisposing cardiac conditions, such as pulmonary hypertension, endocarditis, or left-sided valve disease, often improves the pulmonic regurgitation. As mentioned previously, certain patients may progress to right-heart failure from pulmonic regurgitation following repair of tetralogy of Fallot. These patients may require valve replacement, often with a bioprosthetic valve or pulmonary allograft.

Pulmonic stenosis has been managed with great success by balloon valvuloplasty. Treatment is based on severity of disease: balloon valvotomy is recommended if the RV–to–pulmonary artery peak-to-peak gradient is greater than 30 mm Hg at catheterization in the symptomatic patient, and greater than 40 mm Hg in the asymptomatic patient. Patients with dysplastic valves may not respond to balloon valvuloplasty and may require valve replacement with a bioprosthetic valve. Percutaneous stented pulmonary valve implantation is an alternative to surgical replacement of pulmonic stenosis and regurgitation in selected patients.

Alkashkari W, Alsubei A, Hijazi ZM. Transcatheter pulmonary valve replacement: state of the art. *Curr Cardiol Rep.* 2018;20: 27. [PMID: 29546472]

Prognosis

The prognosis of pulmonic valve disease is generally excellent. With pulmonic regurgitation, clinicians must consider the comorbidities involved (particularly pulmonary hypertension) that may influence prognosis. Patients with congenital pulmonic stenosis can expect a life expectancy comparable to that of the general population.

22 Infective Endocarditis

Michael H. Crawford, MD
Su Aung, MD, MPH

ESSENTIALS OF DIAGNOSIS

- Clinical features: Fever, new valvular regurgitation, embolization, immune complexes, predisposing condition.
- Blood cultures positive for bacteria or fungi.
- Characteristic cardiac lesions on echocardiography or histology.

General Considerations

Infective endocarditis is an infection involving the cardiac endothelium. It remains a challenging disease affecting both adults and children worldwide and is associated with significant morbidity and mortality. Healthy endothelium possesses an effective system of defense against both hemostasis and infection. Infection of the endothelium of blood vessels occurs only at sites markedly altered by disease or surgery, such as the severely atherosclerotic aorta or the suture lines of vascular grafts. By contrast, infection of the cardiac valve leaflet endothelium (endocardium) is not rare and occurs even in the absence of identifiable preexisting valve disease.

Pathophysiology & Etiology

A. Cardiac Infection—Vegetations

1. Precursor lesion and bacteremia—Valve infection probably begins when minor trauma, with or without accompanying valve disease, impairs the antihemostatic function of valve endocardium. Infection usually first appears along the coapting surface of the leaflets, suggesting a role for valve opening and closing. This hypothesis is supported by the observation that the ranking of valves in order of frequency of infection corresponds to the ranking of valves according to the force acting to close the valve (mitral > aortic > tricuspid > pulmonic).

This minor trauma may cause the formation of a microscopic thrombus on the leaflet surface. A small noninfected thrombus on the leaflet is called **nonbacterial thrombotic endocarditis (NBTE)**. The next step is the infection of the fibrin matrix of the thrombus by blood-borne organisms, which appear briefly in blood under many circumstances, such as toothbrushing, defecating, or other mucus membrane manipulation or inflammation. When transient bacteremia coincides with the presence of an NBTE lesion, organisms may adhere to the valve leaflet and begin to proliferate causing additional deposition of platelets and fibrin and forming an infected vegetation. As the infected vegetation grows, the likelihood of severe sepsis and complications increases. The common infecting organisms are those that gain entry to the blood because they colonize body surfaces and are adapted for attachment and proliferation in the NBTE lesion (see Clinical Syndromes).

2. Growth of vegetations—Vegetations begin near the coaptation line of the leaflet on the side that contacts the opposite leaflet during valve closure. Mitral valve vegetations are typically attached within 1–2 cm of the leaflet tip on the left atrial side and prolapse into the left atrium during systole. Aortic valve vegetations usually occur on the left ventricular (LV) side of the mid or distal portions of the aortic cusps and prolapse into the LV outflow tract during diastole. A similar distribution of lesions occurs on the tricuspid and pulmonic valves.

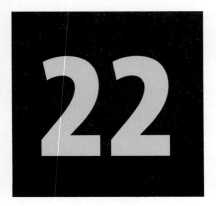

Although the course of cardiac lesions in endocarditis varies, in a typical sequence of events (without treatment), the infection progresses by enlargement of the vegetation and extension of its region of attachment toward the base of the leaflet. Valve regurgitation almost always develops from either destruction of the leaflet tip or scarring and retraction of the leaflet. Erosion of the leaflet may lead to perforation (usually associated with clinically significant regurgitation). Weakening of the leaflet's spongiosum layer may result in a deformity called a leaflet aneurysm. Mitral or tricuspid chordal involvement may cause rupture and acute severe regurgitation. In rare cases (primarily in mitral bioprosthetic endocarditis; see Management of High-Risk Endocarditis), a large vegetation may cause hemodynamically significant valve obstruction and increase the risk of embolization.

3. Metastatic vegetations—These vegetations may form when the regurgitant jet of blood from an infected valve strikes an endocardial surface in the receiving chamber (wall or chordae), producing a small area of denuded endothelium. The thrombus that forms at this site also becomes infected, constituting a secondary vegetation. Such metastatic vegetations most often appear on the ventricular side of the anterior mitral leaflet where it is struck by a regurgitant jet from aortic valve endocarditis. Another common location is on the mitral chordae, also from aortic regurgitation. Metastatic lesions on the mural endocardium of the cardiac chambers can occur as well.

4. Abscess and fistula formation—Organisms eventually invade the valve annulus and adjacent myocardium. Abscess formation can take multiple forms and may occur with or without fistula formation. Aortic annular abscess is an infective mass that burrows into or around the outside of the annulus. The abscess may extend upward to the sinus of Valsalva or ascending aorta (a type of mycotic aneurysm). This extension may lead to a fistulous communication between the aorta and the left atrium or (rarely) the right atrium. In other patients, the abscess extends down through the fibrous trigone and forms a fistula to the LV outflow tract.

A band of fibrous tissue at the base of the anterior mitral leaflet (the intervalvular fibrosa) separates the aortic annulus from the left atrial wall. Infection extending down from the posterior aortic annulus may produce an aneurysm in this area, which may in turn fistulize to the left atrium, aortic root, or into the pericardial space. Infection extending down from the anterior aortic annulus may invade the septal myocardium, causing a block in the conduction system. Evidence of heart block on an electrocardiogram may signal the presence of an aneurysm or abscess.

When mitral valve infection extends to the base of the anterior leaflet, abscess formation involving the fibrous trigone may track upward and become fistulous. Infection from the posterior leaflet may extend to form a myocardial abscess in the LV posterior wall or a fistula around or through the mitral annulus between the left atrium and left ventricle. Infection may even penetrate through the pericardial space, producing purulent pericarditis.

B. Extracardiac Disease

At any time during cardiac infection, extracardiac complications may supervene and dominate the clinical picture. Although these manifestations are emphasized in the medical literature, it should be kept in mind that many patients with endocarditis do not have them, especially at the time of presentation. The extracardiac disease in endocarditis results from immunologic phenomena or from the shedding of bacteria and fragments of infected thrombus from the valve vegetations. Extracardiac foci of infection may vary depending on the patient's risk factors and virulence of the culprit organism.

1. Immune manifestations—The bacteremia accompanying endocarditis presents an antigenic challenge to the immune system. Various antibodies and immune complexes appear in the blood—more so with longer duration of illness or persistent bacteremia. Rheumatoid factors (anti-IgG or IgM antibody) have a low diagnostic value. Other antibodies, such as those that form circulating immune complexes and activate complement, are of major importance because they cause microvascular damage, most frequently glomerulonephritis and vasculitic skin lesions.

2. Systemic and pulmonary emboli—The embolization of fragments of vegetation is a frequent and potentially catastrophic complication of endocarditis. The clinical consequences are highly variable and depend on many factors, including the size of the embolus, the site at which it lodges in the vasculature, the type and quantity of organisms carried, the point during treatment at which embolism occurs, and the host response. Small emboli are likely to present as metastatic infection; the most dreaded of these is brain abscess. Septic embolization may also lead to abscesses in the kidney, liver, bone, and (from the right heart) lung.

Large emboli present with signs and symptoms of major vascular obstruction. For endocarditis of the left heart, the most frequent and serious extracardiac complication is embolism to the brain; these strokes tend to be large, complicating subsequent management, and are associated with high morbidity and mortality. Emboli may also cause infarction of the lung, spleen, liver, kidney, and myocardium. Embolism to large arteries of the extremities is unusual and occurs primarily in fungal endocarditis. Independently, the use of indwelling vascular lines is often necessary for long-term intravenous antibiotic therapy for the treatment of infective endocarditis and poses a risk for development of catheter-associated superficial or deep venous thrombus.

3. Mycotic aneurysms—When infection of the arterial wall results in localized dilatation and progresses to abscess formation, mycotic aneurysms can occur. The cause is thought to be embolization of vegetation that does not obstruct blood flow enough to present clinically as embolism. These lesions frequently occur at vessel branch points. The mycotic aneurysm may produce signs and symptoms many weeks after the diagnosis of endocarditis, and recognition may be difficult. Their effects are especially devastating in the central nervous system. Aneurysms may act as a protected site of infection and cause persistent fever or bacteremia despite appropriate antibiotic therapy. Alternatively, if antibiotic therapy has sterilized the aneurysm, it may present months or years later as unexplained hemorrhage.

C. Clinical Syndromes

Endocarditis can assume any of a wide variety of forms because of the many possible combinations of infecting organisms, portals of entry, and other factors such as the patient's immune status and the presence of concomitant diseases. Although the list of organisms capable of causing endocarditis is very long (and the list of possible combinations of organisms and other factors is even longer), there are several common and distinctive clinical syndromes.

A distinction between the acute and subacute forms of endocarditis has been found to be of some clinical and diagnostic value. The differing characteristics of patients with these two forms are summarized in Table 22–1. Many patients with endocarditis cannot be easily placed into one or the other of these two categories, and there are commonly overlaps. Acute infective endocarditis develops quickly over days to weeks and patients may present with rapid-onset fevers, sepsis, and complications including congestive heart failure, stroke, or pulmonary embolization. A new-onset heart murmur is a hallmark sign of infective endocarditis when accompanied by these clinical signs and symptoms. Subacute infective endocarditis is more difficult to recognize; patients may present with more nonspecific symptoms including low-grade intermittent fevers, fatigue, chills, sweats, malaise, weight loss, dyspnea, back pain, or arthralgias over weeks to months.

D. Microbiology

Gram-positive organisms remain the leading cause of infective endocarditis despite regional variations. The most common bacterial causes are *Staphylococcus* spp., *Streptococcus* spp., and *Enterococccus* spp. In specific populations, drug-resistant pathogens and atypical bacteria must also be considered.

Table 22–1. Characteristics of Acute and Subacute Endocarditis[1]

Acute	Subacute
Symptom onset to diagnosis: ≤ 1 week	Symptom onset to diagnosis: ≥ 4 weeks
Acute malaise	Weight loss
Shaking chills	Fatigue
Fever (may be high)	Night sweats
Tachycardia	Low or no fever
Leukocytosis	Normal white cell count or leukopenia
Normal gamma globulins	Elevated gamma globulins
Rheumatoid factor +	Rheumatoid factor +

[1]Elevated erythrocyte sedimentation rate and anemia common to both syndromes.

1. *Staphylococcus aureus* endocarditis—*S aureus* is the most common cause of endocarditis in the developed world, accounting for approximately a third of all cases and causing substantial morbidity and mortality. Although *S aureus* frequently enters the circulation from the skin or nares, a culprit lesion may not be apparent on examination of these areas. Major risk factors include health care-associated infections, intravenous drug injection, and indwelling vascular devices. Among patients with infective endocarditis and opioid-use disorders in the United States, S aureus is the causative pathogen in more than 50% of cases. Endocarditis should be considered in all patients diagnosed with *S aureus* bacteremia, and infectious disease subspecialty consultation is recommended.

S aureus endocarditis presents as an acute febrile illness with marked constitutional symptoms. Both intracardiac and extracardiac complications are common. *S aureus* tends to cause valve destruction more rapidly than do other organisms; approximately 30% of left-sided cases result in extensive left-heart valve involvement complicated by abscess or fistula formation or pericarditis. *S aureus* endocarditis of the aortic valve is the most common cause of aortic annular abscess, often signaled by the appearance of ECG PR interval prolongation.

A major hallmark of *S aureus* endocarditis is the potential for metastatic infection at any site in the body. For left-sided lesions, central nervous system involvement is present in a third of cases and manifests as cerebral embolization with stroke, mycotic aneurysm with risk for intracranial hemorrhage from rupture, and microscopic or macroscopic brain abscesses. Other significant complications include septic arthritis, vertebral osteomyelitis with or without epidural abscess, and major organ abscesses. Renal involvement, as indicated by an active urine sediment, is present in most cases, and frank renal impairment occurs in approximately 20% of cases. Splenic infarction resulting from emboli may lead to functional asplenia depending on the degree of infarction. Right-sided disease has a better prognosis, but septic pulmonary emboli occur in two-thirds of cases.

S aureus is the most lethal of the organisms commonly causing endocarditis, with mortality rates ranging from 5 to 45%, with the best prognosis in injection drug users with right-sided native valve endocarditis and the worst in those with significant comorbidities, presence of congestive heart failure, severe sepsis with persistent bacteremia, multiple foci of infection, and left-sided prosthetic valve endocarditis. Early surgery, if clinical criteria for this are met, is independently associated with reduced overall mortality.

2. Coagulase-negative *Staphylococcus* endocarditis— Coagulase-negative staphylococci (eg, *Staphylococcus epidermidis and Staphylococcus lugdunensis*) is a rare cause of endocarditis and accounts for approximately 10% of endocarditis cases. However, coagulase-negative staphylococci are emerging as an important cause of both native and prosthetic valve endocarditis both in the community and health-care settings. These organisms colonize the skin and can adhere to indwelling lines and invasive devices. Therefore, individuals with highest risk for coagulase-negative endocarditis include those with a history of injection-drug use, long-term intravascular catheter use, and recent invasive procedures.

Presentation of coagulase-negative Staphylococcal endocarditis can be acute or subacute. Mortality rates associated with coagulase-negative Staphylococcal endocarditis are lower than *S aureus* but higher than endocarditis due to streptococci. Antibiotic sensitivities vary among different coagulase-negative *Staphylococcus* bacteria, and careful attention to antibiotic susceptibility (MIC) data is important for optimal therapy.

3. Streptococcal endocarditis—Endocarditis due to streptococci accounts for about 25% of all cases of endocarditis. These organisms can be divided into three groups: normal human oral flora (also referred to as viridans group *Streptococcus*: *Streptococcus mitis, Streptococcus sanguinis, Streptococcus anginosus, Streptococcus mutans, Streptococcus salivarius,* and nutritionally variant species), inhabitants of the lower gastrointestinal and genitourinary tracts (nonenterococcal group D organisms, of which *Streptococcus bovis* is important), and pyogenic streptococcal species, including *Streptococcus pyogenes*, which are uncommon causes of endocarditis. Other streptococcal species, such as *Streptococcus pneumoniae*, are rarely associated with endocarditis. The main disease caused by the first two groups of streptococci is endocarditis. This predilection appears to stem from bacterial cell wall proteins that bind to fibronectin, platelets, laminin, and other components of blood clots.

Viridans streptococci usually grow slowly, and the patient typically has a febrile illness of at least 10 days in duration and modest intensity; many cases fit the clinical syndrome of subacute bacterial endocarditis. Although valve destruction may be extensive, it is gradual, and abscess formation in the heart or elsewhere is uncommon, except as noted in the following discussion. The renal disease accompanying endocarditis caused by these organisms is usually mild and rarely causes significant renal insufficiency. Viridans streptococcal endocarditis is therefore often treatable medically and has a relatively good prognosis if antibiotic treatment is begun before complications occur.

Endocarditis from *S bovis* is strongly associated with underlying colorectal disease, especially malignancy. Bacteremia with *S bovis* biotype I (*S gallolyticus* subsp. *gallolyticus*) has been strongly correlated with infective endocarditis and colonic neoplasm. Colonization of the gastrointestinal tract by this organism increases with age and with malignancy for reasons that are not well understood. After initial endocarditis treatment, a patient with this disease should undergo colonoscopy.

Extra vigilance for complications is needed when treating patients with endocarditis from certain other streptococci. *Streptococcus anginosus* and *Streptococcus milleri* can cause abscesses in the brain and other major organs, and nutritionally variant streptococci are associated with higher morbidity and mortality rates than other viridans organisms—again for reasons that are not well understood.

Complications from viridans streptococcal endocarditis are almost never due to failure to sterilize vegetations. Nevertheless, the sensitivity of these organisms to penicillin is not uniform and testing for resistance is essential for establishing an appropriate antibiotic regimen.

4. Enterococcal endocarditis—This form accounts for approximately 10% of cases of endocarditis—almost all from *Enterococcus* faecalis and less commonly from *Enterococccus faecium.* Although historically, enterococcal endocarditis was noted in women of childbearing age, modern studies have linked this organism more commonly to urinary or gut sources, particularly in patients undergoing procedures manipulating these areas. Less commonly, this organism has been associated with intravenous drug use, and it also has been linked to prosthetic valve endocarditis and, increasingly, nosocomial cases of endocarditis. An acute or insidious syndrome may be present in patients with enterococcal endocarditis, although the findings typical of subacute bacterial endocarditis are unusual.

Enterococcal endocarditis is especially difficult to treat because of antibiotic resistance (discussed later). It is markedly different in its presentation and outcomes compared with streptococcal endocarditis. Overall mortality is only slightly less than that for staphylococcal endocarditis, and the incidence of major complications and need for valve replacement is approximately 30–40%.

5. Endocarditis from gram-negative bacteria—Gram-negative bacteria rarely cause endocarditis, except for three groups of organisms: the HACEK organisms (*Haemophilus* species, *Actinobacillus* species, *Cardiobacterium hominis, Eikenella corrodens, Kingella* species), *P aeruginosa*, and the enteric organisms (*Escherichia coli, Proteus, Klebsiella,* and *Serratia marcescens*). *Pseudomonas* and *Serratia* are occasional causes of endocarditis in injecting drug users, but the most common risk factor for these gram-negative organisms is health-care contact, especially in the setting of implanted endovascular cardiac device and indwelling catheters. Infective endocarditis from *Pseudomonas aeruginosa* may lead to severe disease. Although rare, *Salmonella* has a predilection for the endovascular space, especially in patients with preexisting aneurysms or cardiac devices.

The HACEK organisms colonize the oropharynx and account for less than 5% of endocarditis and are relatively slow growing. These organisms usually cause a subacute clinical syndrome. Before the introduction of automated blood culture systems, these organisms were often considered as causes of culture-negative endocarditis, but in the modern era, these organisms tend to grow easily within 5 days. Despite the often mild and indolent symptoms and signs of endocarditis caused by these organisms, valve

Table 22–2. Native Valve Endocarditis: Causative Organisms[1]

Organism	Community-Acquired Cases (71%)	Intravenous Drug Users (6%)	Health Care-Associated Cases (23%)
Staphylococcus aureus	20%	80%	40%
Coagulase-negative staphylococci	5%	< 5%	20%
Oral streptococci	25%	5–10%	5–10%
Streptococcus bovis	15%	< 5%	< 5%
Enterococci	10%	5%	20–40%
Pyogenic streptococci	8%	5%	0%
Gram-negative organisms	5%	< 5%	10%
Culture negative Includes zoonotic organisms	15%	5%	10%

[1]May add up to > 100% if multiple organisms are identified.

destruction may be extensive by the time of diagnosis. The HACEK organisms are associated with endocarditis that causes major vessel embolism from large vegetations. The other gram-negative organisms tend to produce an acute clinical syndrome.

6. Fungal endocarditis—Fungal endocarditis is rare, accounting for 1–2% of all cases of endocarditis. Important predisposing factors include immune compromise, injecting drug use, and intravascular and cardiac devices. *Candida* species (especially *Candida albicans*) are the most common organisms, but endemic mycoses, such as *Histoplasma capsulatum,* and molds, including *Aspergillus*, have also been reported. Clinicians must recognize when patients are at risk for fungal endocarditis because the signs and symptoms of the disease often escape notice or lead to misdiagnosis.

The development of symptoms is often insidious, extending over weeks or months. Cardiac involvement is generally limited to the development of vegetations; invasion of the myocardium occurs with a lower frequency than in bacterial endocarditis. The vegetations usually lead to leaflet destruction and valve regurgitation; they may be large and may occasionally cause valve orifice obstruction. The most likely complication of fungal infective endocarditis is embolism, including occlusion of large peripheral arteries from embolization. Ophthalmologic evaluation for endophthalmitis is recommended for patients with fungal endocarditis, particularly involving *Candida* spp.

7. Zoonotic organisms—Zoonotic organisms can rarely cause infective endocarditis and are considered as causes of culture-negative endocarditis. Examples include *Coxiella burnetii* (Q fever) and *Brucella spp* found in farm animals, *Bartonella henselae* in cats, and *Chlamydia psittaci* in birds.

Clinical presentation is often subacute. Symptoms may be nonspecific and develop over weeks to months. Complications such as abscess formation and valve destruction and ensuing heart failure may develop, especially with Brucella endocarditis. Bartonella endocarditis may be associated with other sites of infection including vertebral osteomyelitis and neuroretinitis. A careful social and exposure history is needed to raise clinical suspicion for infective endocarditis involving these organisms.

Table 22–2 lists the approximate frequency of causative organisms in native valve endocarditis.

E. Prosthetic or Device-Related Endocarditis

1. Prosthetic valve endocarditis—The risk of developing endocarditis is higher with prosthetic heart valves than with severely diseased native valves, approximately 0.5% per patient-year. Despite some overlap, there is a clear difference between the causes of disease that develops within 2 months of implantation and the causes of disease occurring later (Table 22–3). The difference is probably due to infection occurring during surgery in early prosthetic endocarditis, with organisms from the skin of the patient and operating room personnel/procedures (*S epidermidis* and *S aureus*) accounting for more than half the cases. The incidence of early prosthetic endocarditis has been greatly reduced by the routine use of prophylactic antibiotics. Prosthetic infection after 2 months usually involves the same mechanism as does native valve endocarditis, except that the causative organisms are those adapted to nonbiologic material.

Infection of a bioprosthesis involves primarily the area of attachment of the sewing ring to the annulus, although vegetations like those of native valve endocarditis can occur. Early in the disease, abscesses may form along the suture line, resulting in fistulization, paravalvular regurgitation, and partial or complete detachment (dehiscence) of the prosthesis.

Similarly, infection of a mechanical prosthesis centers on the sewing ring as well. The inward growth of an infective

Table 22–3. Prosthetic Valve Endocarditis: Causative Organisms

Organism	Early (< 60 days)	Midterm (2–12 months)	Late (> 12 months)
Staphylococcus aureus	35%	7%	25%
Coagulase-negative staphylococci	20%	27%	9%
Oral streptococci	< 5%	7%	11%
Streptococcus bovis	< 5%	7%	9%
Enterococci	8%	7%	20%
Pyogenic streptococci	0%	0%	3%
Other, including gram-negative organisms	0%	33%	12%
Culture negative	30%	12%	12%

mass from the ring frequently causes the occluder to become stuck in a partially open or closed position. In contrast to native valve endocarditis, prosthetic valve infection may be extensive without the clinical signs, such as a murmur of regurgitation, heart failure, or embolism, usually seen in advanced native valve infection. When prosthetic valve dysfunction does occur (especially in a mechanical prosthesis), it tends to be abrupt and severe, as when the occluder becomes fixed in a half-open position (other differences are discussed later in this chapter).

2. Pacemaker or implanted defibrillator endocarditis— Pacemaker endocarditis is infection of the lead or of parts of the heart in contact with the lead (tricuspid valve, right ventricular endocardium). Mortality is high, up to 25%, and the diagnosis is often missed due to the indolent nature of the infection. Most cases are due to contamination at the time of implant or generator change; hematogenous infection of a lead is rare. Most cases present with evidence of present or prior infection at the implant site. Systemic symptoms may be absent. The findings on transthoracic echocardiography (TTE) are often falsely normal. Transesophageal echocardiography (TEE) is the diagnostic test of choice, with a sensitivity of more than 90%. All patients with a cardiac implantable device who have bloodstream infection of unclear etiology should be evaluated for endocarditis.

Staphylococci are the usual infecting organisms, with staphylococci (predominately coagulase-negative strains but with significant *S aureus* contribution as well) accounting for 70% of cases. *Staphylococcus* species produce a slime-like “biofilm” (clustered bacteria embedded in a polysaccharide and proteinaceous matrix) along the lead that protects bacteria from the patient’s immunologic defense as well as from antibiotic therapy. Treatment requires removal of the device. Lead removal can be accomplished percutaneously with reasonable safety if the masses attached to the lead are small (< 1 cm). Surgery is indicated if the lead is fixed, a large mass (> 1 cm) is present (with dislodgement likely to result in severe pulmonary embolism), or tricuspid valve involvement is extensive. Device removal is followed by 6 weeks of antibiotic therapy. Reimplantation, if indicated, can be considered if surveillance blood cultures are negative at 72 hours, if lead vegetations alone were present, or if at 2 weeks a valve vegetation was present. The device should not be reimplanted on the ipsilateral side of previous infection.

F. Endocarditis in Special Populations and Settings

1. Endocarditis in the injection drug user—The mode of infection is a needle contaminated by skin flora, and febrile symptoms often start at 24–48 hours after the last injection. The intravenous injection site may show an abscess or thrombophlebitis. The most likely causative organism is *S aureus*, which, overall, causes 70% of endocarditis in injecting drug users and which, in this setting, has a benign prognosis with only a 2–5% mortality rate. Many other organisms can cause endocarditis in injection drug users, such as gram-negative bacilli, including *P aeruginosa*, fungi, and β-hemolytic streptococci.

Infection of the tricuspid valve occurs in approximately 60% of cases of endocarditis in this population. Significant tricuspid regurgitation may not be clinically apparent. In as many as 40% of cases, the left heart valves alone are infected. Despite its proximity to the portal of entry in injecting drug users, the pulmonic valve is rarely involved, probably because of the low-pressure gradient and low wear and tear of this valve. Chest pain and dyspnea should prompt consideration of septic pulmonary emboli, which occur in 30% of cases of tricuspid valve endocarditis. Radiographic features of this complication include multiple peripheral nodules with occasional cavitation and associated wedge-shaped infarcts. While chest pain, cough, dyspnea, or hypoxemia often prompt this diagnosis, septic pulmonary emboli can be asymptomatic as well.

2. Health care-associated or hospital-acquired endocarditis—Health care-associated endocarditis is a growing problem. Out-of-hospital infections comprise one half of cases of health care-associated native valve endocarditis. Patients develop signs and symptoms consistent with infective endocarditis prior to hospitalization but with extensive contact with health-care services including long-term care facilities, rehabilitation centers, nursing homes, wound care, dialysis, and infusion centers. Hospital-acquired or nosocomial endocarditis is often associated with indwelling catheters. Prosthetic valves are at far greater risk than native valves: endocarditis develops in 15–20% of patients with prosthetic valves who become bacteremic, but most of the hospital-associated endocarditis occurs in patients without underlying valvular disease. Staphylococci, including *S aureus*, and enterococci predominate, but there is an increased likelihood of the presence of unusual or antibiotic-resistant organisms, including *Candida* species. Clinical outcomes for native valve endocarditis are similar between health care-associated and hospital-acquired infections.

Hospital-acquired endocarditis should be suspected when fever develops in a hospitalized patient who has positive blood cultures without an apparent source. Potential culprit catheters should be removed and cultured, followed by echocardiography if additional risk factors for endocarditis exist. Examples of risk factors in this setting include a prosthetic valve, native valve disease predisposing to infection, hemodialysis, or *Candida* or *S aureus* bloodstream infection. Surveillance blood cultures during and after treatment and a repeat echocardiogram should be considered if uncertainty regarding the response to treatment persists. In the case of exposure of a prosthetic valve to bacteremia, blood culture surveillance should be extended for at least 2 months.

Clinical Findings

A. Diagnostic Criteria

In the current era, with the availability of sensitive blood culture techniques and echocardiography, the clinician will rarely need to rely on a formal schema for the diagnosis of endocarditis. The most useful schema is the modified Duke criteria (Table 22–4), which involve two "major" criteria (definite echocardiographic evidence of endocarditis and positive blood cultures with organisms typical for endocarditis) and five "minor" criteria (predisposing cardiac condition, fever, vascular phenomena, immunologic phenomena, and blood cultures not meeting the major criteria) to reach a probable diagnosis. This approach was useful because of the low sensitivity and specificity of individual clinical features by themselves. Now TEE and blood cultures independently have a diagnostic sensitivity of greater than 90%, and TEE has a specificity of greater than 90%. Diagnostic uncertainty may arise when the result of TEE is ambiguous, when adequate blood cultures are not obtained before starting antibiotics, or the culprit pathogen is difficult to identify.

Table 22–4. Modified Duke Criteria for Infective Endocarditis

Major Criteria
Blood culture positive
Typical organisms: Viridans streptococci, *Streptococcus gallolyticus, Staphylococcus aureus*, community-acquired enterococci, and the HACEK group
Evidence of endocardial involvement on echocardiogram
Minor Criteria
Predisposing heart condition, injection drug use
Fever > 100.4°F (38°C)
Valvular phenomena
Major arterial emboli
Septic pulmonary infarcts
Mycotic aneurysm
Intracranial hemorrhage
Conjunctival hemorrhage
Janeway lesions
Immunologic phenomena
Glomerulonephritis
Osler nodes
Roth spots
Rheumatoid factor
Microbiological evidence
Positive blood cultures not meeting major criterion or serologic evidence of active infection with organism consistent with IE
Definite Endocarditis
2 major criteria
1 major and ≥ 3 minor criteria
5 minor criteria
Possible Endocarditis
1 major and 1–2 minor criteria
3–4 minor criteria
Rejected Endocarditis
0 major and 1–2 minor criteria
1 major and 0 minor criteria

HACEK, *Haemophilus* species, *Aggregatibacter actinomycetemcomitans, Cardiobacterium hominis, Eikenella corrodens, and Kingella kingae;* IE, infective endocarditis.

In many such situations, a diagnosis can be reached by gathering more data. For example, if the TEE fails to show endocarditis-specific valve disease and the patient is doing well, discontinuing antibiotics in order to repeat cultures should be considered. Many of the common features of endocarditis—fever, a cardiac murmur, and a set of positive blood cultures—occur frequently in other diseases and are occasionally absent in patients with endocarditis. Other diseases that can mimic endocarditis include malignancy, autoimmune disease, and septicemia. In addition, patients with endocarditis may come to the physician because of a complication of endocarditis so dramatic as to distract attention from the underlying infection. Typical settings in which this error occurs include heart failure, stroke, and myocardial infarction.

The recognition of possible **prosthetic valve endocarditis** may be difficult because the signs of infection may be very subtle or even absent. In early prosthetic valve endocarditis, the symptoms and signs may be incorrectly ascribed to other diseases. Fever and bacteremia during the first few weeks after prosthetic implantation should be considered to indicate prosthetic valve endocarditis until proven otherwise. This is especially important because early prosthetic valve endocarditis appears to follow a more fulminant course than either late prosthetic or native valve endocarditis and may indicate probable causative organisms. These patients often have other potential causes of bacteremia, however, and an effort to prove infection from another site should be pursued vigorously. TEE has a sensitivity of approximately 80% for prosthetic valve endocarditis and should be performed whenever an alternative explanation for fever or bacteremia is not readily apparent. If the TEE findings are normal but bacteremia persists (especially if the organism is a frequent cause of prosthetic endocarditis), prosthetic valve endocarditis should be presumptively treated.

Fungal endocarditis is also often difficult to diagnose. Blood cultures are negative in approximately half of cases caused by *Candida*, most histoplasmosis cases, and almost all cases caused by *Aspergillus*. Histologic examination and culture should be performed whenever possible on specimens of embolic material, oropharyngeal lesions (especially for histoplasmosis), skin lesions (for *Candida* species and *Aspergillus*), liver, bone marrow, and urine (for histoplasmosis). In addition, a careful eye examination should be performed in patients with suspected fungal endocarditis because of the high frequency of anterior uveitis and chorioretinitis.

Tricuspid valve endocarditis (as seen in injecting drug users and patients with indwelling catheters) produces a distinctive picture because of the frequent occurrence of septic pulmonary emboli. Peripheral lung nodules with cavitation, pulmonary edema, and rarely pleural effusions can be seen on chest film and often are accompanied by pleuritic chest pain. The murmur of tricuspid regurgitation may be inaudible or soft because right-heart pressures are normally low, even when tricuspid infection is extensive.

B. Symptoms & Signs

Constellations of certain symptoms should arouse suspicion of endocarditis. One combination of symptoms often seen is constitutional symptoms (eg, fatigue, malaise, headache, arthralgias or myalgias, nausea, anorexia, weight loss) and fever, which can range from mild feverish feelings and night sweats to shaking chills. When these symptoms are chronic or mild, other diagnoses are often also considered, such as malignancy and autoimmune disease.

A high suspicion of endocarditis is warranted when this picture is associated with any symptom pointing to the circulatory system, such as complaints associated with left- or right-heart failure (dyspnea, orthopnea, cough, peripheral edema), vascular occlusion (stroke, systemic embolism), and chest pain.

C. Physical Examination

The physical examination is essential to the treatment of endocarditis. The initial examination assists the clinician in assessing the severity of the illness, extent of heart failure, and evidence of embolic disease. During treatment (or observation for more definite evidence of endocarditis), serial physical examinations are vital for identifying important changes in the patient's status because physical findings may signal the need for surgery.

It is important to caution that most of the physical findings caused by endocarditis are not specific for this diagnosis and should be interpreted in the context of the overall examination and the patient's history. There are also no physical findings that, when absent, are useful for ruling out the diagnosis. A prominent new murmur or skin lesion may arouse a clinical suspicion of endocarditis, but a murmur of valve regurgitation may be absent in patients with endocarditis. Vegetations may be present but may cause only slight regurgitation.

1. Fever—Fever is usually present by the time the patient seeks medical attention, although it may be intermittent or already resolved through inappropriate antibiotic treatment. It may be infrequently masked by severe comorbid conditions, such as alcoholic cirrhosis, immunosuppression, or malnutrition. The diversity of clinical syndromes associated with endocarditis does not permit generalizations about the temporal pattern or degree of fever. Recurrence of fever during treatment of endocarditis is an important problem (see section on failure of antibiotic therapy).

2. Cardiac examination—The cardiac examination in the patient with suspected or known endocarditis focuses on identifying which heart valves are infected, the hemodynamic severity of the resultant regurgitation (or stenosis), and the adequacy of the patient's circulatory state.

At the time of initial evaluation of a patient with suspected endocarditis, the value of a detected murmur may be low because there may be no reliable information about the patient's prior cardiac condition. Systolic murmurs, for example, are common in the general population and very frequent in older or hospitalized patients; they are usually due to LV outflow or degenerative sclerosis of the aortic valve. Because endocarditis rarely causes valve stenosis, a systolic murmur related to endocarditis is almost always regurgitant.

Specific auscultatory features occasionally may be useful in determining how a valve has been damaged by infection. In mitral valve endocarditis, the examination may help identify which mitral leaflet has become partially flail. If the mitral regurgitant murmur radiates to the patient's back, the jet is likely to be directed posteriorly as a result of anterior leaflet prolapse into the left atrium. If the murmur radiates to the upper parasternal area (mimicking aortic stenosis), the posterior leaflet is likely to have lost its support.

It is essential that the examiner carefully note and document the cardiac findings as soon as the diagnosis of endocarditis is suspected. In addition to murmurs, the clinician should pay close attention to those aspects of the examination related to hemodynamic consequences of valvular dysfunction. Signs of pulmonary edema, dysfunction of either ventricle, and a low-output state should be sought.

3. Skin and extremities—Assessment of the severity of extracardiac disease in endocarditis begins with a careful examination of the skin and peripheral circulation for evidence of vasculitis and emboli. Although these findings are not specific for the diagnosis of endocarditis, in the context of probable endocarditis, they strongly support that diagnosis. Their appearance during antibiotic therapy may signal the need for further diagnostic testing or a change in the treatment plan.

A. PETECHIAE—Examine the soft palate, buccal mucosa, conjunctiva, and the skin of the extremities for petechiae, which are often transient, appearing in crops and fading in 2–3 days.

B. SPLINTER HEMORRHAGES—These brown streaks are 1–2 mm in length and found under the fingernails and toenails. Lesions in the proximal nail bed are moderately specific for endocarditis, whereas similar lesions under the distal nails are commonly found in healthy persons with minor trauma to their hands.

C. ROTH SPOTS—Vasculitis affecting small arteries of the retina may, on rare occasions, produce retinal infarction. The resulting funduscopic lesion, usually seen near the optic disc, is a pale retinal patch surrounded by a darker ring of hemorrhage.

D. OSLER NODES—These painful indurated nodules are 2–15 mm in diameter and appear on the palms and soles and often involve the distal phalanges. They are usually multiple and, like petechiae, tend to occur in crops and fade over 2–3 days. Osler nodes are thought to be caused by either vasculitis or septic embolization.

E. JANEWAY LESIONS—These painless, flat red macules are similar in size and location to Osler nodes and usually persist longer than a few days. Their pathogenesis is uncertain but is suspected to be vasculitis.

F. BLUE-TOES SYNDROME—Embolization of small vegetation fragments may cause ischemia in the distal arterial distribution of an upper or lower extremity. The affected finger or toe is tender, mottled, and cyanotic; over a period of days to weeks, the area becomes black and develops dry gangrene. Management is usually conservative (see Embolism section, later in this chapter). Acute arterial occlusive ischemia of a larger portion of an extremity raises the possibility of a large vegetation from fungal endocarditis and is usually managed by embolectomy.

4. Neurologic examination—Neurologic involvement occurs in 15–20% of patients and can include infarct (ischemic or hemorrhagic), mycotic aneurysm, brain abscess, meningitis, or ventriculitis. Cerebral embolization in endocarditis signals a poor prognosis and has a major impact on the overall management approach. The neurologic examination is an integral part of the evaluation of any patient with known or suspected endocarditis. During antibiotic treatment, symptoms that may be of neurologic origin justify careful repeat examination, often with computed tomography (CT) or magnetic resonance imaging (MRI).

5. Abdominal examination—Splenomegaly occurs in patients with endocarditis as part of generalized hyperplasia of the reticuloendothelial system or from splenic infarction. Its presence usually indicates endocarditis of at least 10 days in duration. Marked splenomegaly may be accompanied by abdominal pain and left upper quadrant abdominal tenderness with palpation on physical examination.

D. Diagnostic Studies

1. Detection of blood-borne infection—Bacteremia or fungemia invariably occurs at some point during endocarditis. Bacteremia may be intermittent or of variable intensity depending on the virulence of the causative pathogen, the size of the vegetation, presence of an abscess, or prior treatment.

Blood cultures are integral to the diagnosis of endocarditis, and at least three cultures should be obtained, with the last being at least 1 hour separated in time from the first. Initiation of antibiotic therapy, however, should not be delayed if the suspicion of endocarditis is high and the patient is acutely ill. If there are intravascular lines present, a separate set of blood cultures should be drawn from the line to help differentiate isolated intravascular catheter-associated infection with concomitant peripheral bacteremia.

Blood cultures have been found positive for an infecting organism in 70–95% of cases of endocarditis reported in studies since 1970. Proper technique and timing of blood cultures can improve the positive yield. Potential causes of negative blood cultures in patients with endocarditis are shown in Table 22–5. When blood cultures remain negative at 24–48 hours in a patient with probable endocarditis,

Table 22–5. Causes of Negative Blood Cultures in Endocarditis

Failure to obtain more than one set of blood cultures
Prior antibiotic prescription (normally within 2–3 days of culture)
Organism fails to grow in standard culture (eg, fungi, rickettsiae, Q fever, psittacosis, nutritionally variant streptococci)
Intermittent bacteremia or fungemia (rare)

especially in the absence of recent antibiotic exposure, the most important concern is infection from unusual organisms, such as fungi, HACEK organisms, *Coxiella burnetii* (Q fever), *Chlamydophila psittaci*, or *Bartonella* and *Abiotrophia* species (nutritionally variant streptococci). The laboratory should be notified of the suspected diagnosis, and infectious disease consultation should be obtained. Additional testing that may be considered includes serology and molecular testing, as discussed in the following.

If antibiotics have already been started for another diagnosis, modification of the blood culture technique can increase the positive yield. The importance of recovering the causative organism may warrant stopping all antibiotics and repeating cultures.

If the suspicion for endocarditis remains moderate or high after the initial blood culture sets are drawn, empiric antibiotic therapy should also begin. The antibiotics should be changed according to the blood culture results as soon as these become available. If the initial blood cultures are negative after 24 hours but endocarditis is still suspected, three more sets should be obtained and processed under the guidance of an infectious disease specialist.

2. Serologic testing—Serologic testing can be helpful for identifying certain causes of endocarditis when blood cultures are negative. Positive antibody titers for Q fever (*C burnetii*), *Bartonella*, or *Brucella* in a patient with culture-negative endocarditis identify these organisms as the cause. Histoplasmosis antigen is highly specific for systemic infection by this organism. Although not essential to the diagnosis of endocarditis, nonspecific serologic testing is supportive and can be useful in certain situations. A positive rheumatoid factor is commonly found in patients with endocarditis of longer than 2 weeks in duration. This laboratory abnormality is not specific for endocarditis. When blood cultures are positive but other evidence of endocarditis is lacking or equivocal, a positive rheumatoid factor should prompt careful follow-up and retesting (eg, repeat TEE) for further evidence of endocarditis. Under some circumstances, these positive serologic tests may even warrant extension of antibiotic therapy to treat presumed endocarditis.

3. Additional testing considerations—In the age of molecular testing, broad-based polymerase chain reaction (PCR) and next-generation metagenomic sequencing of the blood or the tissue are increasingly utilized and may play a larger role in diagnosis of endocarditis. If surgery is performed, histology and molecular testing of the tissue can yield further information.

4. Echocardiography

A. Transthoracic echocardiography—Patients with suspected endocarditis should undergo TTE as soon as possible. It is noninvasive and recommended as the initial screening test for evaluation of valvular vegetation. The overall sensitivity of TTE is around 50–70% in native valves and 50% for prosthetic valves. A TTE showing typical vegetations is at least 90% specific for the diagnosis of endocarditis. TTE, however, cannot provide the detailed information regarding the anatomic extent of infection available from TEE. In patients with prosthetic valve endocarditis, the TTE image quality is often limited by the structural components of the prosthesis. In addition, TTE is inadequate for evaluating the perivalvular area and assessing for abscess, fistula, or pseudoaneurysm. According to guidelines from the American Heart Association, endorsed by the Infectious Disease Society of America, TTE alone is adequate in evaluating patients when infective endocarditis is suspected but with low clinical suspicion in a low-risk patient (eg, fever in a patient with known heart murmur and no other stigmata or history of infective endocarditis). In addition, when a vegetation is identified on TTE, subsequent TEE may be deferred if there are no high-risk clinical or TTE imaging features including large or mobile vegetation, valvular insufficiency, perivalvular extension, or secondary ventricular dysfunction. However, when the quality of TTE is suboptimal, clinical suspicion for infective endocarditis is moderate or high, and the patient is at high risk (eg, prosthetic heart valves, congenital heart disease, known cardiac structural defects, previous endocarditis, new murmur, heart failure, or presence of other stigmata of endocarditis), a TEE should be pursued.

TTE has a valuable ancillary role in patients with known endocarditis. It is well suited to assess cardiac chamber dilatation, left and right ventricular dysfunction, and the patient's hemodynamic status. Presystolic closure of the mitral valve on TTE is a sign of elevated LV end-diastolic pressure and is an indication that the patient with aortic regurgitation should be considered for surgery. Similarly, right atrial and pulmonary artery pressures can be estimated by transthoracic Doppler examination. Additional Doppler data are essential to assess the severity and hemodynamic sequelae of mitral regurgitation, including elevated left atrial pressure. Changes in the patient's clinical status during treatment often can be readily diagnosed by comparison of serial TTE studies.

B. Transesophageal echocardiography—With its detailed images of the heart valves and related structures, TEE is highly sensitive and specific for the diagnosis of endocarditis and is essential to defining the extent of disease. A TEE that shows a mass with the characteristics of a vegetation has a specificity of more than 90% for endocarditis (in the absence of a history of endocarditis, since it is difficult to distinguish between old and new vegetations). A normal TEE does not rule out endocarditis, but it has a negative predictive accuracy of at least 90%. Because false-normal TEE studies can occur, however, a patient with a normal study but a high clinical suspicion of endocarditis should be either observed carefully or treated, depending on the clinical severity of the illness. The TEE should be repeated if needed, especially in the setting of clinical signs of worsening cardiac

Table 22–6. Diagnostic Imaging for Infective Endocarditis

Diagnostic Imaging	Native Valve		Prosthetic Valve		Considerations
	Sensitivity	Specificity	Sensitivity	Specificity	
Transthoracic echocardiogram (TTE)	50–70%	90–95%	30–50%	< 30%	Low-risk, noninvasive test. Recommended initial diagnostic imaging for evaluation of IE.
Transoesophageal echocardiogram (TEE)	90–100%	90–100%	80–90%	80–90%	Invasive but with higher sensitivity and specificity for diagnosis of IE, especially for PVE, and recommended for evaluation of complications such as perivalvular abscess
Positron emission tomography-computed tomography (PET-CT)	70–80%	70–85%	75–85%	65–80%	Possible adjunctive diagnostic test for diagnostically challenging cases of IE, especially involving PVE. The test may also detect extracardiac foci of infection.

IE, infective endocarditis; PVE, prosthetic valve endocarditis.

function, persistent bacteremia, or new systemic emboli or foci of infection despite appropriate antimicrobial therapy.

(1) Classification—Transesophageal echocardiographic studies in patients with suspected endocarditis may be classified according to the probability of the disease. A useful scheme is based on four categories: normal, possible, probable, and almost certain. In the **normal** category, no substrate for endocarditis or other abnormalities is present. The TEE findings are classified as **possible endocarditis** in the presence of valve disease, such as a prosthetic heart valve, rheumatic or degenerative valvular sclerosis, or valve regurgitation likely to be pathologic, that predispose the patient to endocarditis—but without evidence of lesions. The classification of **probable endocarditis** is used when less-specific lesions are found. Examples of such abnormalities include localized leaflet thickening or a nonmobile leaflet-related mass (especially if the lesion has the reflectance of soft rather than sclerotic tissue), mitral or aortic valve prolapse, chordal rupture, intracardiac thrombi, and paravalvular regurgitation in patients with prosthetic valves. Patients with no history of endocarditis who have a lesion very strongly associated with infective endocarditis fall into the **almost certain** category. In such cases, TEE shows an intracardiac mass with typical vegetation characteristics—a pedunculated mass attached near the leaflet tip and prolapsing during valve closure into the lower pressure chamber. Vegetations have soft-tissue reflectance (like myocardium) and vibratory or rotatory motion independent of the motion of the leaflet. Vegetations apparent on TEE vary in length from 1 or 2 mm to several centimeters.

Other lesions considered almost certain for endocarditis would be an abscess or fistula, a metastatic vegetation, and an aneurysm of the intervalvular fibrosa. An abscess appears on TEE as an echolucent space adjacent to a valve annulus or prosthetic sewing ring. The abscess often appears to be separated from adjacent structures by a thin septa, and jets of blood flowing into the abscess during systole or diastole (depending on abscess location) may be shown by color Doppler interrogation. The abscess is considered a fistula when there is communication with two or more adjacent cardiac chambers or blood vessels. Metastatic vegetations appear on echocardiography as vibratory or rotatory masses attached to an endocardial surface at a site struck by a regurgitant jet.

It should be noted that this TEE classification scheme is appropriate only in patients with other reasons to suspect endocarditis (eg, unexplained fever, positive blood cultures) and no prior history of endocarditis.

(2) Diagnostic accuracy—Sensitivity and specificity ranges for diagnostic imaging tests are summarized in Table 22–6. Possible causes of false TEE results are shown in Table 22–7. Of particular importance is the possibility that TEE findings may be normal because endothelial infection may be in the vasculature rather than in the heart. Because vascular infection is rare in the absence of prior vascular surgery, the diagnosis is usually suspected based on the patient's

Table 22–7. Causes of False Results of Transesophageal Echocardiography

False-Abnormal
Myxomatous mitral valve disease
Papillary fibroelastomas
Partially flail leaflet
Healed vegetations
Mitral valve strands
Nodules of Arantius (aortic valve)
Lambl excrescences
False-Normal
Aortic valve prosthesis
Mitral valve mechanical prosthesis (includes shadowing of aortic valve by a mitral prosthesis)
Calcified aortic root shadowing tricuspid or pulmonic valves
Mitral annular calcification
Aortic atheroma or aneurysm infection
Study done too early in disease course

history. Nevertheless, the TEE examination in patients with suspected endocarditis routinely includes the thoracic aorta. TEE may identify severe atherosclerosis with mobile atheroma or thrombi. Although these abnormalities are not nearly as specific for infection as are intracardiac vegetations, the clinical picture may justify antibiotic treatment.

In general, less than 10% of TEE results are falsely abnormal. By causing thickened, prolapsing leaflets and ruptured chordae, a myxomatous mitral valve can closely mimic endocarditis. A benign leaflet tumor, called a **papillary fibroelastoma,** may give the appearance of a vegetation. Several other abnormalities seen by TEE have lower specificity for the diagnosis of endocarditis than do typical vegetations; examples include para-aortic cavities (potentially representing either an abscess or an aneurysm of the sinus of Valsalva) and paraprosthetic regurgitation. Clinical context is often crucial to the interpretation of these findings. The paraneoplastic syndrome of myxomas may mimic endocarditis, although usually location and morphologic features of myxomas distinguish them from thrombi or vegetations. Intracardiac thrombi may be innocent bystanders in a patient with a clinical syndrome suggesting endocarditis, or they may be secondarily infected.

Lambl excrescences are thin, strand-like structures extending 1–10 mm from the valve leaflet margins. Because they prolapse and exhibit hypermobility, Lambl excrescences can be mistaken for small vegetations. Nodules of Arantius are similar extensions, not more than a few millimeters in length, from the center of the aortic cusp margin. When the aortic valve is closed, a TEE may show these nodules prolapsing from the center of the valve.

In addition to detecting vegetations, TEE usually provides a detailed picture of the extent of cardiac infection; it is very accurate at assessing the exact size and location of vegetations. Several complicated forms of cardiac involvement are usually identifiable by TEE. Because many of these complex lesions require surgery, TEE should be performed as soon as possible in a patient with a moderate or high suspicion of endocarditis.

Prophylaxis for endocarditis is not indicated prior to TEE.

C. Positron emission tomography-computed tomography (PET-CT)—There is growing evidence for the utility of PET-CT in diagnostically challenging cases of infective endocarditis. Current literature suggests that PET-CT carries sensitivity and specificity rates higher than TTE for both native valve and prosthetic valve endocarditis. In addition, this imaging may detect clinically relevant extracardiac foci of infection. PET-CT may be considered for patients with a high clinical suspicion for endocarditis with negative TTE findings and have relative or absolute contraindications for TEE (eg, structural esophageal conditions such as esophageal stricture or tracheoesophageal fistula).

5. Electrocardiography and chest radiography—The electrocardiogram (ECG) is occasionally useful in alerting the clinician to the severity of endocarditis. In patients with known or suspected aortic valve endocarditis, the PR interval should be monitored closely for prolongation, an indication of aortic annular abscess formation. Less frequently, the ECG may show increased QRS voltage and a precordial strain pattern in patients with either severe aortic or mitral regurgitation and marked LV enlargement. The chest radiograph is primarily useful in evaluating the patient with suspected endocarditis to assess the presence and severity of pulmonary edema and to detect septic pulmonary emboli in patients with possible right-heart endocarditis.

Management

A. Initial Decisions

Management of newly diagnosed endocarditis requires the physician to make two decisions promptly. The first is whether to initiate empiric antibiotic therapy based on available clinical information or to await confirmation of the diagnosis and information about the infecting organism to select the optimal regimen. The second decision is whether valve surgery is indicated immediately or can be deferred to allow assessment of the patient's response to antibiotic therapy.

Both decisions depend on the extent of cardiac infection (usually characterized by TEE), the severity of the patient's symptoms and signs of infection, the patient's circulatory status, the seriousness of extracardiac complications, and the available data about the organism.

Once initial treatment is under way, the physician must maintain a high level of vigilance for evidence of an inadequate response to treatment or the development of complications that will require additional medical or surgical intervention.

B. Antibiotic Therapy

The goal of antibiotic therapy is to sterilize vegetations. For most causative organisms, this is an achievable goal and will cure the patient if cardiac abscess or other complications requiring surgery have not occurred. Vegetations, however, provide proliferating organisms with an environment that is protected against both the patient's immune system and antibiotics. Organisms grow under the surface of the vegetation where phagocytes cannot penetrate, and bacterial metabolism is slowed within the nutrient-poor vegetation, contributing to antibiotic resistance. For these reasons, antibiotic treatment is directed toward achieving bactericidal concentrations of drug within the vegetation over an extended period. It must be noted that certain important aspects of antibiotic dosing, especially in seriously ill patients, are beyond the scope of this text, and infectious disease consultation is advised.

1. Principles of antibiotic therapy

A. In vitro sensitivity testing—The choice of definitive therapy depends on in vitro sensitivity testing of the strain infecting the patient as well as existing data on effective treatment approaches. An organism's sensitivity to an antibiotic is quantified by the minimum inhibitory concentration (MIC). The MIC is defined as the minimum concentration of antibiotic that prevents proliferation of the organism in a standardized culture system. Choice of antibiotic is based on multiple additional factors, such as published data, expert opinion, presence of prosthetic material, and allergic history. Expert consultation should be sought when determining appropriate therapy.

B. Drug combinations—Combinations of drugs with additive, or synergistic, killing power are used frequently for treating endocarditis. A common combination is a β-lactam antibiotic (the penicillins and cephalosporins) with an aminoglycoside. This combination is synergistic because the β-lactam drug damages the bacterial cell wall, which allows more rapid penetration of the aminoglycoside into the cell.

C. Parenteral treatment—Antibiotic treatment must be given parenterally to ensure high and consistent serum drug levels and compliance. Outpatient intravenous drug therapy can be undertaken under specific conditions (see section on Outpatient Treatment). Transition to oral antibiotic therapy after an initial 2–3 weeks of intravenous antibiotics may be considered in low-risk patients with infective endocarditis due to a subset of organisms without complications. The decision to transition to an oral therapy should only be made after consulting with an infectious disease specialist.

D. Prolonged treatment—The duration of antibiotic administration is almost always for a month or more. Prolonged exposure of the patient to antibiotics can lead to frequent side effects and serious toxicity (monitoring antibiotic therapy is discussed in the following section). Duration of therapy is most often defined as the time from first negative blood cultures. If the patient is taken to surgery and valve cultures are positive, the duration of therapy should be counted from the date of surgery. If valve cultures are negative, it is reasonable to count the duration before surgery toward the overall duration of therapy. While initiating treatment for endocarditis, it is important to repeat blood cultures every 48–72 hours until negative.

2. Empiric antibiotic therapy—Empiric antibiotic therapy is the initiation of antibiotics for the purpose of treating endocarditis before identifying the causative organism. Ideally, empiric therapy is needed only briefly until culture and sensitivity data are available. It requires treating the patient broadly for the most likely infecting organisms based on demographic factors and clinical presentation and can subject the patient to the additional risk of receiving multiple antibiotics over a prolonged period. At the minimum, blood cultures should be collected prior to initiating empiric antibiotic therapy.

3. Outpatient treatment—Outpatient parenteral antibiotic therapy (OPAT), now widely used, can provide an excellent outcome while allowing shorter hospital stays. Careful patient selection and management are mandatory. OPAT can be initiated once the patient is clinically deemed appropriate for hospital discharge and can occur within a few days of starting intravenous antibiotic therapy if the patient is at low risk for complications, namely embolic phenomena and heart failure. Factors to consider in making the decision to transition to OPAT include virulence of the organism, blood culture clearance, extent of valve involvement, size of vegetation, and tolerance of therapy.

The dynamics of OPAT care is changing rapidly. OPAT is frequently offered to patients on discharge to home. In home settings, at least once weekly nursing visits are required to check vitals, evaluate the intravenous line and change dressings, and ensure that the patient is not experiencing any complications or side effects. Laboratory monitoring is concurrently done, at least on a once weekly occurrence for close monitoring, and is tailored to the specific antibiotic therapy administered and the patient's baseline results. Access to a health provider, including an infectious disease specialist, and a nearby health-care facility is important in case of any treatment complications that require an urgent evaluation.

4. Monitoring antibiotic therapy

A. Drug levels—Therapeutic drug monitoring is important for certain drugs used for treatment of endocarditis, such as vancomycin and gentamicin, both to ensure therapeutic window and to prevent toxicity. Consultation with an infectious disease specialist is recommended for assistance with dosing and monitoring of these drugs. In general, vancomycin trough levels are measured at steady-state (30 minutes before the fourth dose), with any changes in dosing, and weekly once on stable dosing. Gentamicin trough levels should be measured to monitor for and prevent nephrotoxicity. To ensure therapeutic drug levels, gentamicin peak levels are monitored for thrice-daily dosing and random levels for once-daily dosing.

B. Adverse effects—Adverse effects vary by drug. For β-lactam antibiotics, common adverse effects are allergic reaction, which can be either immunoglobulin E (IgE)-mediated or not, and gastrointestinal upset. In the setting of a rash, systemic involvement or signs of IgE-mediated reaction (hives, anaphylaxis) should be ruled out. If ruled out, it is preferable to continue the antibiotic and treat the symptoms. For patients with a history of β-lactam allergy, a careful history is crucial for determining whether a rechallenge with an alternative β-lactam is safe and appropriate. Skin testing and desensitization are options to allow for treatment of allergic patients with culprit drugs and can be done in consultation with an allergy/immunology specialist. The sodium content of β-lactam antibiotics may require diuretic therapy in patients with heart failure.

For patients receiving vancomycin and gentamicin, renal toxicity is a major concern. Ototoxicity is an idiosyncratic reaction unrelated to aminoglycoside levels that occurs in 10–20% of cases. Baseline audiometry should be obtained for all patients receiving long-term courses of these medications.

All patients on intravenous antibiotics should have complete blood counts and renal function checked at least weekly to evaluate for bone marrow or renal toxicity. As discussed earlier, therapeutic drug monitoring is sometimes indicated as well. Patients receiving daptomycin should have weekly creatinine kinase levels checked. Any patient with a drug rash should have liver biochemical tests (aspartate aminotransferase and alkaline phosphatase) checked to rule out hepatic involvement. Additional laboratory tests may include inflammatory markers including c-reactive protein and sedimentation rate. In general, laboratory monitoring is tailored to the antibiotic prescribed and the patient's baseline results.

Diarrhea may occur during antibiotic therapy; this is usually due to overgrowth of gut organisms competing with those sensitive to the antibiotic. An important consideration is *Clostridium difficile* colitis which requires treatment and does not merit interruption in systemic antibiotic therapy unless the colitis is very severe (eg, megacolon).

Drug fever is a consideration in the patient who is clinically well but remains febrile while receiving antibiotic therapy. This is a diagnosis of exclusion, and treatment failure should be ruled out before invoking this diagnosis.

C. Management of Complications

1. Failure of antibiotic therapy—Changes in the cardiac examination during antibiotic treatment are particularly important in detecting failure of medical therapy. Changes in a regurgitant murmur almost always indicate valve dysfunction, and the appearance of a new murmur may signal metastatic infection of another valve. Such new findings almost always warrant repeat echocardiography and blood cultures. There may also be an increase in the resting sinus rate and the appearance of heart failure. In aortic valve endocarditis, an abrupt increase in the pulse pressure should raise suspicion of worsening or new aortic regurgitation.

Failure of antibiotic therapy is usually heralded by persistent or recurrent fever. Persistent fever is defined as continuing for more than a week during antibiotic treatment. Recurrent fever develops after an afebrile period of several days and occurs at least a week after initiation of antibiotics. Persistent infection is only one cause of fever in this setting; others include hypersensitivity to antibiotics and other drugs, phlebitis, silent emboli (especially pulmonary and splenic), protected foci of infection (eg, epidural abscess or a septic joint that requires irrigation and drainage), intercurrent hospital-acquired infection, or simply a delayed response to antibiotic therapy. Blood cultures should be obtained and efforts made to rule out these possibilities. If blood cultures are negative, and the patient shows no other evidence of deterioration, watchful waiting is appropriate.

Positive blood cultures lasting for more than 1 week of antibiotic therapy strongly suggest persistent infection. The cause may be either antibiotic resistance or a protected site of infection. The site may be an intracardiac annular or myocardial abscess or an extracardiac site of metastatic infection, septic embolization, or mycotic aneurysm. Repeat TTE and/or TEE is strongly indicated. Careful comparison to the studies obtained at the time of initial diagnosis may detect intracardiac suppurative complications; there is a sensitivity range of 80–90%. If TEE findings are abnormal, urgent surgery is indicated. If they are normal, a careful history and physical examination coupled with imaging studies (CT, MRI, or nuclear medicine scan) guided by examination abnormalities and symptoms will often reveal an infective focus.

2. Worsening valve dysfunction and heart failure—At any time during the course of infective endocarditis, heart failure symptoms and signs may appear as a result of worsening regurgitation and failure of ventricular compensatory mechanisms. In fact, heart failure may appear despite effective antibiotic therapy—and even after bacteriologic cure. The onset of heart failure may be insidious and difficult to recognize, or it may be abrupt and catastrophic. Frequent appraisal of the patient's status by history and physical examination is the best way to ensure early detection of heart failure. Any change in the patient's regurgitant murmur during antibiotic therapy usually signifies progression of valvular dysfunction and the likely need for surgery. A persistent tachycardia or slowly increasing heart rate is a useful sign of impending heart failure prior to the appearance of the typical signs such as lung crackles, S_3, and pulmonary vascular redistribution on chest radiograph. In patients with aortic valve endocarditis, the appearance of a widened pulse pressure usually indicates increased valve regurgitation.

Serial TTE or TEE is useful in confirming a suspected change in the patient's hemodynamic status; it may even identify the cause. Worsening of the mitral regurgitant lesion is suggested by an increase in size of the color-flow Doppler jet or an increase in the radius of the flow convergence region on the LV side of the regurgitant orifice. A rise in transmitral early filling velocity (E wave) and a fall in forward systolic pulmonary venous flow (S wave) may indicate a rise in mean left atrial pressure.

In the case of aortic regurgitation, jet enlargement over time is also a useful indicator of worsening regurgitation. Additional indications of severe aortic regurgitation include closure of the mitral valve on M-mode echocardiography prior to the onset of the QRS and shortening of the pressure half-time of the aortic regurgitation velocity, both from a rapid rise of LV pressure to a high level in late diastole. For either mitral or aortic regurgitation, the presence or development of a hyperdynamic left ventricle (increased ejection fraction, stroke volume, or both) and progressive LV dilatation on two-dimensional echocardiography are useful indirect indications of an excessive regurgitant burden. The appearance of pulmonary or right atrial hypertension, as estimated from tricuspid jet velocity and inferior vena cava dynamics, is another sign of hemodynamic decompensation. TEE has the additional major advantage of being able to detect the intracardiac complications accounting for the change in the patient's hemodynamic status.

If heart failure is mild, surgery may be deferred while diuretics and afterload-reducing drugs are given to optimize the patient's hemodynamic status. If the patient responds readily to therapy, surgery might be optional. In most cases, however, surgery should be undertaken as soon as feasible because it is almost certain that valve repair or replacement will be required eventually (for the hemodynamic lesion, if not for infection), and the patient's surgical risk is lowest at this early stage. One clear exception to surgery for mild heart failure is sodium overload (related to antibiotic therapy) and suspected valve dysfunction not confirmed by echocardiography.

If heart failure is moderate or severe, valve surgery should be undertaken immediately while drug therapy is used to stabilize the patient. Because of the difficulty in predicting the rate of progression of valve dysfunction, delaying surgery for hemodynamic optimization is ill-advised. Rapid development of heart failure may signal the occurrence of a major intracardiac complication, such as leaflet perforation, chordal rupture, or fistula formation. Preoperative or intraoperative TEE is usually helpful in guiding surgical planning in this setting.

3. Embolism—Embolism most often occurs early in the course of antibiotic therapy but can occur at any time, even after biologic cure. Suspected cerebral embolism should be evaluated immediately by CT; if necessary, cerebral angiography should be performed in order to rule out an intracranial mycotic aneurysm. Non-hemorrhagic infarcts may warrant measures to reduce cerebral edema.

If the patient is already receiving anticoagulant therapy prior to the development of endocarditis, anticoagulation may be continued. When cerebral embolism in a patient with endocarditis is diagnosed, however, anticoagulation therapy is usually discontinued (if possible) for 14–30 days to reduce the risk of massive intracerebral bleeding. If stroke occurs in mechanical prosthetic valve endocarditis, the balance of risks and benefits of continuing anticoagulation is unknown. In patients with stroke from endocarditis, serial neurologic examinations and (if a change is suspected) repeated CT scans are indicated to permit early detection of brain abscess.

Because no clinically useful means (including echocardiography) has been found to identify patients at high risk for embolism, valve surgery in endocarditis is not indicated to prevent embolism. Surgery may be advised if the patient has had more than one episode and has a persistent vegetation.

Peripheral embolization is managed conservatively and without anticoagulation whenever possible. Vascular surgery to restore the circulation may be indicated if major organ embolization becomes life-threatening. Embolectomy is generally indicated in culture-negative endocarditis to evaluate for a diagnosis; likely organisms include *Aspergillus*, *Candida*, and the HACEK group. Embolectomy is necessary, strictly for treatment, in fungal endocarditis to remove as much infection as possible from the circulation.

4. Mycotic aneurysm—A complaint of severe headache or visual disturbance (especially homonymous hemianopsia) in a patient with endocarditis should prompt an urgent CT scan for the possibility of an expanding intracranial mycotic aneurysm. This catastrophic complication may also present as a subarachnoid or intracerebral hemorrhage, usually massive. If the scan is negative, cerebral angiography is often necessary to confirm or rule out the diagnosis. Treatment may require surgical removal if the patient's condition will allow. Urgent neurosurgical consultation is recommended.

5. Myocardial infarction—Chest pain in the course of infective endocarditis is most likely due to myocardial infarction, pericarditis, or septic pulmonary embolization. Myocardial infarction during infective endocarditis is almost always caused by coronary embolization, although it may occasionally complicate purulent pericarditis or myocardial abscess. In the latter setting, inflammatory thrombosis of the artery probably occurs. Treatment is noninterventional. Anticoagulation is generally not indicated because its benefits for reducing myocardial ischemia in this setting are unknown and the risks of potential cerebral embolization are significant.

6. Pericarditis—The possibility of purulent pericarditis complicating infective endocarditis should be evaluated by TTE. If pericardial fluid is seen, prompt pericardiocentesis is needed. A transudate may be present; in this infrequent case, management can be conservative. Usually, a purulent exudate will be found, necessitating surgical drainage or pericardiectomy. Most importantly, purulent pericarditis may signal the presence of an intracardiac abscess. A TEE is indicated in this setting, and if an abscess is found, surgical drainage and valve surgery should be performed. Fortunately, the treatment of these related problems can be performed in a single operation. If an underlying myocardial abscess is not found, a pericardial window may be sufficient therapy. Continued observation is indicated because of the risk of subsequent additional cardiac or pericardial suppurative complications.

D. Management of High-Risk Endocarditis

1. Prosthetic valve endocarditis—Far higher morbidity and mortality rates are associated with prosthetic valve endocarditis than with native valve endocarditis. Infection of a prosthesis by fungi carries a mortality rate of more than 90%, whereas prosthetic infection from streptococci has a mortality rate of approximately 30%. In addition, the mortality rate from prosthetic valve endocarditis early after implantation is around twice that of late infection (after 2 months). Survival is improved by early operation in most cases when the patient's surgical risk is acceptable. Surgical replacement is necessary in 85% of cases of biologic valve

Table 22–8. Indications for Surgery in Prosthetic Valve Endocarditis

Mechanical prosthesis (almost all cases)
Bioprosthesis if:
New paravalvular regurgitation or fistula
Sewing-ring abscess or dehiscence
Infection from *Staphylococcus epidermidis* or *aureus*, *Enterococcus*, gram-negative bacteria, or fungi
Blood cultures still positive after 1 week of antibiotics
Embolism or other major complication

endocarditis and in almost all cases of mechanical prosthetic infection. Indications for surgery in prosthetic valve endocarditis are summarized in Table 22–8.

Medical treatment can be attempted in mechanical valve endocarditis when the surgical risk is very high and the only evidence of valve involvement (using TEE) is a vegetation in the area of the sewing ring. In such cases, serial TEE may be useful to monitor valve function and the response of the infected mass to treatment. Initial medical treatment of bioprosthetic endocarditis may be attempted when infection is due to a low-risk organism (such as *Streptococcus*) and involvement is limited to a vegetation on either the prosthetic leaflets or sewing ring. Repeat TEE is very useful if the patient does not respond to antibiotics. Blood cultures should be obtained every 4–7 days during treatment and weekly for a month following apparently successful treatment.

2. Fungal endocarditis—Overall mortality rates for fungal endocarditis are more than 80%; they are especially high in cases caused by *Aspergillus* and *Candida* species. Treatment requires the close collaboration of the primary physician, cardiologist, surgeon, and infectious disease specialist. Treatment is almost always a combination of valve replacement and a full course of an antifungal agent. Late relapses are common and require prolonged surveillance for years following successful completion of antifungal therapy. In addition to serologic tests and blood cultures, TEE is useful in monitoring the patient during and after treatment. Some clinicians have advocated long-term suppressive therapy with an oral azole agent if the organism is susceptible for patients who survive the surgical and medical therapies for the acute infection. Involvement of extracardiac sites, particularly endophthalmitis, needs to be carefully evaluated.

3. Endocarditis from gram-negative bacteria—*Pseudomonas* endocarditis carries a mortality rate of almost 80% because of the frequent inability to sterilize vegetations by medical treatment. Among the causes for this inability is the frequent emergence of antibiotic-resistant bacterial strains during therapy. Surgery is usually performed as soon as possible after the diagnosis of *Pseudomonas* endocarditis of the left-sided valves. Surgery is also frequently indicated for endocarditis caused by the HACEK organisms, but here the reason is extensive valvular destruction by the time of diagnosis. In contrast to *Pseudomonas,* infection from HACEK organisms is readily cured by antibiotics. The treatment of endocarditis from enteric gram-negative bacteria should be tailored based on in vitro antibiotic sensitivity testing, and combination therapy may be recommended based on the causative pathogen.

E. Surgery

The indications for valve replacement or repair during infective endocarditis (discussed in the preceding section) are summarized in Table 22–9. The indications and timing of valve surgery are guided by several important principles. Surgical morbidity and mortality rates are much higher if the patient is in even mild heart failure, is hypotensive, or has a low cardiac output when sent to the operating room. Similarly, uncontrolled infection, with its attendant systemic stress and peripheral dilatation, confers a higher surgical risk. Patient's age and comorbidities may prohibit surgery. In the absence of these factors, surgical risk is generally low despite active infective endocarditis. Surgery should not be delayed with the intention of prolonging preoperative antibiotic therapy. It has never been shown that either the risk of reinfection of the new prosthetic valve or surgical complications are reduced by longer preoperative antibiotic treatment but may delay necessary surgery and increase perioperative complications.

The anatomic location and extent of valve involvement and other factors may allow valve debridement and repair rather than replacement. The advantages of valve repair are that future anticoagulation is not needed, and subsequent valve replacement carries a lower risk. The disadvantages of valve repair are the greater possibility of residual infected tissue and significant valve regurgitation. Valve repair is not considered in the presence of abscess or fistula near the valve or when significant leaflet erosion has occurred. As part of a repair, however, leaflet perforation can be patched

Table 22–9. Indications for Valve Surgery in Native Valve Endocarditis

Absolute Indications
Annular or aortic abscess, fistula, or heart block
Left heart failure from severe regurgitation or (rarely) obstruction
Endocarditis caused by *Staphylococcus aureus,* fungi, and highly resistant organisms
Bacteremia despite optimal antibiotic therapy for 5–7 days
Relative Indications
Mild heart failure in an otherwise uncomplicated case
Recurrent embolization with persistent vegetation
Purulent pericarditis
Large (> 10 mm) mobile vegetations
Recurrent life-threatening septic pulmonary emboli
Severe tricuspid regurgitation with a low-output state

and chordal support reconstructed. In general, valve repair is feasible when excision of the infected leaflet with a 2-mm margin of normal tissue will still leave enough normal leaflet to preserve valvular competence. Preoperative or intraoperative TEE is usually indicated for surgical planning and guidance.

For patients with native tricuspid valve endocarditis who are critically ill or with a high preoperative risk, AngioVac may be an effective alternative. AngioVac is a vacuum-based device that uses a venous drainage cannula and extracorporeal circuit to remove vegetations, emboli, or thrombi present in the right heart. This procedure has been used to remove vegetations or debulk large vegetations causing infective endocarditis thereby reducing infectious burden and decreasing further risk of septic embolization.

F. Follow-Up After Endocarditis

Long-term survival of the patient following an episode of endocarditis is much lower than that of the general population. Overall survival following native valve endocarditis is approximately 80% at 5 years and 50% at 10 years. Survival is considerably lower after prosthetic valve endocarditis. The patient remains at risk for three consequences of the disease: relapse of the original infection, noninfective sequelae of the infection, and recurrent endocarditis.

Failure to eradicate infection completely is usually apparent within 2 weeks after antibiotics are discontinued, although relapse has been reported up to 6 months after apparently successful treatment. Relapse rates tend to be low with Viridans streptococci (< 5%), intermediate with enterococci (8–20%), and high with *Pseudomonas* and fungi (> 20%). Relapse of *S aureus* endocarditis is not common (5%) but should prompt a search for an extracardiac source. Treatment of a relapse beyond instituting appropriate antibiotics includes a reassessment of the extent of cardiac infection, and careful consideration for surgery.

After successful treatment of infection, the patient remains at risk for the development of heart failure, stroke, and rupture of a mycotic aneurysm. A new baseline TTE should be obtained after the treatment completion. If the patient had moderate or severe valve regurgitation or an episode of heart failure prior to hospital discharge, the probability of late heart failure is greatly increased. The risk of embolic stroke is very low after the first 4 weeks of antibiotic treatment but may persist for an unknown length of time. Rupture of a mycotic aneurysm after treatment is also rare but should be considered when a patient with stroke has a history of prior endocarditis.

Although estimates vary, recurrent endocarditis, defined as a repeat episode after more than 6 months, occurs in approximately 5–8% of cases. Controversy exists regarding the tendency for the infecting organism and the involved valve to be similar to those of the original episode. The recurrent episode probably carries a higher mortality rate than the original one. Risk factors for recurrent endocarditis include injecting drug use, congenital heart disease, rheumatic and myxomatous disease, existing prosthetic valve, and periodontitis. Any new febrile illness requires three sets of blood cultures before starting antibiotic therapy.

G. Prophylaxis

All patients with endocarditis should have thorough and regular dental evaluation. Patients with a history of prior infective endocarditis involving native or prosthetic valve should receive antibiotic prophylaxis prior to dental procedures involving manipulation of gingival tissue or the periapical region of the teeth or perforation of the oral mucosa. Also, it is reasonable to give antibiotic prophylaxis for those with prosthetic valves or material (eg, patches, closure devices), unrepaired cyanotic congenital heart disease, repaired congenital heart disease with residual shunts, and postcardiac transplant patients with structural valve disease. More controversial is antibiotic prophylaxis for patients with moderate to severe valvular disease. For adults, the recommendation is to administer the antibiotic 30–60 minutes prior to the dental procedure. Recommended therapies are summarized in Table 22–10.

Table 22–10. Prophylactic Antibiotics Prior to Dental Procedures When Indicated

Route	Antibiotic	Dosing; single dose (adults)
No allergies to penicillin or ampicillin		
Oral	Amoxicillin	2 g
Intravenous or Intramuscular[1]	Ampicillin	2 g
	Cefazolin	1 g
	Ceftriaxone	1 g
Allergic to penicillin or ampicillin[2]		
Oral	Cephalexin	2 g
	Azithromycin	500 mg
	Doxycycline	100 mg
Intravenous or Intramuscular	Cefazolin	1 g
	Ceftriaxone	1g

[1]Intravenous and intramuscular antibiotic administration is recommended for patients who cannot take oral medication.
[2]Individuals with severe allergy to penicillin or ampicillin (eg, anaphylaxis), there may be a small risk of cross-reactivity with cephalosporins and detailed allergy history as well as consultation with an allergist is advised when considering this class of medications as an alternative.

Baddour LM, Wilson WR, Bayer AS, et al. Infective endocarditis in adults: diagnosis, antimicrobial therapy, and management of complications: a scientific statement for healthcare professionals from the American Heart Association: endorsed by the Infectious Diseases Society of America. *Circulation.* 2015;132(15):1435–1486. [PMID: 26373316]

Cahill TJ, Prendergast BD. Infective endocarditis. *Lancet.* 2016 Feb 27;387(10021):882–893. [PMID: 26341945]

Iversen K, Ihlemann N, Gill SU, et al. Partial oral versus intravenous antibiotic treatment of endocarditis. *N Engl J Med.* 2019; 380:415–424. [PMID: 30152252]

Pizzi M, Roque A, Fernández-Hidalgo N, et al. Improving the diagnosis of infective endocarditis in prosthetic valves and intracardiac devices with 18F-fluordeoxyglucose positron emission tomography/ compute tomography angiography: initial results at an infective endocarditis referral center. *Circulation.* 2015;132:1113–1126. [PMID: 26276890]

Rao VP, Wu J, Gillott R, Baig MW, Kaul P, Sandoe JAT. Impact of the duration of antibiotic therapy on relapse and survival following surgery for active infective endocarditis. *Eur J Cardiothorac Surg.* 2019;55:760–765. [PMID: 30307552]

Schranz A, Barocas JA. Infective endocarditis in persons who use drugs: epidemiology, current management, and emerging treatments. *Infect Dis Clin North Am.* 2020;34(3):479–493. [PMID: 32782097]

Wang A, Gaca JG, Chu VH. Management considerations in infective endocarditis: a review. *JAMA.* 2018 Jul 3;320(1):72–83. [PMID: 29971402]

Wilson WR, Gewitz M, Lockhart PB, et al. Prevention of viridans group streptococcal infective endocarditis: a scientific statement from the American Heart Association. *Circulation.* 2021 May 18;143(20):e963–978. [PMID: 33853363]

23 Hypertrophic Cardiomyopathy

Karthik Ananthasubramaniam, MD

ESSENTIALS OF DIAGNOSIS

Note: Not all criteria are needed for the diagnosis of hypertrophic cardiomyopathy.

- Asymmetric hypertrophied nondilated ventricle with septal to posterior wall end-diastolic thickness ratio more than 1.3 not explained by other etiologies.
- Ejection murmur that increases with Valsalva with or without concomitant mitral regurgitation murmur and preserved aortic second sound.
- Increased gradients causing obstruction across left ventricular outflow tract and/or mid ventricle with characteristic late peaking "dagger"-shaped Doppler velocity profile.
- Mitral valve apparatus structural abnormalities and systolic anterior motion with varying degree of mitral regurgitation.
- Midsystolic aortic valve closure.
- Impaired diastolic function with decrease in tissue Doppler peak early diastolic velocity (e′) and global longitudinal strain.

General Considerations

A. Definition & Prevalence

Hypertrophic cardiomyopathy (HCM) is a disorder of the myocardium caused by mutations of the sarcomere or sarcomere-associated proteins. It was first brought to attention by the British forensic pathologist Donald Teare in 1958 as a disease manifesting with symmetric or asymmetric left ventricular hypertrophy (LVH) more than 1.5 cm (Figure 23–1) in a nondilated ventricle. Additional observations made by him were myocardial clefts and myocyte disarray seen along with hypertrophy in hearts of young and healthy adults who experienced sudden death. Subsequently, pioneering work by Eugene Braunwald has defined the hemodynamics of the disease process as we know it now. The distribution of hypertrophy is variable, can involve the right ventricle, and is not explained by other causes of LVH (see Table 23–1 for differential diagnosis of LVH).

HCM is relatively common (1:200–1:500) in the general population with about 750,000 people affected in the United States and 15–20 million worldwide. However, only 15–20% of HCM is identified clinically which clearly highlights a troubling reality given that it is the most common cause of sudden cardiac death in individuals less than 35 years of age in North America. On a positive note, most people afflicted with HCM do live a normal life. HCM patients may live well into their sixth to eighth decades, with patients older than age 90 with HCM being reported. Moreover, the first clinical recognition of HCM may occur when patients are in their sixth to eighth decade of life; usually, these patients have milder forms of the disease with the most serious complications being uncommon after age 60. The natural history of HCM can take many paths: sudden cardiac death, symptomatic HCM heart failure, end-stage cardiomyopathy, atrial fibrillation, and stroke. However, if intervened in a timely manner, HCM can potentially have no effect on longevity.

B. Genetics & Histopathology

The genetics of HCM involve an autosomal dominant pattern of inheritance, with 60–70% of patients having an affected family member. HCM is more common in males than females. Offspring of affected individuals have a 50% chance of inheriting mutations and risk of disease. Approximately 70% of genotyped patients have mutations involving β-myosin heavy chain or myosin binding protein C, other mutations include troponin I, and troponin T, but numerous others have been described with over a dozen mutations described in sarcomere-associated proteins. However, in more than 30% of HCM no causal mutations can be identified. The genetic basis of ventricular hypertrophy does not always correlate with prognosis. Patients with tropomyosin

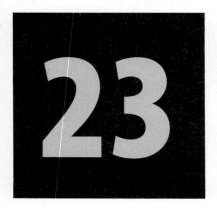

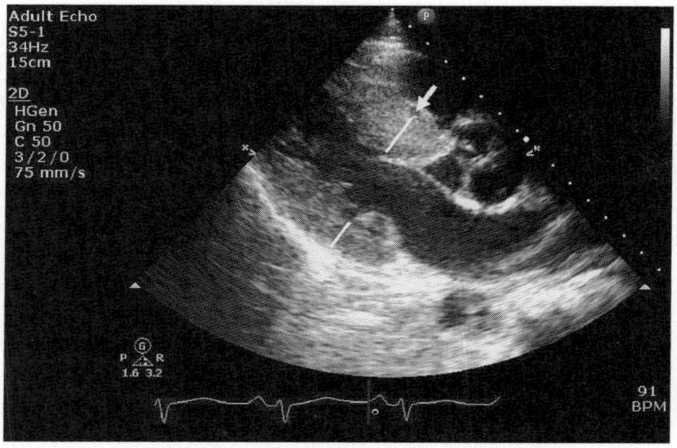

▲ **Figure 23–1.** Echocardiogram parasternal long-axis view in diastole showing asymmetric septal hypertrophy (*white arrow*) compared to the inferolateral wall.

mutations have only a mild degree of ventricular hypertrophy, with little or no left ventricular (LV) outflow tract obstruction, but they still carry a disproportionately high risk for heart failure. Studies to date have not been clearly able to associate certain specific mutations to increased risk of sudden death, although multiple mutations may predict earlier disease expression and progression. Although the majority of modifier genes that influence HCM are unknown, certain modifier genes (ACE, RAAS) appear to influence hypertrophy.

C. Phenotype of Hypertrophic Cardiomyopathy

Mutations of the sarcomeric proteins lead to histopathologic evidence of myocardial disarray, which then leads to pathologic hypertrophy and patchy fibrosis of the myocardium. Intramural vessels are also frequently abnormal in HCM with thrombotic obliteration causing ischemia, which may propagate fibrosis regardless of presence of epicardial coronary disease. Asymmetric hypertrophy is most common but multiple variations of hypertrophy may be present (septal 90%, midventricular 1%, posteroseptal and lateral wall 1%, apical 3%, and symmetric 5%). Asymmetric septal hypertrophy is defined as a septal-to-posterior wall ratio more than 1.3 and, in hypertensive patients, more than 1.5. Massive hypertrophy more than 30 mm is a risk factor for sudden death. Hypertrophy in adults is usually stable but can progress in adolescents and can regress in the subset of patients who develop end-stage heart failure making the diagnosis of HCM in the latter group a challenge. An abnormal mitral valve and its apparatus are commonly seen in HCM. Elongated mitral leaflets and abnormal/anteriorly displaced papillary muscles and direct insertion of papillary muscles to the anterior mitral leaflet can be seen and have now been well defined by cardiac magnetic resonance imaging (Figure 23–2). All these factors may contribute to outflow obstruction.

Table 23-1. Differential Diagnosis of Left Ventricular Hypertrophy

Athlete's heart
Systemic hypertension
Subaortic membrane/ridge
Aortic stenosis
Supravalvular aortic stenosis
Right ventricular hypertrophy
Fabry disease
Glycogen storage disease (PRKAG2 cardiomyopathy, Danon disease, Pompe disease)
Mucopolysaccharide storage disease
Amyloidosis
Sarcoidosis

Pathophysiology

The following processes contribute to the pathophysiology of HCM.

1. Abnormal diastolic function
2. Outflow tract obstruction/systolic anterior mitral valve motion
3. Mitral regurgitation
4. Myocardial ischemia
5. Arrhythmias
6. Abnormal autonomic function

A. Diastolic Dysfunction

Diastolic filling abnormalities, invariably present in almost all patients with HCM, may precede hypertrophy, and as it worsens, an increased dependence on atrial contribution

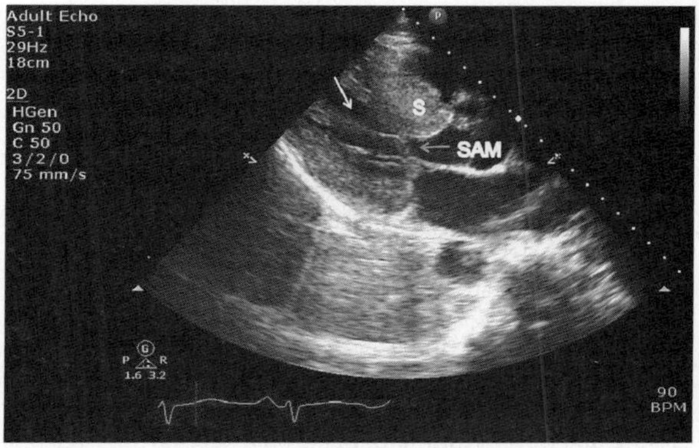

▲ **Figure 23–2.** Echocardiogram parasternal long-axis view still frame in a patient with obstructive hypertrophic cardiomyopathy. Asymmetric septal hypertrophy (S) is noted, along with systolic anterior motion (SAM; *light arrow*) and hypertrophied and anteriorly displaced papillary muscle (*white arrow*) causing further narrowing of left ventricular mid cavity and outflow tract.

to ventricular filling occurs. Mitral inflow parameters demonstrate varying degrees of dysfunction, most impaired relaxation, whereas restrictive filling patterns are less common, but manifest in advanced disease states. Myocardial abnormalities documented by tissue Doppler, speckle tracking echocardiography-based strain, and LV twist and torsion abnormalities have been demonstrated in HCM. Figure 23–3 demonstrates impaired relaxation in mitral inflow, delayed propagation slope on color M-mode, and abnormal tissue Doppler, all indicative of diastolic dysfunction in a patient with HCM.

B. Outflow Obstruction/Systolic Anterior Motion

HCM can be broadly categorized into obstructive and nonobstructive types based on presence or absence of an LV gradient (Figure 23–4). The combination of a hypertrophied septum bulging into the LV outflow tract and abnormal systolic anterior motion of the mitral valve in systole (SAM) contributes to outflow obstruction. Two-dimensional Doppler echocardiography remains the cornerstone for evaluation of HCM and quantifying gradients. About two-thirds of patients with HCM have outflow tract obstruction manifesting as resting or provocable gradients of ≥ 30 mm Hg. However, only 25–30% of patients demonstrate obstruction at rest. Simple maneuvers such as the Valsalva maneuver, standing, or administration of amyl nitrite or exercise echocardiography can provoke or exacerbate outflow tract obstruction and gradients and should be performed as part of clinical and echocardiographic evaluation when HCM is suspected and resting gradients are not observed (Table 23–2, Figure 23–5). Outflow obstruction can contribute to exercise intolerance, angina, syncope, and decreased survival. Patients with obstructive HCM are at higher risk of adverse events (heart failure and death) than those without obstruction.

Although the exact cause of SAM is debated, there are two traditional perspectives for the mechanism of SAM. One is a causal mechanism of SAM precipitated by chordal slackening/anterior displaced mitral valve apparatus leading to "drag forces," and the other explains SAM because of the Venturi effect of accelerated flow across the left ventricular outflow tract (LVOT) (Figure 23–6). However, the "Venturi forces" theory has lately been questioned and increased recognition of anatomic abnormalities of mitral apparatus including elongated mitral leaflets, anterior displacement, anomalous insertion, and bifid papillary muscles all seem to play a role in obstructive physiology and SAM. The severity of obstruction and timing of SAM onset are linearly related. An important caveat is that SAM can be seen in non-HCM states, even when no basal septal hypertrophy is present such as a hyperdynamic small, underfilled ventricle (volume-depleted states), after mitral valve repair, and as a nonspecific finding confined to the chordal apparatus (chordal SAM). More recently increased recognition of dynamic obstructive physiology with SAM has been observed in large

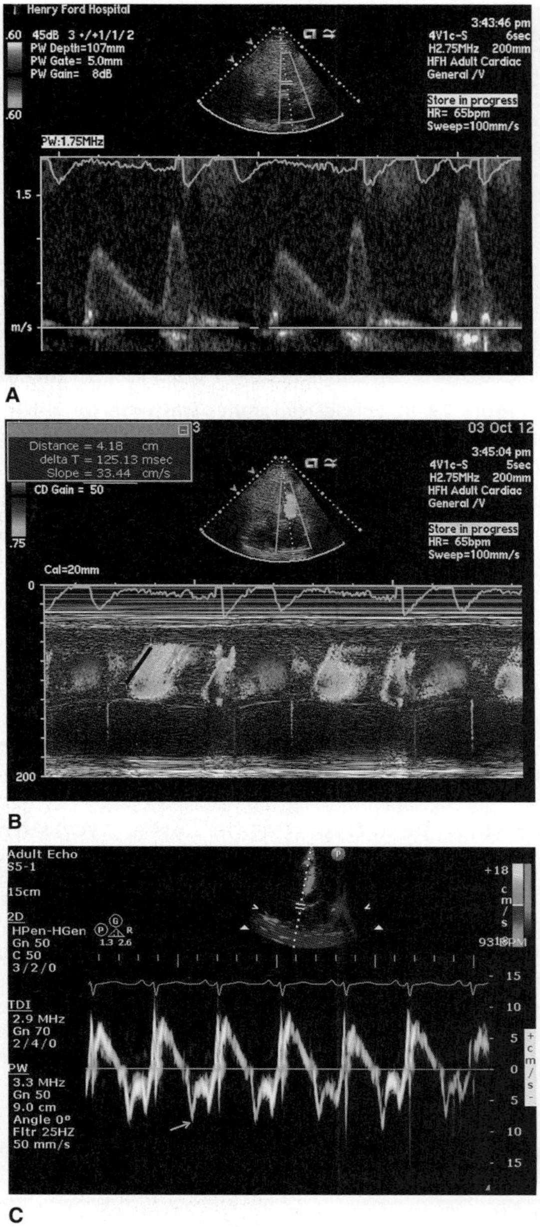

▲ **Figure 23–3.** **A:** Doppler echocardiographic diastolic mitral inflow profile in a 32-year-old patient with hypertrophic cardiomyopathy (HCM) indicating impaired relaxation pattern. **B:** M-mode flow propagation abnormalities in HCM from the same patient. *Black slanted line* indicates propagation slope of < 50 cm/s, indicating impaired relaxation. **C:** Pulsed tissue Doppler of the septal annulus in a 40-year-old patient with HCM and preserved left ventricular ejection fraction showing low e′ velocities suggesting underlying myocardial dysfunction.

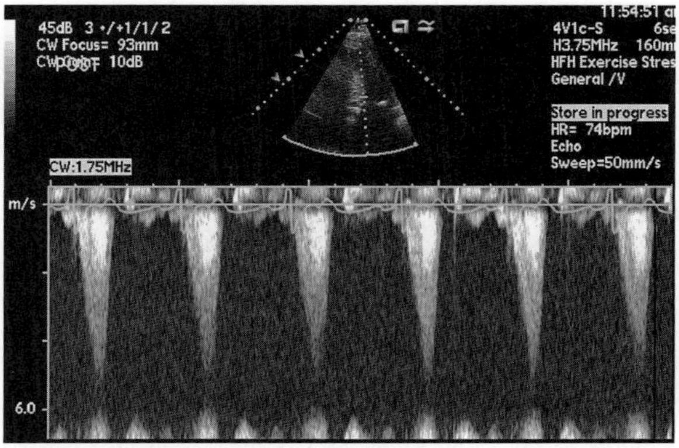

▲ **Figure 23–4.** Continuous wave Doppler across left ventricular outflow tract at rest demonstrates "dagger-shaped" late-peaking velocity consistent with outflow tract obstruction.

anteroseptal infarcts and in Takotsubo cardiomyopathy where the basal septum is hyperdynamic contributing to narrowing of LVOT and drag forces causing SAM and outflow obstruction. Thus, although patients in many different pathophysiologic states may exhibit HCM physiology (gradients, SAM), this does not equate to a diagnosis of HCM.

C. Mitral Regurgitation

The main etiology of mitral regurgitation (MR) in HCM is malcoaptation of the mitral leaflets secondary to SAM. SAM-related MR is posteriorly directed starting in mid-late systole (Figure 23–7). If other MR jet directions are seen, then intrinsic mitral valve disease should be suspected. Concomitant primary mitral valve disease is reported in about 20% of patients with HCM (mitral valve prolapse, ruptured chordae, mitral annular calcification, and anomalous or anteriorly displaced papillary muscle) (see Figure 23–2). If SAM is relieved by either myectomy or septal ablation, posterior MR tends to resolve or diminish. Nonposterior MR may require surgical repair or replacement of the valve, which may be one reason why surgical myectomy is favored over alcohol septal ablation in patients with concomitant mitral valve apparatus abnormalities as a treatment strategy for symptomatic HCM.

A comprehensive echocardiography assessment of MR is important in HCM. The assessment of peak outflow gradients can be challenging in some patients with HCM

Table 23-2. Factors Influencing Obstruction in Hypertrophic Cardiomyopathy

Obstruction worsens (gradient increases and murmur increases)
1. Tachycardia
2. Hypovolemia
3. Standing
4. Valsalva
5. Inotropes, diuretics, vasodilators
Obstruction lessens (gradient decreases and murmur decreases)
1. Negative inotropes
2. Bradycardia
3. Vasoconstrictors
4. Squatting
5. Isometric handgrip

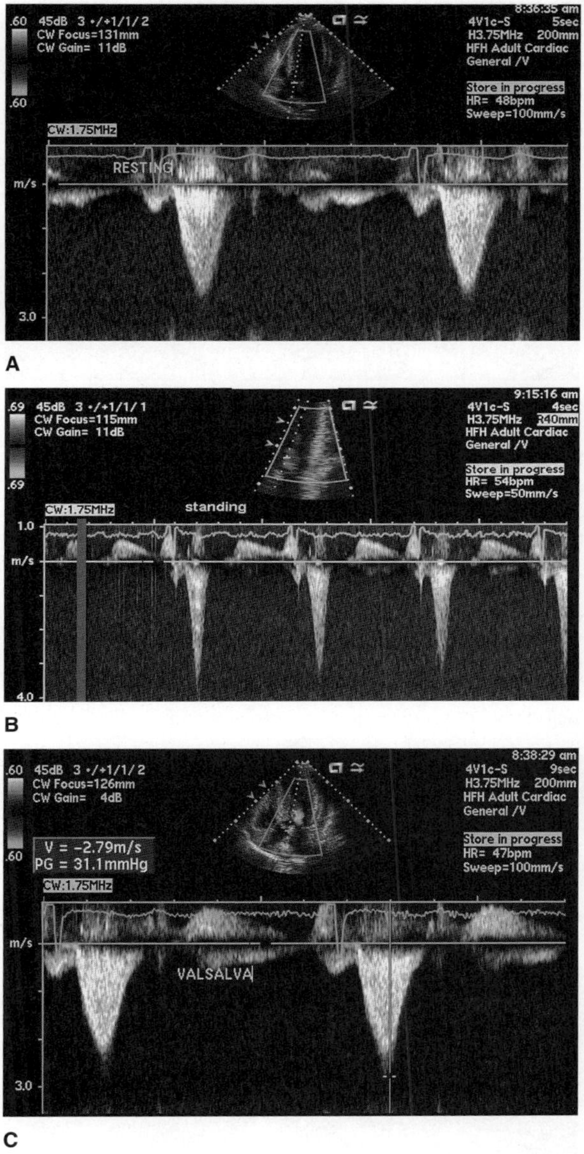

▲ **Figure 23–5.** Hypertrophic cardiomyopathy outflow tract gradient (**A**) at rest, (**B**) standing, and (**C**) with Valsalva.

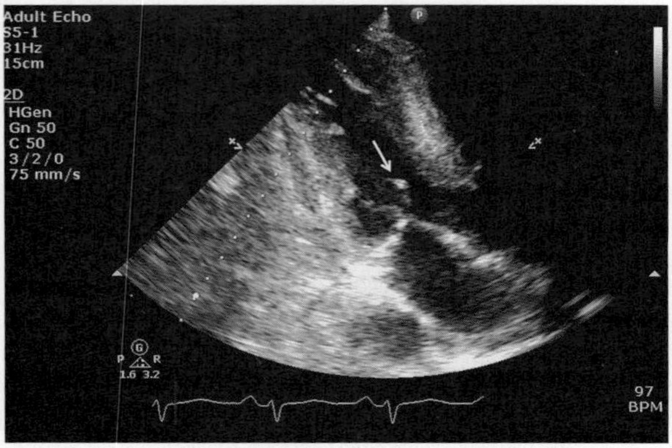

▲ **Figure 23–6.** Echocardiographic apical three-chamber still frame showing systolic anterior motion of mitral valve encroaching on the left ventricular outflow tract creating outflow obstruction physiology (*white arrow*).

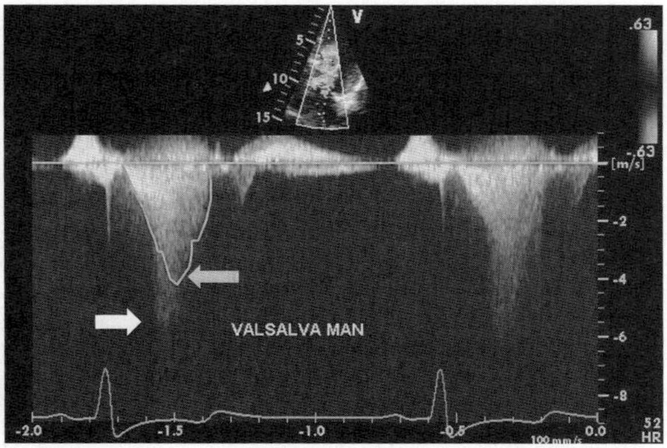

▲ **Figure 23–8.** Continuous wave Doppler evaluation of a patient with hypertrophic cardiomyopathy during Valsalva provocation. Two distinct flow patterns are seen: one of outflow obstruction, which has a late peak (*light arrow*), and a superimposed Doppler profile signal of mitral regurgitation (*white arrow*), making assessment of peak outflow obstruction velocity challenging.

in the setting of MR due to contamination of both jets (Figure 23–8). Careful observation of jet profile and coexistent inflow profile and evaluation of peak gradients from different windows will help to differentiate outflow gradients from MR. Aligning the continuous wave doppler parallel to MR jet and away from LVOT flow acceleration may further help avoid contamination of doppler signals.

D. Myocardial Ischemia

The combination of significant LVH with or without outflow obstruction sets the stage for substantial increases in myocardial oxygen demand and can precipitate angina secondary to myocardial ischemia in HCM. Angina has been reported in approximately 30% of HCM patients, and ischemic perfusion defects on myocardial perfusion imaging can be present in a majority of patients with HCM. Although epicardial coronary disease may cause angina/perfusion defects, a supply-demand mismatch in conjunction with abnormal microvasculature is likely the major contributor. Cardiac positron emission tomography assessment of myocardial blood flow and flow reserve has shed further light on abnormalities in flow and flow reserve causing myocardial ischemia and likely related to microvascular dysfunction in the setting of nonobstructive epicardial arteries.

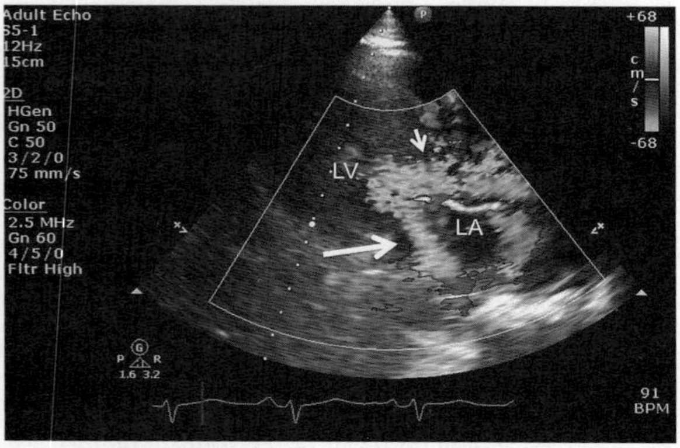

▲ **Figure 23–7.** Echocardiographic parasternal long-axis view still frame with flow velocity mapping illustrating consequence of systolic anterior motion and left ventricular outflow tract (LVOT) obstruction, which leads to turbulent flow across LVOT (*small arrow*) during left ventricular (LV) systole and posterior directed jet of mitral regurgitation (*large thick arrow*) into left atrium (LA).

E. Abnormal Autonomic Tone

About 25% of HCM patients demonstrate abnormalities of autonomic function, which if present, portend a poorer prognosis. Abnormalities with exercise, such as systolic drop in blood pressure of ≥ 20 mm Hg, or failure to augment blood pressure can occur from factors such as outflow obstruction and inappropriate vasodilatation despite an appropriate increase in cardiac output.

▶ Clinical Findings

A. Physical Examination

A general examination is not helpful in diagnosing HCM except when associations with other diseases such as Friedrich ataxia or Noonan syndrome are present. The cardiovascular clinical examination findings of HCM are usually striking unless there is no obstruction at rest. Radial pulse is of brisk character. There is a characteristic brisk carotid upstroke with an abrupt deceleration due to obstruction.

The apical impulse is described as bifid and sustained due to the initial powerful contraction followed by obstruction and then by continued contraction of the left ventricle. A systolic thrill may be felt. The first and second heart sounds are normal. An S_4 may be heard due to atrial contraction against a noncompliant left ventricle.

The systolic murmur in HCM is a harsh and crescendo decrescendo in character. It is heard all over the precordium but usually is not transmitted to the carotids. The murmur increases in intensity with Valsalva, standing, and inhalation of amyl nitrite, due to a drop in preload and decrease in LV cavity size and vasodilation (amyl nitrite), which can worsen outflow obstruction. The murmur intensity decreases with squatting and passive leg raising. A second murmur of mid-late MR can be heard, induced by SAM of the mitral valve. The combination of powerful ejection followed by obstruction and subsequent mitral insufficiency can be aptly described as the "eject-obstruct-leak" triad of hypertrophic obstructive cardiomyopathy (HOCM). The key differentiation of a HOCM murmur is from that of aortic stenosis (AS) and discrete subaortic stenosis. However, the pulse of AS is low amplitude and slow (parvus et tardus) compared to brisk in HCM. Ejection click (with bicuspid etiology) and aortic regurgitation murmur are more common in AS and not typically seen in HCM. The aortic second sound is abnormal in AS and normal in HCM. Finally, an AS murmur decreases with Valsalva in contrast to the murmur of HCM, which increases.

B. Diagnostic Tests

1. Electrocardiogram—More than 90% of patients with HCM exhibit 12-lead electrocardiography (ECG) abnormalities. Common abnormalities include LVH with strain, prominent Q waves, left atrial enlargement, and left-axis deviation. ST elevation or depression or T-wave inversions can also be seen. Specific patterns such as deep symmetric T-wave inversions in lateral precordial leads (suggestive of apical variant HCM) are also well recognized (Figure 23–9). In general, ECG abnormalities are present in more than 80% of HOCM compared to approximately 50% in nonobstructive types of HCM. Preexcitation patterns are also seen in some patients with HCM, and atrial fibrillation has been documented in up to 25–30% of elderly HCM patients. More recently artificial intelligence (AI) has shown great promise in the recognition of patterns associated with HCM. AI-ECG HCM scores correlated with disease status as measured by decreases over time in left ventricular outflow tract gradients and natriuretic peptide (NT-proBNP) levels in

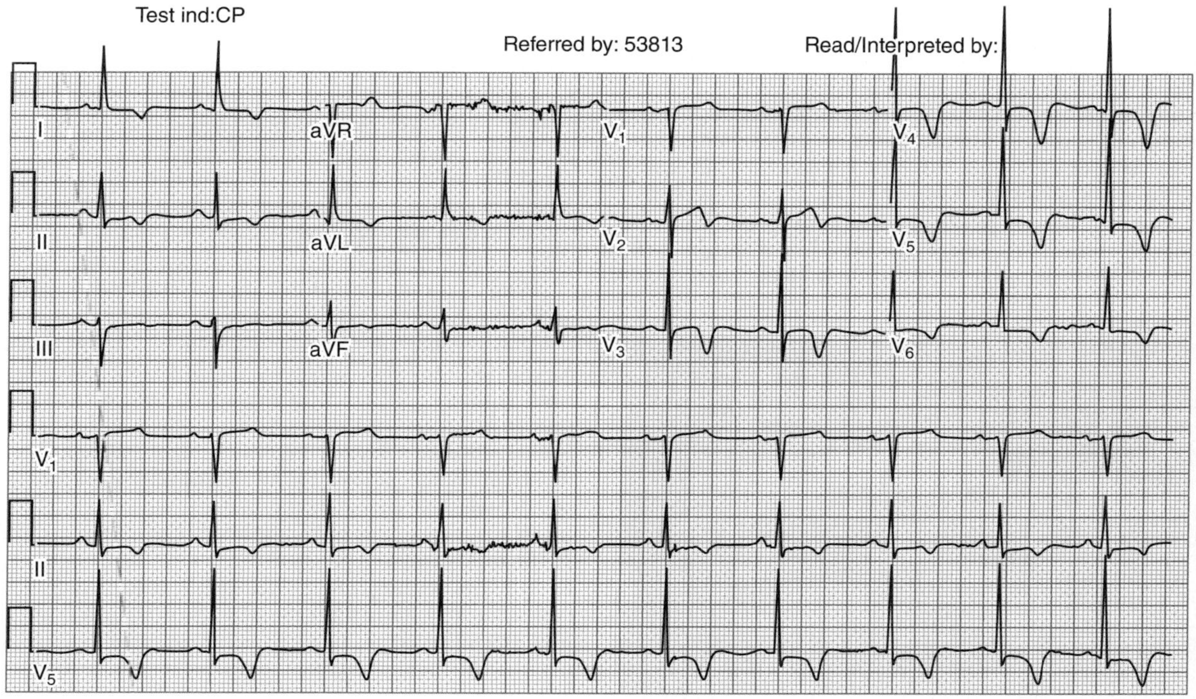

▲ **Figure 23–9.** Twelve-lead electrocardiogram in a patient with palpitations. Note deep symmetric T-wave inversions in the precordial leads. There are also T-wave abnormalities in the limb leads. In the absence of hypertension, these should raise suspicion of hypertrophic cardiomyopathy. Subsequent echocardiography and cardiac magnetic resonance imaging confirmed diagnosis of apical hypertrophic cardiomyopathy.

these patients. The longitudinal associations of the AI-ECG HCM score were significant and likely reflected changes in the raw ECG waveform that were detectable by AI-ECGs and correlated with HCM disease pathophysiology and severity. AI-ECG's potential is enhanced by the advances in that ECGs can now be measured remotely via smartphone-enabled electrodes and may permit remote assessment of disease progression as well as drug treatment response.

Tison GH, Siontis KC, Abreau S, et al. Assessment of disease status and treatment response with artificial intelligence-enhanced electrocardiography in obstructive hypertrophic cardiomyopathy. *J Am Coll Cardiol.* 2022;79:1032–1034. [PMID: 35272798]

2. Echocardiogram—Echocardiography (echo) plays an integral role in diagnosis, follow-up, and management of patients with HCM. Abnormalities can be demonstrated on M-mode echo; two-dimensional (2D) echo; color, pulsed and continuous wave, and tissue Doppler; and strain imaging. Key findings of HCM by echo include the following:

A. M-MODE—Midsystolic notching of aortic valve is seen in HCM (Figure 23–10). SAM of mitral valve can also be assessed, and extent of SAM and SAM-septal contact distance as a marker of severity can be assessed (Figure 23–11). Right ventricular (RV) and LV septal and posterior wall thickness and chamber sizes can be determined.

B. 2D ECHO—Asymmetric septal hypertrophy is the most common pattern, although other patterns can be seen (see Figure 23–1). RV hypertrophy may also be present. Because echo can underestimate or miss hypertrophy confined to the lateral wall and apex, comprehensive multiple nonforeshortened views of LV are needed. Echo contrast imaging can be very useful to assess apical variant HCM. Mitral valve abnormalities can be seen as described previously. SAM can be assessed, and all chamber sizes can be evaluated. Insights from three-dimensional echo reconstructions of the mitral valve

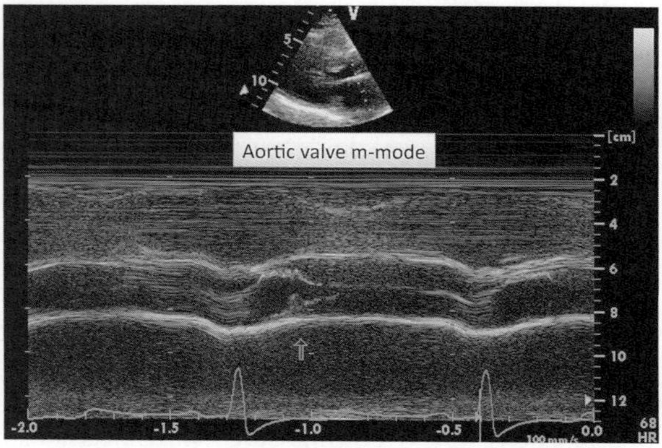

▲ **Figure 23–10.** Midsystolic notching of the aortic valve (*arrow*) is indicative of dynamic left ventricular outflow obstruction.

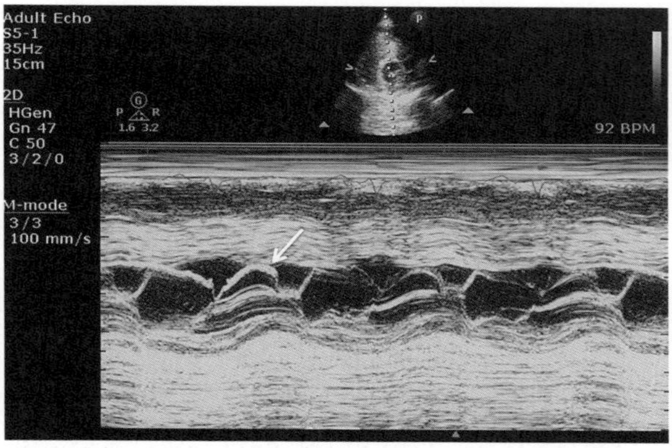

▲ **Figure 23–11.** Systolic anterior motion of mitral valve on M-mode echocardiography. The duration and extent of mitral–septal contact correlate with extent of outflow obstruction.

in HCM show a mitral leaflet area twice that of the normal population, and the indexed mitral valve leaflet area has been shown to be predictive of outflow obstruction. Recently, an enlarged left atrium (indexed volume > 34 mL/m^2) has been shown to be an independent adverse prognosticator in HCM.

C. DOPPLER—Pulsed wave and continuous wave Doppler assessment is integral in establishing the level of outflow obstruction and peak gradients, respectively. The modified Bernoulli equation (4peakV^2) is used to determine peak gradient. The classic late-peaking "dagger-shaped" velocity profile can be seen when outflow obstruction is present (see Figure 23–4). A peak gradient of more than 30 mm Hg is considered evidence for resting outflow obstruction. Gradients should be assessed at rest and with provocation by Valsalva or standing (see Figure 23–5B). If echo features suggest HCM but no or minimal obstruction is demonstrable at rest or Valsalva, exercise echo with peak/immediate post exercise gradient assessment could help unmask HOCM (latent obstruction) and this is recommended in the 2020 ACC AHA guidelines for HCM in all patients with nonobstructive HCM. In contrast the European Society of Cardiology recommendations suggest exercise echocardiography only in symptomatic patients with nonobstructive phenotype and in selected asymptomatic patients where lifestyle or treatment decisions may be impacted (Color Doppler and continuous wave Doppler are very useful to comprehensively assess severity and mechanism of MR. It is important to reliably distinguish the MR signal from the LVOT obstruction signal to avoid overestimation of severity of outflow obstruction. Diastolic function and tissue Doppler abnormalities of myocardial function should be assessed. In particular, average e′ velocities by tissue Doppler of less than 13.5 cm/s predict genotype-positive HCM with a sensitivity of 75% and specificity of 86%. Reduced longitudinal peak systolic deformation (strain) averaged across all walls less than 10.6% (in absolute value) predicts HCM with a sensitivity of 85% and specificity of 100% and helps differentiate it from hypertensive LVH. A combination of septal/posterior wall ratio more than 1.3 and systolic strain assessment yields a predictive accuracy for HCM of 96%. The estimation of filling pressures using E/e′ at best correlates moderately with invasive wedge pressure measurements, although low e′ in itself has independent adverse prognostic value in HCM. Delayed untwisting of LV has been demonstrated by torsion analysis using speckle tracking techniques, again reflecting diastolic dysfunction-related abnormalities seen in HCM.

3. Cardiac magnetic resonance imaging—Cardiac magnetic resonance imaging (CMRI) is rapidly becoming a key component in enhancing diagnostic accuracy, morphology, and more importantly, prognostication due to tissue characterization of fibrosis in HCM. With its superior spatial resolution and indefinite choice of imaging planes, it has demonstrated enhanced accuracy in assessing HCM features and identifying patterns of hypertrophy not well seen on echocardiography. Approximately 6% of patients missed by echo (mainly anterolateral hypertrophy) are diagnosed with HCM by CMRI, and 57% of apical aneurysms missed by echo are identified on CMRI. Assessment of LV mass and end-diastolic wall thickness are more accurate with CMRI than echo. Figures 23–12 and 23–13 show CMRI delineation of septal hypertrophy in HCM.

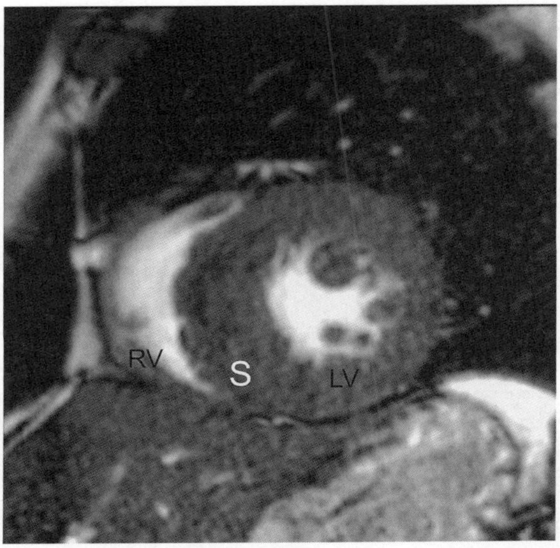

▲ **Figure 23–13.** A still frame from a steady-state free precession short-axis cardiac magnetic resonance study in a patient with suspected hypertrophic cardiomyopathy. There is severe asymmetric left ventricular (LV) hypertrophy involving the septum (S). Multiple papillary muscle heads are also noted in the LV cavity. RV, right ventricle.

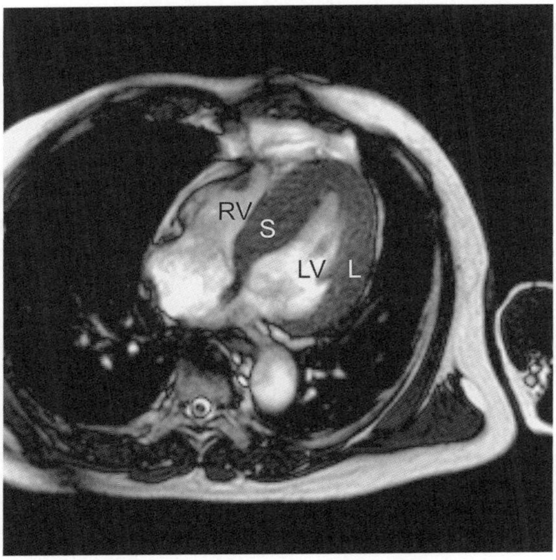

▲ **Figure 23–12.** Steady-state free precession cine sequence still frame (cardiac magnetic resonance imaging) view of left ventricle (LV) and right ventricle (RV) showing significant asymmetric septal hypertrophy (S) compared to lateral wall (L). Note outstanding delineation of the LV blood to endocardial interface enabling accurate measurements of thickness of myocardial walls.

CMRI also provides superb assessment of mitral valve apparatus morphologic abnormalities and gives unparalleled assessment of the right ventricle. The presence of patchy myocardial fibrosis in HCM detected by late gadolinium enhancement techniques in CMRI is increasingly recognized as an adverse prognosticator for arrhythmias and mortality, and ≥ 15% of myocardium with gadolinium enhancement is emerging as a quantitative marker for adverse events. Characteristic patterns include delayed enhancement detected at RV insertion points into the left ventricle, although multiple areas of fibrosis can be seen in the left and/or right ventricle with predominance in the hypertrophied zones of the ventricle (Figure 23–14). CMRI has been used to characterize the presence of "myocardial crypts" or recesses in different areas of the myocardium in phenotype-negative but genotype-positive family members of probands with HCM. Whether these represent early manifestations of an HCM phenotype yet to develop remains to be established, as does any long-term significance.

Kamp NJ, Chery G, Kosinski AS, et al. Risk stratification using late gadolinium enhancement on cardiac magnetic resonance imaging in hypertrophic cardiomyopathy. A systematic review and meta-analysis. *Prog Cardiovasc Dis.* 2021;66:10–16. [PMID: 33171204]

Reichek N. Imaging cardiac morphology in hypertrophic cardiomyopathy: recent advances. *Curr Opin Cardiol.* 2015;30:461–467. [PMID: 26154073]

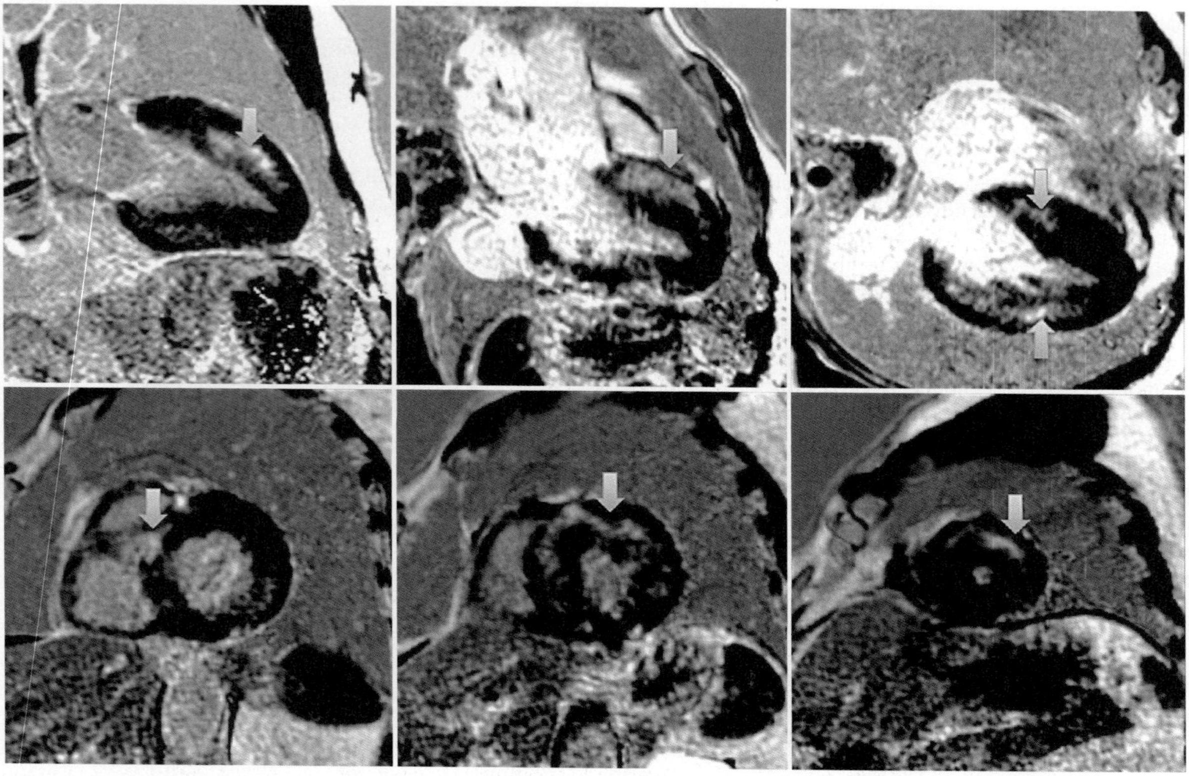

▲ **Figure 23–14.** Gadolinium-based delayed-enhancement cardiac magnetic resonance image showing abnormal enhancement (*arrows*) in multiple areas of the myocardium denoting fibrosis. Note the noncoronary predominant mid-myocardial distribution of hyperenhancement seen in nonischemic etiologies.

4. Cardiac computed tomography angiography, cardiac nuclear perfusion imaging, and positron emission tomography—Cardiac computed tomography angiography (CCTA), cardiac nuclear perfusion imaging, and positron emission tomography (PET) are not routinely used in the assessment of HCM but may be useful in select cases. Retrospective gated CCTA can provide LV function assessment apart from LV morphology and coronary anatomy. CCTA may be useful to define coronary anatomy noninvasively in patients with HOCM. It can also accurately delineate septal perforator course noninvasively as a road map for septal ablation. Single-photon emission computed tomography (SPECT) and PET can demonstrate characteristic intense uptake of radioisotope in hypertrophied zones of myocardium and demonstrate perfusion abnormalities mainly related to microvascular flow reserve abnormalities in HCM (Figure 23–15). Quantitative PET-determined coronary flow reserve abnormalities along with ischemic perfusion defects have been shown to predict adverse outcomes in HCM in limited studies. Most recently, sympathetic innervation imaging (iodine-123 [^{123}I] metaiodobenzylguanidine [MIBG]) has shown that there is sympathetic denervation in hearts of HCM patients (decreased heart-to-mediastinal ratio and increased washout of ^{123}I MIBG) and that this is correlated to septal thickness and outflow obstruction. Whether ^{123}I MIBG denervation imaging predicts sudden death above and beyond other risk markers needs further study.

Shariat M, Thavendiranathan P, Nguyen E, et al. Utility of coronary CT angiography in outpatients with hypertrophic cardiomyopathy presenting with angina symptoms. *J Cardiovasc Comput Tomogr*. 2014;8:429–437. [PMID: 25467830]

Timmer SA, Knaapen P. Coronary microvascular function, myocardial metabolism, and energetics in hypertrophic cardiomyopathy: insights from positron emission tomography. *Eur Heart J Cardiovasc Imaging*. 2013;14:95–101. [PMID: 23152441]

5. Cardiac catheterization—Echocardiography with Doppler is usually sufficient to diagnose HCM, and invasive hemodynamics are usually not necessary. However, if clinical and echo findings are discrepant or the exact severity of obstruction cannot be accurately determined by echo, then catheterization may be needed. A carefully conducted study with continuous documentation of pullback gradients

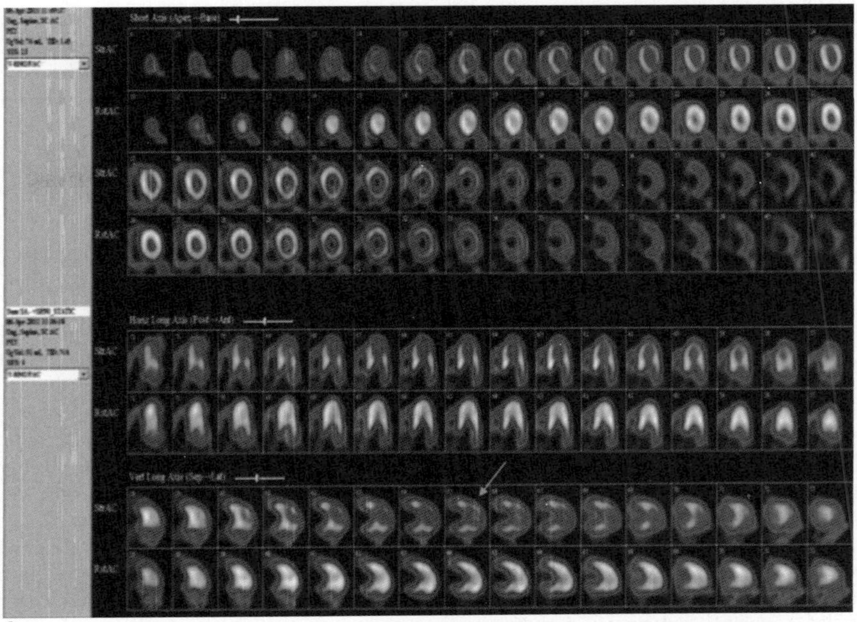

A

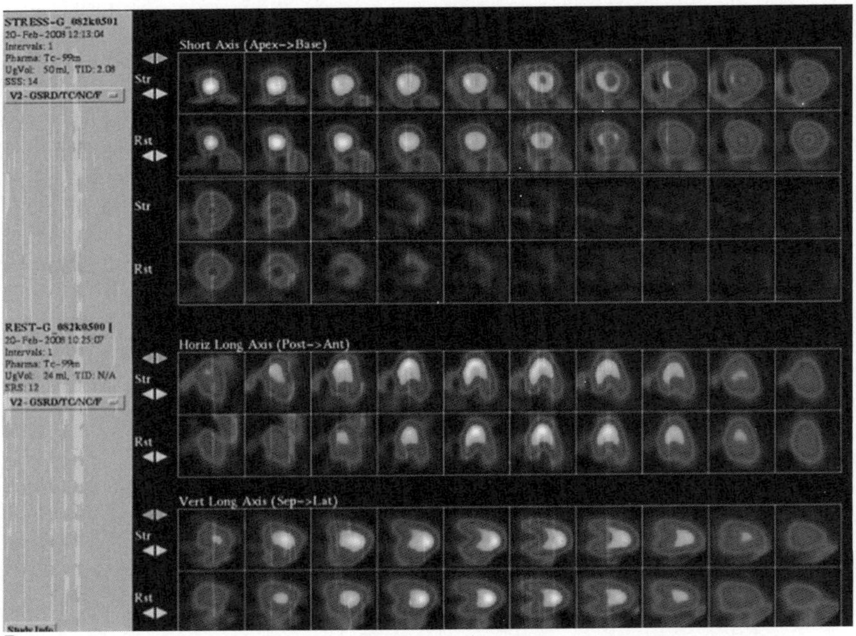

B

▲ **Figure 23–15.** **A:** Regadenoson rubidium-82 rest stress positron emission tomography scan showing moderate reversible ischemic defect (*arrow*) in the mid-distal septum, apex, and distal lateral wall (stress images, *second to last row*). Rest images (*bottom rows*) show intense uptake in mid-distal ventricular walls suggestive of mid-apical hypertrophic cardiomyopathy confirmed by echocardiography and magnetic resonance imaging. Patient had no obstructive coronary artery disease on catheterization. **B:** Regadenoson single-photon emission computed tomography in a patient with new-onset dyspnea. Images show marked increase in uptake of isotope in both stress (*top*) and rest (*bottom*) images in the absence of any ischemia, raising suspicion for mid-apical hypertrophic cardiomyopathy.

will outline the level and severity of obstruction. A classic "spike and dome" arterial pulse waveform can be recorded representing the rapid ejection followed by sudden obstruction. Pulmonary capillary wedge pressure may be elevated, reflecting high filling pressures from diastolic dysfunction, stiff ventricle, and noncompliant atrium. Depending on the severity of MR, a prominent "v" wave can be recorded. Also, the Brockenbrough-Braunwald-Morrow sign can be demonstrated by inducing premature ventricular beats. Following a ventricular extrasystole, an increase occurs in LV systolic pressure, a decrease in ascending aortic pressure, and increase in gradient. Importantly, a drop in pulse pressure is seen in HCM compared to AS where pulse pressure does not change (Figure 23–16).

6. Exercise echocardiography—Exercise echocardiography is recommended to provoke obstruction, which is either absent or minimal at rest (< 30 mm Hg), particularly in symptomatic patients with features of nonobstructive HCM at baseline. Furthermore, exercise can unmask abnormal hemodynamic responses such as failure to augment systolic blood pressure or a drop in systolic blood pressure with exercise. Other abnormal signs with exercise include poor exercise capacity, ventricular arrhythmias, ST depression, and/or ischemic wall motion abnormalities (regardless of presence of epicardial disease). Symptomatic patients with HCM with gradients at rest or with provocation ≥ 50 mm Hg usually require therapy (medical and/or invasive), and hence, exercise testing is not indicated in such patients. However, once medical therapy is maximized in patients with HOCM, repeat exercise echocardiography may be helpful to reevaluate symptoms, exercise hemodynamics, and effects of medical therapy on reduction of outflow obstruction/gradients. Since dobutamine can induce outflow obstruction and gradients, it is not recommended for testing in HCM because it can provoke a similar response even in normal individuals.

7. Genetic testing—Despite initial optimism, the concept of using single-nucleotide sarcomere mutations to identify high-risk patients and prognosticate has not proven useful. The most practical current application for genetic testing in HCM is screening of asymptomatic family members of patients with HCM. If a known mutation exists in HCM patients, focused genetic testing can be done for that mutation in the family. Only about 33% of probands may have a genetic mutation (higher if positive family history). One advantage of genetic testing is identifying the genotype-positive/phenotype-negative family member who may demonstrate subtle ECG or imaging abnormalities and may require closer follow-up to see if he or she progresses to an HCM phenotype. A further use of genetic testing is in differential diagnosis for HCM, including diseases such as *PRKGA2*, *LAMP2* (highly lethal with mortality before 25 years), and Fabry disease, where treatment options such as enzyme replacement are critical. Even if genetic testing is negative in a patient with HCM, continued clinical and surveillance imaging may be needed in at risk relatives. Adolescents and athlete family members should undergo echo annually, and nonathlete family members should undergo echo every 5 years. Pre and post genetic test counselling should be offered to HCM patients undergoing genetic testing. For HCM patients with genetic variants of uncertain significance, serial re-evaluation of test results is recommended

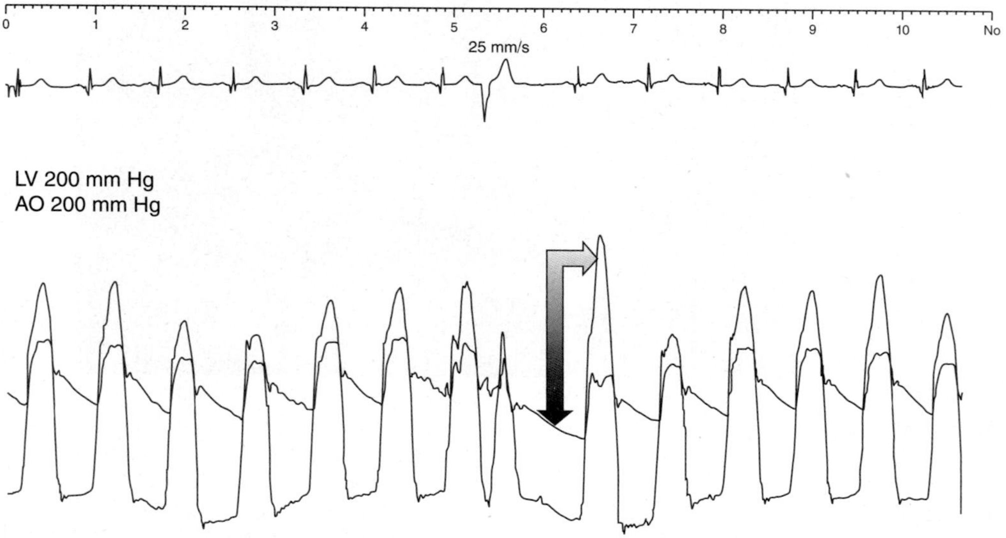

▲ **Figure 23–16.** Brockenbrough-Braunwald-Morrow sign. Following a premature ventricular beat, there is an increase in the gradient but a decrease in aortic and pulse pressure in hypertrophic cardiomyopathy during cardiac catheterization (*double arrow*). AO, aorta; LV, left ventricle.

to assess for variant reclassification, as this may trigger testing for family members. Preconception and prenatal reproductive and genetic counseling should also be offered.

C. Diagnostic Considerations in Hypertrophic Cardiomyopathy Variants

1. Apical HCM—This form of HCM is more frequently reported in Asian populations and is associated with deep symmetric T-wave inversions in the anterior precordial leads (see Figure 23–9). Echo reveals a predominant pattern of hypertrophy distributed toward the apex with relative sparing of the base, although concomitant basal hypertrophy may also be present. In conjunction with the normal contractility, the marked narrowing of the hypertrophied apex in systole produces the "ace of spades" appearance on echo. Apical variant HCM can be missed in echo due to foreshortened views or poor visualization of hypertrophy with low-frequency transducers. Use of higher frequency transducers, color Doppler to delineate full extent of blood flow, and contrast echo can overcome these limitations. CMRI is an excellent alternative to echo and is a superior technique to diagnose apical HCM (Figure 23–17). In general, isolated apical HCM is devoid of outflow obstruction, and these patients have a more benign prognosis than the classical HCM patients.

2. Midventricular HCM—This variant involves predominant hypertrophy of the mid ventricle, resulting in midcavitary obstruction and separation of the ventricle into two compartments in systole. Flow acceleration and obstructive gradients can be demonstrated in the mid-ventricle where most obstruction exists, although concomitant outflow obstruction may be present. Abnormal early diastolic color flow can be seen during isovolumic relaxation due to differential intraventricular pressure gradients across the obstruction. Coexistent hypertension may exacerbate midventricular hypertrophy. In the pure midventricular HCM, SAM may be absent, and no outflow obstruction may be detected. Continuous wave Doppler can delineate maximal obstructive midventricular gradients (Figure 23–18A).

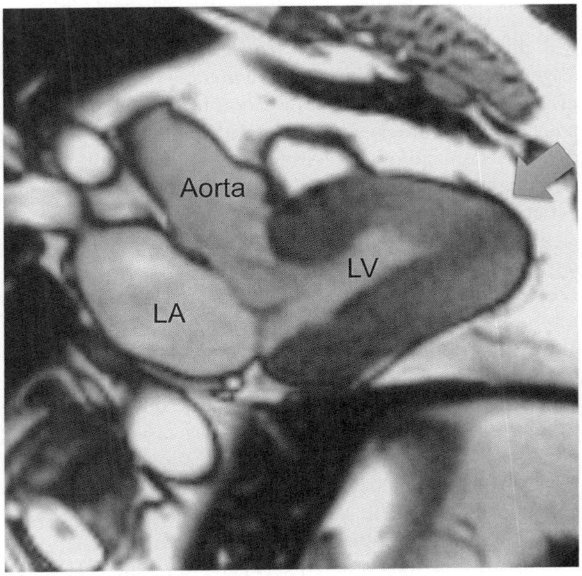

▲ **Figure 23–17.** Steady-state free precession left ventricular (LV) outflow tract view cardiac magnetic resonance imaging still frame showing marked LV myocardial hypertrophy with obliteration of apex in systole (*arrow*). Note characteristic "ace of spades" appearance of LV myocardium in systole. LA, left atrium.

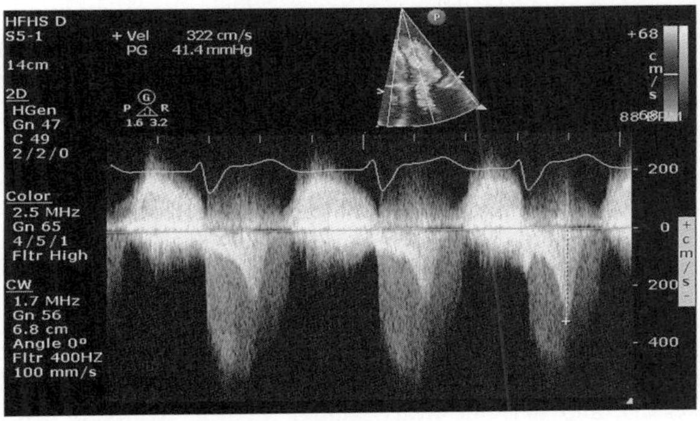

A

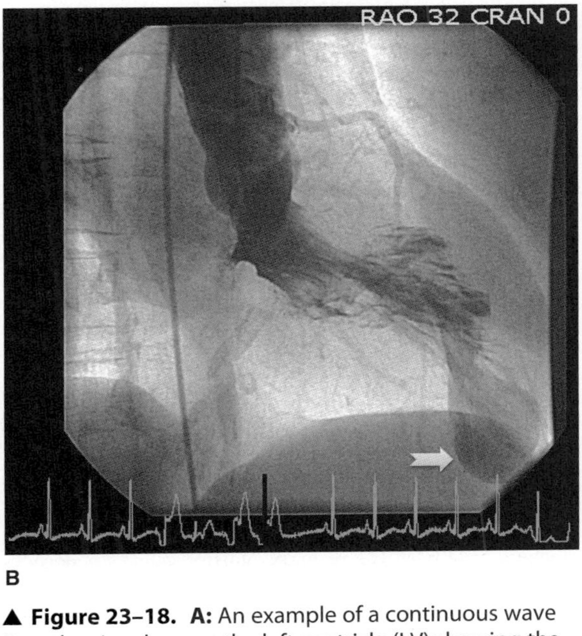

B

▲ **Figure 23–18. A:** An example of a continuous wave Doppler signal across the left ventricle (LV) showing the mitral regurgitation signal and concomitant late-peaking signal of midcavitary obstruction with a peak gradient of 41 mm Hg. **B:** A still frame left ventriculogram in a patient with severe midventricular hypertrophic cardiomyopathy with apical aneurysm outpouching (*arrow*).

Long-standing obstruction in mid ventricle can cause apical necrosis with aneurysm formation due to chronic subendocardial ischemia (Figure 23–18B). This subset of patients is more prone to ventricular arrhythmias and thrombus formation. CMRI is an excellent technique to demonstrate these apical aneurysms, which can be missed by echo.

3. Hypertensive HCM in the elderly—First described in the 1980s, this entity is increasingly recognized more frequently given the growing population of elderly patients with hypertension. Whether this represents a variant of HCM or mimics the physiology of HCM is still debated. Most patients have a long history of hypertension, small, hypertrophied ventricles, a narrow LVOT with mitral annular calcification, and some anterior displacement of the mitral annulus. This constellation can set the stage for acceleration of flow, SAM, and outflow obstruction, although midventricular obstruction may also be present. Treatment is similar to HCM with regard to relief of outflow obstruction with negative inotropic drugs and adequate control of hypertension. Avoidance of excessive diuresis and preload reduction is also a key component.

4. End-stage HCM—Seen in less than 5% of patients, end-stage HCM features ventricular dilation, advanced diastolic dysfunction, and a course predominated with symptoms of systolic and diastolic heart failure. Medical treatment consists of angiotensin-converting enzyme (ACE) inhibitors or angiotensin receptor blockers, β-blockers, diuretics, and spironolactone, as well as nonpharmacologic strategies such as implantable cardioverter-defibrillator (ICD) and biventricular pacing if indicated. In refractory cases, heart transplantation should be considered. Survival after heart transplantation in HCM is comparable to the general population.

Management

Therapeutic strategies in HCM can be divided into pharmacologic and nonpharmacologic strategies. Substantial advances have now been achieved in the medical therapy with HCM.

A. Pharmacologic Strategies

Pharmacologic therapy for HCM is focused on decreasing inotropy, augmenting diastolic filling time, and reducing dynamic outflow obstruction. Resting gradients are not useful to gauge the effectiveness of therapy. Negative inotropic agents such as β-blockers and rate-lowering calcium channel blockers have been the primary "go to" agents for decades and can help diminish gradients and outflow obstruction in HOCM and also decrease myocardial oxygen demand. High doses, such as 200 mg of propranolol or metoprolol or 240–360 mg of verapamil or diltiazem, may be effective. Of note propranolol is the only approved drug by the Food and Drug Administration for use in HOCM although it is not been studied in randomized controlled trials. However, beta blockers do not reduce mortality.

With regards to calcium channel blockers, they can be used as a substitute when beta blockers are not tolerated with verapamil being commonly used (potent negative inotropic effect). However, caution should be used when high resting outflow gradients are present when initiating verapamil, because peripheral vasodilatation may occur, leading to syncope. Calcium channel blockers are also not recommended in conjunction with beta blockers and are contraindicated in setting of hypotension, dyspnea at rest, children less than 6 weeks and resting gradients more than 100 mm Hg. For symptomatic patients with nonobstructive physiology beta-blockers, verapamil or diltiazem is recommended. Disopyramide, a class Ia antiarrhythmic agent with potent negative inotropic effects, can be used as an adjunct to β-blockers or calcium blockers when patient remains symptomatic with obstructive physiology despite initial therapy. Amiodarone, which has β-blocking properties, has been shown to have a favorable effect on prognosis in selected patients with HCM. Pure vasodilators (eg, dihydropyridines, nitrates, hydralazine) should be avoided. β-agonists and digoxin may worsen obstruction by augmenting contractility and should be avoided. Excessive diuresis should also be avoided because it may exacerbate obstruction, although diuretics will be needed to relieve pulmonary congestion in the setting of pulmonary edema. Exercise echocardiography can be used to assess efficacy of treatment and if improvement in provocable gradients happened with therapy.

In nonobstructive variants of HCM, treatments can be targeted for diastolic dysfunction with judicious use of diuretics as needed for elevated filling pressures. In advanced HCM with dilated and dysfunctional ventricles ("burnt out" or end-stage HCM), standard heart failure therapies are indicated as discussed earlier. Atrial fibrillation occurs in 25–30% of elderly patients with HCM, is poorly tolerated, and requires electrical cardioversion and/or aggressive rate control and anticoagulation therapy. Radiofrequency ablation can be offered to some patients with drug-refractory atrial fibrillation.

Recent advances in the understanding of pathophysiology of HCM has led to the development of an entirely new class of therapeutic agents called selective cardiac myosin inhibitors. Specifically mavacamten is now FDA approved and represents a true advance in management of HCM. This agent is indicated in HOCM patients with Class 2–3 symptoms and ejection fraction more than 55%. It has a unique mechanism of action and works by decreasing sarcomeric power and force generation and induction of a negative intotropic effect. Evidence suggests that mavavamten use in conjunction with β-blockers or calcium channel blockers is associated with improvement in exercise capacity, left ventricular outflow tract gradients, NYHA functional class, and patient-reported health issues. Furthermore, mavacamten induces favorable remodeling in myocardial structure as shown by cardiac MRI and more than 80% had complete resolution of SAM with improvements in nt-pro BNP, left ventricular hypertrophy along with diastolic function. These results suggest that mavacamten apart from relieving parameters of obstructive physiology may also have favorable impact in left ventricular remodeling. Mavacamten also appears to show promise in nonobstructive HCM with early evidence showing beneficial effects on myocardial wall stress although definitive evidence is still pending. Finally, preliminary data (unpublished at the time of this update) have shown that patients on mavacamten need less referrals for septal reduction therapies.

As an important note of caution, because of its negative inotropic effects, careful monitoring of ejection fraction is needed with mavacamten and frequent echoes at least once in 4 weeks is required during the initial titration period. The drug is contraindicated if the initial EF is less than 55%.

Olivotto I, Oreziak A, Barriales-Villa R, et al. Mavacamten for treatment of symptomatic obstructive hypertrophic cardiomyopathy (EXPLORER-HCM): a randomized, double-blind, placebo-controlled, phase 3 trial. *Lancet.* 2020;396:759–769. [PMID: 32871100]

B. Nonpharmacologic Therapies

If a HCM patient continues to remain symptomatic despite maximal medical treatment, more aggressive nonpharmacologic therapies should be explored regardless of degree of residual outflow obstruction.

Nonpharmacologic strategies that are clearly shown to be of value are surgical septal myectomy and alcohol septal ablation. Although dual-chamber pacing has been attempted no clear benefit has been demonstrable in controlled trials.

1. Surgical septal myectomy—Septal myectomy is widely regarded as the best treatment for HCM to relief of outflow obstruction, with a 95% success rate. Gradients are often reduced to less than 10 mm Hg after the procedure. In brief, the procedure involves surgical excision of the basal portion of the ventricular septum (5–10 g) to enable a wider outflow tract for exit of blood, thus relieving outflow obstruction. Modifications of this procedure has evolved over the years and now includes wider zones of resection of the ventricular septum up to the level of papillary muscles, resection, and/or reimplantation/realignment of abnormal papillary muscle heads, resection of abnormal septal obstructive bands, plication of anterior mitral leaflet, anterior leaflet extension and mitral valve repair or replacement if needed for associated primary mitral valve disease. To enable pre-procedural planning, CMRI is essential and provides a high-resolution image of the septum and intraventricular anatomy which can enable effective surgical strategy. More recently a novel technique for tackling distal ventricular obstructions where a traditional transaortic approach may not work is to deploy cryoenergy to improve exposure of the interventricular septum enabling surgeons to do extended myectomies deeper in left ventricle. Mortality rate for isolated myectomy is less than 0.5% in experienced centers, with more than 90% of patients experiencing symptomatic relief. Complications occur in less than 1% of patients and include heart block, ventricular septal defect, aortic regurgitation, and conduction delays, most commonly left bundle branch block. Thus, patients with pre-existing right bundle branch block should be informed of the higher likelihood of complete heart block needing permanent pacing and hence this subgroup may warrant consideration of alcohol septal ablation. Myectomy, however has a very low incidence of sustained ventricular arrhythmias (0.2–0.9%/year).

Long-term follow-up data are available for more than 50 years after the procedure, making evidence-based recommendations very strong. Sudden death risk after myectomy is very low. However evidence indicates that centers doing myectomy have very low numbers (median 1/year) and this is associated with fourfold higher mortality, increased length of stay and higher costs compared to more experienced centers with higher volume. This reiterates importance of referral to centers of excellence and the need for adequate heart team learning curve prior to embarking on myectomy.

2. Alcohol septal ablation—Over the past 25 years, a percutaneous solution to HCM-related outflow obstruction has evolved called alcohol septal ablation (ASA). The basic principle is to identify a septal perforator branch (usually from the left anterior descending coronary artery) that supplies the hypertrophied portion of the basal septum and inject absolute ethanol (1–3 mL) via a percutaneous approach under contrast echocardiography guidance and induce a local transmural infarction in that zone (usually an average of 10% of the overall LV wall). This has been shown to reduce outflow gradient and concomitant MR, although frequently a small residual gradient is present. An immediate fall in outflow gradient is observed with successful septal ablation in more than 90% of patients with residual gradients of less than 25 mm Hg. Continued improvement may be seen over ensuing months as the scar forms and retracts and the outflow tract widens. Preprocedural coronary or CT angiography to determine suitable septal perforator artery anatomy and periprocedural contrast echocardiography in the septal perforator to determine myocardial contrast "blush" corresponding to the point of obstruction are important adjuncts to plan the procedure. Also defining accompanying abnormalities like anomalous septal bands, anomalous or dual-headed papillary muscle and other primary mitral valve abnormalities is important as these may not benefit from septal ablation. The likelihood of permanent pacemaker implantation is four to five times higher with septal ablation than with myectomy. A septal thickness of at least ≥ 17 mm is felt to be needed to avoid a procedure-related ventricular septal defect. The hemodynamic and functional improvement over 3–5 years has been shown to be similar overall for ASA and myectomy. Close to 90% of patients are in NYHA Class 1 or 2 after procedure, with relief from LVOT obstruction in 76% and 30-day mortality of 1% in expert centers. Although earlier studies have suggested no difference in the medium-term incidence of sudden cardiac death (SCD) or all-cause mortality between myectomy and ASA, more recent registries have suggested higher event rates long term with ASA so this issue appears to be still controversial. ACC AHA guidelines recommend myectomy over ASA unless the latter is performed in experienced centers or patients who are deemed higher surgical risk due to comorbidities or advanced age. ASA should also be avoided in children, adolescents, and young adults due to lack of long-term data. Massive septal hypertrophy (≥ 30 mm) and concomitant mitral apparatus abnormalities are also unlikely to benefit from septal ablation.

Recently a newer alternative procedure called percutaneous intramyocardial radiofrequency ablation (PIMSRA) has been described. PIMSRA involves a transapical approach with an ablation system using a 17–18-gauge needle is threaded into the myocardium to the targeted area of upper septum and the tip of the needle is used to deliver the radiofrequency. Maximum septal thickness was reduced from 24 to 17 mm Hg, mean gradient was reduced from 79 to 14 mm Hg, and in-hospital mortality was 1%. Permanent right bundle branch block was reported in 2.5% of patients but interestingly this procedure was associated with much lower incidence of need for permanent pacing.

3. Dual-chamber pacing—The physiologic principle underlying dual-chamber pacing (DDD) is the induction of asynchronous contraction of the septum induced by RV pacing. This causes the septum not to bulge into the outflow tract in early-mid systole and thus decreases the outflow obstruction and gradients. However, DDD pacing is no longer considered as a standard HCM treatment option, because most symptomatic improvement reported by patients in initial studies has been deemed to be a placebo effect in subsequent randomized trials. Furthermore, there is no benefit from DDD pacing in reducing risk of SCD, and it has no role in nonobstructive HCM. Figures 23-19 and 23-20 summarize diagnostic approach and treatment options as well as genetic counseling recommendations for HCM.

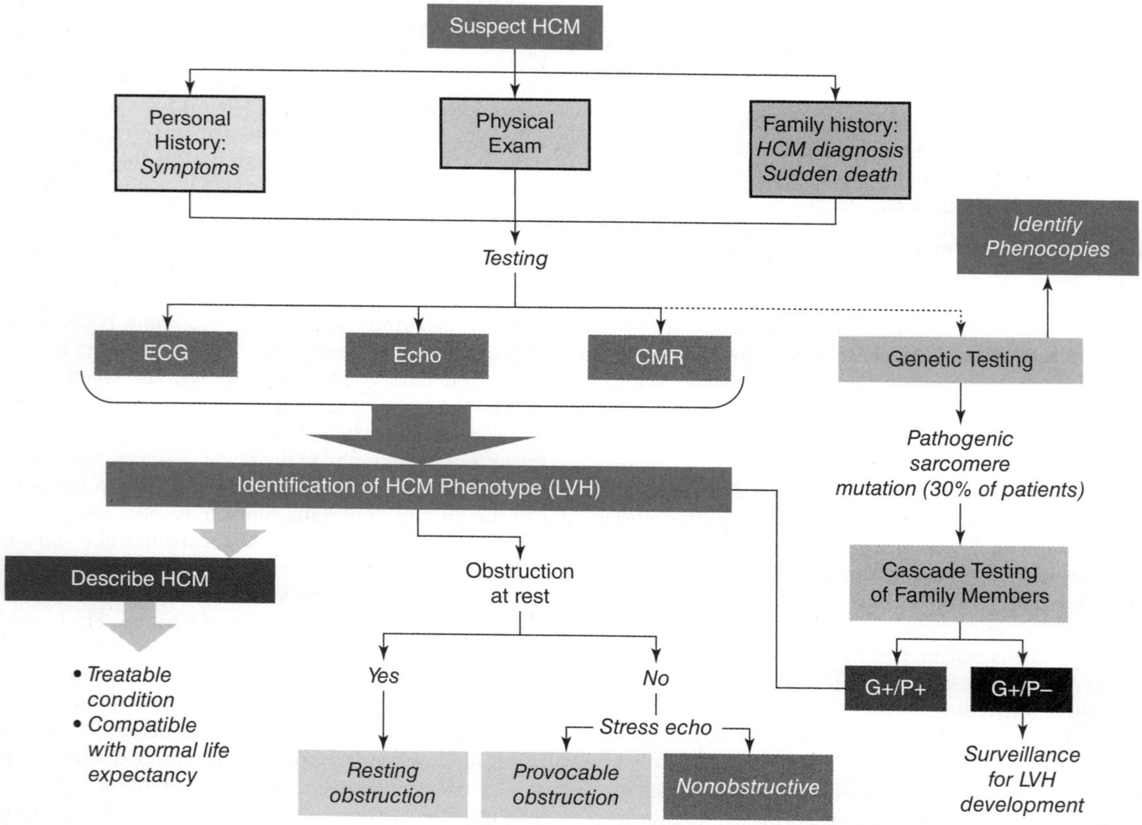

▲ **Figure 23–19.** **Flow diagram outlining the recommended approach to initial clinical assessment and diagnostic categories of hypertrophic cardiomyopathy (HCM). CMR: cardiac magnetic resonance; ECG: electrocardiogram.** (Reprinted from Journal of the American College of Cardiology, 79, Maron BJ, Desai MY, Nishimura RA. et al. *Diagnosis and Evaluation of Hypertrophic Cardiomyopathy JACC State-of-the-Art Review*, 372–389. Copyright 2022, with permission from Elsevier.)

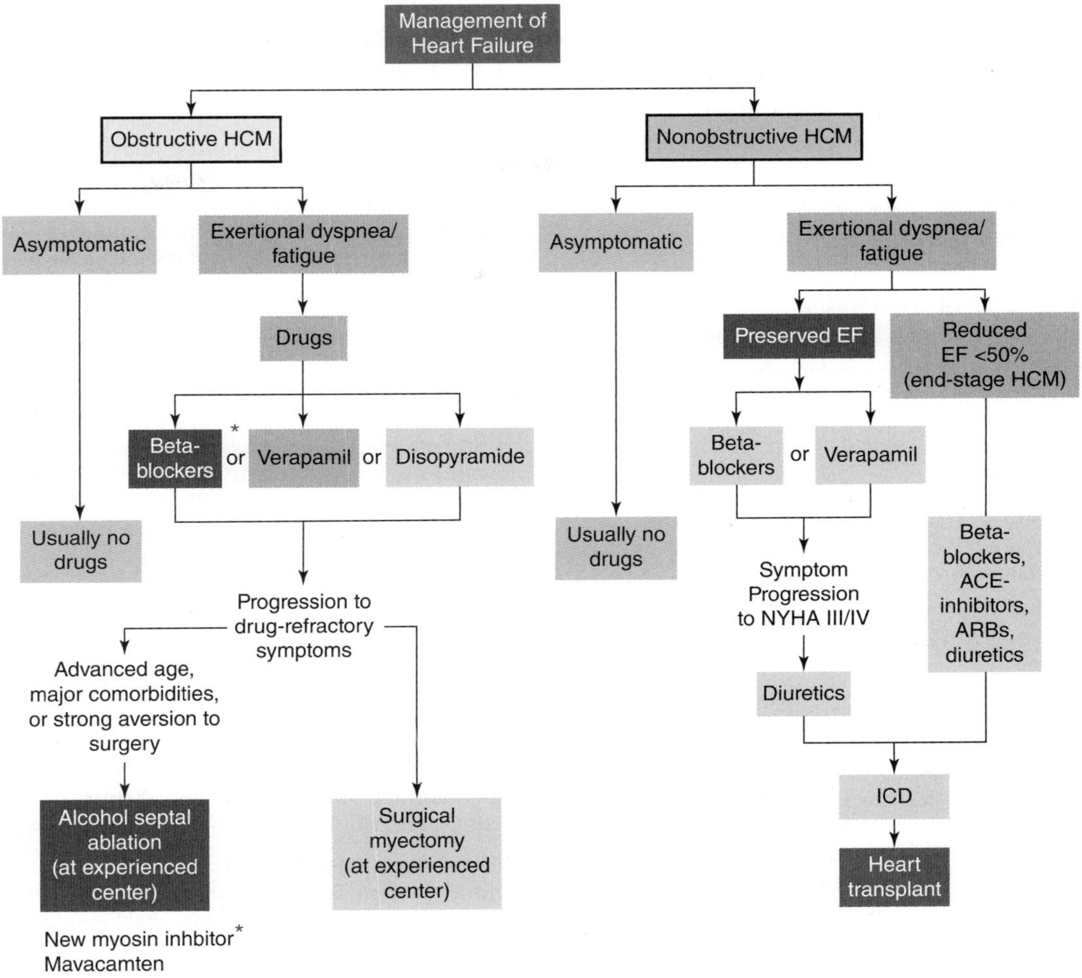

▲ **Figure 23–20.** Flow diagram outlining proposed approach to current treatment strategies of hypertrophic cardiomyopathy (HCM). (Reprinted from Journal of the American College of Cardiology, 79, Maron BJ, Desai MY, Nishimura RA. et al. *Management of Hypertrophic Cardiomyopathy JACC State-of-the-Art Review*, 390–414. Copyright 2022, with permission from Elsevier.)

C. Prevention of Sudden Cardiac Death in Hypertrophic Cardiomyopathy

A subset of patients with HCM is at increased risk of SCD (1%/year). The only effective prevention strategy against SCD for these patients is an implantable cardioverter-defibrillator (ICD). Although ICD recommendations for secondary prevention are usually straightforward (HCM with sudden cardiac death or sustained ventricular tachycardia is a Class 1 indication in 2020 ACC AHA guidelines), the decision as to when to recommend ICD in a primary prevention setting is challenging. Existing evidence suggests a 4%/year ICD intervention rate when used for primary prevention in appropriate high-risk patients.

Listed below are risk factors for SCD that can be used to favor the decision for primary prevention ICD, with special notations as needed. No single factor is an absolute indication and it needs to be evaluated in each patient from a clinical perspective. The more risk factors present, the stronger is the case for primary prevention ICD in HCM. The HCM guidelines consider ICD implantation reasonable for primary prevention (Class 2A, Level of Evidence C) for risk factors indicated with an asterisk. The other factors listed below can also be factored into decision-making if present as supporting evidence. Most importantly shared decision-making and discussion with the patient regarding not only the risk factor, but the magnitude of risk is key as emphasized in the guidelines.

1. Young (age < 30 years)
2. Massive septal hypertrophy (> 30 mm)*
3. Family history of sudden death*
4. Nonsustained ventricular tachycardia on ambulatory ECG monitoring or exercise-induced nonsustained ventricular tachycardia and other SCD risk markers*
5. Prior alcohol septal ablation
6. Certain gene mutations (Arg403Gln) or multiple sarcomere gene mutations
7. Recurrent unexplained syncope*
8. Bradyarrhythmias (occult conduction system disease)
9. Inappropriate blood pressure response (failure to increase by at least 20 mm Hg systolic or a drop of 20 mm Hg systolic with exercise) and other SCD risk markers
10. Marked LVOT gradient at rest (conflicting evidence)
11. Extensive late gadolinium enhancement with CMRI (> 15% of left ventricular myocardium mass. A Class 2b indication if this is only risk factor)*
12. LV apical aneurysm and scarring*
13. Underlying coronary artery disease (modifiable)

The AHA HCM SCD risk calculator can also be used to estimate 5-year SCD risk in patients ≥ 16 years with one major SCD risk factor to further help in guiding shared decision-making toward need for primary prevention of ICD. This calculator should not be used in pediatric patients, elite athletes, HCM related to metabolic or storage diseases or when a clear indication for secondary prevention ICD is indicated in HCM. The online calculator can be accessed at https://professional.heart.org/en/guidelines-and-statements/hcm-risk-calculator

D. Hypertrophic Cardiomyopathy and Athlete's Heart

Physiologic LV remodeling with LVH mimicking HCM can sometimes be seen in athletes, which makes decision-making regarding pathologic versus physiologic LVH challenging. Borderline increase in LV thickness (13–15 mm) is usually seen in elite/endurance athletes (long-distance cycling, cross-country skiing, rowing), but LV thickness more than 15 mm should raise concern for HCM. Women athletes seldom develop LV thickness more than 12 mm, beyond which pathologic hypertrophy should be suspected. Echo plays a key role in helping differentiate physiologic from pathologic hypertrophy. Normal- to small-sized ventricle, diastolic function impairment, tissue Doppler and strain abnormalities, and abnormal mitral valve apparatus all favor HCM. Cardiopulmonary exercise testing may also help because athletes will have high levels of maximal oxygen consumption with excellent exercise capacity compared to HCM, where these parameters will be impaired. CMRI may also help as a complementary imaging modality to make more accurate estimations of LV wall thickness, cavity size, and presence of delayed enhancement. Despite all of these potential parameters used for differentiation between these two entities, sometimes a definitive diagnosis may be elusive and a period of deconditioning for 3 months may be needed with repeat assessment of LV wall thickness/mass. There will be regression of LV thickness and mass in physiologic, but not pathologic, hypertrophy. There has been substantial change in thought process with regard to participation in sport and recreational activities as reflected in recent guidelines. There is no restriction for light to moderate recreational activity participation for athletes with HCM provided they are asymptomatic. Genotype positive–phenotype negative HCM patients can participate in all sport or recreational activities. Participation in high-intensity or competitive sports can be allowed after shared decision-making discussion with an expert who should explain the risks of SCD or ICD firing. Athletes should also undergo periodic re-evaluation.

E. Special Considerations in Hypertrophic Cardiomyopathy

1. Endocarditis prophylaxis—Current ACC/AHA guidelines do not recommend routine antibiotic prophylaxis for HOCM patients unless prior history of endocarditis exists. Overall risk of endocarditis is considered low in HCM unless significant outflow obstruction and abnormal mitral valve structure coexist.

2. Pregnancy and HCM—Asymptomatic HCM is not a contraindication for pregnancy but requires general and genetic counseling prior to planning and careful observation during pregnancy. Pregnancy in the setting of asymptomatic or mildly symptomatic HCM is usually well tolerated and vaginal delivery can be successfully accomplished. Pregnant HCM patients stable on selective β-blockers can have these continued with monitoring of fetus for bradycardia. Severely symptomatic HCM patients who are pregnant require high-risk obstetrics/cardiology care. Pregnancy is discouraged for HCM patients with heart failure due to high maternal and fetal morbidity and mortality. For pregnant HCM patients with atrial fibrillation, low molecular weight heparin or Vitamin K antagonist less than 5 mg total dose can be used for stroke prevention.

3. Atrial fibrillation—Atrial fibrillation is the most common arrhythmia that occur in HCM (in 20–25% of patients). It is poorly tolerated by patients with HCM who are dependent on atrial contribution to a stiff ventricle, and it should be promptly treated with restoration of sinus rhythm after initial rate control. Amiodarone appears to be the most effective agent for pharmacologic restoration of sinus rhythm followed by sotalol, dofetilide, or dronedarone. If this fails or the patient is hemodynamically compromised, electrical cardioversion is indicated. In the long term, if anti-arrhythmics are ineffective, pulmonary vein isolation procedures or surgical maze can be considered. Because of the high risk of systemic emboli and stroke, all HCM patients with atrial fibrillation should be prescribed long-term oral anticoagulant therapy regardless of their CHA_2DS_2VASc score. For HCM patients with atrial fibrillation undergoing myectomy, intrasurgical MAZE procedure can be done.

Ommen SR, Mital S, Burke MA, et al. 2020 ACCF/AHA guideline for the diagnosis and treatment of hypertrophic cardiomyopathy: a report of the American College of Cardiology Foundation/American Heart Association Task Force on Practice Guidelines. *J Am Coll Cardiol.* 2020;76:E159–240. [PMID: 33229116]

Pelliccia F, Alfieri O, Calabro P, et al. Multidisciplinary evaluation and management of obstructive hypertrophic cardiomyopathy in 2020: towards the HCM heart team. *Int J Cardiol.* 2020;304:86–92. [PMID: 31983465]

24 Restrictive Cardiomyopathy

James A. Goldstein, MD

ESSENTIALS OF DIAGNOSIS

- "Restriction" is not a disease per se, but rather a pathophysiological state of predominant ventricular diastolic dysfunction with lesser impairment of systolic performance, resulting in limited preload at an elevated filling pressure.
- Symptomatic presentation:
  - Chronic biventricular "backward failure" manifest as dyspnea and peripheral edema (often hepatomegaly and ascites).
  - Reduced preload limits cardiac output (fatigue).
- Echocardiography: small stiff ventricles, preserved systolic function (until late stages), dilated atria, and diastolic dysfunction by Doppler.
- Many disorders manifest restrictive "physiology" and must be excluded (eg, hypertrophic cardiomyopathy and constrictive pericarditis).
- Cardiac magnetic resonance imaging powerful: delineates myocardial infiltration, inflammation, and fibrosis and assesses pericardium, thereby helping establish underlying disorder.

Overview

Restrictive cardiomyopathies (RCM) are indolent disabling diseases resulting from pathophysiologic processes that induce predominant diastolic chamber dysfunction with lesser impairment of systolic performance. RCM is characterized by small stiff ventricles with progressive impairment of diastolic filling, leading to the hemodynamic conundrum of low preload but high filling pressures (Figure 24–1). This pattern of diastolic dysfunction leads to dilated atria and elevated mean atrial pressures, resulting clinically in biventricular "backward failure" manifest as pulmonary venous congestion (dyspnea) as well as systemic venous pressure elevation (peripheral edema). Systolic function is preserved in most cases, depending on the underlying cause (at least in the presenting stages of most of the underlying diseases). However, despite intact systolic function, the restrictive constraints on true ventricular preload limit stroke volume, thereby resulting in low cardiac output (fatigue) and ultimately hypoperfusion.

It is essential to emphasize that the term "restriction" is not a disease per se, but rather a pathophysiological state of predominant ventricular diastolic dysfunction with lesser impairment of systolic performance, resulting in limited preload at elevated filling pressure. The abnormal diastolic properties of the ventricle are typically attributable to abnormalities of the myocardium (hypertrophy, infiltration, inflammation, or fibrosis) or the endomyocardial surface (inflammation and scarring). RCM classification (Figure 24–2) may be most easily considered based on underlying pathophysiologic process as: (1) *hypertrophic* (eg, hypertension, aortic stenosis); (2) deposition, including both *infiltrative* diseases (eg, amyloidosis) and *storage* disorders (eg, hemochromatosis); (3) *inflammatory* (eg, hypereosinophilic syndrome); and (4) primary or *idiopathic*, including diabetes. It is important to consider the general perception of the "typical" RCM versus the clinical reality; that is, the term RCM tends to conjure cardiac amyloidosis, an infiltrative disease inducing "classic" and dramatic clinical manifestations of RCM. Certainly, identification of specific infiltrative and storage diseases may have important prognostic and therapeutic implications. However, far more prevalent is restrictive "physiology," which most commonly results from hypertrophic states typically seen in patients with advanced hypertension and the elderly (and in more complex forms in cases with aortic stenosis). Such "restrictive physiology" induces clinical manifestations similar and often indistinguishable from other "classic" forms of RCM.

The vast majority of the underlying disease processes are slowly progressive, but by the time patients develop cardiac symptoms, the disease is advanced pathologically, and heart

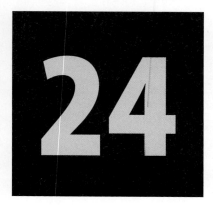

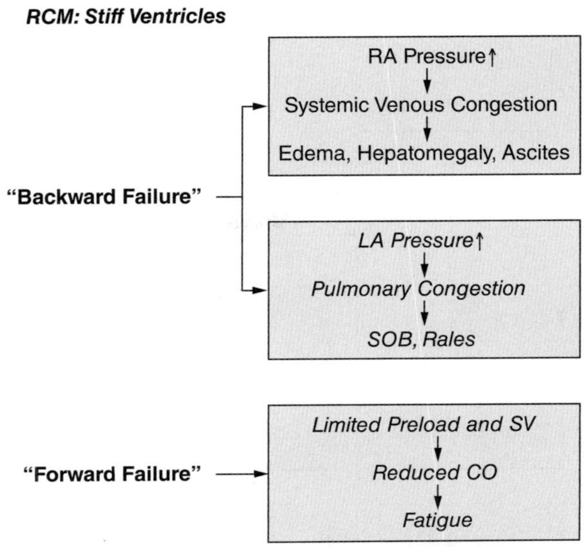

▲ **Figure 24–1.** Pathophysiology of restrictive cardiomyopathy (RCM). CO, cardiac output; LA, left atrium; RA, right atrium; SOB, shortness of breath; SV, stroke volume.

failure progresses rapidly over a short period of time, with the majority of patients dying within a few years following diagnosis.

Pertinent Aspects of Normal Hemodynamics

An appreciation of the physiology of the venous circulations and the dynamic effects of intrathoracic pressure (ITP) and respiratory motion on cardiovascular physiology is critical to understanding the hemodynamic pathophysiology of RCM and differentiating it from other conditions, particularly constrictive pericarditis (CP). Under physiologic conditions, venous return to both atria is biphasic, with a systolic peak determined by atrial relaxation ("X" descent of the atrial and jugular venous pressure [JVP] waveforms) and a diastolic peak determined by tricuspid valve (TV) resistance and right ventricular (RV) compliance ("Y" descent). Respiratory oscillations exert complex effects on cardiac filling and dynamics, with disparate effects on the right and left heart attributable to differences in their anatomic relationships to the respective venous return systems relative to the intrapleural space. Normally, inspiration induces decrements in ITP (−25 to −30 mm Hg), which are transmitted through the pericardium to the cardiac chambers. On the right heart, these decrements in ITP enhance the filling gradient from the extrathoracic systemic veins, thereby augmenting venous return and increasing right-heart filling and output. In contrast, the left heart and its tributary pulmonary veins are entirely intrathoracic. Therefore, inspiratory decrements in ITP are evenly distributed, and thus, mitral valve (MV) flow and left ventricular (LV) filling are essentially unchanged throughout the respiratory cycle.

Pathophysiology

The pathognomonic feature of RCM is stiffness of the ventricular walls, which impairs diastolic filling, resulting in limited ventricular preload (and therefore stroke volume) despite increased diastolic filling pressures. Echocardiography (echo) documents small ventricles, often with thick walls. By invasive hemodynamic assessment, RCM is characterized by elevated ventricular diastolic pressures (Figures 24–3 and 24–4), often with a mild diastolic "dip and plateau" or "square root" pattern, a nonspecific indicator of stiff noncompliant chambers, a phenomenon also seen in other conditions such as CP (discussed later). Echo-Doppler demonstrates classic features of impaired diastolic function (impaired myocardial relaxation with increased early LV filling velocity, decreased atrial filling velocity, and decreased isovolumic relaxation time). Ventricular systolic function is typically preserved until the later stages of the underlying disease. Biatrial enlargement reflects ventricular noncompliance and may also result from primary atrial myocardial involvement by the disease process (eg, amyloidosis). Atrial filling pressures are elevated, and the X and Y descents tend to be relatively blunted; in cases in which the atria are primarily involved by the restrictive process, the A wave may be depressed (see Figure 24–3). In RCM, a pattern of "elevated and equalized" chamber diastolic filling pressures indicating pancardiac "stiffness" is common, but this nonspecific pattern is also seen in other diseases, particularly pericardial constraint conditions (eg, CP). However, in RCM, left-sided pressures are typically somewhat higher than right due to the greater intrinsic stiffness of the LV. This difference may be amplified by maneuvers that augment ventricular filling such as volume infusion, leg-raising, or post–premature ventricular contraction increased filling time. Disproportionate left-heart stiffness may also result in moderate pulmonary hypertension (a subtle distinguishing feature from CP).

In RCM, inspiratory changes in ITP are fully transmitted through the pericardium to the cardiac chambers. However, chamber noncompliance contributes to a relative lack of respiratory variation in cardiac filling, and therefore, mitral and tricuspid flow velocity during respiration are typically decreased. Because of the lack of pericardial constraint and a relatively noncompliant interventricular septum, there is minimal ventricular interdependence, and thus, inspiratory effects on ventricular systolic pressures are concordant (ie, there is little change in peak ventricular systolic pressures with respiration and they move in the same direction) (see Figure 24–4); as will be discussed, the pressure pattern in CP is "discordant." As RCM progresses and right-sided chambers become less distensible, the respiratory swings in pressure diminish further. At its most severe, noncompliance to inflow results in the Kussmaul sign, an inspiratory

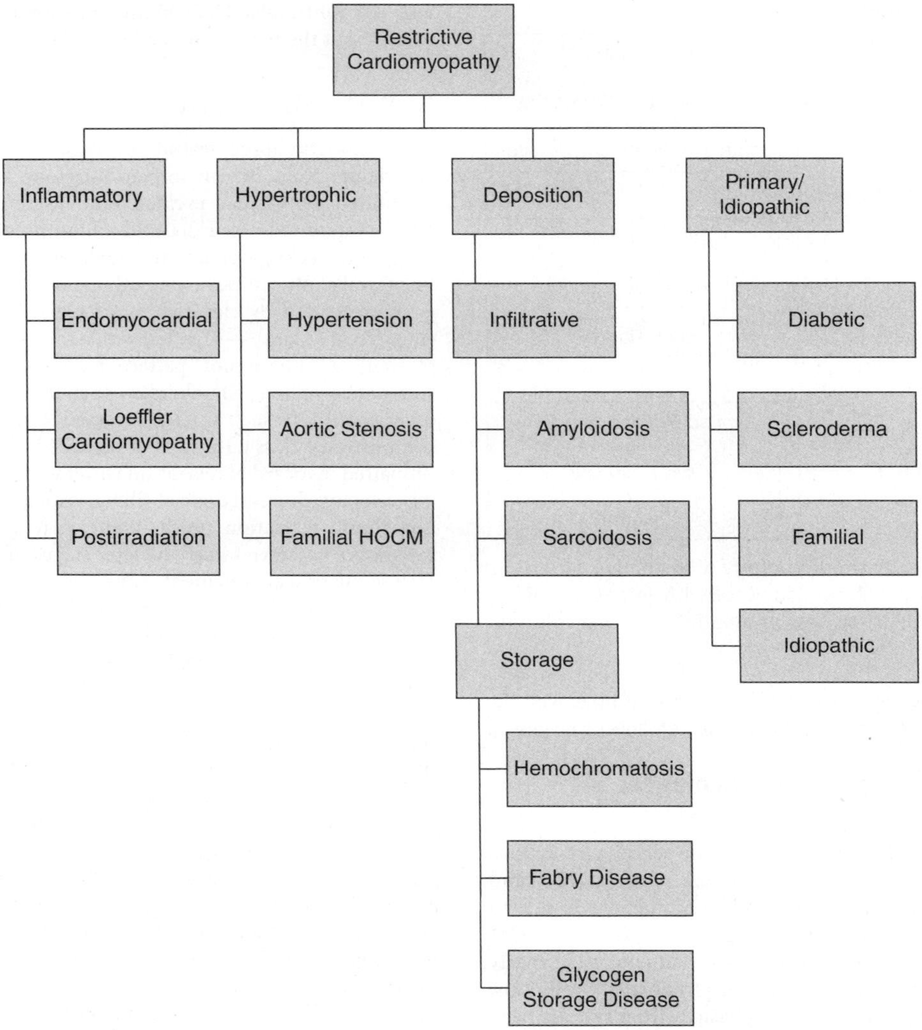

▲ **Figure 24–2.** Classification of restrictive cardiomyopathies. HOCM, hypertrophic obstructive cardiomyopathy.

increase in venous return that cannot be accommodated by the stiff right heart, resulting in inspiratory elevation of JVP (see Figure 24–3). Doppler flow patterns show blunting of the expected physiologic respiratory increases in flow across the TV and minimal change across the MV.

Kusunose K, Dahiya A, Popovic ZB, et al. Biventricular mechanics in constrictive pericarditis comparison with restrictive cardiomyopathy and impact of pericardiectomy. *Circ Cardiovasc Imaging.* 2013;6(3):399–406. [PMID: 23532508]

▶ Clinical Findings

Patients with RCM suffer symptoms attributable to ventricular diastolic dysfunction. Systemic venous congestion related to right heart noncompliance typically predominates, characterized by pedal edema, abdominal swelling, and gastrointestinal symptoms related to hepatic/bowel congestion (loss of appetite). Physical examination reveals elevated jugular venous pressure often with Kussmaul sign, peripheral edema, and ascites; with advancing disease, hepatomegaly, ascites, and anasarca develop. Patients typically are limited by dyspnea on exertion attributable to left-heart diastolic dysfunction. At the bedside, patients will exhibit signs of right heart failure (eg, elevated JVP with edema, ascites), but the precordial examination will be quiet with no evidence of an RV heave, thus pointing away from other causes of right heart failure such as pulmonary hypertension, dilated cardiomyopathy, or TV regurgitation (all of which will manifest an RV heave/lift in the left parasternal area).

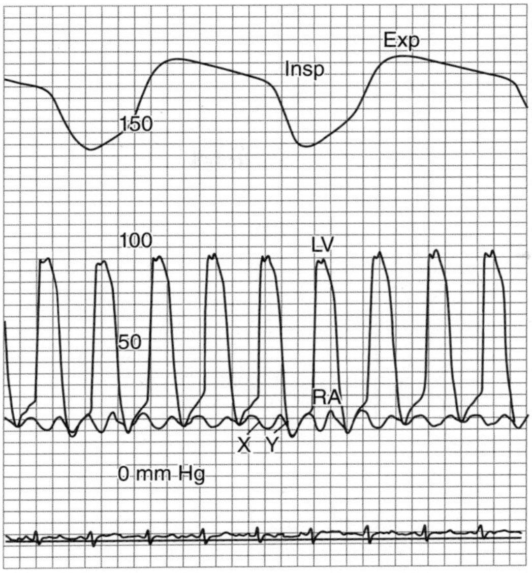

▲ **Figure 24–3.** Simultaneous recordings of left ventricular (LV) and right atrial (RA) pressures. Note the marked "W" or "M" pattern in the RA pressure tracing with prominent X and Y descents and with no fall with inspiration (Kussmaul sign). The nasal respirometer tracing is also shown. Exp, expiration; Insp, inspiration. (Reproduced with permission from Higano ST, Azrak E, et al. Hemodynamic rounds series II: hemodynamics of constrictive physiology: influence of respiratory dynamics on ventricular pressures. *Catheter Cardiovasc Interv*. 1999;46(4):473–486.)

LV diastolic dysfunction manifests as elevated pulmonary capillary wedge pressure and dyspnea, initially at rest but in many cases may precipitate pulmonary congestion. In the classic RCM disease exemplified by infiltrative amyloid disease, there is biventricular diastolic dysfunction resulting in both backward left- and right-heart failure. However, the most common cause of "Restrictive Pathophysiology" is LV hypertrophy (from hypertension and aortic stenosis) which may only manifest in backward left-heart failure and pulmonary congestion, without right heart and systemic venous congestion.

In the early stages of RCM, systolic function is typically preserved, although deterioration in contractility may be observed as the disease progresses; the severity and patterns of dysfunction depend on the specific etiology and severity of the underlying disease entity. Despite preserved systolic ventricular function, impaired diastolic filling limits ventricular preload, thereby rendering the stiff heart limited in its ability to increase cardiac output with exercise, resulting in fatigability. Low output combined with autonomic insufficiency characteristic of some RCMs (eg, amyloidosis) renders patients susceptible to symptoms of orthostatic hypotension. Atrial dilation often leads to atrial fibrillation, which further exacerbates diastolic dysfunction due to high heart rate and loss of atrial contraction.

Etiologies

A. Myocardial Disorders

1. Deposition: infiltrative and storage disorders

A. Cardiac amyloid—Amyloidosis is the prototypical *infiltrative* RCM, arising from a group of disorders characterized as amyloid of immunologic origin (AL) related to plasma cell dyscrasia (which may or may not blossom as frank multiple myeloma with bone marrow involvement), transthyretin (ATTR) amyloidosis (attributable to excessive production of this hepatic-generated protein that carries thyroid hormone) which may be heritable ("mutant" related to genetics with 3% prevalence in African-Americans) or "wild type" also known as "senile" amyloid and predominantly seen in the elderly. Regardless of the etiology, systemic amyloidosis results in infiltrative deposition of these β-pleated sheet proteins, typically with multiorgan involvement. Cardiac amyloid prevalence varies depending on the underlying amyloid precursor protein entity. Cardiac amyloid is typically silent until tissue infiltration is extensive, leading to RCM with symptomatically progressive biventricular diastolic dysfunction. Imaging modalities, biochemical tests, and tissue samples establish a definitive diagnosis. Echo documentation of thick walls, small cavities, and granular speckled "hyperrefractile" myocardial pattern is nearly diagnostic. Cardiac magnetic resonance imaging (MRI) shows diffuse late gadolinium enhancement throughout both ventricles, particularly the subendocardium. To exclude amyloid of the AL type, monoclonal gammopathy may be evident on urine and serum protein electrophoresis, although immunofixation and assays for serum-free light chains are more sensitive. However, it is important to emphasize that advanced imaging with cardiac MRI has dramatically shifted the diagnostic paradigm for cardiac amyloid. To wit, if the heart is thick and MRI confirms a pattern characteristic of amyloid (thick walls, diffuse late gadolinium enhancement), the next step is to perform a technetium pyrophosphate nuclear scan, which if positive definitively establishes the diagnosis of ATTR and precludes the necessity of further diagnostic evaluation; if negative, the MRI still establishes the high likelihood of cardiac amyloid serving, effectively as a "noninvasive biopsy" pointing to the diagnosis which still requires tissue confirmation. An invasive biopsy of the myocardium or other tissue targets (abdominal fat pad) may still be preferred to definitively establish the diagnosis and characterize the immunological protein. Amyloid deposits can be documented by biopsy of myocardium; traditionally by histology, Congo red staining delineates amyloid deposits between cardiac myocytes (now definitively by immuno-histochemical staining and mass spectrophotometric techniques). If AL is confirmed,

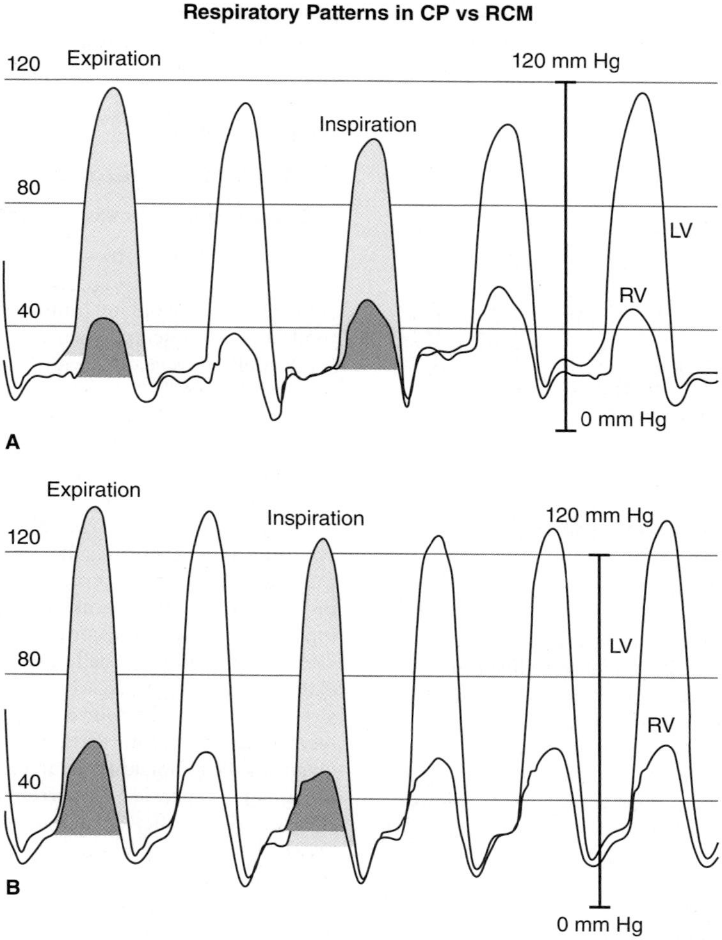

▲ **Figure 24–4.** Left ventricle (LV) and right ventricle (RV) high-fidelity manometer pressure traces from two patients during expiration and inspiration. Note that both patients have early rapid filling and elevation and end-equalization of the LV and RV pressures at end expiration. **A:** A patient with surgically documented constrictive pericarditis (CP). During inspiration, there is an increase in the area of the RV pressure curve (*orange-shaded area*) compared with expiration. The area of the LV pressure curve (*yellow-shaded area*) decreases during inspiration as compared with expiration. **B:** A patient with restrictive cardiomyopathy (RCM) documented by endomyocardial biopsy. During inspiration, there is a decrease in the area of the RV pressure curve (*orange-shaded area*) as compared with expiration. The area of the LV pressure curve (*yellow-shaded area*) is unchanged during inspiration as compared with expiration. (Reproduced with permission from Talreja DR, Nishimura RA, Oh JK, Holmes DR. Constrictive pericarditis in the modern era: novel criteria for diagnosis in the cardiac catheterization laboratory. *J Am Coll Cardiol*. 2008;51(3):315–319.)

hematological evaluation including serum-free light chains bone marrow biopsy should then be pursued.

The general treatment approach is as with any RCM. The mainstay is diuretics to decongest within the limits tolerated by hypotension. These patients are at high risk of thromboembolism, especially with atrial fibrillation, but even in its absence, anticoagulation should be strongly considered. Untreated patients with AL amyloid have a median survival of less than 6 months after onset of heart failure. Aggressive chemotherapy, immunomodulatory drugs (eg, lenalidomide), proteasome inhibitors (eg, Bortezomib), and monoclonal antibodies show potential benefits for the *treatment* of AL *amyloidosis*. Also, stem cell transplantation, followed by cardiac transplantation, has shown promising potential in a small number of cases, but transplantation mortality rate is high, and randomized data are lacking. Transthyretin (ATTR) amyloidosis is increasingly recognized and has a predilection for cardiac involvement but may have a more indolent course, although frequent concomitant autonomic neuropathy predisposes to more hypotension, which complicates management. Recently a few pharmacologic treatments for ATTR have been approved for use, with tafamadis showing improved survival. Liver transplantation is another option.

B. Sarcoidosis—This systemic inflammatory condition results in multiorgan infiltration with noncaseating granulomatous infiltration, typically in the lungs, reticuloendothelial system, and skin. The heart is involved in 20–30% of cases at autopsy, with patchy granulomatous infiltration in discrete areas of the ventricular walls with a predilection for the posterior LV free wall, basal septum, and conduction system. Cardiac infiltrate may result in fibrotic scars and "microaneurysm" formation. Cardiac sarcoid involvement is typically focal and most commonly presents clinically with conduction block or malignant arrhythmias and less commonly with heart failure due to RCM. The electrocardiogram (ECG) may reveal atypical infarction patterns and various degrees of atrioventricular block. Echo varies according to disease activity, with wall thickening due to granulomatous expansion but later wall thinning due to fibrosis. Segmental hypokinesia most commonly localizes to mid and basal segments of the LV free wall and upper septum. Due to patchy involvement, endomyocardial biopsy provides diagnostic evidence in only 25–50% of autopsy-confirmed cases. Cardiac MRI and positron emission tomography (PET) are more sensitive and correlate with disease severity. Treatment is based on the foundation of anti-inflammatory/immunosuppressant therapy initially with corticosteroids induction then weaned to "maintenance," guided by serial PET scanning and echocardiography. Escalated therapies for those not responsive to steroids includes azathioprine and methotrexate, mycophenolate, and infusions of TNF inhibitors. If treated early, when inflammation predominates, and fibrosis is less advanced, pharmacologic therapy may improve cardiac function. Given the arrhythmic complications of sarcoid, referral to an electrophysiologist for pacemaker-defibrillator protection and therapy should be considered.

C. Glycogen storage diseases—RCMs may result from heritable metabolic disorders resulting in myocardial accumulation or infiltration of abnormal metabolic products, producing classic RCM. The recent availability of enzyme replacement in some disorders makes early diagnosis increasingly essential. The most common are glycogen storage disorders (Gaucher and Fabry disease) resulting from lysosomal accumulation in the heart and other organs. Gaucher disease commonly presents with RCM in childhood and is responsive to enzyme replacement therapy or, in extreme cases, hepatic transplantation. In Fabry disease, cardiac involvement is typically manifest in the third or fourth decade of life; the thick ventricular walls mimic hypertrophic cardiomyopathy (HCM); differentiation by MRI may be helpful. Other less common heritable storage disorders that may result in RCM include the mucopolysaccharidoses, myocardial oxalosis (related to underling primary hyperoxaluria), and Friedreich ataxia (an autosomal recessive neurodegenerative disorder associated with RCM and/or dilated cardiomyopathy in 90–100% of cases).

D. Hemochromatosis—Cardiac iron overload, due to heritable disease or chronic and excessive iron administration (eg, transfusions) represents "storage" disorder in which iron deposition with resultant fibrosis is always multiorgan, giving rise to the classic clinical presentation of heart failure, cirrhosis, impotence, and diabetes. At pathology, hearts are dilated, and ventricular walls thickened. Echo shows a nonspecific mixed pattern of systolic and diastolic dysfunction. The condition is commonly complicated by and may be announced by arrhythmias. Laboratory evaluation is usually diagnostic (marked elevations of plasma iron, serum ferritin, and transferrin saturation, but lower normal total iron binding capacity). Cardiac MRI is a sensitive marker of iron deposition and predictive of future events. Endomyocardial biopsy is definitive, but usually not necessary when biochemical testing is diagnostic. Chelation therapy is appropriate and may limit further damage but is unlikely to reverse existing organ dysfunction.

2. Hypertrophic states—LV hypertrophy (LVH) typically results in some degree of diastolic dysfunction; when advanced, "restrictive physiology" results. In fact, LVH is the most common cause of "restrictive pathophysiology." LVH may be acquired (advanced hypertension, aortic stenosis, and the elderly) or heritable (familial HCM). Restrictive physiology from LVH induces clinical manifestations often indistinguishable from other "classic" forms of RCM, characterized by pulmonary congestion due to diastolic dysfunction coupled with restricted filling, leading to low stroke volume and cardiac output and challenging the ability to diurese the patient. Chronic left-sided diastolic pressures commonly induce pulmonary hypertension and right heart failure as well. Restrictive physiology underlies most cases of heart failure with preserved ejection fraction, a disease with near-epidemic proportions in the rapidly growing number of aged patients and those suffering the effects of metabolic syndrome. Restriction is also inherent to the pathophysiology of LV outflow obstruction syndromes, both fixed obstruction in valvular aortic stenosis as well as dynamic obstruction associated with familial hypertrophic obstructive cardiomyopathy. The presence of any obstruction further downstream exacerbates the forward output limitations of the stiff restricted hypertrophic LV. Restrictive physiology underlies the clinical entity of low flow–low gradient aortic stenosis with preserved LV systolic function, wherein profound LV preload limitation reduces stroke volume, which contributes to low gradient despite significant obstruction.

3. Primary and idiopathic RCM—Primary RCM may be due to hereditary contractile protein mutations, representing approximately 50% of cases and occurring more commonly in older women than men. Wall thickness is commonly increased by echocardiography, and biopsy typically reveals myocyte hypertrophy often with patchy endocardial fibrosis involving both ventricles. Diabetics may also develop RCM not related to coronary artery disease or hypertension per se; the LV in such patients shows myocyte hypertrophy and fibrosis by histologic examination. Idiopathic diagnosis can only be established in the absence of other identifiable causes (ie, storage, infiltrative, and inflammatory diseases), many of which induce thick ventricular walls and infiltrative/storage damage on biopsy. Idiopathic RCM characterized by nondilated, nonhypertrophic ventricles with marked biatrial dilatation affects predominantly elderly patients, who suffer systemic and pulmonary venous congestion and atrial fibrillation and have a poor prognosis.

B. Endomyocardial Disease

There are two variants of endomyocardial disease, with different pathogenesis but shared and overlapping features. Endomyocardial fibrosis (EMF) refers to a specific syndrome with characteristic geographic epidemiologic features. Other cardiomyopathy syndromes with similar pathologies include Loeffler endocarditis (also called hypereosinophilic endomyocarditis) and other diseases that induce fibrotic changes of the endocardium (ie, carcinoid heart disease).

1. Endomyocardial fibrosis—EMF occurs primarily in tropical regions and in subtropical zones, presents at a young age, and is the most common form of RCM worldwide. EMF is characterized by fibrosis of the apical endocardium of the ventricles. The clinical manifestations are classic RCM.

2. Loeffler "hypereosinophilic" endomyocarditis—This group of disorders results from sustained overproduction of eosinophils, leading to eosinophilic infiltration and mediator release, which damages multiple organs. Diagnosis is established by eosinophil counts more than 1500 for at least 6 months. The disease may be primary, but it is essential to search for secondary and potentially treatable causes including leukemia, reactive disorders such as parasite infection, allergies, granulomatous syndromes, hypersensitivity, and neoplastic disorders. Eosinophil-mediated heart damage, detected by echo or MRI, evolves through three stages: (1) an acute necrotic stage; (2) an intermediate phase characterized by thrombus formation along the damaged endocardium; and (3) a fibrotic stage. Treatment is aimed at the underlying disease.

3. Carcinoid heart disease—Carcinoid tumors metastatic to the liver elaborating circulating serotonin (and 5-hydroxyindolacetic acid, its primary metabolite) induce fibrous endocardial plaques in 50% of patients. By echo, plaques are typically seen on the endocardium downstream from the liver, commonly resulting in stenotic and regurgitant valvular lesions (especially the tricuspid valve). The observation that the right heart is preferentially affected reflects inactivation of these toxic substances in the lung. Management of the underlying carcinoid is the focus of treatment. Identical pathology results from exposure to the anorectic drug fenfluramine and its related medications.

Baker MC, Sheth K, Witteles R, Genovese MC, Shoor S, Simard JF. TNF-alpha inhibition for the treatment of cardiac sarcoidosis. *Semin Arthritis Rheum*. 2020;50:546–552. [PMID: 31806154]

Bokhari S, Castaño A, Pozniakoff T, Deslisle S, Latif F, Maurer MS. ^{99m}Tc-pyrophosphate scintigraphy for differentiating light-chain cardiac amyloidosis from the transthyretin-related familial and senile cardiac amyloidoses. *Circ Cardiovasc Imaging*. 2013;6(2):195–201. [PMID: 23400849]

Castaño A, Drachman BM, Judge D, Maurer MS. Natural history and therapy of TTR-cardiac amyloidosis: emerging disease-modifying therapies from organ transplantation to stabilizer and silencer drugs. *Heart Fail Rev*. 2015;20(2):163–178. [PMID: 25408161]

Gillmore JD, Maurer MS, Falk RH, et al. Nonbiopsy diagnosis of cardiac transthyretin amyloidosis. *Circulation*. 2016;133(24): 2404–2412. [PMID: 27143678]

Maurer MS, Schwartz JH, Gundapaneni B. Tafamadis treatment for patients with transthyretin amyloid cardiomyopathy. *N Engl J Med*. 2018;379:1007–1016. [PMID: 25408161]

Muchtar E, Blauwet LA, Gertz MA. Restrictive cardiomyopathy: genetics, pathogenesis, clinical manifestations, diagnosis and therapy. *Circ Res*. 2017;121:819–837. [PMID: 28912185]

Ruberg FL, Grogan M, Hanna M, Kelly JW, Maurer MS. Transthyretin amyloid cardiomyopathy: JACC State-of-the-Art Review. *J Am Coll Cardiol*. 2019;73:2872–2891. [PMID: 31171094]

Differentiating Restrictive Cardiomyopathy from Other Disorders

Cardiac chambers with thick walls, small ventricular cavities with intact systolic function, and dilated atria are also typical of conditions with myocyte hypertrophy such as congenital hypertrophic cardiomyopathy (HCM) or acquired hypertensive and valvular heart disease. Coronary artery disease, especially in diabetics, can also mimic clinical RCM. Careful history, physical examination, noninvasive testing, and arteriography can exclude these acquired conditions, whereas differentiating HCM may pose challenges.

Differentiating RCM versus CP poses one of the most challenging clinical hemodynamic conundrums and deserves special consideration. These two conditions are remarkably similar in their hemodynamic pathophysiology, share nearly identical clinical presentation characterized by systemic and pulmonary congestion due to biventricular diastolic dysfunction with limited cardiac output, and appear quite similar by echocardiography, with small ventricles, dilated atria, and intact systolic function. However, they are distinctly different entities in terms of clinical course, management, and prognosis. CP is "curable" through surgical pericardiectomy, whereas RCM is treated by palliative measures and rarely if ever cured. Because of this important distinction, accurate differentiation is crucial.

First, it is essential to appreciate the subtle similarities and differences in hemodynamic pathophysiology of CP compared to RCM. CP is the result of inflammatory fibrocalcification leading to a thick, inelastic pericardium that encases the heart, inducing biventricular diastolic dysfunction. As in RCM, this process is typically indolent and slowly progressive, with clinical manifestations appearing often years after the initial insult. There is substantial overlap in hemodynamic features, which reflect similarities in pathophysiology rather than differences in disease mechanism. In CP, early ventricular filling is resistance free; however, as the ventricles fill, they abruptly meet the inelastic resistance of the stiff pericardium, at which time filling pressure rises rapidly to an elevated plateau, inscribing an RV "dip and plateau" or "square root" waveform pattern, like RCM (see Figure 24–4). In CP, atrial filling pressures are elevated, reflecting both ventricular noncompliance and atrial constraint. The right atrium Y descent is sharper in CP, reflecting the initial rapid, resistance-free early RV filling. In CP, diastolic filling pressures are elevated and equalized, reflecting the common constraining effects of the pericardium. In RCM, the intrinsic cardiac disease more often results in "nearly equalized patterns" with disproportionate elevation of left heart filling pressures. Hemodynamic challenges including rapid volume loading, leg elevation, or exercise to affect a disproportionate rise in LV diastolic pressure suggests RCM but is not diagnostic. The presence of mild-moderate pulmonary hypertension favors the diagnosis of RCM but may occur in constriction due to preexistent left heart or intrinsic pulmonary disease.

The effects of respiration on cardiac dynamics differ between RCM and CP in subtle but complex ways, findings that may help differentiate these conditions. In CP, increased pericardial resistance more tightly couples the two ventricles and increases their interdependence. Pericardial constraint limits total cardiac volume: Consequently, an increase in filling on one side of the heart impedes contralateral filling through intensified septal-mediated interactions. In CP, the inelastic fibrocalcific pericardial shell isolates the heart from the lungs, and therefore, respiratory changes in ITP are not fully transmitted to the cardiac chambers, resulting in dissociation of respiratory effects on ITP and intracardiac flows in the right heart versus the left heart. This represents an important difference compared to RCM. In CP, the inspiratory gradient created between the extrathoracic systemic veins and intrathoracic but extrapericardial cavae augments venous return to the right heart, but the constrictive pericardial shell neither fully facilitates inspiratory augmentation of right heart filling, nor accommodates whatever meager increments in filling occur. The result is an inspiratory increase in jugular venous and right heart filling pressures known as the Kussmaul sign (also seen in RCM). Anatomic–pathophysiologic relationships in the left heart are different: The pulmonary veins are entirely intrathoracic, the left atrium is not fully encased within the pericardium due to the pericardial reflection around the pulmonary veins, but the LV is fully constrained within the pericardium. Therefore, the inspiratory decrement in ITP is exerted on the pulmonary veins, but not transmitted to the LV, resulting in reduced transmitral pressure gradient and flow. Because the rigid pericardium fixes total cardiac volume and induces tight ventricular coupling, there is a reciprocal relation between left- and right-heart filling. This results in inspiratory decrease in LV filling, which allows a small relative increase in tricuspid inflow and RV filling, leading to opposite directional increase in RV but decrease in LV changes in inspiratory ventricular systolic pressures, called "ventricular discordance" (see Figure 24–4), which is indicative of enhanced ventricular interaction and a strong indicator of CP. Analogous findings are evident in Doppler flow velocities including more than 25% expiratory increase in mitral E velocity and expiratory decrease in hepatic vein diastolic flow velocity and more than 25% increase in diastolic flow reversals compared with inspiratory velocity. In contrast, in RCM, inspiratory changes in ITP are fully transmitted through the pericardium to the cardiac chambers, but chamber noncompliance limits respiratory augmentation of cardiac filling, which, together with lack of pericardial constraint and a noncompliant interventricular septum, minimizes ventricular interdependence. The result is blunted respiratory flow velocities by Doppler and "concordant" ventricular systolic pressures. These disparate patterns with respiration have been proposed to differentiate CP versus RCM (see Figure 24–4). However, the overall specificity and sensitivity of these hemodynamic criteria, both alone and in combination, have not been sufficient to provide a basis for definitive diagnosis in individual patients.

Clinical Algorithms to Differentiate Constriction from Restriction

Since the clinical presentation of these two entities is often similar, separating them based on anatomic and physiologic derangements is essential and requires the use of techniques that visualize the cardiac chambers and the pericardium, in conjunction with modalities that delineate the physiologic manifestations of the anatomic abnormalities. Most important, the single distinctive feature differentiating CP from RCM is anatomic, not physiologic: In patients with CP, the pericardium is almost always thickened and motion of the heart within the pericardium constrained, whereas in RCM patients, this is not the case. Therefore, anatomic documentation of pericardial thickness in patients with constrictive-restrictive physiology is crucial in differentiating these conditions (Figure 24–5). However, it must be emphasized that the finding of pericardial thickening should not be construed as the equivalent of a physiologic disorder because a thickened pericardium does not necessarily constrict. For example, pericardial thickening can be present in patients without physiologic constriction, particularly with tuberculosis or after open-heart surgery. Conversely, there can be physiologic pericardial constriction with normal-appearing pericardium by advanced cardiac imaging modalities.

Traditional and advanced cardiac imaging provides valuable information. The chest x-ray in CP may reveal

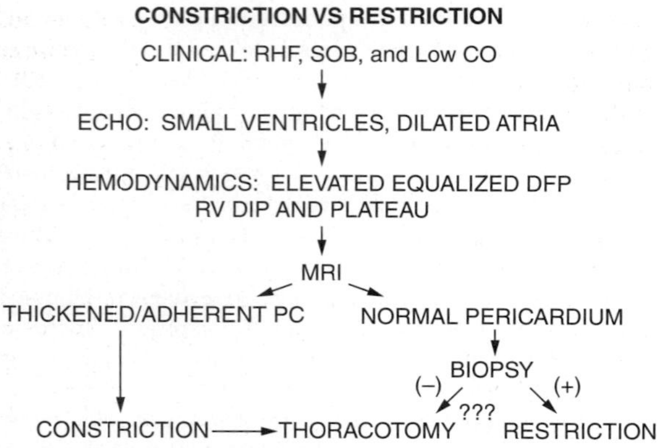

▲ **Figure 24–5.** Clinical algorithm to differentiate constrictive pericarditis versus restrictive cardiomyopathy. CO, cardiac output; DFP, diastolic filling pressure; ECHO, echocardiography; MRI, magnetic resonance imaging; PC, pericardium; RHF, right heart failure; RV, right ventricle; SOB, shortness of breath.

pericardial calcification. In both conditions, the ECG is nonspecific but often reveals diffuse low voltage with nonspecific ST-T changes. By echocardiography, most RCMs exhibit thick walls, whereas CP does not. RCMs, particularly amyloid, result in the paradox of thick walls by echo but reduced voltage on ECG, a pattern not seen in CP. Cardiac MRI is a powerful tool to evaluate patients with RCM in general and to distinguish it from CP. MRI provides data regarding not only chamber size, wall thickness, and ventricular function, but also the presence or absence of myocardial infiltration, inflammation, or fibrosis, patterns which inform the diagnosis of specific forms of RCM. After establishing that the myocardium appears normal, the delineation of pericardial thickness provides a basis for a therapeutic algorithm to definitively delineate CP versus RCM (see Figure 24–5). MRI provides insight not only regarding pericardial thickness, but also the dynamic nature of myocardial-pericardial interactions, specifically whether the pericardial layers are adherent to the heart and whether the heart slides normally in a smooth independent pattern within the pericardium during cardiac motion. Documentation of a thickened pericardium adherent to the epicardium and lack of independent motion are sufficient to diagnose CP, although RCM and CP may coexist (eg, radiation induced).

In patients with a clinical presentation and echo-Doppler findings consistent with either diagnosis, invasive hemodynamics should be performed and documentation of pericardial thickness performed. Employing this strategy, if pericardial imaging is confirmatory and hemodynamic findings consistent, biopsy is unnecessary and surgical exploration and pericardiectomy are warranted. In patients without these findings, assiduous clinical search for disease entities that result in RCM (eg, amyloidosis, hemochromatosis, scleroderma) will often result in delineation of the underlying etiology. Although clinical features and biochemical testing (eg, serum/urine protein electrophoresis, iron studies) may be sufficient, endomyocardial biopsy may be necessary to confirm its presence in the heart. However, if imaging fails to demonstrate constrictive features, then endomyocardial biopsy can be performed at the time of cardiac catheterization. Finally, it is important to emphasize that some patients with severe pericardial constriction proven at surgical exploration may have normal pericardial thickness by imaging techniques. Accordingly, in patients with severe clinical manifestations, lack of increased pericardial thickness, and normal endomyocardial biopsy, thoracoscopy or minimally invasive exploratory thoracotomy with provisional planned pericardiectomy should be considered.

Alajaji W, Xu B, Sripariwuth A, et al. Noninvasive multimodality imaging for the diagnosis of constrictive pericarditis. *Circ Cardiovasc Imaging*. 2021;14:1221–1231. [PMID: 30571315]

Amaki M, Savino J, Ain DL, et al. Diagnostic concordance of echocardiography and cardiac magnetic resonance-based tissue tracking for differentiating constrictive pericarditis from restrictive cardiomyopathy. *Circ Cardiovasc Imaging*. 2014;7(5): 819–827. [PMID: 25107553]

Garcia MJ. Constrictive pericarditis versus restrictive cardiomyopathy. *J Am Coll Cardiol*. 2016;67:2061–2076. [PMID: 27126534]

Geske JB, Anavekar NS, Nishimura RA, Oh JK, Gersh BJ. Differentiation of constriction and restriction: complex cardiovascular hemodynamics. *J Am Coll Cardiol*. 2016;68:2329–2347. [PMID: 27884252]

Treatment

Since few cases of RCM have treatable primary disease etiologies, management is based on diuretics to ameliorate pulmonary and systemic venous congestion. Frustratingly, optimal diuretic doses in RCM may reduce ventricular preload, leading to decreased cardiac output and symptoms of fatigability and light-headedness and even signs of hypotension and hypoperfusion. The development of atrial fibrillation and concomitant loss of atrial contractile contribution to filling of these stiff ventricles may worsen existing diastolic dysfunction and low output; in addition, rapid ventricular response may further compromise cardiovascular function. Thus, it is important to maintain sinus rhythm if feasible. However, digoxin should be used with caution, since it is potentially arrhythmogenic, particularly in patients with amyloidosis; other medications such as amiodarone should be considered. Atrial fibrillation renders patients prone to thromboemboli, and amyloid patients are at particular risk; therefore, anticoagulation should be strongly considered. When systolic dysfunction ensues, vasodilators may be tried, but caution should be employed due to predilection to orthostatic hypotension. Depending on the cause, cardiac transplantation may be considered but is often contraindicated because of the underlying primary disease.

Prognosis

Typically, by the time a patient develops symptoms attributable to RCM, the disease is pathologically advanced and largely irreversible (with few exceptions, ie, acute inflammatory stages of sarcoid responsive to immunosuppression). Clinical progression is typically rapid over a short interval, and although RCM carries a variable prognosis dependent on etiology, most patients die within a few years. The prognosis in amyloid is particularly grim, although the familial transthyretin-related form is more protracted compared with the immunoglobulin-associated disease.

25 Myocarditis, Toxic Cardiomyopathy, & Stress Cardiomyopathy

Mandar Aras, MD, PhD

MYOCARDITIS

ESSENTIALS OF DIAGNOSIS

- Heterogenous clinical presentation including chest pain, heart failure, arrhythmias, or cardiogenic shock.
- A viral prodrome may precede the onset of symptoms.
- Elevated cardiac biomarkers.
- Electrocardiogram may be normal or show nonspecific ST changes, atrial or ventricular arrhythmias.
- Echocardiography demonstrates left ventricular dilation and systolic dysfunction.
- Endomyocardial biopsy reveals cellular infiltrates with associated myocyte damage.

General Considerations

Myocarditis is an inflammatory disease of the myocardium caused by a wide variety of both infectious and noninfectious agents (Table 25–1). Viruses are the most common etiology but other infectious agents including bacteria (such as *Borrelia spp.),* protozoa (such as *Trypanosoma cruzi*), and fungi can also lead to myocarditis. Myocarditis can also be induced by a variety of toxic substances, medications, and systemic immune-mediated diseases. The incidence of myocarditis has increased recently due to (1) reports of acute and chronic/recurrent myocarditis among severe acute respiratory syndrome coronavirus-2 (SARS-CoV-2) infected and recovering individuals and (2) the widespread use of immune checkpoint inhibitors (ICIs) for first-line treatment of numerous cancers, which although effective, can lead to off-target immune-related adverse events including myocarditis. When cardiac dysfunction develops in the setting of myocarditis, the term *inflammatory cardiomyopathy* is often used. The formal diagnosis of myocarditis requires endomyocardial biopsy (EMB) demonstrating typical pathologic changes. However, in practice, the diagnosis is frequently made based on a combination of clinical features, laboratory testing, and imaging.

Tschöpe C, Ammirati E, Bozkurt B, et al. Myocarditis and inflammatory cardiomyopathy: current evidence and future directions. *Nat Rev Cardiol.* 2021;18:169–193. [PMID: 33046850]

Pathophysiology

The pathophysiology of myocarditis is not fully understood. Animal models of viral myocarditis suggest a three-phase response based on both the initial viral infection and subsequent maladaptive immune-mediated response. During the acute phase, virus enters the myocyte via a specific receptor. Once inside the myocyte, viral replication leads to injury and eventual myocyte necrosis. Myocyte necrosis causes exposure of cellular antigens that activate the host immune system. The initial response is composed of natural killer cells and macrophages, followed by T lymphocytes. This acute phase generally lasts 1–7 days and is followed by a subacute phase lasting weeks to months, where host immune reactions predominate. The subacute phase with the activation of the adaptive immune response is characterized by presence of activated T lymphocytes that target the host's organs. Cytokines, including tumor necrosis factor-α and interleukin-1 and 6, aggravate the cardiac damage in some patients and can lead to systolic dysfunction. In most patients, the immune response will decline with elimination of the virus, with recovery of left ventricular (LV) function. However, in some patients, this immune-mediated phase likely persists and leads to a chronic phase characterized by cardiac remodeling and ultimately development of dilated cardiomyopathy (DCM).

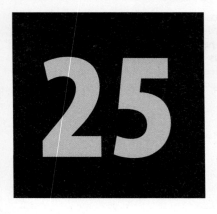

Table 25–1. Causes of Myocarditis

Infectious		Noninfectious
Viral	Bacterial	Toxic
Adenovirus	*Bartonella*	Alcohol
Arbovirus	*Brucellosis*	Amphetamine
Coxsackie (A and B)	*Chlamydia trachomatis*	Anthracycline
Cytomegalovirus	*Clostridium tetani*	Catecholamines
Dengue	*Corynebacterium diphtheriae*	Cocaine
Echovirus	*Coxiella burnetii*	Cyclophosphamide
Epstein-Barr virus	*Francisella tularensis*	Heavy metals
Hepatitis (B and C)	*Haemophilus*	Interferon (alpha-2)
Herpes simplex	*Legionella*	Interleukins
Herpes zoster	*Mycobacterium tuberculosis*	Immune-checkpoint inhibitors
Human herpes virus 6	*Mycoplasma pneumoniae*	Trace metals
HIV	*Neisseria gonorrhoeae*	Trastuzumab
Influenza (A and B)	*Neisseria meningitides*	**Hypersensitivity**
Mumps	*Rickettsia rickettsii*	*Antibiotics* (penicillin, *cephalosporins*)
Parvovirus B19	*Salmonella*	*Benzodiazepines*
Poliomyelitis	*Staphylococcus*	Clozapine
Rabies	*Streptococcus*	Dobutamine
Rubella	*Vibrio cholerae*	Insect bites (bee, spider, scorpion)
Rubeola	**Mycotic**	Lithium
SARS-CoV-2	*Actinomyces*	Snake venom
Varicella	*Aspergillus*	Vaccinations (smallpox)
Variola	*Blastomyces*	**Autoimmune/Systemic**
Yellow Fever	*Candida*	Celiac disease
Spirochetal	*Coccidioides*	Collagen-vascular
Leptospira	*Histoplasma*	Giant cell
Borrelia (Lyme)	*Mucor*	Hypereosinophilia
Treponema pallidum (syphilis)	*Nocardia*	Inflammatory bowel disease
Protozoal	**Helminthic**	Kawasaki disease
Entamoeba histolytica	*Ascaris*	Sarcoidosis
Leishmania	*Echinococcus*	Wegener
Plasmodium (malaria)	*Schistosoma*	
Trypanosoma cruzi (Chagas)	*Strongyloides*	
Toxoplasma gondii	*Trichinella spiralis*	

HIV, human immunodeficiency virus.

Clinical Findings

A. Symptoms & Signs

Myocarditis presents with a wide variety of clinical manifestations, making the diagnosis difficult in some cases. Many patients are asymptomatic or have nonspecific symptoms, and the diagnosis often goes undetected. Early signs and symptoms of myocarditis may also be masked by the symptoms of the initial viral infection, such as fevers and myalgias. When symptoms are present, heart failure is common, often characterized by fatigue and exertional dyspnea. Patients with acute fulminant myocarditis may present with acute decompensated heart failure and cardiogenic shock. Chest pain, often due to associated pericarditis, may be present.

Other presenting symptoms may include presyncope, syncope, palpitations, or sudden cardiac death. While sinus tachycardia is the most common arrhythmia seen in myocarditis, patients may also present with ventricular arrhythmias or high-grade heart block.

B. Physical Examination

Physical examination findings vary widely. Manifestations of the triggering viral illness may dominate early. Tachycardia, hypotension, and fever can all be seen in myocarditis. The tachycardia may be disproportionate to the degree of fever. Bradycardia is less common and may reflect heart block. A pericardial rub may be present in patients with associated pericarditis. When decompensated heart failure develops, patients present with distended neck veins, pulmonary rales, peripheral edema, or cardiac gallops. The most severe cases will present with evidence of cardiogenic shock including hypotension, cool extremities, and somnolence.

C. Diagnostic Studies

1. Electrocardiography—The electrocardiogram (ECG) in myocarditis is often normal or may show nonspecific abnormalities including sinus tachycardia, ST changes, and occasional ectopic beats. Findings consistent with pericarditis may be seen in those with myopericarditis. Some patients with myocarditis may present with ECG findings consistent with acute myocardial infarction including regional ST elevations and Q waves. In several studies, the presence of Q waves or left bundle branch block has been associated with poorer outcomes. Sustained ventricular arrhythmias, atrial arrhythmias (less common), and atrioventricular (AV) block may also be seen.

2. Cardiac biomarkers—Elevation in serum troponin is more common than elevations in creatinine kinase. Serum troponin is elevated in one-third to one-half of patients with myocarditis and is highest early in the disease process. Brain natriuretic peptide (BNP) and N-terminal pro-BNP (NT-proBNP) are sensitive tests when heart failure is present and may be useful when the diagnosis of heart failure is uncertain.

3. Chest radiography—The heart size may be normal or enlarged. Pulmonary venous congestion, frank pulmonary edema, and pleural effusions may be seen in more severe cases. Patients with concomitant pneumonia will have focal pulmonary infiltrates.

4. Echocardiography—There are no pathognomonic findings in myocarditis. Echocardiography is particularly helpful for ruling out other causes of cardiomyopathy such as valvular heart disease in patients with suspected myocarditis. Patients with fulminant myocarditis often have minimal or no LV dilation, and ventricular wall thickening may be seen, likely due to edematous inflammation. Patients with acute myocarditis will have LV dilation and reduced ejection fraction. Systolic dysfunction is usually global but may be regional in some cases. Spherical remodeling may be seen. Patients with relatively normal systolic function at rest may show exercise-induced wall motion abnormalities, thought to reflect microvascular dysfunction. Other findings may include mitral or tricuspid regurgitation, mural thrombi, or pericardial effusion in cases of myopericarditis.

5. Cardiac catheterization—Cardiac catheterization is not required in all patients with myocarditis but may be particularly helpful to evaluate for an acute coronary syndrome in the setting of elevated cardiac biomarkers and/or chest pain. With myocarditis, coronary angiography will show normal coronary arteries or nonobstructive disease. Right heart catheterization often shows elevated intracardiac filling pressures and reduced cardiac index.

6. Endomyocardial biopsy—EMB remains the gold standard for the diagnosis of myocarditis. EMB can also identify the underlying etiology and guide management. The procedure is generally performed via the jugular vein, although the subclavian, brachial, and femoral veins may be used as well. In experienced centers, the complication rate is 0–0.8%. Four to six tissue fragments are obtained and sent for histologic analysis. Findings in myocarditis include histiocytic and mononuclear cellular infiltrates. Myocyte damage may or may not be seen. The Dallas criteria are commonly used to diagnose myocarditis and categorize myocarditis as either active or borderline depending on the extent of inflammation and myocyte injury. Active myocarditis requires the presence of an inflammatory infiltrate with necrosis and/or degeneration of adjacent monocytes. The term *borderline myocarditis* is used when the inflammatory infiltrate is sparse or myocyte injury is not seen. The more recent World Health Organization/International Society and Federation of Cardiology definition for myocarditis includes the Dallas criteria as well as additional immunologic and immunohistochemical criteria.

In addition to evaluating the presence of myocarditis, EMB often provides information regarding the specific etiology. Giant cell myocarditis, granulomatous etiologies,

Chagas disease, Lyme carditis, and others can all be identified from histologic examination. Polymerase chain reaction may identify specific viral pathogens, although the benefit of identifying many pathogens is uncertain at this time.

Although EMB remains the gold standard for diagnosis of myocarditis, it is not required for all suspected cases. After eliminating other potential causes of cardiomyopathy including ischemic and valvular disease, the need for EMB should be determined based on the likelihood that results will impact management. Current guidelines recommend EMB in the following cases:

- New-onset heart failure of less than 2 weeks in duration, associated with a normal size or dilated left ventricle and hemodynamic compromise
- New-onset heart failure of 2 weeks to 3 months in duration associated with LV dilation and either new ventricular arrhythmias, second- or third-degree heart block, or failure to respond to usual care within 1–2 weeks

Patients not meeting these criteria may still benefit from EMB; however, each case needs to be evaluated individually.

7. Cardiac magnetic resonance imaging—Cardiac magnetic resonance (CMR) findings consistent with myocardial inflammation include regional or global myocardial signal intensity increase in T2-weighted images, increased global early gadolinium enhancement between myocardium and skeletal muscle in T1-weighted images, and at least one focal lesion with late gadolinium enhancement in a nonvascular distribution. There is generally good correlation between CMR and EMB-based diagnoses of myocarditis, and CMR may be a reasonable initial evaluation in patients with suspected myocarditis. The Lake Louise Criteria for CMR-based diagnosis of myocarditis include evidence of myocardial edema, hyperemia, and necrosis or scar. When two of the three criteria are present, the CMR is considered consistent with active myocardial inflammation. In one large cohort of biopsy-proven viral myocarditis, the presence of late gadolinium enhancement was the best predictor of all-cause mortality. It should be noted that CMR cannot identify the specific etiology of myocarditis or identify patients who would benefit from disease-specific therapy (eg, those with giant cell myocarditis), and therefore, EMB may still be required.

Ammirati E, Cipriani M, Moro C, et al. Clinical presentation and outcome in a contemporary cohort of patients with acute myocarditis: Multicenter Lombardy Registry. *Circulation*. 2018 Sep 11;138(11):1088–1099. [PMID: 29764898]

Lurz P, Luecke C, Eitel I, et al. Comprehensive cardiac magnetic resonance imaging in patients with suspected myocarditis: The MyoRacer-Trial. *J Am Coll Cardiol*. 2016;67(15):1800. [PMID: 27081020]

Differential Diagnosis

In a patient presenting with new heart failure and cardiomyopathy the differential diagnosis includes ischemic heart disease, valvular heart disease, congenital heart disease, and other forms of cardiomyopathy. Myocarditis may closely resemble acute coronary syndrome with chest pain, ECG abnormalities, elevated cardiac biomarkers, and regional wall motion abnormalities. Coronary angiography is indicated in such scenarios. Depending on the specific presentation, other diagnostic considerations may include arrhythmogenic right ventricular cardiomyopathy or infiltrative cardiomyopathy.

Given the broad clinical presentations, successful prompt diagnosis of myocarditis requires a high index of suspicion. Scenarios that should trigger an evaluation of myocarditis include new, otherwise unexplained heart failure, arrhythmias, or cardiogenic shock. Signs and symptoms of viral illness are absent in many cases, but a patient with new cardiovascular dysfunction with an antecedent viral illness is also a clue to an underlying diagnosis of myocarditis.

Treatment

Hospitalization with cardiac rhythm monitoring is indicated for any patient with suspected acute myocarditis, with close observation for the development of heart failure, arrhythmias, or embolic complications. Physical activity should be restricted until the acute phase has completely resolved, as animal models have shown that exercise intensifies the inflammatory process in the myocardium and increases morbidity and mortality. This includes excluding athletes from competitive sports. Some groups recommend reevaluation at 6 months after the diagnosis of myocarditis before allowing patients to resume unrestricted physical activity.

The role of immunosuppressive therapy depends on the specific type of myocarditis. A controlled trial of prednisone with either cyclosporine or azathioprine failed to show any significant improvement in LV ejection fraction, LV dimensions, or survival at 1 year. Giant cell myocarditis, on the other hand, is routinely treated with immunosuppression. All patients with heart failure should be treated according to standard guidelines. This includes diuretics for fluid overload, angiotensin-converting enzyme (ACE) inhibitors/angiotensin receptor blockers, mineralocorticoid antagonists, and β-blockers. Antiarrhythmic agents may be required for tachyarrhythmias or ventricular arrhythmias, and pacemaker implantation is indicated for patients with high-grade AV block or symptomatic bradycardia.

In patients who fail to improve with initial therapy or in whom cardiac enzymes remain elevated for weeks, repeat EMB should be considered to ensure improvement. Those with acute fulminant myocarditis who develop cardiogenic shock should be evaluated for LV assist device or extracorporeal membrane oxygenation as a bridge to recovery or heart transplantation. Patients treated with full clinical recovery may relapse, sometimes many years after the initial episode. Relapses should be managed in a similar manner as the initial episode.

Prognosis

Prognosis in myocarditis depends on the etiology and clinical presentation. In patients presenting with mild or no symptoms and minimal cardiac dysfunction, the disease is generally self-limited, with no long-term sequelae. However, up to 30% of patients with myocarditis will progress to DCM. One study of 222 patients with biopsy-proven viral myocarditis found a 19.2% rate of all-cause mortality over a median follow-up of 4.7 years, with a 15% cardiac death rate. In addition, 10% of patients had an episode of sudden cardiac death. Presence of late gadolinium enhancement on CMR was the strongest predictor of death. Heart failure on presentation and biventricular dysfunction also predict poor outcome.

Ammirati E, Frigerio M, Adler ED, et al. Management of acute myocarditis and chronic inflammatory cardiomyopathy. *Circ Heart Fail.* 2020 Nov;13(11):e007405. [PMID: 33176455]

Specific Forms of Myocarditis

A. Chagas Disease

Chagas disease is caused by the protozoan *Trypanosoma cruzi*. The organism is endemic to rural areas of Central and South America, and Chagas disease is the most common cause of DCM in Latin America. *T cruzi* is transmitted by reduviid insects, which bite humans during sleep. Chagas disease is divided into two phases: an acute phase and a chronic phase. Acute Chagas will develop in 1% of people bitten by reduviid bugs, approximately 1 week to 4 months after the exposure. Most patients are asymptomatic or experience a mild febrile illness. Because of the nonspecific nature, the diagnosis is rarely established during the acute phase. Serologic testing is often negative during the acute phase, and the diagnosis is made by detecting circulating parasites. Even though most patients are asymptomatic during acute Chagas disease, there is evidence that myocardial involvement is present in many. Echocardiographic and ECG changes are frequent. Following acute Chagas disease, patients enter an indeterminate or latent phase during which there is typically no overt evidence of cardiovascular disease. The latent phase may be diagnosed based on either serologic or parasitologic evidence of *T cruzi* infection. This phase may persist for decades, after which approximately one-third of patients will develop chronic Chagas cardiomyopathy (CCC).

Patients with CCC most often present with heart failure, arrhythmias, or thromboembolism. Biventricular heart failure is common, and echocardiography often shows dilated ventricles with systolic and diastolic dysfunction, wall motion abnormalities, and apical aneurysms. The most common arrhythmias in CCC are heart block and ventricular tachycardia, although atrial fibrillation, sinus node dysfunction, and other arrhythmias may also be seen. Thromboemboli may originate from the ventricular walls, or the atria in patients with atrial fibrillation.

Diagnosis of CCC is made in patients with evidence of Chagas heart disease who have serologic evidence of immunoglobulin G (IgG) antibodies to *T cruzi*. EMB will show evidence of active myocarditis but is generally not required to make the diagnosis.

Treatment for Chagas disease primarily involves standard therapy for systolic heart failure, with anticoagulants and antiarrhythmics as needed. Patients with heart block may require a pacemaker. Antitrypanosomal therapy with benznidazole or nifurtimox is recommended in acute Chagas disease but is not beneficial in CCC. Cardiac transplantation may be considered for advanced cases, with appropriate posttransplant monitoring for reactivation of Chagas disease.

Nunes MCP, Buss LF, Silva JLP, et al. Incidence and predictors of progression to Chagas cardiomyopathy: Long-term follow-up of *Trypanosoma cruzi*-Seropositive individuals. *Circulation.* 2021 Nov 9;144(19):1553–1566. [PMID: 34565171]

B. Giant Cell Myocarditis

Idiopathic giant cell myocarditis (GCM) is a rare cause of myocarditis characterized by multinucleated giant cells within the myocardium. The etiology is not well understood, but an autoimmune component is possible. GCM usually presents as acute or fulminant heart failure due to LV systolic dysfunction. Ventricular tachyarrhythmias and high-grade AV block are especially common in this disease. The prognosis for patients with GCM is significantly worse than for patients with other causes of myocarditis, with a rate of death or heart transplant of 89%. Early recognition is key, and patients with high suspicion for GCM should be considered for early EMB.

One small trial showed that treatment with a combination of immunosuppressive medications may improve prognosis. Treatment regimens usually include cyclosporine and corticosteroid therapy for at least 12 months, with additional agents added in some cases. Using multidrug immunosuppression was associated with transplant-free survival of 77% at 1 year. Patients who fail to improve or deteriorate despite initial therapy should be considered for early consideration of mechanical circulatory support or heart transplantation.

C. Cardiac Sarcoidosis

Sarcoidosis is a heterogenous multisystem inflammatory disease. The pathologic hallmark is the noncaseating granuloma. The granuloma consists of activated helper-induced T lymphocytes, macrophages, and multinucleated giant cells. Granulomas trigger a fibrotic response, resulting in organ damage. The lymphoid, pulmonary, cardiovascular, hepatobiliary, and hematologic systems are most involved, with the lungs affected in more than 90% of patients.

Clinical cardiac disease is reported in 2–5% of patients with sarcoidosis, although the true prevalence of cardiovascular involvement is likely much greater. Involvement of the heart is identified in 27–70% of autopsy cases among patients with sarcoidosis, and cardiovascular disease accounts for 13–25% of sarcoid-related deaths. Cardiac sarcoidosis has varied presentations depending on the extent and location of cardiac granulomas. Patients may have AV block, heart failure, or sudden cardiac death. The disease should be considered especially in young or middle-aged women who present with heart failure and/or AV block or ventricular arrhythmias. Echocardiography may show septal thinning, wall motion abnormalities in a noncoronary distribution, or LV aneurysm. Diagnosis can be made by EMB; however, given the patchy distribution of disease within the myocardium, the sensitivity is only 20–26%. Positron emission tomography and magnetic resonance imaging are both useful modalities for identifying cardiac sarcoidosis. Diagnosis requires a combination of clinical/imaging evidence of cardiac involvement along with tissue diagnosis of extracardiac sarcoid.

Corticosteroids are used routinely for the management of cardiac sarcoid, although there is little consensus opinion regarding dose or duration of therapy. Patients are often started on high-dose prednisone, which is maintained for several months and then tapered. When initiated early, corticosteroids can lead to improvements in symptoms, echocardiographic parameters, and possibly survival. Treatment is much less effective in patients with LV dilation and severe systolic dysfunction. Other considerations include antiarrhythmic drugs and implantable defibrillators in those with reduced ejection fraction or at increased risk for ventricular arrhythmias.

D. Human Immunodeficiency Virus

Infection with human immunodeficiency virus (HIV) is associated with a variety of cardiac complications. Before the widespread use of antiretroviral therapy, both pericardial disease and myocarditis were frequently reported. These complications are now increasingly less common in the developed world, and atherosclerotic disease has become the predominant form of cardiovascular disease observed in HIV-infected individuals. In resource-poor settings, HIV cardiomyopathy is still seen. Patients present with systolic dysfunction, generally later during their HIV and with lower CD4 counts. In these patients, it is important to consider other etiologies of cardiomyopathy including coronary artery disease and opportunistic infections such as coxsackie virus, Epstein-Barr virus, and *Toxoplasma gondii.*

E. Lyme Myocarditis

Lyme disease is a multisystem disease caused by infection with the tick-borne spirochete *Borrelia burgdorferi*. The primary manifestations are myalgias, arthralgias, headache, fever, adenopathy, and erythema chronicum migrans. Symptomatic, though usually transient, cardiac involvement was previously reported in up to 10% of infected patients, although with treatment, the rate of cardiac involvement is now closer to 1%. Conduction abnormalities or fluctuating degrees of AV block may be present. Syncope secondary to complete heart block is common and may require temporary transvenous pacing. LV dysfunction is rare. EMB may reveal active myocarditis. Spirochetes have been isolated from the myocardium in some patients. It is unclear whether the myocarditis of Lyme disease is a direct result of spirochetal infection or the immunologic response to it. The course of the disease is usually benign, and complete recovery is expected. Treatment with penicillin or doxycycline is recommended, but it is unknown if this treatment alters the course of the cardiac disease.

F. Eosinophilic Myocarditis

Eosinophilic myocarditis is a rare condition characterized by eosinophilia and myocarditis with eosinophilic infiltration. Eosinophilic myocarditis can be idiopathic or associated with conditions including Churg-Strauss syndrome, parasitic infection, and malignancy such as chronic eosinophilic leukemia. The presentation depends on the underlying etiology and generally includes biventricular heart failure and arrhythmias. Rash and fever may be present.

G. Immune Checkpoint Inhibitor Myocarditis

ICIs represent a novel category of cancer treatments that help direct the immune system to recognize and target cancer cells. In the last decade, ICIs have been approved for the treatment of many cancer types. The suppression of immune regulation is associated with immune-related adverse events, including myocarditis. ICI-associated myocarditis has emerged as a significant and potentially fatal adverse effect. Data from case series show that prevalence of ICI-myocarditis was 1–3% with a median onset of 34 days, and more likely to occur following combination immune checkpoint inhibitor treatment.

Bonaca MP, Olenchock BA, Salem JE, et al. Myocarditis in the setting of cancer therapeutics: Proposed case definitions for emerging clinical syndromes in cardio-oncology. *Circulation.* 2019 Jul 2;140(2):80–91. [PMID: 31390169]

Mahmood SS, Fradley MG, Cohen JV, et al. Myocarditis in patients treated with immune checkpoint inhibitors. *J Am Coll Cardiol.* 2018 Apr 24;71(16):1755–1764. [PMID: 29567210]

H. COVID-19 Myocarditis

A wide range of cardiovascular complications have been reported in patients hospitalized with the novel coronavirus disease 2019 (COVID-19) pandemic attributed to severe acute respiratory syndrome coronavirus 2 (SARS-CoV-2) infection. Laboratory and imaging evidence of myocardial injury has been observed in both symptomatic and asymptomatic individuals, as well as after the receipt of the COVID-19 mRNA vaccine. The underlying causes of myocardial injury are numerous and include myocarditis, acute coronary syndrome (myocardial infarction type 1), demand ischemia (myocardial infarction type 2), multisystem inflammatory syndrome in children (MIS-C) and multisystem inflammatory syndrome in adults (MIS-A), takotsubo/stress cardiomyopathy, cytokine storm, among others. The definition and approach to diagnosis of myocarditis following SARS-CoV-2 infection continues to evolve and is an active avenue for investigation.

Writing committee. 2022 ACC expert consensus decision pathway on cardiovascular sequelae of COVID-19 in adults: Myocarditis and other myocardial involvement, post-acute sequelae of SARS-CoV-2 infection and return to play: A report of the American College of Cardiology Solution Set Oversight Committee. *J Am Coll Cardiol.* 2022 May 3;79(17):1717–1756. [PMID: 35307156]

TOXIC CARDIOMYOPATHY

ESSENTIALS OF DIAGNOSIS

- Heart failure in a patient with prior or ongoing exposure to agents with known myocardial toxicity, in the absence of alternative explanation.
- Alcohol, cocaine, methamphetamine, and chemotherapeutic agents are all common culprits.
- Echocardiography shows biventricular dilation and systolic dysfunction.
- Biomarkers (BNP) are often elevated.

General Considerations

Toxic cardiomyopathy develops as the result of exposure to cardiotoxic agents. Alcohol and chemotherapeutic drugs are two of the most common etiologies of toxic cardiomyopathy. The pathophysiology is diverse depending on the toxic agent but may include direct myocardial injury and vascular-mediated injury. Patients present with DCM. Diagnosing toxic cardiomyopathy requires first eliminating other common causes of DCM and then identifying a history of toxin exposure and confirming sufficient exposure to result in cardiomyopathy. Prompt diagnosis is important because long-term prognosis is dependent on successful withdrawal of the offending agent.

Clinical Findings

A. Symptoms & Signs

Patients may be asymptomatic at the time of diagnosis, with cardiomegaly detected incidentally or during routine surveillance in the case of patients receiving chemotherapy. When symptoms are present, toxic cardiomyopathy most commonly manifests as heart failure. Patients complain of fatigue, dyspnea, edema, or arrhythmias. Other possible presentations include thromboembolic complications and sudden cardiac death. Symptoms related to noncardiac effects of the offending agent may be present as well.

B. Physical Examination

Clinical findings are like those for other causes of DCM and may include evidence of volume overload (distended neck veins, lower extremity edema, ascites) or a gallop. Patients may also present with arrhythmias. Other stigmata of long-term exposure to the toxin (eg, signs of cirrhosis in patients with alcoholic cardiomyopathy) may also serve as clues to the underlying etiology of a patient's cardiomyopathy.

C. Diagnostic Studies

1. Biomarkers—There is substantial interest in using both troponin and BNP in the diagnosis and monitoring of patients with toxic cardiomyopathy, particularly cardiomyopathies related to chemotherapy. A BNP value more than 200 pg/mL is associated with a 44-fold increased risk of heart failure. However, currently, there are insufficient data to support regular screening of patients receiving chemotherapy with cardiac biomarkers.

2. Chest x-ray—As in other cases of DCM, the chest x-ray may be normal or show cardiomegaly, pulmonary vascular congestion, or pulmonary edema.

3. Echocardiography—Toxic cardiomyopathies are generally characterized by LV dilation, increased LV mass with normal or reduced LV wall thickness, and systolic dysfunction. Diastolic dysfunction may also be present. Right ventricular dilation and systolic dysfunction are often present as well. In alcoholic cardiomyopathy, LV dilation is usually the first sign, preceding the onset of systolic dysfunction.

4. Routine laboratories—Routine laboratory studies may provide clues to chronic alcohol abuse. These include increased mean red cell corpuscular volume and mild thrombocytopenia. The serum aspartate aminotransferase (AST) level is often elevated, and a ratio of AST to alanine aminotransferase (ALT) of greater than two is particularly suggestive of alcohol abuse.

5. Toxicology screen—Serum or urine toxicology screen may be the first clue to a diagnosis of cardiomyopathy due to illicit drug use and should be considered in the workup of new nonischemic cardiomyopathy of unclear etiology. Both cocaine and methamphetamines are included in most screening tests for drugs of abuse.

6. Coronary angiography—Coronary angiography or other diagnostic testing for coronary artery disease should be performed as per standard guidelines for the evaluation of new heart failure based on the patient's age and risk factors. Patients with toxic cardiomyopathy will have little or no coronary artery disease.

Differential Diagnosis

The differential diagnosis includes all causes of DCM including ischemic heart disease, idiopathic DCM, myocarditis, infiltrative disease, and hypertensive cardiomyopathy. Establishing the diagnosis of toxic cardiomyopathy requires that other causes of DCM be excluded. This will often involve evaluation for ischemic heart disease, valvular heart disease, and any other etiologies suggested by the history and initial workup. Once other causes have been excluded and a history of sufficient exposure to the toxic agent has been established, the diagnosis of toxic cardiomyopathy is made.

Treatment

Regardless of the etiology, the first step in the management of toxic cardiomyopathy is withdrawal or minimization of the offending agent. In alcoholic cardiomyopathy, complete abstinence is usually recommended. All patients with reduced ejection fraction should be started on standard therapy for systolic heart failure and titrated to goal doses, and there are data supporting the use of these agents in a variety of toxic cardiomyopathies. One consideration with cocaine cardiomyopathy is the use of β-blocking agents in patients who may continue to use cocaine, because of the potential risk of β-blockade to exacerbate the "unopposed alpha" effect, causing elevated systemic blood pressure and coronary vasospasm during cocaine use. There is no clear evidence that this effect is clinically significant, and the appropriateness of giving β-blockers to cocaine users remains controversial.

Prognosis

For most of the toxic cardiomyopathies, prognosis depends on whether the offending agent is withdrawn. With abstinence, approximately 50% of patients with alcoholic cardiomyopathy will see improvement in the ejection fraction, and even those in whom LV dysfunction persists may see improvement in signs and symptoms of heart failure with abstinence. Even partial reduction in alcohol intake can lead to significant improvement. In anthracycline-associated cardiomyopathy, early detection and prompt initiation of heart failure therapies are associated with improvement in LV systolic function in the majority of patients.

Specific Forms of Toxic Cardiomyopathy

A. Alcoholic Cardiomyopathy

Alcohol is the most frequently consumed toxic substance in the world. Although only a minority of alcoholics will develop cardiomyopathy, given the prevalence of alcoholism, it causes approximately 4% of all cardiomyopathies. The required consumption is thought to be at least 80 g (7–8 standard drinks) daily for at least 10 years. Women only account for approximately 14% of alcoholic cardiomyopathy patients but may be more susceptible at lower lifetime levels of consumption. There is a J-shaped relationship between alcohol consumption and cardiomyopathy, with one study noting that drinking up to 7 drinks per week is associated with a lower risk of future heart failure. Some patients may have a genetic predisposition to developing DCM and heart failure.

The pathogenesis is not fully elucidated. Alcoholic cardiomyopathy was previously thought to be a result of the nutritional deficiencies associated with chronic alcoholism, but now it is appreciated that alcohol itself is toxic to the heart. Proposed mechanisms include altered fatty acid metabolism, decreased myocardial protein synthesis, and impaired mitochondrial function. Ethanol may also cause oxidative stress through the generation of free radicals. Variants in well-characterized DCM-causing genes were more prevalent in patients with alcoholic cardiomyopathy than control subjects, suggesting a role for genetic predisposition.

Clinical manifestations are like those seen in DCM due to other causes. In addition, patients may show noncardiac stigmata of long-term alcohol use. Laboratory studies may show abnormal liver function tests.

The standard recommended treatment for alcoholic cardiomyopathy is total abstinence from alcohol, although studies have suggested that decreasing intake to moderate levels (< 80 g/d) may be sufficient. In addition, patients should receive standard pharmacologic therapy for systolic heart failure, and any nutritional deficiencies should be corrected. With abstinence, the prognosis and likelihood of recovery are equal to or better than what are observed in patients with idiopathic DCM. Even when LV function does not improve, abstinence is generally associated with significant improvement in heart failure symptoms. For those who continue to abuse alcohol, the prognosis is poor, with mortality of up to 50% at 3–6 years. Atrial fibrillation, QRS width more than 120 ms, and absence of β-blocker therapy are associated with worse outcomes.

Guzzo-Merello G, Segovia J, Dominguez F, et al. Natural history and prognostic factors in alcoholic cardiomyopathy. *JACC Heart Fail.* 2015;3(1):78–86. [PMID: 25458176]

Ware JS, Amor-Salamanca A, Tayal U, et al. Genetic etiology for alcohol-induced cardiac toxicity. *J Am Coll Cardiol.* 2018 May 22;71(20):2293–2302. [PMID 29773157]

B. Cocaine Cardiomyopathy

Cocaine use is associated with a variety of cardiovascular effects including myocardial infarction, coronary artery aneurysm, arrhythmias, and stroke. DCM in the absence of coronary artery disease is also reported among cocaine users, with depressed LV systolic function reported in 4–9% of asymptomatic cocaine users. There are several potential mechanisms. Cocaine causes myocarditis and has direct toxic effects on the myocardium. The hyperadrenergic state induced by cocaine may also promote adverse changes. Abstinence from cocaine is associated with reversal of myocardial dysfunction, often returning to normal. However, some patients never recover myocardial function, particularly those with some component of cocaine-induced myocardial infarction. No studies have rigorously evaluated the treatment strategies for cocaine-associated cardiomyopathy. The use of β-blockers in patients with ongoing cocaine use is controversial, although several reports have reported successful use of carvedilol and other β-blocking agents in this population.

C. Methamphetamine Cardiomyopathy

Methamphetamine is currently the second most widely abused illicit drug worldwide, and the association between methamphetamine use and cardiomyopathy is gaining recognition. In one study, methamphetamine users had a 3.7-fold increased risk of developing cardiomyopathy compared to age-matched controls. Potential mechanisms of methamphetamine-associated cardiomyopathy include catecholamine excess, coronary vasospasm, mitochondrial injury, and direct toxic effects. Echocardiography shows ventricular dilation and systolic dysfunction. Those who can quit using methamphetamine generally have significant improvements in both New York Heart Association functional class and ejection fraction, whereas those who continue to use methamphetamine usually worsen over time. Other cardiovascular complications of methamphetamine use include hypertension, arrhythmia, pulmonary arterial hypertension, acute coronary syndrome, and sudden cardiac death.

D. Chemotherapy-Induced Cardiomyopathy

1. Anthracycline cardiomyopathy—Cardiomyopathy due to chemotherapeutic agents is a well-known complication of cancer therapy. As cancer outcomes improve, cardiovascular complications have become increasingly important in cancer survivors. Anthracyclines including doxorubicin (Adriamycin) are frequently used in the management of a variety of cancers, including breast cancer, sarcoma, and lymphoma. The cardiotoxic effects of these agents have been known for decades. The pathophysiology was traditionally thought to be related to the generation of reactive oxygen-free radicals, although more recent evidence suggests cardiotoxicity may be related to targeting of the topoisomerase 2β. Anthracycline-induced cardiotoxicity is dose-dependent. In patients who receive a cumulative dose of 400 mg/m^2, the lifetime risk of cardiomyopathy is 0.14–5%, compared with 18–48% in those receiving 700 mg/m^2. Patients with prior cardiovascular disease, those with prior radiation exposure, and those receiving concurrent treatment with other cardiotoxic agents are all at increased risk.

Three types of anthracycline-induced cardiotoxicity have been described: acute, early-onset chronic, and late-onset chronic. Echocardiography is most used for surveillance of LV ejection fraction (LVEF). Various criteria have been used to diagnose chemotherapy-associated cardiomyopathy, and there is no consensus definition. A 10% decline in LVEF is one commonly used cut point. Strain imaging, cardiac magnetic resonance, and biomarkers may be more useful and are the subject of ongoing clinical research. EMB shows myofibrillar dropout, distortion of Z-lines, and mitochondrial disruption. Biopsy is considered the most sensitive and specific test for anthracycline cardiomyopathy but is rarely used in clinical practice.

Early detection is important for improving outcomes. Although clinical practice varies, most experts recommend baseline measurement of LVEF using echocardiography or radionuclide ventriculography prior to the initiation of chemotherapy. Patients should undergo interval surveillance monitoring of ejection fraction while receiving chemotherapy and whenever symptoms of cardiovascular disease develop. When LV dysfunction or heart failure develops, therapy for heart failure should be initiated promptly, as early initiation of therapies has a significant effect on outcomes. One group performed echocardiograms at baseline and every 3 months during chemotherapy and for the following year in patients receiving anthracyclines. Patients with LV dysfunction detected were started on standard medical therapy for heart failure with ACE inhibitors first as well as β-blockers if tolerated. With this protocol, 82% of patients had at least partial recovery of LV systolic function. Doxorubicin should be discontinued when there is evidence of clinical heart failure, a decline in LVEF of 10% or more to below the lower limit of normal, to 45% or below, or when there is a 20% decline in LVEF at any level. Therapies such as implantable cardioverter-defibrillators can be considered but require consideration of the patient's overall expected survival and quality of life.

A variety of strategies to prevent cardiotoxicity have also been proposed. Limiting the lifetime dose of doxorubicin to less than 450–500 mg/m^2 decreases the risk of cardiotoxicity. Dexrazoxane can be used in patients who have received a cumulative dose of doxorubicin $\geq$ 300 mg/m^2 and has been shown to significantly reduce the incidence of heart failure. Limiting exposure to sequential cardiotoxic therapies (anthracycline followed by HER-2 targeted therapy) will also limit cardiac toxicity. Small studies initially suggesting a benefit from starting prophylactic β-blockers and/or ACE inhibitors in patients at increased risk for chemotherapy-associated cardiomyopathy have not been replicated with clinically significant outcomes in larger studies.

2. Nonanthracycline cardiomyopathy—Many nonanthracycline chemotherapeutic agents also cause cardiotoxicity. These agents include 5-fluorouracil, fludarabine, methotrexate, cytarabine, cyclophosphamide, and the monoclonal antibodies including trastuzumab. Trastuzumab binds to HER2 protein and is used in the treatment of breast cancer. Trastuzumab and other HER2-targeted agents cause a cardiotoxicity that most commonly presents as asymptomatic LV systolic dysfunction, with clinical heart failure being less common. There are many important differences between the cardiotoxicities of trastuzumab and that of anthracyclines. The cardiac dysfunction associated with trastuzumab is generally reversible following treatment discontinuation, and cardiac biopsy shows no evidence of myocyte destruction. Rather, the decline in systolic function is thought to be caused by stunning or myocardial hibernation.

Because of the risk of cardiotoxicity, patients should be evaluated for cardiac dysfunction prior to initiating therapy with trastuzumab or related agents. The optimal surveillance interval during treatment is unknown.

E. Trace Element–Related Cardiomyopathy

Both excess (cobalt, arsenic) or deficiency (selenium) of certain trace elements can lead to cardiomyopathy. Cobalt excess is reported in patients who drink beer containing cobalt sulphate, which is used for foam stabilization, as well as in those with occupational exposures or in patients with cobalt hip prostheses.

Narayan NK, Finkelman B, French B, et al. Detailed echocardiographic phenotyping in breast cancer patients: Associations with ejection fraction decline, recovery, and heart failure symptoms over 3 years follow up. *Circulation.* 2017 Apr 11; 135(15):1397–1412. [PMID: 28104715]

Zhao SX, Seng S, Deluna A, Yu EC, Crawford MH. Comparison of clinical characteristics and outcomes of patients with reversible versus persistent methamphetamine-associated cardiomyopathy. *Am J Cardiol.* 2020 Jan 1;125(1)127–134. [PMID: 31699360]

STRESS (TAKOTSUBO) CARDIOMYOPATHY

ESSENTIALS OF DIAGNOSIS

- Transient regional left ventricular systolic dysfunction, often after exposure to emotional or physical stress.
- Chest pain is the most common presenting symptom, followed by dyspnea.
- Elevated biomarkers.
- ECG most frequently shows ST-segment elevation.
- Coronary angiography without obstructive coronary artery disease.

General Considerations

Stress, or takotsubo, cardiomyopathy was first described in Japan in 1990, and since that time, it has gained increased recognition. The disease is characterized by transient systolic and diastolic LV dysfunction, typically preceded by an emotional or physical trigger. The name *takotsubo* comes from the Japanese word for "octopus pot," in reference to the characteristic LV apical ballooning. The pathogenesis is not well understood, although it is believed that catecholamine excess plays a central role. Both norepinephrine and epinephrine levels are higher in patients with stress cardiomyopathy compared to other patients, including those with acute myocardial infarction. Furthermore, similar clinical manifestations have been seen in patients with other high-catecholamine states including pheochromocytoma. Catecholamines may trigger microvascular spasm and dysfunction, and some patients with stress cardiomyopathy will present with transient myocardial perfusion abnormalities or show coronary artery vasospasm during angiography. Patients with neurologic or psychiatric disorders may be predisposed to stress cardiomyopathy.

Clinical Findings

A. Symptoms & Signs

Stress cardiomyopathy has an abrupt onset, often with a clear trigger. In a recent large international registry, 36% of patients had a physical trigger, 27.7% had an emotional trigger, and 7.8% had both physical and emotional triggers. Common physical triggers include infection, acute respiratory failure, or postsurgical state. Emotional triggers may include interpersonal conflict, anger, grief/loss, or financial stress. In approximately one-quarter of patients, no clear trigger was identified. Patients are more commonly female. The most frequent presenting symptom is substernal chest pain, followed by dyspnea and syncope. The initial presentation may be indistinguishable from an acute coronary syndrome.

B. Physical Examination

There are no physical examination findings pathognomonic for stress cardiomyopathy. Patients may show evidence of heart failure on physical examination, and a minority of patients will present with evidence of cardiogenic shock including cool extremities, abnormal mental status, or hypotension. Tachyarrhythmias, bradyarrhythmias, and mitral regurgitation can also be seen. LV basal hyperkinesis can lead to LV outflow tract (LVOT) obstruction, producing a late-peaking systolic murmur in some cases and contributing to the development of mitral regurgitation. Patients with stress cardiomyopathy are also at increased risk for formation of LV thrombus, which may subsequently embolize, leading to transient ischemic attack or stroke-like symptoms.

C. Diagnostic Studies

1. Electrocardiography—ECG abnormalities are common in stress cardiomyopathy. ST-segment elevation is present in 44% of patients and is most frequently seen in the precordial leads. ST depression may be seen but is less common than in acute coronary syndrome. QT prolongation, Q waves, and T-wave inversions can also be seen.

2. Cardiac biomarkers—Serum levels of troponin are elevated in most patients and, therefore, may not be helpful in early differentiation of stress cardiomyopathy from acute myocardial infarction. The subsequent pattern of troponin levels, however, may be more informative. Serum troponin levels increase by as much as 1.8 times during hospitalization in stress cardiomyopathy, compared to a six-fold rise in patients with acute coronary syndrome. The creatinine kinase is usually not significantly elevated. BNP is elevated in 83% of patients and often markedly elevated, in contrast to patients with acute coronary syndrome.

3. Echocardiography—The hallmark finding of stress cardiomyopathy is transient regional LV systolic dysfunction, usually first identified on either transthoracic echocardiography or left ventriculography. The most common pattern is the apical type, seen in 82% of patients. Apical type is characterized by systolic apical ballooning of the LV, with hyperkinesis of the basal walls, leading to the image resembling the Japanese octopus pot, and hence the name *takotsubo*. The midventricular form is seen in 14.6% of patients, with hypokinesis restricted to the midportion of the ventricle. Less common patterns include basal and focal types. LV systolic function is reduced in most patients, with a mean ejection fraction of 41%. Echocardiography is also useful for identifying the presence of LVOT obstruction, which is present in approximately 20% of patients and an important management consideration. Evaluation for presence of LV thrombus should be performed in all patients.

In addition to the initial evaluation of patients with stress cardiomyopathy, echocardiography is also important for serial evaluation of LV function. Most patients will recover LV systolic function within 4 weeks.

4. Coronary angiography—Coronary angiography is important for patients presenting with findings suggestive of acute coronary syndrome. In patients with stress cardiomyopathy, angiography typically demonstrates normal coronary arteries or mild nonobstructive disease. However, approximately 15% of patients with stress cardiomyopathy will have coronary artery disease.

5. Left ventriculography—Left ventriculography may be useful for identifying the regional wall motion abnormalities required for a diagnosis of stress cardiomyopathy and may be the first diagnostic clue in patients taken for emergent coronary angiography. Like the echocardiographic findings, the majority of patients will have reduced systolic function.

6. Cardiac magnetic resonance—CMR is perhaps the best imaging modality for identifying the segmental wall motion abnormalities associated with stress cardiomyopathy and may be particularly helpful when echocardiography is of poor technical quality or when coronary artery disease is present. Most patients will have evidence of myocardial edema, although this finding is not particularly specific for stress cardiomyopathy. Late gadolinium enhancement is generally absent in stress cardiomyopathy, whereas patients with significant myocardial infarction will show subendocardial or transmural delayed enhancement and those with myocarditis will have patchy, nonvascular patterns of enhancement. When it is present in stress cardiomyopathy, late gadolinium enhancement is associated with an increased frequency of cardiogenic shock.

Differential Diagnosis

The clinical presentation of stress cardiomyopathy may be identical to acute coronary syndromes, including ST-segment elevation myocardial infarction. Suspicion for stress cardiomyopathy should not delay or alter standard evaluation and management of acute coronary syndromes. Myocarditis may also present in a similar fashion, although recovery of systolic function is typically much faster in cases of stress cardiomyopathy. Cocaine-induced acute cardiovascular disease may cause similar findings. Finally, pheochromocytoma may cause a similar clinical picture and should be considered in any patient with findings of stress cardiomyopathy accompanied by headache, diaphoresis, or hypertension.

Treatment

No treatment for stress cardiomyopathy has been evaluated rigorously, and in most cases, treatment is generally supportive because stress cardiomyopathy is a transient disorder. Resolving the trigger often leads to rapid improvement. Patients who develop heart failure or cardiogenic shock require further management. Hemodynamically stable patients with heart failure with reduced ejection fraction are managed according to guideline-based therapy. In one retrospective analysis, the use of ACE inhibitors or angiotensin receptor blockers was associated with improved survival, whereas there was no survival benefit associated with the use of β-blockers. In patients with cardiogenic shock, appropriate management depends on whether dynamic LVOT obstruction is present. Early echocardiography should be used to determine the presence and degree of obstruction. In patients without LVOT obstruction, management of cardiogenic shock centers on optimization of LV filling pressures and inotropic support, keeping in mind that excessive inotropic support may induce LVOT obstruction. Those with LVOT obstruction should not receive inotropic agents, but rather should be managed according to similar algorithms used in the management of patients with hypertrophic obstructive cardiomyopathy. This may include phenylephrine and fluid resuscitation.

The appropriate duration of therapy for patients with stress cardiomyopathy is unknown. All patients should be evaluated for presence of intraventricular thrombus. When identified, anticoagulation with warfarin is recommended, with the duration dependent on the rate of myocardial recovery. For patients with reduced LV systolic function but no documented thrombus, some recommend empiric anticoagulation, although this has not been studied rigorously.

Prognosis

Most patients who survive the acute episode will recover systolic function within 4 weeks. However, the risk of in-hospital complications was 19.1% in one large registry, and in-hospital mortality rates range from 0 to 8%. Risk factors for the development of heart failure include older age, presence of a physical trigger, and ejection fraction less than 40%.

Long term, the rate of death from any cause has been reported as 5.6% per patient-year, and the rate of major adverse cardiovascular or cerebrovascular events is 9.9% per patient-year. Men are at higher risk of death. After surviving an initial episode of stress cardiomyopathy, patients have a 2% annual risk of recurrence. Whether or not long-term medical therapy is effective for reducing this recurrence rate is unknown.

Ghadri JR, Wittstein IS, Prasad A, et al. International expert consensus document on Takotsubo syndrome (Part II): diagnostic workup, outcome, and management. *Eur Heart J.* 2018;39:2047–2062. [PMID: 29850820]

Pelliccia F, Pasceri V, Patti G, et al. Long-term prognosis and outcome predictors in Takotsubo syndrome: A systematic review and meta-regression study. *JACC Heart Fail.* 2019 Feb;7(2):143–154. [PMID: 30611720]

26 Heart Failure with Reduced Ejection Fraction

Sarah Westcott, MD
Liviu Klein, MD, MS

ESSENTIALS OF DIAGNOSIS

- Dyspnea on exertion and at rest, orthopnea, paroxysmal nocturnal dyspnea, and fatigue.
- Elevated jugular venous pressure, crackles throughout both lung fields with wheezing, cardiomegaly, S_3 gallop, hepatomegaly, and bilateral peripheral pitting edema.
- Dilated left ventricle with a reduced ejection fraction on transthoracic echocardiography.
- Elevated left ventricular filling pressures on cardiac catheterization.

General Considerations

Heart failure (HF) is a complex clinical syndrome resulting from any structural or functional myocardial dysfunction that leads to an impaired ability to circulate blood at a rate sufficient to maintain the metabolic needs of internal organs and peripheral tissues. The myocardial dysfunction is often the consequence of long-standing ischemia due to coronary artery disease or loss of myocardial mass due to prior infarction, long-standing myocardial stress due to suboptimally treated hypertension or valvular disease, or direct long-term toxin exposure (alcohol abuse, illicit substance use, or chemotherapeutic agents); rarely, fulminant infections (especially viral) can lead to autoimmune myocardial damage, and in some cases, there is no apparent cause (idiopathic cardiomyopathy, usually related to inherited or spontaneous gene mutations).

The cardinal manifestations of HF are dyspnea and fatigue (which may limit exercise tolerance) and fluid retention (which may lead to pulmonary/hepatic/splanchnic congestion and peripheral edema). Both abnormalities impair the functional capacity and quality of life of affected patients, but they may not necessarily dominate the clinical picture at the same time.

Globally, the prevalence of HF is highest in Central Europe, North Africa, and the Middle East. The lowest rates are observed in Southeast Asia and Eastern Europe. Various HF risk factors predominate in certain geographic regions, with ischemic heart disease being the highest in Europe and North America, valvular heart disease in Asia, and hypertension in Latin America, the Caribbean, and Eastern Europe.

The prevalence of HF in the United States is around 6 million patients, with projections showing a 46% increase from 2012 to 2030 resulting in more than 8 million people with HF. Approximately 50% of those hospitalized with HF have reduced ejection fraction (HFrEF)/systolic dysfunction. Recent data from the Framingham Heart Study have demonstrated that 60% of the middle-aged and older adults had evidence of preclinical HF (AHA/ACC Stage A or B), suggesting a potentially high burden of early HF in the community. There are an estimated one million new HF cases annually in the United States.

In the past 25 years, the residual lifetime risk of developing HF in middle-aged adults increased by about 20% in women and 30% in men. This is likely primarily driven by an increase in both life expectancy and risk factor prevalence (obesity, hypertension, and diabetes). At age 40, the lifetime risk for HF is as high in women as in men and is approximately one in five. Men however have a higher lifetime risk for HFrEF at age 50 compared to women. Although more than 75% of HF patients have antecedent hypertension or coronary artery disease, the population attributable risk is different in men and women; the attributable risk for HF associated with coronary artery disease is 39% in men and 18% in women, whereas the attributable risk associated with hypertension is 39% in men and 59% in women, emphasizing the crucial need for population-based strategies to prevent the development of HF.

Multiethnic epidemiologic studies showed that the highest risk for developing HF is in African Americans (highest in young women and middle-aged men), followed by Hispanics/Latinos, Caucasians, and Chinese. This higher risk likely reflects differences in life expectancies, the prevalence of hypertension and diabetes mellitus and in social determinants of health between different ethnicities.

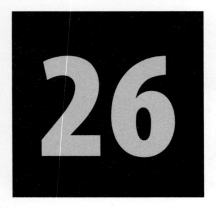

Although the survival after HF diagnosis has improved, the 5-year mortality is still close to 50%, and over a quarter million deaths every year have antecedent HF. In addition, HF is one of the leading causes of hospitalization in the United States, with more than 1 million hospitalizations a year (a figure that has not changed over the past decade). Indeed, 85% of patients diagnosed with HF will be hospitalized at least once, and more than 40% will be hospitalized at least four times. HF accounts for more than 12 million office visits, with an estimated total cost of $30.7 billion, making it a major contributor to total health-care expenditure and the number one health expenditure for Medicare, with projections that it will increase to $69.7 billion by 2030.

Heidenreich PA, Fonarow GC, Opsha Y, et al. HFSA Scientific Statement Committee Members Chair. Economic issues in heart failure in the United States. *J Card Fail.* 2022;28:453–466. [PMID: 35085762]

Savarese G, Lund LH. Global public health burden of heart failure. *Card Fail Rev.* 2017;3:7–11. [PMID: 28785469]

Shah HM, Minhas AMK, Khan MS, et al. Trends and characteristics of hospitalizations for heart failure in the United States from 2004 to 2018. *ESC Heart Fail.* 2022;9:947–952. [PMID: 35098700]

Tsao CW, Aday AW, Almarzooq ZI, et al. Heart disease and stroke statistics - 2022 update: a report from the American Heart Association. *Circulation.* 2022;145:e153–e639. [PMID: 35078371]

Vasan RS, Enserro DM, Beiser AS, Xanthakis V. Lifetime risk of heart failure among participants in the Framingham Study. *J Am Coll Cardiol.* 2022;79:250–263. [PMID: 35057911]

Pathophysiology

When an excessive workload is imposed on the heart by increased systolic blood pressure (pressure overload, such as in chronic hypertension or aortic stenosis), increased diastolic volume (volume overload, such as in progressive dilated idiopathic cardiomyopathy or chronic aortic or mitral regurgitation), or loss of myocardium (acutely in the setting of myocardial infarction, or chronically in the setting of flow-limiting coronary artery disease), normal myocardial cells hypertrophy to increase the contractile force of the unaffected areas. The biochemical, electrophysiologic, and contractile changes that ensue lead to alterations in the mechanical properties of the myocardium. Eventually, the compensatory force of the normal myocardial contraction decreases as cell loss and hypertrophy continue, leading to increased ventricular volume ("cardiac remodeling") and significant geometric ventricular alterations (ellipsoid to spherical shape). After the initial compensatory phase, the increase in ventricular volume is associated with further reductions in the ejection fraction (progressive systolic dysfunction) and with abnormalities in the peripheral circulation from activation of various neurohormonal compensatory mechanisms.

In the United States, coronary artery disease is the underlying etiology for HFrEF in more than half of the cases and a major contributor in another 15–20%. Transient ischemic events may cause prolonged systolic dysfunction that persists even after the ischemic event has resolved (myocardial stunning). The sustained reduction in the coronary blood flow leads to tissue hypoperfusion that is sufficient to maintain viability, but insufficient to maintain a normal contractility (myocardial hibernation). However, hibernation cannot be maintained indefinitely, and myocardial necrosis will ensue if coronary blood flow is not restored. Ischemia and hibernation may lead to myocyte apoptosis, which may result in progression of left ventricular systolic dysfunction characterized by a reduction in cardiac output and/or an increase in wall stress.

These functional and structural myocardial changes result in compensatory activation of neurohormonal systems, such as the renin–angiotensin–aldosterone system (RAAS), the adrenergic system, and the hypothalamic–neurohypophyseal system. The mechanisms for RAAS activation in HF include renal hypoperfusion with decreased filtered sodium reaching the macula densa and decreased stretch of the juxtaglomerular apparatus leading to increased renin release. Renin cleaves four amino acids from circulating angiotensinogen to form the biologically inactive angiotensin I. Angiotensin-converting enzyme (ACE) cleaves two amino acids from angiotensin I to form the biologically active angiotensin II, which binds to vascular angiotensin receptors causing vasoconstriction of the efferent postglomerular arterioles (promoting reabsorption of sodium, urea, and water) and to cardiac angiotensin receptors causing myocyte hypertrophy, apoptosis, and interstitial fibrosis. Increased circulating levels of angiotensin II also promote the release of aldosterone from the adrenal zona glomerulosa, resulting in sodium reabsorption and potassium excretion in the distal nephron, along with myocardial fibroblast proliferation and collagen deposition. The abnormal hypertrophy and fibrosis increase the passive stiffness of the ventricles and arterial bed, interfering with ventricular filling and reducing arterial compliance and, along with myocyte slippage and interstitial growth, result in ventricular remodeling. Finally, angiotensin II may increase the release of arginine vasopressin via a mechanism that does not rely on changes in osmolality, leading to renal free water reabsorption and dilutional hyponatremia seen with severe HF.

In patients with HF, the inhibitory input from high-pressure carotid sinus and aortic arch baroreceptors and low-pressure cardiopulmonary mechanoreceptors decreases, while nonbaroreflex peripheral chemoreceptors and muscle metaboreceptors excitatory input increases, with a net increase in sympathetic nerve traffic and blunted parasympathetic nerve traffic, and a resultant loss of heart rate variability and increased peripheral vascular resistance. As a result of the increase in sympathetic tone, there is an increase in circulating levels of norepinephrine from a combination of increased release from adrenergic nerve endings and its consequent "spillover" into the plasma, with reduced uptake of norepinephrine by adrenergic nerve endings. In patients in early stages of HF, norepinephrine increases heart rate and contractility and may support cardiac function. However, in later stages of HF, cardiac response to norepinephrine is blunted, partly because of the decreased β-receptor density seen in patients with chronic severe HF, where a shift occurs from the normal density (β1/β2 ratio of 70–80%/20–30%) to a more even distribution of 60%/40%. In addition, α-adrenergic receptors increase in the failing heart so that the end result is a more balanced distribution of myocardial α, β1, and β2 receptors. Chronic adrenergic stimulation has been shown to induce expression of proinflammatory cytokines, such as tumor necrosis factor-α, interleukin-1, and interleukin-6. Increased cytokine levels may result in the skeletal muscle myopathy characteristic of HF and cause myocardial inflammation, cell proliferation, and apoptosis, thereby worsening the HF syndrome. Tumor necrosis factor-α also activates transcription factors and enzymes involved in signal transduction, and it induces a number of genes, including the fetal gene program. Peripheral arteriolar tone is also increased in patients with HF (via α-adrenergic receptor stimulation), producing an increase in blood pressure and ventricular afterload and vasoconstriction of the renal efferent arterioles that causes significant sodium and water retention and increases production of renin, angiotensin II, and aldosterone, emphasizing the tight interplay between the adrenergic system and the RAAS. Indeed, ACE inhibition in patients with HF has been found to reduce peripheral sympathetic nerve impulse traffic and cardiac adrenergic drive, and the beneficial effects of ACE inhibitors appear to be especially prominent in patients with increased adrenergic activation. Conversely, β-blockade reduces the secretion of renin, therefore reducing the levels of angiotensin and aldosterone.

In response to cardiac insult, the autonomic nervous system attempts to preserve cardiac output by upregulating sympathetic activity and withdrawing parasympathetic activity. This autonomic imbalance contributes to the pathological left ventricular remodeling, peripheral vasoconstriction, and salt and water retention leading to development and progression of HF. These observations provide the rationale for therapies that block sympathetic activity or enhance parasympathetic activity to treat HF. Such therapies include augmentation of the parasympathetic tone through vagal nerve stimulation, and centrally mediated reduction in sympathetic outflow and increased parasympathetic activity through baroreflex activation therapy.

Arginine vasopressin is synthesized in the hypothalamus, and its release from the hypophysis is enhanced by osmolar stimuli as well as elevated concentrations of norepinephrine and angiotensin II. Increased release of arginine vasopressin in HF causes vasoconstriction and myocardial fibrosis (through binding to vasopressin 1 receptors) and water retention with dilutional hyponatremia (through binding to vasopressin 2 receptors).

The vasodilator peptides, such as atrial natriuretic peptide (ANP) and brain natriuretic peptide (BNP), are overexpressed in HF (as result of increased wall stress) and lead to a lowering of the right atrial, pulmonary artery, and pulmonary artery wedge pressures. In addition, systemic vascular resistance declines and cardiac output improves, circulating aldosterone and norepinephrine levels decrease, and natriuresis and glomerular filtration increase. However, in many patients with HF, the natriuretic peptides become ineffective despite high circulating levels. The profound activation of the RAAS and adrenergic system may overcome the ability of natriuretic peptides to increase sodium excretion or reduce afterload. In addition, most of the circulating natriuretic peptides in advanced HF patients are secreted as biologically inactive ("defective") molecules. Finally, changes in renal hemodynamics and a combination of receptor downregulation and increased cyclic guanosine monophosphate phosphodiesterase activity lead to a decreased natriuretic peptide response with consequent increase in salt retention and further deterioration of renal function and increased vasoconstriction. Neprilysin is a neutral endopeptidase that is responsible for the degradation of natriuretic peptides and angiotensin II and its inhibition enhances endogenous natriuretic peptide levels and activity, counteracting the negative cardiorenal effects of the upregulated RAAS.

The development of myocardial hypertrophy, as consequence of neurohormonal activation, initially represents an important adaptive mechanism to hemodynamic stress and is characterized by structural changes at the myocyte level that are translated into alterations in chamber size and geometry. In addition to myocyte alterations, the cardiac fibroblasts and the increased production of extracellular matrix participate in the remodeling process. Increased hemodynamic stress results in changes in myocardial gene expression leading to an impairment of contractile function. In patients with HF, a marked increase in the ventricular end-diastolic pressure may be responsible for changes in the shape of the left ventricle from an ellipsoid to a more spherical configuration. These changes in ventricular geometry result in papillary muscle rearrangement and secondary mitral regurgitation. In addition, the elevated ventricular end-diastolic pressures cause subendocardial ischemia that is perpetuated by compensatory tachycardia, which shortens the diastole and decreases the coronary filling time. This is reflected at a biochemical level by increased production of lactate, adenosine triphosphate, and creatine phosphate and at a histologic level through fibrosis, lowering the threshold for malignant ventricular arrhythmias.

The myocardial fibrosis and chamber dilatation lead to electrical dyssynchrony by fibrosis of the conduction system that, in turn, results in mechanical dyssynchrony (observed in about 40% of the HFrEF patients). When mechanical dyssynchrony is present, contraction and relaxation of the lateral wall occurs earlier than that of the interventricular septum, leading to decreased stroke volume and cardiac output and eventually to secondary mitral regurgitation.

In HFrEF patients, the decreased cardiac output leads to renal hypoperfusion, and the fluid retention leads to increased venous congestion, resulting in further reduction in the renal blood flow and relative renal vasoconstriction, which further exacerbate the sodium and water retention. In addition, the elevated cytokine levels and relative resistance of the bone marrow to erythropoietin lead to anemia in many HF patients. In these patients, peripheral perfusion decreases as a result of a decreased vascular resistance, leading to neurohormonal activation with subsequent reduction in renal blood flow and kidney function, ultimately resulting in expansion of plasma volumes. The increased plasma volume results in increased cardiac work, which leads to left ventricular hypertrophy and ultimately worsens the cardiac function, which in turn worsens renal function, completing the vicious circle (cardio-renal-anemia syndrome).

The chronic elevation in the left ventricular filling pressures that occurs in the setting of left ventricular remodeling and dilatation will lead to an increase in pulmonary venous pressures and a passive increase in pulmonary artery pressures. Due to the chronic elevation in pulmonary arterial pressures (secondary pulmonary hypertension), the pulmonary vascular resistance increases, increasing the right ventricular afterload and leading to deterioration in the right ventricular function over time (right HF). This eventually leads to a decrease in both right and left ventricular stroke volume, which is associated with signs and symptoms of both congestion (dyspnea, peripheral edema, hepatomegaly, elevated jugular venous pressures) and low cardiac output (mental status changes, renal dysfunction, fatigue).

Eventually, the progressive compensatory mechanisms described earlier are overwhelmed and the patients become symptomatic and present to medical attention, often in a hospital setting. In most patients, the condition is progressive, and further deterioration occurs at a myocardial/renal/hepatic/skeletal muscle level, and patients end up having recurrent hospitalizations. There is clear evidence that each hospitalization for HF leads to further myocardial injury (evidenced by troponin release) and renal injury, which in turn will worsen the overall prognosis and lead to progressive HF and death.

In rare circumstances, a hyperkinetic circulatory state associated with vasodilatation occurs (usually due to an increased demand on the heart from another condition, such as anemia, or thyrotoxicosis) and can trigger HF when superimposed on an underlying heart disease. Fortunately, this is often reversible by prompting and treating the associated triggering condition.

Guazzi M, Ghio S, Adir Y. Pulmonary hypertension in HFpEF and HFrEF. JACC Review Topic of the Week. *J Am Coll Cardiol.* 2020;76:1102–1111. [PMID: 32854845]

Mann DL, Felker GM. Mechanisms and models in heart failure: a translational approach. *Circ Res.* 2021;128:1435–1450. [PMID: 33983832]

Verbrugge FH, Guazzi M, Testani JM, Borlaug BA. Altered hemodynamics and end-organ damage in heart failure: impact on the lung and kidney. *Circulation.* 2020;142:998–1012. [PMID: 32897746]

Clinical Findings

One of the first principles in the clinical evaluation is to determine whether the patient is indeed presenting with HF, since the presenting signs and symptoms are often nonspecific. Despite a careful history and physical examination, additional diagnostic information may be necessary to support the diagnosis and to determine the mechanism of the symptoms, the severity of the condition, and the prognosis for the individual patient (Table 26–1).

A. Symptoms & Signs

The cardinal symptoms of HF are dyspnea and fatigue that occur with exertion and/or at rest, although some patients may present with acute pulmonary edema. **Dyspnea** is a subjective feeling of air hunger and is the most frequent symptom in HF patients. Initially, dyspnea on exertion will be noted by a change in the extent of physical activity that causes the shortness of breath. As the HF worsens, the intensity of exertion required to produce dyspnea will decrease, and eventually the dyspnea will be present at rest. Interestingly, the severity of dyspnea decreases after right ventricular failure develops.

Paroxysmal nocturnal dyspnea occurs after the patient has been in the supine position for some time. The patient wakes up suddenly with a sensation of choking and air hunger and assumes an upright posture to relieve the symptoms. Paroxysmal nocturnal dyspnea usually precedes orthopnea, may be associated

Table 26–1. Clinical Framingham Heart Study Criteria for Heart Failure

Major Criteria	Minor Criteria
Paroxysmal nocturnal dyspnea or orthopnea	Dyspnea on exertion
Elevated jugular venous pressure	Night cough
Hepatojugular reflux	Tachycardia > 120 bpm
Pulmonary crackles	Hepatomegaly
S_3 gallop	Bilateral lower extremity edema
Enlarging heart silhouette on consecutive chest x-rays	Pulmonary vascular engorgement on chest x-ray
Pulmonary edema on chest x-ray	Pleural effusion on chest x-ray
Weight loss on diuretics (> 10 lb in 5 days)	
Increased venous pressure > 16 cm H_2O (assessed via a central line)	

Presence of two major or one major and two minor criteria is required for heart failure diagnosis.

with bronchospasm and wheezing (cardiac asthma), and is caused by a mobilization of interstitial fluid from infradiaphragmatic locations during recumbency with a resultant increase in the circulating blood volume and increased pulmonary venous pressure.

Orthopnea (dyspnea occurring within a few minutes after the patient assumes a supine position) has the same cause as paroxysmal nocturnal dyspnea but represents a more severe cardiac dysfunction. While elevating the head of the bed, sitting up, or standing can improve the symptoms, the most severely affected patients usually sleep sitting upright.

Another manifestation of pulmonary congestion is a dry or nonproductive **cough** (especially at night) that is usually relieved by treating the elevated left-sided filling pressures.

As with dyspnea, the mechanism of **fatigue** in patients with systolic HF is unclear. Although the fatigue was attributed for many years to a low cardiac output, there is mounting evidence of contribution of abnormal skeletal muscle metabolism with shifts in fiber distribution (increase in the percentage of the fast-twitch, glycolytic, easily fatigable fibers) and muscle atrophy, even in the presence of a normal cardiac output. Chronic fatigue begets further inactivity, which leads to further deconditioning and a greater extent of disability.

Other disabling symptoms in HF patients include extreme **thirst** (associated with activation of the arginine–vasopressin system), **nocturia** (due to enhanced urine formation in the recumbent position when renal vasoconstriction decreases and venous return to the heart increases), **oliguria** (usually associated with either increased venous congestion or markedly reduced cardiac output), **cerebral symptoms**—memory impairment, confusion, insomnia—(usually markers of reduced cardiac output), and **ascites and abdominal fullness**, accompanied by **right upper quadrant pain, early satiety, and nausea** (usually related to passive hepatic and splanchnic congestion).

B. Physical Examination

Although most patients with HF appear well nourished, those with more advanced disease (especially in the setting of chronic splanchnic congestion) frequently appear malnourished. This appearance arises from poor caloric intake (due to early satiety and nausea) and impaired absorption of fat and, occasionally, a protein-losing enteropathy, in combination with an increased metabolism due to elevated levels of norepinephrine and tumor necrosis factor-α. The combination of reduced intake and increased energy expenditure leads to a reduction of tissue mass and, in some cases, to **cardiac cachexia**.

Patients with HFrEF frequently show evidence of increased sympathetic activity such as **diaphoresis**, **pallor** and coldness of the limbs, **peripheral cyanosis** of the digits, abnormal distention of the superficial veins, and compensatory **sinus tachycardia** (when the cardiac output is decreased).

Cheyne-Stokes respiration (alternating phases of hyperpnea and apnea in a crescendo-decrescendo manner) can be seen in patients with HFrEF and represents an altered neurogenic control of respiration, facilitated by a combination of pulmonary congestion, prolonged circulation time from lung to the brain, and decreased sensitivity of the respiratory center to hypercapnia and hypoxia.

Cardiomegaly, with a laterally displaced and sustained point of maximal impulse, can be found on physical examination, but this is a nonspecific finding. The decrease in ventricular compliance becomes apparent by the presence of a late diastolic atrial sound (**S_4 gallop**). A protodiastolic sound (**S_3 gallop**), better heard in more tachycardic patients, is caused by acute deceleration of ventricular inflow after the early filling phase and is a marker of increased left ventricular filling pressures. Together with elevated jugular venous pressure, the presence of a third heart sound is a powerful predictor of outcomes and is associated with an increased risk of death and hospitalization for HF. **Systolic murmurs** are common in HF patients and are secondary to functional mitral or tricuspid regurgitation that results from ventricular dilatation.

Pulsus alternans (a regular rhythm of alternating strong and weak pulsations) is common in patients with HFrEF and is due to an alternation in the stroke volume of the left ventricle. If persistent, it usually implies advanced HF and a chronic low output state.

1. Subclinical congestion—Defined as elevated intracardiac filling pressures without obvious clinical signs, subclinical congestion precedes clinical congestion by weeks. This is partly due to the ability of the lymphatic system to accommodate large amounts of fluid before Starling forces are overcome, and manifestations of congestion appear on physical examination. Although difficult to recognize, technological advancements such as hemodynamic sensors have made this important window of therapeutic intervention more apparent to health-care providers.

2. Clinical congestion—Pulmonary crackles can be heard at the lung bases, and they are the result of the transudation of fluid into the alveoli that subsequently moves into the airways. In pulmonary edema, coarse rales and wheezes are heard all over the lung fields and may be accompanied by frothy sputum. With progressive fluid accumulation, pleural effusions occur and will increase the severity of dyspnea by further reducing pulmonary vital capacity. **Dullness on percussion** is the characteristic sign and shifting dullness can be found when the patient moves from the sitting to the lateral decubitus position. Breath sounds over the area of effusion are diminished or absent. The pleural effusions are usually reabsorbed slowly as diuresis ensues, but in many cases, they lag behind for many days after the symptoms disappear.

Symmetric pitting edema is common in HFrEF patients and involves the dependent portions of the body with higher venous pressure: feet and ankles of ambulatory patients and the sacral area of bedridden ones. With progressive, untreated disease, the edema becomes massive and generalized (anasarca), involving the genital area, the upper extremities, and the thoracic and abdominal walls. Occasionally, in massive overload, skin breakdown and extravasation of fluid can occur (weeping). Chronic edema results in increased pigmentation, reddening, and induration of the skin of the lower extremities (**stasis dermatitis**).

An important part of the volume status assessment is detecting the abnormal **distention of the internal jugular veins**. Patients should be examined while they are lying down, with the torso and head tilted at 45 degrees. A persistent elevation of the jugular venous pressure is one of the earliest and most reliable signs of HF and is a powerful prognostic indicator of increased risk of HF hospitalizations and all-cause mortality. The inability of the right ventricle to accept transient increases in venous return (**positive hepatojugular reflux**) is observed during transient compression (30–60 seconds) of the upper abdomen. Passive hepatic congestion is identified by epigastric fullness, **hepatomegaly** and tenderness on palpation, and dullness to percussion of the right upper quadrant. As with the pleural effusions, these findings may persist after other signs of HF have disappeared because it takes longer for hepatic congestion to disappear. Occasionally, systolic pulsations of the liver may be felt in patients with severe tricuspid regurgitation.

Although rarely used, the hemodynamic response to the **Valsalva maneuver** is simple to perform and carries one of the best combinations of specificity (91%) and sensitivity (69%) for the detection of elevated left ventricular filling pressures. The maneuver is performed with the blood pressure cuff inflated 15 mm Hg over the systolic blood pressure. While the physician auscultates over the brachial artery, the patient is asked to perform a forced expiratory effort against a closed airway (the Valsalva maneuver). In a normal response, the Korotkoff sounds disappear during sustained maneuver and reappear after release of the maneuver. An abnormal response, in which blood pressure sounds either do not reappear after the maneuver (absent overshoot) or are maintained throughout the maneuver (square wave), is found in patients with systolic HF and elevated left ventricular filling pressures.

It is important to emphasize that HF is largely a clinical diagnosis, followed by determination of clinical profile (Figure 26–1) and the severity of symptoms (New York Heart Association functional class), which will dictate the subsequent therapy. Recently, there has been a concerted effort to create a universal definition of HF given its high global burden and need for standardization, especially in

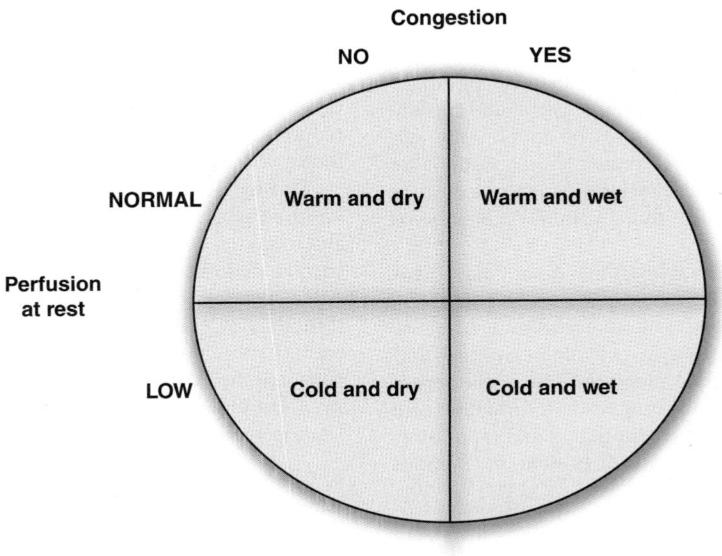

▲ **Figure 26–1.** Presentation of heart failure based on assessment of congestion and perfusion. ACE, angiotensin-converting enzyme.

Signs and symptoms of congestion: orthopnea, paroxysmal nocturnal dyspnea, jugular venous distension, positive hepatojugular reflux, pulmonary crackles, hepatomegaly, symmetric pedal edema, and Valsalva maneuver square wave.

Evidence of impaired perfusion: sleepiness, cool extremities, narrow pulse pressure, low serum sodium, increased serum creatinine, and hypotension with ACE inhibitors.

both diagnosis and research. As part of a consensus document published in the *Journal of Cardiac Failure*, the proposed new definition of HF includes any pathognomonic evidence of HF caused by a structural or functional cardiac abnormality coupled with either elevated natriuretic peptide levels or data indicating cardiogenic pulmonary congestion or systemic congestion. Use of this definition is starting to become more widespread throughout literature and will likely become the standard in future practice.

C. Laboratory Testing

Patients with new-onset HF should undergo routine laboratory tests when the condition is first diagnosed. This is also recommended for patients with chronic HF and acute decompensation, when there is a change in therapeutic intervention, or in periodic monitoring for clinical stability. A basic metabolic profile can show hyponatremia (marker of advanced HF or excessive diuretic use) and signs of renal dysfunction (elevated urea and creatinine). Congestion of the liver is often associated with abnormalities of liver function tests, while hyperglycemia and abnormalities in thyroid-stimulating hormone levels can identify concomitant precipitating conditions (such as diabetes or hyper- or hypothyroidism). The recognition of anemia and iron deficiency in patients with HFrEF is important, as early treatment may reverse these abnormalities.

Determining the level of BNP or of its amino-terminal fragment (NT-proBNP) provides important diagnostic utility for diagnosing HF in the acute clinical setting. BNP levels more than 100 pg/mL and NT-proBNP levels higher than 450 pg/mL in younger patients or higher than 900 pg/mL in patients older than 50 years are highly sensitive and specific for HF when the clinical diagnosis is in doubt. Although several studies have shown the incremental prognostic value of serial natriuretic peptide level determination, the efficacy of natriuretic peptide-guided therapy in HFrEF patients remains controversial.

Serum cardiac troponins (at levels that do not meet myocardial infarction criteria) are detected in over half of HFrEF patients (including in those without significant coronary artery disease) and are usually a sign of volume overload and elevated left ventricular filling pressures. Detectable serum troponin levels carry powerful prognostic information and may help in tailoring therapy (eg, initiation and rapid titration of vasodilators and avoidance of positive intravenous inotropes in hospitalized patients).

D. Diagnostic Studies

1. Electrocardiography—An electrocardiogram should be routinely obtained and examined for evidence of underlying structural alterations (eg, left ventricular hypertrophy, prior myocardial infarctions), for rhythm abnormalities as a cause or consequence of HF decompensation (eg, atrial fibrillation/flutter, frequent ventricular ectopic beats, or sustained arrhythmias), and for the presence of conduction abnormalities (eg, left bundle branch block) that may lead to electrical dyssynchrony. The QT interval should be noted because many therapies can prolong it and provoke lethal arrhythmias. In patients who have undergone cardiac resynchronization therapy (CRT), changes in the QRS complex duration or morphology may provide information about underlying pacing or programming changes.

2. Chest radiography—Careful examination of the cardiac silhouette, as well as the pulmonary vasculature, remains part of routine evaluation in all patients with HFrEF. Cardiomegaly (cardiothoracic ratio > 50%) can be found in almost all patients with chronic HF, but may be absent in those with acute HF due to acute myocarditis or myocardial infarction. In HFrEF, there is progressive vasoconstriction of pulmonary vessels in the lower lobes and redistribution of the pulmonary flow to the upper lobes. Interstitial and perivascular edema develop when the left-sided filling pressures increase above 25 mm Hg and the bronchovascular markings at the bases become prominent. Kerley lines, spindle-shaped linear opacities at the periphery of the lung bases, occur in the later stages of HF. Pleural effusions can also be seen. After lowering the intracardiac filling pressures, there may be a delay of 48 hours before improvement and clearing of pulmonary findings can be seen on chest radiograph.

3. Echocardiography—Echocardiographic evaluation is an essential diagnostic tool for assessing cardiac structure and function. It should be used early in the initial phase of the HF diagnosis to define the syndrome (HFrEF versus HFpEF) to direct therapy, and at any time there is a clinical change that would lead to a change in management. Specifically, recent evidence suggests that a stratification system should define reduced ejection fraction as ≤ 40% and normal as ≥ 55% in men and ≥ 60% in women.

Throughout this evaluation, a careful observer will examine the right and left ventricular size/volume, wall motion abnormalities (including aneurysms), hypertrophy, left ventricular diastolic function, left/right-sided filling pressures, stroke volume, ejection fraction, presence of intracardiac thrombus or shunt, and valvular pathology (morphology, regurgitation, stenosis). A comprehensive examination can elucidate the cardiac component of the HF symptoms and may lead to targeted treatments (eg, diuresis versus vasodilatation versus need for inotropic support).

4. Cardiac magnetic resonance imaging (cMRI)—This newer imaging tool provides in-depth anatomic information and can provide information on the myocardial structure (scarring, fatty infiltration, or iron overload), helping in the noninvasive diagnosis of infiltrative cardiomyopathies (eg, sarcoidosis, amyloidosis), iron overload cardiomyopathies (eg, hemochromatosis), acute myocarditis, or genetic cardiomyopathies (eg, arrhythmogenic right ventricular cardiomyopathy, left ventricular noncompaction cardiomyopathy). In addition, in patients with coronary artery disease, it can relay information on myocardial viability that can be used to decide on percutaneous or surgical revascularization. The major limitations are the use of a magnetic field (which can interfere with cardiac implantable electrical devices that many HFrEF patients have), its relative high cost (limiting its use to major medical centers), and the claustrophobic feeling that many patients experience.

5. Cardiopulmonary exercise stress testing (CPET)—CPET has been shown to add substantial precision in the initial evaluation of patients with HF and in their prognosis over time, especially when advanced therapies are considered. Measurements of the peak oxygen consumption (peak V_{O2}) and the slope of the ratio of ventilation (V_E) to carbon dioxide production (V_{CO2}) (V_E/V_{CO2}) are powerful predictors of prognosis. A peak V_{O2} less than 14 mL/kg/min in patients intolerant of β-blockers (12 mL/kg/min on patients on β-blockers) or less than 50% predicted are considered indications for heart transplantation or left ventricular assist devices implantation. In addition, valuable information regarding chronotropic competence can be gathered from the CPET. Routine assessment of exercise tolerance using the 6-minute walk test can be performed in the office, or at home using mobile smartphone technologies, with similar powerful prognostic implications as the CPET.

6. Cardiac catheterization—Because coronary artery disease is the main cause of HFrEF in the United States, coronary angiography is necessary whenever the suspicion for coronary artery disease as etiologic or aggravating factor of HF is suspected. Research has clearly shown that misdiagnosis of ischemic heart disease among patients with HF is common if angiographic evaluation is not undertaken as part of the initial workup. In addition, surgical revascularization in ischemic HFrEF has been shown to improve cardiovascular outcomes.

Right-heart catheterization may be important in patients who are doing poorly with severe congestion, ascites, or signs and symptoms of low cardiac output or when constrictive physiology or restrictive cardiomyopathy is suspected. Most right-sided heart catheterizations performed in patients with HF today are used to help guide therapy rather than to make a specific diagnosis.

7. Endomyocardial biopsy—The role of diagnostic endomyocardial biopsy in patients with HF has diminished. Although cMRI has replaced many of its uses, endomyocardial biopsy is still used in patients with suspected fulminant myocarditis, giant cell myocarditis, sarcoidosis, or hemochromatosis. In addition, routine surveillance for rejection after cardiac transplantation still uses endomyocardial biopsies (at least for the first 6–12 months).

8. Genetic testing—Clinical genetic testing in HF has become available in many commercial testing laboratories. At present, comprehensive genetic testing is recommended for at-risk individuals (usually first-degree adult relatives of affected persons) for inherited disorders including those with dilated and hypertrophic cardiomyopathies, cardiac conduction disease, or family history of premature unexpected sudden death (< 50 years old). Some argue that this should be expanded to include specific genetic variant testing known to have high prevalence in certain population subgroups. The goal of genetic testing remains to identify those who would benefit from careful evaluation, close monitoring, counseling on risk modification, and possible early intervention with therapeutics and devices.

Significant progress has been made in the last few years on the genes responsible for dilated and hypertrophic cardiomyopathy, where a third to half of individuals with these conditions test positive in genetic screening. Genetic variants that have been implicated in causing dilated cardiomyopathy include Lamin A/C, sarcomeric proteins including titin (*TTN*), various proteins associated with myosin (*MYH6, MYH7, MYBPC3*), troponin (*TNNI3*), tropomyosin (*TPM1*), and proteins integrated in the z-disc (*ACTN2, ANKRD1, CSRP3*). While *MYBPC3* mutations make up a significant portion of those with genetic hypertrophic cardiomyopathy, its involvement has also been associated with the pathogenesis of dilated cardiomyopathy. Mutations in the gene *TTN* have been a particular focus of study. This is because the timing and severity of its presentation can be altered by modifiable HF risk factors. In addition, expression of *TTN* can increase the likelihood of developing HF through pathways outside of the progression of dilated cardiomyopathy. In the future, it is possible that pharmacogenomics-guided therapy will be used to better select HF therapies tailored to specific patient genotypes.

Aimo A, Vergaro G, Gonzalez A, et al. Cardiac remodeling-part 2: Clinical, imaging and laboratory findings. A review from the Study Group on Biomarkers of the Heart Failure Association of the European Society of Cardiology. *Eur J Heart Fail.* 2022;24:944–958. [PMID: 35488811]

Argulian E, Narula J. Advanced cardiovascular imaging in clinical heart failure. *JACC Heart Failure.* 2021;9:699–709. [PMID: 34391742]

Bozkurt B, Coats AJ, Tsutsui H, et al. Universal definition and classification of heart failure: a report of the Heart Failure Society of America, Heart Failure Association of the European Society of Cardiology, Japanese Heart Failure Society and Writing Committee of the Universal Definition of Heart Failure. *J Card Fail.* 2021;27:387–413. [PMID: 33663906]

Buber J, Robertson HT. Cardiopulmonary exercise testing for heart failure: pathophysiology and predictive markers. *Heart.* 2022; in press. [PMID: 35410893]

Cresci S, Pereira NL, Ahmad F, et al. Heart failure in the era of precision medicine. A scientific statement from the American Heart Association. *Circ Genom Precis Med.* 2019;12:458–485. [PMID: 31510778]

Rosenbaum AN, Agre KE, Pereira NL. Genetics of dilated cardiomyopathy: practical implications for heart failure management. *Nat Rev Cardiol.* 2020;17:286–297. [PMID: 31605094]

Treatment

A. Prevention

The burden of HF can be affected only by drastically decreasing its incidence, and as such, it is crucial to identify

Table 26–2. Staging System in the Classification of Heart Failure

ACC/AHA Staging	Clinical Heart Failure	Symptoms (NYHA Functional Class)	Population Estimate from NHANES (millions)[1]	Population Estimate: Adults > Age 45 from Olmsted County (%)[2]
D **Refractory, end-stage** (Marked symptoms despite maximal therapy)	Yes	IIIB–IV	0.3	0.2
C **Symptomatic HF** (Shortness of breath, fatigue, reduced exercise tolerance)	Yes	I–IIIA	5.7	11.8
B **Asymptomatic HF** (Prior myocardial infarction, left ventricular hypertrophy, valvular disease, etc.)	No	None	15	34
A **High Risk for Developing HF** (Hypertension, coronary disease, diabetes, obesity, etc.)	No	None	125	22
None	No	None	185	32

ACC, American College of Cardiology; AHA, American Heart Association; HF, heart failure; NHANES, National Health and Nutrition Examination Survey; NYHA, New York Heart Association.

[1]From Tsao CW, et al. Heart disease and stroke statistics - 2022 update: a report from the American Heart Association. *Circulation*. 2022;145:e153–e639.

[2]From Olmsted country, adapted from Ammar KA, et al. Prevalence and prognostic significance of heart failure stages: application of the American College of Cardiology/American Heart Association heart failure staging criteria in the community. *Circulation*. 2007;115:1563–1570.

the primary drivers for this problem and develop/implement population-level preventive strategies. To aid in this goal, the American College of Cardiology/American Heart Association adopted a stage-based system for the classification of HF in 2001 with revisions in 2022 (Table 26–2). In this approach, stage A or those "at risk" for HF included patients without structural cardiac disorders or HF symptoms, but with risk factors that clearly predispose carriers toward the development of HF (eg, hypertension, coronary artery disease, diabetes). Stage B or those with "pre-HF" included patients without HF symptoms, but with structural cardiac abnormalities (eg, left ventricular hypertrophy, prior myocardial infarction, valvular heart disease), increased filling pressures, or risk factors with additional elevation in natriuretic peptide levels or elevated troponin without another identifiable cause. Stages C and D included the symptomatic HF patients. This classification added a useful dimension to the understanding of HF by recognizing that there are established risk factors and structural prerequisites for the development of the clinical syndrome and that therapeutic interventions performed even before the appearance of left ventricular dysfunction or symptoms can prevent the development of HF.

Because nearly 33% of adults in the United States have hypertension and due to the high attributable risk of hypertension in HF in both men and women, aggressive control of blood pressure is the most effective approach to reduce the incidence of HF. Primary prevention trials have shown up to a 50% reduction in the incidence of HF in patients with hypertension who are treated with thiazide diuretics, ACE inhibitors, angiotensin II receptor blockers (ARBs), and most β-blockers and calcium channel blockers.

The roles of coronary artery disease and myocardial infarction as major antecedents of systolic HF have been well established. Therapy with ACE inhibitors has been shown to reduce the risk of developing HF in patients with stable coronary artery disease, while therapy with ACE inhibitors, ARBs, β-blockers, and mineralocorticoid receptor antagonists (MRAs) have been shown in several randomized trials to reduce the risk of progression to symptomatic HF in patients with myocardial infarction and asymptomatic left ventricular systolic dysfunction.

Diabetes mellitus has been consistently associated with a two- to fivefold increase in the risk of HF, especially in women. Several studies have shown an 8–16% increase in the risk of hospitalizations for HF for every 1% increase in hemoglobin A1c. Outside of the use of sodium/glucose cotransporter-2 (SGLT2) inhibitors in patients with type 2 diabetes, the optimal treatment strategy (eg, insulin versus metformin versus sulfonylureas versus thiazolidinediones) is currently unknown.

Given the high burden of HF risk factors present in the population, multiple risk prediction models have been developed to forecast incidence in various populations. Most of these risk prediction scores incorporate traditional cardiovascular risk factors with the addition of variables easily accessible during an outpatient visit. This includes demographic data, lab findings, echocardiogram and electrocardiogram features, clinical measurements, etc. These scoring systems were developed from specific study subgroups including those with and without cardiovascular disease at baseline with various racial/ethnic and sex makeup. For example, some include the Multi-Ethnic Study of Atherosclerosis (MESA), The Framingham Study, The Health Aging and Body Composition Study, the Prevention of Renal and Vascular End-Stage Disease (PREVEND), and the Atherosclerosis Risk and Communities (ARIC) study. To address generalizability, some of these risk prediction scoring systems have been externally validated by separate cohorts and have proved to be useful in identifying those at high risk. Given the new data surrounding the utility of SGLT2 inhibitors in HF, specific risk models have been created to predict incident HF in individuals with type 2 diabetes with similar external validation measures.

In the 2022 ACC/AHA/HFSA Guidelines on HF, a new recommendation suggested screening patients at risk of developing HF using natriuretic peptide biomarkers. This was based on the results from the STOP-HF study, which showed a reduction in systolic dysfunction and clinical HF in individuals with BNP greater than 50 pg/mL who were followed with an echocardiogram and managed by a multidisciplinary team. Further research is needed on how to integrate this into widespread practice and what individuals would benefit most from screening.

B. Nonpharmacologic Treatment

1. Dietary measures—Given the possibility that increased sodium intake leads to increased fluid retention in HF, it has been assumed that a low-sodium diet would improve outcomes in HF patients. However, the data on which these recommendations are drawn are limited, and the few clinical trials conducted to date have produced inconsistent findings. The 2012 American Heart Association recommendations for 1500 mg/day of sodium for patients with stage A and B were not altered, likely due to a lack of new data surrounding sodium intake with incidence of hypertension and HF. Recent data from the SODIUM-HF trial found that sodium restriction to under 100 mmol (< 1500 mg/day) in ambulatory HF patients with New York Heart Association (NYHA) functional class, 2–3 symptoms did not reduce cardiovascular-related admission to hospital (including Emergency Department visits) or all-cause mortality within 1 year. Furthermore, the GOURMET-HF trial randomized posthospital discharge HF patients to receive 4 weeks of low sodium (< 1500 mg/day) meals and found no significant differences in 30-day readmission rates. Recommendations for fluid restriction in HF remain largely driven by individual practitioner's clinical experience. Most recent recommendations for fluid restriction are 1.5–2 L/day in patients with HF and stage D symptoms.

2. Physical activity and exercise training—For decades, exercise testing and exercise training were considered dangerous in patients with HFrEF because of concerns about exacerbating HF symptoms, potential deleterious effects on ventricular function, and the possibility of severe ventricular arrhythmias and cardiac arrest. Recent work has shown that exercise training in these patients is associated with improved response to pharmacologic vasodilators, improved endothelial function, improved skeletal muscle metabolism and performance, and attenuation of the activation of the overactive muscle ergoreflexes. The large, randomized trial, Heart Failure: A Controlled Trial Investigating Outcomes of Exercise Training (HF-ACTION), showed that in patients with symptomatic systolic HF exercise training was safe (no increase in arrhythmias over usual care) and was associated with a significant decrease in hospitalizations for HF and an improvement in the patients' well-being and in exercise capacity. A recent meta-analysis evaluating the dose-response relationship between physical activity and HF found an inverse, dose-response relationship between physical activity and HF risk with substantial risk reduction in individuals who engaged in physical activity at twice and four times the minimum guideline-recommended levels (ie, 1000 or 2000 MET-min/week). Thus, all patients with HFrEF should be prescribed an exercise-training program in addition to evidence-based pharmacologic therapy. In response to the above data, Center for Medicare and Medicaid Services (CMS) expanded their indications for cardiac rehabilitation in 2014 to include those with HF and an ejection fraction of 35% or less on maximal medical therapy for at least 6 weeks.

3. Treatment of sleep-disordered breathing—Sleep-disordered breathing is common in HFrEF patients, with reported prevalence rates of 50–75% and is associated with poor prognosis. Episodes of apnea and hypopnea during sleep are associated with intermittent hypoxemia and increased sympathetic nervous system activity; therefore, treatments that suppress these have been investigated in patients with HF. Early studies showed improvement in symptoms and ejection fraction with the use of continuous positive airway pressure (CPAP) in obstructive sleep apnea in patients with HF. The recent Treatment of Sleep-Disordered Breathing with Predominant Central Sleep Apnea by Adaptive Servo Ventilation in Patients with Heart Failure (SERVE-HF) showed unexpectedly higher all-cause and cardiovascular mortality in HF patients with central sleep apnea treated with adaptive servo-ventilation (ASV). At present, therapy with CPAP, but not ASV can be recommended for patients with HF and obstructive sleep apnea. A novel approach to central sleep apnea treatment includes transvenous unilateral phrenic nerve stimulation, where its activation normalizes breathing movements of the diaphragm during sleep. This is thought to disrupt the detrimental pattern of Cheyne-Stokes breathing, common in HFrEF patients. Implementation of this nerve stimulation is thought to lead to a reduction of hypercarbia and hypoxemia, arrythmias, decreased activation of the sympathetic nervous system, and normalization of pressures in the systemic and pulmonary vasculature. Preliminary studies have shown its effectiveness in treating central sleep apnea, with an increase in left ventricular ejection fraction, and improvement in HF symptoms. Further research is needed to assess clinical outcomes and possible mortality benefits.

Costanzo MR, Ponikowski P, Coats, et al.; remedē® System Pivotal Trial Study Group. Phrenic nerve stimulation to treat patients with central sleep apnoea and heart failure. *Eur J Heart Fail.* 2018;20(12):1746–1754. [PMID: 30303611]

Cowie MR, Woehrle H, Wegscheider K, et al. Adaptive servo-ventilation for central sleep apnea in systolic heart failure. *N Engl J Med.* 2015;373:1095–1105. [PMID: 26323938]

Ezekowitz JA, Ramirez EC, Ross H, et al. Reduction of dietary sodium to less than 100 mmol in heart failure (SODIUM-HF): an international, open-label, randomised, controlled trial. *Lancet.* 2022;399:1391–1400. [PMID: 35381194]

C. Pharmacologic Treatment: Life-Saving Therapies

The pharmacologic treatment of symptomatic HFrEF has evolved substantially in the past 40 years, with neurohormonal antagonists becoming the mainstay of treatment due to marked improvements in morbidity and mortality.

1. ACE inhibitors—Inhibition of ACE in HF results in an increase in the cardiac output, with concomitant decrease in ventricular filling pressures and pulmonary and systemic vascular resistances, without an increase in the heart rate. Over time, ACE inhibition leads to a decrease in left ventricular end-systolic and end-diastolic dimensions, a reduction in the incidence of ventricular arrhythmias, and continuous and sustained improvements in symptoms (occurring as early as 2 weeks), exercise duration, and quality of life. The most significant benefit of therapy with ACE inhibitors is the 20% increase in survival seen in all patients with HFrEF and in all patients with left ventricular systolic dysfunction after myocardial infarction, even in those without symptoms or signs of HF.

ACE inhibitors should be used in conjunction with β-blockers, MRAs and SGLT2 inhibitors as part of the "quadruple therapy" to achieve the maximal symptomatic improvement and survival benefit, and with a diuretic (as needed) to maintain the sodium balance and prevent the development of fluid overload. The highest tolerated ACE inhibitor dose should be achieved, as clinical trials have shown improved HF outcomes at higher doses. Once the drug has been titrated to achieve blood pressures less than 130/80 (Table 26–3), patients can usually be maintained on long-term therapy with little difficulty. The need to decrease the ACE inhibitor dose due to hypotension and/or renal dysfunction may signal the development of end-stage HF and the need for advanced therapies (ie, ventricular assist devices, heart transplantation). Renal function and serum potassium should be assessed within 2 weeks of initiating therapy and every 3 months thereafter.

The main adverse effects of the therapy are related to the angiotensin suppression (hypotension, increase in serum creatinine and potassium) and bradykinin potentiation (cough and angioedema). The initial hypotension responds to a decrease in the dose of diuretic, liberalization of salt intake, or initiation of a lower dose of ACE inhibitor. Hypotension can be delayed and prolonged with longer-acting ACE inhibitors (enalapril and lisinopril), leading to decreased systemic perfusion and compromise of renal and cerebral functions, but is shorter in duration with captopril, which rarely compromises organ perfusion. Some patients may be very sensitive to the hypotensive effects of ACE inhibitors, particularly end-stage HF patients who are dependent on the RAAS for blood pressure maintenance. In general, treatment should be reassessed if serum creatinine increases above 3 mg/dL or if serum potassium increases above 5.5 mEq/L. Patients should not be given ACE inhibitors if they are pregnant, have a history of angioedema or anuric renal failure during a previous exposure to this class, or are severely hypotensive and at risk of immediate cardiogenic shock.

2. ARBs—These agents block the angiotensin II receptor and inhibit the effects of angiotensin II produced not only through the classical ACE pathway, but also by the chymase pathway. Available ARBs block the angiotensin II type 1 receptors (associated with myocardial hypertrophy and remodeling) and enhance the activation of angiotensin II type 2 receptors, causing vasodilation. In addition, these effects are achieved without the accumulation of bradykinin, which is considered to be responsible for some of the adverse reactions associated with the use of ACE inhibitors, such as cough or angioedema. Although the hemodynamic effects of ARBs are similar to those of ACE inhibitors, the randomized clinical trials have shown a consistent mortality benefit only in patients with HFrEF who are intolerant of ACE inhibitors. Candesartan was the only ARB that showed in clinical trials a 15% reduction in mortality when added to an ACE inhibitor. Use of ARBs in higher doses (see Table 26–3) in addition to ACE inhibitors and β-blockers is associated with symptomatic improvement and an overall modest 15% reduction in HF hospitalizations.

3. Angiotensin Receptor Neprilysin Inhibitors (ARNIs)—A treatment that combines an ARB (ie, valsartan) with a neprylisin inhibitor (ie, sacubitril) and therefore enhances the availability of natriuretic peptides, has been shown to be superior to ACE inhibitors in improving survival and decreasing the HF hospitalization rates in patients with HFrEF.

Table 26–3. Target Doses of Renin–Angiotensin–Aldosterone System Inhibitors in Heart Failure

Agent	Starting Dose (mg)	Target Dose (mg)	Frequency	Trial(s)
ACE inhibitors				
Captopril	6.25	50	Three times daily	SAVE
Enalapril	5	10	Twice daily	SOLVD P/T
Fosinopril	10	40	Daily	FEST
Lisinopril	2.5	40	Daily	ATLAS
Ramipril	2.5	5	Twice daily	AIRE
Trandolapril	1	4	Daily	TRACE
ARBs				
Candesartan	4	32	Daily	CHARM
Losartan	25	150	Daily	HEAAL
Valsartan	40	160	Twice daily	VALHEFT
MRAs				
Eplerenone	12.5	50	Daily	EMPHASIS-HF, EPHESUS
Spironolactone	25	25	Daily	RALES
ARNIs				
Sacubitril/valsartan	24/ 26	97/ 103	Twice daily	PARADIGM-HF, PIONEER-HF

ACE, angiotensin-converting enzyme; AIRE, Acute Infarction Ramipril Efficacy; ARB, angiotensin II receptor blocker; ARNI, angiotensin II receptor blocker–neprilysin inhibitor; ATLAS, Assessment of Treatment with Lisinopril and Survival; CHARM, Candesartan in Heart failure: Assessment of Reduction in Mortality and Morbidity; EMPHASIS-HF, Eplerenone in Mild Patients Hospitalization and Survival Study in Heart Failure; EPHESUS, Eplerenone Postacute Myocardial Infarction Heart Failure Efficacy and Survival; FEST, Fosinopril Efficacy/Safety Trial; HEAAL, Heart Failure End-point Evaluation of Angiotensin II Antagonists Losartan; MRA, mineralocorticoid receptor antagonist; PARADIGM-HF, Prospective comparison of ARNI with ACE inhibitor to Determine Impact on Global Mortality and morbidity in Heart Failure trial; PIONEER-HF, Comparison of Sacubitril/Valsartan Versus Enalapril on Effect on NT-proBNP [N-terminal pro-B type natriuretic peptide] in Patients Stabilized From an Acute HF Episode Trial; RALES, Randomized Aldactone Evaluation Study; SAVE, Survival and Ventricular Enlargement Trial; SOLVD P/T, Studies of Left Ventricular Dysfunction Prevention/Treatment; TRACE, Trandolapril Cardiac Evaluation; VALHEFT, Valsartan Heart Failure Trial.

The sacubitril/valsartan combination is indicated for patients with HFrEF that have NYHA functional class II-IV symptoms, in place of ACE inhibitors or ARBs, in conjunction with other HF therapies. Patients transitioned from ACE inhibitors to ARNIs should do that gradually, with a washout period of 36 hours, and with a stepwise increase in dose, to avoid the significant hypotension associated with the ARNI. Occasionally, it is necessary to decrease or stop the diuretic therapy in HFrEF patients at the time of ARNI initiation, to ensure adequate blood pressure. The PIONEER-HF study demonstrated that it was both safe and effective to initiate sacubitril-valsartan at the time of an acute HF hospitalization in those with HFrEF after initial hemodynamic stabilization. The benefits appeared as soon as 1 week after administration, and adverse event rates did not differ compared to those randomized to receive enalapril. Like ACE inhibitors and ARBs, this medication should be titrated to a blood pressure less than 130/80 mm Hg (Table 26-3). The sacubitril/valsartan combination is contraindicated in patients with a history of ACE inhibitors/ARBs-induced angioedema.

4. MRAs—Despite treatment with ACE inhibitors, ARBs or ARNIs, patients with HF demonstrate elevated aldosterone levels, due to alternative stimuli for aldosterone synthesis (eg, adrenocorticotropic hormone or endothelin), potassium-dependent aldosterone secretion, and reduced aldosterone clearance. Spironolactone is a competitive renal aldosterone antagonist, inhibiting its effect by competing for the aldosterone-dependent sodium–potassium exchange site in the distal tubule cells. Eplerenone is a selective MRA that prevents the binding of aldosterone and is devoid of the painful gynecomastia seen in about 10% of men taking spironolactone. Multiple clinical trials have shown that the use of MRAs in addition to ACE inhibitors and β-blockers in patients with HFrEF and NYHA functional class II-IV leads to a 15–30% decrease in mortality (including a 20% decrease in sudden cardiac death immediately after a myocardial infarction), improvement in HF symptoms, and a 30–40% decrease in hospitalizations for HF. Due to these significant benefits in a variety of HFrEF patients, MRAs should be the drugs of choice in the initial quadruple therapy with ARNIs, β-blockers, and SGLT2 inhibitors (See Table 26–3). The use of MRAs should be restricted to those patients with an estimated glomerular filtration rate above 30 mL/min/1.73 m^2 and with serum potassium below 5 mEq/L; potassium levels should be monitored within a week of initiation and at least every 4 weeks for the first 3 months and every 3 months thereafter. Although low, the risk of hyperkalemia is real with these agents and can lead to a significant increase in morbidity and mortality.

5. β-Adrenergic receptor blockers—β-Blockers act by inhibiting the adverse effects of the sympathetic nervous system activation in patients with HFrEF. Long-term benefits of β-blockade include an increase in ejection fraction, a decrease in left ventricular volumes and in mitral regurgitation, and a reversion of the left ventricle to a more elliptical shape. Administration of β-blockers is associated with an early deterioration in cardiac function (consistent with the negative inotropic effects), followed by return to baseline values after 1 month and an increase in the ejection fraction after 3 months of treatment with further improvement for up to a year. Although the exercise capacity may not be improved by objective assessments (CPET), β-blockers, when added to ACE inhibitors, lead to marked symptomatic improvement, translated in robust 18% decreases in hospitalizations for HF and 35% improvement in survival. Only three β-blockers (bisoprolol, carvedilol, and metoprolol succinate) have been consistently shown to improve symptoms and survival in clinical trials, and therefore, only these should be used in patients with HFrEF. As in the case of ACE inhibitors, use of the highest tolerated β-blocker doses is recommended due to improvement in outcomes. In direct comparison studies, carvedilol was associated with better survival than metoprolol tartrate; in addition, the incidences of myocardial infarction, stroke, atrial fibrillation, and diabetes were lower with the use of carvedilol. In patients with reactive airway disease, bisoprolol has been shown to improve the peak expiratory flow and be better tolerated compared to the other approved β-blockers.

β-Blockers should be prescribed to all patients with asymptomatic left ventricular systolic dysfunction and stable HFrEF unless they have a contraindication. Patients should be clinically stable, receive ARNIs, MRAs, and SGLT2 inhibitors, and receive diuretics as needed to control the fluid retention associated with adrenergic blockade. β-Blockers should be initiated at very low doses (in euvolemic, noninotrope-dependent patients) and increased gradually, typically at 2-week intervals, to achieve the target doses from published clinical trials (Table 26–4).

Treatment with β-blockers can be associated with fatigue and weakness, which usually resolve in a few weeks. Symptomatic bradycardia is a serious adverse effect that requires a decrease in the dose or sometimes cardiac pacing. Hypotension is a side effect seen especially with nonselective blockers such as carvedilol. Usually, it occurs within the first 48 hours of initiation of therapy and subsides with repeated dosing without any change in the dose. Administration of ARNIs and diuretics at a different time of day than the β-blockers can minimize the hypotension and dizziness. Administration of β-blockers is contraindicated in patients with severe bronchospasm, systolic blood pressure below 85 mm Hg, symptomatic bradycardia, or advanced heart block in the absence of a pacemaker.

6. SGLT2 inhibitors—The exact mechanism of benefit of SGLT2 inhibitors in treating HFrEF is unknown; however, basic experimental and clinical studies have pointed to SGLT2 inhibition-related pathways that coincide with HFrEF pathogenesis. It is thought that SGLT2 inhibitors act through three main mechanisms regarding HF. The first is by alternating signaling pathways via upregulation of SIRT1 which reduces oxidative stress. This dampens proinflammatory processes and mitigates maladaptive remodeling. Secondly, this drug class alters the action of the Na-H exchange pump in the heart and kidneys, which could

Table 26–4. Target Doses of β-Blockers in Heart Failure

Agent	Starting Dose (mg)	Target Dose (mg)	Frequency	Trial(s)
Bisoprolol	2.5	10	Daily	CIBIS I, II, III
Carvedilol	3.125	25	Twice daily	CAPRICORN, COPERNICUS, U.S. carvedilol trials
Metoprolol succinate	25	200	Daily	MERIT-HF
Nebivolol[1]	1.25	10	Daily	SENIORS

[1]Approved for use for patients with heart failure and reduced ejection fraction in Europe only.
CAPRICORN, Carvedilol Post-Infarct Survival Control in Left Ventricular Dysfunction; CIBIS, Cardiac Insufficiency Bisoprolol Study; COPERNICUS, Carvedilol Prospective Randomized Cumulative Survival; MERIT-HF, Metoprolol CR/XL Randomised Intervention Trial in Congestive Heart Failure; SENIORS, Study of the Effects of Nebivolol Intervention on Outcomes and Rehospitalisation in Seniors with Heart Failure.

possibly lessen myocyte damage. The third mechanism centers on the reduction of epicardial adipose tissue, with the potential benefit of mitigating the proinflammatory processes and subsequent maladaptive cardiac remodeling. Use of SGLT2 inhibitors reduces incidence of HF in those with type 2 diabetes, reduces mortality in those with HFrEF regardless of whether they have diabetes, and reduces the risk of worsening HF and HF admissions in individuals with or without diabetes. These medications should be prescribed to all patients with HFrEF given their significant mortality benefit and are considered a pillar of quadruple therapy. The adverse effects are mainly related to hypovolemia from diuresis, and rarely complications involving genital mycotic infections. This class of medication should be avoided in patients with severe kidney disease with an estimated glomerular filtration rate below 30 mL/min/1.73 m^2, and type 1 diabetes given its increased risk of diabetic ketoacidosis with normal glucose levels.

7. Hydralazine-nitrates combination—Nitrates have a greater effect on venous capacitance (venodilation) than on the arterial system, while hydralazine is a direct-acting smooth muscle relaxant that seems to dilate arterioles predominantly. Long-term administration of isosorbide dinitrate has been associated with significant improvements in hemodynamic parameters, exercise capacity, and relief of symptoms in moderate-to-severe HFrEF. When used in combination with nitrates, hydralazine has shown a short-term increase in cardiac output and a decrease in ventricular filling pressure. Patients who have dilated left ventricles appear to have a better hemodynamic and clinical response than do patients with lesser degrees of enlargement. The combination therapy was tested in African Americans with HFrEF in the African-American Heart Failure Trial (A-HeFT) and was associated with a significant 43% improvement in survival and a 33% decrease in HF hospitalizations, when used in addition to ACE inhibitors, β-blockers, and spironolactone. These results led to the first approval of a combination drug pill based on self-identified ethnicity. When the endothelial nitric oxide synthase (through which the combination of drugs is thought to work) was genotyped, the benefits of the therapy were evident only in those patients who were homozygous for glutamic acid in position 298 (GLU298GLU). Although 80% of African Americans have this genomic variant (as shown in A-HeFT), studies have shown that up to 40% of Caucasians have the same genotype, leading to intriguing possibilities for future pharmacogenomically targeted therapies. Unfortunately, the therapy is not easily tolerated due to side effects. Nitrates can produce headaches, while hydralazine can be associated with flushing, palpitations, nausea, vomiting, myocardial ischemia, and lupus-like syndrome.

It is paramount that the quadruple guideline-directed medical therapy (GDMT) with ARNIs, β-blockers, MRAs, and SGLT2 inhibitors be started simultaneously in patients with HFrEF. These drugs have additive beneficial effects with results seen within a few weeks of initiation. The side effect profile (eg, fatigue, lowering blood pressure, hyperkalemia) is tolerable and manageable with close monitoring (phone/clinic encounters, blood tests). The simultaneous initiation of GDMT also ensures that the patients are not lost to follow-up and that the full benefit is realized within a few months.

It is important to continue the GDMT even if patients have recovered their ejection fraction. "Recovered" is defined by ejection fractions that were below 40% and have improved above 50% with normalized NT pro-BNP levels, and who are asymptomatic (NYHA functional class I). In the TRED-HF study, patients with HFrEF and dilated cardiomyopathy were observed discontinuing GDMT after initial recovery. The results showed that in just 2 months, patients had developed clinical HF symptoms, a drop in their left ventricular ejection fraction below 50%, and a doubling of their NT-proBNP. As such, patients should be continued on GDMT indefinitely.

Halliday BP, Wassall R, Lota AS, et al. Withdrawal of pharmacological treatment for heart failure in patients with recovered dilated cardiomyopathy (TRED-HF): an open-label, pilot, randomised trial. *Lancet.* 2019;393:61–73. [PMID: 30429050]

McMurray JJV, Solomon SD, Inzucchi SE, et al. DAPA-HF Trial Committees and Investigators. Dapagliflozin in patients with heart failure and reduced ejection fraction. *N Engl J Med.* 2019;381:1995–2008. [PMID: 31535829]

Velazquez EJ, Morrow DA, DeVore AD, et al. PIONEER-HF Investigators. Angiotensin-neprilysin inhibition in acute decompensated heart failure. *N Engl J Med.* 2019;380:539–548. [PMID: 30415601]

D. Pharmacologic Treatment: Symptomatic Therapies

1. Diuretics and aquaretics—Diuretics provide rapid symptomatic relief of congestive symptoms by promoting excretion of sodium and water and lowering plasma volume, thus reducing congestion in the pulmonary and systemic vascular beds and improving symptoms and functional capacity. Diuretics are tightly bound to plasma proteins and are actively secreted into the proximal tubular lumen. Loop diuretics inhibit the sodium/potassium/chloride symporter in the ascending loop of Henle; thiazide-type diuretics affect the sodium/chloride transporter in the distal convoluted tubules; whereas potassium-sparing diuretics work at sites in the collecting duct to inhibit the sodium/potassium transporter.

Loop diuretics increase sodium excretion by 20–25% and enhance free water clearance. Because the plasma half-life of loop diuretics ranges from 1 to 4 hours, once a dose of a loop diuretic has been administered, its effect dissipates before the next dose is given. During this time, the nephron avidly reabsorbs sodium, resulting in rebound sodium retention that nullifies the prior natriuresis. To counteract this, loop diuretics must be given twice daily. Orally dosed furosemide has variable bioavailability (10–100% in patients with HF), whereas bumetanide and torsemide are absorbed more completely, with 80% bioavailability after oral dosing. Currently, there are no data regarding the superiority of any one loop diuretic over another. The TRANSFORM-HF randomized clinical trial is ongoing and is designed to compare outpatient use of furosemide versus torsemide in patients recently hospitalized with HFrEF with a primary endpoint of all-cause mortality.

Thiazides and distal tubule diuretics have longer half-lives that allow them to be given once daily or even every other day. Although thiazide diuretics have a bioavailability of 60–70%, their action is limited if the glomerular filtration falls below 40 mL/min/1.73m^2 (except for chlorothiazide and metolazone). Furosemide and thiazides are renally excreted, whereas the liver metabolizes torsemide and bumetanide.

Diuretics should be used in all patients with evidence of volume overload; in an acutely decompensated state, a higher dose of oral diuretics or intravenous diuretics (starting with twice the home dose) or a combination of loop and thiazide diuretics is needed to achieve euvolemia. Use of inappropriately high doses of diuretics leads to volume contraction and increased risk of hypotension and renal insufficiency with ARNIs. Diuretic resistance can be overcome by the intravenous administration of diuretics (intermittent bolus or continuous infusions have the same efficacy), the use of diuretic combinations (eg, loop and thiazide), or the use of intravenous diuretics with low-dose dopamine. Volume depletion (resulting in hypotension and/or renal failure), hypokalemia, hypomagnesemia, and thiamine deficiency are the most common side effects of diuretics. Diuretics may also cause metabolic alkalosis, carbohydrate intolerance, hyperuricemia, hypersensitivity reactions, and acute pancreatitis.

Tolvaptan is a vasopressin V2 receptor antagonist that selectively blocks the binding of vasopressin to the V2 receptors in the renal collecting ducts, leading to decreased expression and removal of aquaporin-2 from the luminal membrane, resulting in decreased water reabsorption by the kidney. Tolvaptan produces aquaresis, rather than diuresis since it promotes excretion of water without electrolyte loss. As a result, tolvaptan leads to increased serum sodium concentration, correction of hyponatremia, and decreased urine osmolality. Tolvaptan has been shown to improve dyspnea and reduce body weight and edema in patients hospitalized with HFrEF and hyponatremia (serum sodium < 134 mEq/L)

2. Ivabradine—Ivabradine is a specific inhibitor of the I_f current in the sinoatrial node, and, unlike β-blockers, it does not modify myocardial contractility and intracardiac conduction, even in patients with impaired systolic function. The Ivabradine in Stable Heart Failure (SHIFT) trial showed a decrease in mortality and hospital admissions due to HF with ivabradine. However, the drug loses efficacy in patients using more than 50% target doses of β-blockers. In the current ACC/AHA/HFSA Clinical Guidelines for HF, recommendations were changed to reflect that ivabradine can be effective in patients who are on GDMT with β-blockers at the maximum tolerated dose and a heart rate of 70 or greater in sinus rhythm. Full titration of β-blockers remains preferable to initiation of ivabradine given β-blockers' robust survival benefits.

3. Digoxin—Digoxin exerts its effects by inhibiting sodium-potassium adenosine triphosphatase in the myocardium (resulting in an increase in myocardial contraction), in the vagal afferent fibers (sensitizing the cardiac baroreceptors and reducing the sympathetic outflow), and in the kidney (reducing the renal tubular reabsorption of sodium). These observations have led to the hypothesis that the beneficial effects of digoxin in HF are due to the attenuation of the activation of neurohormonal systems. Clinically, the beneficial effects in patients with HFrEF and sinus rhythm include improved HF symptoms, increased exercise time, modestly increased ejection fraction, enhanced cardiac output, and decreased HF hospitalizations. The benefits of digoxin are higher in patients with more symptomatic HF (NYHA functional class IV), cardiomegaly (greater cardiothoracic ratio on chest x-ray), or an ejection fraction below 25%. However, due to its narrow therapeutic index, digoxin has a bidirectional effect with improvement in HF mortality and increase in the non-HF (presumed arrhythmic) mortality. Retrospective analyses of the Digitalis Investigation Group (DIG) trial have suggested an increased mortality with serum concentration above 1 ng/mL, especially in women. Due to these considerations, digoxin has been reserved in HFrEF patients in sinus rhythm who are still symptomatic despite quadruple GDMT. In patients with HFrEF and atrial fibrillation, digoxin can be used to decrease the ventricular response, usually associated with improved symptoms. Although rarer than in prior decades, digitalis intoxication may occur in patients hospitalized for HF. Common findings are nausea, vomiting, anorexia, malaise, drowsiness, headache, insomnia, altered color vision, or arrhythmia. Cardiac arrhythmias (most commonly premature ventricular beats, junctional tachycardia, paroxysmal atrial tachycardia with block, bidirectional ventricular tachycardia) can be caused by digitalis and are facilitated by hypokalemia. Digoxin toxicity is usually confirmed by the reversal of symptoms or cessation of arrhythmias after withdrawal of digoxin therapy. Severe toxicity can be reversed quickly with digoxin immune Fab.

4. Soluble Guanylate Cyclase (sGC) stimulators—The mechanism of vericiguat, an oral sGC stimulator, is to increase activity of the cGMP pathway independent of nitric oxide. In HF, reactive oxygen species are pathologically high, which work to decrease concentrations of nitric oxide. Vericiguat has been shown to increase cardiac output and decrease systemic vascular resistance. In the Vericiguat Global Study in Subjects with Heart Failure with Reduced Ejection Fraction (VICTORIA) trial, vericiguat modestly reduced the combined end point of cardiovascular death or

HF hospitalizations compared to placebo. No differences on mortality alone were observed. This medication should be avoided in patients who have severe refractory anemia or are currently taking other nitrates, as adverse effects common to these medications (headache, syncope, hypotension, gastrointestinal distress, etc.) can be compounded. Current clinical practice guidelines reserve this drug to a limited number of patients who are still symptomatic despite quadruple GDMT and are at high risk for HF hospitalizations. Its exact role in the future of HF therapies is unknown, and further research is needed on what type of HF patients it may benefit the most.

Armstrong PW, Pieske B, Anstrom KJ, et al. VICTORIA Study Group. Vericiguat in patients with heart failure and reduced ejection fraction. *N Engl J Med*. 2020;382:1883–1893. [PMID: 32222134]
Felker GM, Ellison DH, Mullens W, Cox ZL, Testani JM. Diuretic therapy for patients with heart failure: JACC State-of-the-Art Review. *J Am Coll Cardiol*. 2020;75:1178–1195. [PMID: 32164892]
Greene SJ, Velazquez, Anstrom KJ, et al. Pragmatic design of randomized clinical trials for heart failure: rationale and design of the TRANSFORM-HF Trial. *JACC Heart Fail*. 2021;9:325–335. [PMID: 33714745]

E. Pharmacologic Treatment: Other Therapies

1. Antiarrhythmic agents—More than 80% of HFrEF patients have frequent and complex ventricular arrhythmias as documented by Holter monitoring, and 50% have frequent nonsustained ventricular tachycardia. In addition, 35–40% of patients have paroxysmal or persistent atrial fibrillation that can lead to HF exacerbation. Patients with HFrEF frequently require some antiarrhythmic drugs to stabilize these arrhythmias. Due to the structural heart disease seen in HF, only some of the class III anti-arrhythmic drugs (ie, dofetilide and amiodarone) are safe to use.

Although clinical trials have shown that amiodarone per se does not improve prognosis in HFrEF patients, they have also shown that it is a rather safe option. It can be administered acutely to control ventricular response in HF patients with atrial fibrillation, and its long-term use may restore and maintain sinus rhythm. Amiodarone may also be used to suppress symptomatic ventricular tachycardia in combination with β-blockers, especially in patients who are receiving frequent defibrillator shocks. Close monitoring for the myriad of side effects is required.

Dofetilide was shown to be effective in restoring sinus rhythm in patients with HFrEF and atrial fibrillation without adverse effects on overall survival. Treatment with dofetilide also decreased the overall HF hospitalizations in the Danish Investigations of Arrhythmia and Mortality on Dofetilide (DIAMOND) study. However, dofetilide dosing must be closely titrated, based on creatinine clearance and QT interval, requiring 72-hour inpatient monitoring. Dronedarone is a benzofuran-derivative class III antiarrhythmic drug with pharmacologic properties like amiodarone and should not be used in patients with HFrEF due to the increased mortality risk associated with the drug.

2. Antithrombotic therapy—In patients with HFrEF and sinus rhythm, antithrombotic therapy has traditionally been considered for those with very low ejection fraction. However, a multitude of clinical trials have failed to show a clear benefit of this strategy in preventing strokes in these patients. A post-hoc analysis of the COMMANDER-HF trial examined whether rivaroxaban was associated with a significant reduction in thromboembolic events in patients with coronary disease and worsening HF. When excluding sudden and or unwitnessed deaths from its composite score of thromboembolic events, no difference was observed compared to placebo. As such, the decision to use an antiplatelet or anticoagulant must be individualized, considering the comorbidities of the patient (eg, presence of concomitant coronary artery disease or peripheral vascular disease). All patients with systolic HF and atrial fibrillation (even paroxysmal) should be anticoagulated with direct anticoagulants (preferred over warfarin) to prevent strokes.

3. Statins (3-hydroxy-3-methyl-glutaryl–coenzyme A reductase inhibitors)—Statins are the cornerstone of primary and secondary prevention for patients with coronary artery disease or vascular disease. Paradoxically, even though 70% of HFrEF patients have coronary artery disease, the role of statins in HFrEF is only marginal. Two large randomized clinical trials testing the role of rosuvastatin in this setting failed to show a benefit on mortality. Patients with underlying coronary artery disease experienced a reduction in cardiovascular hospitalizations, presumably by averting small myocardial infarctions due to plaque destabilization. As such, statins should only be used in patients with HFrEF and clinical coronary artery disease.

4. Omega-3 polyunsaturated fatty acids—The use of omega-3 polyunsaturated acids in HFrEF patients leads to small improvements in left ventricular ejection fraction, reduction in left ventricular end systolic volumes and functional capacity, and a small 10% decrease in cardiovascular mortality and 7% decrease in risk for cardiovascular hospitalizations. The dose used in clinical trials of 1 g (850–882 mg eicosapentaenoic acid and docosahexaenoic acid as ethyl esters in the average ratio of 1:1.2) is much smaller than the dose used to treat hypertriglyceridemia and, therefore, more likely to be tolerated by patients.

5. Intravenous iron therapy—Iron deficiency is quite frequent in patients with HFrEF, and several studies have shown improvements in symptoms, exercise capacity, and quality of life with intravenous ferric carboxymaltose. In the AFFIRM-HF study, iron-deficient patients with ejection fractions less than 50% who were repleted with ferric carboxymaltose after a HF hospitalization had fewer HF hospitalizations and a reduction in time to first HF hospitalization or cardiovascular death. Intravenous iron therapy (there are several preparations available) is relatively safe and should be used for all patients with HFrEF who are iron deficient even in the absence of anemia (ferritin level < 100 mcg/L or 100–299 mcg/L if the transferrin saturation is < 20%).

Although anemia is common and portends poor prognosis in HFrEF, treatment with **darbepoetin** was not associated with improved survival or decrease in hospitalization in these patients. Moreover, patients treated with darbepoetin experience more thromboembolic events, and thus, the erythropoiesis-simulating agents should not be used or should be used very cautiously in HFrEF patients. In patients with decompensated HF and hemoglobin level < 10 g/dL, careful transfusion with packed red blood cells, while giving diuretics, has been shown to improve outcomes.

6. Myotropes—Omecamtiv mecarbil is a selective cardiac myosin activator and works as an inotrope by increasing the available number of myosin heads that can bind to actin filaments, thus augmenting sarcomere function by increasing the force of the power stroke during cardiac contraction. In phase 2 studies, this drug has been shown to increase stroke volume, decrease heart rate, and lengthen systolic ejection time. The GALACTIC-HF trial examined outcomes on both inpatient and outpatient participants with a diagnosis of HFrEF at or less than 35%. Results showed a small reduction in the composite of HF-related hospitalizations or cardiovascular death, with no benefits on survival of more than 24 weeks. In a predetermined subgroup analysis, treatment benefit had its greatest effect in patients with lower ejection fractions and blood pressures. No differences in adverse effects were observed compared to placebo, including hypotension, kidney injury, and ischemic or ventricular arrhythmic events. Given that this drug does not significantly alter blood pressure, this therapy could theoretically be useful in GDMT titration that is limited in patients with symptomatic hypotension. However, further research is needed on the role this medication will take in the current HFrEF therapeutics landscape.

Greenberg B, Neaton JD, Anker SD, et al. Association of rivaroxaban with thromboembolic events in patients with heart failure, coronary disease, and sinus rhythm: a post hoc analysis of the COMMANDER HF Trial. *JAMA Cardiol.* 2019;4:515–523. [PMID: 31017637]

Ponikowski P. AFFIRM-AHF investigators. Ferric carboxymaltose for iron deficiency at discharge after acute heart failure: a multicentre, double-blind, randomised, controlled trial. *Lancet.* 2020;396:1895–1904. [PMID: 33197395]

Teerlink JR, Diaz R, Felker GM, et al. Cardiac myosin activation with omecamtiv mecarbil in systolic heart failure. *N Engl J Med.* 2021;384:105–116. [PMID: 33185990]

F. Pharmacologic Treatment: Specific Therapies in Hospitalized Patients

Most hospitalized patients with HFrEF are volume overloaded and may require **vasodilators** to decrease the filling pressures and improve dyspnea. For faster action, intravenous options such as sodium nitroprusside or nitroglycerin are available. Due to the frequent titration needed, sodium nitroprusside and nitroglycerin can only be used in the intensive care setting.

A minority of hospitalized HFrEF patients presents with very low cardiac output ("cold" profile) and require **intravenous inotropes** to maintain perfusion and diuresis. The two most frequently used agents are dobutamine and milrinone. Dobutamine augments cardiac contractility primarily via stimulation of β-adrenergic receptors and is a modest vasodilator, whereas milrinone exerts potent inotropic and direct vasodilator effects via phosphodiesterase inhibition in the myocardium and vasculature. While these agents are fairly effective, their use is associated with further myocardial injury (evidence of troponin release even in nonischemic cardiomyopathy), and they can precipitate fatal ventricular arrhythmias. Studies have not shown superiority in milrinone versus dobutamine, and selection is mostly directed by their specific agent-related adverse effects. Their use is best reserved for patients in need of a bridge to mechanical circulatory support or transplant or in those patients where palliative home hospice is entertained. Of note, many trials have failed to show mortality benefit with inotropes in clinical scenarios outside of cardiogenic shock.

Ahmad T, Miller PE, McCullough M, et al. Why has positive inotropy failed in chronic heart failure? Lessons from prior inotrope trials. *Eur J Heart Fail.* 2019;21:1064–1078. [PMID: 31407860]

Lewis TC, Aberle C, Altshuler, Piper GL, Papadopoulos J. Comparative effectiveness and safety between milrinone or dobutamine as initial inotrope therapy in cardiogenic shock. *J Cardiovasc Pharmacol Ther.* 2019;24:130–138. [PMID: 30175599]

G. Electrical Treatment

The majority of patients with HFrEF experience ventricular arrhythmias, and as many as 50% of all deaths in this population are sudden in nature. Findings from large clinical trials have shown that **implantable cardioverter-defibrillators** (ICDs) are the most effective therapy available to prevent sudden cardiac death in these patients at risk, and ICD treatment has become standard therapy for primary and secondary prevention of sudden cardiac death in addition to optimal medical therapy in patients with left ventricular ejection fraction below 35%. Only about 10% of patients implanted with ICDs have appropriate discharges (highlighting the poor predictive value of current selection algorithms based solely on ejection fraction), with another 20% of patients experiencing inappropriate shocks (leading to an increase in mortality), and with the vast majority not using them at all. Fortunately, better discrimination algorithms for supraventricular tachycardia and the optimal use of ventricular antitachycardia pacing have markedly decreased the frequency of inappropriate shocks in these patients. The role of ICDs in the current setting of quadruple GDMT has been questioned, as the combination of these specific agents has a marked effect in reducing sudden death.

A third of HFrEF patients experience intraventricular conduction abnormalities (eg, left bundle branch block) that lead to mechanical dyssynchrony and adversely affect the cardiac performance. Several clinical trials have shown that **CRT** as standalone treatment or combined with ICD in patients with HFrEF and ejection fraction below 35% significantly improves the ejection fraction, decreases ventricular volumes, improves HF symptoms, improves exercise tolerance, and decreases the hospitalization rate for HF, as well as cardiovascular and all-cause mortality. These benefits are seen across the spectrum of HF patients (NYHA functional class I–IV) and are more evident in patients in sinus rhythm, with a left bundle branch block pattern, QRS duration greater than 150 ms, and an ejection fraction below 35%. Proper patient selection to meet these strict criteria, together with selection of a viable (noninfarcted) lateral wall, optimal placement of the coronary sinus pacing lead, and use of quadripolar leads, can markedly decrease the frequency of CRT "nonresponders" (estimated at about 40% of the population implanted). The value of periodic CRT optimization by adjusting the atrioventricular and intraventricular timing for pacing (either via device-specific algorithms or echocardiography) is still a matter of debate, although in several studies it has been shown to improve symptoms and ventricular remodeling parameters, and most recently to decrease hospital readmissions for HF.

Cardiac contractility modulation was developed to target a subset of HF patients who do not qualify for CRT but still have reduced ejection fraction. Cardiac contractility modulation augments cardiomyocyte contraction by delivering nonexcitatory electrical signals during the cardiac absolute refractory period. This technology has been shown to reduce HF hospitalizations, improve exercise tolerance (measured through pVO_2), and improve the quality of life in patients with an ejection fraction between 25% and 45% with QRS durations less than 130 ms. However, due to the lack of randomized data on HF hospitalizations and mortality, the therapy is not yet recommended in the latest HF guidelines, albeit being FDA-approved.

Baroreflex activation therapy delivers electrical stimulation of carotid baroreceptors, resulting in centrally mediated reduction in sympathetic outflow and increased parasympathetic activity. This leads to increased arterial and venous compliance and reduced peripheral resistance. A single randomized control trial showed improvements in functional status, quality of life and exercise capacity for patients with HFrEF and NYHA functional class III symptoms. Although FDA approved, the current clinical HF guidelines do not recommend this therapy, in the absence of clinical data on HF hospitalization or mortality.

Augmentation of the parasympathetic tone through vagal nerve stimulation has been evaluated as a potential therapy to normalize the autonomic imbalance that leads to the progression of HF. To date, three clinical trials of vagal nerve stimulation showed contradictory results. The large ANTHEM-HFrEF (AutoNomic Regulation Therapy to Enhance Myocardial Function in Heart Failure with Reduced Ejection Fraction) ongoing trial is assessing its effect on mortality and HF hospitalizations in patients with HFrEF.

Abraham WT, Kuck KH, Goldsmith RL, et al. A randomized controlled trial to evaluate the safety and efficacy of cardiac contractility modulation. *JACC Heart Fail.* 2018;6:874–883. [PMID: 29754812]

Fudim M, Abraham WT, von Bardeleben RS, et al. Device therapy in chronic heart failure: JACC State-of-the-Art Review. *J Am Coll Cardiol.* 2021;78:931–956. [PMID: 34446165]

Zile MR, Lindenfeld J, Weaver FA, et al. Baroreflex activation therapy in patients with heart failure with reduced ejection fraction. *J Am Coll Cardiol.* 2020;76:1–13. [PMID: 32616150]

H. Interventional Treatment

Several percutaneous treatment options have recently been approved or are in development for the treatment of HFrEF. Many patients with HFrEF develop functional mitral regurgitation as a result of left ventricular enlargement. **Transcatheter edge-to-edge (TEER) mitral valve repair** is a viable option for those HFrEF patients that have moderate to severe symptomatic mitral regurgitation. The COAPT trial demonstrated a mortality benefit and reduction in HF hospitalizations compared to medical therapy alone for more than 24 months. These results remained significant among various subgroups, including those with ischemic and nonischemic HF, and thus TEER should be offered to all those patients with HFrEF with symptomatic severe mitral regurgitation who are optimized on medical therapy.

The creation of **intratrial shunts** to potentially reduce left atrial pressure has become a focus of study in populations with HFrEF. Specifically, unilateral left to right intraatrial valves have shown preliminary data to be positive, demonstrating an increase in quality of life and functional status with good safety outcomes. Although limited, most data on this intervention exists in the realm of HFpEF, where trials in HFrEF populations are ongoing. The long-term implications of increased right-heart loading and potential need for thromboembolic prophylaxis with these interventions are unknown.

Given its widespread prevalence, HF and atrial fibrillation have large overlaps in this patient population. The role of **ablation** in those with atrial fibrillation and HFrEF was studied in the CASTLE-HF trial. Patients with symptomatic paroxysmal or permanent atrial fibrillation and HF who were unable to or had no response to antiarrhythmic drugs were randomized to ablation versus medical therapy alone. The results showed a reduction in all-cause mortality, mostly from cardiovascular-related death in the ablation group with additional reductions in HF hospitalization. The current 2022 HF guidelines recommend catheter ablation for patients with atrial fibrillation, HF, and ejection fraction below 50%, who have high ventricular rates and have failed rhythm control strategies.

Brachmann J, Sohns C, Andresen D, et al. Atrial fibrillation burden and clinical outcomes in heart failure: The CASTLE-AF Trial. *JACC Clin Electrophysiol.* 2021;7:594–603. [PMID: 33640355]

Fudim M, Abraham WT, von Bardeleben RS, et al. Device therapy in chronic heart failure: JACC State-of-the-Art Review. *J Am Coll Cardiol.* 2021;78:931–956. [PMID: 34446165]

Stone GW, Lindenfeld J, Abraham WT, et al. COAPT Investigators. Transcatheter mitral-valve repair in patients with heart failure. *N Engl J Med.* 2018;379:2307–2318. [PMID: 30280640]

I. Surgical Treatment

Cardiac surgical approaches for patients with HFrEF have changed and matured over the last decade due to improved surgical techniques and as a result of several randomized clinical trials. The Surgical Treatment of Ischemic Heart Failure (STICH) trial showed a 19% decrease in cardiovascular mortality and a 15% decrease in cardiovascular hospitalizations in patients undergoing **coronary artery bypass surgery** in addition to optimal medical therapy when compared to optimal medical therapy alone. Thus, patients with ischemic HFrEF and ejection fraction below 35% should be evaluated for surgical (or possibly percutaneous) revascularization.

Many HF patients with decreased systolic function and coronary artery disease have apical aneurysms as a result of prior myocardial infarctions. Based on case series, surgical aneurysm reduction was thought to be beneficial by making the left ventricular contraction more efficient; however, data from the STICH trial showed that the improvement in ventricular volume with **surgical ventricular restoration** did not translate into a measurable clinical benefit for the patients.

While data are more convincing for concomitant **mitral valve replacement** at the time of coronary bypass surgery, several large case series showed that even in nonischemic patients, mitral valve repair with an undersized complete rigid annuloplasty ring and without alteration of the subvalvular apparatus can be performed safely with low operative mortality. At present, it is unknown if this operation will translate into reverse remodeling or improved clinical outcomes. Recently, percutaneous plication or repair of the mitral valve has become possible and may replace surgical approaches in the future.

Patients with advanced HFrEF who are not amenable to conventional pharmacologic, electrical, or surgical therapies should be considered for advanced surgical options. Although with the current advances in immunosuppression therapy, the 1-year survival after **cardiac transplantation** is more than 90% and 50% of patients survive more than 13 years; only about 3300 adult patients will get transplanted every year due to the lack of available organs. The strict evaluation of candidates for heart transplantation will address comorbid diseases such as pulmonary hypertension, kidney disease, diabetes, chronic obstructive lung disease, and cancers to identify the candidates most likely to benefit long-term from this therapy. Novel technologies for organ procurement and preservation, as well as the expansion of extended criteria donors will likely increase the availability of organs in the future.

Left ventricular assist device implantation has been used as a bridge to recovery (in patients with acute myocarditis or postpartum cardiomyopathy), a bridge to transplant (for patients likely to wait extended period for an available organ) or destination therapy. The only device in current commercial use, Thoratec HeartMate III is a third-generation device with excellent reliability and low adverse events profile and has transformed the field of mechanical circulatory support. While the surgical operation itself has become standardized, the long-term postoperative care is complex, and the use of assisted circulation is associated with risk of complications such as gastrointestinal bleeding, right-sided HF, renal insufficiency, infection, and thromboembolic events.

Howlett JG, Stebbins A, Petrie MC, et al. STICH Trial Investigators. CABG improves outcomes in patients with ischemic cardiomyopathy: 10-year follow-up of the STICH Trial. *JACC Heart Fail.* 2019;7:878–887. [PMID: 31521682]

Mehra MR, Uriel N, Naka Y, et al. MOMENTUM 3 Investigators. A fully magnetically levitated left ventricular assist device - Final Report. *N Engl J Med.* 2019;380:1618–1627. [PMID: 30883052]

Disease Management

Disease management programs are an important part of the care for patients with HFrEF and include a broad range of health services, such as home health care, visiting nurses, and rehabilitation. The goal of these programs is to offer a combination of treatment, complication prevention, and education (about medications, diet, symptoms, etc.) in a variety of settings. However, systematic research has shown that monitoring technologies using weights and symptoms check fails to show a decrease in hospitalizations or improvement in survival. In contrast, using implantable hemodynamic monitors (eg, CardioMeMS) and monitoring pulmonary artery pressures, has been successful in reducing HF hospitalizations in patients with NYHA functional class II-III symptoms. Implantable hemodynamic sensors (eg, CardioMEMS, Cordella, Vectorius), are the only available and validated tools to monitor subclinical congestion. Other novel devices that monitor hemodynamic congestion include cardiovascular implantable electronic devices (eg, HeartLogic), wearable technologies, and lung impedance/radar technologies. Most of these technologies are undergoing investigation in clinical trials. These sensors provide a crucial opportunity for health-care providers to intervene early and thus reduce HF hospitalizations by identifying and trending hemodynamic congestion.

Proper utilization of telehealth has been an attractive concept for HF management given both the scale and cost associated with HF clinic visits. Few data existed before the COVID-19 pandemic due to regulatory roadblocks inhibiting robust implementation of this resource. Since the COVID-19 pandemic started, telehealth has assumed a more prominent role in medical management and further research concerning telehealth's value in HF management is ongoing.

Lindenfeld J, Zile MR, Desai AS, et al. Haemodynamic-guided management of heart failure (GUIDE-HF): a randomised controlled trial. *Lancet*. 2021;398:991–1001. [PMID: 34461042]

Prognosis

Prognostication is critical in patient management, and patients deserve careful, thoughtful, and compassionate analysis of the data and information that will guide them through the important challenges of self-care. Although many demographic and clinical variables have been shown to predict survival in epidemiologic studies and clinical trials, the clinician is faced with the almost impossible task of juggling all these variables at the hospital bedside or in the office when seeing a patient. During day-to-day management of individuals with HFrEF, the physician should focus attention on readily available clinical information that includes symptom severity (usually NYHA functional class, distance walked in 6 minutes, or oxygen consumption on CPET), left ventricular ejection fraction, routine biochemical markers (serum sodium, creatinine, blood urea nitrogen, and uric acid levels), and select neurohormones such as natriuretic peptides, especially at times of discharge from a HF hospitalization. Several algorithms have been developed and tested to assist in determining which patients might benefit from advanced HR options such as assist devices or cardiac transplantation. The models that are most used are the Heart Failure Survival Score (using presence of ischemia, resting heart rate, left ventricular ejection fraction, presence of a QRS duration > 200 ms, mean resting blood pressure, peak oxygen uptake, and serum sodium level) and the Seattle Heart Failure Model (using 25 different demographic and clinical variables). Both models have been extensively validated and can give a fairly accurate survival estimate. When such evaluation indicates a poor prognosis, the clinician needs to have an in-depth discussion with the patient and their family, where all the options (including palliative care) should be discussed.

Heidenreich PA, Bozkurt B, Aguilar D, et al. 2022 AHA/ACC/HFSA Guideline for the Management of Heart Failure: A Report of the American College of Cardiology/American Heart Association Joint Committee on Clinical Practice Guidelines. *J Am Coll Cardiol.* 2022;79:e263–e421. [PMID: 35379503]

27 Heart Failure with Preserved Ejection Fraction

Jonathan D. Davis, MD, MPHS
Sanjiv J. Shah, MD

ESSENTIALS OF DIAGNOSIS

- Preserved left ventricular ejection fraction (LVEF ≥ 50%).
- Presence of the signs and symptoms of heart failure resulting from any structural or functional impairment of ventricular filling or ejection of blood, such as:
  - Abnormal cardiac chamber enlargement, echocardiographic evidence of left ventricular diastolic dysfunction, moderate/severe ventricular hypertrophy or moderate/severe valvular obstructive or regurgitant lesion.
- Evidence of spontaneous or provokable increased LV filling pressures, such as:
  - Elevated natriuretic peptide level (eg, BNP, NT-proBNP).
  - Noninvasive and invasive hemodynamic measurement.

General Considerations

Heart failure with preserved ejection fraction (HFpEF) is an increasingly recognized, debilitating syndrome, and carries a high rate of morbidity and mortality. HFpEF accounts for more than 50% of all hospitalizations for heart failure (HF). Survival for all HF patients is equally as poor regardless of underlying ejection fraction, especially after HF hospitalization. It is a heterogeneous syndrome, and categorizing patients based on their underlying pathophysiology and comorbidities is the key to treatment.

HFpEF is the preferred term for patients with a normal ejection fraction who have the syndrome of HF because HFpEF highlights the fact that HF is a syndrome and not a distinct clinical or pathophysiologic entity. The terminology of "diastolic heart failure" and "systolic heart failure" is now obsolete. By calling HFpEF "diastolic HF," clinicians may not consider the entire differential diagnosis and syndrome of HFpEF. HFpEF has also previously been called "HF with preserved systolic function" or "HF with normal systolic function." Patients with HFpEF have abnormalities in longitudinal systolic function (as defined by tissue Doppler imaging and speckle-tracking echocardiography) despite a normal ejection fraction, and patients with HF with reduced EF (HFrEF) often have abnormal diastolic function.

In 2021, the Heart Failure Society of America (HFSA), the Heart Failure Association of the European Society of Cardiology (HFA-ESC), and the Japanese Heart Failure Society (JHFS) jointly published a new *Universal Definition and Classification of Heart Failure*. Patients with HF are classified based on ejection fraction into three categories: reduced ejection fraction (< 40%), mildly reduced ejection fraction (40–50%), and preserved ejection fraction (> 50%). Further, to capture improvements in ejection fraction seen with contemporary guideline-directed medical therapy (GDMT), they introduced "HF with improved EF" as HF with a baseline LVEF ≤ 40%, a ≥ 10-point increase from baseline LVEF, and a second measurement of LVEF more than 40%.

In 2022, the American College of Cardiology (ACC), the American Heart Association (AHA), and the HFSA released an updated Guideline for the Management of Heart Failure. This guideline statement serves as a key reference for the prevention, diagnosis, and management of patients with heart failure. To have a diagnosis of HFpEF, patients must have evidence of increased LV filling pressures at rest, exercise, or other provocations. This is manifested by invasive hemodynamic measurement at rest or exercise, echocardiographic diastolic parameters (eg, $E/e' \geq 15$) or other evidence of elevated filling pressures, or elevated levels of natriuretic peptides (eg, BNP, NT-proBNP). Evidence of structural heart disease (eg, LV structural or functional alterations), most notably an increase in left atrial size and volume (left atrial volume index) and/or an increase in LV mass (LV mass index), may be used to further support the diagnosis of HFpEF.

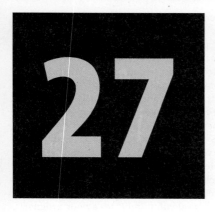

Bozkurt B, Coats AJ, Tsutsui H, et al. Universal definition and classification of heart failure: a report of the Heart Failure Society of America, Heart Failure Association of the European Society of Cardiology, Japanese Heart Failure Society and Writing Committee of the Universal Definition of Heart Failure. *J Card Fail.* 2021 Feb 7;S1071–S9164(21)00050-6. [PMID: 33662581]
Heidenreich PA, Bozkurt B, Aguilar D, et al. 2022 AHA/ACC/HFSA Guideline for the Management of Heart Failure: A Report of the American College of Cardiology/American Heart Association Joint Committee on Clinical Practice Guidelines. *J Am Coll Cardiol.* 2022 May;79(17):e263–e421. [PMID: 35379503]
Shah KS, Xu H, Matsouaka RA, et al. Heart failure with preserved, borderline, and reduced ejection fraction: 5-year outcomes. *J Am Coll Cardiol.* 2017 Nov;70(20):2476–2486. [PMID: 29141781]

Pathophysiology

HFpEF is the end result of heterogeneous pathophysiologic processes with no single mechanism. Patients typically have one or more of the following underlying pathophysiologic processes acting in concert: (1) diastolic dysfunction due to impaired left ventricular (LV) relaxation, increased LV diastolic stiffness, or both; (2) LV remodeling (typically concentric remodeling or concentric hypertrophy); (3) abnormal ventricular-arterial coupling with increased ventricular systolic stiffness and increased arterial stiffness; (4) right ventricular HF due to pulmonary venous hypertension with or without superimposed pulmonary arterial hypertension; (5) chronotropic incompetence; (6) endothelial dysfunction; (7) skeletal muscle abnormalities; and (8) extracardiac causes of volume overload. In addition, coronary artery disease can be an important contributor to the pathophysiology of HFpEF.

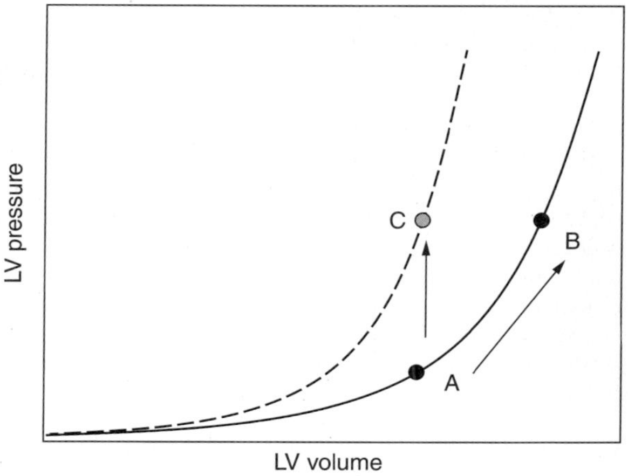

▲ **Figure 27–1.** In patients who have a noncompliant left ventricle (LV), the end-diastolic pressure–volume relationship (EDPVR) is displaced upward and to the left; therefore, there is diminished capacity to fill at low LV filling pressures. A = normal LV compliance; B = stiff, noncompliant LV with upward and leftward-shifted EDPVR; C = normal LV compliance with volume overload (note that the EDPVR curve does not shift but LV filling pressure is increased). It is difficult to distinguish scenario A from scenario C on echocardiography alone (ie, both scenarios could result in grade II diastolic dysfunction on echocardiography). Thus, "diastolic dysfunction" determined by echocardiography can help diagnose elevated LV filling pressures (and impaired LV relaxation), but it is harder to diagnose reduced LV compliance by echocardiography alone.

A. Diastolic Dysfunction

Diastolic dysfunction occurs when the ventricle loses its normal ability to suction blood from the left atrium. When the ventricle relaxes abnormally, filling is delayed and left atrial emptying is incomplete. An abnormally stiff ventricle worsens the problem by also impeding left atrial emptying. The result is abnormally high left atrial and LV diastolic pressures. The LV loses its suction, and instead of "pulling" blood from the left atrium and pulmonary veins, it now relies heavily on left atrial contraction so that the LV can fill and distend appropriately and recoil in systole. This is one reason why atrial fibrillation is tolerated so poorly in patients with advanced LV diastolic dysfunction with resultant elevation of left atrial pressure, pulmonary vascular congestion, and poor cardiac output.

In patients with HFpEF who have substantial diastolic dysfunction as a cause of their symptoms, the end-diastolic pressure-volume relationship is shifted up and to the left (Figure 27–1). In these patients, even small increases in central blood volume or vascular (arterial or venous) tone can result in significant increases in left atrial volume and pulmonary venous pressures. Patients with an upward and leftward shift in the LV end-diastolic pressure–volume relationship tend to have a high relative wall thickness (high LV mass/volume ratio); increased diffuse interstitial fibrosis of the LV myocardium (or increased stiffness without fibrosis due to abnormal functioning of titin, the protein in cardiomyocytes that serves as a molecular "spring"); and impaired active relaxation of the myocardium (due to abnormal myocyte calcium homeostasis).

B. Left Ventricular Remodeling

Among patients with HFpEF, LV geometry varies but tends to involve concentric remodeling (increased relative wall thickness and normal LV mass index) or concentric hypertrophy (increased relative wall thickness and increased LV mass index). These geometries contrast with the eccentric hypertrophy found in HFrEF and are likely caused by differing stimuli leading to a pathologically distinct cardiomyocyte structure at the level of the sarcomere. Whereas in HFpEF the sarcomeres are added in parallel leading to a shorter, thicker myocyte, in HFrEF, sarcomeres are added in series, leading to a longer, thinner myocyte with increased mass. The concentric hypertrophy of HFpEF is thought to be initiated by increased systolic wall stress encountered with elevated aortic impedance due to hypertension, loss of arterial elasticity, or both. The hypertrophic changes, adaptive at first, eventually lead to myocyte degeneration and death that contributes to fibrosis, myocardial dysfunction, and clinical heart failure. Furthermore, because of increased LV wall thickness, the subendocardium is especially vulnerable to ischemia in patients with and without epicardial coronary disease due to decreased coronary blood flow during exercise. Subendocardial ischemia can cause both systolic and diastolic dysfunction in these patients and further exacerbate HFpEF.

C. Abnormal Ventricular-Arterial Coupling

Ventricular-arterial coupling describes the interaction between ventricular stiffness and central arterial stiffness. In healthy patients, young and old, arterial and ventricular elastance (stiffness) are matched to maintain optimal cardiac efficiency. However, with increasing age, ventricular stiffness is elevated and results in decreased contractile reserve, thereby rendering elderly patients susceptible to HF, blood pressure lability, and decreased exercise tolerance. Some patients with HFpEF appear to be particularly susceptible to abnormal ventricular-arterial coupling. These patients have the age-related increases in ventricular stiffness described earlier, but instead of matched ventricular and arterial stiffness, ventricular stiffness rises out of proportion of arterial stiffness, which results in poor cardiac efficiency. These patients tend to have high pulse pressure, and they tend to be most sensitive to diuretics whereby small changes in blood volume result in large changes in blood pressure (either significantly hypertensive or hypotensive).

D. Right Heart Failure

Elevated pulmonary artery systolic pressure (PASP) on echocardiography is present in more than 75% of patients with HFpEF and is a marker of worse outcomes in HFpEF. In addition, elevated PASP is the echocardiographic finding that has the best test characteristics for differentiating patients with HFpEF from those with systemic hypertension without HF. It is not surprising that elevated PASP and pulmonary hypertension are common in HFpEF since elevated left atrial pressure (at rest and/or with exercise) is present almost universally in these patients. Elevated left atrial pressure results in increased pulmonary venous pressures, thereby causing pulmonary hypertension. Significant systemic hypertension, which also occurs commonly in HFpEF, is also associated with high PASP, likely due to a shared pathophysiology of arterial stiffness in the systemic and pulmonary circulations. Thus, pulmonary venous hypertension, defined invasively as mean pulmonary artery pressure (mPAP) more than 25 mm Hg with a pulmonary capillary wedge pressure (PCWP) more than 15 mm Hg, is common in HFpEF and contributes to right ventricular hypertrophy, dysfunction, and eventual right HF. Some patients (most likely < 5–10% of HFpEF) develop superimposed pulmonary arterial hypertension (on top of pulmonary venous hypertension [also known as combined post- and precapillary pulmonary hypertension]) either as an extension of their severe pulmonary venous hypertension or due to other risk factors such as chronic thromboembolic disease, chronic hypoxemic lung disease, or obstructive sleep apnea. The best invasive marker for differentiating pulmonary venous hypertension from superimposed pulmonary arterial hypertension is not the transpulmonary gradient (mPAP-PCWP) or pulmonary vascular resistance; rather, it is the diastolic pulmonary gradient (pulmonary artery diastolic pressure [PADP]-PCWP). If the PADP-PCWP gradient is more than 5–7 mm Hg, pulmonary arterial hypertension is present; if the PADP and PCWP are equalized (ie, PADP-PCWP < 5 mm Hg), only pulmonary venous hypertension is present, and there is no significant superimposed pulmonary arterial hypertension.

E. Chronotropic Incompetence

A high proportion of patients with HFpEF have evidence of chronotropic incompetence. The inability to increase heart rate with exercise causes exercise intolerance. Patients with advanced HFpEF, such as those with restrictive cardiomyopathy, severe LV hypertrophy, or severe coronary artery disease, have a very stiff LV and are unable to augment stroke volume with exercise. Thus, these patients rely on increasing heart rate to augment cardiac output with exercise. If chronotropic incompetence is present, exercise capacity will be very limited in these types of patients.

F. Coronary Artery Disease

Approximately 50% of patients with HFpEF have concomitant coronary artery disease. In these patients, coronary disease is often severe, involving multiple epicardial coronary arteries. Patients with prior myocardial infarction, ongoing ischemia, or stable chronic coronary disease can all present with HFpEF. Myocardial ischemia causes calcium sequestration in diastole, which results in impaired LV relaxation and increased LV filling pressures. In areas of prior infarction or ongoing ischemia, regional systolic dysfunction and dyssynchrony can further exacerbate abnormal loading conditions and create a mixture of systolic and diastolic dysfunction. Furthermore, patients with chronic coronary artery disease often have LV remodeling with resultant ventricular enlargement, a known risk factor for increased mortality and HF, regardless of ejection fraction. Preservation of ejection fraction can occur in some patients with prior infarction due to hypertrophy and hyperdynamic function of noninfarcted areas.

Patients with coronary disease suffer from a vicious cycle of abnormalities that contribute to HFpEF. As noted earlier, ischemia can cause impaired LV relaxation and increased

LV filling pressures. Impaired LV relaxation in turn can also adversely affect coronary blood flow and coronary flow reserve, which exacerbates ischemia. Increased LV filling pressures results in extravascular compression of the small intramyocardial coronary vessels, which can cause subendocardial ischemia. Increased LV end-diastolic pressure can also result in poor epicardial coronary blood flow. Thus, ischemia begets worsening LV diastolic function, which begets more ischemia.

G. Endothelial Dysfunction

There is now ample evidence that underlying comorbid states including, but not limited to, obesity, diabetes mellitus, hypertension, iron deficiency, chronic kidney disease, and chronic obstructive pulmonary disease lead to a systemic proinflammatory state that results in impaired cardiac mechanics. The presence of elevated circulating proinflammatory cytokines including interleukin-6 and tumor necrosis factor-α leads to the increased production of reactive oxygen species (ROS) from coronary microvascular endothelial cells. The production of ROS decreases nitric oxide bioavailability for cardiomyocytes, which in turn leads to low protein kinase G (PKG) activity. PKG plays several roles in the cardiomyocyte, and its reduced activity has been shown to accelerate cardiomyocyte hypertrophy (leading to concentric LV remodeling) and cardiomyocyte stiffening due to hypophosphorylation of titin. Such a state of reduced nitric oxide availability has also been implicated as a primary driver of the blunted vasodilator response to exercise exhibited by patients with HFpEF.

Borlaug BA. The pathophysiology of heart failure with preserved ejection fraction. *Nat Rev Cardiol.* 2014;11(9):507–515. [PMID: 24958077]

Obokata M, Reddy YNV, Bourlaug BA. Diastolic dysfunction and heart failure with preserved ejection fraction: understanding mechanisms by using noninvasive methods. *J Am Coll Cardiol Img.* 2020 Jan;13(1 Part 2):245–257. [PMID: 31202759]

Clinical Findings

The first step in caring for a patient with HFpEF is to ensure the correct diagnosis (see later section on Differential Diagnosis). The diagnosis of HFpEF requires signs and symptoms of HF with objective evidence of preserved LV ejection fraction (≥ 50%) and either elevated natriuretic peptide levels or objective evidence of cardiogenic pulmonary or systemic congestion.

A. Risk Factors

1. Age—The prevalence of HFpEF increases with age, though the phenotype of HFpEF changes with age, too. Younger patients are more often male, obese, and of Asian or Black race whereas older patients are more often female, Caucasian, and tend to have more comorbidities (eg, diabetes mellitus, hypertension, chronic kidney disease, and atrial fibrillation). Aging has several pertinent effects on cardiovascular structure and function. Aging reduces the diastolic filling rate as a result of prolonged relaxation, which results in left atrial overload and pulmonary venous hypertension. Arterial stiffness increases with age, resulting in increased afterload and load-dependent diastolic dysfunction. In addition, stiffening of the central arteries (which is especially common in women) leaves them less capable to handle changes in blood volume, thereby increasing susceptibility to hypotension, lightheadedness, and dizziness. Finally, aging reduces exercise capacity by increasing ventricular end-systolic chamber elastance (stiffness), which results in decreased ability to augment contractility with exercise.

2. Hypertension—Hypertension is the most important risk factor for HFpEF and is present in most patients with HFpEF. Hypertensive emergency with flash pulmonary edema is a common presentation of HFpEF. Hypertension leads to LV hypertrophy, which causes impaired relaxation, poor coronary flow reserve, and increased diastolic stiffness, all of which exacerbate HFpEF. Hypertension is also a potent risk factor for epicardial coronary disease, which often complicates HFpEF. Ischemia causes both increased LV stiffness and impaired LV relaxation. Many patients with HFpEF have symptoms of chronic angina. Alternatively, recurrent HF may be an anginal equivalent in many patients with concomitant HFpEF and coronary disease.

3. Obstructive sleep apnea—Obstructive sleep apnea is a common comorbidity in patients with HFpEF, and it can result in worsening LV hypertrophy and pulmonary hypertension. In addition, patients with HFpEF may also have sleep-disordered breathing (such as Cheyne-Stokes respirations) due to their HF. Finally, increased upper airway edema due to generalized HF may cause obstructive sleep apnea, a finding that has been shown to improve with diuretic therapy. All of the above contribute to nocturnal microarousals and hypoxia, which result in poor sleep quality, which in turn worsens daytime fatigue and exercise intolerance. Therefore, there should be a low threshold to perform overnight polysomnography on the patient with HFpEF.

4. Other clinically important risk factors—Other clinically important risk factors for HFpEF include coronary artery disease, diabetes, chronic kidney disease, obesity, atrial fibrillation, anemia, and chronic obstructive pulmonary disease. All of these comorbidities have their own signs and symptoms that can complicate presentations of HFpEF and add to diagnostic, prognostic, and therapeutic complexities.

B. Symptoms & Signs

HF is a clinical syndrome of dyspnea and fluid retention independent of ejection fraction. Symptoms include dyspnea, fatigue, orthopnea, and peripheral edema and signs include jugular vein distention and hepatojugular reflux.

Exercise intolerance and acute decompensated HF are two common presentations of HFpEF.

1. Exercise intolerance—Exercise intolerance is one of the main symptoms of HFpEF and one of the most debilitating. In patients with HFpEF, there are many reasons for exercise intolerance, including the following:

- Almost all patients with HFpEF have increased LV diastolic or left atrial pressures, or both. These pressure increases are transmitted to the pulmonary veins, which can cause decreased lung compliance, which is exacerbated by exercise.
- Increased LV diastolic pressure during exercise can limit subendocardial blood flow at a time when there are increased myocardial demands, thereby worsening diastolic function. Poor myocardial perfusion is even worse in patients with LV hypertrophy, which is very common in patients with HFpEF.
- Patients with HFpEF have an abnormal stroke volume response to tachycardia with blunted increase in cardiac output with exercise. Inadequate cardiac output can increase lactate production and worsen muscle fatigue.

2. Acutely decompensated HFpEF—The most common factor in acute decompensation is uncontrolled, severe hypertension. Other common clinical findings associated with acute decompensated HFpEF include arrhythmias; noncompliance with medications or salt restriction, or both; acute coronary syndrome; renal insufficiency; valvular regurgitation or stenosis; and infection (eg, pneumonia, urinary tract infection). It is important to recognize the clinical factors associated with acute decompensation because preventing hospitalization is one of the most important goals in patients with HFpEF.

C. Diagnostic Studies

Diagnosing HFpEF begins with careful patient history, physical examination, ECG, and labs to establish the presence of the syndrome of heart failure. The diagnosis of HFpEF involves three pieces: (1) preserved left ventricular ejection fraction (LVEF ≥ 50%); (2) presence of the signs and symptoms of heart failure resulting from any structural or functional impairment of ventricular filling or ejection of blood. This may include abnormal cardiac chamber enlargement, echocardiographic evidence of left ventricular diastolic dysfunction, moderate/severe ventricular hypertrophy or moderate/severe valvular obstructive or regurgitant lesion; and (3) evidence of spontaneous or provokable increased LV filling pressures, as evidenced by elevated natriuretic peptide level (eg, BNP, NT-proBNP) or noninvasive (eg, echocardiography) or invasive (eg, pulmonary artery catheter) hemodynamic measurement. Once diagnosed, it is then necessary to determine the key comorbidities driving the pathophysiology.

Echocardiography is a key diagnostic test because it allows the determination of LV ejection fraction and cardiac structural and functional abnormalities. However, it is critical to note that while moderate or greater diastolic dysfunction can help rule in the diagnosis of HFpEF, the presence of "diastolic dysfunction" on echocardiography is not synonymous with a diagnosis of HFpEF. In patients in whom the diagnosis is in question, invasive hemodynamic testing can be helpful to establish the presence of elevated LV filling pressures at rest or with exercise. Table 27–1 lists a standardized battery of diagnostic and prognostic tests for patients being evaluated for HFpEF.

Table 27–1. Diagnostic Evaluation of Heart Failure with Preserved Ejection Fraction

Cardiac imaging
Two-dimensional/M-mode echocardiography
Doppler echocardiography
Tissue Doppler imaging
Contrast-enhanced cardiac MRI
Laboratory testing
Complete blood count with evaluation of anemia (if present)
Comprehensive chemistry panel (including liver function tests, albumin, total protein)
Fasting glucose, hemoglobin A_{1c}
Fasting lipid panel
B-type natriuretic peptide (or NT-proBNP)
Urine microalbumin
Serum immunofixation and urine protein electrophoresis
Exercise testing
Cardiopulmonary exercise testing
Noninvasive evaluation of coronary artery disease (eg, stress echocardiography)
Diastolic stress echocardiography
Cardiac catheterization
Coronary angiography (if pretest probability is high or if stress test is abnormal)
Invasive hemodynamic testing to confirm elevated LV diastolic pressure, evaluate for constriction versus restriction, evaluate for pulmonary hypertension, and dynamic testing (systemic or pulmonary vasodilator challenge, fluid challenge, exercise testing)
Endomyocardial biopsy (in selected cases)
Other
Pulmonary function testing
Overnight polysomnography

1. Echocardiography—Echocardiography is the most important initial tool in diagnosing evidence of elevated filling pressure in diastole and evaluating for etiologies of HFpEF, such as myocardial (eg, infiltrative), valvular, pericardial, and coronary diseases. All patients with possible or confirmed HFpEF should undergo comprehensive Doppler echocardiography with tissue Doppler imaging. Besides assessment of diastolic function (see later), all patients should be evaluated for increased LV mass and increased relative wall thickness (= [2 × posterior wall thickness]/LV end-diastolic dimension) more than 0.45. Assessment of PASP; right atrial pressure (from size and collapsibility of the inferior vena cava); and right ventricular size, function, and wall thickness is important in evaluation of pulmonary hypertension.

It is critically important to understand that no one abnormality on echocardiography can diagnose HFpEF, and age and comorbidities must be factored into the diagnosis. Specifically, diastolic dysfunction on echocardiogram is not synonymous with HFpEF. While the proper combination of echocardiographic abnormalities can make the diagnosis of diastolic dysfunction, this does not by extension denote the presence of HFpEF.

Although echocardiography guidelines have evolved over time to weigh increased left atrial volume more heavily in the diagnosis of diastolic dysfunction. The presence of left atrial enlargement, reduced e′ velocity (septal e′ < 7 cm/s; lateral e′ < 10 cm/s), and/or elevated E/e′ (> 15 or > 12 at the septal or lateral mitral annulus, respectively) is the first clue to the presence of diastolic dysfunction, though estimated right atrial pressure (eRAP) and LV wall thickness are also important. Compared to eRAP less than 3, eRAP ≥ 8 mm Hg has been shown to be associated with more severe LV diastolic dysfunction as well as worse right-heart structure and function. Elevated eRAP has been shown to be independently associated with higher rates of cardiovascular death or HF hospitalization, with an incremental prognostic value over E/e′ ratio.

The next step in evaluating diastolic function by echocardiography is to examine mitral inflow. In most patients, a ratio of early (E) to late (A) mitral inflow velocities (E/A ratio) less than 0.8 signifies impaired relaxation (grade I diastolic dysfunction), especially if the patient is younger than 70 years and tissue Doppler e′ velocity is less than 10 cm/s at the lateral annulus. In these patients, exercise stress echocardiography (see following discussion) can help evaluate the functional significance of impaired LV relaxation. If the E/A ratio is more than 1.5 and early mitral inflow deceleration time is less than 150 ms in an elderly patient, the diagnosis is grade III diastolic dysfunction. These patients universally should have an e′ velocity less than 10 cm/s at the lateral mitral annulus.

If the E/A ratio is 0.8–1.5 or if the E/A ratio is more than 1.5 and early mitral deceleration time is more than 150 ms, the question of normal versus pseudonormal mitral inflow arises. In these cases, an E/e′ ratio more than 15 or e′ velocity less than 10 cm/s usually signifies pseudonormal mitral inflow (grade II diastolic dysfunction). In these patients, left atrial volume index should be increased (> 34 mL/m^2). Left atrial volume index less than 34 mL/m^2 should cause reconsideration of the diagnosis of diastolic dysfunction. In patients who do not meet these criteria, further evaluation with Valsalva maneuver, pulmonary venous flow, or flow propagation velocity can all be used to help differentiate normal versus pseudonormal mitral inflow. Even with all these criteria for LV diastolic dysfunction, there is a subset of patients in whom diastolic function is indeterminate. In addition, there are patients in whom diastolic function is difficult or impossible to assess noninvasively. These patients include those with moderate or greater mitral regurgitation, any degree of mitral stenosis, severe mitral annular calcification, a mitral annuloplasty ring, or mitral valve prosthesis. In patients with atrial fibrillation, although diastolic function grade is difficult to determine, an E/e′ ratio more than 11, using e′ velocity from the septal mitral annulus, signifies elevated LV filling pressures.

It is important to note that although Doppler echocardiography is a powerful noninvasive tool for the assessment of diastolic function, as mentioned earlier, diastolic dysfunction is not synonymous with HFpEF. Many asymptomatic patients have abnormal diastolic function, but in the absence of the signs and symptoms of HF, they should not be diagnosed with HFpEF. In addition, all Doppler echocardiographic variables for the assessment of diastolic function are load sensitive, and therefore convey more information about preload and afterload than true intrinsic diastolic stiffness. Even tissue Doppler e′ velocity is somewhat load dependent. Therefore, it is always important to consider all clinical data, including clinical history and physical examination, when making the diagnosis of HFpEF.

2. B-type natriuretic peptide (BNP)—The use of BNP to assist in the diagnosis of heart failure is a class I American College of Cardiology (ACC)/American Heart Association (AHA) clinical guideline. However, its use in the diagnosis of HFpEF is not entirely straightforward. On average, BNP levels are significantly lower in patients with HFpEF than in those with HFrEF. This finding can likely be attributed to several factors, including: (1) reduced diastolic wall stress in HFpEF compared with HFrEF, and (2) higher frequency of comorbid obesity in HFpEF patients (which reduces ventricular BNP production and increases BNP clearance by peripheral adipocytes). Contemporary studies of patients with HFpEF demonstrate that BNP does not have good negative predictive value in patients with HFpEF. Therefore, BNP, like Doppler echocardiography findings, must be considered within the context of the patient and cannot be used as a stand-alone diagnostic test for HFpEF.

3. Exercise testing—Since exercise intolerance is a key symptom in HFpEF, exercise testing is extremely valuable in these patients. Although many patients who are being evaluated for HFpEF may not be able to withstand a Bruce protocol exercise test given their advanced age and multiple comorbidities, low-intensity treadmill and bicycle stress protocols are very feasible. There are two exercise tests that are helpful in evaluating patients with HFpEF: cardiopulmonary exercise testing (CPET) and diastolic stress echocardiography. Studies have shown that on CPET, patients with HFpEF have reduced exercise tolerance, low peak workload, and low peak oxygen consumption (Vo_2). Exertional dyspnea is prominent in HFpEF, and a Vo_2 provides objective evidence of reduced exercise tolerance. In addition, CPET is useful in differentiating cardiac from pulmonary components of dyspnea and decreased exercise tolerance. Often, CPET is coupled with pulmonary function testing, which also helps evaluate for pulmonary dysfunction, which is very common in elderly patients with HFpEF.

Stress echocardiography for the evaluation of diastolic function aims to look for increases in LV filling pressures with exercise. The diastolic evaluation stress can be combined with traditional exercise stress echocardiography. Therefore, one test can diagnose coronary disease and exercise-induced LV diastolic dysfunction. Patients are either tested with a treadmill or bicycle stress protocol. Baseline images are obtained in the parasternal long axis, parasternal short axis, and apical two-chamber, four-chamber, and three-chamber (long-axis) views for assessment of wall motion. Baseline images should also include Doppler assessment of early mitral inflow (E) and tissue Doppler imaging of the septal mitral annulus e′. At peak stress, wall motion analysis should come first, after which the patient should undergo repeat assessment of mitral inflow and mitral annular velocities. In patients with exercise-induced diastolic dysfunction, LV filling pressures remain elevated for several minutes, which is advantageous since the heart rate must come down to below 100 bpm to prevent E and A (and e′ and a′) merging on mitral inflow and tissue Doppler imaging, respectively. At peak exercise, an E/e′ ratio more than 13 (using e′ at the septal annulus) suggests exercise-induced increase in LV filling pressures and is diagnostic of exercise-induced diastolic dysfunction.

4. Stress testing for the evaluation of coronary artery disease—All patients with HFpEF should undergo evaluation for coronary artery disease. Exercise stress echocardiography is ideal since patients can be evaluated for the presence of coronary artery disease and exercise-induced diastolic dysfunction with one test. However, adenosine or regadenoson pharmacologic stress imaging is the test of choice in patients who cannot exercise and in institutions where nuclear myocardial perfusion imaging is superior. Dobutamine stress echocardiography can be performed, but in patients with significant LV hypertrophy, this test may have reduced sensitivity for the detection of wall motion abnormalities.

5. Cardiac catheterization—In patients with an intermediate or high pretest probability for coronary artery disease and in patients with abnormal results of stress testing, coronary angiography should be performed. LV diastolic pressures should be measured in all patients to confirm the diagnosis of elevated LV pressures. Simultaneous right- and left-heart catheterization can be extremely valuable in the assessment of patients with HFpEF and is often underutilized. Invasive assessment in the cardiac catheterization laboratory is currently the gold standard for hemodynamic assessment, allows accurate assessment of cardiac output, and can be very helpful in evaluating for restrictive cardiomyopathy, constrictive pericarditis, or pulmonary hypertension. In addition, dynamic maneuvers such as exercise, fluid challenge, nitroprusside challenge, and pulmonary vasodilator testing (with inhaled nitric oxide or intravenous adenosine) can be valuable in specific circumstances.

6. Cardiac magnetic resonance imaging (MRI)—Cardiac MRI can be extremely helpful in the evaluation of patients with HFpEF. Cardiac MRI is the gold standard for assessment of LV and right ventricular volumes, left atrial volume, and LV mass. In addition, cardiac MRI can evaluate for focal and diffuse areas of fibrosis (late gadolinium hyperenhancement and extracellular volume fraction via T1 mapping, respectively), aortic enlargement and dissection (which is important because most patients with HFpEF have significant hypertension), infiltrative cardiomyopathies, and pericardial thickness/enhancement.

7. Endomyocardial biopsy—If the cardiac MRI or echocardiogram shows significant LV hypertrophy (LVH) but either the ECG or the patient does not have a long-standing history of hypertension, it is important to evaluate for evidence of an infiltrative cardiomyopathy. This may require endomyocardial biopsy.

8. H_2FPEF predictive nomogram—A recently developed scoring system for the probability of a patient's dyspnea being due to HFpEF has shown good discrimination from noncardiac etiologies of dyspnea. The score was derived from right-heart catheterization hemodynamic data of patients presenting with dyspnea in the absence of ejection fraction less than 50% (current or prior), significant valvular heart disease (> mild stenosis, > moderate regurgitation), pulmonary arterial hypertension, constrictive pericarditis, primary cardiomyopathies, or heart transplant. The H_2PEF score is comprised of being **H**eavy (BMI > 30 kg/m^2; 2 points), **H**ypertension (two or more antihypertensive medications; 1 point), atrial **F**ibrillation (paroxysmal or persistent; 3 points), **P**ulmonary hypertension (PASP > 35 mm Hg; 1 point), **E**lder (age > 60 years; 1 point), and elevated **F**illing pressure (Doppler echocardiography E/e' > 9; 1 point). The probability of HFpEF ranged from 0.25 (1 point) to 0.55 (3 points) to 0.95 (7 points).

Mitter SS, Shah SJ, Thomas JD. A test in context: E/A and E/e' for the echocardiographic assessment of diastolic dysfunction. *J Am Coll Cardiol.* 2017;69:1451–1464. [PMID: 28302294]

Nagata R, Harada T, Omote K, et al. Right atrial pressure represents cumulative cardiac burden in heart failure with preserved ejection fraction. *ESC Heart Fail.* 2022 Feb 15. [PMID: 35166056]

Reddy YNV, Carter RE, Obokata M, Redfield MM, Borlaug BA. A simple, evidence-based approach to help guide diagnosis of heart failure with preserved ejection fraction. *Circulation.* 2018 Aug 28;138(9):861–870. [PMID: 29792299]

Differential Diagnosis

When considering the etiology of a patient's HFpEF, it is important to first make sure that the diagnosis of HF is correct. Mimickers of HF include pulmonary disease, obesity,

Table 27–2. Selected Potential Causes of Elevated Natriuretic Peptide Levels

Cardiac Causes
HF, including RV HF syndromes
Acute Coronary Syndrome
Heart muscle disease, including left ventricular hypertrophy
Valvular heart disease
Pericardial disease
Atrial fibrillation
Myocarditis
Cardiac surgery
Cardioversion
Toxic-metabolic myocardial insults, including cancer chemotherapy
Noncardiac Causes
Advancing age
Anemia
Renal failure
Obstructive sleep apnea
Severe pneumonia
Pulmonary embolism
Pulmonary arterial hypertension
Critical illness
Bacterial sepsis

and anemia, all of which can cause shortness of breath and exercise intolerance. As these comorbid conditions can also coexist with HFpEF, the presence of these comorbidities alone should not exclude the diagnosis. Edema, whether confined to the lower extremity or more generalized, has a large differential diagnosis beyond HF, and includes venous insufficiency or obstruction (eg, venous thrombosis), liver disease, renal disease (eg, nephrotic syndrome), thyroid disease, and protein-losing enteropathies. Further, causes of elevated natriuretic peptide levels other than primary diagnosis of heart failure include cardiovascular etiologies and noncardiovascular etiologies (Table 27–2).

Once the diagnosis of HF is confirmed, it is important to make sure that the LVEF has been accurately measured and that ejection fraction is truly preserved. A multiplanar imaging modality (most commonly two-dimensional echocardiography) with quantitative measurement of ejection fraction (ie, biplane method of discs) is essential for ensuring accurate quantitation of global LV systolic function. An increasingly common group of patients with HF are those with a prior history of HFrEF who have improved ejection fraction with medical and/or device therapies. Patients may still have symptoms (ACC/AHA Stage C, Persistent HF) or be asymptomatic (ACC/AHA Stage C, HF in Remission). These patients with improved EF are distinct from patients with HFpEF. Regardless of symptoms, patients in whom the EF has improved back to the normal range continue to be treated with HFrEF GDMT indefinitely.

Once the diagnosis of HFpEF is made, the list of potential contributors is broad. Table 27–3 lists the various causes of HFpEF. It is important to recognize common comorbidities in patients with HFpEF, which may act in concert to cause signs and symptoms of HF. The most important comorbidities include hypertension, diabetes mellitus, coronary artery disease, chronic kidney disease, obesity, anemia, and atrial fibrillation, and it is common for multiple comorbidities to coexist in a single patient with HFpEF. Furthermore, many patients have more than one of the etiologies of HFpEF. For example, in clinical practice, it is not uncommon to encounter an elderly patient who has HFpEF with hypertension, diabetes mellitus, chronic kidney disease, severe coronary artery disease, and moderate mitral regurgitation.

All patients should be evaluated by echocardiography for the diagnoses of infiltrative cardiomyopathy and constrictive pericarditis. Clues on echocardiography for infiltrative

Table 27–3. Etiologies of Heart Failure with Preserved Ejection Fraction

HFpEF with abnormal diastolic function
Hypertensive heart disease
Coronary artery disease
Prior myocardial infarction
Inducible myocardial ischemia
Severe, chronic, stable multivessel coronary disease
Restrictive cardiomyopathy
Radiation-induced cardiac injury
Infiltrative diseases (amyloidosis, sarcoidosis, hemochromatosis)
Metabolic storage diseases (eg, Fabry disease)
Endocardial fibrosis
Primary diabetic cardiomyopathy (in the absence of hypertension and coronary disease)
Idiopathic
Hypertrophic cardiomyopathy
Obstructive
Nonobstructive
Other causes of HFpEF
Primary valvular heart disease
Aortic stenosis
Aortic regurgitation
Mitral stenosis
Mitral regurgitation
Mimickers of obstructive valvular disease (eg, left atrial myxoma, cor triatriatum)
Pericardial disease
Constrictive pericarditis
Cardiac tamponade
Primary right ventricular dysfunction
Pulmonary arterial hypertension
Right ventricular myocardial infarction
Arrhythmogenic right ventricular dysplasia
Congenital heart disease
High-output cardiac failure
Severe anemia
Thyrotoxicosis
Cirrhosis
Arteriovenous fistulae

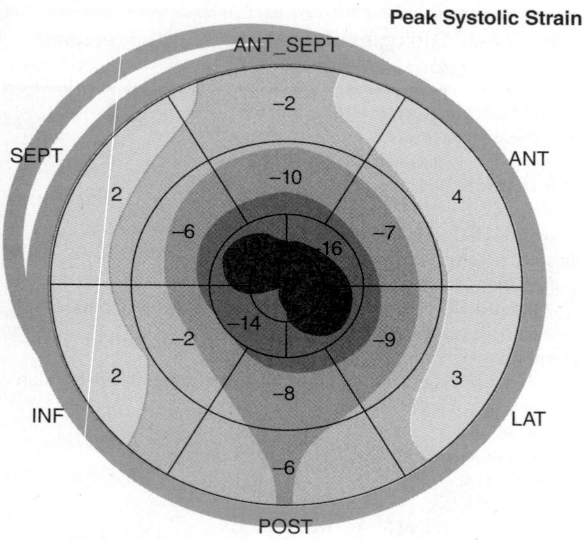

▲ **Figure 27–2.** Speckle-tracking echocardiography bullseye map of longitudinal strain of the left ventricle (17-segment model) in a patient with transthyretin cardiac amyloidosis. The basal and mid segments of the left ventricle demonstrate severely reduced longitudinal strain (*light-blue color*), whereas the apical segments demonstrate relative preservation of strain (*red color*). This pattern is highly specific for the diagnosis of cardiac amyloidosis but cannot differentiate primary (AL) amyloidosis from transthyretin amyloidosis.

cardiomyopathy include: (1) severe (grade III) diastolic dysfunction (especially if present in a young patient without end-stage renal disease or severe coronary artery disease); (2) absence of LVH on electrocardiography with increased LV wall thickness on echocardiography; (3) severely reduced longitudinal tissue velocities; and/or (4) relative apical sparing of longitudinal strain on speckle-tracking analysis ("cherry-on-the-top" sign; Figure 27–2).

Clues for the diagnosis of constrictive pericarditis include: (1) history of radiation to the chest wall, cardiac surgery, connective tissue disease, acute pericarditis, or rheumatic heart disease; (2) markers of diastolic dysfunction on mitral inflow and pulmonary vein flow with preserved or increased tissue Doppler e′ velocities; (3) increased respiratory variation in the mitral inflow Doppler tracing; and (4) diastolic interventricular septal "bounce."

Prevention

HFpEF often represents the culmination of several underlying comorbidities such as hypertension, diabetes, coronary artery disease, chronic kidney disease, and obesity. Therefore, it is imperative to aggressively treat these risk factors in all patients, particularly before they develop HF. Aggressive control of hypertension is probably the most important factor in preventing HFpEF and is a class I ACC/AHA recommendation for treatment and prevention of HFpEF.

The Valsartan in Diastolic Dysfunction (VALIDD) trial showed that improvement in diastolic function is related to decreases in blood pressure irrespective of type of antihypertensive therapy, and these findings underscore the importance of aggressive blood pressure control in patients with hypertension to improve diastolic function. Many studies have shown that lowering blood pressure reduces HF events, and VALIDD adds to these studies by showing improvement in diastolic function with aggressive control of hypertension. Furthermore, the ALLHAT-HFpEF substudy showed that chlorthalidone outperformed other antihypertensives in reducing incident HFpEF.

Poor control of diabetes mellitus has been associated with increased incidence of HF (regardless of type of HF). Although there is a tight association between poor glycemic control and incidence of HF, it is unclear whether tight control of diabetes will reduce HFpEF. In the absence of randomized controlled data, patients with diabetes should be treated aggressively with tight glycemic control, although vigilance is needed to prevent hypoglycemic episodes. Tight glycemic control results in the prevention of microvascular complications, particularly diabetic nephropathy, which can result in fluid overload and HF.

Treatment of ischemia is an attractive target for prevention of HFpEF. However, there is little data on whether there is a benefit of revascularization. In the Coronary Artery Surgery Study (CASS) database, patients with HFpEF had a higher mortality compared with those with preserved ejection fraction but no HF. Despite these findings, there were no differences in survival between patients with HFpEF in CASS who underwent surgical revascularization and those who underwent medical therapy for multivessel coronary disease. Therefore, patients with symptomatic angina and significant coronary disease should be treated with medications or revascularization, or both, but whether doing so will prevent HFpEF remains to be seen.

Treatment

A. Nonpharmacologic Therapy

All patients should keep a diary of daily weight and blood pressure. These two parameters are of extreme importance in evaluating for under diuresis and over diuresis. When patients are educated about looking for increased weight gain and increasing blood pressure, they can alert their health-care provider in a timely fashion to allow for intervention prior to progression of HF, which invariably leads to hospitalization.

Several studies have now shown that patients with HFpEF benefit from exercise training. Thus, in symptomatic HFpEF patients who can exercise, prescribed exercise training should be considered. In addition to exercise, in obese patients with HFpEF, a recent randomized controlled trial demonstrated the benefits of caloric restriction in increasing exercise capacity. Thus, a healthy lifestyle with sodium restriction, caloric restriction, and exercise training is likely to be beneficial in these patients.

There are few data to guide whether patients with HFpEF who have coronary artery disease should be revascularized. In a retrospective study of 376 patients with HFpEF, Hwang and colleagues found that 68% of the patients had coronary artery disease, and in these patients, complete coronary revascularization was associated with less deterioration in LVEF and lower mortality compared with patients who were not completely revascularized, independent of other predictors (hazard ratio, 0.56; 95% confidence interval, 0.33–0.93; $P = 0.03$). Therefore, although data are limited, coronary revascularization should be considered in patients with HFpEF and significant coronary disease.

B. Pharmacologic Therapy

Until recently, the pharmacologic treatment of HFpEF has been largely empiric and focused on treating patients' comorbidities. The publication of The Empagliflozin Outcome Trial in Patients with Chronic Heart Failure with Preserved Ejection Fraction (EMPEROR-Preserved) in 2021 marked the first HFpEF pharmacologic trial to meet its primary end point. The primary outcome of this randomized, placebo-controlled, double-blind trial of the sodium–glucose cotransporter 2 inhibitor (SGLT2i) empagliflozin versus placebo was a composite of adjudicated cardiovascular death or hospitalization for HF. This occurred in 13.8% (415 of 2997 patients) in the empagliflozin group and in 17.1% (511 of 2991 patients) in the placebo group (hazard ratio, 0.79; 95% confidence interval, 0.69 to 0.90; P < 0.001). Though reduction in hospitalization for HF drove the primary composite outcome, it marked a milestone in the treatment of HFpEF. The United States Food and Drug Administration in 2022 approved empagliflozin for the use in the treatment of HF irrespective of ejection fraction.

Dapagliflozin, the other SGLT2i with a Class I recommendation for the treatment of HFrEF, has also shown promise in the treatment of HFpEF. PRESERVED-HF was a multicenter, double-blind trial that randomized 324 HFpEF patients to dapagliflozin or placebo. The primary endpoint was whether dapagliflozin improves quality of life in HFpEF patients as measured by the Kansas City Cardiomyopathy Questionnaire Clinical Summary Score (KCCQ-CS), a measure of heart failure-related health status. At 12 weeks after treatment initiation, dapagliflozin improved KCCQ-CS (effect size, 5.8 points (95% confidence interval [CI] 2.3–9.2, P = 0.001), meeting the predefined primary endpoint, due to improvements in both KCCQ total symptom score (KCCQ-TS) (5.8 points [95% CI 2.0–9.6, P = 0.003]) and physical limitations scores (5.3 points [95% CI 0.7–10.0, P = 0.026]). DELIVER, an international, multicenter, parallel group, event-driven, randomized, double-blind trial in patients with chronic HF and LVEF more than 40%, comparing the effect of dapagliflozin 10 mg once daily versus placebo has completed enrollment. The primary outcome is to determine whether dapagliflozin is superior to placebo, when added to standard of care, in reducing the composite of CV death and HF events (hospitalization for HF or urgent HF visit) in patients with HFpEF. Results are forthcoming.

Numerous prior randomized trials have evaluated in HFpEF patients the efficacy of pharmacologic therapies that have proven effective in HFrEF, including digoxin, β-blockers, renin–angiotensin–aldosterone system (RAAS) antagonism, and nitrates. The major trials include PARAMOUNT, PARAGON-HF, DIG-PEF, CHARM-Preserved, I-PRESERVE, PEP-CHF, SENIORS, RELAX, TOPCAT, and NEAT-HFpEF.

In PARAMOUNT, a phase II randomized controlled trial (N = 301) of the angiotensin receptor neprilysin inhibitor (ARNI) sacubitril-valsartan versus placebo, patients with HFpEF randomized to ARNI had greater reduction in NT-proBNP and left atrial volume at 3 months compared to placebo. ARNI was well tolerated, and there were also less serious adverse outcomes in the ARNI arm, although this finding did not reach statistical significance (15% vs. 30%, $P = 0.32$).

PARAGON-HF, a randomized controlled trial of ARNI versus valsartan in patients (N = 4822) with EF ≥ 45%, narrowly missed meeting its primary outcome composite of total hospitalizations for heart failure and death from cardiovascular causes (rate ratio, 0.87; 95% confidence interval, 0.75 to 1.01; $P = 0.06$). Among 12 prespecified subgroups, there was suggestion of benefit with ARNI in patients with ejection fraction below 57% (median EF for clinical trial) and in women. Subsequent pooled analysis of 13,195 patients from PARADIGM-HF and PARAGON-HF in which EF was assessed as a continuous variable demonstrated consistent benefit of ARNI in men with EF up to normal and in women through the upper limit of normal. The United States Food and Drug Administration in 2021 approved sacubitril/valsartan for the treatment of HF with below normal ejection fraction. ARNI now carries a IIb recommendation for the reduction in hospitalization risk in HFpEF patients from the ACC/AHA/HFSA.

RAAS antagonism was studied in the TOPCAT trial (N = 3445), which evaluated the efficacy of the mineralocorticoid receptor antagonist spironolactone versus placebo. Although the trial failed to show benefit in reducing cardiovascular death, there was a reduction in heart failure hospitalization among patients with HFpEF. Further analysis demonstrated that, unfortunately, patients recruited in Russia and Georgia (49% of enrollment) neither had HFpEF nor received spironolactone. When analysis was restricted to the Americas, there was a clearer benefit for spironolactone in HFpEF, with reduced cardiovascular mortality and HF hospitalization. Given these findings, spironolactone carries a IIB recommendation in patients with HFpEF, provided the potassium and renal function are closely monitored.

In the DIG trial, digoxin did not decrease mortality, and although there was a trend toward decreased hospitalization, there was also a trend toward increased unstable angina. Digoxin increases systolic energy demand and adds to calcium overload in diastole and may be deleterious to patients with HFpEF; therefore, it is generally not recommended. If digoxin is necessary for rate control in patients with HFpEF who have atrial fibrillation, digoxin concentration should be kept at 0.5–0.9 ng/mL since higher concentrations were associated with increased mortality in the DIG trial.

In the CHARM-Preserved trial of mostly male patients with ejection fraction more than 40%, candesartan, an angiotensin receptor blocker, was associated with a slight decrease in time to first hospitalization but no difference in mortality when compared with placebo. The large I-PRESERVE trial (N = 4128) enrolled HFpEF patients who more closely matched with those encountered in clinical practice (60% female with a mean age of 72 years). However, I-PRESERVE, which studied irbesartan versus placebo, also found no improvement in outcomes with angiotensin receptor blocker therapy in HFpEF.

The PEP-CHF trial, which studied perindopril (an angiotensin-converting enzyme inhibitor [ACEI]), and SENIORS, which studied nebivolol (a vasodilating β-blocker), both included patients with HF and preserved or relatively preserved ejection fraction, and both did not show major benefits in terms of improved hard outcomes, although PEP-CHF did show improvements in exercise capacity with perindopril.

The RELAX trial (N = 216) examined sildenafil, a phosphodiesterase-5 (PDE-5) inhibitor, to determine whether it could improve exercise capacity in patients with HFpEF with New York Heart Association class II–III symptoms. Smaller randomized controlled trials performed previously had suggested a beneficial role for PDE-5 inhibition; however, the use of sildenafil for a total of 6 months in RELAX did not result in improved exercise capacity, as measured by peak oxygen consumption compared with placebo, or improvement in the secondary end points of cardiovascular/renal hospitalization, quality-of-life questionnaire results, or imaging indices of ventricular remodeling/diastolic function.

Isosorbide mononitrate was studied in NEAT-HFpEF (N = 110) to evaluate whether the drug would result in increased activity levels as measured by accelerometers worn by study participants. When compared with placebo, 1 month of nitrate therapy was not associated with increased activity level or improvement in 6-minute walk test, BNP levels, or quality-of-life scores. Furthermore, there was a trend toward decreased exercise levels in patients taking isosorbide mononitrate compared with placebo.

For symptomatic relief, the most important first step is to reduce the congestive state. Salt restriction diuretics and other forms of fluid removal (eg, dialysis, ultrafiltration) are often needed, but as the acute congestive episode resolves, it is important to minimize diuretic therapy, since overdiuresis activates a heightened neurohormonal response and aggravates the cardiorenal syndrome.

C. Atrial Fibrillation

From an electrophysiologic standpoint, it is important, whenever possible, to maintain atrial contraction and atrioventricular synchrony. Though this has yet to be studied in a prospective, randomized trial, we recommend patients with HFpEF and atrial fibrillation or atrial flutter be treated with a rhythm control strategy rather than just heart rate control.

In some patients with HFpEF, it is ideal to promote bradycardia and avoid tachycardia. Tachycardia increases myocardial oxygen demand and decreases coronary perfusion time, which promotes diastolic dysfunction due to ischemia even in the absence of epicardial coronary disease. In addition, the time allotted for LV relaxation is decreased and diastolic filling time is decreased when tachycardia is present. By inducing relative bradycardia (eg, heart rate 50–60 bpm), coronary perfusion is optimized, and LV relaxation and diastolic filling time are both increased. Patients who benefit most from this type of treatment are most likely those who have impaired LV relaxation and prolonged early mitral inflow deceleration times. When necessary, patients should undergo pacemaker therapy to ensure atrioventricular synchrony or to treat chronotropic incompetence.

Alternatively, in patients with more severe, end-stage HFpEF, such as severe restrictive cardiomyopathy, increased heart rate may be the most important factor maintaining cardiac output, since stroke volume is often decreased and fixed. These patients invariably have a very high early mitral inflow velocity and short deceleration time. Although excessive tachycardia should be avoided, heart rates of 80–90 bpm are often required to maintain adequate cardiac output. In these patients, overzealous β-blockade or nondihydropyridine calcium channel blocker therapy can result in a precipitous decline in cardiac output.

When considering pharmacologic agents for rate control in HFpEF, a good rule of thumb to follow when choosing β-blockers is that metoprolol succinate is a good agent in patients who have problems with rate control (eg, atrial fibrillation) and those with low or normal blood pressure. In patients who have severe hypertension, carvedilol is the agent of choice since it has potent antihypertensive effects due to its α-adrenergic blockade properties. Most patients with HFpEF have significant hypertension; thus, carvedilol is typically a first-line drug for most HFpEF patients.

D. Other Considerations

As stated earlier, all patients should be evaluated for myocardial ischemia, and when present, ischemia should be treated aggressively. Hypertension should be treated aggressively with goal blood pressure less than 130/80 mm Hg. Control of hypertension is the only proven therapy for prevention of HFpEF and is therefore essential in all patients.

HFpEF patients commonly have severe hypertension. In patients with severe, resistant hypertension the following steps should be taken: (1) ensure medication compliance, (2) ensure euvolemia since fluid overload will exacerbate hypertension, and (3) look for causes of secondary hypertension. Besides beneficial antihypertensive effects, ACEIs, angiotensin receptor blockers, and spironolactone may prevent fibrosis and may promote regression of LV hypertrophy. Statins may have pleiotropic benefit in HF, and all HFpEF patients with dyslipidemia or coronary risk factors should be treated with a statin.

1. Categorization of HFpEF subtype—As stated earlier, HFpEF is a heterogeneous syndrome. Once the HFpEF syndrome is diagnosed, patients can be further categorized clinically into etiologic and pathophysiologic subtypes to help guide therapy above and beyond the recommendations listed earlier. Table 27–4 summarizes these HFpEF subtypes and provides guidance to HFpEF subtype-specific treatment options.

2. Caveats—Some patients with HFpEF live a delicate balance between symptomatic congestion (due to inadequate diuresis) and poor cardiac output (due to overdiuresis). The latter causes lightheadedness, dizziness, fatigue, and worsening renal dysfunction due to decreased renal perfusion. Patients with HFpEF who have significant diastolic dysfunction rely on increased LV filling pressures to maintain cardiac output, and they tend to be very sensitive to overdiuresis, with small decreases in LV diastolic pressure resulting in large decreases in stroke volume. Therefore, it is important to start low and go slow with diuretic therapy. Many patients typically require frequent visits to find a diuretic regimen that results in optimal symptom control without exacerbating the cardiorenal syndrome.

In patients with hypertrophic cardiomyopathy, nondihydropyridine calcium channel blockers (verapamil, diltiazem) can be beneficial and therefore may be used as first-line therapy before β-blockade. Thiazide diuretics can exacerbate hyperglycemia and hyperuricemia, which are often present in elderly patients with HFpEF. Positive inotropes should be avoided in general because they promote calcium influx into cardiac myocytes, which worsens diastolic function. In addition, many of these patients have hypercontractile ventricles with small LV volumes. Therefore, positive inotropes frequently cause cavity obliteration with resultant obstruction of forward flow and decreased cardiac output. In patients with HFpEF who have non-ST elevation acute coronary syndromes, mortality is increased, and patients are often undertreated. Therefore, all efforts should be made to treat this high-risk group (including an early invasive approach) using evidence-based guidelines.

Aside from treatment of hypertension, coronary disease, and atrial fibrillation (as listed earlier), it is important to treat other underlying comorbidities such as diabetes, metabolic syndrome, obesity, chronic kidney disease, and anemia. In addition, many patients with HFpEF have concomitant chronic obstructive pulmonary disease, which should also be treated aggressively to improve symptoms of breathlessness.

Table 27–4. Treatment of Heart Failure with Preserved Ejection Fraction: Treatment Approaches by Subtype

"Garden variety" HFpEF: See Table 27–5 for general recommendations; several medications are often required for control of blood pressure. Treatment of comorbidities is essential.

Coronary artery disease HFpEF: These patients typically have multivessel coronary artery disease and/or a history of prior coronary artery bypass graft. Treatment of these patients involves revascularization (if indicated to improve symptoms), β-blocker, ACEI or angiotensin receptor blocker, statin, nitrate, and antiplatelet therapy.

Atrial arrhythmia-predominant HFpEF: In these patients, blood pressure is typically easy to control, but atrial arrhythmias can be difficult to control and result in HF exacerbations. Here, treatment with long-acting metoprolol succinate, a nondihydropyridine calcium channel blocker, and/or amiodarone (or other antiarrhythmic, if not contraindicated) can be helpful. Some patients may require further intervention with either catheter-based or surgical treatment of atrial arrhythmias.

Right heart failure HFpEF: These patients typically have right ventricular dysfunction and pulmonary hypertension that predominates their clinical course. Right heart catheterization should be performed to exclude pulmonary arterial hypertension or superimposed pulmonary arterial hypertension (on top of pulmonary venous hypertension). In patients with advanced right ventricular failure, cardiac output is reduced and systemic blood pressure can be low. Treatment is challenging and often requires a combination of diuretics (or ultrafiltration for refractory cases), digoxin (for right ventricular inotropy), and phosphodiesterase-5 inhibition (eg, sildenafil). Midodrine, an α-agonist, can be useful to support the systemic blood pressure if hypotension occurs during diuresis.

Hypertrophic cardiomyopathy (HCM)-like HFpEF: These patients are typically elderly with long-standing hypertension. They have echocardiographic characteristics that mimic HCM (moderate or severe LV hypertrophy [with or without asymmetric septal hypertrophy] and LV outflow tract or intracavitary obstruction). These patients should be treated like younger patients with genetic HCM. Treatment includes metoprolol succinate and/or nondihydropyridine calcium channel blockers, control of atrial arrhythmias, and avoidance of vasodilators. Diuretics should be used sparingly and with caution to avoid hypotension or syncope.

High-output HFpEF: Treatment of the underlying cause of the high-output state is essential. Diuretics will be the mainstay of treatment for fluid overload.

Rare causes of HFpEF: Treat the underlying cause of HFpEF and understand the caveats of treatment (eg, for cardiac amyloidosis, the most common cause of infiltrative cardiomyopathy, besides working up and treating the underlying type of amyloidosis, certain drugs [eg, digoxin, nondihydropyridine calcium channel blockers, ACEIs/angiotensin receptor blockers] should be avoided, and all patients should be evaluated for anticoagulation given the high risk of atrial thrombi).

Table 27–5. Treatment of Heart Failure with Preserved Ejection Fraction: General Principles

Treat underlying causes and precipitating factors
Treat congestion and edema
Diuretics
Ultrafiltration or dialysis (when diuretics are insufficient)
Sodium restriction
Vasodilator therapy
Aggressively treat hypertension
Use vasodilating β-blockers (eg, carvedilol), ACEIs or angiotensin receptor blockers, and thiazide diuretics whenever possible
Avoid clonidine
Control heart rate and rhythm
Goal heart rate ~60 bpm (use caution in patients with advanced diastolic dysfunction or restrictive cardiomyopathy who require increased heart rates to maintain cardiac output because of fixed stroke volume, and also consider the diagnosis of chronotropic incompetence in patients who do not tolerate heart rate–lowering agents)
Maintain sinus rhythm (cardioversion, ablation)
Pacemaker therapy (when necessary) to maintain atrioventricular synchrony or for patients who have chronotropic incompetence
Treat comorbidities
Myocardial ischemia (medications, revascularization)
Dyslipidemia (preferably with statins for pleiotropic benefit)
Anemia
Chronic kidney disease
Nonpharmacologic therapy
Instruct patients to keep diary of daily weight and blood pressure
Prescribe exercise training (cardiac rehabilitation) in mild to moderate heart failure to improve functional status and decrease symptoms
Treat obstructive sleep apnea, sleep-disordered breathing, and nocturnal hypoxia

3. Drugs to avoid—In all patients with HFpEF, it is important to avoid polypharmacy since adverse events increase and compliance decreases with increased numbers of medications. In addition, medications should always be scrutinized as causes of signs and symptoms of HF. For example, dihydropyridine calcium channel blockers (eg, amlodipine and nifedipine) and thiazolidinediones (eg, pioglitazone) can cause significant edema, nonsteroidal anti-inflammatory drugs (NSAIDs) can cause renal failure, and hydroxychloroquine (which is frequently used in rheumatologic diseases such as systemic lupus erythematosus and rheumatoid arthritis) can cause a restrictive cardiomyopathy. In the elderly cohort of patients with HFpEF, medications for Parkinson disease are common, and these agents have been shown to cause valvular disease. Certain foods and herbal supplements can also be deleterious in patients with HFpEF. Licorice can cause mineralocorticoid excess, ginseng interferes with warfarin, and ginseng also falsely elevates digoxin levels. Treatment of gout is difficult since NSAIDs are contraindicated in patients with HFpEF. In these patients, corticosteroid injection directly into the involved joint, a short pulse of oral corticosteroids, and colchicine 0.6 mg three times a week or allopurinol for maintenance therapy may be the best treatment options.

E. Societal Guidelines

In April 2022, the ACC, AHA, and HFSA jointly published updated guidelines for the management of heart failure. As has been discussed, HFpEF is a heterogenous disorder whose treatment is based on addressing the contributory comorbidities, such as hypertension, coronary artery disease, diabetes mellitus, atrial fibrillation, chronic kidney disease, and obesity. The new guideline statement provides new recommendations based on recent clinical trial data.

1. Pharmacologic management—For symptomatic heart failure with EF with EF ≥ 50%, diuretics as needed remain the only pharmacologic treatment with a Class I recommendation. SGLT2i now has a 2a recommendation to reduce the risk of HF hospitalization and cardiovascular mortality. ARNI, MRA, and ARB all carry 2b recommendations for reduction in hospitalization risk. Greater benefit is seen with these agents in patients with EF closer to 50%.

2. Nonpharmacologic management—Optimal hypertension treatment in accordance with published clinical practice guidelines retains a Class I recommendation to prevent morbidity. Other Class I recommendations include SGLT2i use in patients with HF and diabetes mellitus Type II to reduce HF-related morbidity and mortality, multidisciplinary management of patients with HF attributable to valvular heart disease or cancer treatment, and systemic anticoagulation in select patients with HF and atrial fibrillation. Management of atrial fibrillation (including ablation) to improve symptoms, formal sleep assessment in those with suspected sleep-disordered breathing, and CPAP use for patients with obstructive sleep apnea all carry a Class IIa recommendation. Routine use of nitrates or phosphodiesterase-5 inhibitors to increase activity or QOL is ineffective (Class III).

Table 27–4 lists important treatment priorities for patients with HFpEF.

Anker SD, Butler J, Filippatos G, et al. Empagliflozin in heart failure with a preserved ejection fraction. *N Engl J Med.* 2021;385:1451–1461. [PMID: 34449189]

Heidenreich PA, Bozkurt B, Aguilar D, et al. 2022 AHA/ACC/HFSA Guideline for the Management of Heart Failure: A Report of the American College of Cardiology/American Heart Association Joint Committee on Clinical Practice Guidelines. *J Am Coll Cardiol.* 2022 May;79(17):e263–e421. [PMID: 35379503]

Hwang SJ, Melenovsky V, Borlaug BA. Implications of coronary artery disease in heart failure with preserved ejection fraction. *J Am Coll Cardiol.* 2014;63(25 Pt A):2817–2827. [PMID: 24768876]

Nassif M, Windsor SL, Borlaug BA, et al. The SGLT2 inhibitor dapagliflozin in heart failure with preserved ejection fraction: a multicenter randomized trial. *Nat Med.* 27(11):1954–1960. [PMID: 34711976]

Solomon SD, McMurrray JJV, Anand IS, et al. Angiotensin–Neprilysin inhibition in heart failure with preserved ejection fraction. *N Engl J Med.* 2019;381:1609–1620. [PMID: 31475794]

Solomon SD, Vaduganathan M, Claggett BL, et al. Sacubitril/Valsartan across the spectrum of ejection fraction in heart failure. *Circulation.* 2020;141:352–361. [PMID: 31736342]

Prognosis

Patients with HF have a poor prognosis, irrespective of ejection fraction. In risk-adjusted survival analysis, both HFrEF and HFpEF groups had similar 5-year mortality of about 75%. Interestingly, echocardiographic global longitudinal strain (GLS) has been shown to be a better predictor of mortality than ejection fraction. BNP or NT-proBNP levels are also of predictive value.

Comorbidities typically drive the cause of death in HFpEF. Studies have demonstrated a shift in cause of death from the youngest to oldest. Sudden death was the most common cause of death in the youngest patients and decreased in prevalence as patients aged. The most common cause of death in the eldest group was noncardiovascular causes, and this decreased in prevalence in younger ages. Given the multifactorial causes of death in HFpEF, it is important for health-care providers to understand the importance of comorbidities in the prognosis of these patients. Therefore, although evaluation of treatment of HFpEF itself is extremely important, attention to comorbidities and a multidisciplinary approach to patients with HFpEF will likely lead to the best possible outcome in these patients.

Park JJ, Park JB, Park JH, Cho GY. Global longitudinal strain to predict mortality in patients with acute heart failure. *J Am Coll Cardiol.* 2018 May;71(18):1947–1957. [PMID 29724346]

Shah KS, Xu H, Matsouaka RA, et al. Heart failure with preserved, borderline, and reduced ejection fraction: 5-Year outcomes. *J Am Coll Cardiol.* 2017 Nov;70(20):2476–2486. [PMID: 29141781]

Tromp J, Shen L, Jhund PS, et al. Age-related characteristics and outcomes of patients with heart failure with preserved ejection fraction. *J Am Coll Cardiol.* 2019 Aug 6;74(5):601–612. [PMID: 31370950]

28 Pericardial Diseases

Massimo Imazio, MD

General Considerations

A. Normal Pericardial Anatomy & Physiology

The pericardium consists of two layers: a serous visceral layer, which is intimately adherent to the heart and epicardial fat, and a fibrous parietal layer. The pericardium encloses the greater part of the surface of the heart, the juxtacardial portions of the pulmonary and systemic veins, and the proximal segments of the great vessels. A significant portion of the left atrium, however, is not enclosed within the pericardium. The pericardium is not essential for sustaining life or health, as evidenced by the preservation of cardiac function even if the pericardium is congenitally absent or surgically removed. The pericardium plays a role in normal cardiovascular function, however, and can be involved in a number of important disease states. The normal functions of the pericardium include maintaining an optimal cardiac shape, promoting cardiac chamber interaction, preventing the overfilling of the heart, reducing friction between the beating heart and adjacent structures, providing a physical barrier to infection, and limiting displacement during the cardiac cycle.

B. Pericardial Pressure & Normal Function

The bulk of current evidence indicates that with normal cardiac volumes, the effective pericardial pressure ranges from 0–1 mm Hg to (at most) 3–4 mm Hg. The pericardial space between the parietal and visceral layers normally contains 15–50 mL of fluid, and the reserve volume of the pericardium is relatively small. The pericardium has a limited distensibility essentially determined by the histologic composition of the parietal pericardium with a limited amount of elastic fibers and more collagen fibers. However, if pericardial fluid accumulates slowly, a remodeling of pericardial connective tissue may allow pericardial distension with an accumulation of 1000–1500 mL of fluid, and occasionally up to 2000 mL. Normally, acute tamponade occurs with rapid accumulation of less than 250 mL of fluid. The pressure–volume relation of normal pericardium is a J-shaped curve. After an initial short shallow portion, which allows the pericardium to prevent cardiac chamber dilatation in response to physiologic events such as posture changes, there is a minimal increase in pericardial pressure. Thereafter, the pressure increase is extremely steep for sudden, acute changes of volume. Thus, an acute increase of 100–200 mL may greatly elevate pericardial pressure to 20–30 mm Hg and be responsible for cardiac tamponade. On the contrary, a slowly increasing pericardial volume is accompanied by only modest increase of pericardial pressure until 1000–2000 mL before the development of cardiac tamponade.

Etiology & Pathogenesis

Pericardial diseases are relatively common in clinical practice and may have different presentations either as an isolated disease or manifestation of a systemic disorder. Although the etiology is varied and complex (Table 28–1), the pericardium has a relatively nonspecific response to these different causes. On this basis, there are a few main clinical presentations including pericarditis, pericardial effusion, cardiac tamponade, and constrictive pericarditis. Causes are essentially divided as infectious or noninfectious.

A. Infectious Pathogens

1. Viruses—Viruses are considered the most common causes of pericardial diseases in developed countries with a low prevalence of tuberculosis. Unidentified viral infections are considered the most common cause of idiopathic pericarditis. The possibility of a viral cause is suggested when pericarditis occurs in the absence of other factors, and it is usually preceded by an upper respiratory tract infection or gastroenteritis 1–2 weeks before or prodromic symptoms. The viral agents most commonly associated with pericarditis include Coxsackie viruses, Epstein-Barr virus, parvovirus, and human immunodeficiency virus (HIV). Although a wide range of viral agents has been implicated, no specific

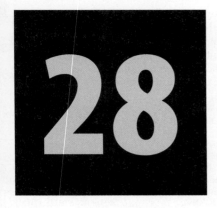

Table 28–1. Etiology of Pericardial Diseases (with most common causes in bold)

Infectious causes:
Viral (coxsackievirus, influenza, **Epstein-Barr virus,** cytomegalovirus, adenovirus, varicella, rubella, mumps, hepatitis B virus, **hepatitis C virus, HIV, parvovirus B19,** coronavirus, and human herpes virus 6)
Bacterial (tuberculosis, *Coxiella burnetii*, other bacterial rare may include pneumo-, meningo-, gonococcosis, *Haemophilus*, streptococci, staphylococci, *Chlamydia*, *Mycoplasma*, *Legionella*, *Leptospira*, *Listeria*)
Fungal (rare: *Histoplasma* more likely in immunocompetent patients; aspergillosis, blastomycosis, *Candida* more likely in immunosuppressed host)
Parasitic (very rare: *Echinococcus*, *Toxoplasma*)

Noninfectious causes:
Autoimmune:
Pericardial injury syndromes (postmyocardial infarction syndrome, ***postpericardiotomy syndrome***, posttraumatic including forms after iatrogenic trauma; ***postinterventions***: eg, coronary percutaneous intervention, pacemaker lead insertion, and radiofrequency ablation).
Systemic autoimmune and autoinflammatory diseases (systemic lupus erythematosus, Sjögren syndrome, rheumatoid arthritis, systemic sclerosis, systemic vasculitides, Behçet syndrome, sarcoidosis, familial Mediterranean fever)
Neoplastic:
Primary tumors (rare, above all pericardial mesothelioma)
Secondary metastatic tumors (common, above all ***lung and breast cancer, lymphoma***)
Metabolic (uremia, myxedema, other rare)
Traumatic and iatrogenic:
Direct injury (penetrating thoracic injury, esophageal perforation, iatrogenic)
Indirect injury (nonpenetrating thoracic injury, radiation injury)
Drug-related (procainamide, hydralazine, isoniazid, and phenytoin as lupus-like syndrome, penicillins as hypersensitivity pericarditis with eosinophilia, doxorubicin and daunorubicin [often associated with a cardiomyopathy, may cause a pericardiopathy])

antiviral therapy has been shown to be effective in immunocompetent patients or to change the evolution of the disease.

2. Bacterial pericarditis—Bacterial infection of the pericardium is uncommon beyond tuberculosis. It can occur following thoracic surgery; as a result of a contiguous pleural, mediastinal, or pulmonary infection; as a complication of bacterial endocarditis; or as a result of systemic bacteremia. Direct extension from pneumonia or empyema with staphylococci, pneumococci, and streptococci accounts for most cases. However, the most important bacterial agent is *Mycobacterium tuberculosis*, especially in developing countries. In developed countries, bacterial pericarditis is rare (< 5%), but the relative frequency is expected to increase following increased immigration from developing countries and in specific ethnic groups. Preexisting pericardial effusions and immunosuppressed states are important predisposing factors. HIV infection is often associated with tuberculous pericarditis and effusions in developing countries (eg, countries in Africa).

3. Tuberculous pericarditis—Although several decades of effective antituberculous therapy and public health measures have brought about a declining rate of tuberculous pericarditis, this condition remains a major problem in immunocompromised persons and in developing countries, especially in association with HIV infection. Thus, HIV-associated tuberculosis is a common cause of symptomatic pericardial effusion and effusive-constrictive pericarditis.

4. HIV and acquired immunodeficiency syndrome (AIDS)—The most common pericardial abnormality encountered in AIDS is an asymptomatic pericardial effusion. Before highly active antiretroviral therapies, symptomatic pericardial effusion with or without chest pain, friction rub, and electrocardiogram (ECG) changes was caused by a variety of opportunistic infections and neoplasms in patients with HIV infection and AIDS. The most common infectious pathogens identified in symptomatic pericardial effusion are *M tuberculosis* and *Mycobacterium avium-intracellulare*. The HIV virus itself can cause an effusion. Lymphomas and Kaposi sarcoma are the most common neoplasms associated with effusion. Pericarditis or symptomatic pericardial effusion in a patient with AIDS should therefore prompt an immediate search for infection or neoplasm. Pericardial effusion in HIV disease usually occurs in the context of full-blown AIDS and is strongly associated with a shortened survival time independent of the CD4 count. The mortality rate at 6 months for patients with effusion was nine times greater than for patients without effusion. After the introduction of highly active antiretroviral therapy, the etiologic spectrum of the HIV-infected patient has become similar to that of noninfected patients.

B. Iatrogenic Causes

Iatrogenic causes of pericardial diseases are emerging in developed countries due to the aging of the population and the widespread use of percutaneous interventions. Such forms are usually reported as **postcardiac injury syndromes**, reflecting the fact that the offending agent may involve not only the pericardium but also the myocardium and whole heart.

1. Surgery-related syndromes—Several distinct pericardial syndromes may occur after heart surgery.

Cardiac tamponade may occur during in-hospital recuperation, most commonly in the first 24 hours due to hemopericardium. It is identified by the hemodynamic perturbations typical of tamponade. The sudden cessation of previously brisk bleeding from drains should alert the physician to the possibility of clogging. Therapy consists of prompt surgical exploration and evacuation.

Cardiac tamponade is less common after the first 24 hours, with fewer typical clinical manifestations, and symptoms may consist largely of nonspecific generalized complaints. Two-dimensional echocardiography establishes the presence of a significant effusion and may delineate its anatomic distribution. Pericardial effusions in this setting are often loculated and may compress only one cardiac chamber. The approach to drainage is largely dictated by the location of the effusion.

Early pericarditis, consisting of fever, chest pain, pericardial friction rubs, and typical ECG features, is common. In most cases, the syndrome resolves spontaneously, and nonsteroidal anti-inflammatory drugs (NSAIDs) with colchicine are effective treatment. Corticosteroids are also very efficacious in this setting.

Postpericardiotomy syndrome is reported in 10–40% of patients, depending on the type of surgery and the adopted diagnostic criteria. This syndrome, which usually occurs during the first postoperative weeks, consists of fever, pleuritis, and pericarditis. Diagnosis proceeds by exclusion, and treatment consists of administering NSAIDs and colchicine; sometimes corticosteroids are used, especially to avoid interference of aspirin or a NSAID with oral anticoagulant therapy.

Constrictive pericarditis occurs rarely as a complication of cardiac surgery. Its incidence is estimated to only be 0.2–0.3% of cardiac operations. However, cardiac surgery is emerging as an important cause of constrictive pericarditis because so many cardiac surgeries are performed in the United States annually. The risk of constriction has been estimated at 2–5% in patients with acute pericarditis due to a postcardiac injury syndrome. Constrictive pericarditis has been reported to occur at times ranging from 2 weeks to 21 years after the surgery. Because of the relative rarity of this complication, it has been difficult to identify specific predisposing procedural factors; however, bleeding in the pericardium is presumed to be a major trigger. Occasionally, constrictive pericarditis appears within days or weeks after surgery. These cases appear to respond well to a course of corticosteroids. With this exception, the mainstay of therapy for postsurgical constrictive pericarditis is pericardiectomy.

2. Trauma—Traumatic hemorrhagic pericardial effusions, which can result from blunt or penetrating injuries of the chest, can also be caused by a variety of iatrogenic causes such as cardiac catheterization and coronary interventional procedures, pacemaker insertion, arrhythmia ablation procedures, endoscopy, and closed-chest cardiac massage. The rapidity with which pericardial fluid can accumulate can quickly cause hemodynamic compromise. Hypotension in this setting should prompt both an immediate echocardiographic search for pericardial fluid and swift evacuation of any significant effusions. Delayed manifestations may include recurrent pericardial effusions and constrictive pericarditis, especially with bloody pericardial effusions.

3. Radiation therapy—The incidence of pericardial injury from therapeutic radiation is related to dose, duration, and technical features. Pericardial damage from radiation may appear during the course of therapy or following it. The syndrome that appears during radiation therapy is acute pericarditis. The onset of clinical manifestations in the delayed form is usually within 12 months but may take many years. The clinical features of the late form range from asymptomatic pericardial effusions to acute pericarditis or constrictive pericarditis. Radiation therapy is now one of the leading causes of constrictive pericarditis. Moreover, radiation therapy may affect coronary arteries, cardiac valves, and the myocardium, worsening the prognosis of these patients.

C. Connective Tissue Disorders

Connective tissue vascular diseases are a common cause of pericardial diseases. A number of rheumatic diseases can involve the pericardium, especially systemic lupus erythematosus, Sjögren syndrome, rheumatoid arthritis, progressive systemic sclerosis, mixed connective tissue disease, polyarteritis, giant cell arteritis, other systemic vasculitides, and familial Mediterranean fever.

Symptomatic pericarditis can occur with all of these disorders, during the active phase of the systemic disease. In other cases, pericardial involvement may be subclinical with a clinically silent pericardial effusion. In unselected series of patients, acute pericarditis occurred in 2–7% of cases. However, in many cases, the diagnosis of a connective tissue disease was already known at the time of the diagnosis of pericarditis.

D. Other Causes

1. Myocardial infarction—Clinical evidence of pericarditis can be found in 7–20% of patients within the first week after myocardial infarction, although autopsy series suggest a significantly higher incidence of clinically silent, localized fibrinous pericarditis. The incidence is greatest with large, ST-segment elevation myocardial infarctions. Anticoagulant therapy and antiplatelet therapy administered in conjunction with percutaneous revascularization procedures do not appear to increase the incidence of pericardial effusions after myocardial infarction. While it is theoretically possible that these drugs may increase the chance of hemorrhage into the pericardial space if an effusion does occur, they are not generally considered to be contraindicated in the setting of early postmyocardial infarction pericarditis. Thrombolytic therapy has been associated with a decreased incidence of pericarditis in placebo-controlled studies. In contemporary series of patients with ST-segment elevation acute myocardial infarctions (AMIs) treated with primary percutaneous coronary intervention, pericarditis has become less common. Early post-AMI pericarditis has been reported in 4–5% with an increasing prevalence according to presentation delay: less than 2% for less than 3 hours, 5–6% for 3–6 hours, and 10–15% for more than 6 hours. Identified risk factors for early post-AMI pericarditis include presentation times more than 6 hours and primary percutaneous coronary intervention failure. Although pericarditis is associated with a larger infarct size, in-hospital and 1-year mortality and major adverse cardiac events are similar in patients with and without pericarditis. Treatment is based on the use of high-dose aspirin and colchicine.

Dressler syndrome (postmyocardial infarction syndrome) occurs from 1 to 6 weeks after myocardial infarction and consists of fever, pleuropericardial pain, malaise, and evidence of pleural and pericardial effusions. The syndrome has been considered a **contraindication to anticoagulant therapy**. However, because a real increase in the likelihood of pericardial hemorrhage and tamponade has not been demonstrated, there are few data to support this precaution. The incidence of this syndrome has been decreasing in recent years. Dressler syndrome has become rare in the primary percutaneous coronary intervention era and is reported in less than 0.5% of cases. It is believed to have an autoimmune cause due to sensitization to myocardial cells at the time of necrosis. Antimyocardial antibodies have been demonstrated in patients with Dressler syndrome. Treatment is based on high-dose aspirin and colchicine as the first option.

2. Malignancy—A variety of hematologic and solid malignancies (especially lung and breast cancer, lymphomas) can cause pericardial metastases that are more frequently revealed during autopsy rather than during life. Malignant tumors can spread to the pericardium through the lymphatics (mainly lung and breast carcinomas, and other carcinomas with lung metastases), through the coronary arteries (leukemia, lymphomas, and melanomas), or by direct local invasion (lung or mediastinal neoplasms). Neoplastic involvement of the pericardium can cause pericarditis, pericardial effusion with or without cardiac tamponade, and constrictive pericarditis. Primary tumors of the pericardium are rare; most are mesotheliomas and may be relatively frequent in some areas where asbestos is extracted or used in industry. Neoplastic pericarditis is responsible for 4–7% (approximately 5%) of unselected cases of pericarditis.

Typically, the diagnosis of malignancy has already been established in the patient with a malignant pericardial effusion, and other sites of metastatic spread are evident. On rare occasions, tamponade from the malignant effusion is the first manifestation of a tumor. Approximately two-thirds of cases of pericardial effusions are not related to cancer in oncology patients. It is important to distinguish malignant effusions from other causes of effusion, such as radiation, infection, and uremia, because the management and prognosis of malignant and nonmalignant effusions in cancer patients differ substantially.

3. Renal failure—Pericardial involvement in patients with renal failure can take several forms. Pericardial effusions can be found on an echocardiogram in many patients with chronic kidney disease who are asymptomatic. These effusions, which are typically small, are related more closely to the patient's volume status than other variables and usually warrant no intervention beyond clinical vigilance.

The incidence of uremic pericarditis has been decreasing for years, a trend attributable to earlier and more intensive dialysis. Uremic pericarditis typically occurs before the initiation of long-term dialysis; its development is related, in part, to the elevation of absolute levels of blood urea nitrogen (BUN) and serum creatinine, and it almost always responds to dialysis. Although uremic pericarditis can lead to tamponade, it is more commonly associated with the slow accumulation of large, low-pressure pericardial effusions.

4. Drug-related causes—A number of pharmacologic agents have been implicated in pericardial disease, although this etiology is rare. Pericarditis can occur as a feature of drug-induced systemic lupus erythematosus syndrome caused by procainamide, hydralazine, diphenylhydantoin, reserpine, methyldopa, and isoniazid. In addition to their propensity for causing myocardial inflammation, anthracycline antineoplastic agents can cause acute pericarditis. Methysergide can cause pericardial constriction as part of the syndrome of mediastinal fibrosis, and pericarditis can be part of a hypersensitivity reaction to penicillin. Minoxidil has been reported to cause pericarditis and tamponade; the mechanism is unknown.

5. Hypothyroidism—Pericardial effusion can be found in one-third of patients with myxedema. The frequency of pericardial involvement is related to both the severity and duration of hypothyroidism. The accumulation of pericardial fluid in this condition appears to be a result of a combination of increased capillary permeability and retarded lymphatic drainage. Because the pericardial fluid accumulates slowly, tamponade is rare. If pericardiocentesis is required before the diagnosis of hypothyroidism is made, the diagnosis can be suspected if the fluid is yellow and contains a high level of cholesterol. Pericardial disease in hypothyroidism reliably responds to thyroid hormone replacement therapy.

Furqan MM, Verma BR, Cremer PC, Imazio M, Klein AL. Pericardial diseases in COVID-19: a contemporary review. *Curr Cardiol Rep*. 2022;23:90. [PMID: 34081219]

Imazio M, Gaita F, LeWinter M. Evaluation and treatment of pericarditis: a systematic review. *JAMA*. 2015;314(14):1498–1506. [PMID: 26461998]

ACUTE PERICARDITIS

ESSENTIALS OF DIAGNOSIS

- Central chest pain aggravated by coughing, inspiration, or recumbency.
- Pericardial friction rub on auscultation.
- Characteristic ECG changes (widespread ST-segment elevation or PR depression).
- Pericardial effusion (new or worsening).

General Considerations

Acute pericarditis is an inflammatory condition of the pericardium that can be caused by virtually any of the conditions just discussed. As discussed earlier, a viral infection is the most common cause in developed countries (North America and Western Europe), while tuberculosis is the most common cause of pericarditis and pericardial diseases in developing countries and all over the world. This epidemiologic background should be kept in mind when managing a single patient, since immigration may lead to an increase in less common infectious causes, especially tuberculous pericarditis.

Clinical Findings

A. Symptoms & Signs

The primary symptom of acute pericarditis is chest pain whose location, intensity, and nature are variable. The pain may be described as sharp or dull. Most often it is precordial or retrosternal in location and may be referred to the trapezius ridge, which is almost pathognomonic for pericarditis. It is characteristically aggravated by inspiration, coughing, or recumbency and lessened by sitting upright and leaning forward. Although it typically takes an hour or two to develop fully, the pain can sometimes appear remarkable abruptly. Many patients relate prodromal symptoms suggestive of a viral infection (respiratory infections or gastroenteritis). Bacterial pericarditis may present with high fever, chills, night sweats, and dyspnea.

B. Physical Examination

Patients with pericarditis may be febrile (but high fever > 38°C is usually associated with a bacterial or immune-mediated form) and show tachycardia. The pericardial friction rub—the characteristic auscultatory finding—is typically scratchy and may have three components corresponding to atrial contraction, ventricular systole, and early diastole. It is not unusual for only one or two components to be audible; the systolic component is most consistently present. It has been reported in about one-third of patients. Exercise may facilitate the identification of all three components. Because the friction rub may be evanescent, varying widely in intensity even in the course of a single day, repeated auscultation is important. Furthermore, because posture can affect the pericardial rub, auscultation with the patient in several positions (eg, supine, sitting) is often helpful. When the intensity of the rub is modulated significantly by respiration, it is termed a "pleuropericardial friction rub."

C. Diagnostic Studies

Evaluation of a patient with suspected pericarditis should routinely include an ECG, complete blood count, markers of inflammation (ie, erythrocyte sedimentation rate and C-reactive protein), markers of myocardial lesion (ie, troponins), echocardiography, and a chest radiograph. Additional diagnostic laboratory tests should be tailored to the clinical presentation. High-risk features at presentation include high fever (> 38°C), subacute course, large pericardial effusion, cardiac tamponade, and lack or incomplete response to empiric anti-inflammatory therapy after 7–10 days (Figure 28–1). Echocardiography is a sensitive test for detecting pericardial effusion; however, pericardial effusion can occur in the absence of pericardial inflammation, and pericarditis may occur without a pericardial effusion. About 60% of patients with acute pericarditis show pericardial effusion at presentation, generally mild (< 1 cm). The clinical diagnosis of acute pericarditis is made with the presence of at least two of four clinical diagnostic criteria: (1) pericarditic chest pain, (2) pericardial rubs, (3) typical ECG findings (widespread ST-segment elevation or PR depression) (Figure 28–2), and (4) pericardial effusion. Elevation of markers of inflammation (eg, C-reactive protein) or evidence of pericardial inflammation by an imaging technique (eg, computed tomography or cardiac magnetic resonance) may confirm the diagnosis in atypical or doubtful cases.

1. Electrocardiography—Serial ECGs are valuable in diagnosing pericarditis. Four classical stages of ECG changes have been described (Table 28–2). In stage I, the changes accompany the onset of chest pain and consist of widespread ST-segment elevation (see Figure 28–2). The ST segment is concave upward (in distinction to the elevation in myocardial infarction). ST-segment elevation is typically present in all leads except aVR and V_1, where ST-segment depression is often present. The T waves are upright in the leads with ST elevation. The stage I pattern of pericarditis may be difficult to distinguish from the normal variant of early repolarization. A differentiating point that may be useful is the ST:T ratio in V_6. A T-wave apex four times (or greater) higher than the height of the ST segment is more likely to indicate early repolarization; if this ratio is less than 4, pericarditis is more likely. In addition, pericarditis causes other changes in the ECG that distinguish it from early repolarization. Often PR-segment depression is noted in the inferior leads and P-R elevation in aVR. In stage II, typically occurring several days later, the ST segments return to baseline, and the initially upright T waves flatten. In stage III, the T waves invert, and the ST segments may become depressed; these changes may persist indefinitely. Finally, in stage IV, which may occur weeks or months later, the T waves revert to normal. All four stages can be serially identified in about 60% of patients. ECG changes are reported in about 60% of cases with pure pericarditis and are more common with concomitant myocarditis since the pericardium is electrically silent and ECG changes reflect subepicardial involvement rather than simple pericarditis. These findings are confirmed by uremic pericarditis with pure serosal involvement where ECG changes are usually absent. On this basis the finding of ECG changes, especially ST-segment elevation should prompt the exclusion of concomitant myocarditis.

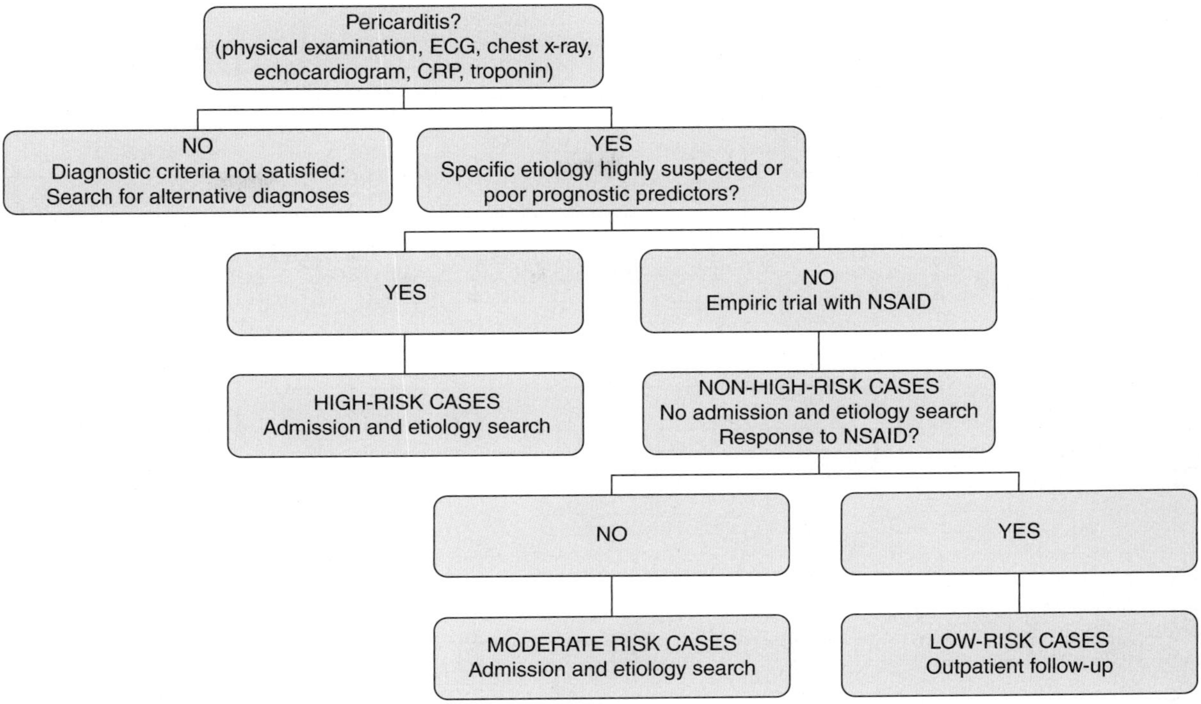

▲ **Figure 28–1.** Triage of acute pericarditis. Red flags include high fever (> 38°C), subacute course, large pericardial effusion, cardiac tamponade, and lack or incomplete response to empiric anti-inflammatory therapy after 7–10 days. If at least one is present, the patient should be admitted to hospital and complete etiology search performed. Otherwise, low-risk pericarditis may be managed as outpatient. CRP, C-reactive protein; ECG, electrocardiogram; NSAID, nonsteroidal anti-inflammatory drug. (Reproduced with permission from Imazio M, et al. Controversial issues in the management of pericardial diseases. *Circulation*. 2010;121(7):916–928.)

2. Other tests—Laboratory evidence of inflammation, such as mild leukocytosis and an elevated erythrocyte sedimentation rate and C-reactive protein, is common in acute pericarditis. These findings are less consistent in pericarditis associated with uremia or connective tissue disorders. Cardiac enzymes may be slightly elevated when the inflammatory process involves subepicardial myocardium. Alternatively, some cases occur in conjunction with a true viral myocarditis with more substantial elevations in creatine kinase and troponin. Although the chest radiograph most often reveals no abnormalities in uncomplicated pericarditis, it may occasionally show evidence of pericardial effusion (discussed in the following section). Cases with acute pericarditis (according to clinical criteria) and troponin elevation, but normal ventricular function and wall motion, are usually referred to as **myopericarditis**. They have a generally good prognosis, and management mimics that are reported for acute pericarditis. When myocardial inflammatory involvement is prevalent (as generally manifested by troponin elevation, wall motion abnormalities, and/or mildly reduced ventricular function), the term generally used in the literature is **perimyocarditis** (Figure 28–3). The only way to make the diagnosis of bacterial pericarditis is to analyze pericardial fluid, which should include Gram staining, acid-fast staining, fungal staining, and culture to identify the responsible organism. In addition, blood cultures should be always considered in patients with high fever (eg, > 38°C). In suspected tuberculous pericarditis, polymerase chain reaction can be used to detect *M tuberculosis* DNA in the pericardial fluid.

▶ Treatment

The management of pericarditis associated with an identifiable etiology is directed primarily to the underlying cause. In the usual case of idiopathic acute pericarditis, treatment with any of the NSAIDs usually suppresses the clinical manifestations within 24–48 hours—and frequently more rapidly. Because of its excellent side-effect profile, ibuprofen, 600–800 mg orally three times a day for 10–14 days, has been recommended. Aspirin, 750–1000 mg three times a day, is equally efficacious and may be favored in patients who already are taking it or need it for other indications (ie, ischemic heart disease). An alternative regimen, especially useful in systemic inflammatory diseases and in recurrences,

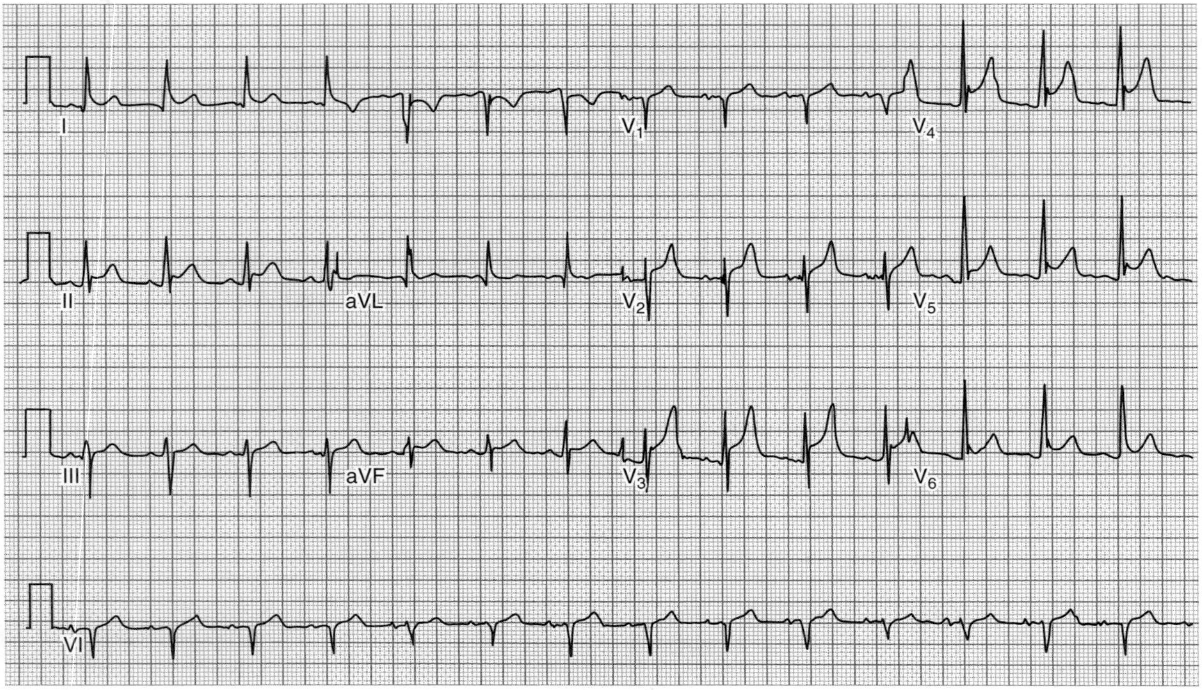

▲ **Figure 28–2.** Electrocardiogram of the first stage of pericarditis demonstrating diffuse ST-segment elevation and upright T waves. Also, subtle P-R segment depression can be seen best in leads II and aVF, with P-R elevation in aVR.

is indomethacin, 25–50 mg three times a day (Table 28–3). The initial dose is given every 8 hours to achieve good symptom control throughout the whole day. Tapering may be considered when the patient is asymptomatic and markers of inflammation are normalized. C-reactive protein may be helpful to confirm the clinical suspicion of pericarditis and to individualize the length of the initial dose as recently demonstrated in acute pericarditis. Colchicine is now recommended as an adjunct to aspirin or a NSAID in all cases with acute or recurrent pericarditis to hasten the response to anti-inflammatory therapy, improve remission rates at 1 week, and halve the recurrence rates. The loading dose should be avoided to improve patient tolerance. Weight-adjusted doses of 0.5–0.6 mg once daily for patients ≤ 70 kg or 0.5–0.6 mg twice daily for patients more than 70 kg have been recommended for 3 months in acute pericarditis and for 6 months for recurrences. At these low doses, the drug is safe and well tolerated. Gastrointestinal intolerance, especially diarrhea, is the main side effect, and has been reported in about 8% of cases.

A short course of corticosteroids is very effective in ameliorating the pain of acute pericarditis. However, their use is rarely required, and recent evidence suggests they

Table 28–2. Serial Electrocardiographic Changes in Pericarditis

Stage	ST Segment	T Waves
I	Elevated	Upright
II	Isoelectric	Upright → flat
III	Isoelectric	Inverted
IV	Isoelectric	Upright

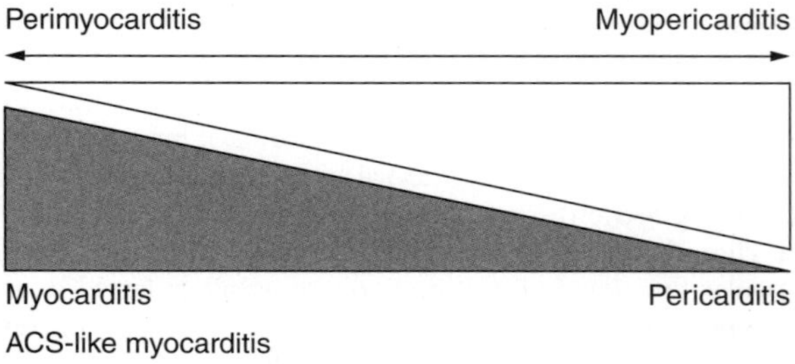

▲ **Figure 28–3.** Spectrum of myopericardial inflammatory syndromes ranging from pure pericarditis to pure myocarditis through intermediate stages: prevalent pericarditis (myopericarditis) or prevalent myocarditis (perimyocarditis). ACS, acute coronary syndrome.

Table 28–3. Empiric Anti-Inflammatory Therapy of Pericarditis

Drug	Attack Dose and Tapering
Aspirin	975 mg every 8 hours for 1–2 weeks then tapered (ie, 650 mg every 8 hours for 1–2 weeks, then 325 mg every 8 hours for 1–2 weeks)
Ibuprofen	600 mg every 8 hours for 1–2 weeks, then tapered every week (ie, 600 mg + 400 mg + 600 mg for 1 week, then 600 mg + 400 mg + 400 mg for 1 week, then 400 mg every 8 hours for 1 week)
Indomethacin	50 mg every 8 hours for 1–2 weeks, then tapered every week (ie, 50 mg + 25 mg + 50 mg for 1 week, then 50 mg + 25 mg + 25 mg for 1 week, then 25 mg every 8 hours for 1 week)
Prednisone	0.2–0.5 mg/kg/day for 2–4 weeks, then slow tapering
Colchicine	0.5–0.6 mg every 12 hours for 3–6 months (halved doses if < 70 kg: 0.5–0.6 mg once a day for 3–6 months)

may increase the chance of recurrence. Accordingly, corticosteroids should be avoided unless absolutely necessary to control severe symptoms that do not respond to other measures. If used, low to moderate doses (ie, prednisone 0.2–0.5 mg/kg/day; ie, a prednisone dose of 25 mg for the average man of 70 kg) should be used instead of high doses (ie, prednisone 1 mg/kg/day). Specific indications for the use of corticosteroids include pregnancy, systemic inflammatory diseases when steroids are needed, pericarditis in patients with renal failure, and postpericardiotomy syndromes to avoid interference of aspirin or NSAID with concomitant oral anticoagulant therapies.

In about 85–90% of patients, a single course of NSAID therapy will effectively control the illness, and pericarditis will resolve without sequelae. In about 30% of patients, a recurrence may develop over a period of weeks or months after the initial episode, generally within 18 months from the index attack. Recurrences can be managed with repeated courses of an NSAID plus colchicine. In difficult cases of recurrent pericarditis, prolonged colchicine therapy has demonstrated efficacy in prophylaxis and should be strongly considered. Although in general corticosteroids should be avoided in patients with chronic recurrent pericarditis, occasional patients can be managed best with corticosteroids. Full doses are maintained for 2–4 weeks and then tapered very slowly (ie, reducing the dose by 2.5 mg every 2–4 weeks) (Table 28–4). Triple therapy (aspirin or an NSAID plus low-dose corticosteroid plus colchicine) may be used in more difficult cases to better control symptoms. Additional therapies may be considered in colchicine-resistant cases. In patients with an inflammatory phenotype (eg, fever and C-reactive protein elevation), corticosteroid-dependence and colchicine resistance, growing evidence suggests the use of anti-IL1 agents (anakinra and rilonacept). Currently the FDA has approved rilonacept (320 mg as attack dose followed by a weekly administration of 160 mg sc for adults) to treat recurrent pericarditis and reduce the risk of recurrence in adults and children 12 years and older.

Table 28–4. Prednisone Tapering for Patients with Recurrent Pericarditis

Prednisone Daily Dose (mg)	Tapering: Daily Dose to Be Reduced at Weekly Intervals as Indicated Below[1]
> 50	10 mg/day every 1–2 weeks
25–50	5–10 mg/day every 1–2 weeks
15–25	2.5 mg/day every 2–4 weeks
< 15	1.25–2.5 mg/day every 2–6 weeks

[1]Every decrease should be done only if the patient is asymptomatic and markers of inflammation are within the normal reference values.

Additional therapies may be considered for those without evidence of systemic inflammation at presentation, including human intravenous immunoglobulins (400–500 mg/kg/day intravenously for 5 days in a single cycle that can be repeated if necessary after 1 month) and azathioprine (usually 2 mg/kg/day for several months) as a steroid-sparing agent; however, these therapies have a weaker reported evidence base.

Intravenous antimicrobial therapy should be started as soon as the diagnosis of purulent pericarditis is suspected. Although high intrapericardial antibiotic levels are achievable, prompt percutaneous or surgical drainage is essential. Cardiac tamponade may occur rapidly and resemble septic shock. In countries where tuberculosis is not endemic, only patients with proven or very likely tuberculous pericarditis should be treated.

In rare cases, frequent and severe recurrences despite aggressive medical therapy have prompted pericardiectomy. Pericardiectomy is the last option to be considered in patients who are refractory to medical therapy and should be performed in experienced cardiac surgery centers.

The most feared complication of pericarditis is the development of constrictive pericarditis. The risk is related to the etiology and not the number of recurrences. Idiopathic and viral pericarditis has a low risk (< 1%); immune-mediated (systemic inflammatory diseases and postcardiac injury syndromes) and neoplastic pericardial diseases have an intermediate risk (2–5%), whereas the highest risk has been reported for bacterial etiologies, especially tuberculosis and purulent forms (20–30%). The risk of constrictive evolution is negligible in idiopathic recurrent pericarditis.

Adler Y, Charron P, Imazio M, et al. 2015 ESC guidelines for the diagnosis and management of pericardial diseases: the Task Force for the Diagnosis and Management of Pericardial Diseases of the European Society of Cardiology (ESC) endorsed by: the European Association for Cardio-Thoracic Surgery (EACTS). *Eur Heart J.* 2015;36(42):2921–2964. [PMID: 26320112]

Brucato A, Imazio M, Gattorno M, et al. Effect of anakinra on recurrent pericarditis among patients with colchicine resistance and corticosteroid dependence: the AIRTRIP randomized clinical trial. *JAMA.* 2016 Nov 8;316(18):1906–1912. doi: 10.1001/jama.2016.15826. [PMID: 27825009]

Imazio M, Andreis A, De Ferrari GM, et al. Anakinra for corticosteroid-dependent and colchicine-resistant pericarditis: the IRAP (International Registry of Anakinra for Pericarditis) study. *Eur J Prev Cardiol.* 2019;27(9):956–964. doi: 10.1177/2047487319879534. [PMID: 31610707]

Klein AL, Imazio M, Cremer P, et al; RHAPSODY Investigators. Phase 3 Trial of interleukin-1 trap rilonacept in recurrent pericarditis. *N Engl J Med.* 2021 Jan 7;384(1):31–41. doi: 10.1056/NEJMoa2027892. Epub 2020 Nov 16. [PMID: 33200890]

PERICARDIAL EFFUSION

ESSENTIALS OF DIAGNOSIS

- Echocardiographic demonstration of pericardial fluid.

General Considerations

Pericardial effusion can develop as a result of pericarditis or an injury of any kind to the pericardium. It can be encountered in the absence of pericarditis in many clinical settings, such as uremia, cardiac trauma or chamber rupture, malignancy, AIDS, and hypothyroidism.

Clinical Findings

A. Symptoms & Signs

Clinical manifestations of pericardial effusion are directly related to the absolute volume of the effusion and the rapidity of accumulation. Small, incidental effusions rarely, if ever, cause symptoms or complications, and patients with slowly developing pericardial effusions can accumulate large volumes of fluid without symptoms. With a very slowly accumulating effusion, the pericardium can accommodate 1–2 L or more of fluid without a clinically significant elevation of intrapericardial pressure. Many of these large effusions are discovered incidentally when a chest radiograph is performed. Some may become clinically manifest by compression of adjacent structures or by causing dysphagia, cough, dyspnea, hiccups, hoarseness, nausea, or a sense of abdominal fullness. It is exceedingly rare for a specific cause of large, incidentally discovered effusions to be identified. In contrast, more rapid accumulation of even modest fluid volumes can be associated with increased intrapericardial pressures and life-threatening hemodynamic compromise.

B. Physical Examination

On examination, signs of pericardial effusion are absent in patients who have small effusions without increased pressure. Large effusions may muffle the heart sounds or cause left lower lobe lung dullness to percussion of the chest and egophony (Ewart sign) as a result of compression of lung parenchyma, or dullness to percussion in the right fifth interspace adjacent to the sternum (Rotch sign).

C. Diagnostic Studies

1. Electrocardiography—The ECG may be entirely normal. Large effusions can cause both reduced voltage (Figure 28–4) and electrical alternans—alternating QRS voltage as a result of a swinging motion of the heart that characteristically occurs at a frequency of half the heart rate. If pericarditis coexists with effusion, the usual findings may be present.

2. Chest radiography—An increase in the cardiac silhouette combined with clear or oligemic lung fields suggests the presence of a significant pericardial effusion (> 250–300 mL) (Figure 28–5), although the chest radiograph can appear entirely normal in the presence of a small to moderate effusion. Very rapidly accumulating fluid may result in only the subtlest of changes in the cardiac silhouette. With slowly accumulating fluid, the cardiac silhouette may assume a globular shape that has been likened to a water bottle with clear lungs. Radiographic differentiation of pericardial effusion and cardiac enlargement may not be possible. Occasionally, the presence of an effusion may cause increased posterior displacement of the epicardial fat pad (fat pad sign).

3. Echocardiography—Transthoracic echocardiography is the fastest and most accurate means of diagnosing and estimating the size of a pericardial effusion, but it is not accurate in assessing pericardial thickness. The effusion appears as an echo-free space between the moving epicardium and the stationary parietal pericardium. Although M-mode echocardiography can identify as little as 15 mL of pericardial fluid, which is within the normal range (15–50 mL). Usually if the effusion is seen predominantly in systole and less than 2 mm in diastole it is within the normal range. Two-dimensional echocardiography has the advantage of demonstrating the full distribution of the effusion and identifying loculated effusions. Quantification of the volume of effusion by echocardiography is not always precise. Semiquantitative assessment is practical. Large pericardial effusions (> 20 mm posteriorly in the parasternal long-axis view) have been associated with a higher risk of nonidiopathic etiologies and complications during follow-up (Figure 28–6). Small effusions (< 10 mm)

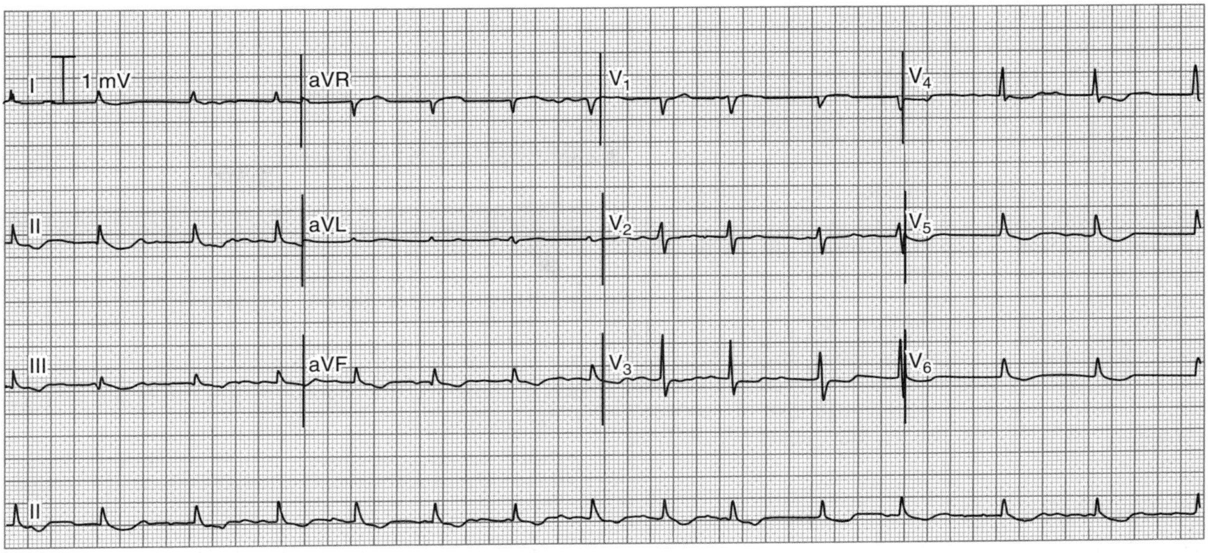

▲ **Figure 28–4.** Reduced QRS voltages (the amplitudes of QRS complexes are < 5 mm in the limbs leads and < 10 mm in all but one of the precordial leads) and atrial fibrillation in a patient with a chronic, large pericardial effusion.

tend to be imaged only posteriorly, whereas an anterior echo-free space, however, may reflect subepicardial fat rather than pericardial effusion. Larger effusions are usually distributed both anteriorly and posteriorly. A moderate effusion is considered with the widest diastolic echo-free space between 10 and 20 mm. On occasion, large effusions (> 20 mm) are associated with an excessive swinging motion of the heart within the fluid-filled pericardium. Transesophageal echocardiography is particularly useful in quantifying the anatomic distribution of effusions, especially when loculated, and is superior to transthoracic echocardiography in imaging the thickness of the pericardium.

4. Cardiac magnetic resonance imaging and computed tomography—Both of these modalities provide highly accurate imaging of pericardial effusions but, in most cases, are not necessary if echocardiographic images

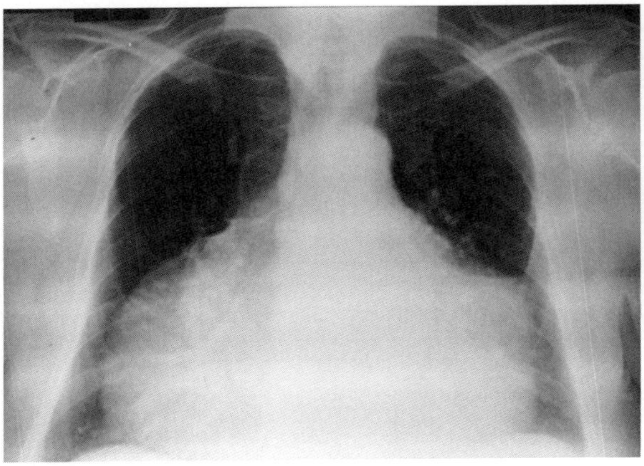

▲ **Figure 28–5.** Large pericardial effusion on chest x-ray with water bottle heart shape.

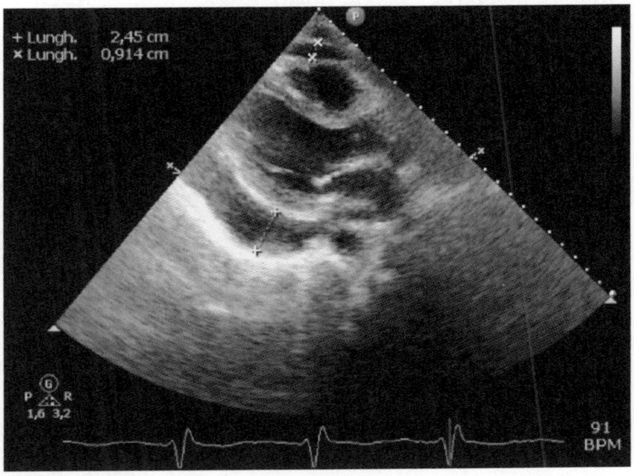

▲ **Figure 28–6.** Semiquantitative assessment of pericardial effusion. The largest diastolic width of echo-free space is measured by M-mode or two-dimensional echocardiography using different echocardiographic views, also off-axis if needed. The largest size is used to estimate the effusion as mild (< 10 mm), moderate (10–20 mm), or large (> 20 mm).

are technically satisfactory. However, they are the most accurate methods for delineating the size of effusions, their anatomic distribution, and the thickness of the pericardium. Thus, they are often valuable adjuncts to echocardiography and may help to characterize the nature of the effusion.

5. Triage of pericardial effusion—In clinical practice, most cases with pericardial effusion (> 60%) have a known underlying medical condition or systemic disease that may explain the presence of the effusion. Pericarditis with elevation of markers of inflammation should be ruled out, and if present, the management of the effusion should follow the recommendations for pericarditis. In the absence of inflammation and systemic conditions, large effusions with cardiac tamponade are associated with a high risk of neoplastic etiologies, especially lung cancer, that should be ruled out (Figure 28–7).

Treatment

The management of a pericardial effusion is largely dictated by its size, the presence or absence of hemodynamic compromise from increased intrapericardial pressure (see next section), and the nature of the underlying disorder (discussed earlier). In most cases, a small or incidentally discovered effusion warrants no specific intervention. At the same time, it should be recalled that once an effusion reaches a certain magnitude, even small additional amounts of fluid can cause a marked increase in intrapericardial pressure and rapid clinical deterioration; these patients must be monitored closely. Very large, chronic effusions (> 3 months) discovered accidentally usually do not progress. However, some of these (up to one-third) will eventually result in cardiac tamponade. Therefore, elective, closed pericardiocentesis may be recommended in these cases. Interestingly, these effusions typically do not recur following the removal of the fluid.

CARDIAC TAMPONADE

ESSENTIALS OF DIAGNOSIS

- Increased jugular venous pressure with an obliterated y descent.
- Pulsus paradoxus.
- Echocardiographic evidence of right atrial and ventricular collapse.
- Equal diastolic pressures in all four cardiac chambers.

General Considerations

Cardiac tamponade exists when increased intrapericardial pressure from accumulation of fluid compromises the filling of the heart, thereby impairing cardiac output. Whether the intrapericardial pressure rises to a level that impedes filling depends on both the rapidity of accumulation and the volume of the effusion. Severe tamponade may thus ensue in the setting of a traumatic effusion where a modest volume of blood fills the pericardial space in a brief time. Conversely, in settings such as myxedema or chronic idiopathic effusions, a slowly accumulating effusion may reach a remarkably large volume without raising the intrapericardial pressure.

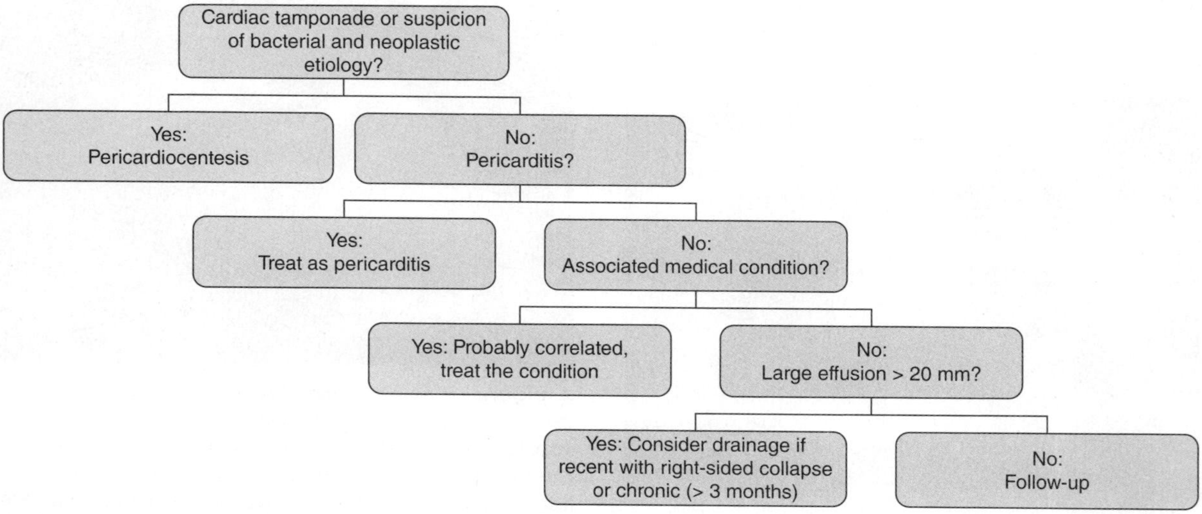

▲ **Figure 28–7.** Triage for pericardial effusions of unknown origin. (Reproduced with permission from Imazio M, et al. Controversial issues in the management of pericardial diseases. *Circulation*. 2010;121(7):916–928.)

Clinical Findings

A. Symptoms & Signs

Patients with cardiac tamponade may complain of dyspnea and chest discomfort, but dyspnea has been reported as the symptom with the highest sensitivity (85–90%). In more severe cases, consciousness may be impaired, and there may be signs of reduced cardiac output and shock. The systemic arterial pressure is typically low, although it may be surprisingly well-preserved on occasion; pulse pressure is usually diminished. The patient with tamponade is typically tachycardiac and tachypneic, although bradycardia may ensue in terminal stages. Patients with tamponade are almost always more comfortable sitting upright. If pericarditis coexists, typical pain and a friction rub may be present.

1. Pulsus paradoxus—Pulsus paradoxus, defined as an abnormally large decline (> 10 mm Hg) in systolic arterial pressure during inspiration, is present in most cases. This is the most accurate physical sign with a high sensitivity (70–90%) and specificity (70–80%). The term is actually something of a misnomer because the paradoxical pulse represents an exaggeration of the normal small decline in systolic arterial pressure that occurs during inspiration. In the presence of cardiac tamponade, the volume that can be occupied by cardiac chambers becomes fixed. During inspiration, the increase of venous return and thus right ventricle volume can occur only at the expenses of a reduced left ventricular volume. This phenomenon is also referred as ventricular interdependence. On echocardiography, mitral peak E waves show a marked respiratory variation more than 25% of their values.

Pulsus paradoxus is evaluated through careful auscultation of the Korotkoff sounds as the cuff pressure is slowly released. It is measured as the difference in cuff pressure from the point at which sounds are initially heard intermittently during expiration and the point at which the sounds are audible throughout the respiratory cycle and with each ventricular systole. A pulsus paradoxus greater than 10 mm Hg is considered abnormal. In severe tamponade, the peripheral pulse reveals an obvious decrease in the stroke volume and may even disappear on inspiration. The presence of an abnormal pulsus paradoxus is not essential to the diagnosis of cardiac tamponade, and it may be absent in clinical situations where tamponade coexists with cardiac volume overload lesions, such as atrial septal defect or aortic insufficiency. The absence of a pulsus paradoxus in these settings should not dissuade the physician from the correct diagnosis. In addition, pulsus paradoxus can be present when the inspiratory decrease in intrapleural pressure is exaggerated, as in obstructive airway disease. Reversed pulsus paradoxus—a fall in pressure with expiration—can be seen in patients on positive pressure respirators.

2. Jugular venous pressure—The venous pressure is usually markedly elevated, and examination of the jugular venous pulse wave reveals obliteration of the normal y descent. In patients with low-pressure tamponade (see section on cardiac catheterization), the venous pressure may actually be normal or only mildly elevated.

3. Other findings—Diminished heart sounds can be heard in one-third of cases; a pericardial friction rub may be heard but is absent in most patients. The concept of an inverse relation between the intensity of a pericardial rub (when present) and the size of the effusion cannot be used in assessing individual patients; the relationship is too variable to be reliable.

B. Diagnostic Studies

1. Electrocardiography—ECG may offer no specific diagnostic clues, although the ECG abnormalities described in pericarditis and pericardial effusion may be seen. The development of electrical alternans almost always indicates a hemodynamically significant effusion. However, low QRS voltages and electrical alternans have a low reported sensitivity (< 50%).

2. Chest radiography—Chest radiography offers no specific diagnostic signs of tamponade. As mentioned earlier, the cardiac silhouette may be remarkably normal in size in cases where a modestly sized effusion accumulates rapidly. A pericardial fat pad sign is diagnostic of pericardial effusion but does not necessarily indicate tamponade. The lung fields are frequently oligemic. Occasionally, the chest radiograph offers clues to important coexisting conditions, such as aortic dissection or malignancy.

3. Echocardiography—Echocardiography is an invaluable adjunctive tool. It confirms the presence of pericardial fluid and can provide evidence of increased intrapericardial pressure. The most useful echocardiographic sign is diastolic collapse of the right atrium and right ventricle. Although these changes are neither completely sensitive nor specific, they first occur when the pericardial pressure transiently exceeds the intracardiac chamber pressure. They can therefore be useful in identifying patients whose pericardial pressure level should be of concern. Echocardiography is also extremely useful as a guide in pericardiocentesis. The cardiac chambers are small in tamponade, and as discussed earlier, in extreme cases, the heart swings anteroposteriorly within the effusion. Distention of the caval vessels that does not diminish with inspiration is another useful sign.

Doppler velocity recordings demonstrate exaggerated respiratory variation in right- and left-sided venous and valvular flow, with marked inspiratory increases on the right (> 35%) and decreases on the left (> 25%). Loss of the y descent in the jugular venous pressure is caused by reduced systemic venous inflow during early diastole. Correspondingly, Doppler evaluation reveals that most caval and pulmonary venous inflow occurs during ventricular systole. These flow patterns were found to have a sensitivity of 75% and a specificity of 91% for diagnosing tamponade. The absence of chamber collapse is especially useful in excluding tamponade in patients with effusions, but its presence is less well-correlated with tamponade than abnormal venous flow patterns. Newer techniques such as tissue Doppler do not yet have a well-defined, additive role in cardiac tamponade. Inferior vena cava plethora with reduced or absent respiratory changes of size have been typically reported in cardiac tamponade.

4. Cardiac catheterization—In the patient with tamponade, cardiac catheterization reveals a depressed cardiac output as well as elevated and equal or near-equal filling pressures in all four chambers (difference < 5 mm Hg). Examination of the atrial pressure waveforms reveals the loss of the normal y descent. The initial presentation and hemodynamic profile of tamponade may, however, be altered by a concomitant state of intravascular volume depletion, a scenario that has been called **low-pressure cardiac tamponade.** This term underscores an important feature of the pathophysiology of pericardial effusions; the hemodynamic effect is a function of both the intrapericardial pressure and the intravascular volume. Although this syndrome typically occurs in patients undergoing dialysis for chronic renal failure, it can be encountered in any setting of increased intrapericardial fluid and intravascular volume depletion. In these patients, the effusions are ordinarily insufficient to cause major hemodynamic embarrassment, but they become significant when intravascular volume is depleted. The diagnosis should be considered in patients who become unusually hypotensive during dialysis. In some cases, volume expansion will result in more typical hemodynamic findings.

Treatment

Drainage of pericardial fluid is the cornerstone of therapy; reflecting the small pericardial reserve volume, draining even modest amounts (100–200 mL) of fluid may result in striking improvement. Drainage is most commonly achieved by subxiphoid percutaneous pericardiocentesis. Although the procedure is effective and safe, there may be complications; the most common serious complication is laceration or puncture of the heart, typically the right ventricle, because of its anterior location. Echocardiography, by confirming the presence of a sufficiently large volume of fluid in an anterior location, can decrease the risk of cardiac puncture. The presence of at least 1 cm of echo-free space anterior to the heart has been recommended as a guideline for the minimum volume of fluid that should be present before percutaneous pericardiocentesis is undertaken. In addition, the patient should be positioned in a semi-upright position to allow inferior pooling of the effusion. An apical approach using echocardiographic guidance is preferred by some.

Several aspects of the performance of pericardiocentesis also contribute to a safe and successful outcome. The procedure is ideally carried out in the cardiac catheterization laboratory with fluoroscopic guidance and concomitant right-heart catheterization. The latter allows for hemodynamic confirmation of the diagnosis and assessment of the response to therapy. Occasionally, performance of emergency pericardiocentesis may be required at the bedside; however, it is rare for circumstances to be so critical as to preclude confirming the diagnosis with echocardiography.

Intravenous fluids and vasopressors can be administered as temporizing measures until the procedure can be performed. These modalities usually will not significantly improve the clinical status, however, and should never be used in place of or allowed to interfere with prompt evacuation of the fluid. Diuretics are contraindicated in this setting because they have the potential to markedly worsen the hemodynamic status.

Pericardial fluid can also be evacuated through a subxiphoid surgical pericardiotomy performed under local anesthesia; this procedure also permits pericardial biopsy in cases of suspected malignant effusion. The pericardial fluid should be sent for cultures and cytologic examination except when the tamponade is clearly traumatic. The gross appearance of the fluid is not helpful in establishing the cause, and cell counts and chemistries are also of limited value. The risks of pericardiocentesis must therefore be weighed against the likely benefits before performing the procedure solely for diagnostic purposes. Usually, a pericardial biopsy is most useful when the diagnosis is unclear.

In some cases, a single pericardiocentesis alleviates the effusion fully, but in most cases, a pericardial catheter should be left in place for continued drainage, typically for 24–48 hours. The catheter can be removed when the rate of drainage decreases and plans for definitive management of the pericardial disease are in place. Subsequent management is largely dictated by the specific cause of the effusion (discussed earlier).

Definitive management of pericardial fluid accumulation in some conditions may require surgical removal of the pericardium or the surgical creation of an opening between the pericardium and left pleura (a pericardial window). A percutaneous balloon technique for creating a pleuropericardial opening has also been described. If tissue is not required for diagnostic purposes, this may be the preferred technique for draining a chronically recurring effusion and preventing tamponade. Pericardial windows can close in patients with intense inflammation, and pericardial stripping or sclerosis may be required.

Lazaros G, Vlachopoulos C, Lazarou E, Tsioufis K. New approaches to management of pericardial effusions. *Curr Cardiol Rep.* 2022;23:106. [PMID: 34196832]

CONSTRICTIVE PERICARDITIS

ESSENTIALS OF DIAGNOSIS

- Markedly elevated jugular venous pressure with accentuated x and y descents and Kussmaul sign.
- Pericardial knock on auscultation.
- Magnetic resonance, computed tomography, or echocardiographic imaging showing a thickened pericardium.

General Considerations

Constrictive pericarditis can develop as the aftermath of virtually any pericardial injury or inflammation. Cardiac surgery, radiation therapy, and idiopathic causes are currently the most common. Tuberculous constriction, a leading cause in previous decades, is now rare in most of the industrialized world, but it remains significant in underdeveloped countries and may reappear in developed countries if tuberculosis continues to increase. A highly variable length of time—sometimes many years—can elapse between the initial insult and the development of constriction and its clinical manifestations. Recently the risk of evolution to constrictive pericarditis has been evaluated in 500 consecutive patients with acute pericarditis. The risk is essentially related to the etiology and not to the number of recurrences. Idiopathic and viral pericarditis has a low risk (< 1%), immune-mediated and neoplastic etiology has an intermediate risk (2–5%), and bacterial etiologies, especially tuberculosis and purulent forms, have the highest risk (20–30%).

The major physiologic perturbation of constrictive pericarditis is thickening (80% of cases, but 20% may have normal pericardial thickness), fibrosis, and (especially with tuberculosis) calcification of the pericardium, causing it to encase the heart in a solid, noncompliant envelope that impairs diastolic filling. In early diastole, the ventricles fill normally until the volume limit of the noncompliant pericardium is attained. At that point, diastolic filling halts abruptly. At the same time, the rigid pericardium markedly increases the intracardiac filling pressures. Because contractile function is usually normal, constrictive pericarditis can be considered an extreme example of heart failure that is caused by diastolic dysfunction.

Clinical Findings

A. Symptoms & Signs

Many symptoms of constrictive pericarditis are nonspecific and are related to chronically elevated cardiac filling pressures and chronically depressed cardiac output; symptoms secondary to venous congestion are most common and may simulate right heart failure. Ascites, peripheral edema, and symptoms referable to congestion of the gastrointestinal tract and liver (eg, dyspepsia, anorexia, postprandial fullness) usually develop. Cardiac cirrhosis may be present in extreme cases. Symptoms of left-sided congestion, such as exertional dyspnea, orthopnea, and cough, are uncommon. The chronically low cardiac output results in fatigue and, in conjunction with the effects of visceral congestion, wasting.

B. Physical Examination

The patient may have a striking body habitus with a marked contrast between a massively swollen abdomen and edematous lower extremities and a cachectic, wasted upper torso. Ascites, hepatomegaly with prominent hepatic pulsations, and other signs of hepatic failure are common.

Patients with constrictive pericarditis **have marked elevation of the jugular venous pressure.** In contrast with cardiac tamponade, the x and y descents are prominent, typically resulting in an M or W shape of the venous waves. Kussmaul sign—the loss of normal inspiratory decrease in the jugular venous pressure or even a frank increase with inspiration—may be present. The arterial pulse pressure may be diminished or normal. A pulsus paradoxus is present in perhaps one-third of cases.

Auscultation of the heart can reveal a characteristic early diastolic sound—the pericardial knock, which is caused by the sudden halt in ventricular filling by the thickened pericardium. The knock occurs slightly earlier in diastole than a third heart sound and has a higher acoustic frequency.

C. Diagnostic Studies

1. Electrocardiography—Characteristic ECG abnormalities in constrictive pericarditis are nonspecific and include low-voltage, T-wave inversions, and P mitrale or atrial fibrillation. Atrioventricular and intraventricular conduction delays or the development of Q waves are related to the extension of calcification into the myocardium and surrounding the coronary arteries.

2. Chest radiography—The cardiac silhouette on chest radiograph can be small, normal, or enlarged. The presence of pericardial calcifications (in no more than one-third of cases) is helpful because a number of patients with constriction have pericardial calcification. Conversely, a calcified pericardium does not always indicate constriction (Figure 28–8).

3. Echocardiography—Echocardiography may suggest pericardial thickening in most cases of constriction, although transthoracic echocardiography is not reliable to measure pericardial thickness. Transesophageal echocardiography is more reliable than transthoracic echocardiography for imaging pericardial thickness. Echocardiography may be useful in first raising the suspicion of constrictive pericarditis in a patient with right-heart failure signs and symptoms, by demonstrating preserved left ventricular ejection fraction, and normal or small cardiac chamber sizes. In cases with extreme limitation of cardiac filling or when pericardial calcification extends into the myocardium, left ventricular ejection may be impaired. Thus, preserved systolic function is not a prerequisite for diagnosis. A characteristic echocardiographic feature of constrictive pericarditis is the septal "bounce," a stuttering motion of the septum during diastole. A variety of indices using Doppler echocardiography to assess ventricular filling in various stages of diastole have been proposed to distinguish between constrictive pericarditis and restrictive cardiomyopathy. Those that appear most useful are exaggerated respiratory variations of transmitral flow velocity (> 25%), increased diastolic hepatic vein flow reversal in expiration, and inferior vena cava plethora. These findings are present in constriction but absent in restrictive cardiomyopathy. Also, tissue Doppler examination

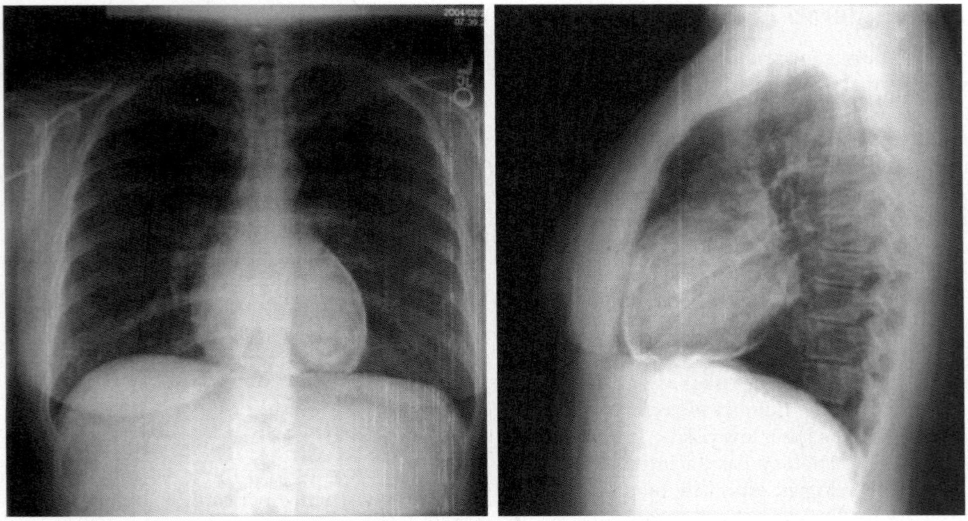

▲ **Figure 28–8.** Chest radiograph showing a heavily calcified pericardium in constrictive pericarditis. (Reprinted by permission from Cavendish JJ, et al. Constructive pericarditis from a severely calcified pericardium. *Circulation*. 2005;112:e137.)

reveals increased E′ velocity of the mitral annulus as well as septal abnormalities analogous to the "bounce" in constriction. Tissue Doppler appears to be at least as sensitive as conventional echocardiography Doppler for diagnosing constriction.

Specific echocardiographic criteria for the diagnosis of constrictive pericarditis have been recently proposed by the Mayo Clinic and include septal bounce or ventricular septal shift with either medial e′ > 8 cm/s or hepatic vein expiratory diastolic reversal ratio > 0.78 (sensitivity of 87%, specificity of 91%; specificity may increase to 97% if all criteria are present with a corresponding decrease of sensitivity to 64%).

4. Magnetic resonance imaging and computed tomography—Both of these methods are especially useful for imaging the pericardium. They are more accurate than echocardiography in this regard and provide a much more complete assessment of the appearance of the entire pericardium. Figure 28–9 is an example of a computed tomographic scan from the same patient whose chest radiograph is shown in Figure 28–8. Computed tomography is the best imaging technique to assess the presence and extent of calcifications and is especially useful for the surgical plan for pericardiectomy. Magnetic resonance imaging can be used to discern features of constrictive pericarditis such as the septal bounce and exaggerated interventricular interdependence (Figure 28–10). Although the presence of pericardial thickening ordinarily is a key point in distinguishing constrictive pericarditis, occasional cases of constriction in the absence of thickening have been reported (up to 20% of cases). Evidence of inflammation on CMR (evidence of pericardial edema and/or LGE) strongly supports a trial of empiric anti-inflammatory therapy before pericardiectomy since 40–60% of cases may be cured with medical therapy for pericarditis with regression of constriction following the resolution of pericarditis.

5. Cardiac catheterization—Cardiac catheterization can help establish the correct diagnosis. It confirms elevated—and usually virtually equal—diastolic pressures in both ventricles. The diastolic pressure waveform has been described as a square root sign, or dip and plateau: an exaggerated early diastolic downward deflection (the dip) followed by a rapid early pressure rise and plateau. This waveform, however, is not pathognomonic for constriction; it can also be found in restrictive cardiomyopathy. Examination of the right and left atrial waveforms reveals prominent x and y descents. As with the jugular venous waveform, the appearance of the atrial pressure recording has been likened to a W or an M shape. Several hemodynamic criteria are useful in distinguishing constrictive pericarditis from restrictive cardiomyopathy (Table 28–5). Although the accuracy of any one of these criteria is far from perfect, the concordance of all three criteria favoring constriction renders the diagnosis 91% certain. Similarly, if none or only one hemodynamic criterion in favor of constriction is met, the patient has restriction with 94% certainty. One-fourth of patients with the appropriate physiology will meet two criteria, making their chances of either diagnosis approximately equal.

As an expression of exaggerated interventricular interdependence, the ventricular pressure tracings show marked changes with respiration. Typically with constrictive pericarditis, the right ventricular pressure increases with inspiration and the LV pressure decreases, which is considered a discordant response. In restrictive

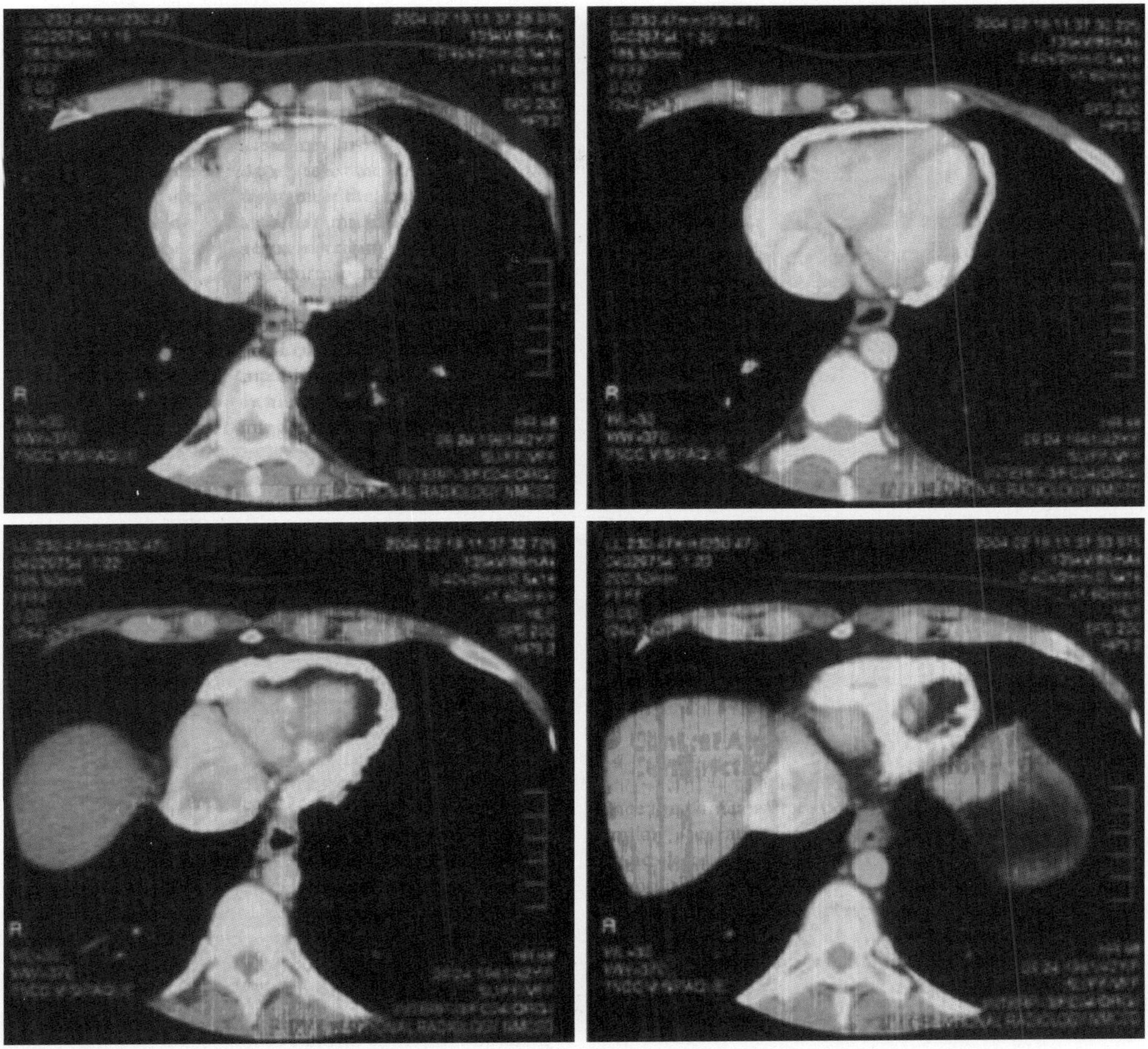

▲ **Figure 28–9.** Computed tomography scan from same patient as in Figure 28–8 showing a heavily calcified pericardium. (Reprinted by permission from Cavendish JJ, et al. *Circulation*. 2005;112:e137.)

cardiomyopathy, the two pressures change in the same direction with inspiration or a concordant response. The discordant response has a high predictive accuracy for constrictive pericarditis.

Differential Diagnosis

With the combined use of Doppler echocardiography, magnetic resonance imaging or computed tomography to image the pericardium, careful hemodynamic studies, and endomyocardial biopsy, it should be possible in the great majority of cases to distinguish constrictive pericarditis from restrictive cardiomyopathy. This distinction is not always possible, however, and such differentiation can sometimes be a major diagnostic challenge. Restrictive cardiomyopathy is a condition that is most commonly caused by infiltrative diseases of the myocardium such as amyloidosis, sarcoidosis, and hemochromatosis—or, in Africa, by endocardial fibroelastosis. Both constrictive pericarditis and restrictive cardiomyopathy are characterized by impaired diastolic filling of the ventricles. The two differ, however, in the degree of impairment of various phases of diastole. Unlike the

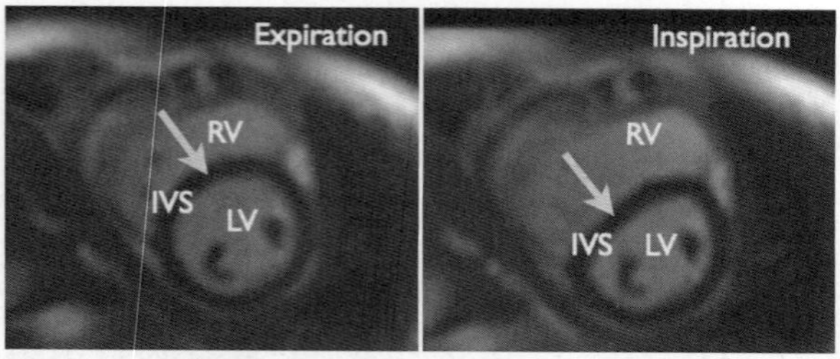

▲ **Figure 28–10.** Real-time cine magnetic resonance imaging of a short axis of the two ventricles during respiratory phases: it is evident that a septal bulge has been caused by the increased right ventricle volume (RV) during inspiration (see *white arrows*). IVS, interventricular septum; LV, left ventricle.

rapid early diastolic filling and abrupt halt of constrictive pericarditis, ventricular filling in restrictive cardiomyopathy is impaired uniformly throughout diastole. This physiologic difference underlies many of the features that help distinguish the two diagnoses. Other useful distinguishing features are biatrial enlargement, which is usually striking in restrictive cardiomyopathy and absent in constriction, and markedly increased ventricular wall thickness, which is the rule in most cases of restrictive cardiomyopathy. Last, brain natriuretic peptide levels are helpful; they are elevated in restrictive cardiomyopathy and normal in constriction. The correct differentiation of these two conditions is of paramount importance: Constrictive pericarditis is an eminently treatable disease; cardiac restriction of almost any cause carries a limited prognosis—despite therapy. When the distinction between constriction and restriction remains ambiguous, it may be necessary to proceed to thoracoscopy to permit direct inspection of the pericardium. Pulmonary hypertension causing right-heart failure has several similarities with both constrictive pericarditis and restrictive cardiomyopathy. Measurement of the pulmonary artery pressure and vascular resistance establishes the diagnosis of pulmonary hypertension.

Table 28–5. Hemodynamic Criteria Differentiating Constrictive Pericarditis from Restrictive Cardiomyopathy

Criteria Favoring Constriction	Predictive Accuracy (%)
Difference between LVEDP and RVEDP < 5 mm Hg	85
RV systolic pressure < 50 mm Hg	70
RVEDP:RV systolic pressure ratio > 0.33	76
Discordant RV, LV pressure changes with inspiration	100

LVEDP, left ventricular end-diastolic pressure; RV, right ventricle; RVEDP, right ventricular end-diastolic pressure.

At the bedside, constrictive pericarditis is sometimes difficult to distinguish from more common causes of congestive heart failure. Disproportionate right-sided failure or ascites out of proportion to peripheral edema may be clues to the presence of constriction. Because of the relative rarity of constriction, it is often not suspected, and congestive heart failure or even noncardiac cirrhosis is diagnosed instead. Because the primary form of therapy for constriction is surgical, it is essential to be sure that the diagnosis of constriction is correct.

Treatment

Although intensive medical management may effectively control symptoms, the long-term prognosis with medical therapy alone is limited. The natural history in most cases is one of advancing severity.

Pericardiectomy is the definitive treatment for chronic constrictive pericarditis. The only exception is early post-surgical constriction which, as discussed earlier, responds well to a course of corticosteroids. Clinicians should also be cautious in any case of newly diagnosed "constrictive pericarditis," since cases of transient constriction have been described, especially in the setting of pericarditis with effusion. Such cases can be identified by evidence of systemic inflammation (ie, elevated C-reactive protein) and pericardium enhancement by magnetic resonance imaging. Empiric anti-inflammatory therapy may be useful in this setting, and disappearance of constrictive features has been reported in 1–3 months. Careful observation is needed in these cases, and pericardiectomy is indicated only for persistent, chronic (> 3 months) cases.

In most cases, the procedure is straightforward, and the surgical mortality rate in recent series has ranged from 4% to 11%. Occasionally, however, the dense fibrosis and calcification extend into the epicardium, making identification of a cleavage plane impossible. The operation in this case is associated with excessive hemorrhage and an inability to relieve the compression completely. In other patients, hepatic or cardiac failure may be irreversible. The myocardium may undergo atrophy as a result of long-standing compression, and a low-cardiac-output state may persist after pericardiectomy. Such patients may require positive inotropic support for days to weeks after surgery.

In most cases, patients will exhibit dramatic and sustained improvement, although full improvement may occur only after several months. When symptoms are persistent or recurrent, three possibilities should be considered: myocardial dysfunction resulting from severe, prolonged constriction; incomplete or inadequate pericardiectomy; and recurrence of the constriction. In some cases, the inflammatory and fibrotic process involves the epicardial layers and progresses after the pericardium has been removed, leading to a recurrence of constrictive physiology and symptoms.

The combination of constrictive pericarditis and occlusive coronary artery disease is especially difficult to manage.

In some cases, the coronary lesions are due to the visceral pericardial process and stripping the pericardium may damage the coronary arteries. Bypass surgery can be extremely difficult in the presence of dense calcium. If the coronary obstructions are not corrected, however, the increased myocardial oxygen demands of increased cardiac filling following pericardiectomy may cause postoperative ischemia, which may severely complicate recovery from the surgery.

Chetrit M, Xu B, Kwon DH, et al. Imaging-guided therapies for pericardial diseases. *JACC Cardiovasc Imaging.* 2019;13(6):1422–1437. [PMID: 31734199]

EFFUSIVE-CONSTRICTIVE PERICARDITIS

ESSENTIALS OF DIAGNOSIS

- ► Echocardiographic demonstration of pericardial fluid.
- ► Persistence of elevated intracardiac filling pressures following pericardiocentesis.

Effusive-constrictive pericarditis combines features of pericardial effusion and constrictive pericarditis. The syndrome is dynamic and may represent an intermediate stage in the development of constrictive pericarditis. The most common causes of effusive-constrictive pericarditis are uremia and metastatic pericardial disease, but any cause of pericarditis can produce this condition. Echocardiography usually shows a small-to-moderate-sized effusion with strands of solid material between the visceral and parietal pericardium. Although effusive-constrictive pericarditis may be suspected on clinical grounds, the diagnosis is established through cardiac catheterization and characterization of the hemodynamics. Effusive-constrictive pericarditis can present as frank tamponade. As the effusion is drained during pericardiocentesis, elevation of intracardiac filling pressures persists and the recorded waveforms may exhibit the classic appearance of constriction.

Although pericardiocentesis may be associated with an improved cardiac output and diminished symptoms, subsequent management is essentially that for pericardial constriction. Thoracotomy with pericardiectomy is indicated to relieve the constriction in symptomatic patients who do not have diagnoses with a very poor short-term prognosis, such as advanced metastatic cancer.

Janus SE, Hoit BD. Effusive-constrictive pericarditis in the spectrum of pericardial compressive syndromes. *Heart.* 2021 Jan 15; doi: 10.1136/heartjnl-2020-316664. Epub ahead of print. Erratum in: *Heart.* 2021 Nov;107(22):e17. [PMID: 33452122]

29 Pulmonary Embolic Disease

Connor G. O'Brien, MD
Christopher F. Barnett, MD, MPH

ESSENTIALS OF DIAGNOSIS

- Otherwise unexplained dyspnea, tachypnea, or chest pain.
- Clinical, electrocardiogram, radiographic or echocardiographic evidence of acute right ventricular failure.
- Positive computed tomographic pulmonary angiography scan.
- High-probability ventilation-perfusion lung scan or high-probability perfusion lung scan with a normal chest radiograph.
- Positive venous ultrasound of the legs with a convincing clinical history and suggestive lung scan.
- Positive invasive pulmonary angiogram.

General Considerations

The term "venous thromboembolism" (VTE) encompasses both pulmonary embolism (PE) and deep venous thrombosis (DVT) and is a common cause of hospitalizations. Pulmonary embolism leads to or contributes to at least 100,000 deaths per year in the United States. With the widespread availability of computed tomographic pulmonary angiography (CT-PA) in mainstream clinical practice, a larger proportion of PE cases are now being diagnosed. The estimated incidence of PE has approximately doubled since the introduction of CT-PA in routine clinical practice, from 62.1 to 112.3 cases per 100,000 individuals in the United States. At the same time, the mortality of PE has decreased 33% from about 12% to 8%. Much of this effect can be attributed to increased recognition of low to moderate risk PEs. High-risk and intermediate high-risk PEs still carry significant morbidity and mortality. Risk stratification is now a central feature of society guidelines: attempting to minimize cost by encouraging outpatient treatment of low-risk VTE while promoting diagnostic vigilance in high- and intermediate-risk VTE. Improvements in noninvasive diagnostics now facilitate early recognition and intervention of high-risk PE, but realizing the benefits of these advancements is contingent on physicians being savvy with the interpretation of CT-PA and echocardiographic features of right ventricular (RV) failure. Improved noninvasive diagnostics also help identify and monitor disabling long-term complications of VTE like chronic thromboembolic pulmonary hypertension (CTEPH) and chronic venous insufficiency. Direct oral anticoagulants (DOACs) have created opportunities for improving outcomes and reducing costs via improved safety profiles and ease of administration, but DOACs have shortcomings in certain disease states of which providers must be aware. Lastly, VTE events raise important considerations like whether an occult malignancy is present, future risk of VTE, and whether risk extends to family members via inherited traits.

Etiology

"Primary" PE occurs in the absence of surgery or trauma. Patients with this condition often have an underlying hypercoagulable state, although a specific thrombophilic condition may not be identified. A common scenario is a clinically silent tendency toward thrombosis, which is precipitated by a stressor such as prolonged immobilization, oral contraceptives, pregnancy, or hormone replacement therapy. Recently, there has been an increased appreciation of the risks of VTE among patients with medical illnesses, including cancer (which itself may be associated with a hypercoagulable state), congestive heart failure, chronic obstructive pulmonary disease, and infectious diseases like COVID-19.

The prevalence of "secondary" PE is high among patients undergoing certain types of surgery, especially orthopedic surgery of the hip and knee, gynecologic cancer surgery, major trauma, and craniotomy for brain tumor. PE in these patients may occur as late as a month after discharge from the hospital.

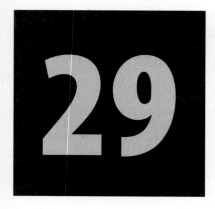

A. Thrombophilia

A thorough history should be obtained, including history of prior VTE, family history of VTE, history of frequent miscarriages, past history of cancer, recent history of heparin use (suggestive of heparin-induced thrombocytopenia), and history of prothrombotic conditions (myeloproliferative disease, nephrotic syndrome, collagen-vascular disease, and congestive heart failure). An acquired or heritable risk factor is found in as many as 50% of patients who present with an initial VTE. Principal thrombophilic risk factors for VTE are listed in Table 29–1. The two most common genetic mutations that predispose to VTE are the factor V Leiden and the prothrombin gene. Both are autosomal dominant. Whether factor V Leiden predisposes to recurrent VTE after anticoagulation is discontinued remains controversial. The prothrombin gene mutation is associated with an increased risk of recurrent VTE after discontinuation of anticoagulation, especially in patients who have coinherited the factor V Leiden mutation.

Laboratory screening for inherited thrombophilia does not always impact the treatment plan and therefore is not always indicated. Regardless of whether a risk factor is identified, just the history of having had a VTE event is the most significant risk factor for predicting future recurrence. Screening for deficiencies of antithrombin III, protein C, and protein S is a low-yield strategy that produces positive findings in less than 5% of patients. Heparin decreases the antithrombin III level, whereas warfarin, pregnancy, and oral contraceptives decrease the protein C and S levels, thereby resulting in potentially spurious diagnoses of these hypercoagulable states. There are no data supporting screening for or treating hyperhomocysteinemia in the setting of VTE. A positive finding of inherited thrombophilia does not necessarily imply that the patient is at higher risk for recurrent VTE or would benefit from an extended duration of anticoagulation. Therefore, the 2016 American College of Chest Physicians (ACCP) guidelines did not find that testing for inherited thrombophilic disorders should be a major determinant of VTE treatment. However, in patients with a strong family history of VTE, or based on strong patient preferences, screening can be considered for the patient and first-degree relatives, particularly if it may impact decisions about oral contraceptive use.

In contrast to screening for inheritable disorders, because malignancy is a hypercoagulable state and because VTE may be the first presenting symptom of malignancy, age-appropriate cancer screening after VTE is prudent.

Table 29–1. Thrombophilic Risk Factors for Venous Thromboembolism

Common
Factor V Leiden
Prothrombin gene mutation
Anticardiolipin antibodies (including lupus anticoagulant) as a feature of the antiphospholipid antibody syndrome
Hyperhomocysteinemia (usually due to folate deficiency)
Uncommon
Antithrombin III deficiency
Protein C deficiency
Protein S deficiency
Mutations of cystathionine β-synthase or methylene tetrahydrofolate reductase (MTHFR)
High concentrations of factors VIII or XI (or both)

B. Women's Health

PE poses a unique threat to women because VTE is associated with the use of oral contraceptives, pregnancy, and hormone replacement therapy.

One-third of pregnancy-related VTE occurs postpartum. The risk of DVT is present throughout pregnancy and is highest during the third trimester. After delivery, two of the most important risk factors for VTE are increased maternal age and cesarean section. Emergency cesarean section increases the VTE risk by about 50% compared with elective cesarean section.

Among women with a history of VTE during pregnancy or puerperium in one study, the prevalence of factor V Leiden was 44% and the prevalence of the prothrombin gene mutation was 17%. Compared with controls, the Leiden mutation increased the risk of VTE ninefold, and the prothrombin gene mutation increased the risk by a factor of 15. The combination of the Leiden and prothrombin gene mutations increased the VTE risk to more than 100 times that seen in the controls. Irrespective of factor V Leiden, pregnancy itself causes hypercoagulability because it induces a relative state of activated protein C resistance.

Hormone replacement therapy also predisposes to VTE. As with oral contraceptives, the risk of VTE peaks during the first year of hormone replacement therapy. Recent ESC guidelines now dictate that continuation of oral contraceptives is acceptable after VTE as long as therapeutic anticoagulation is in place. Women who experience VTE of oral contraceptives are recommended to take VTE prophylaxis in the antepartum and postpartum periods for future pregnancies.

Barco S, Valerio L, Ageno W, et al. Age-sex specific pulmonary embolism-related mortality in the USA and Canada, 2000-18: an analysis of the WHO Mortality Database and of the CDC Multiple Cause of Death database. *Lancet Respir Med.* Jan 2021;9(1):33–42. [PMID: 33058771]

Benjamin EJ, Muntner P, Alonso A, et al. Heart Disease and Stroke Statistics-2019 Update: A Report From the American Heart Association. *Circulation.* 2019;139(10):e56-e528. [PMID: 30700139]

Robert-Ebadi H, Elias A, Sanchez O, et al. Assessing the clinical probability of pulmonary embolism during pregnancy: The Pregnancy-Adapted Geneva (PAG) score. *J Thromb Haemost.* 2021;19:3044–3050. [PMID: 3449621]

Van Es N, Le Gal G, Otten HM, et al. Screening for occult cancer in patients with unprovoked venous thromboembolism. *Ann Intern Med.* 2017;167:410–417. [PMID: 28828492]

Clinical Findings

PE is often difficult to diagnose due to its variable clinical presentation. Acute PE can manifest clinically as high-risk, intermediate high-risk, intermediate low-risk, or low-risk based on the severity of the clinical presentation. This nomenclature is likely to replace the previous labels of massive, submassive, and nonmassive PE as these terms lack consensus definitions and lead to vague patient classifications in the medical literature. High-risk PE is a life-threatening condition characterized by sudden onset of chest pain/pressure, hypotension, hypoxemia, and distended neck veins, and it needs to be differentiated quickly from other potentially lethal conditions including acute myocardial infarction, tension pneumothorax, or pericardial tamponade. Despite the availability of chest computed tomography (CT) scanning and pulmonary angiography, many pulmonary emboli are not discovered until postmortem examination. Appreciation of the clinical settings that make patients susceptible to PE and maintenance of a high degree of clinical suspicion are of paramount importance.

A. Symptoms & Signs

The most common symptoms or signs of PE are nonspecific: dyspnea, tachypnea, chest pain, or tachycardia. Patients with life-threatening or high-risk PE commonly present with dyspnea, syncope, or cyanosis rather than chest pain. Less than one-third of patients with PE have symptoms of a DVT. High-risk PE should be suspected in hypotensive patients who have evidence of or predisposing factors for venous thrombosis and clinical findings of acute right ventricular failure, such as distended neck veins, a right-sided S_3 gallop, a right ventricular heave, tachycardia, or tachypnea. The definition of high-risk PE proposed by the European Society of Cardiology is: an acute PE with sustained hypotension (systolic blood pressure < 90 mm Hg for at least 15 minutes or requiring inotropic support, not due to a cause other than PE, such as arrhythmia, hypovolemia, sepsis, or left ventricular dysfunction), PESI score ≥ III or sPESI ≥ 1 (see Table 29–5), evidence of right ventricular dysfunction on TTE or CT, and positive biomarkers for myocardial injury. Intermediate high-risk PE has been defined as an acute PE without systemic hypotension but with PESI score ≥ III or sPESI ≥ 1, evidence of right ventricular dysfunction, and myocardial injury. Intermediate low-risk differs from intermediate high-risk in that there is no evidence of right ventricular dysfunction by TTE or CT scan. Low-risk PE is defined as an acute PE without the presence of hemodynamic instability, right ventricular dysfunction, or myocardial necrosis.

Patients with severe chest pain or hemoptysis usually have anatomically small PE near the periphery of the lung. This is where innervation is greatest and where pulmonary infarction is most likely to occur from a dearth of collateral bronchial circulation.

Decision algorithms have been developed to help determine the probability of PE based on clinical symptoms and signs and to guide the selection of diagnostic tests to make a rapid and accurate diagnosis and thus initiate treatment without delay. To this end, an integrated diagnostic approach for cases of suspected PE, as shown in Figure 29–1, has been shown to be useful. The diagnostic workup should begin by quantifying the clinical suspicion with a precise clinical scoring algorithm.

Traditionally, the clinical likelihood of PE has been estimated subjectively by "gestalt" as low, intermediate, or high. However, to better define the clinical probability of PE in a given patient, quantitative clinical scoring systems have been devised to provide the clinician with a standardized and objective approach.

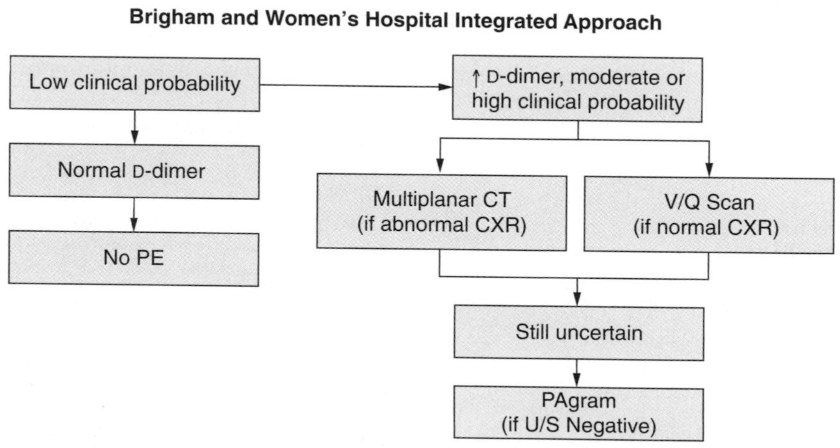

▲ **Figure 29–1.** Strategy for diagnosing pulmonary embolism. CT, computed tomography; CXR, chest x-ray film; PAgram, pulmonary angiogram; PE, pulmonary embolism; U/S, ultrasound.

Table 29–2. Ottawa (Modified Wells) Scoring System

Signs or Symptoms	Points
Hemoptysis	1.0
Malignancy (on treatment, treated in the last 6 months or palliative)	1.0
Heart rate > 100 bpm	1.5
Immobilization or surgery in the previous 4 weeks	1.5
Previous DVT or PE	1.5
Clinical signs and symptoms of DVT (minimum of leg swelling and pain with palpation of the deep veins)	3.0
An alternative diagnosis is less likely than PE	3.0
Risk level	**Score**
Low	0.1
Intermediate	2.6
High	≥7

DVT, deep vein thrombosis; PE, pulmonary embolism.

One of the most widely used clinical scoring systems is the Ottawa Scoring System (also known as the modified Wells index), which has a maximum of 12.5 points (Table 29–2). The greatest emphasis is placed on the presence of signs or symptoms of DVT (3 points) and whether an alternative diagnosis is unlikely (3 points). If the score exceeds 4 points, the overall likelihood of PE being confirmed with imaging tests is 41%. However, if the score is 4 points or less, the likelihood of PE is only 8%. Although this scoring system has the advantage of simplicity and rapidity, it offers a somewhat subjective approach with regard to the important, heavily weighted category of "alternative diagnosis unlikely."

In clinical settings such as outpatient clinics or emergency departments where the overall prevalence of PE is low but many patients have symptoms such as chest pain or shortness of breath, the Pulmonary Embolism Rule-out Criteria (PERC) may be used to exclude a PE without additional diagnostic testing. The eight factors that constitute the PERC are age less than 50 years, heart rate less than 100 bpm, oxygen saturation ≥ 95%, no hemoptysis, no estrogen use, no prior history of PE or DVT, no unilateral leg swelling, and no surgery or trauma needing hospitalization within the past 4 weeks. If a patient does not have any of the PERC criteria *and* has a low clinical suspicion of PE using clinical gestalt or the modified Wells index, then the diagnosis of PE can likely be excluded without additional diagnostic testing. This approach has been validated in a multicenter cohort study of more than 8,000 emergency department patients, but it should only be used in a setting where the prevalence of acute PE is low.

B. Diagnostic Studies

1. Non-imaging Studies

A. ELECTROCARDIOGRAPHY—Electrocardiograms (ECG) may show evidence of acute cor pulmonale, manifested by a new S_1 Q_3 T_3 pattern, new incomplete right bundle branch block, right axis deviation, or right ventricular ischemia or strain with ST-segment depressions in the right precordial leads. However, these changes are usually only seen in patients with acute high-risk PE, and therefore, absence of these ECG changes in a patient with suspected PE should not preclude additional diagnostic testing. Some ECG findings that have been associated with an adverse prognosis in patients with acute PE include atrial arrhythmias, right bundle branch block, Q waves in the inferior leads III and aVF, and ST-segment changes and T-wave inversions in the precordial leads.

B. ARTERIAL BLOOD GASES—Neither measurement of room air arterial blood gases nor calculation of the alveolar-arterial oxygen gradient is useful in excluding the diagnosis of PE. Among patients in whom PE is suspected, neither test helped differentiate patients with a confirmed PE at angiography from those with a normal pulmonary angiogram. Therefore, arterial blood gases should not be obtained as a screening test for suspected PE.

C. PLASMA D-DIMER ENZYME-LINKED IMMUNOSORBENT ASSAY—Endogenous fibrinolysis, although ineffective in preventing PE, almost always causes the release of D-dimers from fibrin clot in the presence of established PE. However, an elevated D-dimer test is not specific and may occur in a variety of other conditions including acute comorbid illnesses, such as acute myocardial infarction, metastatic cancer, sepsis, or recent surgery. A normal (< 500 ng/mL) result virtually excludes the diagnosis of PE in those less than 50 years old: among patients with a normal D-dimer level, the likelihood of PE is less than 5%. In patients older than 50 years, age-adjusted D-dimer thresholds should be used (age × 10 ng/mL). Despite its sensitivity, in patients with a very high clinical suspicion of PE, the D-dimer should not be used in isolation to exclude PE. The combination of low clinical suspicion, ideally quantified with a validated scoring system, and a normal D-dimer enzyme-linked immunosorbent assay makes PE exceedingly unlikely.

D. TROPONIN LEVELS—Screening for troponins is now the standard blood test for cardiac injury, and it is obtained routinely when acute myocardial infarction or unstable angina is suspected. Circulating troponin indicates irreversible myocardial cell damage and is much more sensitive than creatine kinase or its myocardial muscle isoenzyme. Cardiac markers of injury should not be used, however, as a primary diagnostic test for acute PE. Nevertheless, elevation of cardiac troponin is an adverse prognostic factor in patients with acute PE and is associated with a markedly increased mortality rate and requirement for inotropic support and

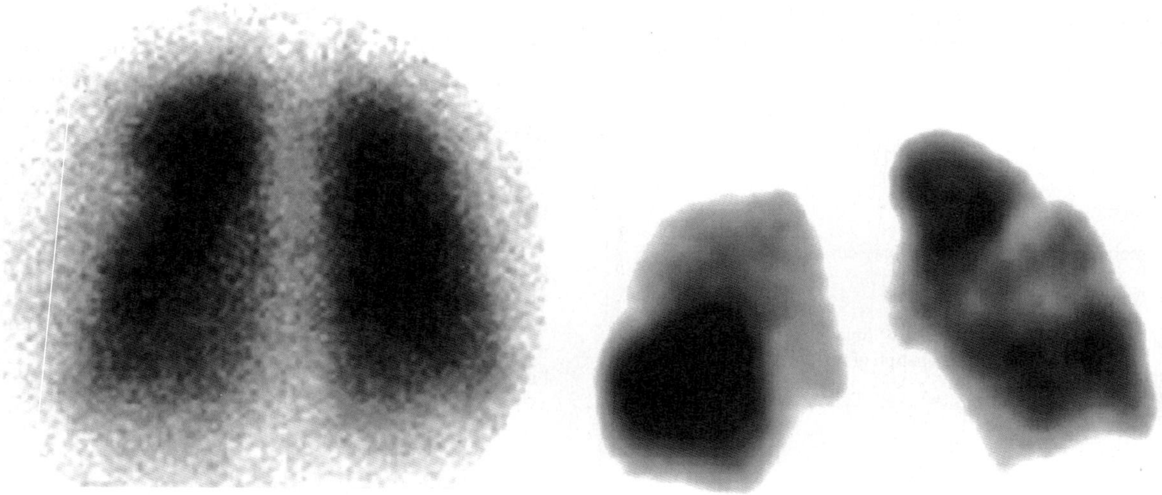

▲ **Figure 29–2.** Lung scan for a 63-year-old woman who presented with idiopathic pulmonary embolism. The lung scan showed (**A**) normal ventilation and (**B**) multiple segmental perfusion defects, indicating a ventilation-perfusion mismatch and high probability of pulmonary embolism.

mechanical ventilation. Troponin elevation also correlates with ECG evidence of right ventricular strain. This suggests that the release of troponin from the myocardium during PE may result from acute right ventricular microinfarction due to pressure overload, impaired coronary artery blood flow, or hypoxemia caused by the PE. A meta-analysis of 20 observational studies showed that patients with acute PE with elevated troponin T or troponin I levels had a fivefold higher risk of short-term mortality and a ninefold increased risk of death due to PE.

E. Brain natriuretic peptide (BNP) levels—As with cardiac troponins, measurement of BNP levels or N-terminal proBNP (NT-proBNP) levels should not be used to diagnose an acute PE. However, elevation of BNP or NT-proBNP levels may reflect right ventricular dysfunction in the setting of an acute PE and therefore may have prognostic value. In a meta-analysis of 16 studies of patients with acute PE, in-hospital or short-term mortality was increased sixfold in those with a BNP level more than 100 pg/mL and 16-fold among those with an NT-proBNP level more than 600 ng/L.

2. Diagnostic Studies

A. Chest radiography—Chest radiography can help exclude diseases such as lobar pneumonia, pneumothorax, or cardiogenic pulmonary edema, which can have clinical presentations that mimic acute PE. However, patients with these disorders can also have concomitant PE.

B. Radionuclide lung scanning—This study previously served as the principal diagnostic imaging test for PE but has been replaced by chest CT scanning. Lung scanning is most useful when unequivocally normal or when highly suggestive of PE (Figure 29–2). Neither intermediate nor low-probability scans (in the presence of high clinical suspicion) exclude PE. For example, with the combination of a low-probability scan and high clinical suspicion for PE, the likelihood of PE is 40%. When lung scanning is performed, the ventilation scan is being used less frequently than previously because its contribution to the diagnostic decision is only marginally better than the combination of a perfusion scan and chest radiograph.

C. Chest CT scanning—The CTPA is the gold standard modality for diagnosing PE. PE is diagnosed by visualization of an intraluminal pulmonary arterial filling defect surrounded by contrast. CT scanning has significant advantages over other diagnostic modalities by allowing for direct visualization of thrombus, estimation of thrombus burden, identification of high venous filling pressures and RV distension suggestive of RV failure, and establishment of additional or alternative pulmonary, thoracic, and cardiac pathology.

CTPA, multidetector CT, or dual-energy CT are now the preferred standard scanning modalities. Both modalities acquire high-resolution cuts ranging from 5 mm to 1.25 mm providing excellent visualization of subsegmental vessels. Multirow detector scanners provide 80–90% sensitivity for the diagnosis of acute PE (Figure 29–3).

Occasionally, determining whether a pulmonary embolus represents the residua of prior PE or a new event may be challenging. A systematic review of the literature has shown that over half of patients with PE will still have a defect

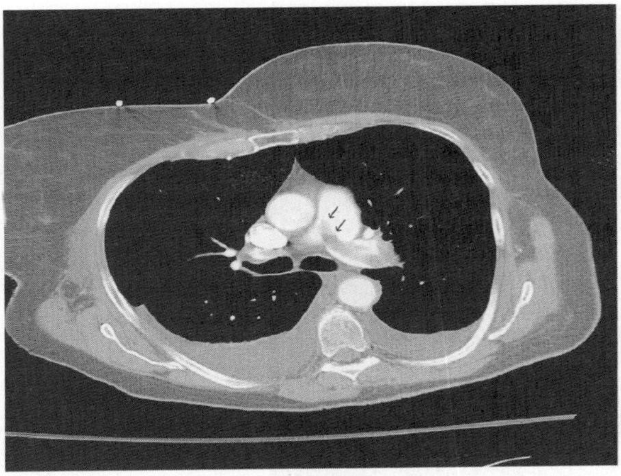

▲ **Figure 29–3.** Spiral computed tomography scan of high-risk bilateral pulmonary arterial filling defects (*arrows*) in the main pulmonary arteries of a 72-year-old woman who suffered acute pulmonary embolism after general surgery.

on either CT scan or radionuclide imaging 6 months after diagnosis.

D. Venous ultrasonography—In combination with color Doppler imaging, venous ultrasonography is known as duplex sonography and is the principal diagnostic imaging test for suspected acute DVT. Sonographic evaluation uses compression ultrasound along the full length of the femoral, popliteal, and calf veins. The transducer is held transverse to the vein and, normally, the vein collapses with gentle compression with the ultrasound probe. The compressed vein appears as if it is winking. The main criterion for diagnosing DVT is the inability to obliterate the lumen of a deep vein with compression. This diagnosis can be confirmed by direct visualization of thrombus on ultrasound or by abnormal venous flow on Doppler examination (eg, loss of physiologic respiratory variation or loss of the expected augmentation of blood flow during calf compression).

Among symptomatic patients, duplex sonography is very accurate, with high sensitivity and specificity. Its sensitivity decreases when assessing asymptomatic patients. Major limitations include an inability to image pelvic vein thrombosis directly, lower sensitivity for diagnosing isolated calf DVT, and difficulty diagnosing an acute DVT superimposed on a chronic one. Magnetic resonance imaging may be useful under these circumstances.

Importantly, many patients with PE do not have evidence of leg DVT, probably because the thrombus has already embolized the pulmonary arteries. Therefore, PE is not necessarily ruled out if the clinical suspicion is high and imaging evidence of DVT is lacking.

E. Echocardiography—Echocardiography should not be used routinely to diagnose suspected PE because most patients with PE have normal echocardiograms. However, the echocardiogram, like the troponin level, is an excellent tool for risk stratification and prognostication. Echocardiography is useful diagnostically when the differential diagnosis includes pericardial tamponade, right ventricular infarction, and dissection of the aorta as well as PE.

Imaging a normal left ventricle in the presence of a dilated, hypokinetic right ventricle strongly suggests the diagnosis of PE (Figure 29–4). The presence of right ventricular mid-free wall akinesis with sparing of the apex (the McConnell sign) has been found to be highly specific for acute PE. Occasionally clot in transit can also be identified by echo, helping identify acute risk for further embolism

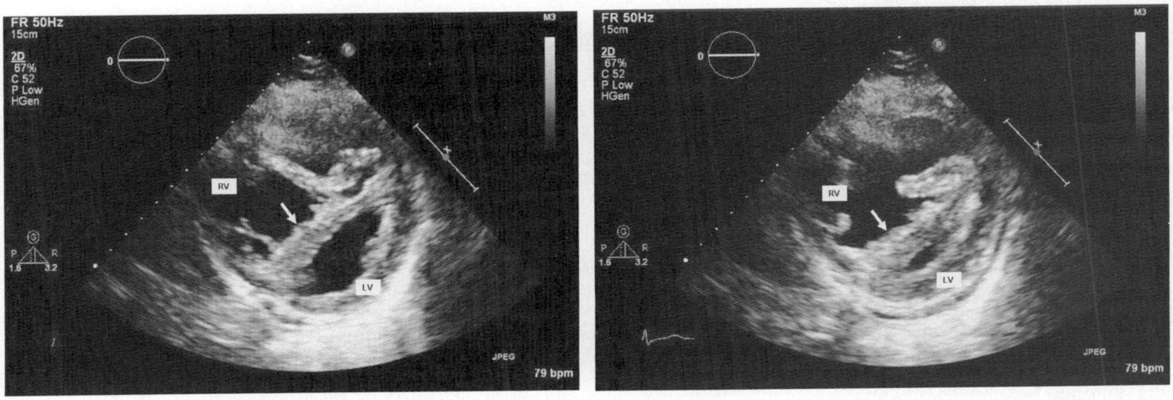

A B

▲ **Figure 29–4.** Parasternal short-axis views of the right ventricle (RV) and left ventricle (LV) in (**A**) diastole and (**B**) systole. Diastolic and systolic bowing of the interventricular septum (*arrows*) into the LV is evident, which is compatible with RV volume and pressure overloads, respectively. The RV is appreciably dilatated and markedly hypokinetic, with little change in apparent RV area from diastole to systole.

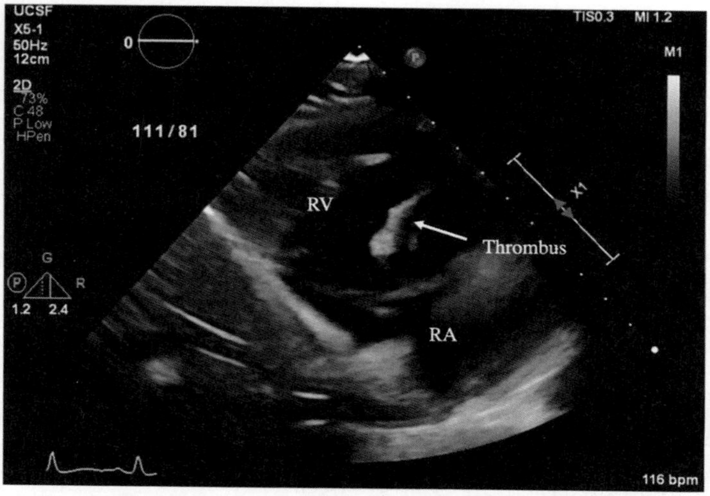

▲ **Figure 29–5.** Right ventricular inflow view showing a large clot in transit in the right ventricle. Thrombus is pinned between the lateral leaflet of the tricuspid valve and the right ventricular free wall.

(Figure 29–5). Echocardiographic findings in PE patients are summarized in Table 29–3.

The pulmonary arterial systolic pressure can be estimated by measuring the peak velocity of the tricuspid regurgitant jet obtained with Doppler echocardiography. The gradient across the tricuspid valve can be estimated by using the modified Bernoulli equation, $P = 4V^2$, where V is the peak velocity of the regurgitant jet, and P represents the peak pressure difference between the right atrium and right ventricle. The estimated right atrial pressure is added to the gradient to obtain an estimate of pulmonary arterial systolic pressure. The pulmonary artery systolic pressure may be low, normal, or mildly elevated in the setting of acute PE. Significant pulmonary hypertension suggests a subacute or chronic process. The incidence of chronic thromboembolic pulmonary hypertension following the first episode of PE is low overall (~1%), but in patients with unexplained persistent dyspnea after PE, the incidence may be as high as 4% after

Table 29–3. Abnormal Echocardiographic Findings in Pulmonary Embolism

Abnormal Finding	Description
Right ventricular dilatation and hypokinesis	Associated with leftward septal shift; the ratio of the RVEDA to LVEDA exceeds the upper limit of normal (0.6). Associated with right atrial enlargement and tricuspid regurgitation.
Septal flattening and paradoxical septal motion	Right ventricular contraction continues even after the left ventricle starts relaxing at end-systole; therefore, the interventricular septum bulges toward the left ventricle.
Diastolic left ventricular impairment with a small difference between left ventricular area during diastole and systole, indicative of low cardiac output	Due to septal displacement and reduced left ventricular distensibility during diastole; consequently, Doppler mitral flow exhibits a prominent A wave, much higher than the E wave, with an increased contribution of atrial contraction to left ventricular filling.
Direct visualization of PE	Only if PE is large and centrally located; much more easily visualized on transesophageal than on transthoracic echocardiography.
Pulmonary arterial hypertension detected by Doppler flow velocity in the right ventricular outflow tract	Shortened acceleration time, with peak velocity occurring close to the onset of ejection. Biphasic ejection curve, with midsystolic reduction in velocity.
Right ventricular hypertrophy	With mildly increased right ventricular thickness (often about 6 mm, with 4 mm as upper limit of normal); clear visualization of right ventricular muscle trabeculations.
Patent foramen ovale	When right atrial pressure exceeds left atrial pressure, the foramen ovale may open and cause worsening hypoxemia or stroke.

LVEDA, left ventricular end–diastolic area; PE, pulmonary embolism; RVEDA, right ventricular end–diastolic area.

2 years. Echocardiography to measure pulmonary artery pressure and exclude chronic thromboembolic pulmonary hypertension should be obtained for patients with persistent unexplained dyspnea following treatment of PE.

Transesophageal echocardiography for suspected PE is best reserved for critically ill patients. Transesophageal echocardiography diagnoses PE by direct visualization of thrombus, assesses its extent, and provides guidance regarding its surgical accessibility. Transesophageal echocardiography may also have a valuable role in detecting unexplained sudden cardiac arrest and pulseless electrical activity due to acute PE. In a series of 1,246 patients who suffered cardiac arrest, 5% of cases were caused by PE; of those with PE, 63% of cardiac arrest cases were caused by pulseless electrical activity. Therefore, when pulseless electrical activity is present, the possibility of an acute PE should be considered.

F. Pulmonary angiography—Pulmonary angiography was considered to be the "gold standard" diagnostic modality for the diagnosis of acute PE. This imaging method is rapidly becoming a lost art and is being undertaken primarily for therapeutic interventions rather than to solve diagnostic dilemmas. Most diagnostic questions can be resolved with the new-generation chest CT scanners, which provide resolution to subsegmental branches. A constant intraluminal filling defect seen in more than one projection is the most reliable angiographic diagnostic feature for PE.

Pulmonary angiography can almost always be accomplished safely, although the risk may be increased in patients with severe pulmonary hypertension. Selective angiography should be performed, with the equivocal portion of the perfusion lung scan or chest CT scan serving as a road map. To avoid damaging the intima of the pulmonary artery, soft, flexible catheters with side holes should be used, rather than stiff catheters with end holes. Low-osmolar contrast agents minimize the transient hypotension, heat, and coughing that often occur with conventional radioactive contrast agents.

Boon G, Verhaar YME, Beenen LFM, et al. Prediction of chronic thromboembolic pulmonary hypertension with standardised evaluation of initial computed tomography pulmonary angiography performed for suspected acute pulmonary embolism. *Eur Radiol.* Apr 2022;32(4):2178–2187. [PMID: 34854928]

Kearon C, de Wit K, Parpia S, et al. Diagnosis of pulmonary embolism with D-dimer adjusted to clinical probability. *N Engl J Med.* 2019;381:2125–2134. [PMID: 31774957]

Klok FA, Ageno W, Ay C, et al. Optimal follow-up after acute pulmonary embolism: a position paper of the European Society of Cardiology Working Group on Pulmonary Circulation and Right Ventricular Function, in collaboration with the European Society of Cardiology Working Group on Atherosclerosis and Vascular Biology, endorsed by the European Respiratory Society. *Eur Heart J.* Jan 25 2022;43(3):183–189. [PMID: 34875048]

Le Roux PY, Robin P, Tromeur C, et al. Ventilation/perfusion SPECT for the diagnosis of pulmonary embolism: A systematic review. J. Thromb. Haemost. 2020;18:2910–2920. [PMID: 33433051]

Robert-Ebadi H, Robin P, Hugli O, et al. Impact of the age-adjusted D-dimer cutoff to exclude pulmonary embolism: a multinational prospective real-life study (the RELAX-PE Study). *Circulation.* 2021:1828–1830. [PMID: 33939529]

Valerio L, Turatti G, Klok FA, et al. Prevalence of pulmonary embolism in 127 945 autopsies performed in cancer patients in the United States between 2003 and 2019. *J Thromb Haemost.* Jun 2021;19(6):1591–1593. [PMID: 34047011]

Prevention

PE is easier and less expensive to prevent than to diagnose or treat; therefore, virtually all hospitalized patients should receive prophylaxis against VTE. Unfortunately, such prophylaxis is underutilized, even for high-risk patients. Furthermore, prophylaxis, even when instituted, may not be effective. Nonetheless, prevention programs should be established at all hospitals to ensure that adequate measures are implemented. Nurses and physicians must collaborate to achieve this goal by instituting standardized protocols. In addition, quality assurance personnel should adopt a proactive stance to encourage the development of such programs.

The preventive measures should be based on an assessment of the patient's level of risk for PE and whether the optimal strategy will be nonpharmacologic, pharmacologic, or combined modalities. Because the risk of PE continues after discharge from the hospital, prophylaxis should be continued at home among those patients at moderate or high risk for VTE.

A. Nonpharmacologic Prevention

The most commonly used nonpharmacologic measures are graduated compression stockings (GCS) and intermittent pneumatic compression devices (IPC or "SCD boots"). Vascular compression with either GCS or IPC is effective among surgical patients because it counters the otherwise-unopposed perioperative venodilation that appears causally related to postoperative venous thrombosis. Even among low-risk general surgery patients, graduated compression stockings can substantially reduce the frequency of venous thrombosis and should therefore be considered first-line prophylaxis against PE in all hospitalized patients, except those with peripheral arterial occlusive disease whose condition may be worsened by vascular compression. GCS are not, however, recommend for the prevention of post-thrombotic syndrome after the development of a DVT.

IPC boots, which provide intermittent inflation of air-filled cuffs, prevent venous stasis in the legs; they also appear to stimulate the endogenous fibrinolytic system. Because it appears that GCS and IPC boots work through somewhat different—although complementary—mechanisms, these modalities can be used in combination in patients at moderate or high risk for venous thrombosis.

B. Pharmacologic Prevention

Anticoagulant drugs can be used instead of—or in addition to—nonpharmacologic prophylaxis. Several agents are used for prophylaxis against VTE in patients at high risk for thrombosis. These include unfractionated heparin (usually administered at a dose of 5,000 units subcutaneously twice or thrice daily), low-molecular-weight heparins (LMWHs) such as enoxaparin or dalteparin, and antithrombin-binding pentasaccharides such as fondaparinux. Other agents have recently been recommended for use for VTE prophylaxis in selected patient populations, such as vitamin K antagonists and direct oral anticoagulants (DOACs), including dabigatran, rivaroxaban, apixaban, and edoxaban.

The American College of Chest Physicians, European Society of Cardiology, and American Society of Hematology have all published clinical guidelines for the use of thromboprophylaxis in hospitalized patients. All critically ill patients should receive thromboprophylaxis with either LMWH (such as enoxaparin or dalteparin) or low-dose unfractionated heparin, unless they are actively bleeding or are at high risk of major bleeding, in which case they should receive nonpharmacologic prophylaxis with GCS or IPC devices until the bleeding risk is reduced. For acutely ill, nonsurgical hospitalized patients who are at high risk for thrombosis, pharmacologic prophylaxis is recommended with LMWH, low-dose unfractionated heparin (at a dose of 5,000 units two to three times per day), or fondaparinux. For nonsurgical hospitalized patients with high risk for thrombosis who are bleeding or are at risk for major bleeding, nonpharmacologic prophylaxis should be used. Hospitalized patients at low risk for thrombosis should not receive any thromboprophylaxis, and early and frequent ambulation is desirable in these patients.

The ACCP clinical guidelines also provide detailed recommendations for the use of thromboprophylaxis for patients undergoing orthopedic and non-orthopedic surgery. Table 29–4 lists the various pharmacologic agents that are recommended for use in patients undergoing orthopedic

Table 29–4. Food and Drug Administration–Approved Low-Molecular-Weight Regimens for Orthopedic and General Surgery Prophylaxis

Indication	Drug and Dose	Duration	Timing of Initial Dose
Hip replacement ("USA-style") with enoxaparin	Enoxaparin 30 mg q12h or 40 mg q24h	≤ 14 days	12–24 h postoperatively, providing that hemostasis has been achieved
Hip replacement ("European style") with enoxaparin	Enoxaparin 40 mg q24h	≤ 14 days	12 h ± 3 h preoperatively
Hip replacement with dalteparin (option #1)	Dalteparin 2500 units preoperatively and first dose postoperatively, followed by 5000 units q24h	≤ 14 days	First dose within 2 h preoperatively; second dose at least 6 h after the first dose, usually on the evening of the day of surgery; omit second dose on the day of surgery if surgery is done in the evening
Hip replacement with dalteparin (option #2)	Dalteparin 5000 units q24h	≤ 14 days	First dose on the preoperative evening; second dose on the evening of the day of surgery (unless surgery is done in the evening)
Extended hip prophylaxis	Enoxaparin 40 mg q24h	An additional 3 weeks after initial hip replacement prophylaxis	After the initial hip replacement prophylaxis regimen has been completed
General surgery with enoxaparin	Enoxaparin 40 mg q24h	≤ 12 days	2 h preoperatively
General surgery with dalteparin (moderate risk for venous thromboembolism)	Dalteparin 2500 units q24h	5–10 days	1–2 h preoperatively
General surgery with dalteparin (high risk for venous thromboembolism: option #1)	Dalteparin 5000 units q24h	5–10 days	Preoperative evening
General surgery with dalteparin (high risk for venous thromboembolism: option #2)	Dalteparin 2500 units preoperatively and first dose postoperatively, followed by 5000 units q24h	5–10 days	First dose 1–2 h preoperatively; second dose 12 h later

and general surgery. In patients undergoing total hip or total knee arthroplasty, the ACCP recommends the use of one of the following agents for thromboprophylaxis for a minimum of 10–14 days: LMWH (enoxaparin or dalteparin), fondaparinux, apixaban, dabigatran, rivaroxaban, low-dose unfractionated heparin, adjusted-dose vitamin K antagonist (warfarin), aspirin, or an IPC device. In patients undergoing major orthopedic surgery who have an increased risk of bleeding, they recommend the use of an IPC or no prophylaxis rather than pharmacologic treatment. Patients undergoing general and abdominal-pelvic surgery at very low or low risk for VTE should receive nonpharmacologic prophylaxis using IPC devices and early ambulation, whereas those at moderate to high risk for VTE but not at high risk for major bleeding should receive pharmacologic prophylaxis with LMWH or low-dose unfractionated heparin, along with the use of nonpharmacologic agents such as IPC devices in high-risk patients.

C. Future Directions

Many hospitals routinely use protocol-driven prophylaxis for all hospitalized patients, especially for medical patients hospitalized in intensive care units. Decision support tools being integrated into electronic medical record via admission and discharge order sets prompting providers to consider DVT prophylaxis. These decision support tools can integrate risk calculators like the Padua Prediction Score (for medical population) or Caprini Score (for surgical population) to help determine the appropriate prophylaxis strategy both during admission as well as on hospital discharge. Orders to prescribe prophylactic measures are then suggested to the provider improving standardization of care. Treatment recommendations and metrics will likely change in coming years as the role of DOACs expands both for inpatient and outpatient populations.

Schünemann HJ, Cushman M, Burnett AE, et al. American Society of Hematology 2018 guidelines for management of venous thromboembolism: Prophylaxis for hospitalized and nonhospitalized medical patients. *Blood Adv*. 2018;2:3198–3225. [PMID: 30482763]

Risk Stratification

Diagnostic and therapeutic advances have facilitated the creation of robust risk stratification tools. Low-risk PE, in particular, carries strong evidence describing a reliable treatment pathway allowing early discharge and outpatient management with DOACs. More intermediate and intermediate high-risk pulmonary embolisms are now being identified with the expanded use of CT, more frequent biochemical testing for myocardial injury or strain, and increased reporting of radiographic evidence for RV dysfunction.

The Pulmonary Embolism Severity Index (PESI) is a clinical scoring system that uses a total of 11 weighted parameters, including demographic characteristics (age and male sex), comorbid illnesses (cancer, heart failure, and chronic lung disease), and clinical findings (heart rate, systolic blood pressure, respiratory rate, body temperature, alteration of mental status, and arterial oxygen saturation) that has been shown to predict 30-day mortality in patients with acute PE. PESI scores range from 0 to 5. Scores are divided into five risk classes (Class I–V), I (0–1.6%) being associated with lowest and V (10–24.5%) highest 30-day mortality. PESI can help discriminate low versus intermediate versus high-risk PEs. A simplified version of the PESI (sPESI) has also been validated. sPESI is a simple, unweighted, 8-point index, but only differentiates high (> 8.8% 30-day mortality) from low (< 1.1% 30-day mortality). The simplified PESI score is summarized in Table 29–5. It is important to recognize the limitations of PESI and sPESI and that evaluation of the right ventricle and biochemical markers or RV injury should be considered even with a low-risk PESI or sPESI score. Studies have shown a modest but significant increase in 30-day mortality for patients with sPESI scores of 0 but evidence of RV dysfunction either by CT or echocardiography suggests these patients should be considered at low-intermediate risk.

A comprehensive evaluation for hemodynamic compromise is now recommended for all patients diagnosed with a pulmonary embolism. Early identification of high-risk and intermediate high-risk PEs is essential to optimizing outcomes. Previously the gold standard for identification of RV dysfunction was echocardiography. Acute RV pressure overload can be identified by echocardiography. Free-wall hypokinesis with apical buckling (McConnell's sign) is a specific but not sensitive sign for pulmonary embolus. The accepted mechanism behind McConnell's sign is pressure overload drives acute spherical remodeling and ischemia of the RV free wall. The 60:60 rule can also describe acute compromise of RV performance through a reduced RVOT VTI acceleration time of less than 60 ms and PASP of less than 60 mm Hg. LVOT VTI less than 15 cm has also been shown

Table 29–5. Simplified Pulmonary Embolism Severity Index (PESI)

		Points
Age > 80		1
Cancer		1
Chronic cardiopulmonary disease		1
Systolic blood pressure < 100 mm Hg		1
Oxygen saturation ≤ 90%		1
Severity Class	**Points**	**30-day Mortality**
Low risk	0	1%
High risk	≥ 1	>8.8%

Data from Jimenez D, et al. *Arch Intern Med*. 2010;170:1383–1389.

to predict poor outcomes in PE. While LV performance is preserved, a low VTI suggests a reduced LV stroke volume arising from compromised right to left flow.

Advancements in CT scan technology now allow for interpretation of interventricular size relationships and contrast distribution. RV:LV intracavitary diameter ratio more than 0.9 has been shown to predict hemodynamic instability and poor outcomes in PE. Some studies have suggested that an RV:LV ratio of more than 1.0 may have greater specificity for high-risk pulmonary embolism. Evidence of reflux of contrast into the IVC and liver can further support a diagnosis of RV dysfunction and systemic congestion. Given widespread access to CT, use of radiographic evidence of RV dysfunction can be useful in early identification of high-risk and intermediate high-risk PE.

Biomarkers that reflect right ventricular pressure overload or ischemia carry prognostic value. Elevations in BNP, NT-proBNP, and/or troponin are associated with worse outcomes across all PE risk classes, and normal enzyme levels in low-risk PE have a high negative predictive value for poor outcomes. Guideline organizations now recommend the routine use of natriuretic peptides and troponin to risk stratify PEs, and elevated enzyme levels should prompt evaluation of right ventricular function.

Any signs of right ventricular dysfunction or strain should prompt admission for observation. Evidence suggests that intermediate high-risk patients remain at risk for hemodynamic compromise for 2–3 days.

Barco S, Mahmoudpour SH, Planquette B, Sanchez O, Konstantinides SV, Meyer G. Prognostic value of right ventricular dysfunction or elevated cardiac biomarkers in patients with low-risk pulmonary embolism: a systematic review and meta-analysis. *Eur Heart J*. 2019;40(11):902–910. [PMID: 30590531]

Prosperi-Porta G, Solverson K, Fine N, Humphreys CJ, Ferland A, Weatherald J. Echocardiography-derived stroke volume index is associated with adverse in-hospital outcomes in intermediate-risk acute pulmonary embolism: a retrospective cohort study. *Chest*. 2020;158:1132–1142. [PMID: 32243942]

Yurtiditsky Y, Mitchell OJL, Sista AK, et al. Right ventricular stroke distance predicts death and clinical deterioration in patients with pulmonary embolism. *Thromb Res*. 2020;195:29–34. [PMID: 32652350]

Treatment

The treatment of PE must be initiated as soon as possible, and the timing of initiation of therapy depends on the clinical suspicion of PE and the expected delay between ordering a diagnostic test and making a definitive diagnosis of acute PE. The clinical suspicion of acute PE should be informed by the use of a validated clinical scoring system. If there is strong clinical suspicion of acute PE, empiric treatment with a parenteral anticoagulation agent should be started while waiting for the test results to arrive. In patients with intermediate clinical suspicion for acute PE in whom the test results are expected to be delayed for 4 hours or more, empiric anticoagulation should be initiated. In patients with a low clinical suspicion for acute PE, empiric anticoagulation should not be given until the test results are obtained, provided the results are available within 24 hours. However, in patients in whom the risk of major bleeding is moderate or high, the decision to initiate anticoagulation should be made on a case-by-case basis considering the overall clinical picture, as well as the patient's preferences and values. If anticoagulation is contraindicated and an acute PE is confirmed, the patient should be considered for placement of an inferior vena cava (IVC) filter, as detailed later.

LMWH or fondaparinux are recommended as first-line agents for most patients with acute PE, as studies have shown they are either equivalent or superior in efficacy to unfractionated heparin, have lower rates of heparin-induced thrombocytopenia and major bleeding, have more predictable pharmacokinetics, and do not require frequent monitoring of the activated partial thromboplastin time (aPTT) or heparin activity level (antifactor Xa level). DOACs have been shown to have comparably reliable pharmacokinetics and pharmacodynamics to LMWH and are appropriate alternatives for low- and intermediate-risk PEs.

A. Heparin

Although unfractionated heparin has served as the standard foundation of PE treatment for more than 40 years, this anticoagulant has important limitations. Variable protein binding leads to an often unpredictable dose response, which can delay the achievement of therapeutic anticoagulation or provoke major bleeding at supratherapeutic doses. Serum depletion of antithrombin III can also render patients resistant. Antithrombin III can be depleted in patients who are critically ill, post-cardiopulmonary bypass, experiencing disseminated intravascular coagulation, and with liver disease and is not routinely checked until heparin resistance is observed.

Unfractionated heparin for PE treatment is usually ordered as an intravenous bolus followed by a continuous intravenous infusion. Heparin is usually administered as a bolus of 5,000–10,000 units (80 units/kg) followed by a weight-based hourly infusion (18 units/kg/h), which is titrated based on the aPTT or anti-Xa level measured every 4–6 hours (Table 29–6). In patients at low to moderate risk of bleeding, the target partial thromboplastin time is 60–80 seconds or anti-Xa level of 0.3–0.7 IU/mL.

Unfractionated heparin is now only recommended as first-line therapy in the following clinical situations: patients with increased risk of bleeding (due to its shorter half-life); patients with morbid obesity or severe anasarca (due to concern about adequate subcutaneous absorption); patients with severe renal insufficiency (since most LMWHs are renally excreted); and patients being considered for surgical embolectomy, mechanical circulatory support, or thrombolytic therapy.

Patients being treated with heparin who have a subsequent drop in platelet count should be evaluated for

Table 29–6. Unfractionated Heparin Weight-Based Nomogram for Acute Venous Thromboembolism

PTT	Repeat Bolus	Stop Infusion (min)	Rate Change	Repeat PTT (h)
< 35	70 units/kg[1]	0	Increase 3 units/kg/h	6
35–59	35 units/kg[2]	0	Increase 2 units/kg/h	6
60–80 target	0	0	No change	6
81–100	0	0	Decrease 2 units/kg/h	6
> 100	0	60	Decrease 3 units/kg/h	6

[1]Maximum bolus 10,000 units.
[2]Maximum bolus 5000 units.
PTT, activated partial thromboplastin time; measured in seconds.

heparin-induced thrombocytopenia (HIT). The platelet count may decline within hours or, more commonly, 5–10 days after exposure to heparin. Falling platelet counts within the first 48 hours commonly reflects HIT type 1 precipitated by platelet activation by heparin. Platelets generally recover within days with continued heparin administration. A drop in platelet count after 48 hours is more commonly HIT type 2, the immune-mediated process associated with thrombosis. Patients with known or suspected HIT type 2 should be treated with either direct thrombin inhibitors (such as lepirudin, argatroban, or bivalirudin) or heparinoids (such as danaparoid). Heparin, LMWH, and warfarin monotherapy should be avoided in the setting of known or suspected heparin-induced thrombocytopenia.

B. Low-Molecular-Weight Heparin

LMWHs have revolutionized the initial management of VTE (Table 29–7) allowing for shorter hospital stays and simple outpatient management. LMWHs are considered first-line agents for the initial treatment of acute PE and are the preferred agents for long-term anticoagulation for PE patients who are pregnant or have underlying cancer. In the United States, two LMWHs are commonly used for the treatment of PE: enoxaparin and dalteparin. The U.S. Food and Drug Administration–approved dose of enoxaparin is 1 mg/kg actual body weight given subcutaneously twice daily, or a once-daily subcutaneous dose of 1.5 mg/kg actual body weight. Dalteparin is administered subcutaneously at a dose of 100 IU/kg actual body weight twice daily or 200 IU/kg actual body weight once daily, up to a maximum daily dose of 18,000 IU per day. Tinzaparin is administered once daily at a dose of 175 IU/kg actual body weight but is contraindicated in patients older than 70 years with renal insufficiency. Patients with cancer, extensive clot burden, or obesity (actual body weight > 100 kg or a body mass index of 30–40) preferably should be treated with enoxaparin at the 1 mg/kg twice-daily dose.

LMWHs appear to be safer than unfractionated heparin carrying lower rates of osteopenia and HIT. They have a more predictable dose response than unfractionated heparin and can usually be administered based on weight alone, without any blood testing to modify the dose. They have a minimal effect on the partial thromboplastin time. Renal insufficiency (particularly a creatinine clearance [CrCl] < 30 mL/min), low body weight, morbid obesity (BMI ≥ 40 kg/m^2), elderly age, and pregnancy increase the risk of incorrect dosing, resulting in either

Table 29–7. Comparison of Unfractionated Heparin (UFH) Versus Low-Molecular-Weight Heparin (LMWH)

Characteristic	UFH	LMWH
Molecular weight (average in daltons)	15,000	5000
Ratio of anti-Xa to anti-IIa (thrombin) activity	1	> 1
Metabolism	Hepatic	Renal
Bioavailability	Fair	Excellent
Frequency of subcutaneous administration	2–3×/day	1–2×/day
Frequency of heparin-induced thrombocytopenia	1–2%	0.1–0.2%
Osteoporosis after prolonged exposure	Rare	Very rare
Laboratory assay of anticoagulant effect	Activated partial thromboplastin time or Anti-Xa level	Anti-Xa level
Reversal of anticoagulant effect	Protamine	Protamine
Spinal or epidural anesthesia	Okay	Heed the FDA warning

FDA, Food and Drug Administration.

Table 29–8. Low-Molecular-Weight Heparin Weight-Based Nomogram for Enoxaparin in the Presence of Renal Insufficiency or Marked Obesity

Renal Insufficiency Creatinine Clearance (mL/min)	Enoxaparin Dose	Anti–Xa Monitoring (Heparin Level)[1]
> 70	1 mg/kg q12h	None
35–69	0.75 mg/kg q12h	3–6 h after the third injection
< 35	1 mg/kg q24h	3–6 h after the third injection
Obese Weight	**Enoxaparin Dose**	**Anti–Xa Monitoring (Heparin Level)[1]**
< 100 kg	1 mg/kg q12h	None
100–130 kg	1 mg/kg q12h	3–6 h after the first injection
> 130 kg	130 mg q12h	3–6 h after the first injection

[1]Therapeutic level is 0.5–1.0 units/mL.

over- or under-anticoagulation. Avoidance of LMWH, dose-adjustment, or monitoring of anti-factor Xa activity may be necessary for these patients (Table 29–8). Even though dose adjustment is not recommended for patients with mild to moderate renal insufficiency (CrCl ≥ 30 mL/min), spontaneous bleeding from standard weight-based dosing of LMWHs may develop in such patients.

In a meta-analysis of randomized DVT treatment trials comparing LMWHs with unfractionated heparin, LMWHs were found to be more effective and safer. Their use resulted in fewer recurrent thromboemboli, less bleeding, less thrombocytopenia, and an improved quality of life and patient satisfaction. The strategy of using LMWHs was also more cost-effective. The ACCP and ESC guidelines recommend the preferential use of subcutaneous LMWH or fondaparinux over intravenous or subcutaneous unfractionated heparin for patients diagnosed with acute PE.

C. Fondaparinux

Fondaparinux is a subcutaneously administered synthetic pentasaccharide that contains the antithrombin-binding domain found in heparin and LMWH, which binds to antithrombin and inactivates factor Xa, leading to formation of a covalent antithrombin–Xa complex. Subcutaneous fondaparinux has been shown to be noninferior to intravenous unfractionated heparin for treatment of acute PE and has the advantages of not requiring dose adjustment and a lower risk of thrombocytopenia.

Fondaparinux has almost complete bioavailability after subcutaneous administration, a predictable anticoagulant response, and a long half-life, making it amenable to once-daily, fixed-dose administration. Fondaparinux is given at a dose of 7.5 mg subcutaneously once daily for patients with a body weight of 50–100 kg, 5 mg once daily for those with body weight less than 50 kg, and 10 mg once daily for those with body weight more than 100 kg.

However, fondaparinux is cleared almost exclusively by the kidneys and is thus contraindicated in patients with renal insufficiency (CrCl < 30 mL/min). The dose should be reduced by 50% in patients with mild to moderate renal insufficiency (CrCl 30–50 mL/min). Most patients do not need monitoring of factor Xa levels while on fondaparinux, but in those who do, fondaparinux-specific factor Xa assays are needed. If uncontrollable bleeding occurs with the use of fondaparinux, recombinant factor VIIIa may be used since protamine sulfate is ineffective.

D. Thrombolysis

Though thrombolysis has never been shown to improve mortality in a double-blind, randomized control trial in high-risk pulmonary embolism, current AHA/ACC (evidence class IIa), ACCP, ACP, ASH, and ESC guidelines (evidence class Ib) recommend their use. Thrombolysis has been shown to reduce right ventricular strain, improve pulmonary artery patency, and reduce pulmonary vascular resistance faster than parenteral anticoagulation justifying their use in the setting of hemodynamic instability. Rapid reduction in pulmonary vascular resistance and reduced right ventricular strain likely reducing the risk of progressing down the spiral of RV ischemia and hemodynamic collapse is depicted in Figure 29–6. Given the hemorrhage risk of systemic thrombolytic therapy, bleeding risk should be assessed prior to administration. Trial data informing bleeding risk and indications for catheter-directed thrombolysis will be discussed in the coming paragraphs.

Thrombolysis for intermediate high-risk PE remains a topic of study and debate. Thrombolysis for intermediate high-risk PE with adverse prognostic features (respiratory insufficiency, severe right ventricular dysfunction, or biochemical evidence of RV pressure overload) is an ACC/AHA Class IIb indication but is not directly addressed by 2019 ESC guidelines. Two major trials guide decision-making

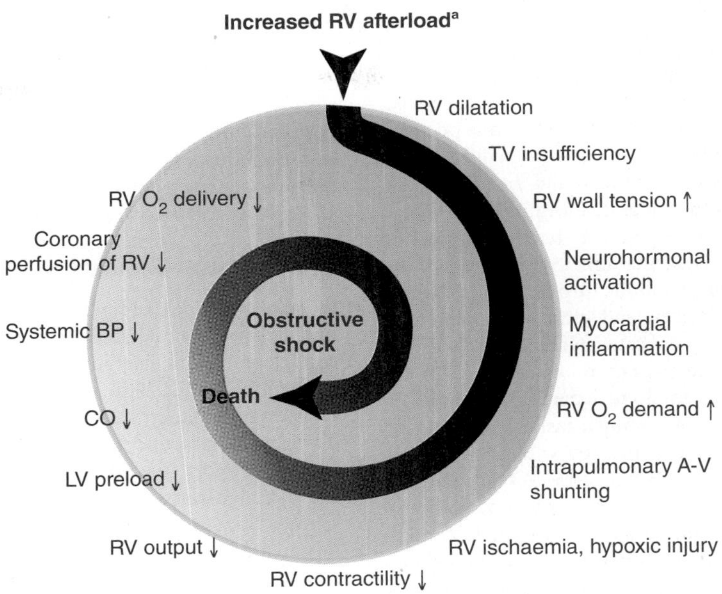

▲ **Figure 29–6.** Key factors contributing to hemodynamic collapse and death in acute pulmonary embolism. A-V: arterio-venous, BP: blood pressure, CO: cardiac output, LV: left ventricular; O_2: oxygen; RV: right ventricle; TV: tricuspid valve. [a]The exact sequence of events following an increase in RV afterload is not fully understood.

in this population: PEITHO and TOPCOAT. PEITHO, the largest of the trials, demonstrated a reduction in the risk of death or hemodynamic decompensation of 3% and OR 0.44 (95% CI 0.23–0.87). This was predominantly driven by a reduction in hemodynamic decompensation (1.6% vs 5.0%, thrombolysis vs parenteral anticoagulation) while mortality had a nonsignificant reduction (1.2% vs 1.8%). There was also a trend toward fewer recurrent pulmonary embolism (OR 0.20, 95% CI 0.02–1.68). These benefits came at the expense of increased major bleeding (11.5% vs 2.4%) and hemorrhagic stroke (2.0% vs 0.2%). There was a total of 10 hemorrhagic strokes, four of which were fatal. Patients aged 75 or older and women demonstrated greater propensity for bleeding in the trial (OR 20.38 and 11.49, respectively). When interpreting these results, it should be noted that 4.6% of patients in the placebo arm received thrombolytic therapy for other indications. These data suggest a role for thrombolysis in intermediate high-risk PE in a selected population.

Identifying at-risk patients within the intermediate high-risk cohort is a topic of active research. For hemodynamically stable patients with intermediate high-risk pulmonary embolisms, a comprehensive evaluation and close clinical monitoring are recommended. The identification of the following objective findings may help identify patients at risk for deterioration who may benefit from thrombolytics: a left ventricular outflow tract velocity time integral less than 15 cm (excluding patients with prior LV failure), RVOT VTI less than 10 cm, persistent respiratory distress more than 24 hours, a high thrombus burden in deep veins, and systolic pulse pressure variation greater than 10%. Massive elevations in troponin, BNP, and/or NT-proBNP may also help identify high-risk patients, but cutoffs are not established. Current evidence only supports the assertion that higher concentrations of troponin and/or natriuretic peptide are associated with worse outcomes.

A careful assessment of the risks of bleeding must be made before the decision to use thrombolytic therapy is made. Contraindications to the use of systemic thrombolytic therapy in patients with acute PE include the presence of an intracranial neoplasm, recent intracranial surgery or head trauma within the past 2 months, history of internal bleeding within the past 6 months, history of a hemorrhagic stroke, history of nonhemorrhagic stroke within the past 2 months, any surgery within the past 10 days, history of a bleeding diathesis, thrombocytopenia (< 100,000/mm^3), or uncontrolled hypertension (systolic blood pressure > 200 mm Hg or diastolic blood pressure > 110 mm Hg). Thrombolytics also pose greater bleeding risk to patients 75 years of age or older and female sex.

If a decision to use thrombolytic therapy is made, the ESC and ACCP recommend infusion of 100 mg of recombinant tissue-type plasminogen activator (rtTPA) via a peripheral vein for more than 2 hours. rtTPA is preferred as it can be administered concomitantly with heparin. Streptokinase or urokinase may also be used, but heparin must be discontinued. Reduced dose rtTPA has been studied, but studies are small and difficult to generalize. Reduced dose rtTPA appears to have noninferior outcomes, but biochemical assessment of fibrinolysis shows lower concentrations of fibrin split products with lower doses. Rates of bleeding are similar between higher and lower doses suggesting there is no safety benefit and potential for inferior effect. It bares mentioning that PEITHO and mOPETT studied reduced dose rtTPA in intermediate-high-risk PE with positive effects suggesting that there may be a role for reduced dose rtTPA in a subset of this population with high risk for hemodynamic collapse and low to moderate bleeding risk.

There are several invasive catheter-based approaches for delivery of thrombolytic agents directly into the pulmonary embolus, including intraembolic thrombolytic delivery, rheolytic and rotational devices, and ultrasound-enhanced thrombolysis. These are sophisticated techniques that may necessitate transport of the patient to a facility with an experienced interventional radiology department. Studies of catheter-directed therapies have shown faster resolution of RV function compared to monotherapy with anticoagulation. Rates of major bleeding were ~10% but intracranial bleeding was rare. These results should, however, be interpreted with caution as the studies are from single centers and represent small cohorts. The ACCP and ESC guidelines suggest the use of catheter-directed thrombolysis in patients with acute PE associated with hypotension in whom systemic thrombolysis is contraindicated or has failed and that it should only be performed in centers with adequate resources and expertise in these techniques.

E. Embolectomy

Patients at high risk for an adverse outcome with anticoagulation alone should be considered for embolectomy if they have contraindications to thrombolytic therapy. Embolectomy can be performed as a catheter-based procedure in the interventional laboratory or in the operating room. Recent phase I/II studies with novel catheters have demonstrated significant success in debulking thrombus and normalizing PA pressures. Phase II/III trials are underway but impact on mortality and hard outcomes has yet to be established.

Surgical embolectomy for acute PE can be considered for patients who have contraindications to thrombolysis. The operation is best performed by median sternotomy with continuous transesophageal echocardiogram monitoring. The embolus should be removed under direct visualization, never "blindly." With experience, all lobar and most segmental pulmonary artery branches can be visualized. It is crucial to refer high-risk PE patients as soon as their poor candidacy for anticoagulation is established.

To manage severe *chronic* thromboembolic pulmonary hypertension (CTEPH) due to a prior PE, a separate and more technically challenging operation can be performed—a pulmonary thromboendarterectomy. This operation is recommended by the ACCP, ESC, and ACC/AHA guidelines by an experienced thromboendarterectomy team for selected patients with CTEPH who have central disease. If successful, this operation can reduce and possibly cure pulmonary hypertension. This surgery requires careful dissection of the old thrombus, which has turned whitish and hardened, from the walls of the pulmonary arteries. Complications include pulmonary arterial perforation and hemorrhage; pulmonary steal syndrome, in which blood rushes from previously well-perfused lung tissue to newly perfused tissue; and reperfusion pulmonary edema. For patients who are not candidates for pulmonary thromboendarterectomy, balloon pulmonary angioplasty can be considered.

F. Mechanical Circulatory Support

In cases of active or impending circulatory collapse, utilization of mechanical circulatory support (MCS) should be considered. Venoarterial extracorporeal membrane oxygenation (VA ECMO) carries the most data describing encouraging outcomes. While RCTs are missing, case series describe hospital and 1-year survival rates above 90% when ECMO support is used to support patients through treatment of high-risk PE.

VA ECMO can be used to support patients through any treatment modality. In the era of expanded procedural treatment options, VA ECMO can support patient hemodynamics and oxygenation to survive transport to tertiary centers. VA ECMO can provide support to allow adequate time to plan for less readily available procedures like catheter directed or surgical embolectomy. VA ECMO can even be used in conjunction with thrombolysis though the risk of bleeding complications is high.

Case reports of RP ImpellaÔ being used to support high-risk PE have also been published. This carries the advantage of only requiring venous access, but has the disadvantage of sitting in the pulmonary artery potentially obstructing thrombectomy devices. It should be noted that experience is extremely limited and that H:Q curves of microaxial devices suggest the device support may be attenuated in a high afterload environment.

Careful conversations about treatment plans should be between the primary, MCS cannulation, and other treatment teams to ensure MCS placement does not complicate planned procedures and is timed around administration of thrombolytics.

G. Pulmonary Embolism Response Team (PERT)

Modern management of high-risk pulmonary embolism requires rapid mobilization of complex resources. In recent years, experiences from PERTs have been published showing increased utilization of recommended therapies. PERT members and protocols vary between institutions. Activation of the team leads to a multidisciplinary video or phone conference between a critical care physician, hematologist, interventional radiologist, and cardiothoracic surgeon. The PERT discusses and implements appropriate stepwise interventions. Unfortunately, PERTs, though effective, have struggled to remain active due to complex staffing needs and poor reimbursement. The ESC and ACCP both recommend utilization of PERTs when possible.

H. Inferior Vena Cava Filters

There are two indications for placing an IVC filter for patients with acute PE associated with acute proximal DVT: (1) concomitant major bleeding requiring transfusion, intracranial hemorrhage, or any absolute contraindication to the use of anticoagulant therapy; and (2) recurrent PE despite prolonged intensive anticoagulation. Other situations in which an IVC filter may be considered are patients with high-risk PE or CTEPH in whom another embolic event would be devastating; a proximal DVT in a patient with poor cardiopulmonary reserve; or DVT in a patient with a high bleeding risk. Although IVC filters reduce the frequency of PE, they do not halt the thrombotic process and are associated with a doubling of the rate of DVT. If the contraindication to anticoagulation is expected to be short-term, a retrievable IVC filter can be placed, and removal can be assessed periodically after 3–12 months. If the patient becomes a candidate for anticoagulation after an IVC filter has been placed, the patient should be preferentially anticoagulated and filter removal should be considered.

I. Warfarin

Warfarin was previously the gold standard for long-term anticoagulation in PE but has been largely replaced by DOACs due to less major bleeding and ease of administration. Warfarin dosing is adjusted according to a standardized prothrombin time by using the international normalized ratio (INR). For PE and DVT, the target INR is ordinarily between 2.0 and 3.0. Warfarin can be started on the same day or after the initiation of heparin or fondaparinux, and patients should have an overlap of at least 5 days or until the INR has been within the therapeutic range for at least two consecutive days. Warfarin should not be initiated before the administration of heparin or fondaparinux, because it can cause a transient hypercoagulable state and has been associated with a threefold increased risk of recurrent PE or DVT when used alone without "bridging." This effect is driven by depletion in protein C and S before other procoagulation factors.

Unfortunately, warfarin treatment is limited by a narrow therapeutic window. Too little anticoagulant effect leads to thromboembolism, and excessive anticoagulation leads to bleeding. The drug is plagued by a long list of interactions with other drugs that either decrease or increase warfarin's anticoagulant effect. The consumption of vitamin K–containing foods such as green leafy vegetables decreases the anticoagulant effect, whereas the ingestion of alcohol increases the likelihood of hemorrhage. Working closely with a coumadin clinic or pharmacy team can improve outcomes and limit untoward effects stemming from challenges in warfarin dosing.

J. Direct Oral Anticoagulants (DOACs)

All DOACs (dabigatran, rivaroxaban, apixaban, and edoxaban) have been shown in phase III RCTs to be noninferior to a standard treatment approach (enoxaparin followed by warfarin or acenocoumarol titrated to an INR of 2.0–3.0) for treating VTE and preventing recurrence. DOACs are safer in terms of major bleeding complications, particularly intracranial and fatal hemorrhage. They are recommended as first-line therapy by ASH, ACC/AHA, ACCP, and ESC guidelines.

DOACs have revolutionized treatment of acute PE. Previously, most patients diagnosed with acute PE were admitted to the hospital for initiation of anticoagulation. Now, patients with low-risk pulmonary embolisms can initiate therapy with a DOAC and discharge directly from home from clinic or the emergency department. The Hestia score (Table 29–9) is a validated risk calculator that identifies patients at low risk for complications from anticoagulant therapy and hemodynamic collapse who are candidates for outpatient management of their PE. A score of ≥ 1 indicates need for admission while a score of zero suggests the patient has a 0% chance of mortality and less than 2% chance of recurrence.

K. Adjunctive Measures

Occasionally, PE patients will require ventilatory assistance for respiratory failure. Most patients with acute PE, however, can be cared for in an intermediate-care or step-down unit. Most will benefit from supplemental oxygen. Opioids usually do not relieve the chest discomfort. Nonsteroidal anti-inflammatory agents are often effective and combining them with anticoagulation usually does not pose an undue risk of bleeding complications.

L. Duration of Treatment of Acute Pulmonary Embolism

The ACC/AHA, ACCP, ASH, and ESC guidelines recommend anticoagulation be continued for ≥3 months for VTE due to transient risk factors (such as postoperative state) or idiopathic disease. The more than 3-month treatment recommendation is long-standing and based on older VKA trials showing no difference in risk for recurrent PE between patients treated for 3–6 months versus 12–24 months. Treatment extending beyond 3 months has been shown to significantly reduce recurrent VTE (≥ 90%), but bleeding risk increases commensurate with duration of therapy.

In the DOAC era, longer-term treatment strategies have been reconsidered. DOACs are associated with lower rates of life-threatening hemorrhage (~1% per year) and non-major bleeding (~6% per year) compared to VKAs, but bleeding risk is not uniform across patients. Patients older than 75 years, with chronic liver disease, chronic kidney disease, active cancer, history of bleeding, prior stroke, serious chronic illness, and concomitant antiplatelet carry higher bleeding risk.

While data guiding specific recommendations for extended duration anticoagulation are lacking, professional

Table 29–9. Hestia Score

		Points
Hemodynamically unstable (SBP <100, HR>100, requiring ICU care)		1
Thombolysis or embolectomy needed		1
Active bleeding or high risk for bleeding		1
> 24 hours of supplemental O_2 to maintain sat > 90%		1
PE diagnosed while on anticoagulation		1
Severe pain requiring IV pain medication for > 24 hours		1
Creatine clearance < 30 mL/min by Crockoft Gault		1
Medical or social reason for admission >24hrs		1
Pregnant		1
Severe liver impairment		1
History of HIT		1
Severity Class	**Points**	**30-day Mortality**
Low risk	0	0% mortality, 2% recurrent VTE risk, candidate for at-home anticoagulation therapy
Not Low	≥ 1	Not a candidate for at-home anticoagulation therapy

Data from Zondag et al. *J Thom Haemo*. 2011, 9(8):1500–1507.

organizations have published expert consensus based on pooled risk offering guidance for patient-centered decision-making. While each guideline offers slightly different guidance, a common theme runs throughout. Given the reduced bleeding risks associated with DOAC therapy, professional societies currently favor long-term therapy for secondary prevention for more patients when bleeding risk is favorable.

The 2019 ESC guidelines describe the data informing recurrent VTE risk by dividing patients into three categories: low (< 3% per year), moderate (3–8% per year), and high risk (> 8% per year). Low-risk patients are those with significant reversible insults: patients exposed to surgery more than 30 minutes, hospitalized more than 3 days, and trauma or fractures. Moderate risk are VTE patients who suffered VTE without identifiable risk factors, chronic inflammatory conditions, or minor immobility/insults like long flights, oral estrogens, short surgery, and minor trauma. Patients are at high risk for recurrent VTE or those with prior recurrent VTE, antiphospholipid syndrome, symptomatic inherited thrombophilia, and/or active cancer. Providers can use the categories to weigh bleeding risk against the patient-specific risk of recurrent VTE as well as physiologic significance for that specific patient.

ASH guidelines simplify recommendations for secondary prevention further than ESC. ASH guidelines recommend indefinite secondary prevention for patients who have developed either unprovoked VTE or VTE provoked by a chronic risk factor when the bleeding profile is favorable. This recommendation is graded as of moderate certainty based on evidence and may be subject to modification.

Providers should be aware that this guidance may evolve as more data about low-dose DOACs are published. Trials comparing reduced dose rivaroxaban (10 mg vs 20 mg) and apixaban (2.5 mg vs 5 mg) demonstrate similar efficacy in minimizing recurrent VTE. Bleeding rates are similar in initial trials, but further study is needed. Lower doses for treatment durations ≥ 6 months may prove adequate.

M. Venous Thromboembolism in Pregnancy

The risk of VTE is increased fivefold during pregnancy and is one of the leading causes of maternal mortality. There is insufficient evidence to definitively guide the management of VTE during pregnancy, as most of the evidence comes from retrospective studies. Warfarin should be avoided in early pregnancy because it may lead to embryopathy between 6 and 12 weeks of gestation. On the other hand, unfractionated heparin and LMWH are not associated with embryopathy because they do not cross the placenta.

However, prolonged unfractionated heparin use may lead to osteoporosis, may lead to HIT, and is inconvenient to use due to the need for frequent aPTT testing to titrate the dose. LMWHs are more convenient to use, are associated with a lower risk of thrombocytopenia, and may also carry a lower risk of osteoporosis. However, the correct dosing of LMWH may also be difficult to determine by weight during pregnancy; thus, anti-factor Xa levels may need to be monitored periodically to ensure adequacy of dosing. Single-dose, prefilled vials of LMWH that are preservative-free should be preferably used in pregnant patients, as some preservatives used in multidose vials may have adverse fetal effects.

The ACCP guidelines recommend the use of LMWH over unfractionated heparin for both prevention and treatment of VTE during pregnancy. LMWH should be stopped at least 24 hours before induction of labor or induction of epidural anesthesia or cesarean section. Heparin can be started 6 hours after vaginal delivery or 12 hours after a cesarean section if there is no significant bleeding risk. Patients may then be transitioned to warfarin with discontinuation of heparin once the INR is within the therapeutic range. DOACs have not been studied in pregnancy or in the postpartum period and are not recommended for breastfeeding patients.

Counseling

Although PE can be as devastating emotionally and physically as myocardial infarction, the burden on individual patients may be even greater because the public does not have as good an understanding of PE, particularly in terms of the potential incomplete recovery from it and long-term disability it engenders. Young patients with PE repeatedly voice a common theme. Although they appear healthy, they have suffered a life-threatening illness. Because of their youth and healthy appearance, others may not empathize with their fears and feelings about the illness. Virtually all patients with PE will wonder why they were stricken with the illness and whether they harbor an underlying coagulopathy (or "bad" gene) that predisposed them. When anticoagulation is discontinued after an adequate course of therapy, patients are often fearful of recurrent PE. It is therefore essential to have an open discussion about the various treatment options available, the adverse effect profile of the drugs used, and the recommended duration of treatment using evidence-based clinical guidelines, and to understand the patient's values and expectations for treatment, to make balanced, collaborative treatment choices that both the patient and the treating clinician can agree on. A close collaboration with an experienced clinical pharmacist is also of benefit to assist with long-term management of patients on anticoagulant therapy. Regular assessments and ongoing discussions with the patient about the risks and benefits of ongoing treatment are essential, especially in those on long-term anticoagulation.

Follow Up

As treatment of VTE migrates toward an outpatient treatment pathway, follow-up and protocolized care become of increased importance to ensure safe resumption of activities, mitigation of bleeding risk, and adherence to therapy. First and foremost, age-appropriate cancer screening should be performed as this can both be lifesaving and influence duration of anticoagulation.

After the first 2–3 weeks of treatment have passed, patients should be screened for antiphospholipid syndrome. Should testing yield a positive result, an appropriate transition to VKA therapy should be made as DOAC will likely be the prescribed treatment for most patients not diagnosed as an inpatient. As stated above, routine screening for genetic thrombophilia is not recommended.

Efforts should be made to minimize bleeding risk. For patients being treated beyond 3 months, interval bleeding risk assessments should be performed. Reduced dose DOAC therapy may be considered in the future should data infer a lower bleeding risk. Importantly, concomitant antiplatelet medications greatly increase bleeding risk. Antiplatelet therapy may be dose reduced or discontinued in the setting of chronic anticoagulation on a case-by-case basis. Efforts to avoid NSAID therapy should also be taken.

Patients should be encouraged to gradually resume exercise. Cardiac rehab may be appropriate in cases of moderate to severe RV dysfunction. For patients with moderate to severe RV dysfunction, expert consensus now recommends confirming recovery of function prior to resuming full exercise. For patients who remain symptomatic after 3 months of therapy, cardiopulmonary testing is recommended to help identify patients at risk for CTEPH.

Bledsoe JR, Woller SC, Stevens SM, et al. Cost-effectiveness of managing low-risk pulmonary embolism patients without hospitalization. The low-risk pulmonary embolism prospective management study. *Am J Emerg Med.* Mar 2021;41:80–83. [PMID: 33388651]

Klok FA, Ageno W, Ay C, et al. Optimal follow-up after acute pulmonary embolism: A position paper of the European Society of Cardiology Working Group on Pulmonary Circulation and Right Ventricular Function, in collaboration with the European Society of Cardiology Working Group on Atherosclerosis and Vascular Biology, endorsed by the European Respiratory Society. *Eur Heart J.* 2022;43:183–189. [PMID: 34875048]

Konstantinides SV, Meyer G, Becattini C, et al. 2019 ESC Guidelines for the diagnosis and management of acute pulmonary embolism developed in collaboration with the European Respiratory Society (ERS): The Task Force for the diagnosis and management of acute pulmonary embolism of the European Society of Cardiology (ESC). *Eur Heart J.* 2019;41(4):543–603. [PMID: 31473594]

Ortel TL, Neumann I, Ageno W, et al. American society of hematology 2020 guidelines for management of venous thromboembolism: treatment of deep vein thrombosis and pulmonary embolism. *Blood Adv.* 2020;4:4693–4738. [PMID: 33007077]

Rivera-Lebron B, McDaniel M, Ahrar K, et al. Diagnosis, treatment and follow up of acute pulmonary embolism: Consensus Practice from the PERT Consortium. *Clin Appl Thromb Hemost*. Jan-Dec 2019;25:1076029619853037. [PMID: 31185730]

Roy PM, Penaloza A, Hugli O, et al. Triaging acute pulmonary embolism for home treatment by Hestia or simplified PESI criteria: The HOME-PE randomized trial. *Eur Heart J*. 2021;42:3146–3157. [PMID: 34363386]

Stevens SM, Woller SC, Kreuziger LB, et al. Antithrombotic Therapy for VTE Disease: Second Update of the CHEST Guideline and Expert Panel Report. *Chest*. Dec 2021;160(6):e545–e608. [PMID: 34352278]

Valerio L, Barco S, Jankowski M, et al. Quality of life 3 and 12 months following acute pulmonary embolism: analysis from a prospective multicenter cohort study. *Chest*. Jun 2021;159(6):2428–2438. [PMID: 33548221]

Pulmonary Hypertension

30

Christopher F. Barnett, MD, MPH
Teresa De Marco, MD

ESSENTIALS OF DIAGNOSIS

Pulmonary hypertension

- ▶ A loud pulmonic valve closure sound (P_2), a right-sided S_4, or a right ventricular heave.
- ▶ Electrocardiographic evidence of right ventricular hypertrophy.
- ▶ Presence of sustained elevation in mean pulmonary artery pressure ≥ 20 mm Hg.

Pulmonary arterial hypertension

- ▶ A subset of pulmonary hypertension.
- ▶ Elevated mean pulmonary artery pressure ≥ 20 mm Hg and pulmonary arterial wedge pressure ≤ 15 mm Hg and PVR > 2 Wood units.
- ▶ Appropriate clinical context.

Pulmonary hypertension (PH) describes the finding of a mean pulmonary artery pressure (mPAP) ≥ 20 mm Hg and may occur in many settings. In most cases, PH results from a left heart disease (LHD) that increases pulmonary artery pressure (PAP) by transmission of elevated left heart filling pressures or from lung disease causing hypoxia-mediated pulmonary vasoconstriction. The term *pulmonary arterial hypertension* (PAH) describes a specific group of diseases characterized hemodynamically by an mPAP ≥ 20 mm Hg and normal left heart filling pressures (pulmonary artery wedge pressure [PAWP] ≤ 15 mm Hg) resulting from vasoconstriction and arteriopathy of the precapillary pulmonary arterioles. PAH may be idiopathic or associated with one or more underlying diseases such as connective tissue disease, human immunodeficiency virus (HIV) infection, or portal hypertension. In patients clinically suspected of having PH, echocardiography is often the first test performed to estimate PAP and evaluate right ventricular function. Further comprehensive testing is required to make a diagnosis and establish the etiology of PH.

PH commonly occurs in patients with LHD and hypoxia from lung disease. The development of PH in patients with heart or lung disease is an ominous sign and is generally associated with reduced survival. Treatment in such cases is directed at the underlying condition (ie, bronchodilators, supplemental oxygen, valve repair, or heart failure treatment). The use of PAH-specific therapy in this setting is generally not beneficial and can worsen symptoms and mortality. In patients with PAH, vasoconstriction and pulmonary vascular arteriopathy cause increased pulmonary vascular resistance (PVR) and increased PAP, ultimately causing right heart failure and death. In this setting, PAH-specific therapy improves symptoms, exercise tolerance, and survival. Selection of PAH therapies is complex, and the prescriber must consider PAH severity, associated diseases, toxicities, and drug interactions and provide close follow-up. Early referral and collaboration with a PH specialty center are recommended for confirmation of diagnosis, initiation of appropriate therapy, and monitoring of response to treatment. Despite significant advances in understanding of the clinical profile, pathobiology, and treatment of PAH, delays in diagnosis remain common and patient outcomes remain poor.

▶ General Considerations

PH is defined as a sustained elevation in the mPAP of ≥ 20 mm Hg at rest. This contrasts with a normal mPAP of 12–16 mm Hg. In healthy humans, the small arteriovenous pressure gradient generated by blood flow across the pulmonary circulation results from the large total vascular surface area and high pulmonary vascular compliance. The PVR is quantified using **Ohm's law** (PVR = [mPAP – PAWP]/cardiac output [CO]) and describes the relationship between the pressure gradient and blood flow.

▶ Classification & Pathogenesis

The clinical classification of PH was updated in 2022 (Table 30–1). A hemodynamic approach to classification

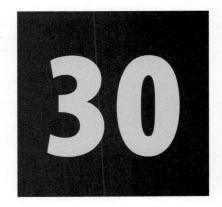

Table 30–1. Classification System for Pulmonary Hypertension

Group 1: Pulmonary arterial hypertension
• Idiopathic
• Heritable
• Drug and toxin-induced
• Associated with:
Connective tissue disease
HIV infection
Portal hypertension
Congenital heart disease
Schistosomiasis
• Long-term responders to calcium channel blockers
• Pulmonary veno-occlusive disease and/or pulmonary capillary hemangiomatosis
• Persistent pulmonary hypertension of the newborn
Group 2: Pulmonary hypertension due to left heart disease
• Heart failure with preserved ejection fraction
• Heart failure with reduced ejection fraction
• Congenital/acquired cardiovascular conditions leading to postcapillary pulmonary hypertension
Group 3: Pulmonary hypertension due to lung disease and/or hypoxia
• Obstructive lung disease
• Restrictive lung disease
• Other lung disease with mixed restrictive/obstructive pattern
• Hypoxia without lung disease
• Developmental lung disorders
Group 4: pH due to pulmonary artery obstructions
• Chronic thromboembolic PH
• Other pulmonary artery obstructions (tumors, arteritis, congenital stenosis, infection)
Group 5: Pulmonary hypertension with unclear multifactorial mechanisms
• Hematological disorders
• Systemic and metabolic disorders
• Others
• Complex congenital heart disease

of PH is illustrated in Figure 30–1. PH severity is graded by the value of the mPAP: mild (20–40 mm Hg), moderate (41–55 mm Hg), or severe (> 55 mm Hg).

A. Pulmonary Arterial Hypertension

Pathologic abnormalities in PAH are localized to the precapillary pulmonary arterioles, resulting in a characteristic hemodynamic profile that can be identified during right heart catheterization (RHC) (see Figure 30–1). Hemodynamically, PAH is defined by a sustained elevation of the mPAP ≥ 20 mm Hg and a PAWP or left ventricular end-diastolic pressure ≤ 15 mm Hg (normal PAWP, 8–12 mm Hg) and a PVR >2 Wood units (WU).

PAH is caused by a disparate group of diseases that have in common vasoconstriction and arteriopathy with remodeling of the precapillary pulmonary arterioles (see Table 30–1). Chronically elevated PAP leads to right ventricular failure and death. Although the prognosis for patients with PAH varies with the underlying cause, overall survival is poor even with modern therapies.

The prevalence of PAH in the United States is estimated to be between 50,000 and 100,000 cases. Of these, only 15,000 to 25,000 cases are appropriately diagnosed and treated. Multicenter registry data suggest that most patients with PAH are women (with a 2:1 female-to-male ratio), with a mean age of 50 years. Seventy-five percent of patients with PAH have symptoms at rest or with minimal exertion. The mean duration of symptoms prior to diagnosis is 24 months.

Three processes contribute to pulmonary artery luminal narrowing in PAH: vasoconstriction, arterial remodeling, and thrombosis in situ (Figure 30–2). In susceptible individuals, pulmonary vascular injury leads to disruption of the homeostatic balance present in the healthy pulmonary arteries. Upregulation of vasoconstrictive and proproliferative mediators (ie, endothelin-1, serotonin, and thromboxane) and downregulation of vasodilatory and antiproliferative mediators (ie, nitric oxide, prostacyclin, and smooth muscle cell potassium channels) lead to increased vasoconstriction and disordered cell proliferation. In situ thrombus formation occurs as a result of increased platelet activation, increased blood stasis, upregulation of plasminogen activator inhibitor-1, and reduced fibrinolytic activity.

PAH is termed idiopathic if no disease associated with PAH is present and heritable if there is a genetic predisposition or familial occurrence of PAH. Idiopathic PAH and heritable PAH are rare disorders with a prevalence of 15–50 cases per million per year and an incidence of 6 cases per million per year. Idiopathic and heritable PAH afflict predominantly young women, with a mean age at diagnosis of 35 years. These are progressive disorders with a high mortality (untreated median life expectancy of 2.8 years from diagnosis).

Pathogenic variants in the bone morphogenetic protein receptor (*BMPR*)*-2* gene have been identified in approximately 50% of patients with heritable PAH. Those who inherit the mutation have a 10% risk of developing PAH. The genetic pattern of inheritance is autosomal dominant with incomplete penetrance and anticipation (subsequent generations manifest the disease at an earlier age). A mutation in the activin receptor-like kinase type 1 (*ALK-1* or endoglin), often with coexistent hereditary hemorrhagic telangiectasia, may also be identified in patients with PAH. Both *BMPR-2* and *ALK-1* are members of the transforming growth factor-β signaling pathway. Continued discovery of deleterious genetic variants is likely to result in the movement molecular genetic testing into PH clinics where it will be used to select targeted PAH therapies.

Diseases associated with PAH include connective tissue disease, congenital systemic-to-pulmonary shunts, portal hypertension, HIV infection, drug and toxin exposures, and other disorders as delineated in Table 30–1.

Development of PAH has been associated with nearly all types of connective tissue disease but is most common in patients with systemic sclerosis. When PAH develops secondary

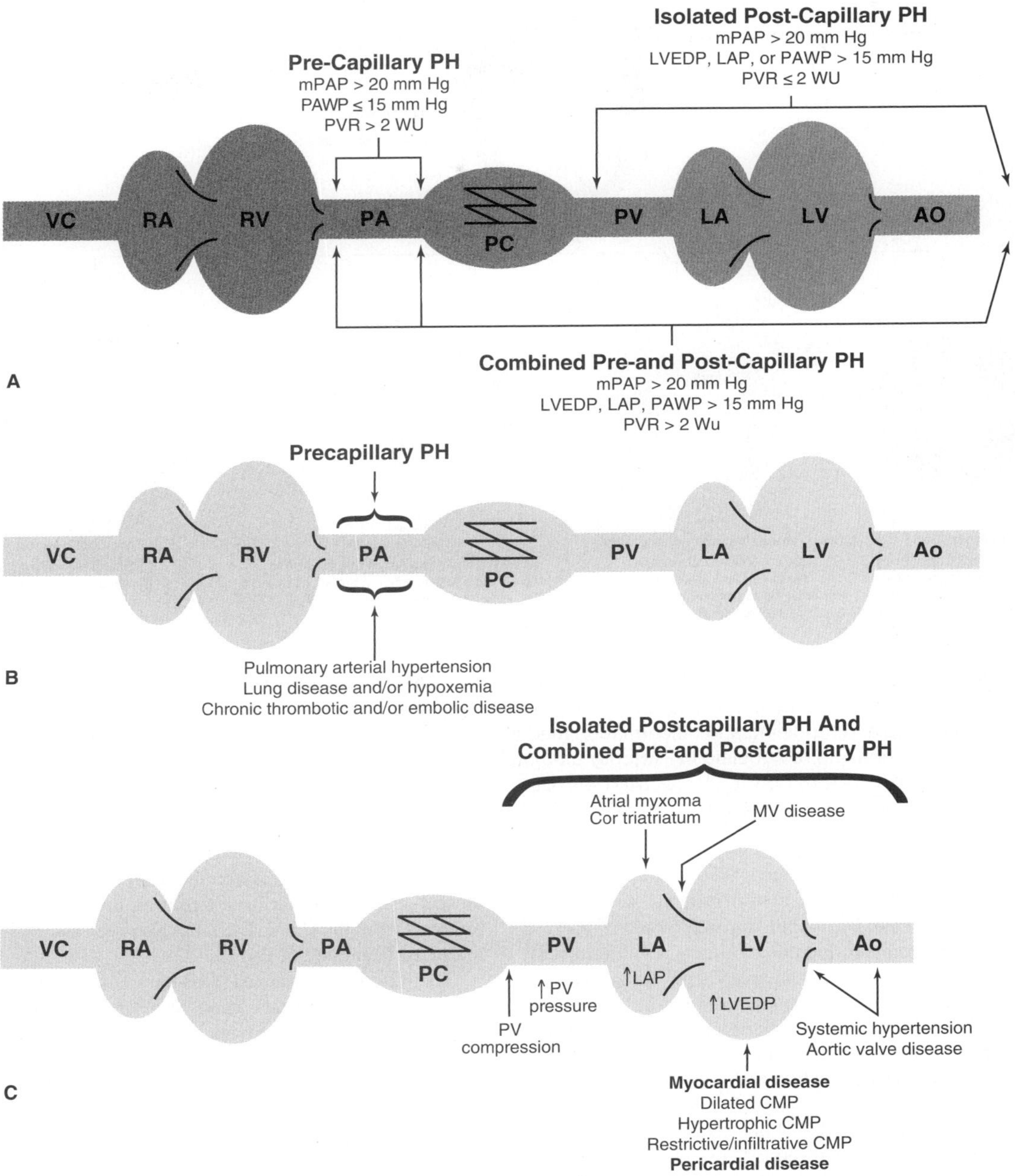

▲ **Figure 30–1.** Hemodynamic classification of pulmonary hypertension (PH). **A:** Pulmonary hypertension may result from pathology in precapillary or postcapillary pulmonary circulation. **B:** Common causes of precapillary PH. **C:** Common causes of postcapillary and mixed PH. Ao, aorta; CMP, cardiomyopathy; DTPG, diastolic transpulmonary gradient; LA, left atrium; LV, left ventricle; LVEDP, left ventricular end-diastolic pressure; PA, pulmonary artery; PAWP, pulmonary arterial wedge pressure; PC, pulmonary capillaries; PV, pulmonary veins; PVR, pulmonary vascular resistance; RA, right atrium; RV, right ventricle; TPG, transpulmonary pressure gradient; VC, vena cava. (Reproduced with permission from De Marco T, et al. Pulmonary hypertension in left heart disease—systolic, diastolic, valvular. In: Kirklin JK (ed), *Pulmonary Hypertension and Right Heart Failure: ISHLT Monograph Series*. Vol 9. 2015.)

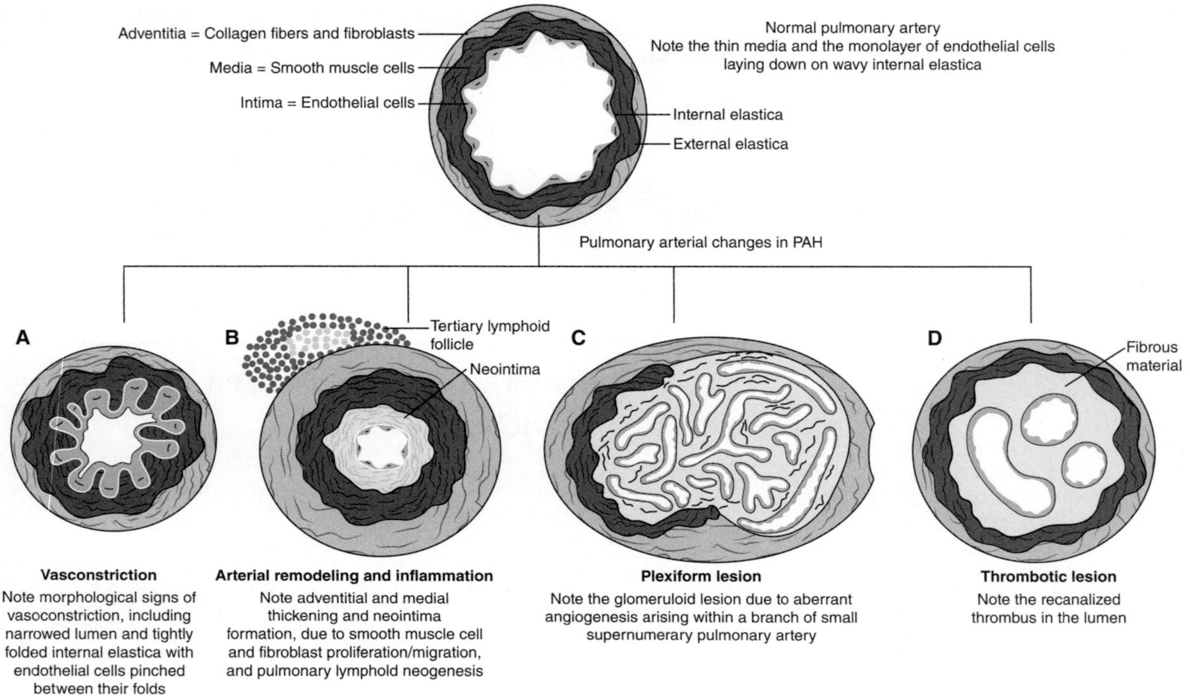

▲ **Figure 30–2.** Pathobiology of pulmonary arterial hypertension (PAH). **A:** Vasoconstriction secondary to vasodilator-vasoconstrictor imbalance and endothelial dysfunction is an early event in pulmonary arterial hypertension. **B:** Pulmonary vascular remodeling and inflammation mediated by cytokines, chemokines, serotonin, and other growth factors. **C:** Proliferation and remodeling in PAH may ultimately results in plexiform lesions. **D:** Endothelial dysfunction in PAH may lead to local thrombosis. (Reproduced with permission from McLaughlin VV, et al. Management of pulmonary arterial hypertension. *J Am Coll Cardiol*. 2015;65(18):1976–1997.)

to connective tissue disease, the prognosis is extremely poor. In patients with PAH associated with systemic sclerosis, for instance, the 1-year survival is approximately 50%.

Congenital systemic-to-pulmonary shunts result from ventricular or atrial septal defects, anomalous pulmonary venous drainage, patent ductus arteriosus, or an aortopulmonary window. Systemic-to-pulmonary shunts expose the pulmonary vasculature to a persistent high-flow state. This can lead to pulmonary artery endothelial dysfunction, mediator activation, and reactive vasoconstriction. Vascular remodeling ensues and can progress to the point that shunt reversal occurs (Eisenmenger syndrome). Shunt reversal worsens hypoxemia and further exacerbates PAH. PAH may also develop many years after the repair of a congenital shunt as a long-term consequence of vascular injury sustained prior to shunt repair.

PAH develops in approximately 5–10% of patients with portal hypertension. Portopulmonary hypertension can interfere with eligibility for liver transplantation because it is associated with high perioperative mortality.

It is estimated that PAH develops in 1 of every 200 patients with HIV infection. Those patients with HIV in whom PAH develops have a particularly poor prognosis. Methamphetamine use is also associated with the development of PAH. The diet drug fenfluramine, which has been removed from the U.S. market, has also been associated with increased likelihood of PAH.

The disorders discussed thus far, while distinct, similarly result in pulmonary endothelial and vascular smooth muscle cell dysfunction, maladaptive arterial remodeling, and increased vascular resistance causing increased PAP and right heart failure. Although the prognosis of PAH varies based on the underlying disease, presence of PAH significantly increases the morbidity and mortality of all associated conditions.

B. Pulmonary Hypertension with Left-Sided Heart Disease

Elevation of left-sided cardiac filling pressures can lead to PH through passive congestion and retrograde transmission of elevated pressure to the pulmonary artery tree. This is termed *isolated postcapillary pulmonary hypertension* (IPC-PH) (see Figure 30–1). IPC-PH is characterized hemodynamically by an mPAP greater than 20 mm Hg, PAWP greater than 15 mm Hg, and a PVR ≤ 2 WU. With chronic elevation of pulmonary venous pressures, upregulation of inflammatory cytokines, as well as vasoconstrictive and proproliferative mediators, may eventually cause pathologic pulmonary vascular remodeling. This entity is referred to as combined pre- and post-capillary PH (CPC-PH) and is characterized hemodynamically by an mPAP greater than 20 mm Hg, PAWP greater than 15 mm Hg, and a PVR > 2 WU.

Elevation of left-sided cardiac filling pressures may result from aortic or mitral stenosis or regurgitation, heart failure with reduced or preserved ejection fraction (HFrEF or HFpEF, respectively), pericardial disease, atrial myxoma with obstruction, or pulmonary vein compression. In most patients with LHD, PH is a direct result of elevated left heart filling pressures and PAP will normalize with appropriate therapies that lower left heart filling pressures. The presence of PH in patients with mitral or aortic valve disease is frequently an indication for valve repair with either surgical or percutaneous intervention. Patients with HFrEF should receive maximal guideline-recommended treatment. Optimal management of important comorbidities such as hypertension and atrial fibrillation may be beneficial. In both HFrEF and HFpEF, optimal volume management with diuretics reduces left heart filling pressures and lowers PAP. Patients being considered for heart transplantation with PH must undergo testing with short-acting vasodilators such as nitroprusside to determine whether PAP can be reduced when CPC-PH is present (reversible CPC-PH). If PAP cannot be adequately lowered with vasodilators, heart transplant is contraindicated due to the risk of acute right ventricular failure after transplant. In this case, left heart unloading with long-term inotrope infusions or placement of a ventricular assist device may convert fixed CPC-PH to reversible CPC-PH or reduce PAP, permitting heart transplantation.

C. Pulmonary Hypertension Associated with Lung Diseases and Hypoxemia

Chronic lung diseases causing hypoxemia, such as chronic obstructive pulmonary disease (COPD) and interstitial lung disease (ILD), are common causes of PH, as are sleep-disordered breathing, alveolar hypoventilation disorders, and prolonged exposure to high altitude.

Multiple mechanisms contribute to PH in these patients. The primary mechanism is hypoxia-mediated vasoconstriction of the pulmonary arteries, which results in a hemodynamic profile that is similar to that of PAH (see Figure 30–1). Hypoxia also induces pulmonary vascular remodeling by upregulation of proproliferative mediators. Destruction of lung parenchyma and pulmonary capillary networks results in a decrease in the overall surface area of the pulmonary vascular bed and thereby increases PVR. Hyperviscosity secondary to hypoxia-induced erythrocytosis can also worsen PH.

Treatment of these disorders is based on optimal treatment of parenchymal lung disease, primarily involving supplemental oxygen to avoid hypoxemia. Inhaled treprostinil was approved by the FDA in 2022 to improve exercise tolerance in patients with ILD and is under investigation in patients with COPD. However, other PAH therapies studied have been either ineffective or harmful in patient with PH from lung disease and should generally not be prescribed. Because the development of PH in patients with parenchymal lung disease is associated with high mortality, expedited lung transplant evaluation is recommended in patients who may be candidates.

D. Chronic Thromboembolic Pulmonary Hypertension

Chronic thromboembolic PH (CTEPH) occurs in up to 4% of patients following acute pulmonary embolism (PE) or 10% following recurrent PE. However, 50% of patients diagnosed with CTEPH have no antecedent history of a deep vein thrombosis or PE. Why some patients develop CTEPH is not well understood. Surgical specimens from patients undergoing pulmonary endarterectomy (PEA) demonstrate organization of thromboembolic material as well as vascular remodeling characterized by intimal thickening with deposition of collagen and hemosiderin, atherosclerosis, and calcification (Figure 30–3). Vasculopathy and pathologic remodeling of unobstructed downstream pulmonary arterioles like that which occurs in idiopathic PAH may also develop.

Excluding CTEPH as a cause of PH is important because mortality is high without appropriate surgical management. Excluding CTEPH as a cause of PH requires evaluation with a ventilation-perfusion scan followed by confirmatory conventional pulmonary angiography. Computed tomography (CT) pulmonary angiography is insensitive and does not exclude the diagnosis. If a diagnosis of CTEPH is suspected, early referral to a specialized center where PEA is performed is recommended. Balloon pulmonary angioplasty (BPA) may be of benefit in selected patients.

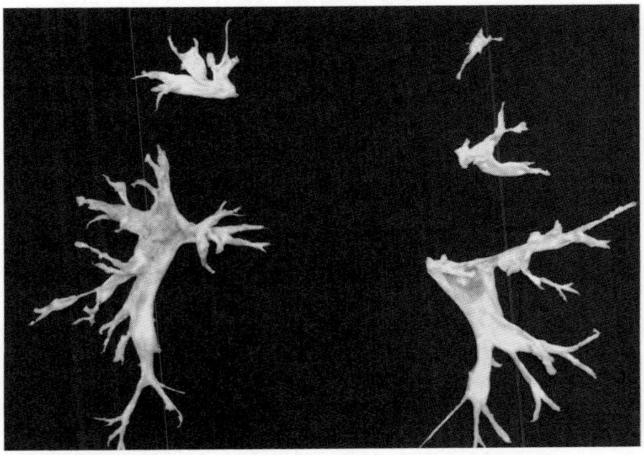

▲ **Figure 30–3.** Surgical specimens obtained during pulmonary endarterectomy for the treatment of chronic thromboembolic pulmonary hypertension. (Reproduced with permission from Kim Kerr, MD, Professor of Medicine, UCSD.)

E. Pulmonary Hypertension with Unclear and Multifactorial Mechanism

This category of PH encompasses a diverse group of disorders that cause PH by mechanisms that are not easily characterized.

F. Right Ventricular Failure Resulting from Pulmonary Hypertension

PH increases the afterload of the right ventricle, resulting in compensatory right ventricle hypertrophic remodeling so that the right ventricle can maintain the CO. Early on, the right ventricle can have supernormal function and normal-to-reduced chamber dimensions. Chronic right ventricular pressure overload results in persistent upregulation of pro-proliferative neurohormones, endothelin-1, and cytokines. These mediators contribute to the development of maladaptive hypertrophy with fibrosis and diastolic dysfunction (Figures 30–4 and 30–5).

If exposure to elevated PAP continues, the right ventricle dilates. This is an ominous sign because it signifies the presence of increased right ventricular wall stress. Increased wall stress, when coupled with increased heart rate, results in increased myocardial oxygen demand. This develops in concert with a reduction in the epicardial-to-endocardial coronary perfusion gradient secondary to increased right ventricular end-diastolic pressure. In sum, these changes result in a myocardial oxygen supply-demand mismatch and right ventricular ischemia. Right ventricular ischemia worsens systolic function, increases end-diastolic pressure, and promotes further ventricular enlargement. Tricuspid regurgitation secondary to annular dilatation often occurs and serves to further reduce effective right ventricular forward output.

Right ventricular dilation, in the setting of an intact pericardium, results in a shift of the interventricular septum toward the left ventricle. This, especially when coupled with increased intrapericardial pressure, impedes left ventricular filling (preload). In turn, when left ventricular filling is impaired, systemic CO is reduced.

Multiple mechanisms contribute to the development of hypoxemia in PH, even when intrinsic pulmonary disease is absent. Pulmonary vascular remodeling and in situ thromboses disrupt normal capillary-alveolar gas exchange and raise the alveolar-to-arterial oxygen gradient. Increased pulmonary pressures can increase right atrial pressure and cause shunting through a patent foramen ovale.

Humbert M, Guignabert C, Bonnet S, et al. Pathology and pathobiology of pulmonary hypertension: state of the art and research perspectives. *Eur Respir J*. Jan 2019;53(1):1801887. [PMID: 30545970]

Humbert M, et al. 2022 ESC/ERS Guidelines for the diagnosis and treatment of pulmonary hypertension. Eur Heart J. Aug 26 2022;[PMID: 36017548]

Huston JH, Shah SJ. Understanding the pathobiology of pulmonary hypertension due to left heart disease. *Circ Res*. Apr 29 2022;130(9):1382–1403. [PMID: 35482841]

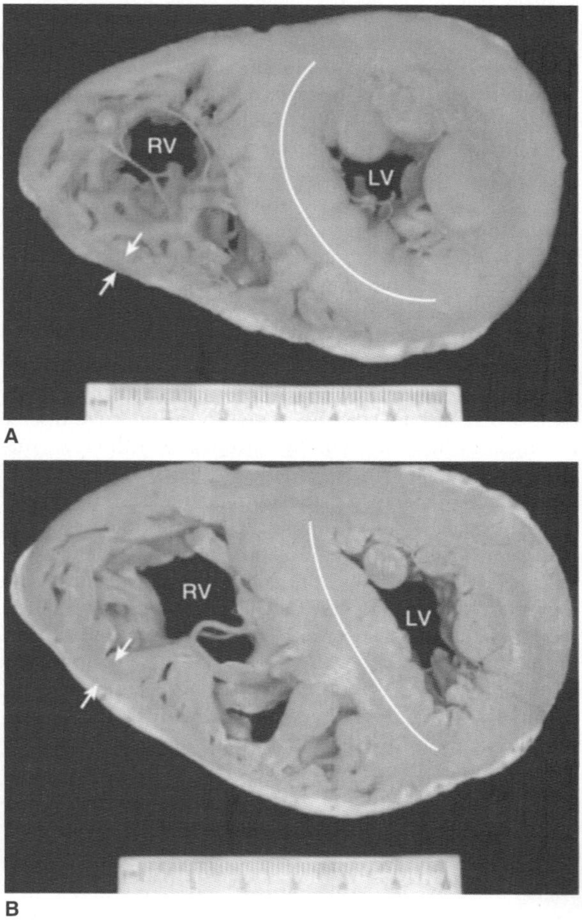

▲ **Figure 30–4.** Appearance of the right ventricle in pulmonary hypertension. **A:** A transverse section through a normal heart illustrates a crescentic right ventricular cavity, thin right ventricular free wall (*arrows*), and round left ventricular cavity (*line*). **B:** A transverse section of a heart from a patient who had severe pulmonary hypertension showing dilation of the right ventricular cavity giving the right ventricle a more spherical shape than in the normal heart. Also seen is thickening of the right ventricular free wall (*arrows*) and flattening of the interventricular septum (*line*). LV, left ventricle; RV, right ventricle. (Reproduced, with permission, from Barnett CF, et al. Pulmonary hypertension due to lung disease. In: Broaddus VC, et al, eds. *Murray and Nadel's Textbook of Respiratory Medicine*, 6th ed. Philadelphia: W.B. Saunders; 2016:1050–1065. e1055. Copyright © Elsevier.)

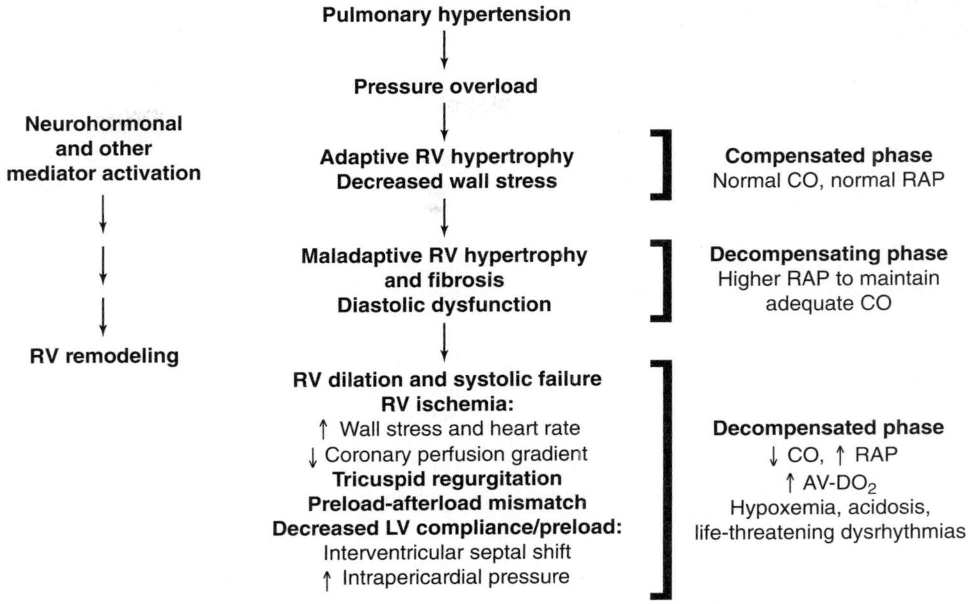

▲ **Figure 30–5.** Pathophysiology of right ventricular dysfunction in pulmonary hypertension. AV-DO_2, arteriovenous oxygen differential; CO, cardiac output; LV, left ventricular; RAP, right atrial pressure; RV, right ventricular.

Papamatheakis DG, Poch DS, Fernandes TM, Kerr KM, Kim NH, Fedullo PF. Chronic thromboembolic pulmonary hypertension: JACC Focus Seminar. *J Am Coll Cardiol.* Nov 3 2020; 76(18):2155–2169. [PMID: 33121723]

Singh N, Dorfmuller P, Shlobin OA, Ventetuolo CE. Group 3 pulmonary hypertension: from bench to bedside. *Circ Res.* Apr 29 2022;130(9):1404–1422. [PMID: 35482836]

Southgate L, Machado RD, Graf S, Morrell NW. Molecular genetic framework underlying pulmonary arterial hypertension. *Nat Rev Cardiol.* Feb 2020;17(2):85–95. [PMID: 31406341]

Vonk Noordegraaf A, Chin KM, Haddad F, et al. Pathophysiology of the right ventricle and of the pulmonary circulation in pulmonary hypertension: an update. *Eur Respir J.* Jan 2019;53(1): 1801900. [PMID: 30545976]

Clinical Findings

A. Symptoms & Signs

PAH frequently presents with nonspecific symptoms such as dyspnea on exertion, fatigue, or chest pain. These symptoms are often attributed to other diseases such as asthma, anxiety, or, if present, connective tissue disease or HIV. Exertional presyncope or syncope, edema, and ascites develop in more advanced right heart failure. A modified New York Heart Association (NYHA) classification system is used to describe patients with PH (Table 30–2).

B. Physical Examination

Physical examination of the patient with PH can reveal clues not only about the presence or severity of PH but also about the underlying cause. Classic examination findings that occur late with markedly elevated PAP include a loud pulmonic valve closure (P_2) or an early systolic ejection click. A right-sided S_3 or S_4 gallop is heard in patients with significant elevation in the right ventricular end-diastolic pressure. With right ventricular hypertrophy and enlargement, a left parasternal lift can be palpated.

Table 30–2. New York Heart Association (NYHA) and World Health Organization (WHO) Functional Classes in Pulmonary Hypertension

Class	Symptoms/Function
NYHA I/WHO I	No limitation in physical activity. Ordinary physical activity does not cause undue dyspnea, fatigue, chest pain, or near-syncope.
NYHA II/WHO II	Slight limitation in physical activity. Ordinary physical activity causes undue dyspnea, fatigue, chest pain, or near-syncope.
NYHA III/WHO III	Marked limitation in physical activity. Less than ordinary physical activity causes undue dyspnea, fatigue, chest pain, or near-syncope.
NYHA IV/WHO IV	Inability to carry out any physical activity without symptoms. Patients manifest signs of right heart failure. Dyspnea and/or fatigue may be present at rest.

Table 30–3. Electrocardiographic Criteria for Right Ventricular Hypertrophy

Right axis deviation (axis > +90 degrees)
R/S amplitude ratio in lead V_1 > 1.0 mm
R-wave amplitude in V_1 ≥ 7 mm
S-wave amplitude in V_1 < 2 mm
qR pattern in precordial lead V_1
R-wave amplitude in lead V_1 + S-wave amplitude in V_5 or V_6 > 10.5 mm
R/S amplitude ratio in V_5 or V_6 < 1.0 mm

Often the holosystolic murmur of tricuspid regurgitation (although frequently without the classically described respiratory variation) and the less common diastolic murmur of pulmonic insufficiency are noted in patients with PH. Cool extremities, diminished peripheral pulses, jugular venous distention, peripheral edema, and ascites develop with progressive right heart failure.

A murmur of mitral or aortic stenosis or a left-sided S_3 or S_4 gallop suggests left-sided heart disease, whereas wheezing and diminished breath sounds may be clues to the presence of pulmonary parenchymal disease. Jaundice and spider angiomata may point to the presence of cirrhosis and portal hypertension. Connective tissue diseases may present not only with signs of PH but also with Raynaud phenomenon, arthritis, rashes, or other skin changes such as sclerodactyly.

C. Diagnostic Studies

1. Electrocardiography—The electrocardiogram (ECG) in patients with significant PH typically shows right ventricular hypertrophy. Classic ECG findings include right axis deviation and right atrial enlargement. Incomplete or complete right bundle branch block is also common. The ECG criteria for right ventricular hypertrophy and a typical ECG in a patient with PH are shown in Table 30–3 and Figure 30–6, respectively. However, the ECG is not sensitive enough to exclude a diagnosis of PH.

2. Chest radiography—The chest radiograph in a patient with PAH may show enlargement of the main pulmonary artery and its major branches with a reduction in the number of distal vessels referred to as pruning. A lateral image will show filling of the retrosternal space, which signifies right ventricular enlargement. Pulmonary venous congestion and left atrial or left ventricular enlargement suggest the presence of a left-sided cause of PH. Hyperinflated lung fields or bullous changes point to PH from lung disease. A classic chest radiograph of a patient with PAH is shown in Figure 30–7.

3. Echocardiography—Echocardiography is often the first test ordered in a patient with suspected PH and may reveal direct or indirect evidence of elevated PAP. Echocardiography is used to estimate the pulmonary artery systolic pressure (PASP). The peak velocity (v) of the tricuspid regurgitant (TR) jet is determined from the continuous wave spectral Doppler signal and entered into the modified Bernoulli equation along with the right atrial pressure (RAP), estimated by evaluating respiratory change in the inferior vena cava diameter: $PASP = 4v^2 + RAP$ (Figure 30–8). Echocardiographic estimates of PASP are often inaccurate, especially if the TR jet is minimal or eccentric. Therefore, a low estimated PASP does not exclude PH in patients in whom PH is clinically suspected.

Structural changes seen on echocardiography may suggest that PH is present. Over time, elevated PAP results in right atrial or right ventricular enlargement, right ventricular hypertrophy, and pulmonary artery enlargement. Ventricular interdependence results in flattening or leftward shift of the interventricular septum and, if seen during systole, suggests pressure overload or, if seen during diastole, suggests volume overload of the right ventricle. The left ventricle is often small and underfilled in PH, with normal systolic function (Figure 30–9). Accurate assessment of the right ventricular systolic function in patients with PH is important because impaired function is a predictor of poor

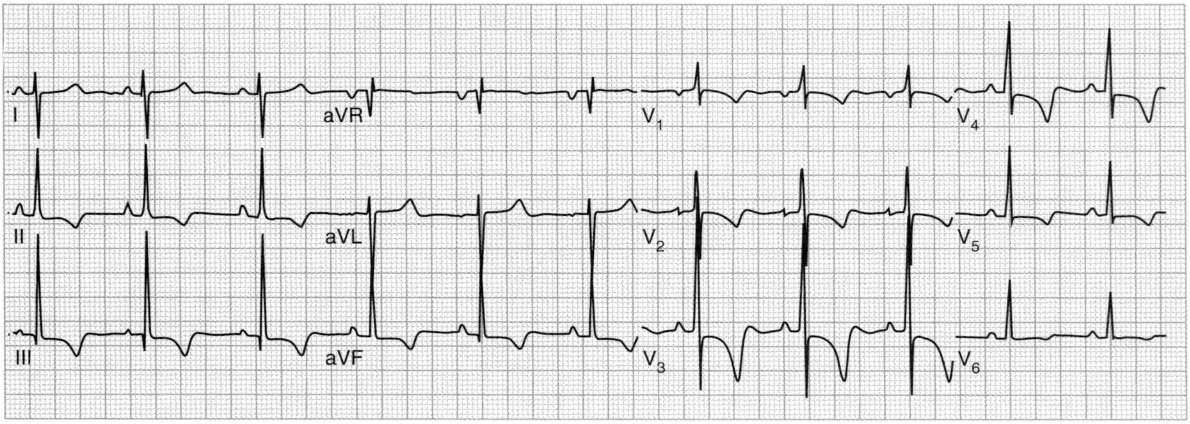

▲ **Figure 30–6.** Electrocardiogram in a patient with pulmonary arterial hypertension and right ventricular hypertrophy.

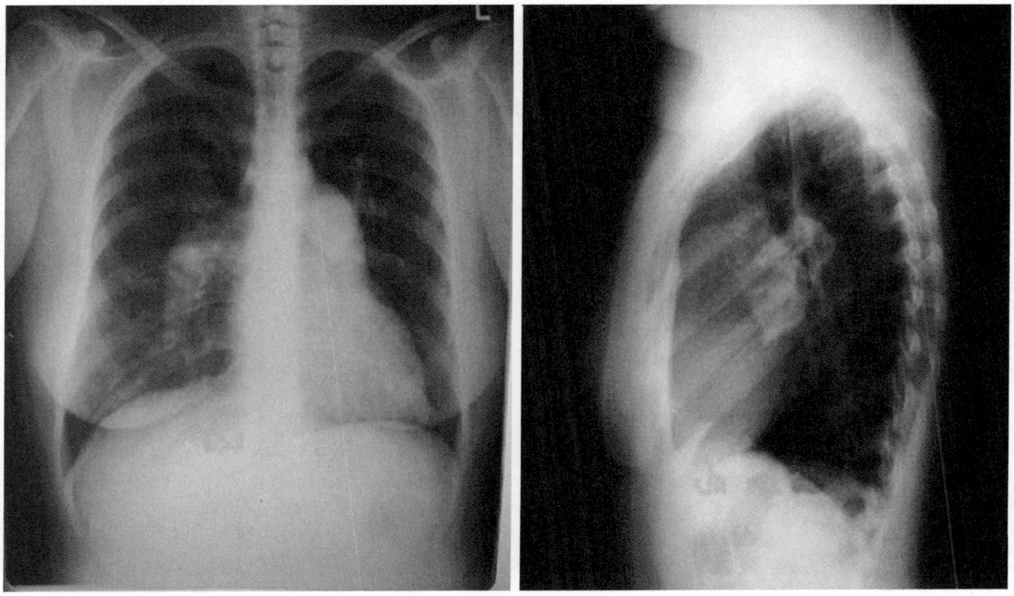

▲ **Figure 30–7.** Chest radiograph in pulmonary arterial hypertension demonstrating enlargement of the central pulmonary arteries with peripheral pruning of the pulmonary vasculature. Also notable is the reduction in the retrosternal air space on the lateral view and the distinct lack of pulmonary pathology.

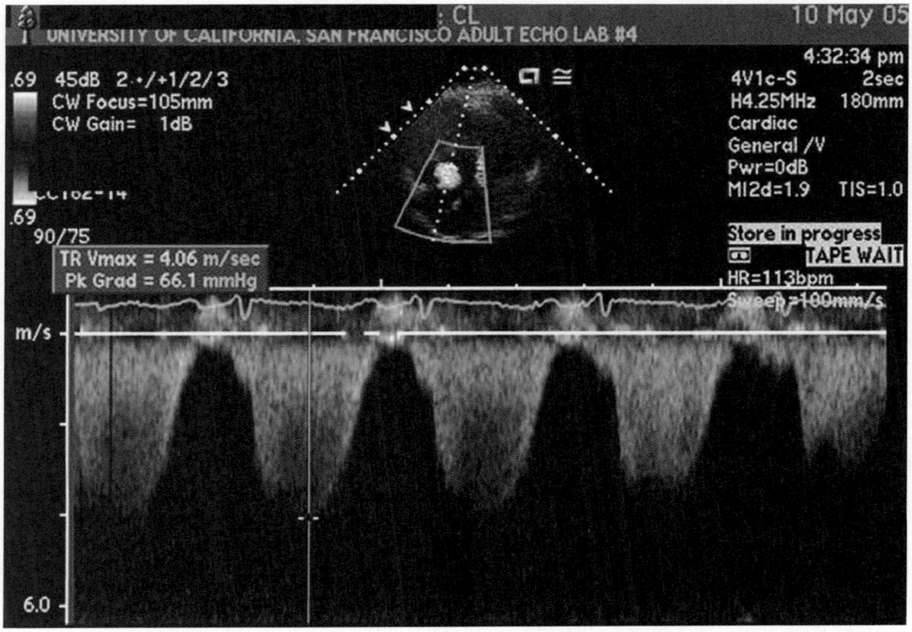

▲ **Figure 30–8.** A continuous wave Doppler recording of the tricuspid regurgitation velocity. The pulmonary artery systolic pressure is calculated by entering the peak tricuspid velocity into the modified Bernoulli equation and adding the right atrial pressure (PASP = $4v^2$ + RAP). PASP, pulmonary artery systolic pressure; v, peak tricuspid regurgitant velocity; RAP, right atrial pressure.

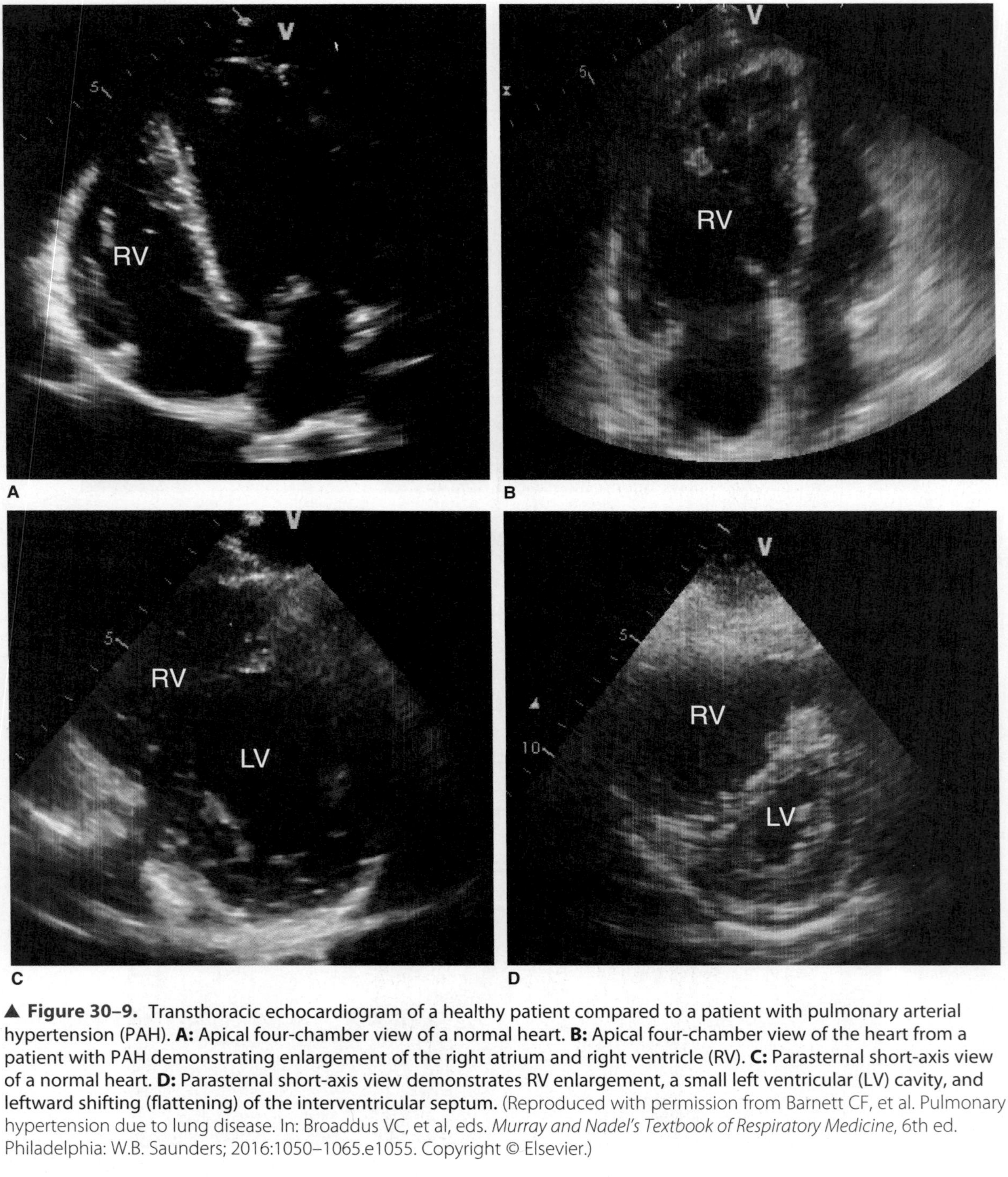

▲ **Figure 30–9.** Transthoracic echocardiogram of a healthy patient compared to a patient with pulmonary arterial hypertension (PAH). **A:** Apical four-chamber view of a normal heart. **B:** Apical four-chamber view of the heart from a patient with PAH demonstrating enlargement of the right atrium and right ventricle (RV). **C:** Parasternal short-axis view of a normal heart. **D:** Parasternal short-axis view demonstrates RV enlargement, a small left ventricular (LV) cavity, and leftward shifting (flattening) of the interventricular septum. (Reproduced with permission from Barnett CF, et al. Pulmonary hypertension due to lung disease. In: Broaddus VC, et al, eds. *Murray and Nadel's Textbook of Respiratory Medicine*, 6th ed. Philadelphia: W.B. Saunders; 2016:1050–1065.e1055. Copyright © Elsevier.)

survival. Approaches to right ventricular function assessment are described; however, they are subject to multiple technical limitations so that the opinion of an experienced echocardiographer is necessary (Figure 30–10).

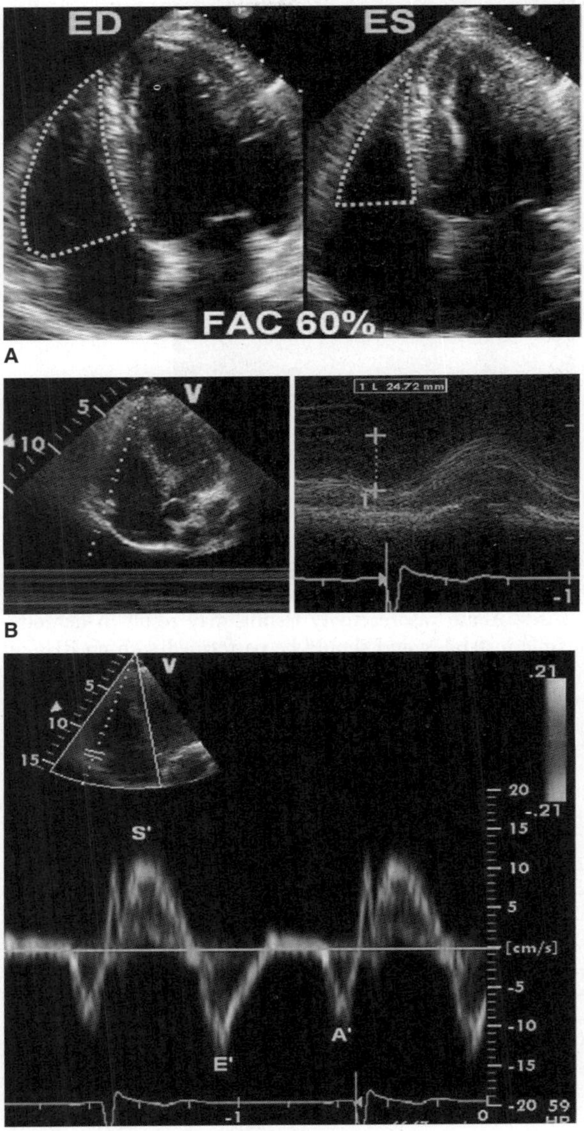

▲ **Figure 30–10.** Approach to assessment of right ventricular function in patients with pulmonary hypertension. **A:** Right ventricular fractional area change (FAC). **B:** Tricuspid annular plane systolic excursion **C:** Tissue Doppler of tricuspid annular systolic velocity (S′). ED, end diastolic; ES, end systolic; E′, tricuspid annular plane early diastolic; A′, late diastolic velocities.

The careful review of the echocardiogram is required to exclude LHD as a cause of PH. HFrEF and valvular heart disease are generally easily diagnosed on a routine echocardiogram. Diagnosing HFpEF is more challenging and should be suspected when PH is seen in a patient with left atria or left ventricular enlargement or left ventricular hypertrophy. Additional maneuvers, such as injection of agitated saline, should be performed to identify cardiac and intrapulmonary shunts.

4. Ventilation-perfusion lung scintigraphy—Ventilation-perfusion (V/Q) lung scintigraphy is required to exclude CTEPH as the etiology of PH because CT pulmonary angiography is insensitive to this diagnosis. In PAH, the V/Q scan may reveal a normal perfusion pattern, or it may show diffuse, patchy perfusion defects. Parenchymal lung disease can also result in perfusion scan abnormalities, but typically, these are matched by ventilatory defects. In CTEPH, the lung perfusion scan demonstrates one or more segmental defects mismatched by the ventilation scan (Figure 30–11). An abnormal V/Q scan should prompt referral to a CTEPH center and conventional pulmonary angiography to confirm the diagnosis of CTEPH and consideration for surgical PEA.

5. Pulmonary function testing—Pulmonary function testing is helpful in PH because it can establish the diagnosis of underlying obstructive or restrictive pulmonary disease. Interpretation of pulmonary function test results should be tempered by an awareness that PAH can reduce diffusing capacity of carbon monoxide. If the total lung capacity is less than 70% of predicted, a high-resolution CT scan should be considered to evaluate for ILD.

6. Computed tomography and magnetic resonance imaging—Chest CT or magnetic resonance imaging (MRI) scans may reveal other causes of PH such as fibrosing mediastinitis and cystic fibrosis, as well as infiltrative or granulomatous lung diseases. Findings on CT pulmonary angiography may suggest a diagnosis of CTEPH; however, the test is not sensitive enough to exclude the diagnosis of CTEPH.

7. Cardiac catheterization and pulmonary angiography—RHC represents the gold standard test to establish the diagnosis of PH, ascertain its etiology, establish severity and prognosis, evaluate vasoreactivity, and guide therapy. RHC should be performed by a clinician with experience in the evaluation and management of patients with PH.

During RHC, hemodynamic measurements should include right atrial pressure, right ventricular pressure, PAP, PAWP, and the CO (Figure 30–12). The PVR is calculated using the following equation (mPAP – PAWP)/CO. Arterial and venous oxygen saturations obtained during RHC are used to detect and determine the presence and severity of shunts. An elevated PAWP suggests LHD, such as aortic or mitral valve disease, HFrEF, or HFpEF as the cause of PH. In elderly patients with diabetes, hypertension, left ventricular hypertrophy, or left atrial enlargement, administration of a

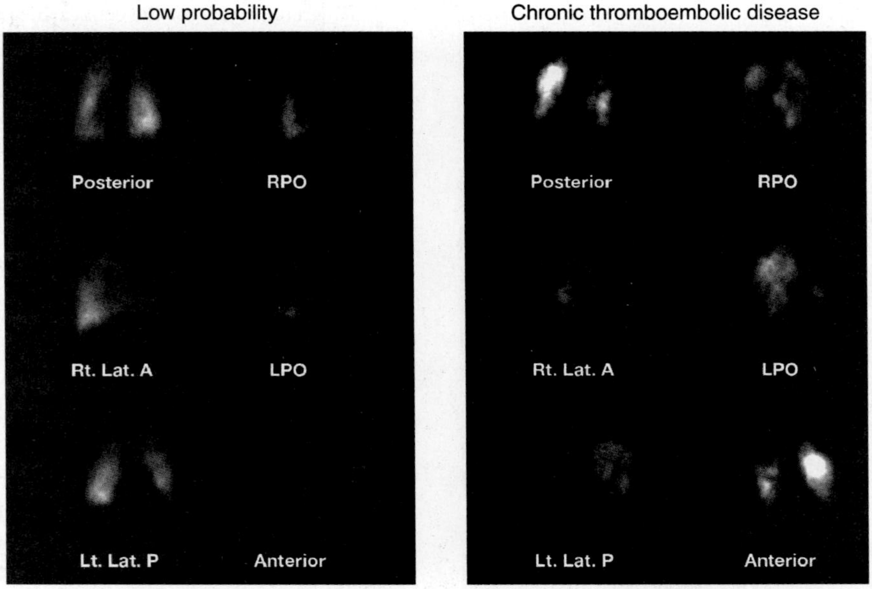

▲ **Figure 30–11.** Perfusion lung scans from a normal patient and a patient with chronic thromboembolic disease. The scan on the left shows uniform perfusion. The scan on the right shows multiple perfusion defects consistent with the diagnosis of chronic thromboembolic disease. LPO, left posterior oblique; RPO, right posterior oblique.

fluid bolus or exercise during RHC should be considered to exclude the presence of otherwise unrecognized HFpEF.

Vasoreactivity testing during RHC is used to identify the small proportion of patients with idiopathic or heritable PAH who can be successfully treated with calcium channel blockers and is not useful in patients with PAH from other underlying causes. Acute vasoreactivity testing may result in hemodynamic instability and should be performed with an RHC in

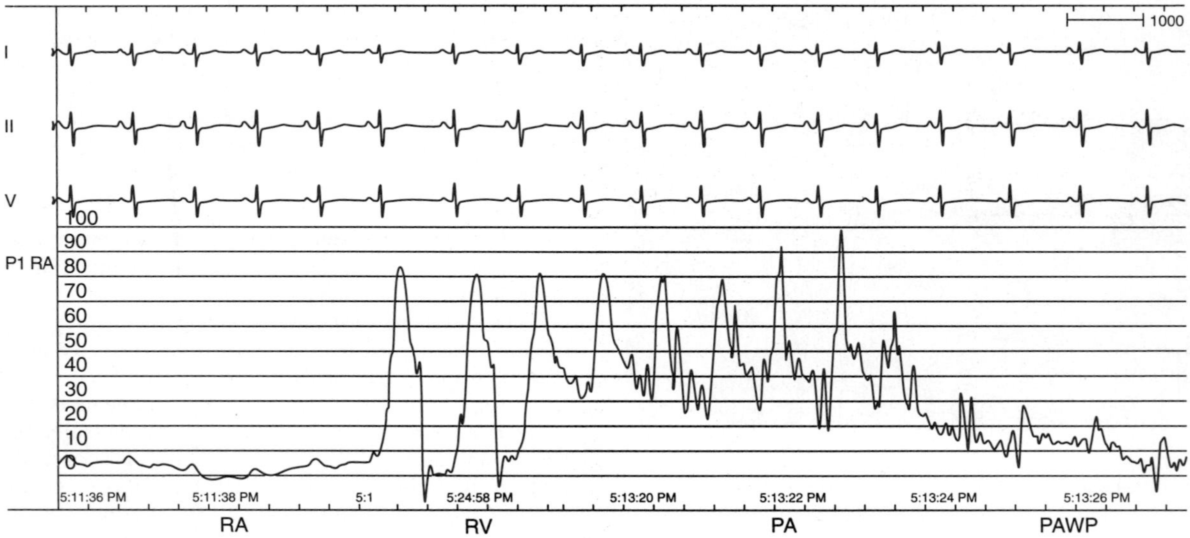

▲ **Figure 30–12.** Hemodynamic tracing from a patient with pulmonary hypertension. Waveforms that are obtained as the catheter passes from the right atrium (RA) through the right ventricle (RV), pulmonary artery (PA), and into the pulmonary artery wedge position. Notable findings include the markedly elevated pulmonary artery pressure and the normal pulmonary artery wedge pressure (PAWP).

place in a monitored setting with the supervision of experienced physicians. Vasodilator testing is usually performed by administering inhaled nitric oxide at a dose of 20 parts per million for 10 minutes. A reduction in mPAP greater than 10 mm Hg with a final mPAP ≤ 40 mm Hg without a reduction in the CO or increase in the PAWP identifies patients who can be treated with calcium channel blockers.

Although not routinely performed, pulmonary angiography is useful to confirm the diagnosis of CTEPH and to determine if surgical PEA can be performed.

8. Lung biopsy—Lung biopsy rarely provides useful diagnostic information and is associated with significant risk in patients with PH. When performed, lung biopsy may reveal findings such as injected particulate matter in injection drug users, arterialization of pulmonary venules in pulmonary veno-occlusive disease, or typical findings of ILD. Typical pathologic findings of PAH are illustrated in Figure 30–13.

9. Functional capacity and exercise testing—Determination of each patient's World Health Organization functional classification and symptom-limited exercise testing should be performed during the evaluation of all patients with PH. Exercise testing, particularly the 6-minute walk (6MW) test, has been shown to predict mortality and allows for objective assessment of symptom burden. Exercise tolerance should be assessed prior to initiation of therapy with the 6MW test, which is then repeated often to monitor response to treatment.

10. Other studies—Overnight pulse oximetry should be performed to identify patients who require supplemental oxygen to treat nocturnal hypoxemia. If sleep-disordered breathing is suspected, a full sleep study should be performed. Testing of liver enzymes and liver ultrasound is used to look for evidence of liver dysfunction and portal hypertension. Screening for connective tissue diseases including scleroderma, rheumatoid arthritis, systemic lupus erythematosus, mixed connective tissue disease, and polymyositis should be performed with appropriate serologic and immunogenetic studies. Thyroid function and HIV testing should also be performed in all patients. Schistosomiasis can cause PAH and should be excluded in patients from endemic areas with PAH.

Farrell C, Balasubramanian A, Hays AG, et al. A clinical approach to multimodality imaging in pulmonary hypertension. *Front Cardiovasc Med.* 2021;8:794706. [PMID: 35118142]

Maron BA, Kovacs, Vaidya A, et al. Cardiopulmonary hemodynamics in pulmonary hypertension and heart failure: JACC Review Topic of the Week. *J Am Coll Cardiol.* 2020 Dec 1; 76(22):2671–2681. [PMID: 33243385]

Remy-Jardin M, Ryerson CJ, Schiebler ML, et al. Imaging of pulmonary hypertension in adults: a position paper from the Fleischner Society. *Eur Respir J.* Jan 2021;57(1):2004455. [PMID: 33402372]

Ruopp NF, Cockrill BA. Diagnosis and treatment of pulmonary arterial hypertension: a review. *JAMA.* Apr 12 2022; 327(14): 1379–1391. [PMID: 35412560]

Differential Diagnosis

Determining if a patient has PAH versus PH from heart disease, lung disease, or CTEPH is critically important due to significant differences in management and survival (see Table 30–1). For example, endothelin receptor antagonists

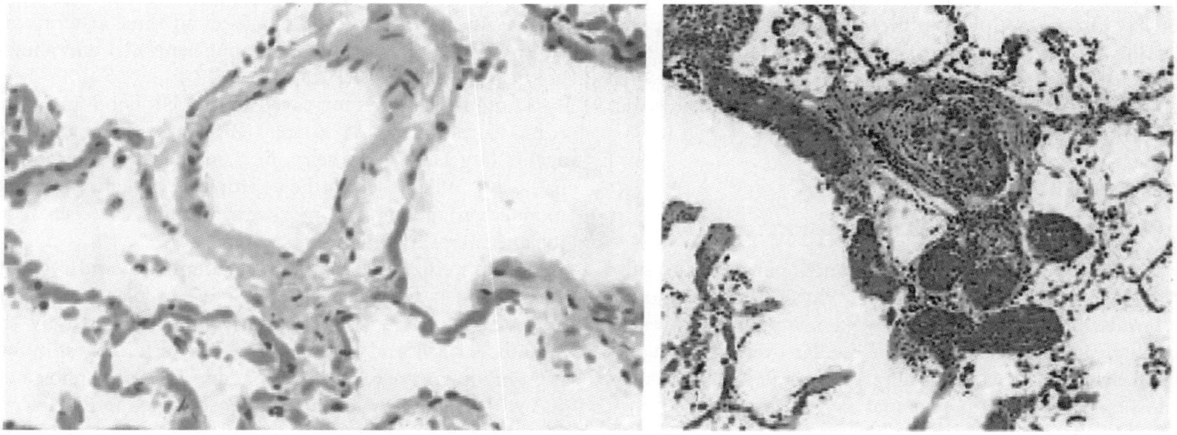

A B

▲ **Figure 30–13.** Pathologic appearance of a normal pulmonary arteriole compared to a pulmonary arteriole in pulmonary arterial hypertension. **A:** Normal pulmonary arteriole. **B:** Pulmonary arteriole from a patient with pulmonary arteriole hypertension demonstrating a vascular endothelial cell proliferation and smooth muscle cell hypertrophy and a plexiform lesion. (Reprinted, with permission, from Barnett CF, et al. Pulmonary hypertension due to lung disease. In: Broaddus VC, et al, eds. *Murray and Nadel's Textbook of Respiratory Medicine*, 6th ed. Philadelphia: W.B. Saunders; 2016:1050–1065.e1055. Copyright © Elsevier.)

significantly improve outcomes in patients with PAH, whereas, by contrast, they worsen symptoms and increase hospitalization in patients with LHD and ILD. A comprehensive diagnostic evaluation that integrates findings from the patient history and physical examination as well as the results of all diagnostic tests is mandatory so that underlying diseases can be correctly identified and treated and so that optimal therapy for PAH, if present, can be chosen. The diagnostic approach currently recommended in PH is shown in Figure 30–14.

In many cases, an elevated PAP is first noted on echocardiography that is performed to evaluate symptoms of exertional dyspnea, edema, chest pain, presyncope, or syncope. LHD is the most common cause of PH, and often, HFrEF or severe valvular heart disease will be evident on the initial echocardiogram so that no further evaluation will be required.

Pulmonary disease is the second most common cause of PH and may be suggested by findings on chest radiograph, arterial oxygen saturation measurement, pulmonary function testing, sleep study, and chest CT scan.

A V/Q scan should be performed, and diagnosis of CTEPH should be considered in all patients with PH because it may coexist with PH from heart or lung disease.

A diagnosis of PAH is typically reached when other more common causes of PH have been excluded. Patients then undergo evaluation for secondary causes of PAH by performing serologic testing for connective tissue diseases, thyroid disease, and HIV. Imaging studies should be reviewed to exclude evidence of portal hypertension.

RHC is a required test in all patients in whom a diagnosis of PAH is being considered to confirm the diagnosis as well as determine prognosis and select initial therapy. RHC is also sometimes required to exclude a diagnosis of HFpEF. Reaching a final diagnosis requires integrating features of the clinical presentation together with hemodynamic findings and results of the entire diagnostic evaluation.

Treatment

A. Pulmonary Arterial Hypertension

Improvement in exercise capacity, functional class, and survival are the goals of PAH treatment. Physical activity should be limited below levels that provoke symptoms. However, low-intensity physical activity or regular exercise to maintain skeletal muscle conditioning and overall cardiovascular fitness is beneficial. Supplemental oxygen should be administered to all patients to maintain an oxygen saturation more than 92% with exertion, as well as for travel to high altitudes and for air travel. Immunization against influenza and pneumococcus is recommended. Oral anticoagulation is no longer recommended in all forms of PAH. Anticoagulation can be considered in patients with idiopathic, heritable PAH, and drug-induced PAH on a case-by-case basis after an individualized risk-benefit analysis. Treatment is generally with warfarin adjusted to an international normalized ratio (INR) of 1.5–2.5.

Pregnancy in patients with PAH is associated with high mortality, so women of childbearing potential should be counseled to avoid pregnancy and should be prescribed appropriate contraception. Hemoglobin levels should be monitored regularly. In patients with Eisenmenger syndrome, erythrocytosis should be treated with phlebotomy if symptoms of hyperviscosity develop. Patients with PAH should not smoke. Sodium restriction is often necessary to minimize fluid retention.

Diuretic therapy is necessary for most patients to maintain euvolemia. Furosemide, even at high doses, may be inadequate due to poor absorption and variable pharmacodynamics. Alternative loop diuretics such as bumetanide and torsemide and combination with thiazide diuretics are often necessary. Atrial arrhythmias are best treated with digoxin, which is tolerated better than calcium channel blockers or β-blockers.

In patients with PAH and decompensated right heart failure, strategies to improve right ventricular function and restore end-organ perfusion include (1) afterload reduction with pulmonary vasodilators, such as oxygen, inhaled nitric oxide, prostanoids, endothelin receptor antagonists, and phosphodiesterase inhibitors; (2) preload reduction with diuretics; and (3) augmentation of right ventricular function with intravenous inotropic drugs such as dobutamine or milrinone.

A small percentage of patients (< 10%) with idiopathic or heritable PAH can be successfully treated with high-dose calcium channel blocker therapy. These patients can be identified by a reduction in mPAP of at least 10 mm Hg to ≤ 40 mm Hg without a reduction in CO or an increase in PAWP. In patients who do not meet all these criteria, calcium channel blocker therapy is not beneficial and should not be used to treat PAH.

Multiple therapies approved by the US Food and Drug Administration (FDA) to treat PAH are available. These agents target the endothelin, nitric oxide, and prostacyclin pathways. When used in the appropriate patient, these pulmonary vasodilators can improve symptoms, exercise capacity, and mortality (Table 30–4).

Prostacyclin (PGI_2) is a direct pulmonary and systemic vasodilator as well as an inhibitor of vascular remodeling and platelet aggregation. Prostacyclin is secreted by the endothelial cell and exerts its vascular effect by stimulating smooth muscle cell cyclic adenosine monophosphate (cAMP). The PGI_2 pathway is downregulated in PAH.

Epoprostenol was the first available PAH-specific therapy approved in 1996 following a landmark 12-week trial that showed a marked improvement in mortality with epoprostenol treatment. Epoprostenol remains the gold standard treatment for PAH and is the treatment of choice for patients at high risk of death. Due to its short half-life, epoprostenol must be administered by continuous intravenous (IV) infusion, and treatment can be difficult given the

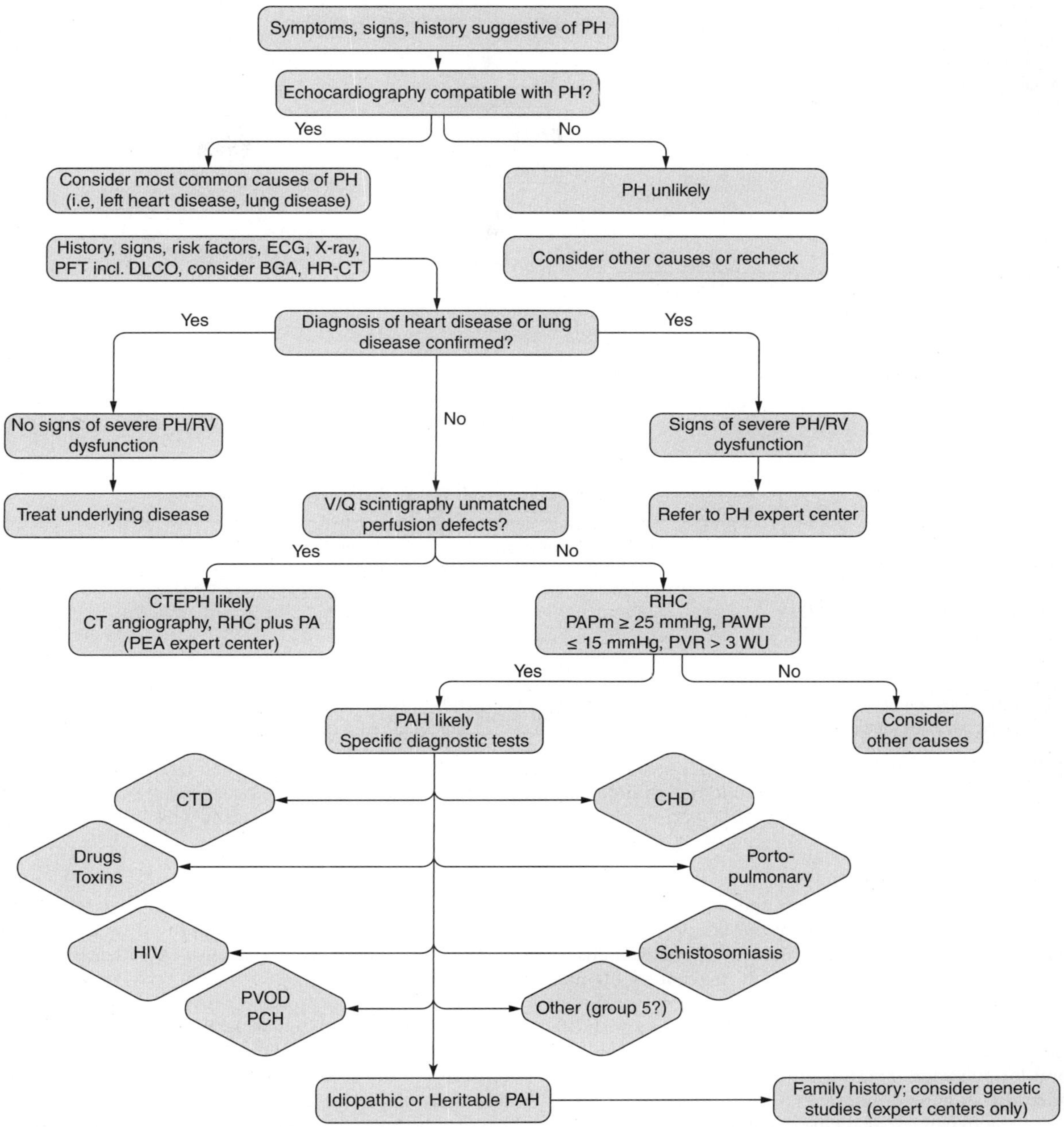

▲ **Figure 30–14.** Diagnostic algorithm for pulmonary arterial hypertension updated at the Fifth World Symposium on Pulmonary Hypertension. BGA, blood gas analysis; CHD, congenital heart disease; CTD, connective tissue disease; CTEPH, chronic thromboembolic pulmonary hypertension; DLCO, diffusion capacity of the lung for carbon monoxide; ECG, electrocardiogram; HR-CT, high-resolution computed tomography; PA, pulmonary angiography; PAH, pulmonary arterial hypertension; PAPm, mean pulmonary artery pressure; PAWP, pulmonary arterial wedge pressure; PCH, pulmonary capillary hemangiomatosis; PEA, pulmonary endarterectomy; PFT, pulmonary function testing; PH, pulmonary hypertension; PVOD, pulmonary veno-occlusive disease; PVR, pulmonary vascular resistance; RHC, right heart catheter; RV, right ventricle; V/Q, ventilation/perfusion; WU, Woods units; x-ray, chest radiograph. (Reproduced with permission from Hoeper MM, et al. Definitions and diagnosis of pulmonary hypertension. *J Am Coll Cardiol*. 2013;62[25 Suppl]:D42–D50.)

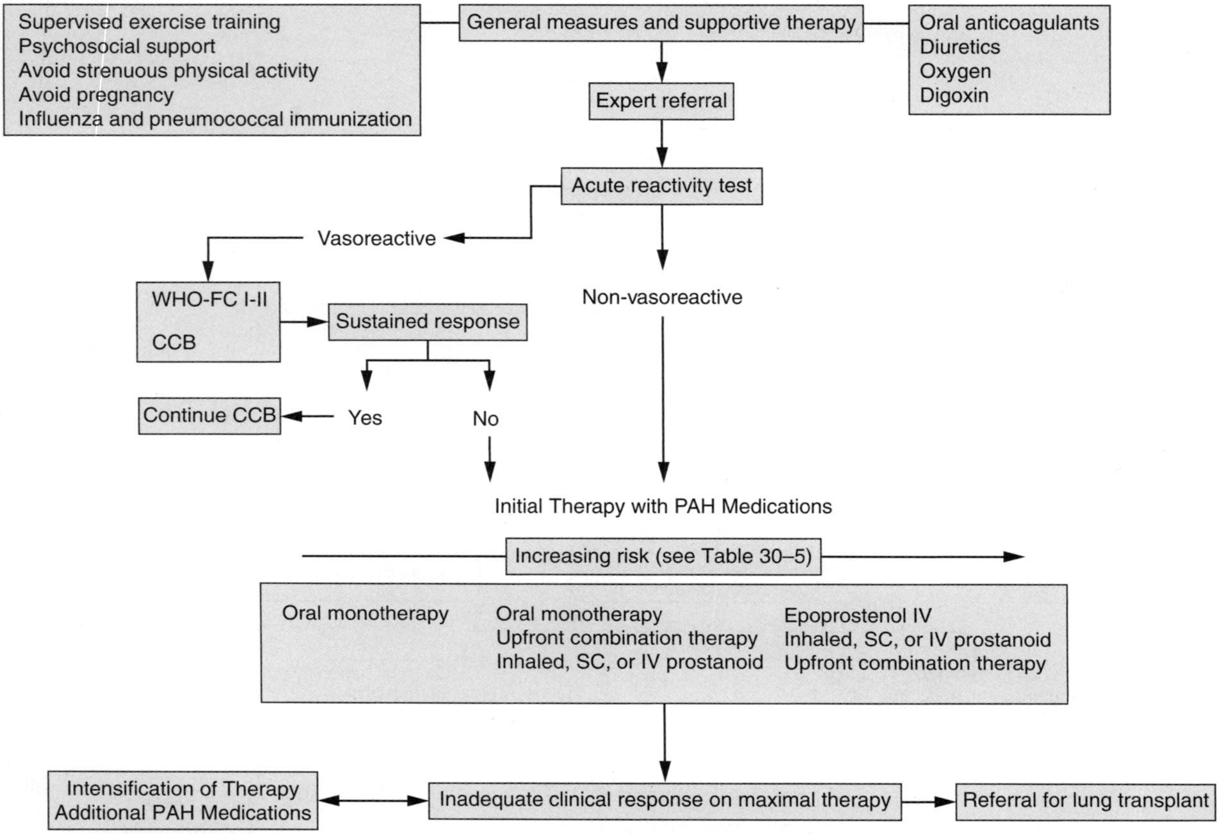

▲ **Figure 30–15.** **Pulmonary arterial hypertension (PAH) treatment algorithm. CCB, calcium channel blocker; IV, intravenous; SC, subcutaneous; WHO-FC, World Health Organization functional classification.** (Reproduced with permission from Galiè N, Corris PA, Frost A, et al. Updated treatment algorithm of pulmonary arterial hypertension. *J Am Coll Cardiol.* 2013;62[25 Suppl]:D60–D72.)

required complex delivery system and associated complications including central venous catheter infection, thrombosis, and pump malfunction. Even brief interruptions of the epoprostenol infusion can result in rebound PH and cardiopulmonary collapse.

Treprostinil is a prostanoid with a 4- to 6-hour half-life that is available in IV, subcutaneous (SC), inhaled, and oral formulations. Treprostinil was first approved for SC administration and improves 6MW distance, dyspnea, and hemodynamics. SC delivery eliminates the need for a central venous catheter; however, difficult-to-manage pain surrounding the SC infusion site is common, and superficial infection can occur. Dosing is equivalent, so that IV and SC treprostinil are interchangeable. The longer half-life of treprostinil reduces the potential adverse outcomes of infusion interruptions. Inhaled treprostinil confers similar benefits and is delivered using a proprietary inhaler device four times daily. Oral treprostinil is also available and improves 6MW distance in treatment-naïve patients but is of unclear utility in patients already receiving other PAH therapy. Treprostinil was approved by the FDA in 2022 to improve exercise tolerance in patients with PH caused by ILD.

Iloprost is another prostanoid that is delivered by inhalation; however, its use is limited by the need for frequent dosing and an expensive and difficult-to-use nebulizer device.

Selexipag is a first-in-class prostacyclin IP receptor agonist approved by the FDA in December 2015 based on a large study showing that, when used alone or added to other therapies, it improved exercise tolerance, reduced disease progression, and reduced mortality.

Dose-limiting side effects are common during prostanoid treatment and often include headaches, flushing, nausea, vomiting, diarrhea, arthralgias, myalgias, and jaw pain. Side effects can often be managed with lifestyle modification and treatment with agents such as gabapentin. Side effects can be minimized and higher doses achieved by very slowly increasing the dose of prostanoids.

Table 30–4. U.S. Food and Drug Administration–Approved Drugs for the Treatment of Pulmonary Hypertension

Drug	Study Characteristics	Positive Results	Disadvantages
Endothelin Receptor Antagonists (ERAs)			
Bosentan (A and B)	*Name*: BREATHE-1 *Design*: Double-blind *Number*: 213	Improved 6-minute walk distance Improved dyspnea Delayed clinical worsening	Hepatic toxicity Teratogenic Fluid retention, peripheral edema, anemia, nasal congestion, sinusitis, flushing Monthly transaminase monitoring required
Ambrisentan (A)	*Name*: ARIES-1 *Name*: ARIES-2 *Design*: Double-blind *Number*: 202 and 192, respectively	Improved 6-minute walk distance Delayed clinical worsening Improved hemodynamics Transaminase monitoring not required	Teratogenic Fluid retention, peripheral edema, anemia, nasal congestion, sinusitis, flushing
Macitentan (A and B)	*Name*: SERAPHIN *Design*: Double-blind *Number*: 742	Reduced incidence of composite end point of death, atrial septostomy, lung transplantation, IV or SC prostanoid therapy, or worsening PAH	Teratogenic Headache, nasopharyngitis, anemia
Phosphodiesterase-5 (PDE-5) Inhibitors			
Sildenafil	*Name*: SUPER-1 *Design*: Double-blind *Number*: 278	Improved 6-minute walk distance Improved dyspnea Improved hemodynamics	No delay in clinical worsening end point Headache, flushing, dyspepsia, epistaxis, visual disturbance Interactions with protease inhibitors
Tadalafil	*Name*: PHIRST *Design*: Double-blind *Number*: 405	Improved 6-minute walk distance Improved time to clinical worsening Improved hemodynamics Improved quality of life	Headache, myalgias, flushing, dyspepsia, epistaxis, visual disturbance
Soluble guanylate cyclase agonists			
Riociguat	*Name*: PATENT-1 and -2 *Design*: Double-blind *Number*: 443	Improved 6-minute walk distance Improved hemodynamics Improved time to clinical worsening Improved quality of life Reduced brain natriuretic peptide Improved WHO class Improved dyspnea	Teratogenic Headache, dyspepsia, edema, dyspepsia, nausea, dizziness Severe hypotension with PDE-5 inhibitors
Riociguat	*Name*: CHEST-1 and -2 (Group 4 PH-CTEPH) *Design*: Double-blind *Number*: 261	Improved 6-minute walk distance Improved hemodynamics Reduced brain natriuretic peptide Improved WHO class	Teratogenic Severe hypotension with PDE-5 inhibitors
Prostanoids			
Epoprostenol, intravenous	*Design*: Open-label *Number*: 81	Improved 6-minute walk distance Improved dyspnea Improved hemodynamics Improved survival	Indwelling central line Pump malfunction Flushing, jaw pain, thrombocytopenia, headache, dizziness, nausea/vomiting/diarrhea, abdominal pain, hypotension, rash
Treprostinil, intravenous or subcutaneous	*Design*: Double-blind *Number*: 470	Improved 6-minute walk distance Improved dyspnea Improved hemodynamics	Indwelling central line or subcutaneous catheter Pain, erythema at infusion site (subcutaneous) Flushing, jaw pain, thrombocytopenia, headache, dizziness, nausea/vomiting/diarrhea, abdominal pain, hypotension, rash

(*Continued*)

Table 30–4. U.S. Food and Drug Administration–Approved Drugs for the Treatment of Pulmonary Hypertension (*Continued*)

Drug	Study Characteristics	Positive Results	Disadvantages
Treprostinil, inhaled	*Name*: TRIUMPH *Design*: Double-blind *Number*: 470	Improved 6-minute walk distance Improved quality of life Administration 4 times daily	No delay in clinical worsening or dyspnea No change in functional class Cough, headache, nausea, dizziness, flushing, throat irritation or pain
Treprostinil, inhaled	*Name*: INCREASE (Group 3 PH-ILD) *Design*: Double-blind *Number*: 326	Improved 6-minute walk distance Improved time to clinical worsening Reduced brain natriuretic peptide	Cough, headache, dyspnea, dizziness, nausea, fatigue, and diarrhea
Treprostinil, oral	*Name*: FREEDOM-M *Design*: Double-blind *Number*: 349	Improved 6-minute walk distance	No additional benefits when added to PDE-5 or ERA Headache, nausea, diarrhea, jaw pain
Iloprost, inhaled	*Design*: Double-blind *Number*: 203	Improved composite end point of 6-minute walk distance and dyspnea	Administration 6–9 times daily Cough, headache, nausea, dizziness, flushing, throat irritation or pain
IP Prostacyclin Receptor Agonist			
Selexipag	*Name*: GRIPHON *Design*: Double-blind *Number*: 1156	Reduced incidence of composite end point of any complication of PAH or death	Headache, diarrhea, nausea, jaw pain

IV, intravenous; PAH, pulmonary arterial hypertension; SC, subcutaneous; WHO, World Health Organization.

Endothelin-1 is secreted by vascular endothelial cells and is a potent vasoconstrictor and mediator of smooth muscle cell proliferation. In addition, endothelin-1 enhances vascular fibrosis, increases platelet aggregation, promotes cardiac myocyte hypertrophy, and increases aldosterone production. Endothelin-1 is secreted in response to a variety of stimuli, including hypoxemia, endothelial sheer and pulsatile stress, and neurohormonal activation, as well as PH-related growth factors and cytokines.

Three endothelin receptor antagonists are now available for the treatment of PAH. Bosentan is an endothelin-A and -B receptor antagonist that has been shown to increase 6MW distance, decrease symptom burden, and delay clinical worsening in patients. Ambrisentan is an endothelin-A receptor antagonist that improves exercise capacity, delays time to clinical worsening, and improves cardiopulmonary hemodynamics. Macitentan is unique because it was shown to improve exercise tolerance and reduce mortality. Macitentan is also FDA approved for the treatment of CTEPH.

Endothelin receptor antagonists are teratogenic, so patients of childbearing potential must reliably use approved contraception and undergo monthly pregnancy testing. Reversible transaminitis requiring liver function test monitoring occurs in patients treated with bosentan but not with ambrisentan or macitentan. Other common endothelin receptor antagonist side effects include nasal congestion, flushing, anemia, and lower extremity edema.

Nitric oxide is secreted by the endothelial cell and diffuses to the smooth muscle cell where it mediates vasodilation and exerts an antiproliferative effect via activation of the cyclic guanosine monophosphate (cGMP) pathway. Nitric oxide effects can be augmented by inhibiting, degradation of cGMP with phosphodiesterase-5 (PDE-5) inhibitors or by direct activation of guanylate cyclase.

Sildenafil and tadalafil are oral PDE-5 inhibitors. When administered long term, both agents improve exercise capacity, reduce symptom burden, and improve hemodynamics. Tadalafil but not sildenafil has been shown to delay clinical worsening. Tadalafil is dosed once daily compared to three times daily dosing for sildenafil. PDE-5 inhibitors can cause headache, flushing, dyspepsia, epistaxis, and visual changes.

Riociguat is an oral guanylate cyclase stimulator. It has the theoretical advantage that its efficacy does not depend on endogenous nitric oxide production, which is reduced in PAH. Riociguat improves exercise tolerance and reduces clinical worsening in patients with PAH. Riociguat is approved for use in CTEPH but should only be considered in patients who are not candidates for PEA. Riociguat cannot be used in combination with sildenafil or tadalafil because it may precipitate severe hypotension.

Sotatercept is the first in a new class of drugs for PAH that acts by rebalancing growth-promoting and growth-inhibiting signaling made abnormal by defects in the

Table 30–5. Characteristics Associated with High Risk of Poor Outcome in Pulmonary Arterial Hypertension

Determinant	Higher Risk
Syncope	Yes
Disease progression	Rapid
World Health Organization functional class	IV
6-Minute walk distance	< 300 m
Cardiopulmonary exercise testing	Peak VO_2 < 10.4 mL/kg/min
Brain natriuretic peptide	>180 pg/mL
Echocardiographic findings	Pericardial effusion Right ventricular dysfunction TAPSE(tricuspid annular plane systolic excursion) < 1.8 cm
Hemodynamics	Right atrial pressure > 15 mm Hg Cardiac index ≤ 2 L/min·m^2

BMPR-II signaling pathway. In a phase 2 trial, sotatercept improved hemodynamics and exercise tolerance compared with placebo. A phase 3 trial is underway.

Initial treatment choice is determined by disease severity. In patients with high-risk features and in critically ill patients, IV prostacyclin is generally the treatment of choice (Table 30–5). Individual patient factors, such as comorbidities (ie, liver disease), concomitant drug therapy, or a history of medication nonadherence, may all influence treatment choice (Figure 30–15).

Recent improvements in medical therapy have minimized the role of invasive PAH treatments; however, lung transplantation, combined heart–lung transplantation, and atrial septostomy remain useful options in patients unresponsive to medical treatment. Mortality among PAH patients awaiting lung transplantation is high, so patients who are unresponsive to medical therapy should be referred early for lung transplant evaluation. Combined heart and lung transplantation is most often performed in patients with congenital heart disease. Atrial septostomy is performed at some expert centers as a palliative treatment for severely symptomatic PAH. The resulting right–left shunt improves left ventricular filling and CO; however, it can also worsen hypoxemia and increase the risk of paradoxical embolization.

B. Pulmonary Hypertension with Left-Sided Heart Disease

PH occurs in 25–30% of patients with LHD and is the most common cause of PH. When PH develops as a complication of LHD, it is associated with worse outcomes. In addition to optimal guideline-recommended therapy, diuretics should be used to achieve euvolemia in patients with HFrEF and HFpEF, which may require guidance with invasive assessment of PAP. Valvular heart disease and coronary artery disease should be aggressively treated in accordance with guideline recommendations.

There is currently no role for PAH therapies to patients with PH-LHD. IV prostacyclin increases mortality in patients with HFrEF and endothelin receptor antagonists worsen heart failure and increase mortality. Although short-term hemodynamic improvements are described, treatment with PDE-5 inhibitors does not yield improvement in clinically meaningful end points in HFrEF and HFpEF patients. In highly selected patients, long-term infusion of inotropes and vasodilators, ventricular assist devices, or PDE-5 inhibitors may be used to lower PAP to facilitate heart transplantation.

C. Pulmonary Hypertension Associated with Lung Disease or Hypoxemia

Lung disease is the second most common cause of PH and, in most cases, results primarily from hypoxic pulmonary vasoconstriction. Correction of hypoxemia and optimal treatment of the underlying lung disease are generally the appropriate treatments. Comorbid conditions that can cause or worsen PH from lung disease, such as HFpEF and CTEPH, are common and should be identified and treated. Inhaled treprostinil was approved to treat patients with PH from ILD in 2022. However, other PAH therapies should generally not be used because they have not been shown to improve PH from lung disease and may worsen outcomes. Sildenafil is known to worsen gas exchange, and macitentan increases exacerbations of ILD. Because development of PH in patients with lung disease is associated with increased mortality, patients who might be lung transplant candidates should undergo expedited evaluation.

D. Pulmonary Hypertension due to Chronic Thrombotic or Embolic Disease

Mortality in patients with CTEPH who do not undergo surgical PEA is high, so CTEPH should be excluded in all patients undergoing evaluation for PH. Patients with suspected CTEPH should be referred to a CTEPH expert center for confirmatory conventional pulmonary angiography and surgical evaluation (Figure 30–16). At experienced centers, perioperative mortality following PEA is as low as 4.4%, and surgery may be possible in patients previously considered inoperable. Following PEA, most patients experience marked improvement in PAP, right heart function, NYHA class, and exercise capacity. Riociguat and macitentan have been approved for the treatment of inoperable CTEPH; however, it is important that this drug not be considered an alternative to surgical PEA. Percutaneous treatment of CTEPH with BPA is now offered in some CTEPH centers.

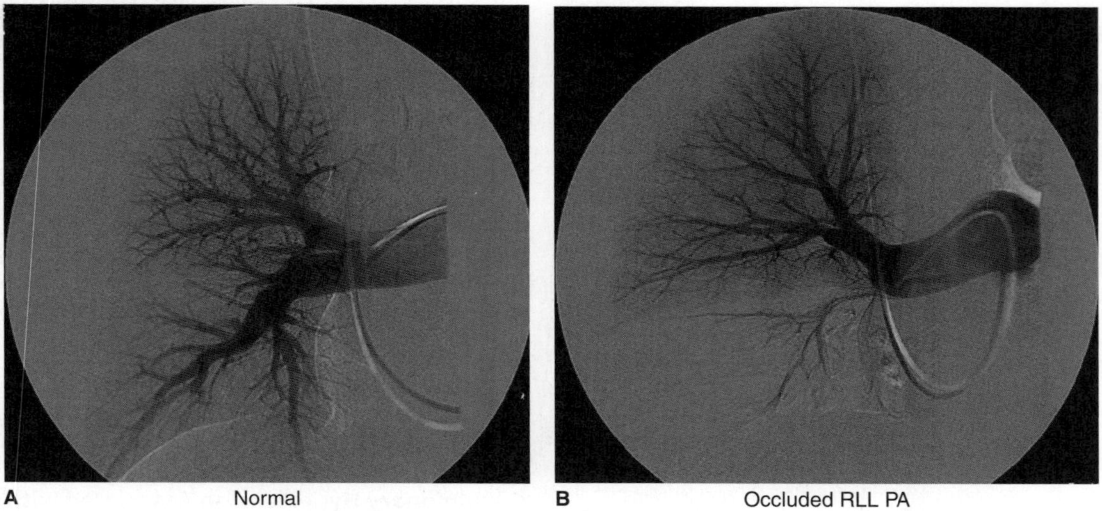

▲ **Figure 30–16.** Conventional pulmonary angiography. **A:** Normal pulmonary angiogram. **B:** Pulmonary angiogram from a patient with chronic thromboembolic pulmonary hypertension demonstrating occlusion of the right lower lobe pulmonary artery (RLL PA). (Reprinted, with permission, from Barnett C, et al. Cardiac catheterization in the patient with pulmonary hypertension. In: Yuan JXJ, et al, eds. *Textbook of Pulmonary Vascular Disease*. New York: Springer US; 2011: 1387–1402. Copyright © Springer Science+Business Media, 2011.)

Barnett CF, O'Brien C, Marco TD. Critical care management of the patient with pulmonary hypertension. *Eur Heart J Acute Cardiovasc Care*. Jan 12 2022;11(1):77–83. [PMID: 34966914]

Galiè N, Channick RN, Frantz RP, et al. Risk stratification and medical therapy of pulmonary arterial hypertension. *Eur Respir J*. Jan 2019;53(1):1801889. [PMID: 30545971]

Ghofrani HA, Simonneau G, D'Armini AM, et al. Macitentan for the treatment of inoperable chronic thromboembolic pulmonary hypertension (MERIT-1): results from the multicentre, phase 2, randomised, double-blind, placebo-controlled study. *Lancet Respir Med*. Oct 2017;5(10):785–794. [PMID: 28919201]

Humbert M, McLaughlin V, Gibbs JSR, et al. Sotatercept for the treatment of pulmonary arterial hypertension. *N Engl J Med*. Apr 1 2021;384(13):1204–1215. [PMID: 33789009]

Ruopp NF, Cockrill BA. Diagnosis and treatment of pulmonary arterial hypertension: a review. *JAMA*. 2022 Apr 12;327(14): 1379–1391. [PMID: 35412560]

Waxman A, Jaramillo RR, Thenappan T, et al. Inhaled treprostinil in pulmonary hypertension Due to Interstitial Lung Disease. *N Engl J Med*. Jan 28 2021;384(4):325–334. [PMID: 33440084]

Prognosis

PH is a progressive disorder associated with a high mortality rate. The underlying cause of the PH is a key factor in determining the prognosis and natural history of the disease (see Table 30–1). Patients with PAH associated with connective tissue disease and those with PAH and HIV have the worst prognosis. Patients with congenital heart disease, by contrast, have the best prognosis. Even for patients with PH due to lung disease or hypoxemia, survival rates vary widely. Patients with PH and emphysema have a 6-month survival of 81%, whereas patients with PH and ILD have a 6-month survival of 38%.

Clinical features and hemodynamic parameters also strongly influence survival. Markers of poor prognosis in PH include advanced functional class (NYHA III–IV) (see Table 30–2), poor exercise capacity (reduced 6MW distance), and resting hemodynamics consistent with right ventricular failure (high right atrial pressure, low CO), elevated B-type natriuretic peptide, and presence of a pericardial effusion or significant right ventricular dysfunction on echocardiogram (see Table 30–5).

Benza RL, Maitland MG, Elliott CG, et al. Predicting survival in patients with pulmonary arterial hypertension: The REVEAL Risk Score Calculator 2.0 and Comparison With ESC/ERS-Based Risk Assessment Strategies. *Chest*. Aug 2019;156(2): 323–337. [PMID: 30772387]

Humbert M, Faber HW, Ghofrani HA, et al. Risk assessment in pulmonary arterial hypertension and chronic thromboembolic pulmonary hypertension. *Eur Respir J*. Jun 2019;53(6):1802004. [PMID: 30923187]

Congenital Heart Disease in Adults

31

Aarthi Sabanayagam, MD
Ian S. Harris, MD

General Considerations

Congenital cardiac anomalies are the most common birth defects in humans, affecting approximately 0.8 in 100 live births. While the incidence of congenital heart disease (CHD) is expected to decline as a consequence of improved prenatal diagnosis, the number of patients surviving with CHD, both in the United States and worldwide, has increased significantly over the past three decades. More than 85% of infants born with cardiovascular anomalies now can expect to reach adulthood. Reduced mortality rates can be attributed to improved diagnostic abilities, enhanced surgical and nonsurgical therapies, and improvements in intensive care. Once the province of pediatric cardiology, CHD is now largely an adult phenomenon. As of 2010, 66% of patients with CHD in North America are adults.

The increase in the number of adults with CHD requires that internists and adult cardiologists develop a more sophisticated knowledge of the anatomy and physiology of these defects. These patients fall into several broad categories: those surviving into adulthood without intervention and perhaps without clinical recognition, those surviving with curative surgical or nonsurgical intervention, and those surviving with palliative surgical or nonsurgical intervention. Nonsurgical interventions may include catheter-based valvuloplasty, stenting, coiling, or device occlusion. The patients who are today making the transition into the adult CHD population have hemodynamic and cardiac problems differing from those in previous eras. Surgical techniques have evolved, intervention occurs earlier and is often definitive rather than palliative, and a greater number of patients with complex single-ventricle physiology and various modifications of cavopulmonary anastomoses (Glenn shunt, Fontan procedure) will reach adulthood. Because of the unique clinical conditions and needs of these patients, the American College of Cardiology and the American Heart Association have recommended that all patients with moderate or complex CHD be evaluated at least once by a physician with specialized training and expertise in adult CHD. Furthermore, it is recommended that diagnostic and interventional cardiac catheterization and electrophysiologic and surgical procedures in these patients be performed in regional adult CHD centers.

ACHD AP (ANATOMIC AND PHYSIOLOGIC) CLASSIFICATION

Acquired heart disease patients with heart failure have been classified based on the traditional staging system that doesn't necessarily apply to the adult congenital heart disease (ACHD) population. Hence in the 2018 ACC/AHA Guidelines on ACHD, an anatomic and physiologic (AP) classification was described taking into account a patient's specific anatomy (mild, moderate, severe), with their physiologic stage identified based on their current functional status (eg, NYHA classification) as well as aortic enlargement, end-organ involvement, degree of cyanosis or shunting, arrhythmias, and pulmonary hypertension (see Table 31–1). This allowed for the physiologic stage to be modified based on improvements after transcatheter or surgical intervention that provided better prognostication going forward. For example, a patient with repaired Tetralogy of Fallot (TOF), NYHA class II symptoms, and mild pulmonary regurgitation would be classified as II b based on the ACHD AP classification.

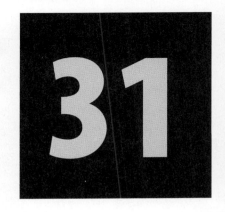

Table 31–1. CHD Anatomy

Simple (I)	Moderate (II)	Severe (III)
Isolated ASD, VSD, PDA	Repaired or unrepaired conditions	Pulmonary atresia (all forms)
Mild pulmonic stenosis	Tetralogy of Fallot	Transposition of the great arteries
Previously ligated PDA	AV canal defects	Truncus arteriosus
Repaired secundum ASD/SVASD/VSD without residual chamber enlargement or shunt	Ebstein anomaly	ventricular inversion etc.
	Coarctation of aorta	single ventricle palliated with Fontan circulation
	Anomalous coronaries	double outlet ventricle (DORV)
	Congenital mitral or aortic valve disease	Interrupted aortic arch

ASD, atrial septal defect; CHD, congenital heart disease; PDA, patent ductus arteriosus; SVASD, sinus venosus atrial septal defect; VSD, ventricular septal defect.

Stout K, et al. AHA/ACC Guidelines for the Management of Adults with Congenital Heart Disease: A Report of the American College of Cardiology/American Heart Association Task Force on Clinical Practice Guidelines. *Circulation*. 2019;139:e698–e800. [PMID: 30121239]

ACYANOTIC CONGENITAL HEART DISEASE

The most common acyanotic congenital heart defects include abnormalities of the heart valves and great vessels, ventricular or atrial communications with left-to-right shunting, and such lesions as partial anomalous pulmonary veins and anomalous coronary arteries.

CONGENITAL AORTIC VALVULAR DISEASE

ESSENTIALS OF DIAGNOSIS

- History of murmur since infancy, coarctation repair, or endocarditis.
- Early systolic ejection sound, harsh crescendo-decrescendo systolic, or early decrescendo diastolic murmur.
- Left ventricular hypertrophy.
- Abnormal bicuspid or dysplastic aortic valve with stenosis or regurgitation on Doppler echocardiography.

General Considerations

Congenital aortic stenosis is the most common anomaly encountered in the adult population and constitutes approximately 7% of all forms of CHD. The male-to-female ratio is approximately 2–3:1. The term "bicuspid aortic valve" is actually a misnomer; a raphe caused by commissural fusion of two leaflets usually exists. The valve is often dysplastic, with thickened, rolled, and calcified leaflets. The predominant pathophysiology results from mildly obstructed nonlaminar (disturbed) flow across the abnormal valve. A left ventricle-to-aorta pressure gradient of variable severity occurs, setting the stage for the inevitable deterioration of the valve with long-term calcium deposition and progressive stenosis or regurgitation. The valve is also at risk for endocarditis, which can lead to early destruction and regurgitation. Congenital aortic valve disease frequently occurs as a developmental "triad" with coincident aortopathy and coarctation, and these conditions should be sought clinically and by echocardiograhy in patients with congenital aortic valve disease. Familial congenital aortic valve disease occurs occasionally. While the genetics of this are incompletely understood, mutations in the gene encoding Notch 1 have been implicated in a subset of these patients.

Clinical Findings

A. Symptoms & Signs

The individual with congenital aortic stenosis is usually asymptomatic unless hemodynamically significant stenosis or regurgitation is present. Routine physical examination reveals a normal carotid pulse contour and left ventricular (LV) impulse, a normal S_2, an early systolic sound, and an early-peaking systolic murmur. Identifying these patients in the asymptomatic stage is important. Current guidelines do not recommend endocarditis prophylaxis for the native valve. Refraining from high-level isometric exercise is generally believed to preserve valve function and limit valve regurgitation. The presence of a diastolic murmur of aortic regurgitation in a patient with a febrile illness should alert the clinician to the possibility of endocarditis and prompt the performance of appropriate diagnostic tests (eg, blood cultures, echocardiogram).

Congenital aortic stenosis is progressive; once hemodynamically significant valvular disease develops in a patient, generally in the fifth or sixth decade of life, the symptoms and signs are identical to those of a patient with acquired aortic valvular disease. Dyspnea, chest pain, and exertional syncope are the classic presenting symptoms. When stenosis predominates, the carotid upstroke is delayed and diminished in volume, the systolic click is no longer present, S_2 is single, and the systolic murmur is crescendo-decrescendo, peaking in late systole. The murmur of aortic regurgitation is often present. The finding of upper extremity hypertension should alert the examiner to the possibility of concomitant aortic coarctation.

B. Diagnostic Studies

1. Electrocardiography and chest radiography—The major electrocardiographic (ECG) findings occur in the presence of hemodynamically significant disease and include left ventricular hypertrophy (LVH) with high QRS voltage, left-axis deviation, and repolarization changes; left atrial enlargement may also be present. The chest radiographic findings are nonspecific. With predominant valvular aortic stenosis, the cardiothoracic ratio may be normal, but LV enlargement and calcification may be evident in the region of the aortic valve on the lateral film. A dilated ascending aorta or a prominent aortic knob may be seen. The cardiac silhouette is enlarged in patients with predominant aortic regurgitation. Pulmonary vasculature may be prominent in the presence of congestive heart failure (CHF).

2. Echocardiography—In the child and younger adult, the abnormally thickened leaflets of the congenitally abnormal valve are readily seen, and the bicuspid valve with its ovoid appearance in systole is apparent (Figure 31–1). On M-mode echocardiography, the point of closure may be eccentric. Heavy calcification often obscures the original valve morphology in the older individual with stenosis. The peak systolic gradient in severe aortic stenosis is usually greater than 64 mm Hg (peak velocity > 4 m/s by continuous wave Doppler). Aortic valve area can be accurately calculated by the continuity equation. Severe aortic stenosis is defined as a valve area of less than 1.0 cm^2 or 0.5 cm^2/m^2. The LV shows concentric hypertrophy with thick walls and normal cavity dimensions, and the LV ejection fraction is usually normal. In cases with reduced ejection fraction, however, the peak gradient across the aortic valve is generally lower.

In hemodynamically significant aortic regurgitation, the high-velocity diastolic color-flow jet is broad at its site of origin below the aortic valve. Spectral Doppler imaging demonstrates a dense diastolic velocity signal with a short pressure half-time (< 400 ms), and diastolic flow reversal can be recorded in the descending aorta. The LV shows eccentric hypertrophy with normal LV wall thickness and a dilated cavity.

In occasional patients with poor precordial windows, transesophageal echocardiography (TEE) may be required to define valve anatomy by demonstrating commissural fusion and asymmetric sinuses of Valsalva. Systolic doming of the leaflets can be easily seen in the long axis view of the LV outflow tract, which also allows measurements to be taken of the aortic valve annulus, sinuses of Valsalva, sinotubular ridge, and ascending aorta.

Cardiac magnetic resonance angiography (MRA) is a possible alternative imaging technique.

3. Cardiac catheterization—Indications for cardiac catheterization in congenital aortic valve disease have changed significantly because most of the diagnostic data are now available noninvasively. According to current guidelines, however, cardiac catheterization is indicated when noninvasive tests are inconclusive or when there is a discrepancy between noninvasive tests and clinical findings regarding severity of aortic stenosis. It is also indicated preoperatively in patients at risk for atherosclerotic coronary artery disease (men age 35 years or older, premenopausal women age 35 years or older who have coronary risk factors, and postmenopausal women) and in patients for whom a pulmonary autograft (Ross procedure) is contemplated and if the origin of the coronary arteries was not identified by noninvasive techniques

4. Magnetic resonance imaging—Serial imaging with magnetic resonance imaging (MRI) permits accurate and reproducible follow-up of aortic dilatation and is accepted as the standard of care for follow-up of repaired coarctation, a frequent association with a bicuspid aortic valve.

Differential Diagnosis

Valvular aortic stenosis should be distinguished from subaortic stenosis, which may be due to an obstructing fibrous membrane in discrete subaortic stenosis, which is more frequently encountered in adults, or by a tubular fibromuscular channel that usually presents in childhood. Aortic regurgitation, commonly associated with discrete membranous subaortic stenosis (in approximately 60% of cases), increases in frequency with age. Regurgitation may occur due to leaflet thickening induced by direct trauma to the aortic leaflets from the high-velocity jet or by interference with leaflet closure from the membrane. The aortic valve appearance and the severity and mechanism of aortic regurgitation must be carefully assessed.

Recurrent stenosis caused by regrowth following surgical resection of the fibromuscular ridge is sometimes encountered in the adolescent or adult. Discrete subaortic stenosis and congenital valvular aortic stenosis must also be distinguished from dynamic LV outflow-tract obstruction caused by hypertrophic cardiomyopathy (see Chapter 23). Supravalvular aortic stenosis is frequently seen in patients with Williams syndrome.

When aortic regurgitation is the predominant lesion and ascending aorta dilatation is present, the condition must be distinguished from Marfan syndrome and other genetic aortopathies. This latter condition is characterized by dilatation of the aortic root at the level of the sinuses of Valsalva (Figure 31–2). The aortic valve leaflets are not thickened,

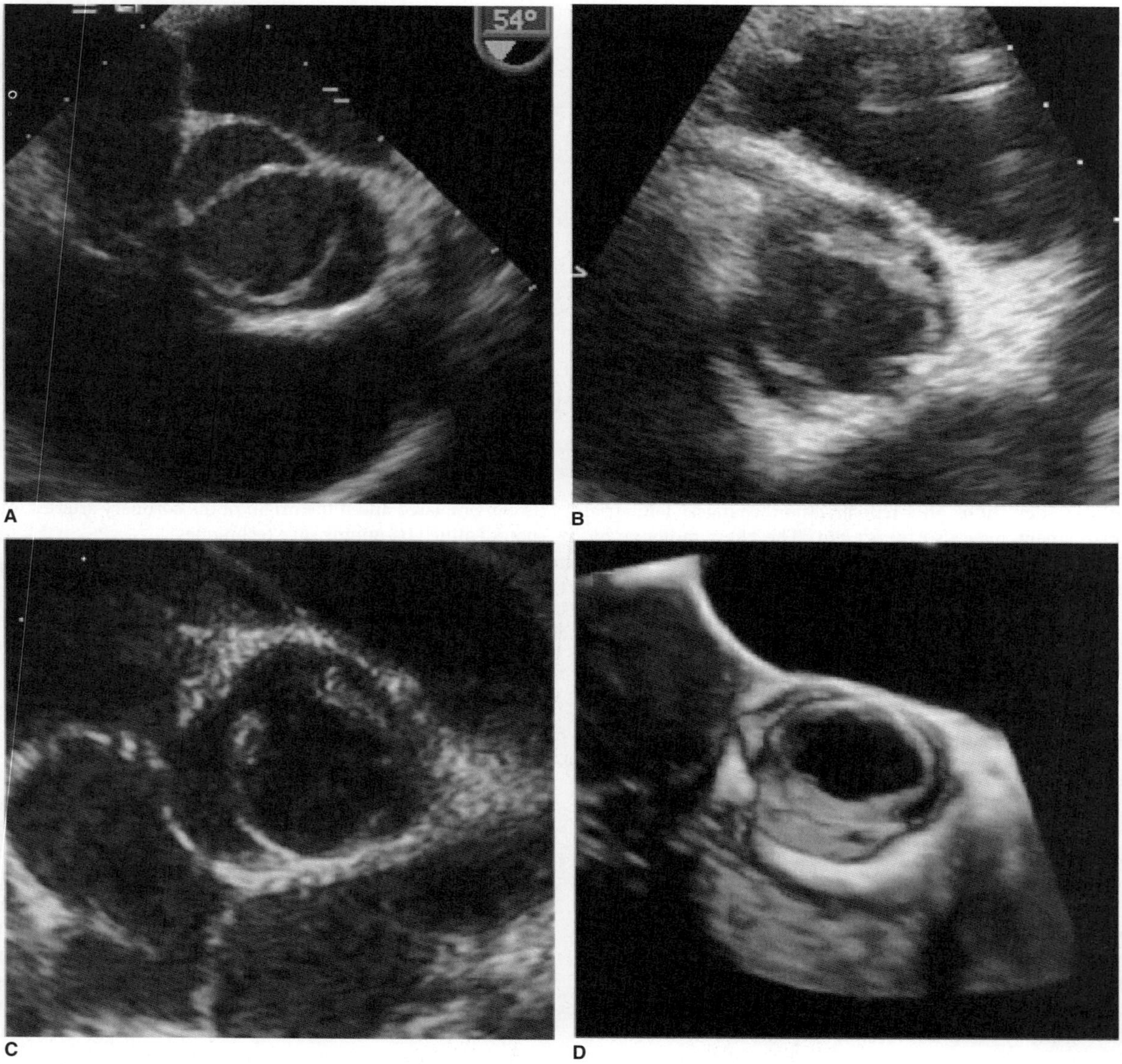

▲ **Figure 31–1.** Transesophageal echocardiographic views of a patient with bicuspid aortic valve. **A:** Systolic frame showing two leaflets of the aortic valve with an ovoid opening. **B:** Bicuspid valve with fusion of the right and left coronary cusps. **C:** Unicuspid valve with a key hole appearance. **D:** Three-dimensional view on transesophageal echocardiography of a bicuspid valve.

and regurgitation is caused by failure of leaflet coaptation caused by the root dilatation. With valvular stenosis, the aorta narrows toward normal at the sinotubular junction, and the descending thoracic aorta is spared. In some patients with a bicuspid aortic valve, an underlying abnormality of the medial layer of the aorta above the valve predisposes to the dilatation of the aortic root, which may progress to aneurysm formation or rupture and places the patient at risk for aortic dissection. All components of the vessel wall, smooth muscle, elastic fibers, collagen, and ground substance can be affected and should be recognized as a potential risk in the surgical patient.

Prognosis & Treatment

The natural history of aortic stenosis presenting in childhood depends largely on the severity of the stenosis at

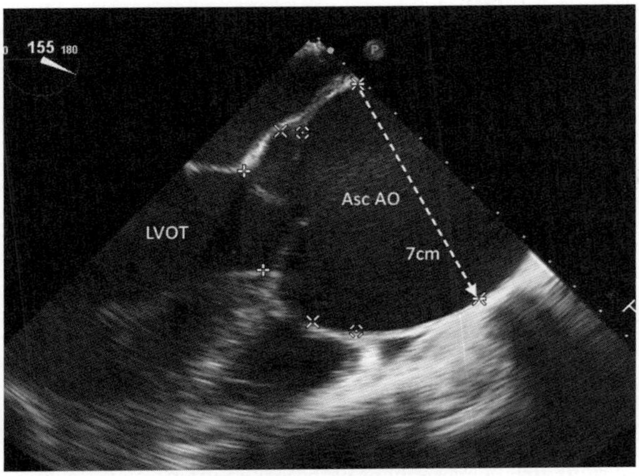

▲ **Figure 31–2.** Transesophageal echocardiographic (TEE) views of the ascending aorta (Asc Ao) measuring 7 cm in a patient with Marfan syndrome. LVOT, left ventricular outflow tract.

the time of diagnosis. During a 25-year follow-up period, approximately one-third of the children with a peak systolic gradient of less than 50 mm Hg who were treated medically required surgery, in contrast to 80% of those with an intermediate gradient (50–79 mm Hg). Of those treated surgically for a gradient of more than 79 mm Hg, approximately one-fourth required reoperation; reoperation was more common in those treated with initial valvotomy (30%) than aortic valve replacement (5%). The overall 25-year survival rate is approximately 85%; sudden death accounts for approximately half of the cardiac-related deaths. There is no clear role for the use of aspirin, β-blockers, or statins in the medical management of these patients.

Once symptoms of aortic stenosis develop, the prognosis without valve replacement is poor; the 5-year mortality rate is approximately 90%. Although percutaneous valvuloplasty has been successful in children and adolescents, the results in adults (even those with congenitally abnormal valves) have been disappointing. Therefore, surgery with aortic valve replacement, rather than percutaneous valvuloplasty, is generally mandated. Surgery is indicated in the symptomatic patient with a valve area of less than 1.0 cm^2 (or $< 0.5\ cm^2/m^2$). It should be considered in the asymptomatic patient with critical stenosis when the patient requires cardiac surgery (eg, coronary artery bypass surgery) for another lesion. A particularly difficult management decision ensues in the asymptomatic woman with severe aortic stenosis who is contemplating pregnancy. Valve replacement prior to pregnancy should be considered when there is evidence of LV dysfunction or reduced exercise tolerance on objective stress testing.

Patients with a bicuspid aortic valve and concomitant annuloaortic ectasia may show a more rapid progression of aortic regurgitation and require surgical intervention earlier than patients with pure aortic stenosis. Composite aortic root and valve replacement should be considered in patients requiring valve replacement with an aortic root diameter exceeding 4.5 cm, and in patients with an aortic root diameter exceeding 5.0 cm in the absence of significant valve dysfunction.

An ideal substitute for replacing the aortic valve does not exist. Homografts and bioprosthetic valves can develop rapid calcific degeneration, causing valve dysfunction, particularly in the younger cohort of patients. Mechanical valves, although extremely durable, require anticoagulation to reduce the complication of thromboembolism. The risks associated with long-term anticoagulation have made surgical options to avoid the use of mechanical valves desirable alternatives. This is particularly germane to the choice of prosthetic valve in young women of childbearing age, in whom management of anticoagulation can be problematic. Recent advances in transcatheter aortic valve replacement have introduced the possibility that patients who opt for a bioprosthetic valve will later be candidates for these newer techniques and avoid open heart surgery. The Ross procedure (in which the autologous pulmonary valve replaces the aortic valve, and an aortic or pulmonary homograft replaces the pulmonary valve) has been increasingly performed for a variety of LV outflow tract diseases, including aortic insufficiency and valvar aortic stenosis with or without other forms of obstruction (eg, subaortic stenosis, supravalvar stenosis, and arch hypoplasia). Although the Ross procedure is more complex than simple aortic valve replacement, it can be performed with a low mortality rate in selected patients. Advantages of the pulmonary valve autograft include freedom from anticoagulation and the absence of compromise from host reactions and autograft growth, making it an attractive option for aortic valve replacement in infants and children. It is recognized, however, that the pulmonary homograft will require replacement for degenerative disease and size restriction in children. In adults who are confronting surgery for a stenotic aortic valve in the fifth or sixth decade of life, the Ross procedure has shown to be an acceptable alternative to the usual mechanical or bioprosthetic valve. However, recently recognized problems associated with the Ross procedure include progressive dilatation of the neo-aortic root, pulmonary conduit stenosis, and neo-aortic valve regurgitation. Contraindications to the Ross procedure include advanced three-vessel coronary artery disease, poor LV function, a severely calcified or dilated aortic root, or pulmonary valve pathology.

PULMONARY VALVE STENOSIS

ESSENTIALS OF DIAGNOSIS

- History of systolic murmur since infancy.
- Systolic ejection sound and an early systolic murmur in the second left intercostal space with transmission to the back. S_2 may split widely.

- ECG evidence of right ventricular hypertrophy.
- Dilatation of main and left pulmonary arteries on chest radiograph.
- Right ventricular hypertrophy, systolic doming of the pulmonary valve, and a transpulmonic gradient by Doppler echocardiography.

General Considerations

Pulmonary valve, or pulmonic stenosis (PS), is the second most common form of CHD in the adult. Although many cases are so mild that they require no treatment, it often coexists with other congenital cardiac abnormalities (atrial septal defect [ASD], ventricular septal defect [VSD], patent ductus arteriosus, or TOF). Pulmonary valve stenosis is characterized by a conical or dome-shaped pliant valve with a narrow outlet at its apex. Right ventricular (RV) outflow is obstructed depending on the size of the orifice, and RV stroke volume may not rise appropriately during exercise. In response to the pressure overload, the RV hypertrophies, with an increase in wall thickness. This compensatory hypertrophy can involve the infundibulum and potentially lead to reversible dynamic subpulmonic stenosis once the valvular stenosis is relieved. If severe stenosis remains untreated, RV failure may ensue. It is important to differentiate pulmonary valve stenosis from stenoses of the peripheral pulmonary arteries and primary infundibular stenosis, often associated with VSD (see Tetralogy of Fallot). Pulmonary stenosis from a thickened, dysplastic valve is seen in patients with Noonan syndrome (a heterogeneous malformation syndrome with autosomal dominant inheritance).

Clinical Findings

A. Symptoms & Signs

The patient with PS usually has exercise intolerance in the form of exertional fatigue, dyspnea, chest pain, or syncope. RV failure with systemic venous congestion occurs late in the course of the disease. If the foramen ovale is patent or a concomitant ASD exists, shunting of blood from the right atrium to the left may occur, causing cyanosis and clubbing. The volume overload of pregnancy may precipitate right heart failure in patients with severe PS, although mild stenosis and even moderate stenosis are usually well tolerated.

In significant PS, the physical examination demonstrates a parasternal RV heave, a delayed and diminished or absent P_2, and a late-peaking crescendo-decrescendo murmur that increases in volume with inspiration. If the valve is pliable, an ejection sound precedes the murmur. This pulmonic ejection sound, best heard in the second left intercostal space, is the only right-sided event that decreases in intensity during inspiration and increases during expiration. As the stenosis becomes more severe, the systolic murmur will peak later in systole and the ejection sound moves closer to the first heart sound, eventually becoming superimposed on it. The jugular venous pulse shows a prominent *a* wave, as a result of the diminished RV compliance, but jugular venous pressure is increased only in the late stages when RV failure occurs. Similarly, there may be an RV S_4 gallop early in the course of the disease and a right-sided S_3 in the later stages.

B. Diagnostic Studies

1. Electrocardiography and chest radiography—The ECG demonstrates evidence of right ventricular hypertrophy (RVH) with right-axis deviation, prominent R waves in the right precordial leads, and deep S waves in the left precordial leads (Figure 31–3). There may also be evidence of right atrial enlargement with peaked inferior (II, III, aVF) P waves.

The cardiac silhouette on the chest radiograph is normal in mild-to-moderate PS but may become enlarged in severe stenosis when right heart failure occurs. The main and left pulmonary arteries are often dilated. In addition to this "poststenotic dilatation," dilatation may be seen even in cases of mild PS and may be related to intrinsic abnormalities of the pulmonary artery (idiopathic pulmonary artery dilatation).

2. Echocardiography—The poor near-field resolution of transthoracic echocardiography (TTE) often limits definition of pulmonary valve morphology in the adult patient. When examined from the parasternal short-axis view, the valve may appear thickened (rarely calcified) and usually manifests systolic doming. In the absence of right heart failure, the RV dimension is normal or only mildly increased, but the RV wall thickness is increased (> 5 mm). In severe cases, the septum may be deviated toward the LV from the pressure overload of the RV. The right atrium and ventricle dilate late in the course of the disease. Saline contrast echocardiography should be performed in all patients with pulmonary valve stenosis to exclude an ASD or a patent foramen ovale.

Color-flow Doppler imaging demonstrates high-velocity flow within the pulmonary artery and is helpful in excluding a VSD or a patent ductus arteriosus. Continuous wave Doppler demonstrates a high-velocity jet across the RV outflow tract (Figure 31–4B). This signal is best obtained from the parasternal short-axis or subcostal short-axis views where flow is axial to the Doppler beam. PS is classified as mild when the RV systolic pressure is less than 50 mm Hg, moderate when the gradient is 50–79 mm Hg, and severe when the gradient is greater than 80 mm Hg. Unfortunately, because of the lack of range resolution, continuous wave Doppler cannot localize the level of the obstruction. The morphology of the valve by echocardiography and pulsed wave Doppler mapping may provide localizing information, but additional diagnostic procedures are often necessary.

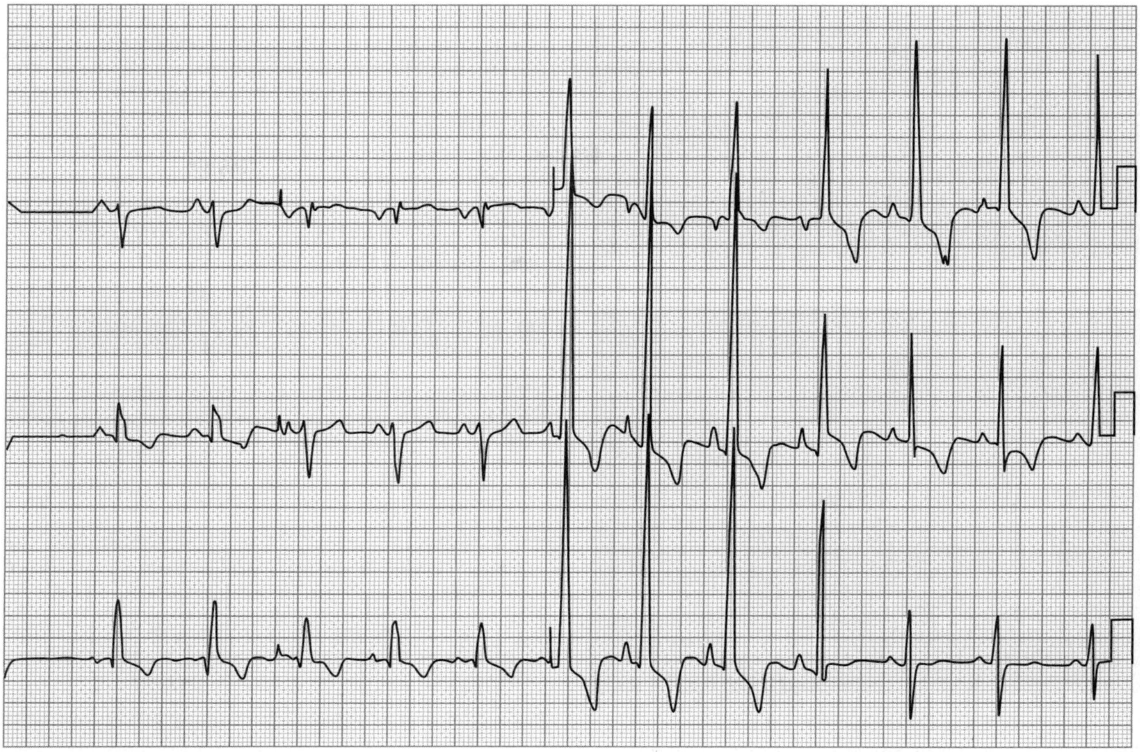

▲ **Figure 31–3.** Electrocardiograph in congenital pulmonic stenosis with severe right ventricular hypertrophy and marked right-axis deviation.

TEE provides excellent definition of the RV outflow tract and pulmonary valve in the basal longitudinal views and excellent images of the atrial septum. As a result, noninvasive methods may now be adequate for establishing the diagnosis, even in adults.

3. Cardiac catheterization—In most patients, cardiac catheterization is therapeutic as well as diagnostic because percutaneous balloon valvuloplasty has virtually replaced surgery for treatment of pulmonary valve stenosis (see later). During right-heart catheterization, the level of the stenosis can be confirmed by pressure monitoring during pullback from the pulmonary artery and supplemented by RV angiography. In valvular stenosis, there is a rise in peak systolic pressure as the catheter tip passes from the pulmonary artery into the infundibulum. In contrast, when the stenosis is in the infundibulum, the systolic pressure increases when the catheter is pulled into the body of the RV. As mentioned earlier, in PS, secondary hypertrophy may result in some degree of infundibular stenosis, and a pressure differential may be demonstrated at both levels on pullback (Figure 31–5). If the level of obstruction is still uncertain, cineangiography may show the hypertrophied infundibulum or, alternatively, the domed and thickened pulmonary valve. Of course, both levels of obstruction may coexist.

Unlike aortic valve stenosis, the valve area is not calculated from the Doppler or invasive hemodynamic data, and the gradient alone is used to determine the severity of the obstruction and guide therapy.

Prognosis & Treatment

In severe untreated pulmonary valve stenosis, the average life expectancy is approximately 30 years. The natural history of medically treated mild (gradient < 50 mm Hg) or moderate (gradient 50–79 mm Hg) PS and surgically treated severe (gradient > 80 mm Hg) PS is excellent, with a 25-year survival rate of 95%. Surgical valvotomy via a pulmonary artery incision has been extremely effective in long-term relief of pulmonary valve obstruction. Although approximately 50% of patients have mild-to-moderate regurgitation following surgery, it is seldom of hemodynamic significance, and reoperation is rarely necessary.

In children treated conservatively for PS, the likelihood of eventually requiring surgery is dependent on the initial gradient: less than 25 mm Hg, 5%; 25–49 mm Hg, 20%; and 50–79 mm Hg, 76%. In the adult, the indication for treatment of pulmonary valve stenosis is a peak systolic gradient in excess of 50 mm Hg. When the gradient is between 40 and

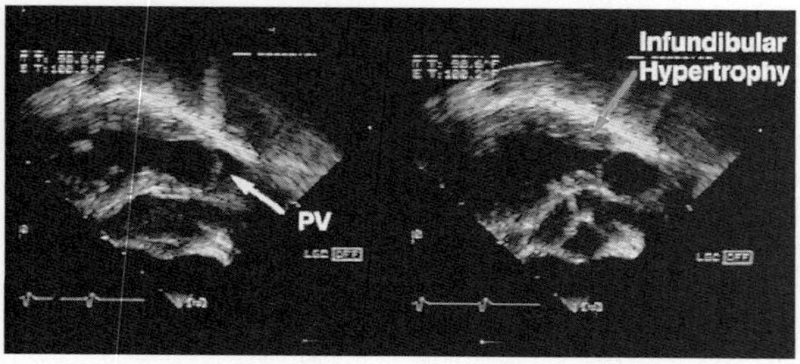

A

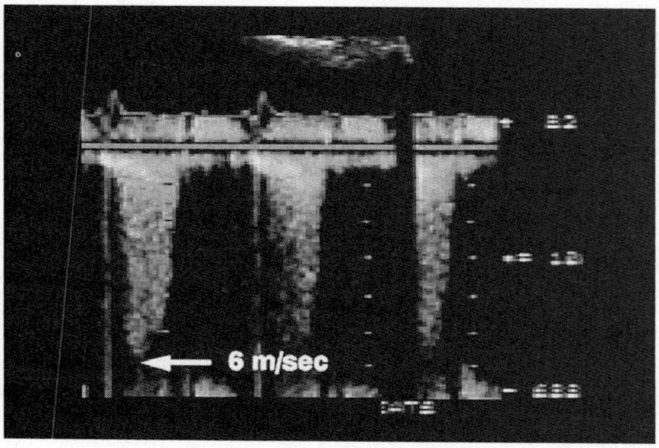

B

▲ **Figure 31–4. A:** Transesophageal echocardiographic views of a pregnant woman with severe pulmonary valve (PV) stenosis. The left image demonstrates the doming pulmonary valve in systole. The right frame illustrates the severe infundibular hypertrophy. **B:** Continuous wave Doppler recording from the same patient demonstrated a peak velocity of 6 m/s corresponding to a peak transvalvular gradient of 144 mm Hg.

50 mm Hg, the decision to treat is based on the presence of symptoms, the age of the patient, and the degree of RVH (by echocardiography or ECG). Echocardiography, before and after exercise, may be an important technique to assess RV function in the presence of an increased gradient.

As mentioned earlier, most patients (including adults) with pulmonary valve stenosis are currently treated with percutaneous balloon valvuloplasty. The Registry of the Valvuloplasty and Angioplasty of Congenital Anomalies has listed 35 patients over the age of 20, among them a 76-year-old man. No significant complications occurred in adult patients, and the gradient was reduced from approximately 70 to 30 mm Hg, with about 50% of the residual gradient caused by infundibular hypertrophy. Ongoing assessment of these patients indicates sustained long-term relief of the pulmonary valve gradient with progressive infundibular remodeling causing further reduction in the outflow tract gradient over time. Recent technical improvements leading to the development of low-profile balloons have decreased the risk of pulmonary regurgitation after dilatation. Based on these results, percutaneous balloon valvuloplasty appears to be the treatment of choice in adults with pulmonary valve stenosis. Results in recent studies have been similar in both children and adults. Severe pulmonary valve insufficiency after either balloon or surgical valvotomy is uncommon, but patients should be evaluated every 5–10 years for this complication. Even when PS is associated with severe infundibular stenosis and tricuspid regurgitation, the long-term results from balloon valvuloplasty are excellent.

ATRIAL SEPTAL DEFECT

ESSENTIALS OF DIAGNOSIS

- A widely split S_2 without respiratory variation ("fixed split") and a midsystolic murmur are characteristic.
- RV conduction delay ("incomplete right bundle branch block") with vertical QRS axis (ostium secundum ASD) and superior axis (ostium primum ASD) on ECG.
- Prominent pulmonary arteries and RV enlargement (decreased retrosternal air space) on chest radiograph. Increased pulmonary vascular markings.
- RV dilatation, increased pulmonary artery flow velocity, and left-to-right atrial shunt by contrast and Doppler echocardiography.
- Oxygen step-up within the right atrium; right-sided catheter can pass into the left atrium across the defect.

General Considerations

ASDs make up 10% of CHD cases in newborns and are regularly encountered as new diagnoses in adults. The defects vary in size from the smallest fenestrated ASD (a few millimeters) to the largest defect—the complete absence of the atrial septum, or common atrium. The most common interatrial communication is a patent foramen ovale that is anatomically and physiologically not classified as an ASD.

Classification of ASDs is according to location (Figure 31–6): ostium secundum in the region of the fossa ovalis, ostium primum in the lower portion of the atrial septum (actually part of an atrioventricular [AV] canal defect, discussed later), sinus venosus in the upper part of the septum near the entrance of the superior vena cava or at the entrance of the inferior vena cava, and unroofed coronary sinus (communication between the coronary sinus and left atrium). Important associated abnormalities include anomalous drainage of the right upper pulmonary vein into the superior vena cava associated with a superior sinus venosus ASD, a persistent left superior vena cava draining to the coronary sinus with secundum or primum ASDs, and a cleft anterior mitral leaflet and mitral regurgitation

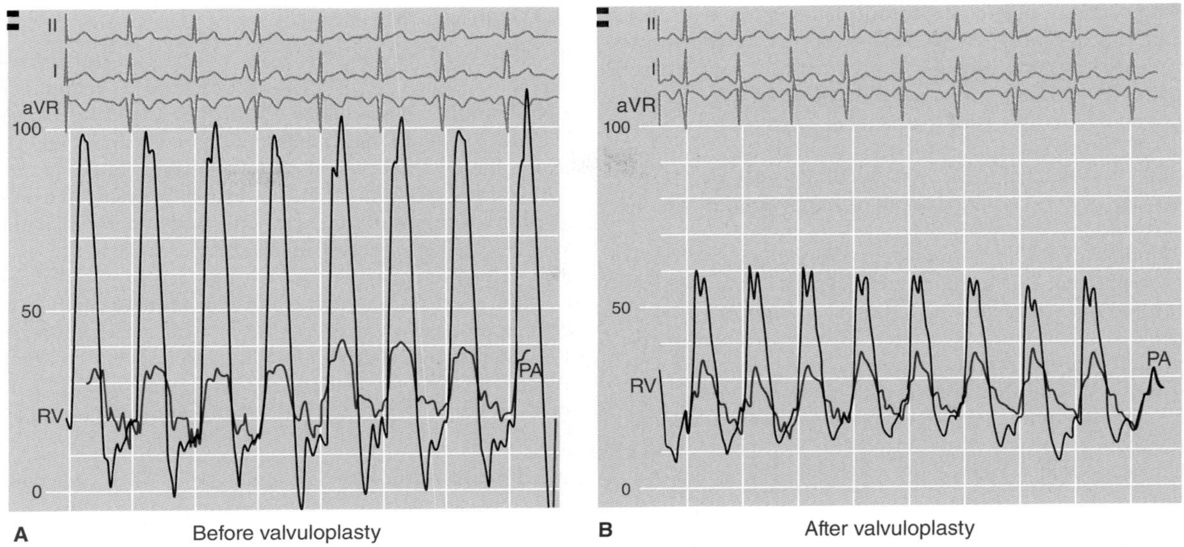

▲ **Figure 31–5.** Hemodynamic tracings in pulmonic stenosis. **A:** Predilation: Peak gradient of 65 mm Hg between right ventricle (RV) and pulmonary artery (PA). **B:** Postdilation: Residual gradient of 20 mm Hg between RV infundibulum and pulmonary artery.

associated with an ostium primum ASD. Ostium primum ASD is a common cardiac anomaly in trisomy 21 (Down syndrome) and is part of the spectrum of AV septal "canal" defects (discussed later). There is an approximately 2:1 female predominance for ostium secundum ASDs, while the sex ratio for ostium primum and sinus venosus ASDs is approximately 1:1. An autosomal dominant inheritance pattern has been demonstrated in some patients with ostium secundum ASD with associated first-degree AV block, and cases of ASD in monozygotic twins have been reported. Recent studies have implicated mutations in the genes *gata4* and *nkx2-5* in nonsyndromic ASDs, whereas point mutations in the gene *tbx5* are known to cause the Holt-Oram syndrome (ASD and limb defects).

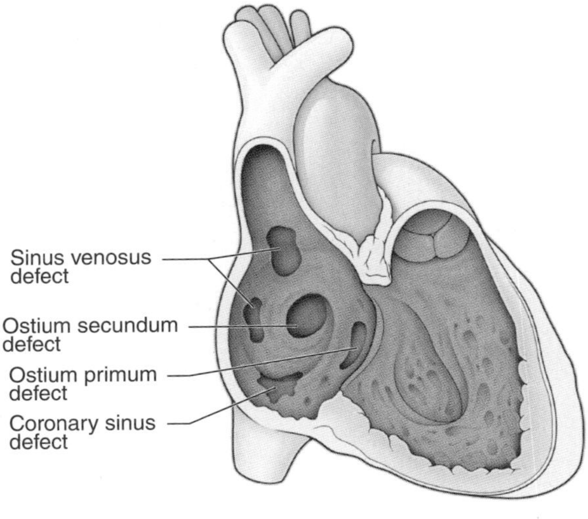

▲ **Figure 31–6.** Anatomic location of atrial septal defects.

The pathophysiologic consequences of an ASD depend on the quantity of blood shunted from the systemic to pulmonary circulation. The size of the shunt is in turn dependent on the size of the defect and the relative compliance of the RV and LV. Little or no shunting occurs immediately after birth because of the high pulmonary vascular resistance (PVR), but as resistance falls, the more compliant RV receives the shunted blood mainly in diastole, when all four chambers are in communication. In the compensated patient with ASD, pulmonary resistance is usually low. The older adult with the LV diastolic abnormalities of hypertension, coronary artery disease, and aging may experience increased left-to-right shunting and, consequently, right heart failure. While pulmonary resistance may increase, the development of Eisenmenger physiology is unusual after the age of 25. Atrial arrhythmias, especially atrial fibrillation, are common over the age of 50 and may be the presenting symptom.

Clinical Findings

A. Symptoms & Signs

The young adult with an uncorrected ASD and normal pulmonary artery pressures is usually asymptomatic, with normal or minimally diminished exercise tolerance. After the age of 30, however, exertional dyspnea and atypical chest pain increase in frequency. As mentioned earlier, the frequency of atrial arrhythmias increases with age and occurs in a high percentage of patients over the age of 50 who have not been treated surgically. Signs and symptoms of RV failure may occur because of pulmonary hypertension or as a result of long-standing volume overload.

Important findings of the physical examination in an uncomplicated ASD include a prominent RV impulse along the lower left sternal border; a palpable pulmonary artery; a systolic ejection murmur, caused by increased flow across the pulmonic valve, which does not vary in intensity with respiration; and the almost pathognomonic fixed split second heart sound. When the ratio of pulmonic to systemic flow exceeds from 1:5 to 2:1, there may be an associated right-sided diastolic flow rumble and S_3 gallop from increased flow across the tricuspid valve. The patient with ostium primum ASD usually has a holosystolic murmur of mitral regurgitation. If pulmonary hypertension is present, P_2 is increased and a high-pitched murmur of pulmonary regurgitation (Graham Steell murmur) may be audible. Signs of RV failure with elevated jugular venous pressure and venous congestion may be apparent in the later stages of this disease.

B. Diagnostic Studies

1. Electrocardiography and chest radiography— The ECG shows an RV conduction delay (“incomplete right bundle branch block” [IRBBB]) in 90% of cases (Figure 31–7). In ostium secundum and sinus venosus ASDs, the QRS axis is vertical or rightward. In the patient with ostium primum ASD, the axis is superior and leftward. Abnormal sinus node function in patients with sinus venosus ASD often results in an ectopic atrial rhythm with a superior P-wave axis.

The chest radiograph shows prominent main and branch pulmonary arteries with a small aortic knob and RV enlargement. The right atrium may appear enlarged. In the absence of pulmonary hypertension, the lung markings are increased as a result of increased pulmonary blood flow.

2. Echocardiography—The findings on TTE include right-heart enlargement and increased pulmonary artery flow. Color-flow Doppler often can identify the interatrial flow, especially in the subcostal four-chamber view. An intravenous saline contrast injection should be used in all patients with these findings to exclude an unsuspected ASD. In the presence of an ASD, a negative contrast effect can be seen in the right atrium as the unopacified left atrial blood is shunted from left to right. A small degree of bidirectional

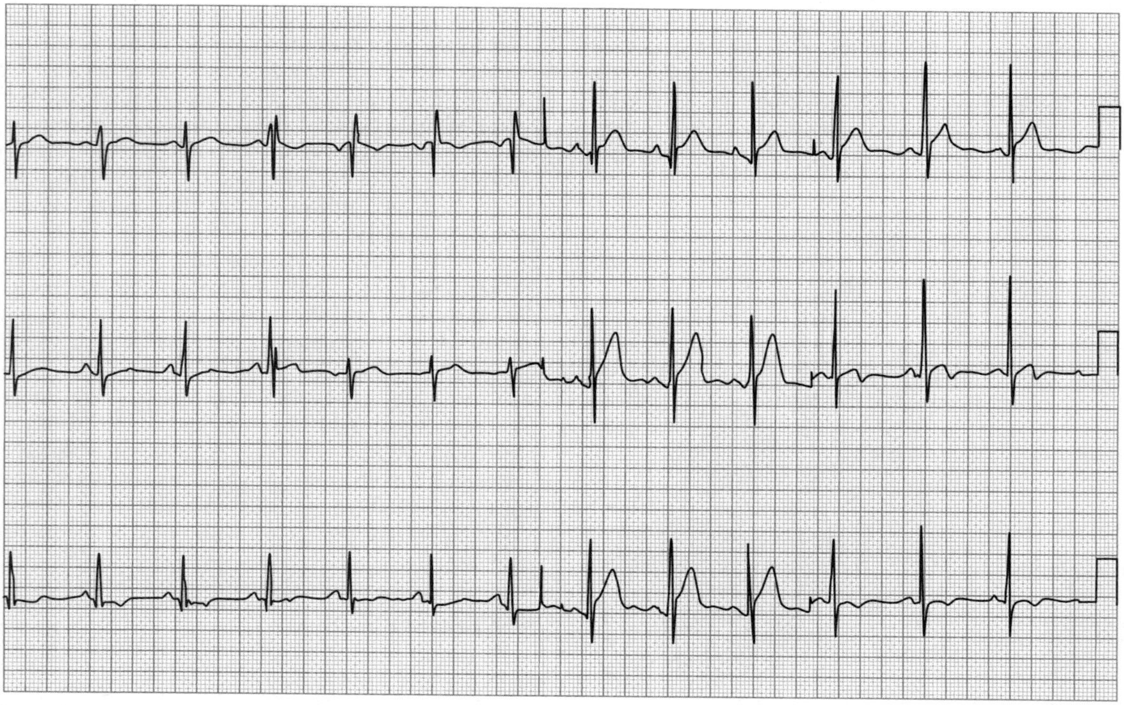

▲ Figure 31–7. Electrocardiograph in atrial septal defect with right-axis deviation, incomplete right bundle branch block, and right ventricular hypertrophy.

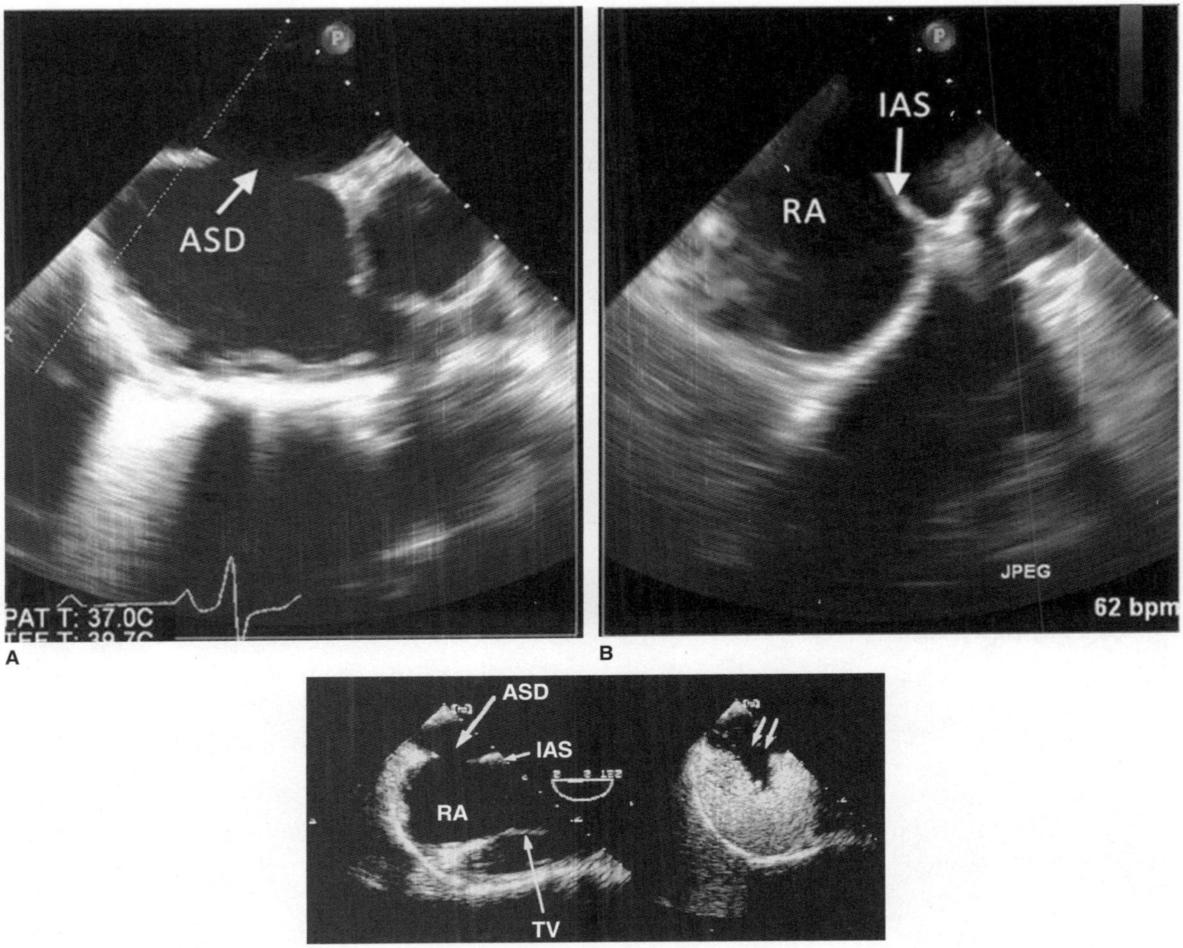

A B C

▲ **Figure 31–8. A:** Transesophageal echocardiogram in a patient with an ostium secundum atrial septal defect (ASD). **B:** The image clearly demonstrates the position of the ASD in the midportion of the interatrial septum (IAS). **C:** The image is obtained after intravenous injection of agitated saline, which opacifies the right atrium (RA). The negative contrast effect produced by the unopacified left atrial blood entering the RA is clearly demonstrated (*double arrow*). TV, tricuspid valve.

shunting nearly always is present, and microbubbles can be seen in the left atrium as a result of right-to-left shunting. The shunting across a patent foramen ovale is purely right to left and occurs only during transient (eg, Valsalva maneuver, coughing) or persistent elevations in right atrial pressure.

Pulmonary artery pressure can be estimated from the peak velocity of the tricuspid regurgitant jet. Echocardiographic measurements may be used to determine shunt flow, eliminating the need for an invasive assessment. In adults, however, the TTE is somewhat limited in quantifying the magnitude of shunts and the size of the defect and in locating sinus venosus defects or anomalous pulmonary veins. As noted earlier, TEE has been found to be more accurate in determining the size and location of atrial communications (Figure 31–8). Biplanar and three-dimensional transesophageal views are particularly useful in identifying sinus venosus–type ASD and associated anomalous pulmonary veins (Figure 31–9).

3. Cardiac catheterization—In some younger individuals with unequivocally large defects on noninvasive imaging, diagnostic cardiac catheterization may be avoidable. In others, however, invasive studies may be necessary to accurately quantitate the shunt, measure PVR, and exclude coronary artery disease. Right-heart catheterization with repeated blood sampling for oxygen saturation demonstrates an oxygen

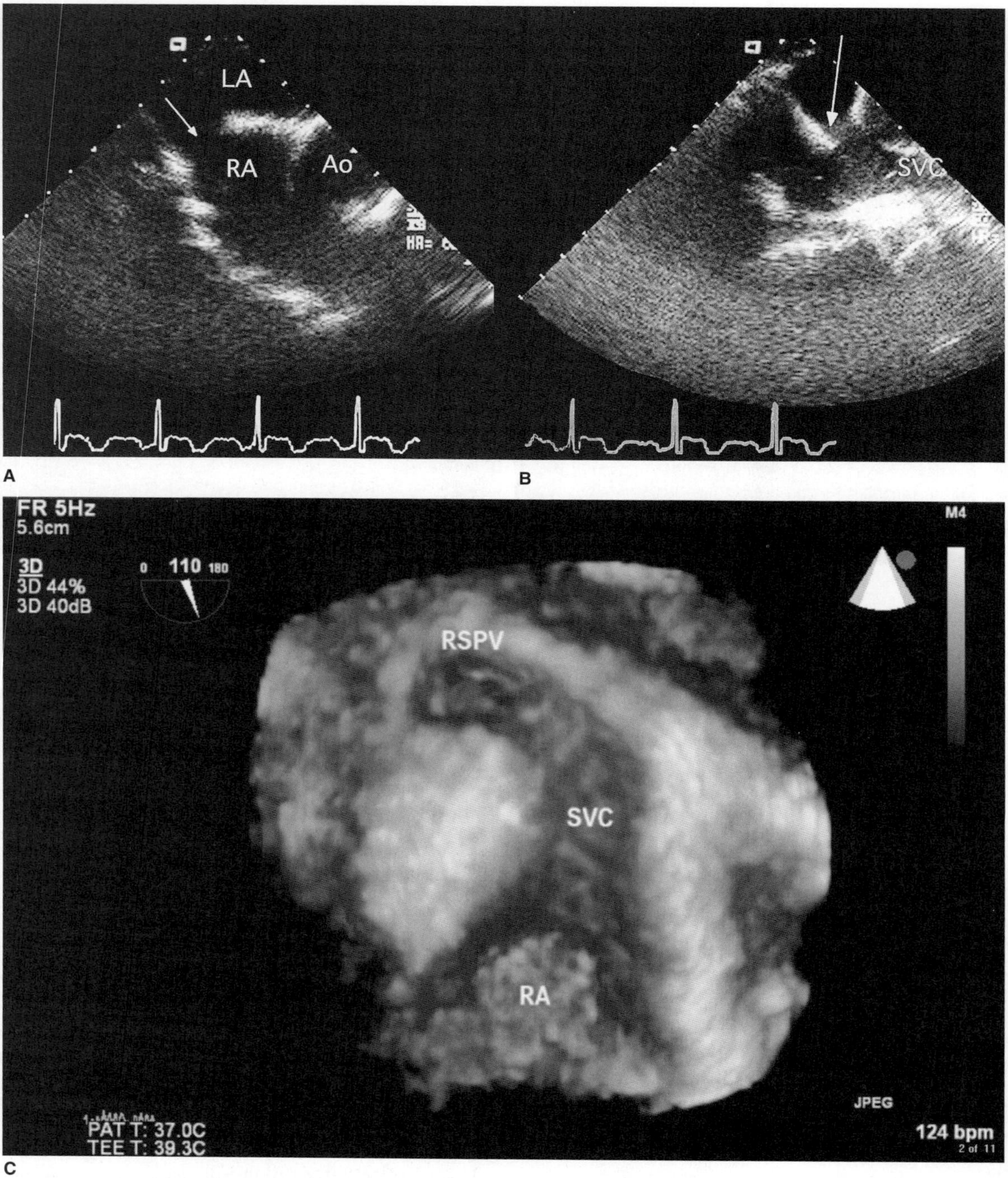

▲ **Figure 31–9.** Transesophageal echocardiography in a 50-year-old man with a sinus venosus atrial septal defect. **A:** Horizontal view showing the defect (*arrow*) in the superior portion of the interatrial septum. **B:** The defect (*arrow*) is clearly demonstrated in this longitudinal plane view. **C:** Three-dimensional transesophageal echocardiogram demonstrating anomalous connection of the right superior pulmonary vein (RSPV) to the superior vena cava. Ao, aorta; LA, left atrium; RA, right atrium; SVC, superior vena cava.

step-up (ie, an increase in saturation) from the vena cava to the right atrium. In general, the higher the pulmonary arterial oxygen saturation, the greater is the shunt, with a value greater than 90% suggesting a large shunt. The ratio of pulmonary to systemic flow can be calculated by the following formula:

$$\frac{Q_P}{Q_S} = \frac{(SAO_2 - MVO_2)}{(PVO_2 - PAO_2)}$$

where SAO_2, MVO_2, PVO_2, and PAO_2 are systemic arterial, mixed venous, pulmonary venous, and pulmonary arterial blood oxygen saturations, respectively. MVO_2 is calculated using the Flamm equation, [(3 × SVC) + IVC]/4, where SVC is the oxygen saturation of blood from the superior vena cava and IVC is the oxygen saturation of blood from the inferior vena cava.

A PVR that is more than 70% of the systemic vascular resistance suggests significant pulmonary vascular disease, and closure is best avoided. Pulmonary vasodilator therapy may be used, and occasionally, pulmonary resistance decreases enough to consider closure.

Prognosis & Treatment

Although patients with an uncorrected ostium secundum ASD generally survive into adulthood, their life expectancy is not normal; older natural history studies showed a 50% survival beyond age 40. The mortality rate after the age of 40 is about 6% per year. Small ASDs (a Q_p:Q_s < 1.5–2:1) may cause problems only in the advanced years, when hypertension and coronary artery disease cause reduced LV compliance, resulting in increased left-to-right shunting, atrial arrhythmias, and potential biventricular failure. Severe pulmonary hypertension develops during young adulthood in only 5–10% of patients with large shunts (Q_p:Q_s > 2:1). Although most adults with ASDs have mild-to-moderate pulmonary hypertension, the late development of severe pulmonary hypertension in older adults appears to be quite rare. Pregnancy, in the absence of pulmonary hypertension, is usually uncomplicated. Another potential complication of ASD (including even the smallest patent foramen ovale) in the adult patient is paradoxical embolization. Endocarditis is rare in patients with ASD, and prophylaxis is not routinely recommended unless associated lesions with higher risk exist.

The natural history of sinus venosus ASDs is similar to that of ostium secundum defects, although many of these patients have associated partial anomalous pulmonary venous connection. Adults with an ostium primum ASD are less commonly encountered and may have additional complications resulting from mitral regurgitation caused by the cleft leaflet (see the discussion on AV canal defects, later in this chapter).

Ostium secundum ASDs have been surgically repaired for more than 40 years. There were no late cardiac deaths and overall good survival in those who had early surgical repair of ASDs (before the age of 18) among patients in large registries. However, the right ventricle needs to be monitored long term because a third of patients may have decline in function, although functional status remains good. Patients with elevated pulmonary systolic pressure (> 40 mm Hg) at the time of surgery have the poorest survival rate, especially if they are older than 40 at the time of operation.

Despite the poorer surgical results in adults older than 40 years, closure is superior to medical therapy and is recommended in patients with predominant left-to-right shunts (Q_p:Q_s > 1.5–2:1) and PVR less than 10 Wood units/m^2. Although mortality rates increase when the resistance exceeds this level, surgery can be performed safely in many patients with PVR between 10 and 15 Wood units/m^2; pulmonary vasodilator therapy should be considered in these patients before closure. Surgery will improve functional class and eliminate the risk of paradoxical embolization, but closure does not reduce the incidence of atrial arrhythmias.

Percutaneous device closure is widely available, and retrospective studies have suggested comparable results with device closure and surgical closure. Therefore, device closure with the assistance of TEE has become the standard of care for appropriately selected adolescents and adults with ostium secundum defects. While sinus venosus defects have traditionally been closed surgically, there has been recent single center publications looking at transcatheter closures of these defects in high-risk cases with comorbidities who cannot undergo surgery. This is performed after obtaining cross-sectional imaging and ex vivo simulation using printed or virtual three-dimensional models to assess anatomy and, if favorable, to proceed with intervention. If so, stents are placed within the SVC extending inferiorly in such a manner as to cover the defect and redirect the anomalous vein (Figure 31–10).

Adult patients with initially small shunts (Q_p:Q_s < 1.5) should undergo continued echocardiographic surveillance because the shunt may increase over time owing to a progressive decline in LV compliance.

In patients with patent foramen ovale who have suffered embolic phenomena, device closure has become a standard intervention.

Hansen JH, Duong P, Jivanji SGM, et al. Transcatheter correction of superior sinus venosus atrial septal defects as an alternative to surgical treatment. *J Am Coll Cardiol.* 2020 Mar 24;75(11):1266–1278. [PMID: 32192652]

VENTRICULAR SEPTAL DEFECTS

ESSENTIALS OF DIAGNOSIS

- History of murmur appearing shortly after birth.
- Holosystolic murmur at left sternal border radiating rightward.
- Left atrial and LV or biventricular enlargement.
- High-velocity color-flow Doppler jet across VSD.
- Increased pulmonary flow velocities.

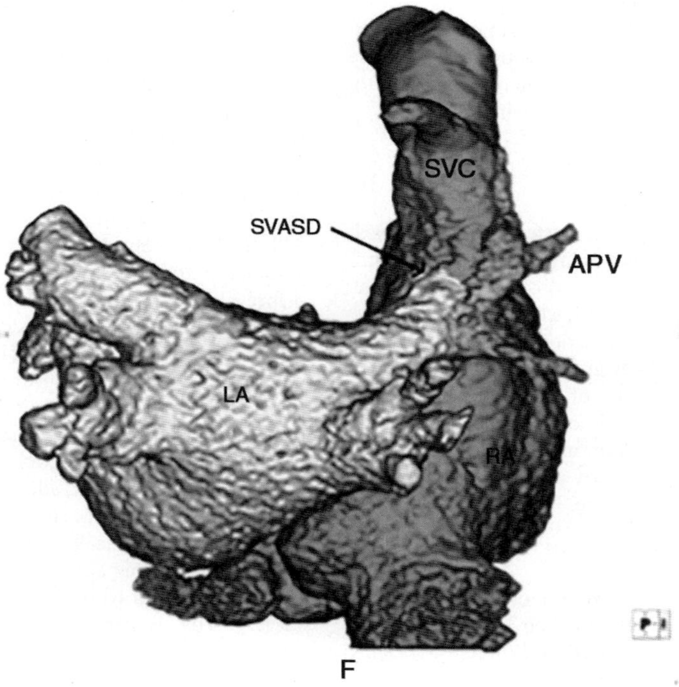

▲ **Figure 31–10.** Three-dimensional imaging of a sinus venosus atrial septal defect (SVASD) to assess if anatomy is amenable for transcatheter closure. APV, anomalous pulmonary vein; LA, left atrium; RA, right atrium; SVC, superior vena cava.

General Considerations

Because of the tendency for many VSDs to close spontaneously (see later discussion) and the tendency of larger defects to produce CHF in early childhood, it is relatively uncommon to encounter adults with previously undiagnosed VSDs of hemodynamic consequence. In adults, VSDs are usually either small and hemodynamically insignificant or large and associated with Eisenmenger syndrome. The importance of identifying the former is that they pose an ongoing risk of endocarditis and the potential complication of progressive aortic regurgitation. Eisenmenger syndrome is discussed later in this chapter.

Classifications of VSDs can be based on anatomic location or physiology. The anatomic classification includes defects of both the membranous and muscular portions of the ventricular septum (Figure 31–11). Membranous VSDs can be subdivided into supra-cristal (also known as doubly committed sub-arterial), peri-membranous (the inlet portion of the membranous septum), and malalignment (found in TOF with an overriding aorta) defects. The muscular VSDs, often multiple, may be located in the inlet or outlet regions or within the trabecular portion of the septum. Classifying VSDs physiologically is based on the size of the defect as well as the relative vascular resistances within the

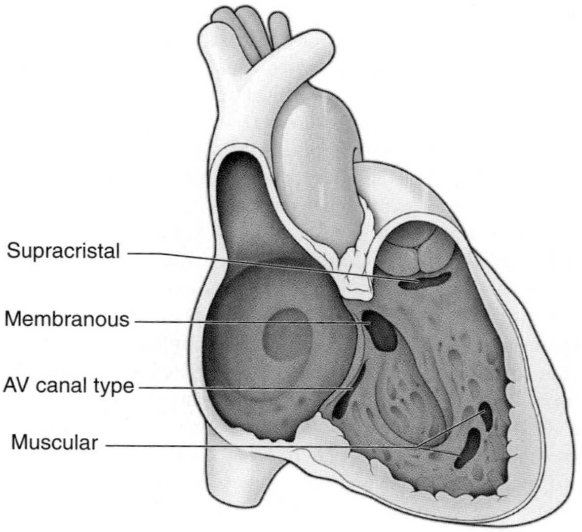

▲ **Figure 31–11.** Anatomic location of ventricular septal defects (VSDs). AV, atrioventricular.

systemic and pulmonary circulation. A high-pressure gradient exists across a small restrictive VSD, with normal or mildly elevated pulmonary artery pressure and predominant left-to-right shunting. A large nonrestrictive VSD permits equalization of RV and LV pressures with obligatory pulmonary hypertension (in the absence of RV outflow tract obstruction) and bidirectional shunting. The smallest VSD (maladie de Roger) is characterized by a hemodynamically insignificant shunt, a loud murmur, and an intermediate to high risk of endocarditis.

In the infant, left-to-right shunting occurs only when PVR falls below systemic vascular resistance, and the murmur usually becomes audible in the first month of life. With a large nonrestrictive defect, PVR may not fall; if the defect is not surgically closed by age 2, irreversible pulmonary hypertension may ensue. The volume overload caused by a large restrictive VSD may cause CHF in the first 6 months of life. Approximately 40% of VSDs close spontaneously by age 3, and a smaller percentage close before age 10. Generally, the smaller defects are more likely to close, but even in infants with heart failure, 7% will experience spontaneous closure.

Three late complications of VSD are worth mentioning. Tricuspid regurgitation may rarely result when the septal leaflet of the tricuspid valve is deformed by the ventricular septal aneurysm that causes spontaneous closure of a perimembranous VSD. Aortic regurgitation is common in patients with doubly committed sub-arterial VSDs (supracristal, or outlet, VSDs), as a result of herniation of the right aortic sinus into the defect; it also occurs in those with perimembranous VSDs. Infundibular PS from hypertrophy of the RV outflow tract can develop, functionally dividing the RV into inflow and outflow segments, a condition termed "double-chambered right ventricle." If a sufficient pressure gradient develops, RV systolic pressure can exceed LV systolic pressure, and right-to-left shunting can occur across the VSD. The resultant hypoxia may only occur during exercise.

Clinical Findings

A. Symptoms & Signs

The young adult with an uncorrected VSD and normal pulmonary artery pressures is usually asymptomatic, with normal or minimally diminished exercise tolerance. Like those with ASDs, exertional dyspnea often develops in patients with VSDs after the age of 30 when the Q_p:Q_s exceeds 2–3:1. Individuals with smaller shunts rarely report symptoms. The most disabled group with pulmonary hypertension and cyanosis (Eisenmenger physiology, or syndrome) will be discussed later.

Physical findings depend on the size of the VSD. The patient with uncomplicated VSD is acyanotic, and the LV apical impulse is displaced laterally, suggesting LV volume overload, and may be hyperdynamic. A holosystolic murmur occurs, often associated with a systolic thrill, heard best in the fourth or fifth intercostal space along the left sternal border, with radiation to the right parasternal region. Because of the increased flow across the mitral valve, an S_3 gallop and a diastolic rumble may be present. Additional signs of tricuspid insufficiency (prominent jugular venous *v* wave and systolic murmur) or aortic valve regurgitation (diastolic blowing murmur, increased arterial pulses) will be present in patients with these complications.

B. Diagnostic Studies

1. Electrocardiography and chest radiography—In the presence of a large shunt, the ECG is suggestive of LVH or biventricular hypertrophy, with biphasic QRS complexes in the transitional precordial leads. Evidence of left or right atrial enlargement is present in only about 25% of patients.

Cardiac enlargement with an increased cardiac silhouette is evident on chest radiograph only in the presence of a large left-to-right shunt. In the absence of pulmonary hypertension, there is evidence of pulmonary vascular engorgement with a plethora of the peripheral vasculature as well as enlargement of the proximal vessels. Left atrial enlargement may be evident on the lateral chest radiograph.

It is important to remember that in most adults with a small VSD (> 1.5–2:1 shunt), both the ECG and radiograph are normal, even in the presence of a loud murmur. On the other hand, the presence of pulmonary hypertension alters the ECG and radiograph findings.

2. Echocardiography—Two-dimensional and Doppler echocardiography can usually define the location and often the size of a VSD, although accurate Doppler shunt quantitation may not be possible in the adult. There is evidence of left atrial and LV dilatation. The right-heart chamber dimensions are usually normal, although the main pulmonary artery may appear dilated. The presence of RVH usually signifies pulmonary hypertension or associated PS (with right-to-left shunting and cyanosis). Usually only the largest defects, often located in the membranous septum, can actually be visualized on echocardiography (Figure 31–12). The aneurysmal pouch of a ventricular septal aneurysm may be seen in the parasternal short-axis view just below the aortic valve in the inlet portion of the septum near the septal leaflet of the tricuspid valve. Saline contrast administration shows a negative contrast effect within the RV, and a small degree of bidirectional shunting is sometimes present, with microbubbles appearing in the LV.

Color-flow Doppler imaging demonstrates a high-velocity (aliased) systolic jet across the ventricular septum into the RV. The location of the jet provides the best guide to the location of the defect. In the parasternal short-axis view, the jet from a membranous VSD may be seen in the region of the tricuspid valve (peri-membranous) or toward the pulmonary artery (doubly committed sub-arterial, or supra-cristal). Muscular VSD jets are best seen in the apical or subcostal four-chamber views (Figure 31–13).

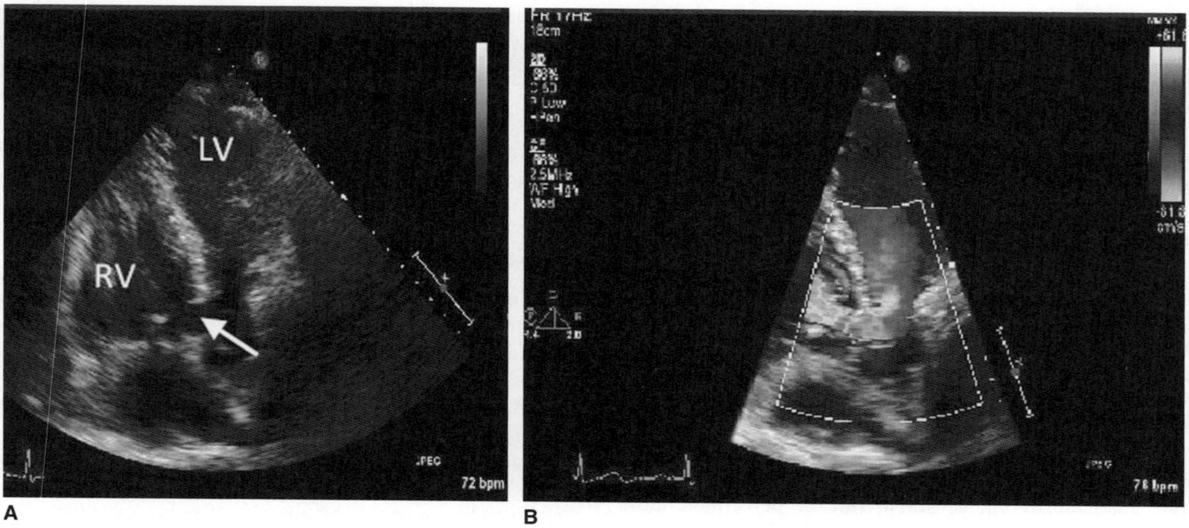

▲ **Figure 31–12. A:** Transthoracic echocardiogram in a 30-year-old woman with a large membranous ventricular septal defect (*arrow*). **B:** There is left-to-right shunting seen on color-flow Doppler. LV, left ventricle; RV right ventricle.

In continuous wave Doppler, the peak velocity of the jet across the ventricular septum provides the peak systolic LV-RV gradient (using the modified Bernoulli equation). Subtracting this gradient from the systolic blood pressure gives the peak RV systolic pressure. In the absence of a pressure gradient across the RV outflow tract—including the pulmonary valve (which should be carefully sought)—the RV systolic pressure is equivalent to the pulmonary artery systolic pressure. Additional Doppler evidence of the left-to-right shunt is found in the increased pulmonary artery flow velocity.

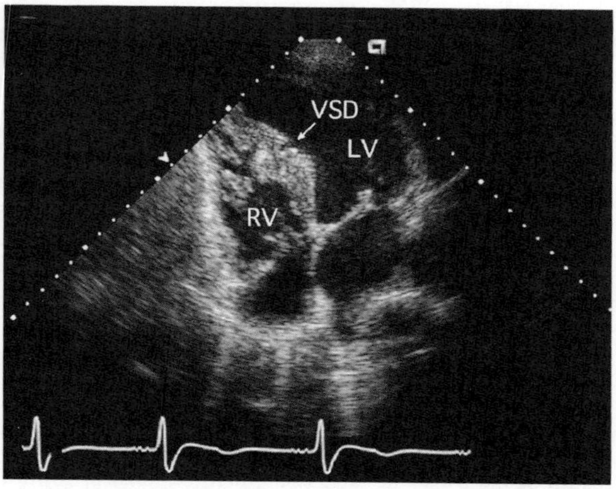

▲ **Figure 31–13.** Transthoracic echocardiogram in a 45-year-old woman with a small muscular ventricular septal defect (VSD). LV, left ventricle; RV, right ventricle.

In the post repair patient, the VSD patch may or may not be apparent, depending on the size of the original defect. Once endothelialized, the patch may not cause acoustic shadowing (or distal echo blackout). Color-flow Doppler may demonstrate patch leaks at the peripheral suture lines of the patch in a small percentage of patients. Spontaneous closure of a VSD involving juxtaposed tricuspid valve tissue may cause significant tricuspid regurgitation. Varying degrees of aortic regurgitation may be present and are most often associated with membranous or supracristal VSDs.

3. Cardiac catheterization—Although the diagnosis is often made noninvasively, the decision to close a VSD rests on accurate measurements of the shunt ratio and the level of PVR. Catheterization is therefore often necessary for therapeutic decision-making.

Right-heart catheterization with sequential measurements of oxygen saturation reveals a step-up within the body of the RV. As with an ASD, the higher the RV oxygen saturation, the greater is the degree of shunting. For the calculation of Q_p:Q_s, the same formula is used as for ASD, except that the mixed venous blood sample is drawn from the right atrium. Pulmonary artery pressures and vascular resistance should be measured, and a gradient across the RV outflow tract, including the infundibulum and the pulmonary valve, must be excluded. Left ventriculography in the cranial left anterior oblique projection will reveal the location of the defect as contrast enters the RV.

Prognosis & Treatment

As previously mentioned, adults with large, uncorrected VSDs are uncommonly encountered. With an uncorrected VSD, the overall 10-year survival rate after initial presentation is 75%. Survival is adversely affected by functional class greater than New York Heart Association class I, cardiomegaly, and elevated pulmonary artery pressure (> 50 mm Hg). As in patients with ASD, surgery is generally recommended when the magnitude of the systemic-to-pulmonary-shunt ratio exceeds 2:1. Other indications for surgery may include recurrent endocarditis and progressive aortic regurgitation.

In patients with small VSDs treated either conservatively or with surgery, outcomes are identical for patients with a Q_p:Q_s less than 2.0, normal PVR, no LV volume overload or VSD-related aortic regurgitation, and no symptoms of exercise intolerance.

Surgery for closure of VSDs has been available for more than 50 years, and long-term follow-up data are available. Surgery prior to age 2—even in infants with a large VSD, high pulmonary blood flow, and preoperative pulmonary hypertension—almost always prevents the development of pulmonary vascular obstructive disease. In patients who underwent surgery during the 1960s and 1970s, there is an approximately 20% incidence of residual left-to-right shunt and a persistent risk of endocarditis. Ventricular arrhythmias and right bundle branch block (RBBB) are more common with a repair performed via right ventriculotomy (eg, muscular or sub-arterial VSD); when possible, the right atrium is the preferred approach. The risk of sudden death and complete heart block is low. Most patients who have VSDs repaired in childhood survive to lead normal adult lives.

Devices have been developed for percutaneous closure of both muscular and peri-membranous VSDs. Muscular VSD occluders have been approved by the U.S. Food and Drug Administration and are commercially available in the United States. Initial case series suggest high success rates and low complication rates. Reported complications (in nine patients) include conduction anomalies and aortic or tricuspid regurgitation. More extensive follow-up data are needed before device implantation becomes routine.

PATENT DUCTUS ARTERIOSUS

ESSENTIALS OF DIAGNOSIS

- Continuous machinery-like murmur, loudest below the left clavicle.
- Left ventricular hypertrophy.
- Pulmonary plethora, left atrial and ventricular enlargement, and in older adults, calcification of the ductus on chest radiograph.
- Left atrial and ventricular dilatation with normal right-heart chambers on echocardiography.
- Continuous high-velocity color Doppler jet with retrograde flow along lateral wall of main pulmonary artery near left branch.

General Considerations

The patent ductus arteriosus (PDA) is a remnant of the normal fetal circulation. In the fetal circulation, superior vena cava blood enters the right atrium and characteristically is directed across the tricuspid valve into the RV. It is then delivered into the systemic circulation via the ductus arteriosus, which connects the left pulmonary artery to the descending aorta just distal to the insertion of the left subclavian artery (Figure 31–14). In the normal full-term newborn, the ductus closes within the first 10–15 hours following birth. If the ductus fails to close after birth when PVR falls, the direction of blood flow within the ductus reverses, producing a left-to-right shunt. CHF usually develops within the first year of life in patients with nonrestrictive PDA (large left-to-right shunts). As with VSD, it is relatively unusual—but by no means rare—to encounter an adult with uncorrected PDA.

An anatomic variant of the PDA is the aortopulmonary window (see Figure 31–14), which is usually a relatively large communication between the ascending aorta and the main pulmonary artery. The pathophysiology is similar to that of the PDA and is dependent on the size of the shunt and the level of PVR. The degree of pulmonary hypertension depends on the directly transmitted aortic pressure, which in turn depends on the size of the channel and the amount of pulmonary blood flow. If LV failure occurs, pulmonary venous hypertension may contribute further to the pulmonary hypertension. In a small number of patients, PVR rises above systemic vascular resistance and the shunt reverses. Because the site of the PDA is distal to the left subclavian, the head and neck vessels continue to receive oxygenated blood—but the descending aorta receives the desaturated blood, with the development of differential cyanosis.

When present in isolation, the PDA may lead to heart failure from pulmonary over-circulation. In conjunction with other defects, however, it may represent the sole pulmonary (eg, pulmonary atresia with intact ventricular septum) or systemic (eg, aortic atresia) blood supply, and survival may depend on persistent patency.

Clinical Findings

A. Symptoms & Signs

The mothers of patients with PDA may have a history of maternal rubella, and the patient may have had a murmur since infancy. If CHF has not developed by age 10, most patients will be asymptomatic as adults. CHF develops in a

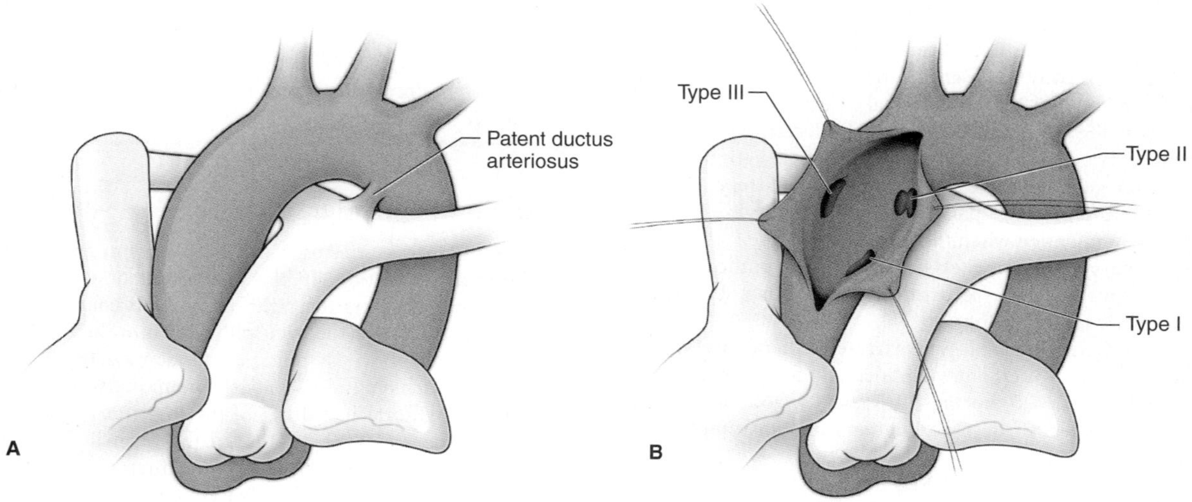

▲ **Figure 31–14.** Anatomic locations of patent ductus arteriosus (PDA) (**A**) and aortopulmonary window (**B**), with multiple distinct anatomic locations possible.

few patients in their 20s and 30s, however, and presents as exertional dyspnea, chest pain, and palpitations.

The patient is almost always acyanotic; but when cyanosis and clubbing are present, the upper extremities are usually spared. Thus, the lower extremities and sometimes the left hand may show clubbing and cyanosis, but the right hand and head are always pink. The pulse pressure may be widened, and the pulses are collapsing. The LV impulse is hyperdynamic and often laterally displaced. The classic murmur of the uncomplicated PDA is best heard below the left clavicle and gradually builds to its peak in late systole; it is continuous through the second heart sound and wanes in diastole. There may be a pause in late diastole or early systole. With a significant LV volume overload caused by a large shunt, an S_3 gallop and a diastolic murmur of relative mitral stenosis (similar to that of the large VSD) may be present. The murmur varies as PVR increases and shunting reverses, first with a decrease in the diastolic component and then a decrease in the systolic component. Finally, the murmur is silent and the physical findings are consistent with pulmonary hypertension (see Eisenmenger Syndrome).

B. Diagnostic Studies

1. Electrocardiography and chest radiography—The ECG is normal when the shunt is small; it shows left atrial and ventricular hypertrophy in the presence of a large shunt. When pulmonary hypertension is present and the shunt is predominantly right to left, the ECG may show P-pulmonale, right-axis deviation, and evidence of RVH.

The chest radiograph is also normal in the presence of a small shunt. With a significant shunt, LV prominence is evident with an enlarged cardiac silhouette and pulmonary vascular plethora. In the presence of pulmonary hypertension, pruning of the peripheral pulmonary vessels is present, with prominence of the central pulmonary arteries. The ductus may be calcified in the older adult.

2. Echocardiography—The two-dimensional echocardiogram shows left atrial and ventricular enlargement, but imaging of the ductus itself is usually difficult in the adult. Color-flow Doppler imaging is diagnostic and reveals continuous high-velocity flow within the main pulmonary artery near the left branch. Flow is predominantly retrograde within the pulmonary artery and can be detected by continuous wave Doppler. In an aortopulmonary window, continuous color flow is detected, but it is most often antegrade, which distinguishes it from the flow through a PDA. Pulmonary artery pressure can be estimated from the almost ubiquitous tricuspid regurgitant jet.

3. Cardiac catheterization—Right-heart catheterization is performed to measure the pulmonary artery pressure, PVR, and flow ratio (Q_p:Q_s). The oxygen step-up is at the level of the pulmonary artery, and when the ductus is large enough, the descending aorta can be entered from the pulmonary artery. The ductus can also be seen during aortography in the left lateral projection. Because echocardiography is noninvasive and diagnostic, cardiac catheterization may become exclusively therapeutic in the future. Techniques for coil and, more recently, device occlusion are well established and currently represent the treatment of choice for simple PDAs in many institutions. Thus, catheterization should be combined with a therapeutic intervention.

Prognosis & Treatment

Patients who survive into adulthood with a large uncorrected PDA generally have CHF or pulmonary hypertension (with right-to-left shunting and differential cyanosis) by about age 30. Most adults with PDA and normal or only mildly elevated PVR (< 4 Wood units) are either asymptomatic or mildly impaired and can undergo surgical ligation or percutaneous closure with good results. In the group with severely elevated PVR (> 10 Wood units/m^2), survival is poor. Approximately 15% of patients older than 40 years may have calcification or aneurysmal dilatation of the ductus, which can complicate surgery. Surgical ligation or percutaneous coil or device occlusion of a PDA can be performed with low morbidity and mortality and is recommended—independent of the size of the shunt—because of the high risk of endocarditis in uncorrected cases. Division of an isolated restrictive PDA in childhood can be curative of CHD. If repaired after childhood, the morbidity and mortality rates depend on the degree of pulmonary hypertension, LV volume overload, and calcification of the ductus. Unless persistent shunting is present following a surgical ligation, endocarditis prophylaxis is not recommended after the sixth postoperative month.

COARCTATION OF THE AORTA

ESSENTIALS OF DIAGNOSIS

- Elevated systolic blood pressure in the upper extremities (always in right arm); normal or diminished systolic blood pressure in lower extremities (and often left arm); radial-femoral pulse delay.
- LVH, LV prominence, "3" sign, rib notching on chest radiograph.
- Visualization of the coarctation by imaging.
- Distal aortic pressure drop by Doppler echocardiography or catheterization.

General Considerations

Coarctation of the thoracic aorta predominates in males, is often associated with a congenitally abnormal aortic valve, and is a congenital narrowing of the aorta, usually in the region of ductal insertion. The most common location is distal to the origin of the left subclavian artery (postductal; Figure 31–15), but the narrowing may also be proximal (preductal). Infrequently, a preductal coarctation is present in combination with an anomalous origin of the right subclavian artery, causing reduced pressures in the right upper extremity. There is considerable variability in the degree and extent of narrowing, ranging from a localized shelf to a long tubular narrowing. Multiple discrete sites are rarely encountered. Coarctation of the abdominal aorta is less common than that of the thoracic aorta; it is found equally in males and females and presents with symptoms of claudication. Additional coexisting problems may include congenital mitral valve disease and aneurysms of the circle of Willis (the latter are present in approximately 25% of patients with coarctation). Coarctation is frequently seen as part of a syndrome. Approximately 50% of patients have an associated bicuspid aortic valve. Long, tubular narrowing should alert the clinician to the possibility of Williams syndrome, whereas preductal coarctation is frequently seen in Turner syndrome. Collateral circulation to the distal aorta develops mainly via the subclavian and intercostal arteries, in addition to the vertebral and anterior spinal arteries.

Aortic coarctation is usually diagnosed during childhood in the asymptomatic phase by routine examination of blood pressure and femoral pulse palpation. Aortic coarctation is approximately two to five times more common in boys than in girls. In cases of severe obstruction, infants may have CHF. Symptoms may arise in the adult during the 20s and 30s, and evidence of coarctation should always be sought in patients of this age group presenting with hypertension. Early detection and repair are highly desirable because repair forestalls the associated accelerated development of coronary artery disease.

Clinical Findings

A. Symptoms & Signs

The adult with uncorrected coarctation is usually asymptomatic. When symptoms occur, they are nonspecific: exertional dyspnea, headache, epistaxis, and leg fatigue. CHF can occur in the adult with long-standing hypertension secondary to coarctation. Additional significant complications, usually occurring between the ages of 15 and 40, include aortic rupture or dissection of the proximal thoracic aorta or an aneurysm distal to the coarctation, infective endocarditis on an associated bicuspid aortic valve or endarteritis at the site of coarctation, and cerebrovascular accidents, which are most often due to rupture of an aneurysm of the circle of Willis.

The systolic blood pressure is elevated in the right arm and often the left arm, with reduced systolic blood pressures in the lower extremities. Diastolic blood pressures are not usually affected. Simultaneous palpation of the radial and femoral pulses reveals delayed arrival of the femoral pulse. Adult patients with highly developed collateral circulation may no longer exhibit these signs, however, and a clinically recorded difference between upper and lower extremity blood pressure will underestimate the coarctation gradient. The jugular venous pulse is normal, the carotid upstroke is usually brisk, and the aorta may be palpable in the suprasternal notch. Cardiac examination reveals a nondisplaced, but forceful, LV impulse. The first heart sound is normal, and the aortic component of the second heart sound may be accentuated. A late systolic murmur is present (as a result of

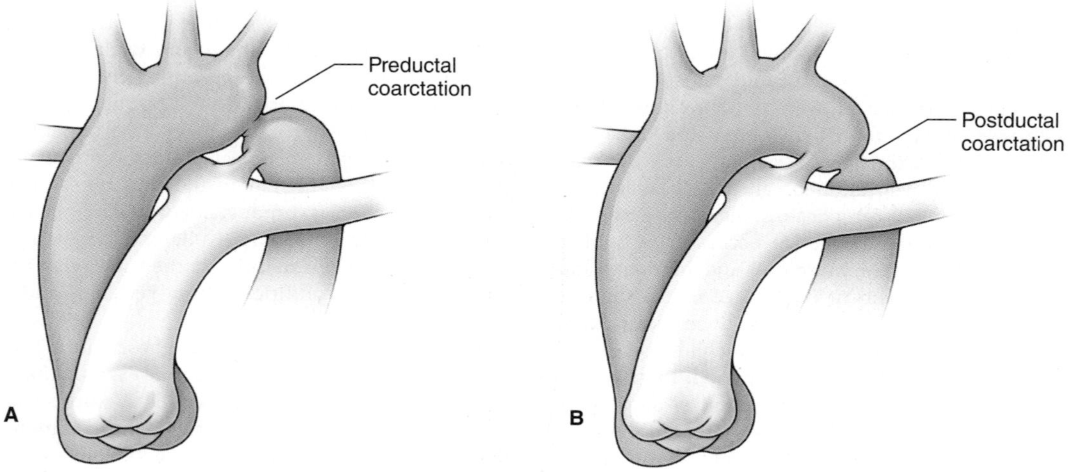

▲ **Figure 31–15.** Anatomic features of aortic coarctation. **A:** Preductal coarctation, in which differential cyanosis may occur. **B:** Postductal coarctation.

the coarctation) that is best heard between the scapulae to the left of the spine. The murmur caused by collateral flow through the intercostal and internal mammary arteries is longer, but it is not necessarily continuous. An ejection click and systolic murmur as well as a blowing diastolic murmur of aortic regurgitation may be associated with a bicuspid aortic valve.

B. Diagnostic Studies

1. Electrocardiography and chest radiography—The ECG is nonspecific, with LVH and, in the later stages, left atrial enlargement. As in other patients with long-standing hypertension, atrial fibrillation may occur.

On the other hand, the radiograph finding of rib notching is highly specific, although it is not 100% sensitive even in adults. Notching is present on the bottom of the rib where the intercostal arteries are located. In preductal coarctation (ie, proximal to the left subclavian artery), the rib notching is present only on the right side, and in abdominal coarctation, it is limited to the lower ribs. Another classic radiograph finding is the "3" sign, with the aortic arch and dilated left subclavian artery forming the upper curvature and the dilated distal aorta forming the lower. There may be radiologic evidence of LV and atrial enlargement.

2. Ambulatory BP monitoring and exercise testing—A significant number of patients especially those who are repaired late in life develop systemic hypertension. In these patients 24-hour ambulatory BP monitoring can be useful for diagnosis or management of hypertension. Another reasonable approach is to perform exercise testing in evaluating exercise-induced hypertension which may necessitate the use of antihypertensives in a select patients with abnormal imaging findings.

3. Echocardiography—It is extremely difficult to identify the actual site of the coarctation in the adult patient with precordial two-dimensional echocardiography. Doppler evidence of flow acceleration in the descending aorta from the suprasternal notch, however, can often identify obstruction even when images are suboptimal. The peak systolic velocity can be used to estimate the gradient, but the presence of persistent antegrade flow in diastole (Figure 31–16A) and decreased acceleration time beyond the coarctation provide additional confirmation of hemodynamic significance. Further localization of the coarctation is now possible with imaging of the descending aorta in the longitudinal plane during multiplanar TEE. The anatomy of the aortic valve should be carefully defined, and careful Doppler interrogation for evidence of stenosis or insufficiency is essential.

4. Magnetic resonance angiography and computed tomography angiography—MRA can localize and define the extent of narrowing with a high degree of accuracy (Figure 31–16C) and provides estimates of the presence of collateral flow to the distal aorta. Aneurysmal dilatation is visible, and postoperative evaluation is possible. Computed tomography (CT) angiography provides excellent anatomic definition but cannot provide any physiologic information.

5. Cardiac catheterization—Aortography is necessary only when the diagnosis is not adequately confirmed clinically, or the anatomy cannot be fully defined noninvasively. Premature coronary disease is common, and if it is clinically suspected, coronary arteriography should be performed. Balloon dilatation with or without stent placement across

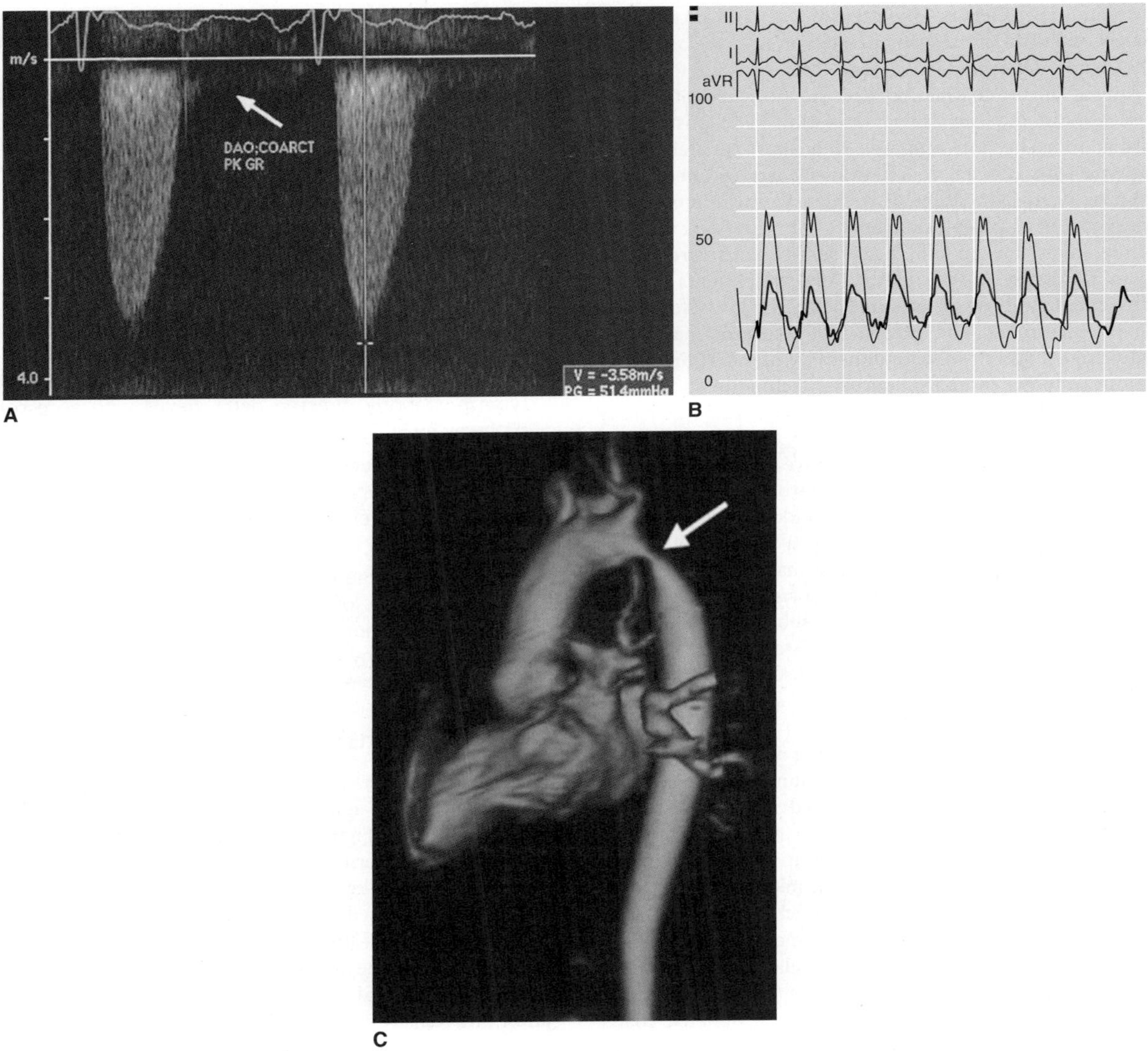

▲ **Figure 31–16.** **A:** Continuous wave Doppler from transthoracic echocardiogram in a patient with coarctation of the descending aorta (DAO). There was a peak gradient (PK GR) of 51.4 mm Hg with runoff in diastole (*arrow*). **B:** Right heart catheterization confirming the gradient between the right ventricle (*red*) and the pulmonary artery (*black*). **C:** Magnetic resonance imaging of coarctation of the aorta (*arrow*).

native and recurrent coarctation has been attempted in cases of discrete narrowing (see later discussion).

Prognosis & Treatment

The importance of identifying coarctation in adults lies in the tendency toward LVH and CHF, premature coronary artery disease, and cerebral hemorrhage. In an autopsy series of uncorrected coarctation, 50% of patients had died by about age 30 and 90% by age 60. Proximal aortic rupture, aortic dissection, and cerebral hemorrhage often occur before the age of 30, and the incidence of CHF continues to increase after the age of 40.

Surgery for correcting coarctation presents a considerable challenge in patients over the age of 15 years because of large intercostal aneurysms and atheromatous changes in the aorta near the shelf. It should be noted that surgical repair even in childhood is often only palliative, and these patients require continued surveillance, particularly in the presence of associated cardiac lesions or preoperative systemic hypertension. Hypertension persists in approximately one-third of patients operated on after the age of 14. The major determinants of long-term survival following repair of aortic coarctation are the presence of associated lesions and the age at operation. The postsurgery cardiac mortality rate after age 20 is approximately 5% in patients with isolated coarctation. Causes of late cardiovascular deaths (in order of frequency) include coronary artery disease, sudden death, aortic regurgitation and heart failure, hypertension and heart failure, and cerebrovascular accidents. Approximately 10% of patients require subsequent cardiovascular surgery, the majority for aortic valve replacement. The incidence of recurrent coarctation requiring surgery or percutaneous intervention varies significantly depending on surgical technique and can be 16–60%, with the highest re-coarctation rates generally associated with earlier operation.

The surgical methods of repair have undergone considerable evolution since their initial introduction in the late 1950s. In part, this is due to the considerable morphologic variability that has precluded using a single method for correction. The removal of the abnormal coarctation tissue as occurs in an end-to-end anastomosis is most desirable, but depending on other factors, a subclavian flap repair or an interposition graft may be necessary. Less reliance is placed on the patch angioplasty because long-term studies have shown late aneurysm formation due to thinning of the posterior wall.

Over the past 10 years, endovascular repair of coarctation has become a popular treatment option. Furthermore, the advent of balloon-expandable covered stents has reduced the complication rate associated with balloon angioplasty alone. Complications of stent implantation can be classified into three categories: technical (stent migration or fracture, balloon rupture, and overlap of the brachiocephalic vessels), aortic (intimal tear, dissection, and aneurysm formation), and peripheral vascular (cerebral vascular accident, peripheral embolization, and injury to access vessels). Compared with surgical therapy, endovascular stenting of native coarctation has a similar morbidity and mortality but is associated with a significantly higher incidence of re-coarctation, need for reintervention, and persistent hypertension. In light of these differences, there is ongoing controversy about the best treatment approach for adults and adult-sized adolescents with native coarctation of the aorta. There is general agreement, however, that re-coarctation in adults can be managed by percutaneous transluminal balloon angioplasty, with or without stent implantation.

Because of the risk of re-coarctation and of complications such as aortic aneurysm, periodic surveillance with MRI or with CT aortography is recommended in the adult after repair, irrespective of technique. It is essential to screen women of childbearing age for post repair aortic dilatation because the risk of aortic dissection or rupture during pregnancy is high. The need to screen for intracranial aneurysms is controversial.

EBSTEIN ANOMALY

ESSENTIALS OF DIAGNOSIS

- History of dyspnea, atypical chest pain, or intermittent cyanosis.
- Palpitations associated with supraventricular arrhythmias and preexcitation syndrome.
- Right parasternal lift, widely split S_1, systolic clicks, and systolic murmur of tricuspid regurgitation (without inspiratory accentuation).
- Right atrial enlargement, RV conduction defect of RBBB type, posteriorly directed delta waves with accessory pathway by ECG. Frequent first-degree AV block.
- Normal or reduced pulmonary vascularity without pulmonary artery enlargement, right atrial enlargement, normal left-sided cardiac silhouette on chest radiograph.
- Apical displacement of septal tricuspid valve leaflet; variable degrees of tricuspid regurgitation originating from apical portion of RV; and enlarged right atrium on echocardiography.

General Considerations

Ebstein anomaly is characterized by deformity of the tricuspid valve with apical displacement of the septal and posterior leaflets (Figure 31–17) and their adhesion to the RV wall. The anterior leaflet is elongated and has been described as sail-like. Tricuspid regurgitation arises from the apically displaced site of leaflet coaptation with considerable variability in the extent of tricuspid leaflet displacement and the degree of tricuspid regurgitation. The portion of the RV proximal to the leaflets is atrialized (thinned), and if the remaining RV is diminutive in size, pump function may be inadequate. Cyanosis may be present as a result of right-to-left shunting across an ASD or patent foramen ovale in the presence of significant tricuspid regurgitation or elevated right atrial pressures. Interatrial septal defects, including patent foramen ovales, are the most common associated anomaly, occurring in 80–90% of patients with Ebstein anomaly.

Tremendous variability exists in the morphologic abnormalities and clinical presentation of patients with Ebstein anomaly. In severe cases, CHF or cyanosis may be present during infancy. At the opposite end of the spectrum, a mildly affected adult may be asymptomatic or symptomatic only because of supraventricular tachyarrhythmias. The latter are an important feature of Ebstein anomaly, which is associated with preexcitation in 25–30% of patients. The accessory pathway is usually posteroseptal or posterolateral in location.

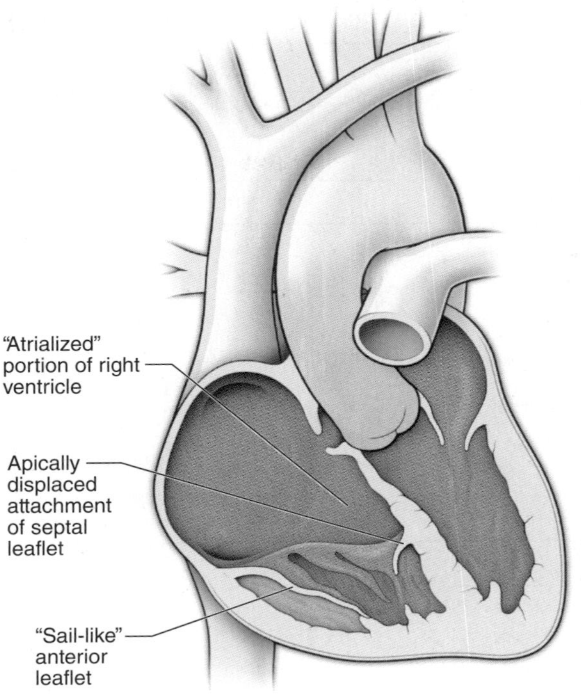

▲ **Figure 31–17.** Anatomy of Ebstein anomaly.

Clinical Findings

A. Symptoms & Signs

Cyanosis may be the most important clinical feature in early life, but in older patients, long-standing RV volume overload and right atrial distention result in CHF. Dysrhythmias, including the Wolff-Parkinson-White syndrome, are frequent. Adult patients may have dyspnea, arrhythmias, decreased exercise tolerance, and intermittent or exercise-induced cyanosis (with associated right-to-left shunting across an ASD or patent foramen ovale).

Physical examination reveals right parasternal lift, widely split S_1, systolic clicks (from delayed tricuspid valve closure, the "sail" sounds), and the systolic murmur of tricuspid regurgitation. The latter does not usually increase in intensity during inspiration, because the noncompliant RV cannot accept an increase in venous return. On the other hand, the right atrium is compliant, and systemic venous congestion is uncommon; the jugular venous pulse is therefore usually normal. S_3 and S_4 gallops may be present, as may an early diastolic snap from the opening of the elongated anterior leaflet.

B. Diagnostic Studies

1. Electrocardiography and chest radiography—The ECG shows evidence of right atrial enlargement and an RV conduction defect of the RBBB type. The PR interval may be prolonged, except in the presence of an accessory pathway. In 25–30% of patients, ECG findings are consistent with Wolff-Parkinson-White syndrome; the PR interval is short, and delta waves from a posterolateral or posteroseptal bundle of Kent are evident (Figure 31–18). Atrial fibrillation may be present in older patients.

The chest radiograph shows normal or reduced pulmonary vascularity without pulmonary artery enlargement; it also shows cardiac enlargement to the right of the sternum caused by right atrial enlargement. The LV and left atrium are normal in size.

2. Echocardiography—The classic M-mode description of this anomaly included increased excursion of the anterior tricuspid valve leaflet and delayed tricuspid valve closure (> 40 ms) following mitral valve closure. Two-dimensional and Doppler echocardiography are diagnostic in most adults. The four-chamber apical and subcostal views provide most of the necessary information. The right atrium is enlarged and the RV is usually small, consisting of the atrialized portion and the remaining pumping chamber. The septal, and possibly the posterior, leaflet of the tricuspid valve is apically displaced, and color-flow Doppler imaging shows the regurgitant jet arising from the apical point of coaptation (Figure 31–19). The degree of tricuspid regurgitation can be estimated from the extent of right atrial filling by color flow and from the density of the continuous wave Doppler signal. The pulmonary artery systolic pressure estimated from the continuous wave tricuspid regurgitation jet is nearly always normal.

Although color-flow imaging may reveal a patent foramen ovale or an ASD, it is mandatory to perform a saline contrast examination to reliably exclude these sources of right-to-left shunting. When precordial echocardiography is inadequate, TEE can be used to exclude associated lesions of the atrial septum.

3. Cardiac catheterization—During right-heart catheterization, simultaneous recordings of an RV electrogram and a right atrial pressure tracing are obtained with a catheter in the atrialized portion of the RV. This finding is considered pathognomonic of Ebstein anomaly, but catheterization is rarely necessary for diagnosis.

Prognosis & Treatment

The chance of surviving up to age 50 is about 50%, with survival dependent on the degree of the anatomic and physiologic abnormalities. As mentioned, 25–30% of patients have supraventricular arrhythmias, many associated with accessory pathways that are now amenable to catheter ablation. Evaluation of these patients with an electrophysiology study prior to consideration for surgery may be necessary. Tricuspid annuloplasty and repair with RV plication have been challenging. The success of these approaches has traditionally been limited, with approximately 50% of patients

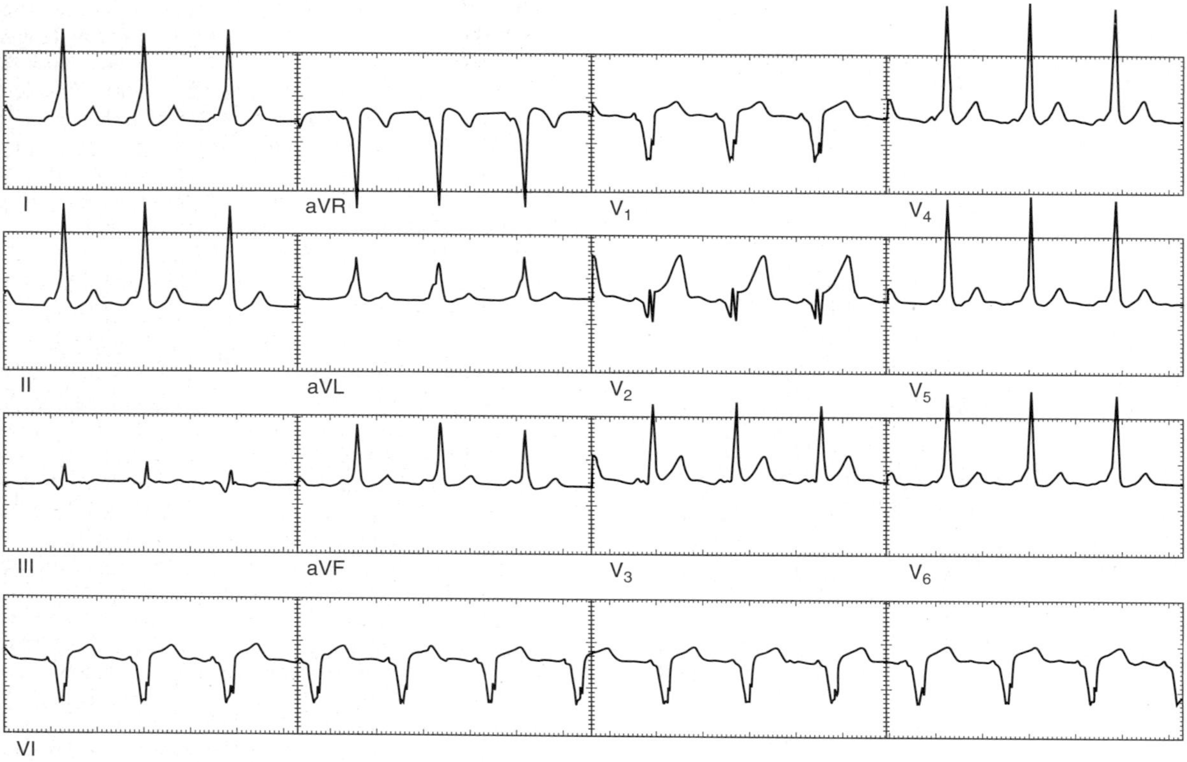

▲ **Figure 31–18.** Electrocardiogram in Ebstein anomaly with associated Wolff-Parkinson-White syndrome.

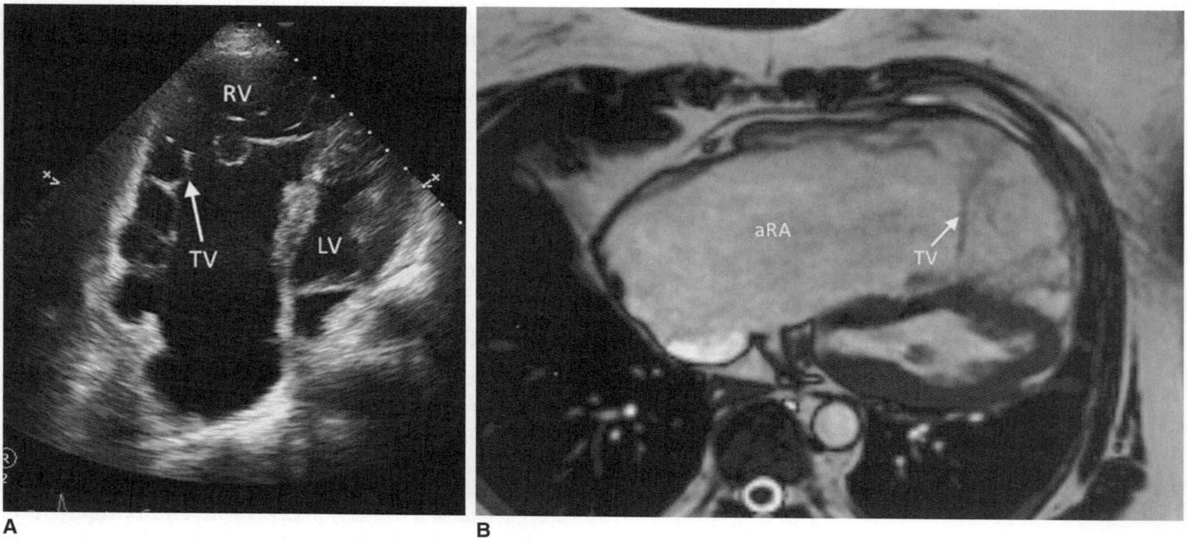

▲ **Figure 31–19. A:** Transthoracic echocardiogram in a 56-year-old woman with Ebstein anomaly. This four-chamber view shows the apically displaced tricuspid valve (TV) in relation to the normal mitral valve (lower part of left ventricle [LV]). **B:** Off-axis magnetic resonance imaging of the right ventricle (RV) showing the large atrialized right atrium (aRA).

requiring tricuspid valve replacement. Newer techniques, such as the Carpentier and "cone" techniques, promise to reduce further the need for valve replacement. Improvement in exercise tolerance following tricuspid valve replacement or repair has been observed, especially in patients with associated ASD. In patients with severe morphologic variants, a Fontan-like procedure (see Palliative Surgical Procedures) may be the only suitable choice. In patients who are symptomatic predominantly based on exercise-induced cyanosis, device closure of the interarterial septal defect may be adequate treatment.

CONGENITALLY CORRECTED TRANSPOSITION OF THE GREAT ARTERIES

ESSENTIALS OF DIAGNOSIS

- Prominent left parasternal impulse, soft S_1, accentuated A_2, soft or inaudible P_2.
- PR prolongation, variable degrees of AV block, Q waves in right precordial leads with absence in left precordial leads on ECG.
- Absence of left-sided aortic knob on chest radiograph.
- Rightward and posterior pulmonary artery with leftward and anterior aorta, apical displacement of right-sided AV valve, coarsely trabeculated left-sided systemic ventricle with moderator band (the morphologic RV) on cardiac imaging.

General Considerations

In congenitally corrected transposition of the great arteries (CC-TGA, also abbreviated as l-TGA), the visceroatrial relationship is normal with the right atrium to the right of the left atrium (Figure 31–20). The systemic venous blood drains into the right atrium and through a bileaflet (mitral) valve into a morphologic LV pumping into a posterior and rightward pulmonary artery. The pulmonary venous blood drains into the left atrium and through a trileaflet tricuspid valve into a morphologic RV pumping into an anterior and leftward aorta. This occurs because of atrial-ventricular discordance (ventricular inversion), which causes the RV to be located to the left of the LV. The great arteries are transposed, with the aorta arising from the RV and the pulmonary artery rising from the LV. The result is physiologic correction of the circulation, in that oxygenated blood comes into the left atrium, goes to the anatomic right ventricle, and then flows out of the aorta. The patient is acyanotic, and early symptoms typically result from associated lesions such as PS, VSD, and heart block.

The most common complications are complete heart block (occurring with an incidence of approximately 2% per year) and other associated anomalies, most commonly VSD, subvalvular PS, and abnormalities of the systemic AV valve. Coronary anomalies are uncommon, and the coronary circulation is usually concordant; that is, a right coronary artery supplies the RV. Eventually, the systemic ventricle (a massively hypertrophied RV) is subject to pump failure, even in cases of isolated CC-TGA. The relative degree of PS and the size of the VSD determine whether cyanosis is present. In the absence of PS, the patient with a large VSD may have CHF due to the volume overload of the systemic ventricle and is at risk for pulmonary vascular disease.

The male-to-female ratio is approximately 1.5:1. Although familial recurrence has been reported, no genetic linkage has been identified.

Clinical Findings

A. Symptoms & Signs

Most patients with isolated CC-TGA are asymptomatic in childhood and young adulthood, although formal cardiopulmonary exercise testing typically reveals lower VO_{2max} than in healthy controls. The highly prevalent complication of complete heart block may present with syncope, sudden death, or, less dramatically, exercise intolerance. More often, the clinical picture is dominated by associated lesions.

Exertional dyspnea and easy fatigability may develop with systemic AV valve regurgitation, which may be functional, due to annular dilatation, or related to intrinsic dysplasia of the valve. Pulmonary venous congestion from pump failure of the anatomic RV may occur in middle age.

The physical examination depends largely on the associated anomalies. The left parasternal impulse is prominent as a result of the hypertrophied systemic ventricle. In the presence of a prolonged PR interval, S_1 is diminished in intensity. The proximity of the aorta to the chest wall causes an accentuated A_2; conversely, the posterior displacement of the pulmonary valve causes a soft or inaudible P_2. Systolic thrills occur in the presence of PS, with and without VSD. If PS is present, the murmur is best heard in the third left intercostal space, radiating to the right. The murmur of a VSD is usually typical, but the murmur of left-sided AV valve regurgitation radiates to the left sternal border in CC-TGA.

B. Diagnostic Studies

1. Electrocardiography and chest radiography—The ECG and radiologic findings of CC-TGA are dominated by its associated lesions. The ECG shows variable degrees of AV block, from simple PR prolongation to complete heart block. The absence of Q waves in leads I, V_5, and V_6 or the presence of Q waves in leads V_4R or V_1 is characteristic of the condition. This pattern results because the ventricular septal depolarization proceeds from the morphologic LV to RV (Figure 31–21). The typical chest radiograph finding in isolated CC-TGA is a straight, left upper cardiac border,

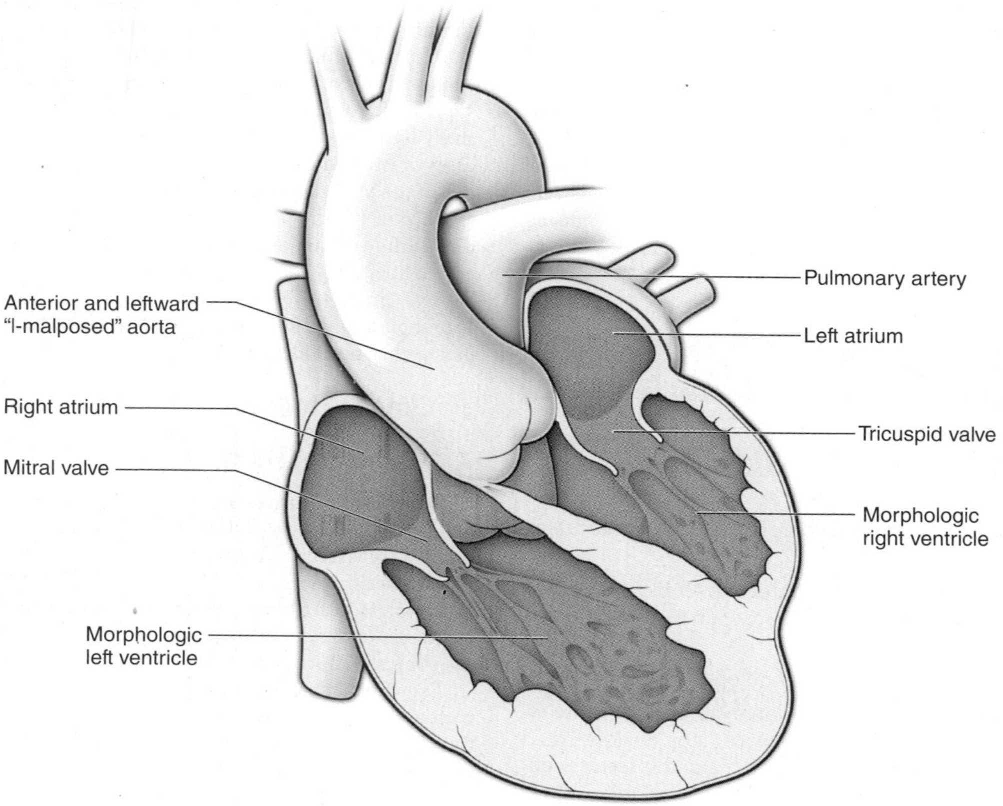

▲ **Figure 31–20.** Anatomy of congenitally corrected transposition of the great arteries.

formed by the ascending aorta and loss of the pulmonary trunk contour.

2. Echocardiography—The anatomic features of isolated CC-TGA are usually apparent by TTE, even in adults. TEE may be useful in defining the anatomy of associated lesions such as infundibular obstruction and the severity of left-sided AV valve regurgitation. In the basal parasternal short-axis view, the aortic valve is anterior and usually to the left of the pulmonic valve. Because the two great arteries arise in parallel, there is a "figure-eight" appearance, rather than the usual arrangement of the pulmonary artery in long axis surrounding the aortic valve. On careful inspection, the coronary arteries can be identified as they emerge from the aortic root. In the long-axis view (obtained from a more vertical and leftward scan), the aorta arises from the posterior ventricle, and its valve is not in fibrous continuity with the AV valve. The heavily trabeculated and hypertrophied RV with its moderator band is posterior and to the left, and the smoothly trabeculated LV is anterior and to the right (Figure 31–22). The systemic AV (anatomically a tricuspid) valve has three leaflets and septal attachments, is apically displaced, and may show variable degrees of regurgitation, often as a consequence of an "Ebstein-like" displacement of the septal leaflet. In contrast, the subpulmonary AV (anatomically a mitral) valve has two leaflets and no septal attachments.

It is essential to identify associated lesions because these are the primary determinants of survival, specifically a VSD and infundibular pulmonary valve stenosis. Doppler echocardiography should be used to determine the pulmonary valve gradient and to identify any pulmonary hypertension. Autopsy studies of patients with CC-TGA have documented abnormalities of the pulmonary venous AV valve in greater than 90% of cases. The most common of these is an Ebstein-like deformity. The leaflets of this systemic tricuspid valve are displaced apically, and the chordae tendineae are short and thickened. Clinically significant tricuspid systemic AV valve regurgitation has been reported in 20–50% of patients with CC-TGA.

3. Cardiac catheterization—When noninvasive data are diagnostically conclusive, the role of cardiac catheterization is for preoperative evaluation in patients with surgically remediable lesions. The pulmonary artery may be difficult to enter; fluoroscopically, the venous catheter is noted to enter a posterior and rightward vessel. The PVR must be measured to rule out irreversible pulmonary vascular disease

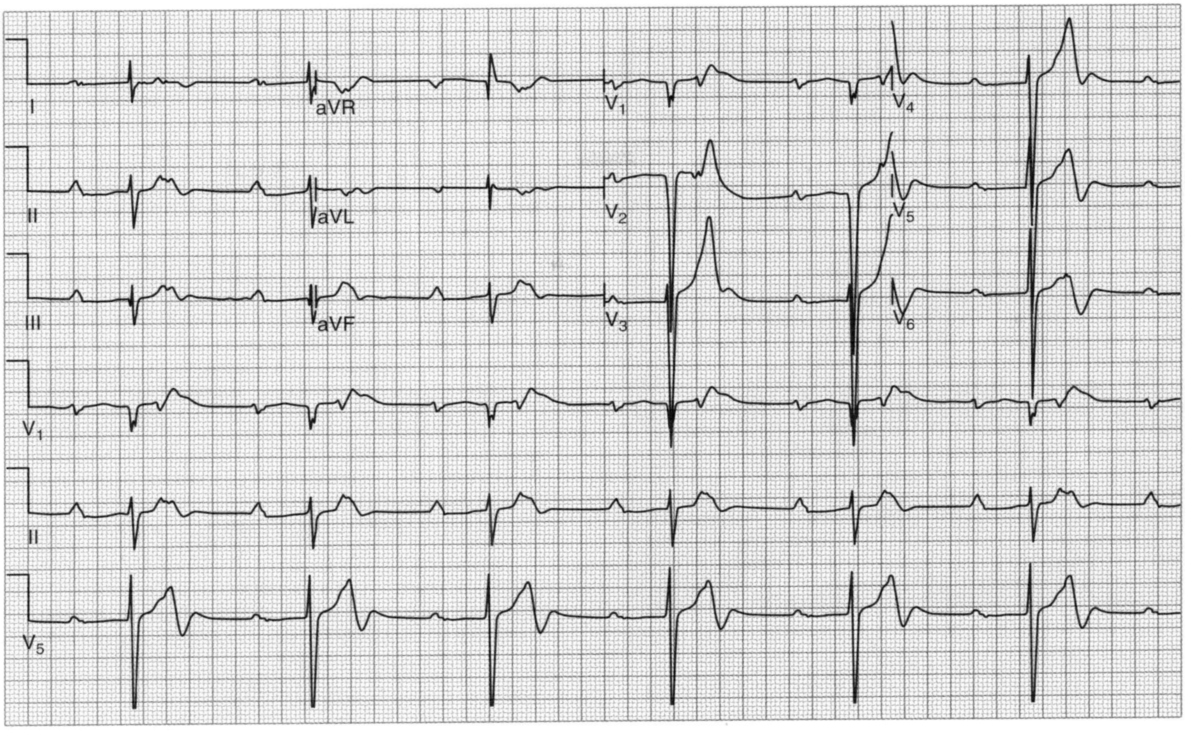

▲ **Figure 31–21.** Electrocardiograph in congenitally corrected transposition of the great arteries with associated pulmonic stenosis and ventricular septal defect. Note the 2:1 AV block and the Q waves in aVR and V_1.

in patients with VSD. Although angiography can indicate the abnormally positioned great arteries, it is important only for identification of anomalous coronary arteries, which are infrequently encountered.

Prognosis & Treatment

Survival in CC-TGA is usually determined by other associated lesions, but even in its isolated form, survival may not be normal. The natural history and postoperative outcome of patients with CC-TGA and the commonly associated lesions of VSD and PS are known to be less satisfactory than those of patients with normal AV connections and similar intracardiac lesions. The propensity for AV conduction abnormalities and for tricuspid valve dysfunction and the much-debated capability of the RV to function adequately in the systemic circulation may all affect survival.

A frequent feature of CC-TGA is the development of complete heart block, estimated to occur at a rate of about 2% per year. AV conduction abnormalities of varying degrees are seen in nearly 75% of patients with this anomaly; many will require permanent pacemaker insertion. Periodic surveillance for the development of high-degree AV block is important: sudden death may be the first manifestation of this complication. However, it is the morphologic abnormalities of the tricuspid valve resulting in severe valvular dysfunction/regurgitation that have been shown to be the most critical determinant for survival. The systemic RV in CC-TGA appears to be less tolerant than an anatomic LV of similar degrees of valvular incompetence, and there is an acceleration of the usual vicious cycle of ventricular remodeling, hypertrophy, and dysfunction in response to volume overload. The RV's inability to cope with significant tricuspid regurgitation leads to decreased contractility and annular dilation that, in turn, exacerbates the degree of regurgitation. Theoretically, the anatomic RV is subject to progressive pump failure from the obligatory pressure overload of the systemic circulation, potentially hastened by systemic hypertension, coronary artery disease, and volume overload from a regurgitant AV valve. Because the circulation is functionally corrected, the indications for surgery are those of the associated lesion requiring surgery (eg, VSD with a Q_p:Q_s of 2:1, VSD with PS causing cyanosis). Repair or replacement of the tricuspid valve may be indicated; however, 10-year survival after surgical intervention is low. A "double switch" operation has been proposed for patients whose tricuspid valves are severely insufficient. An atrial switch combined with an arterial switch (see the section on Transposition of the Great Arteries) in the absence of LV outflow obstruction or with a **Rastelli** procedure (RV to

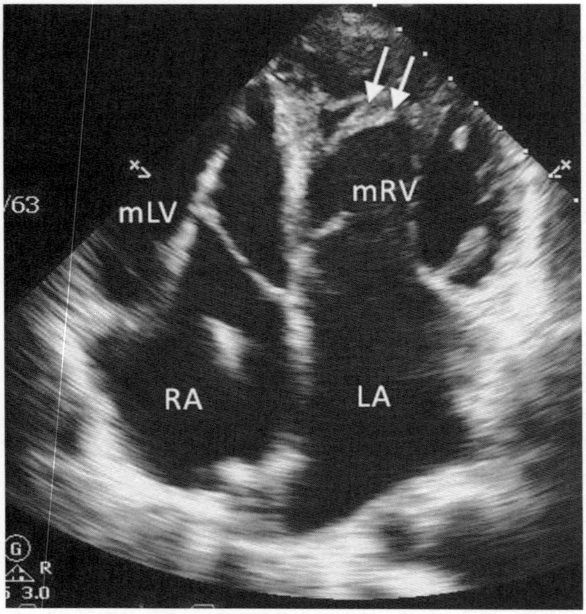

▲ **Figure 31–22.** Apical transthoracic echocardiographic views in a patient with congenitally corrected transposition of the great arteries. The moderator band is clearly visualized (*double arrow*) in the left-sided morphologic right ventricle (mRV). The right ventricle is spherically dilated, reflecting the pressure overload of this chamber. The left ventricle is smaller, and a pacemaker lead is visualized within. The left-sided atrioventricular (AV) valve is a morphologic tricuspid valve and is more apically displaced than the right-sided AV valve which is a morphologic mitral valve. LA, left atrium; mLV, morphologic left ventricle; RA, right atrium.

pulmonary artery conduit) has been successfully performed. After surgery, the LV and mitral valve are restored to systemic circulation. Improvement in tricuspid valve function in a low-pressure RV has been documented after these operations. This procedure carries significant risk, and late complications relating to the atrial switch component (baffle obstruction, sick sinus syndrome) are of additional concern. Heart transplantation remains the final option for patients with CC-TGA, intractable tricuspid regurgitation, and RV failure.

OTHER ACYANOTIC CONGENITAL DEFECTS

Partial anomalous pulmonary venous return usually involves abnormal drainage of the right upper pulmonary vein into the superior vena cava and is often associated with sinus venosus ASD. Other sites of drainage include the coronary sinus and the inferior vena cava (scimitar syndrome). The need for surgical correction depends on the presence or degree of pulmonary venous obstruction and on the size of the shunt, which in turn is related to the number of pulmonary veins draining into the pulmonary circulation. As a rule, more than one anomalously draining pulmonary vein is required to produce a hemodynamically significant shunt.

AV septal defects (also known as **endocardial cushion defects** or **AV canal defects**, both terms referring to abnormalities of derivatives of the endocardial cushions of the embryonic AV canal) are particularly common in children born with trisomy 21. These defects include an ostium primum ASD, a membranous VSD, and a mitral valve malformation, consisting of a cleft in the anterior leaflet or anterior and posterior bridging leaflets (Figure 31–23). Irreversible pulmonary vascular disease with shunt reversal may lead to cyanosis (see section on Eisenmenger Syndrome) and is extremely common in the adult who has had no attempt at repair. Residual mitral regurgitation is often encountered following repair. Even when the valve is competent in the early postoperative period, late regurgitation occurs in a small percentage of patients.

Coronary artery anomalies are seen not uncommonly as an isolated defect in the adult patient. They are found in approximately 1% of patients undergoing coronary arteriography and in approximately 0.3% of autopsies. An anomaly of particular importance is the left main coronary artery arising from the pulmonary trunk. This may present in infancy as cardiomyopathy and CHF from myocardial ischemia and systolic dysfunction. Sufficient myocardial collaterals from the right coronary artery may develop in a small

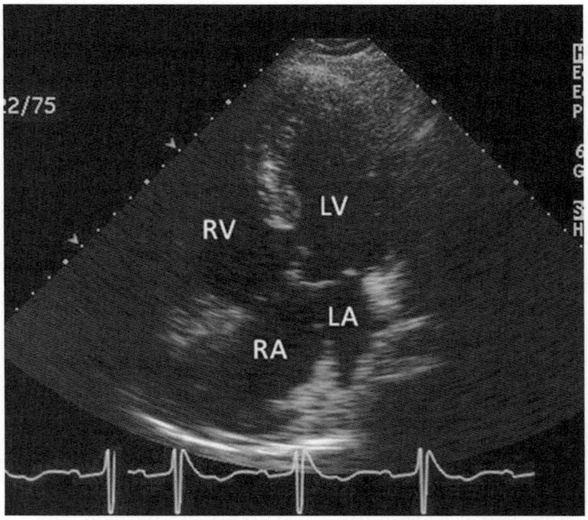

▲ **Figure 31–23.** Apical four-chamber view from a transthoracic echocardiogram in a patient with atrioventricular septal defect and Down syndrome. The crux of the heart is missing, and a large ostium primum atrial septal defect and large ventricular septal defect are evident. LA, left atrium; LV, left ventricle; RA, right atrium; RV, right ventricle.

number of patients, which allows survival into adulthood. Physical examination may reveal a continuous murmur, and clinical assessment may be remarkable for angina pectoris, myocardial infarction, dyspnea, syncope, and sudden death. Treatments include surgical closure of the left main artery with possible bypass to the left anterior descending artery or primary re-anastomosis of the anomalous artery from the pulmonary artery to the aorta or the subclavian artery. There are many anatomic variations of the less severe coronary anomalies. When the left coronary artery arises from the right or noncoronary cusp and passes between the aorta and pulmonary artery, however, the patient is at increased risk for ischemia and sudden death. This diagnosis should be considered in young patients with exertional chest pain. TEE may identify anomalous coronary ostia. Although MRA or CT angiography may be diagnostic in skilled hands, coronary angiography is currently the diagnostic gold standard. The role for surgery in these patients is controversial and is usually reserved for patients with unequivocal evidence of ischemia and for young, athletic patients, who are at the highest risk for sudden cardiac death.

Coronary arteriovenous fistulas are more likely than serious coronary anomalies to permit survival to adulthood. Large fistulas draining into the right side of the circulation may be associated with a sizable shunt and can rarely present with CHF in infancy. Coronary steal may occur, leading to myocardial ischemia. In the adult, there may be a history of exertional dyspnea or chest pain and a continuous murmur on physical examination. TTE detects the dilated fistulous coronary artery in approximately 50% of patients. Abnormal continuous jets within the cardiac chambers (RV is most common) or in the pulmonary artery seen in color-flow Doppler should suggest this diagnosis. Cardiac catheterization showing the dilated coronary artery and fistulous communication confirms the diagnosis.

Congenital **sinus of Valsalva aneurysms** may coexist with supracristal VSDs and have the potential for catastrophic rupture with development of acute severe aortic regurgitation or pericardial tamponade. Although the perforation may be subacute with mild regurgitation, it nonetheless poses an ongoing risk for endocarditis. Echocardiography, with a transesophageal approach if necessary, is diagnostic. Surgical repair with a pericardial patch is indicated when rupture is present.

CYANOTIC CONGENITAL HEART DISEASE

Patients with cyanotic CHD have arterial oxygen desaturation resulting from the shunting of systemic venous blood to the arterial circulation, or from cardiac anatomy that mandates mixing of systemic and pulmonary venous blood. The shunting can occur at the level of the atrium (ASD), the ventricle (VSD), or the great vessels (PDA or aortopulmonary window), or in the lungs (pulmonary arteriovenous malformations or venovenous collaterals). If a right-to-left shunt is present, it implies a right-sided obstruction distal to that level or the presence of pulmonary vascular obstructive disease causing reversal of flow through a previously left-to-right shunting lesion.

There are many specific congenital cardiac lesions that cause cyanosis, and each of the specific diagnoses may have its own variations, making memorization of a comprehensive list of diagnoses difficult. However, the spectrum of basic cyanotic congenital lesions can be remembered as the "5 Ts": TOF, (complete) transposition of the great vessels, total anomalous pulmonary venous return, tricuspid atresia, and truncus arteriosus communis. The many remaining lesions can generally be thought of as variants of these basic diagnoses. The pathophysiology of each of these lesions is discussed in the respective section. Untreated cyanotic heart disease carries an extremely high mortality rate in the infant and child; therefore, most patients reaching adulthood have had reparative or palliative surgery. Those who reach adulthood without surgery are usually those with TOF or irreversible pulmonary vascular disease (eg, Eisenmenger syndrome) from underlying congenital cardiac lesions.

The importance of recognizing cyanotic heart disease in the adult lies not only in the potential for possible surgical or nonsurgical intervention but is also important for appropriate management of the extracardiac manifestations of long-standing cyanosis. The systemic complications of cyanotic heart disease include the development of hematologic and metabolic disorders. Neurologic abnormalities include infectious, hemorrhagic, and hypoxic disorders.

Hematologic disorders in adults with cyanotic CHD can significantly influence morbidity and mortality rates. Secondary erythrocytosis has been classified as either **compensated** or **decompensated**. Patients with compensated erythrocytosis are in equilibrium with stable hematocrits, no evidence of iron depletion, and few (if any) symptoms of hyperviscosity. Even with hematocrits above 70%, they do not appear to be at increased risk for cerebrovascular accidents and do not require phlebotomy. Patients with decompensated erythrocytosis have increased hematocrits (> 65%) with symptoms. Because iron deficiency and dehydration may also produce hyperviscosity, these conditions should be excluded and, if present, treated before phlebotomy is undertaken. Generally, phlebotomy is not recommended for patients with hematocrits of less than 65%. A bleeding diathesis is also associated with cyanotic heart disease; it is usually mild and requires no specific therapy except for the avoidance of heparin and aspirin. Because severe life-threatening bleeding can occur during surgical procedures, preoperative phlebotomy to attain a hematocrit just below 65% is recommended. Associated abnormalities include thrombocytopenia and hyperuricemia secondary to increased red cell turnover. Urolithiasis and urate nephropathy rarely occur, but gout is common. The last problem can be managed with conventional therapy, taking care to avoid the antiplatelet properties of anti-inflammatory agents. In managing CHF in cyanotic patients, diuretics must be used judiciously to avoid dehydration, which may exacerbate hyperviscosity, and thrombotic risk. These patients may also be more susceptible to digoxin toxicity.

Counseling of the young adult with reference to contraception, pregnancy, and exercise is especially important in this group of patients.

Palliative surgical procedures for complex cyanotic CHD performed during infancy or childhood in the early years of pediatric cardiothoracic surgery were associated with unique physical findings and specific complications. These procedures, such as aortopulmonary anastomoses (Waterston, Potts, Blalock-Taussig) and atrial switches (Senning and Mustard), are still commonly encountered in adult patients. These procedures may produce unique physical findings and specific complications, which are discussed later (see Palliative Surgical Procedures). Most of these procedures are no longer performed in children, since surgical techniques that optimize physiology and reduce complications have evolved over the years.

TETRALOGY OF FALLOT & PULMONARY ATRESIA WITH VENTRICULAR SEPTAL DEFECT

ESSENTIALS OF DIAGNOSIS

- History of exercise intolerance and squatting during childhood.
- Central cyanosis, mildly prominent RV impulse, murmur of PS (with sufficient pulmonary blood flow) and absent P_2.
- Mild RVH; occasionally, LVH.
- Chest radiograph shows classic boot-shaped heart (coeur en sabot) in severe cases without left-to-right shunt; LV enlargement and poststenotic pulmonary artery dilatation in milder cases; right-sided aortic arch in approximately 25% of patients.
- Echocardiogram shows RVH, overriding aorta, large peri-membranous VSD, and obstruction of the RV outflow tract (subvalvular, valvular, supravalvular, or in the pulmonary arterial branches).
- Gradient across pulmonary outflow tract, normal pulmonary artery pressures, equalization of RV and LV pressures.
- Possibly anomalous branches of right coronary artery crossing RV outflow tract on coronary angiography.

General Considerations

TOF is the most common form of cyanotic CHD. Without surgical intervention, most patients die in childhood; however, occasionally an acyanotic patient with only mild-to-moderate PS and minimal right-to-left shunting is encountered (pink TOF). Although it is called a tetralogy, only the membranous nonrestrictive VSD, PS, and dextroposition of the aorta contribute to the pathophysiology of this disorder (Figure 31–24). The severity of PS determines the RV systolic pressure and thus the degree of right-to-left shunting. The PS can be valvular or, more commonly, infundibular with an obstructing muscular band in the RV outflow tract. The other two components of the tetralogy include the aortic override and the secondary RVH. Both cyanotic and acyanotic patients are at high risk for endocarditis, much like patients with complicated VSD.

Common associated anomalies include ASD (15%; the pentalogy of Fallot or Cantrell), right-sided aortic arch (25%, most commonly seen in pulmonary atresia with VSD), and anomalous coronary distribution (about 10%). It is important to identify the origin of the left anterior descending artery from the right coronary cusp preoperatively because the artery courses over the RV infundibulum, a potential incision site for the repair. TOF is a form of conotruncal malformation that may occur in conjunction with DiGeorge syndrome. The chromosome 22q11.2 microdeletion is present in as many as 8–35% of patients with TOF, and routine screening for the deletion is now recommended for affected patients to guide appropriate management and identify those patients whose offspring will be at increased risk for CHD. In addition, mutations in the genes encoding the cardiac transcription factor NKX2-5 and the Notch-1 ligand Jagged have been reported in patients with TOF.

Clinical Findings

A. Symptoms & Signs

The patient with TOF was typically a blue baby, cyanotic at birth. There is usually a history of exercise intolerance and squatting during childhood. Characteristic "tet spells," which are typified by episodic faintness and worsening cyanosis, are believed to be due to infundibular spasm and are generally diminished or absent by adulthood. Worsening cyanosis also occurs during exercise because of the associated systemic vasodilation and increased right-to-left shunt.

In severe cases of PS or atresia, the patient may have had life-saving surgical palliation with an aortopulmonary shunt. In the past, total repairs were not attempted until school age, but they are now being performed in infancy in most centers.

Physical examination reveals cyanosis and, less frequently, clubbing. The precordium is generally quiet, although a mild RV heave may be present. The intensity and duration of the pulmonic flow murmur vary with the degree of PS; P_2 is usually absent. In cases of pulmonary atresia with VSD (an extreme form of TOF), P_2 is absent by definition, and a continuous murmur may be audible over the back due to aortopulmonary collaterals. Patients who have had a "classic" Blalock-Taussig shunt, anastomosis of the subclavian to the side of the pulmonary artery, will have an

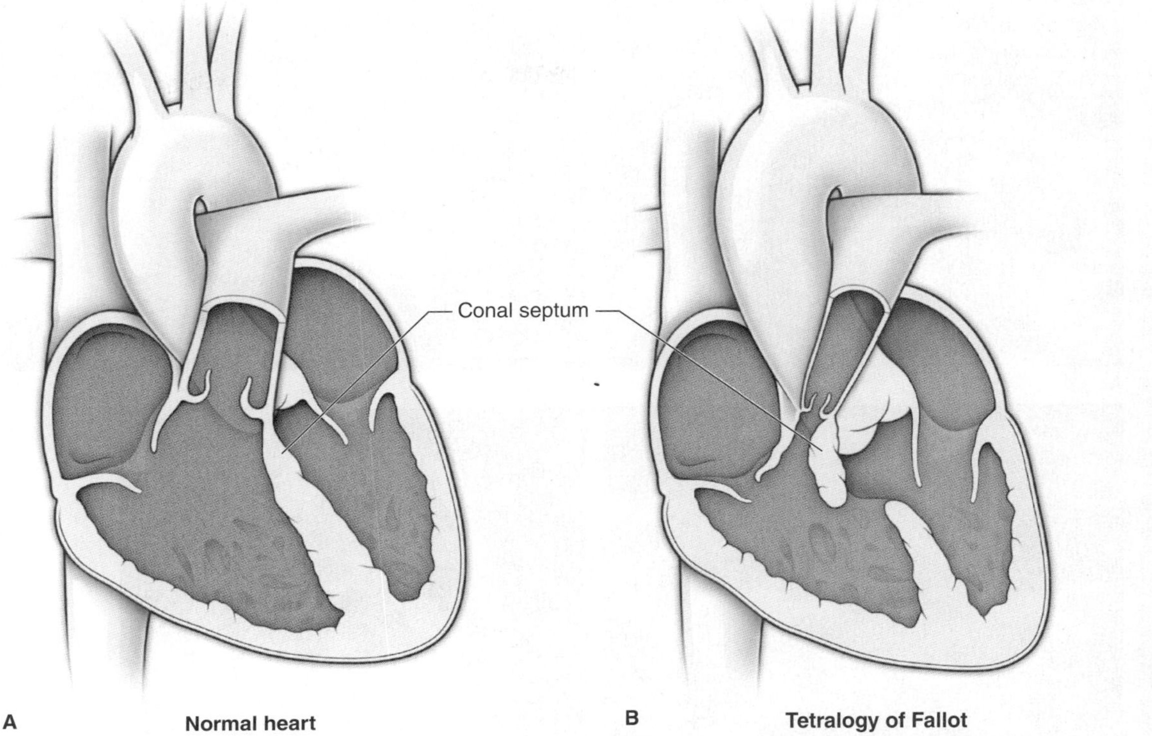

▲ **Figure 31–24.** Anatomy of tetralogy of Fallot (TOF). Note that in TOF, the conal septum is displaced anteriorly and to the right, resulting in a smaller pulmonary artery orifice and subpulmonic obstruction.

absent pulse in the ipsilateral arm and a continuous murmur as long as the shunt is patent and functioning properly. A "modified" Blalock-Taussig shunt, interposing a small Gore-Tex tube between the subclavian artery and the pulmonary artery, preserves the brachial pulse and is easily occluded at the time of intracardiac repair. In patients who have had intracardiac repair, a low-pitched pulmonary regurgitation murmur is commonly audible. When the murmur occurs only in early diastole, it suggests clinically important residual regurgitation.

B. Diagnostic Studies

1. Electrocardiography and chest radiography—The ECG findings depend on the severity of the PS and the relative degree of shunting. If PS is severe, RVH is usually evident. If the PS is mild and the shunt is predominantly left to right, LVH may be evident. P waves are usually normal. Following intracardiac repair with infundibular resection, RBBB and varying forms of heart block are common. Postoperative atrial and ventricular arrhythmias are well-recognized complications. A QRS duration of greater than 180 ms has been shown to correlate with significant RV dilatation due to pulmonic regurgitation after surgical repair and to predict sudden cardiac death in patients with repaired TOF.

The radiographic findings also depend on the underlying individual pathophysiology. The typical boot-shaped (coeur en sabot) is seen when PS is severe and the LV is small. In these cases, pulmonary blood flow is reduced. Post stenotic pulmonary artery dilatation and a right-sided aortic arch may be visible on chest radiograph.

2. Echocardiography—Transthoracic two-dimensional and Doppler echocardiography demonstrates the features of this defect in its native and repaired state. The typical findings in patients with unrepaired TOF include severe RVH and a thickened, malformed pulmonary valve with post stenotic dilation. Alternatively, the level of stenosis may be primarily infundibular, with marked hypertrophic narrowing of the RV outflow tract (Figure 31–25). Systolic color-flow aliasing and a continuous wave Doppler gradient are detectable across the RV outflow tract or pulmonic valve. Two-dimensional imaging reveals a peri-membranous VSD with evidence of right-to-left shunting by color-flow imaging; the peak velocity of the VSD jet seen by spectral Doppler is usually low, reflecting the low interventricular gradient. The aortic root is variably enlarged and overrides the VSD.

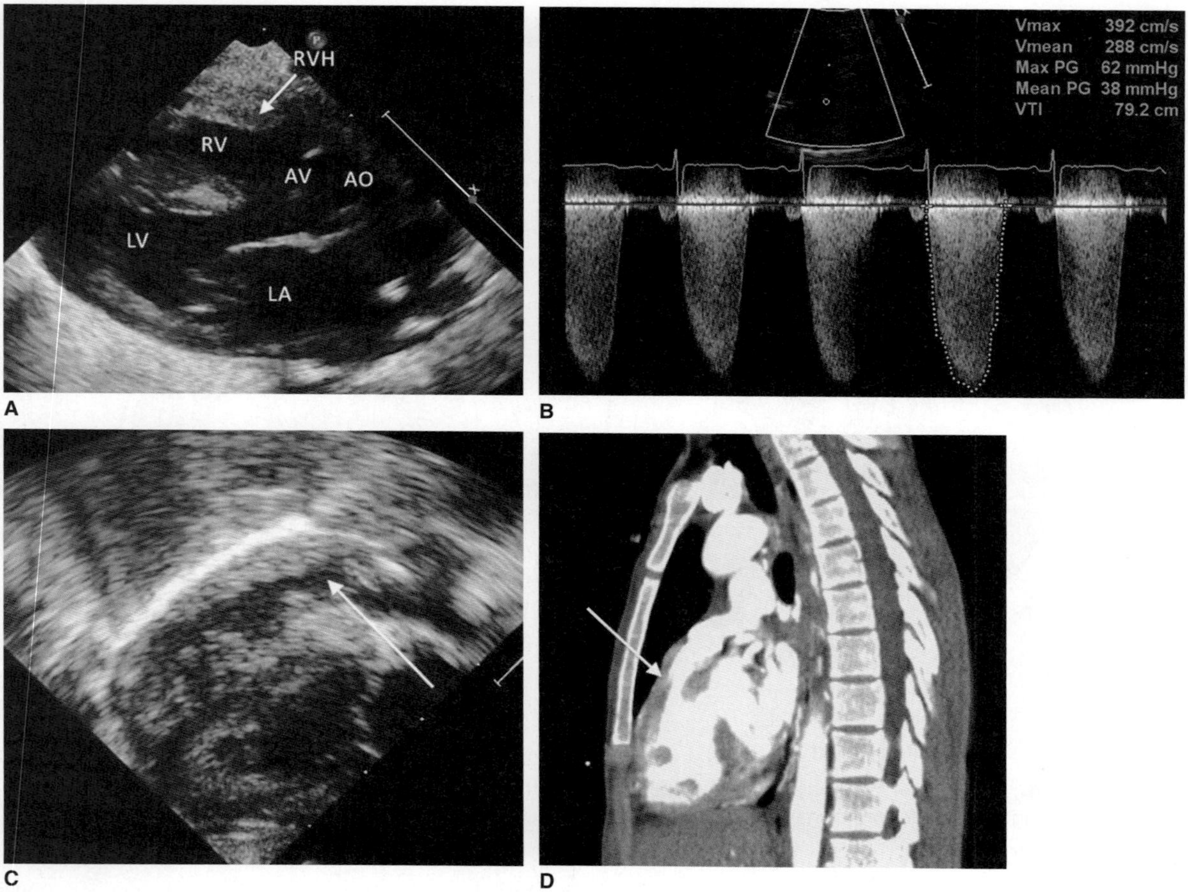

▲ **Figure 31–25.** Transthoracic echocardiogram in patient with tetralogy of Fallot. **A:** The parasternal long-axis view shows the ventricular septal defect, overriding aorta. **B:** Continuous wave Doppler signal across the right ventricular outflow tract shows a high velocity. This demonstrates severe outflow tract obstruction. **C and D:** Echocardiography and computed tomography showing the severe infundibular hypertrophy (*arrows*). AO, aorta; AV, aortic valve; LA, left atrium; LV, left ventricle; Pk, peak; RV, right ventricle; RVH, right ventricular hypertrophy.

Aortic insufficiency, usually mild, may be present. Multiplanar TEE is particularly suited to define the anatomy of the RV outflow tract and the pulmonary valve when precordial imaging is difficult. In pulmonary atresia with VSD, aortopulmonary collaterals arising from the descending aorta can also be imaged by TEE.

Complications of TOF repair that can be detected noninvasively by echocardiography include residual outflow obstruction, pulmonary valve regurgitation, RV outflow tract aneurysms, and VSD patch leak. In rare cases, an anomalous left anterior descending artery that was severed during surgery results in an LV apical aneurysm. Late LV systolic dysfunction has been increasingly recognized after TOF repair and is a risk factor for sudden cardiac death.

3. Magnetic resonance imaging—MRI has become an important noninvasive imaging modality in the assessment of patients with cono-truncal anomalies, including TOF. Advantages include the ability to obtain accurate measurements of RV size and ejection fraction and pulmonic regurgitant fraction.

4. Cardiac catheterization—Cardiac catheterization reveals a gradient across the pulmonary outflow tract, usually normal pulmonary artery pressure, and equalization of RV and LV pressures. Angiography may better define the anatomy of the RV outflow tract and the size of the VSD (this information is usually available noninvasively). Coronary arteriography may demonstrate anomalous origins of the left coronary artery.

5. Other laboratory findings—Arterial saturation is variably reduced, and secondary erythrocytosis is present in the adult who has had no reparative surgery. In those with adequate surgical repair, arterial saturation should be normal.

Prognosis & Treatment

Only 11% of individuals born with this lesion survive without palliative surgery beyond the age of 20, and only 3% survive beyond the age of 40. Because the PS protects TOF patients from the development of pulmonary hypertension, however, they are almost always surgical candidates as adults. Medically, it is important to avoid systemic vasodilator therapy in the patient whose TOF is uncorrected because a reduction in arterial blood pressure can increase right-to-left shunting. Endocarditis is relatively common in unrepaired TOF.

Total intracardiac repair with closure of the VSD and correction of the pulmonary or infundibular stenosis is indicated in the cyanotic patient to reduce symptoms and forestall complications attributable to cyanosis. The infundibulum is incised and resected to alleviate obstruction, with patching of the RV outflow tract or pulmonary annulus when necessary. The indications for surgery in the occasional acyanotic patient with TOF are similar to those of a patient with VSD. Important considerations prior to surgery include the presence of anomalies in the pulmonary and coronary arteries (approximately 15% and 35%, respectively). In pulmonary atresia with VSD, survival depends on the presence of well-developed bronchopulmonary or systemic-to-pulmonary collaterals. In the rare adult with uncorrected pulmonary atresia with VSD, surgical repair is either more complicated, requiring multiple procedures, or is not feasible.

In patients who undergo intracardiac repair for TOF, potentially significant postoperative anatomic sequelae are possible, including residual outflow obstruction, pulmonary valve regurgitation, RV aneurysms, and VSD patch leak. Pulmonary regurgitation may develop as a consequence of surgical repair of the RV outflow tract as well as with placement of a patch to enlarge the pulmonary artery annulus (transannular). Although even substantial regurgitation can be tolerated for long periods, enlargement of the RV eventually occurs, with resultant RV dysfunction, and replacement of the pulmonary valve is frequently required. The development of transcatheter pulmonic valve replacement techniques in recent years has permitted a nonsurgical approach in a large number of patients.

A recent large retrospective study of risk stratification for arrhythmia and sudden death in these patients underscores the importance of vigilant assessment of ECG parameters (QRS duration) and hemodynamic characteristics (pulmonary regurgitation/obstruction) with timely intervention as a means of modifying the risk for sudden cardiac death in these patients. Appropriately timed surgical replacement of the regurgitant pulmonic valve has been shown to stabilize QRS prolongation and to reduce the incidence of ventricular arrhythmias when combined with cryoablation. It is hoped that two current trends in surgery will further reduce the incidence of arrhythmias. The first is avoidance of RV outflow tract incisions by either a transatrial or transpulmonary approach. Second, earlier surgical intervention may allow less time for the development of ventricular fibrosis. Given the frequency of ventricular tachycardia and sudden cardiac death in these patients, clinicians should remain vigilant for symptoms of palpitations and syncope. Some experts advocate routine annual screening with ambulatory ECG monitoring. Referral for electrophysiologic study on finding nonsustained ventricular tachycardia or complex ectopy maybe reasonable to risk stratify for sudden cardiac death.

EISENMENGER SYNDROME

ESSENTIALS OF DIAGNOSIS

- History of murmur or cyanosis in infancy, symptoms of dyspnea and exercise intolerance since childhood.
- Hemoptysis, chest pain, and syncope in the adult.
- Clubbing, cyanosis, and prominent P_2.
- Compensatory erythrocytosis, iron deficiency, and hyperuricemia.
- RVH; large central pulmonary arteries with peripheral pruning on chest radiograph.
- Severe RVH and right atrial enlargement, elevated pulmonary artery pressures, pulmonary regurgitation.
- Detection of bidirectional shunt.

General Considerations

Three related, but not identical, clinical terms bear the name of Eisenmenger. The development of pulmonary hypertension in the presence of increased pulmonary blood flow is called the **Eisenmenger reaction. Eisenmenger syndrome** is a general term applied to pulmonary hypertension and shunt reversal in the presence of a congenital defect, including VSD, ostium primum ASD, AV canal defect, aortopulmonary window, or PDA. **Eisenmenger complex**, as originally described, is the association of a VSD with pulmonary hypertension and shunt reversal. The pulmonary hypertension usually develops before puberty; however, pulmonary vascular disease and the Eisenmenger reaction can occasionally develop after puberty in patients with ostium secundum ASDs.

In approximately 10% of patients with nonrestrictive VSDs, the pulmonary artery pressure does not fall normally in the neonatal period. Therefore, a large left-to-right shunt and CHF are not present. If the VSD goes undetected and the problem is not repaired before the infant reaches the age of 1 year, irreversible pulmonary vascular disease may result. The same is true for the other lesions associated with Eisenmenger syndrome. In patients with ostium secundum ASD, PVR almost always falls to normal levels in the neonatal period, and the development of irreversible pulmonary hypertension is far less common.

Clinical Findings

A. Symptoms & Signs

Patients usually have a history of murmur during infancy, and cyanosis occurs later in childhood. Exertional dyspnea is the most commonly encountered symptom. Chest pain, hemoptysis, and presyncope are less common. Transient bacteremia can result in brain abscess as a result of right-to-left shunting and entry of bacteria into the cerebral circulation without the normal filtering through the pulmonary circulation.

Physical examination reveals cyanosis (involving the legs when the cause is PDA); cardiovascular examination is most remarkable for findings associated with pulmonary hypertension. The LV impulse is not displaced and an RV parasternal heave is present. The jugular venous pressure may be elevated in the presence of RV failure, and the *a* wave may be prominent. The first heart sound is normal, and P_2 is markedly accentuated. A systolic murmur of tricuspid regurgitation may be present, and a high-pitched diastolic murmur of pulmonary regurgitation (Graham Steell murmur) is common. In the presence of RV failure, hepatomegaly, ascites, and peripheral edema may be present.

B. Diagnostic Studies

1. Electrocardiography and chest radiography—The ECG shows evidence of right atrial enlargement and RVH with a rightward axis (Figure 31–26A). The presence of a leftward or superior axis suggests an ostium primum ASD or AV canal defect as the underlying cause (Figure 31–26B). Chest radiograph findings include RV enlargement with filling in of the retrosternal air space, prominent proximal pulmonary arteries with pulmonary oligemia, and pruning of the peripheral pulmonary vessels.

2. Echocardiography—Severe RVH and right atrial enlargement are evident (Figure 31–27A). RV function may be normal until the late stages of the disease, at which time the right atrium enlarges. The LV appears small and underfilled; the septum deviates toward the LV. The level of shunt can be determined by two-dimensional imaging, aided by color-flow Doppler and saline contrast injection (Figure 31–27B). When a VSD is present, the flow velocity across the defect is low because of pressure equalization between the two ventricles. On the other hand, the tricuspid regurgitant velocity is increased and can be used to estimate the peak RV systolic pressure (Figure 31–27C). Pulmonary insufficiency with a high-velocity regurgitant jet is a frequent finding. Other valvular lesions are uncommon except in ostium primum ASD or AV canal defects, when mitral regurgitation is commonly present.

Eisenmenger syndrome can usually be differentiated from primary pulmonary hypertension noninvasively by TTE, although shunting across a patent foramen ovale may mimic an ASD with Eisenmenger syndrome and a PDA may be missed on color-flow Doppler in the presence of severe pulmonary hypertension. In these cases, further investigation with TEE or cardiac catheterization and sometimes cardiac MRI/MRA may be indicated.

3. Cardiac catheterization—The pathognomonic hemodynamic findings are elevated pulmonary artery pressure, increased PVR, and right-to-left shunting. The degree of residual left-to-right shunt should be measured. Oxygen should be administered during catheterization to determine whether pulmonary vascular reactivity persists. If PVR falls during oxygen or nitric oxide administration, increased left-to-right shunting can be measured. In this case, the patient may be a candidate for pulmonary vasodilator therapy and surgical repair.

4. Other laboratory findings—The arterial oxygen saturation by pulse oximetry or arterial blood gas measurements is markedly decreased. The hematocrit is elevated, with an overall increase in red cell mass. Iron deficiency is common, particularly after injudicious phlebotomies. Hyperuricemia caused by increased red cell turnover may be present.

Prognosis & Treatment

Life expectancy is markedly shortened in patients with Eisenmenger syndrome; however, patients with preserved right ventricular function have a better life expectancy and some patients can surprisingly live for several decades. The causes of death include uncontrollable hemoptysis (due to pulmonary infarction or pulmonary arteriolar rupture), arrhythmias with sudden death, progressive RV failure, and brain abscess.

The availability of a range of pulmonary vasodilators has revolutionized the management of Eisenmenger syndrome. Treatment with pulmonary vasodilators has been shown in a large clinical trial to improve the functional status of these patients (see Chapter 30).

Surgical repair is contraindicated when the pulmonary vascular disease is fixed; that is, pulmonary resistance does not fall in response to oxygen or nitric oxide inhalation. In these patients, closure of the VSD (or other defects) increases the work of the RV, with a resultant excessively high mortality rate. Heart-lung transplantation offers hope for the adolescent and young adult with Eisenmenger syndrome, but the results support only guarded optimism, and the current practice has in general moved away from this option given the reported survival outcomes post combined heart-lung transplant. In addition, some centers are considering the feasibility of intracardiac repair in children after treatment with pulmonary vasodilator therapy to decrease the PVR.

Careful medical management of the complications of cyanotic CHD is crucial in these patients (see earlier section, Cyanotic Congenital Heart Disease). Counseling regarding contraception is also crucial in these patients; pregnancy is accompanied by an unacceptably high rate of maternal and fetal mortality and is virtually contraindicated in patients with Eisenmenger syndrome (see later discussion).

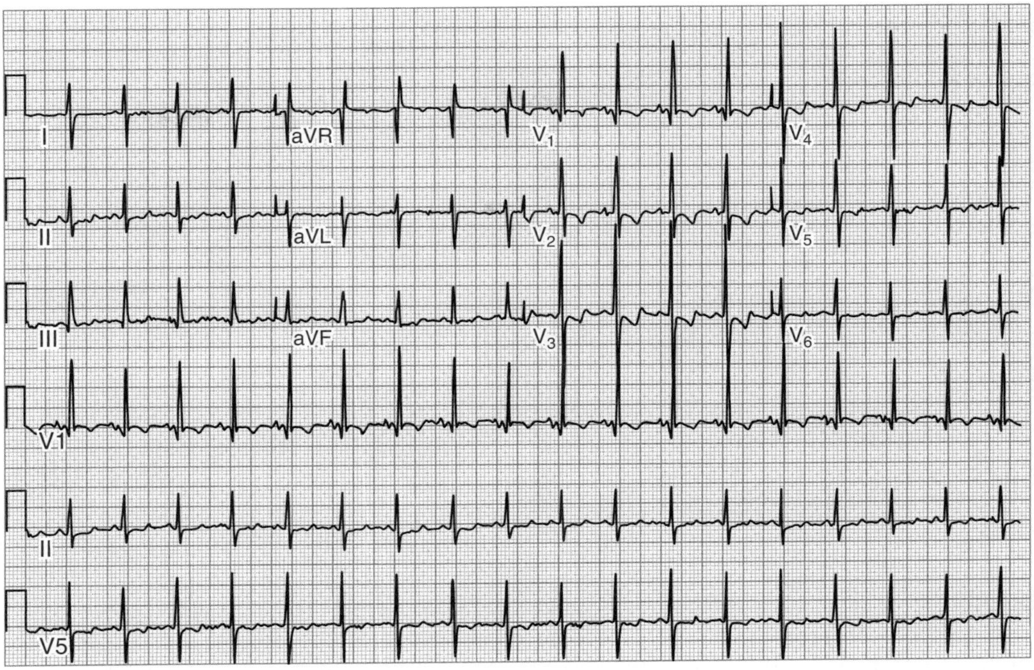

A

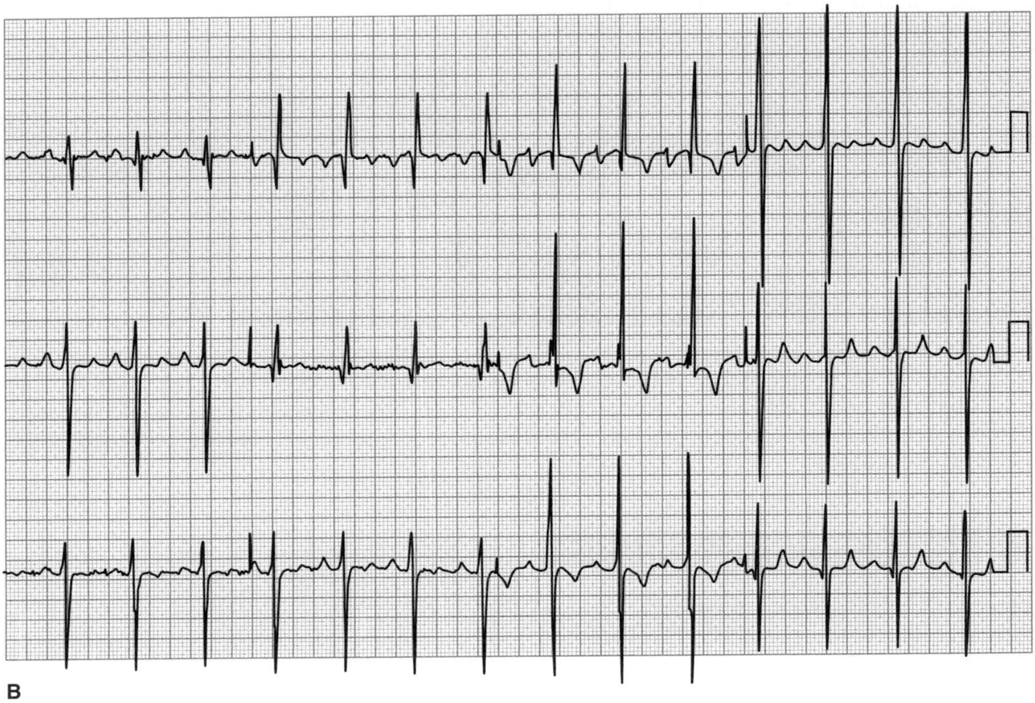

B

▲ **Figure 31–26.** **A:** Electrocardiograph in Eisenmenger syndrome from ostium secundum atrial septal defect with right ventricular hypertrophy and right-axis deviation. **B:** Electrocardiograph in Eisenmenger syndrome and atrioventricular canal defect with right ventricular hypertrophy and left anterior hemiblock.

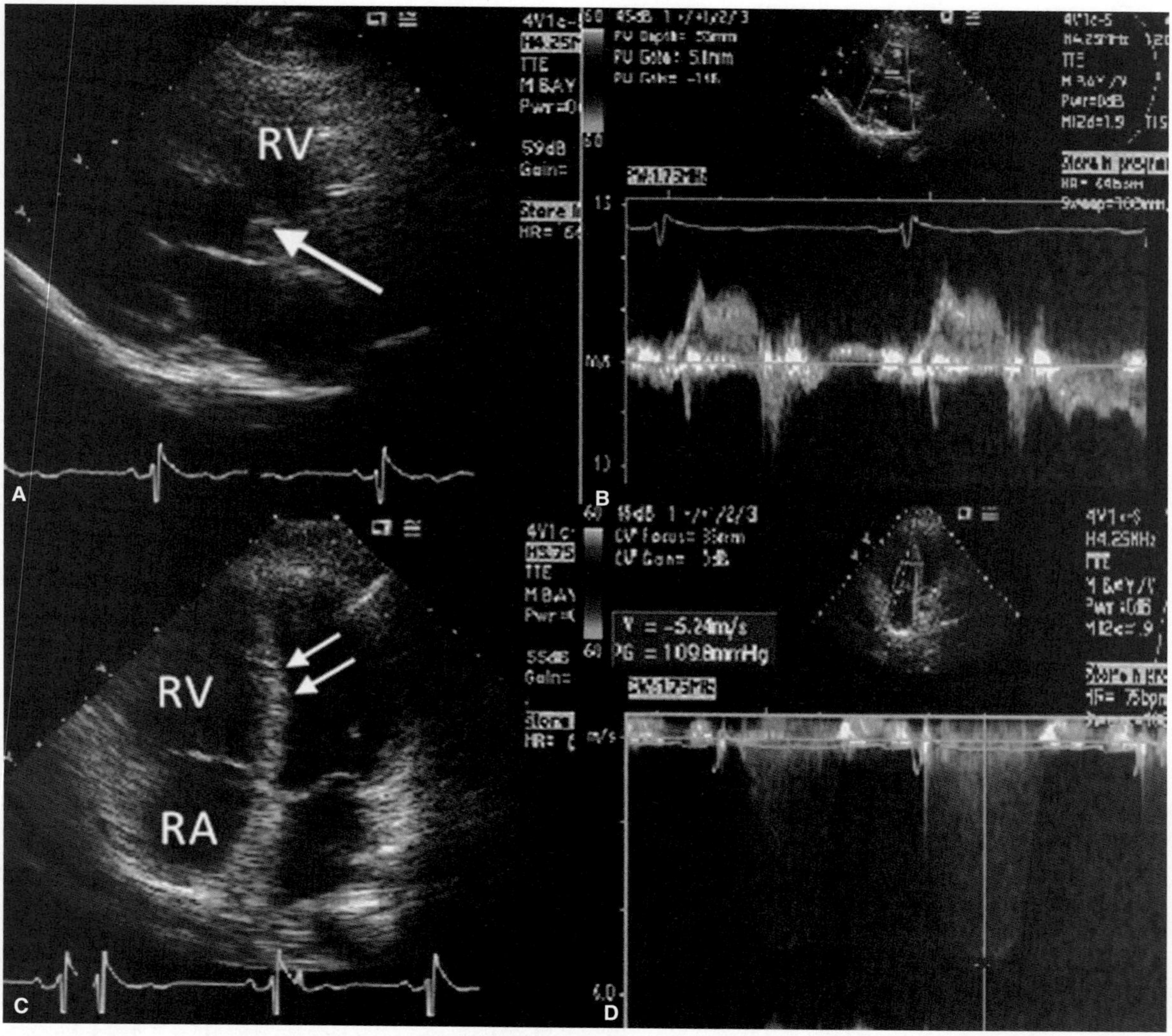

▲ **Figure 31–27.** **A:** Transthoracic echocardiogram in a 29-year-old patient with a large perimembranous ventricular septal defect (*arrow*). **B:** With bidirectional shunting. **C:** There is bowing of the septum to the left (*double arrows*), a dilated right atrium (RA), and dilated and hypertrophied right ventricle (RV). **D:** Systemic right ventricular pressures were estimated from a continuous wave Doppler tracing of the tricuspid regurgitation jet. Pressure gradient (PG) 109.8 mmHg plus RA pressure = RV pressure.

TRANSPOSITION OF THE GREAT ARTERIES

ESSENTIALS OF DIAGNOSIS

- History of cyanosis that worsens shortly after birth at the time of ductal closure.
- Prominent RV impulse, palpable and delayed A_2; murmurs from associated defects (eg, VSD, PS).
- Chest radiograph shows narrowing at base of heart in region of great vessels; prominent pulmonary vascularity unless PVR is increased.
- Right atrial enlargement, RVH; occasionally biventricular hypertrophy (with an associated VSD).
- Great arteries discordant with anterior and rightward aorta arising from the RV and leftward and posterior pulmonary artery arising from the LV. Atria and ventricles usually in normal position with severe RVH.

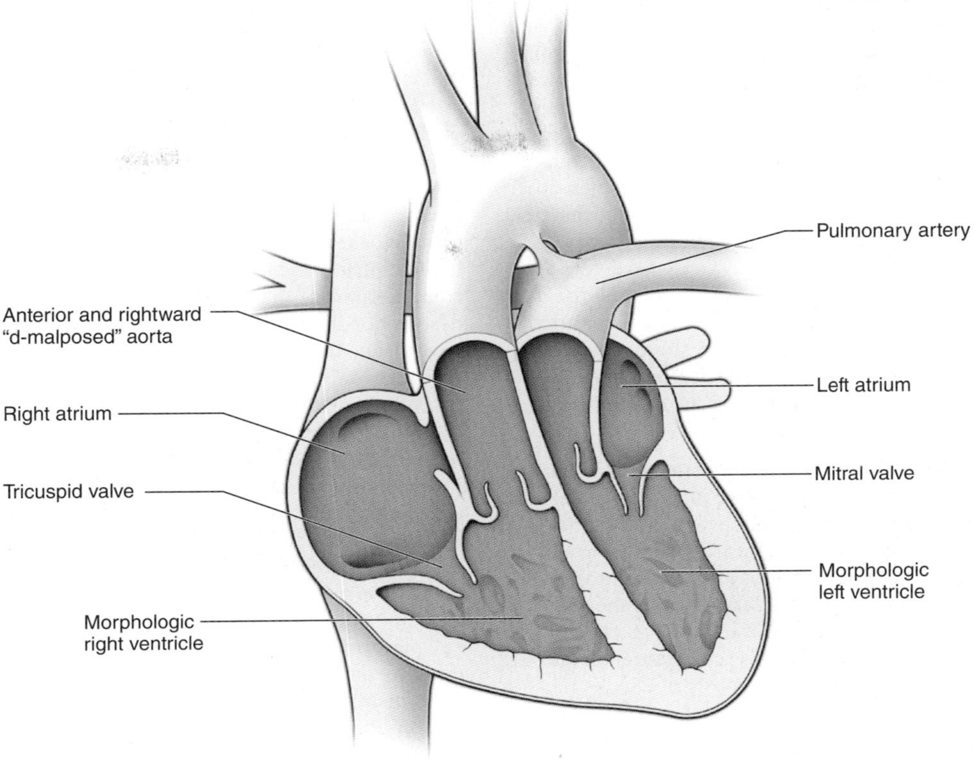

▲ **Figure 31–28.** Anatomy of transposition of the great arteries (D-TGA).

General Considerations

The key to the pathophysiology of transposition of the great arteries (D-TGA) is that the pulmonary and systemic circulations exist in parallel rather than in the normal series relationship (Figure 31–28). Survival after birth therefore depends on mixing saturated and desaturated blood via a PDA or an ASD or VSD. If an ASD or VSD does not coexist with D-TGA, an atrial communication must be created (usually percutaneously via an atrial balloon septostomy [the Rashkind procedure]) to permit survival in the newborn once the ductus closes. Prostaglandin E_1 may be given to restore or maintain patency of the ductus arteriosus; however, this does not always provide adequate mixing. When a VSD is present, the physiologic consequences depend largely on whether associated PS is present. In the absence of PS, there is a risk of pulmonary vascular disease because of the increased pulmonary blood flow; in the presence of PS, an aortopulmonary shunt may be necessary to increase pulmonary blood flow.

Clinical Findings

A. Symptoms & Signs

More males than females (3:1) are affected by this condition. There is a history of cyanosis at birth that worsens shortly thereafter when the ductus closes. In the infant with a large VSD, heart failure can occur with lesser degrees of cyanosis. In addition to profound central cyanosis, physical examination reveals a prominent RV impulse and murmurs caused by associated defects (eg, VSD, PS). A_2 is typically loud and often palpable, as a consequence of the anterior malposition of the aortic valve. A_2 may also be delayed as a consequence of volume overload or RV dysfunction. The findings usually associated with a large PDA (see previous discussion of PDA) may be absent. The physical examination is often nondiagnostic and may actually provide more information about associated anomalies than about the presence of transposition.

B. Diagnostic Studies

1. Electrocardiography and chest radiography—The ECG usually demonstrates right atrial enlargement, a rightward QRS axis, and RVH. In the presence of a VSD, biventricular hypertrophy may be evident. The chest radiograph shows narrowing at the base of the heart in the region of the great vessels. In the newborn, prior to surgery, pulmonary vascularity is prominent unless pulmonary blood flow is limited by PS or, in older individuals, the PVR is increased by the associated pulmonary vascular disease. The RV and right atrium are prominent.

2. Echocardiography—The atria and ventricles are usually in the normal position with severe RVH. The great vessels are discordant with the anterior and rightward aorta arising from the RV, and leftward and posterior pulmonary artery arising from the LV. In the newborn, complete examination, using combined two-dimensional and color-flow Doppler imaging should confirm or exclude the presence of an associated ASD, VSD, or PS. In patients who have had an atrial switch operation, baffle obstruction and leaks can be detected by color-flow Doppler and contrast echocardiography. Late obstruction of the superior vena cava can be detected by contrast echocardiography with agitated saline injected into an arm vein, opacifying the inferior vena cava. After arterial switch procedures, echocardiography may show regurgitation of the neoaortic valve or stenosis of the neo-pulmonary valve or branches. MRI may also be helpful in determining the anatomy of the vena cava and pulmonary veins.

3. Cardiac catheterization—Invasive studies confirm the noninvasive diagnosis and the presence of associated defects. In the newborn, catheterization with a percutaneous atrial balloon septostomy is therapeutic and usually life-saving as well as diagnostic. The administration of intravenous prostaglandin E_1 to maintain ductal patency may preclude the need for an atrial septostomy if the oxygen saturations are adequate. In the adult with associated VSD, cardiac catheterization may be indicated to determine PVR or the severity of PS.

Prognosis & Treatment

Without treatment, isolated D-TGA carries a mortality rate of greater than 90% in the first year of life. Infants with an ASD, a VSD, or a large PDA have higher oxygen saturations and better survival rates, but early surgery is indicated to prevent the development of irreversible pulmonary vascular disease.

Definitive repair of this defect was first undertaken in the early 1960s. The atrial switch operation (Mustard or Senning) redirects the pulmonary and systemic venous return at the atrial level. The atrial septum is excised, and using either a pericardial or prosthetic baffle, the systemic venous return is directed across the mitral valve into the left ventricle and the pulmonary venous return flows across the tricuspid valve into the RV. The postoperative physiology after an atrial switch procedure is similar to that of patients with CC-TGA, in that the RV continues to supply the systemic circulation. Many of these patients have survived to lead productive lives; however, they are potentially faced with significant late postoperative complications, including sinus node dysfunction, atrial and ventricular tachyarrhythmias, baffle obstruction and leaks (approximately 15%), and systemic ventricular dysfunction (10–15%). The late (30-year) mortality rate is approximately 20%. Sudden (presumed arrhythmic) death and systemic ventricular failure are the most common causes of late death. Atrial arrhythmias are particularly common. In a large cohort study, sinus rhythm was present in 77% of patients at 5 years and only 40% of patients at 20 years. Atrial flutter, which may signal a higher risk for sudden death, was present in 14% of patients. Pacemaker implantation, which can pose technical challenges after atrial switch, was required in 11% of patients.

Over the last decade the number of patients living with atrial switch type of repair has significantly declined in favor of the arterial switch (pioneered by Jatene) that has been adopted since the early 1980s. The Jatene procedure involves switching the position of the great vessels and reimplanting the coronary arteries with the use of "coronary buttons." The obvious benefit of this repair re-establishes the LV as the systemic ventricle and has ameliorated many of such long-term complications of the atrial switch such as arrhythmias, RV dysfunction, baffle stenosis, and tricuspid regurgitation that have plagued those with the atrial switch causing significant morbidity and mortality.

Follow-up of patients after arterial switch procedures is now available. The late mortality rate is low, and studies have reported normal LV function of 98% in these patients. Postoperative aortic regurgitation is seen in ~6% of patients and the potential for development of coronary artery ostial stenosis and late supravalvular narrowing at the anastomotic sites are concerns that require ongoing assessment and possibly intervention. These may be done by periodically assessing for symptoms suggestive of angina and if present performing physiological assessments with the use of exercise or pharmacological stress testing or anatomical assessments with computed tomography or cardiac catheterization (Figure 31–29).

Tyson AF, Buratto E, Weintraub RG, et al. Long-term outcomes of the arterial switch operation. *J Thoracic Cardiovasc Surg.* 2022;163(1):212–219. [PMID: 3375839]

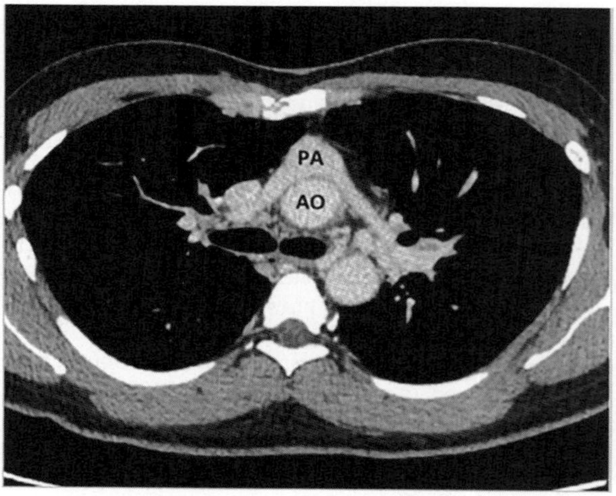

▲ **Figure 31–29.** Computed Tomography showing cross-sectional imaging of a patient with transposition of the great arteries. PA, pulmonary arteries "straddle"; AO, aorta after the Lecompte maneuver (moving the main PA anterior to the AO) at the time of an arterial switch.

TRICUSPID ATRESIA

ESSENTIALS OF DIAGNOSIS

- History of either cyanosis (70%) or CHF (30%).
- Cyanotic patient with absent RV impulse and prominent LV impulse.
- Oligemic lung fields, right atrial and LV without RV enlargement in retrosternal airspace on chest radiograph.
- Evidence of LVH, absent or atretic tricuspid valve, ASD, small RV.

General Considerations

Tricuspid atresia represents a spectrum of congenital defects characterized by the absence of connection between the right atrium and RV. In these patients, the tricuspid valve is absent or imperforate, the RV is hypoplastic, and the inflow portion of the RV is absent. Although an atrial communication is invariably present, the additional associated anomalies determine the ultimate pathophysiology and clinical presentation (Figure 31–30). Tricuspid atresia is usually classified according to the presence or absence of pulmonary stenosis and of malposition of the aorta and pulmonary artery. The great arteries are normally related in about 70% of the cases and are transposed in 30%. Pulmonary blood flow is supplied by either a PDA or aortopulmonary collaterals. Palliative surgery in this group is aimed at increasing pulmonary blood flow by a systemic venous or an arterial-to-pulmonary-artery shunt (see Palliative Surgical Procedures). A minority of patients will have a sufficiently large PDA to provide unrestricted pulmonary blood flow at the expense of ventricular volume overload, CHF, and the development of pulmonary vascular disease. In the 30% of patients born with tricuspid atresia and associated transposition of the great vessels, a VSD is usually present and no pulmonary obstruction is evident. These infants have CHF; pulmonary banding in the first year of life may prevent the development of irreversible pulmonary vascular disease and allow a later intracardiac repair to be performed.

Adult survival without surgical intervention is rare. The clinical condition at presentation depends on the patient's

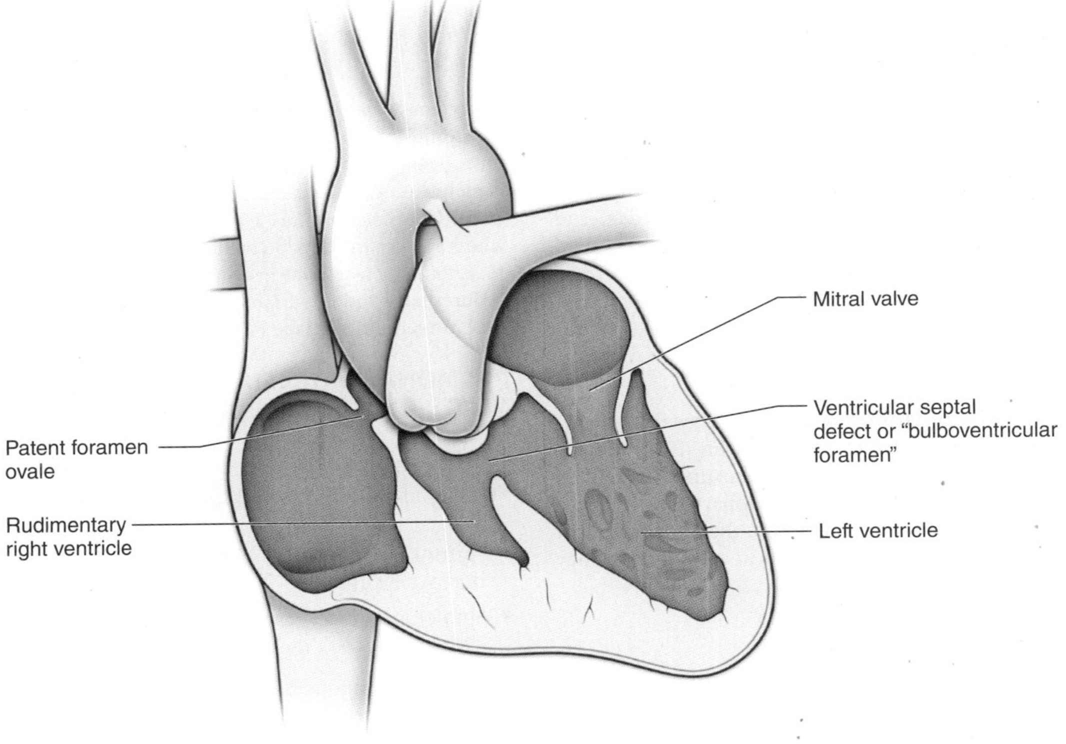

▲ **Figure 31–30.** Anatomy of tricuspid atresia.

underlying anatomy as well as the adequacy of the palliative procedure.

Clinical Findings

A. Symptoms & Signs

A history of cyanosis predominates in patients with normally related great arteries, restrictive VSD, or PS or atresia. Patients with associated transposition of the great vessels and nonrestrictive VSD usually have a history of CHF from LV volume overload.

Physical examination is highly variable, but the absence of an RV impulse with a prominent LV impulse in a cyanotic patient suggests tricuspid atresia. The first heart sound is single, and the second heart sound often is as well. A continuous murmur may be present as a result of aortopulmonary collaterals or a Blalock-Taussig shunt.

B. Diagnostic Studies

1. Electrocardiography and chest radiography—The ECG reveals right atrial enlargement, LVH, and the absence of right-sided precordial forces. This is the only cyanotic lesion associated with LVH at birth. In the adult, the chest radiograph usually shows oligemic lung fields and right atrial and LV prominence without RV enlargement in the retrosternal airspace.

2. Echocardiography and magnetic resonance imaging—Constant echocardiographic features include an absent or atretic, imperforate tricuspid valve, ASD, and a small RV. More variable features include the size of the RV, the presence and size of a VSD, the presence of pulmonary atresia or stenosis, and relationship of the great vessels (normal or transposed). Doppler examination can estimate the degree of PS and the gradient across the VSD. When PS is not present, the VSD gradient can be subtracted from the systolic arterial pressure to estimate the pulmonary artery systolic pressure. Color-flow Doppler imaging is helpful in confirming the pattern of flow and the site of the VSD (Figure 31–31). MRI can also be helpful in defining the anatomy.

3. Cardiac catheterization—Cardiac catheterization is used to determine operability by measuring PVR and the size of the pulmonary arteries. The RV cannot be entered through the right atrium, and the pulmonary artery (in the absence of atresia) must be entered from the LV through the VSD. Catheterization can also be used to assess the patency of palliative shunts.

Prognosis & Treatment

Adults with tricuspid atresia will almost uniformly have undergone one or more operations to separate the pulmonary and systemic circulations. Patients with reduced pulmonary blood flow generally undergo a bidirectional Glenn procedure (superior vena cava to right pulmonary artery anastomosis) followed by a complete cavopulmonary anastomosis (Fontan procedure). Patients with increased pulmonary blood flow (typically those with associated d-malposition) may undergo pulmonary arterial banding as an initial procedure. The 1-year survival rate among patients who have not undergone palliative surgery is approximately 10%. Patients who have had successful modified Fontan procedures have widely variable outcomes, but routinely survive well into adulthood (see Palliative Surgical Procedures).

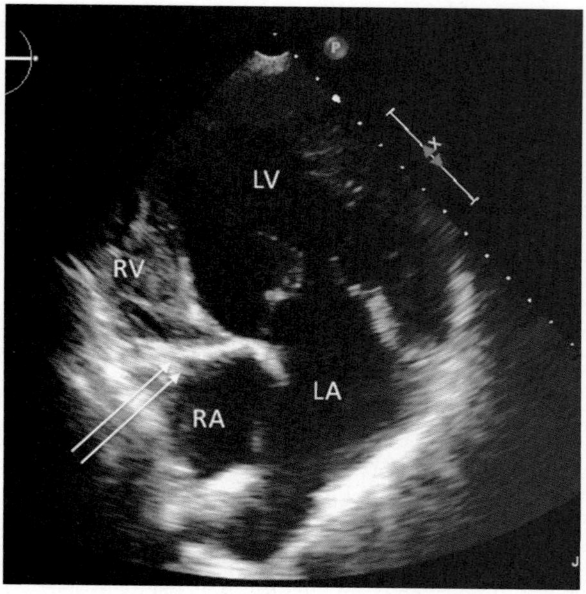

▲ **Figure 31–31.** Transthoracic echocardiogram in a 40-year-old woman with unpalliated tricuspid atresia. This four-chamber view demonstrates the plate-like imperforate tricuspid annulus (*double arrows*). The right ventricle (RV) is hypoplastic. LA, left atrium; LV, left ventricle; RA, right atrium.

PULMONARY ATRESIA WITH INTACT VENTRICULAR SEPTUM

ESSENTIALS OF DIAGNOSIS

- History of cyanosis at birth, worsening at the time of ductal closure.
- Single S_2; continuous murmur is rare.
- Prominent LV forces.
- Oligemic lung fields, enlarged cardiac silhouette on chest radiograph.
- ASD, small RV, absent pulmonary valve. In adults, a palliative shunt or RV-to-pulmonary-artery conduit.

General Considerations

Pulmonary atresia with intact ventricular septum is rarely encountered as an unpalliated defect in the adult population. The pulmonary valve is absent or imperforate, and blood flow is entirely through a PDA in the newborn. As in tricuspid atresia, an atrial communication exists through which the left atrium receives all of the systemic and pulmonary venous return. The volume-overloaded LV pumps the total blood flow into the aorta, and in most cases, all the pulmonary blood flow is received retrograde via the ductus. When the ductus closes, cyanosis may worsen acutely, and pulmonary blood flow must be restored by a palliative shunt. The RV may be diminutive, normal, or increased in size, and the tricuspid valve is, respectively, atretic, normal, or severely regurgitant. The high pressure in the RV is decompressed through dilated coronary circulation (ie, coronary sinusoids) into the left or right coronary artery. The presence of the sinusoids directly relates to RV pressure and inversely to the amount of tricuspid regurgitation. These factors largely determine the clinical and echocardiographic findings.

Clinical Findings

Patients have a history of cyanosis at birth that worsens shortly afterward, at the time of ductal closure. The physical examination is variable, and the findings depend on the size of the RV and the presence of tricuspid regurgitation. The chest radiograph may reveal oligemic lung fields and an enlarged cardiac silhouette, caused by the enlargement of the LV. The main pulmonary artery segment is concave. The echocardiogram most commonly shows an ASD; a hypertrophied RV wall with a small cavity; a patent but small tricuspid valve; and a thickened, immobile, atretic pulmonary valve with no Doppler evidence of blood flow through it. The ductus arteriosus is seen running vertically from the aortic arch to the pulmonary artery (ie, vertical ductus). In adults, a palliative shunt (see section on Tricuspid Atresia) or an RV-to-pulmonary-artery conduit is almost always present. Cardiac catheterization reveals systemic or suprasystemic RV pressures, and the catheter cannot be passed from the RV to the pulmonic artery. Angiography of the RV fails to opacify the pulmonary arteries, and contrast may fill the sinusoidal vessels that often communicate with the coronary arteries.

Prognosis & Treatment

Three categories of surgical intervention exist for infants with pulmonary atresia with intact ventricular septum. The intervention selected depends on the size of the RV and the presence or absence of coronary sinusoids or coronary artery anomalies. When the RV is of adequate size for anticipated future growth, a connection is established between the RV and main pulmonary artery to prepare for a two-ventricle repair. A systemic-to-pulmonary-artery shunt is performed at the same time. Generally, an RV-to-pulmonary-artery conduit (with or without a valve) can be placed in the older child. Problems from valvular obstruction or degeneration and conduit obstruction caused by pseudo-intimal thickening can be detected by Doppler echocardiography. A two-ventricle repair is not possible in the subset of these patients with severely hypoplastic RVs. Therefore, a systemic-to-pulmonary-artery shunt without the connection to the RV is performed, with anticipation of a Fontan procedure at a later date. Patients who have a rudimentary RV and sinusoidal channels serving as the major source of coronary circulation, with perfusion by desaturated blood, represent a special problem. Decompression of the RV by connection with the pulmonary artery may result in a reversal of coronary flow into the RV, thereby producing myocardial ischemia. If coronary anomalies are identified by an aortogram, the sinusoids are left alone, and a systemic-to-pulmonary-artery shunt is performed in anticipation of a future Fontan-type operation. Overall, the prognosis in pulmonary atresia is limited, and although palliative surgery improves longevity, these patients require careful surveillance for complications of the surgery in addition to the underlying cyanotic heart disease. An exciting therapeutic innovation of recent years for patients with a well-formed but imperforate pulmonic valve is the development of radiofrequency-assisted valve perforation followed by balloon valvotomy. This has permitted completely percutaneous repair of the defect, provided that there is a patent infundibulum and a non–RV-dependent coronary circulation. The first patients to have undergone this procedure will be entering adulthood shortly.

OTHER CYANOTIC CONGENITAL HEART DEFECTS

It is increasingly common to encounter adults with complex forms of cyanotic CHD who have had some sort of palliative surgery. In addition to the conditions already discussed, there are many variants of the single-ventricular and double-outlet-ventricular anomalies. Most common among these are the **double-inlet LV, double-outlet RV**, and **hypoplastic left heart**. The anatomic features of the dominant ventricle that identify it as a right or left ventricle on echocardiography include the trabeculae (coarse in an RV, smooth in an LV), the presence of the moderator band (RV), the presence of septal attachments of the AV valve (RV), and the presence of conus tissue between the annuli of the AV and subarterial valves (RV). Sometimes, a rudimentary second ventricle is present. In the absence of pulmonary or infundibular stenosis, pulmonary vascular disease is prevalent; subaortic stenosis and AV valve regurgitation are also common. Cyanosis is invariably present as a consequence of mixing of systemic and pulmonary venous blood. Survival into adulthood is more likely in patients with PS.

The defect in **truncus arteriosus communis** arises from a failure of the single truncus in the embryo to divide into pulmonary and aortic vessels; and the pulmonary artery, aorta, and coronary arteries arise from a single main trunk. Although the anatomy of this lesion varies, a VSD is always present. The single semilunar valve, often with more than three cusps, is usually incompetent. The LV is faced with not only the volume overload of both pulmonary and systemic circulations, but also that caused by truncal valve regurgitation. Cyanosis is present as a consequence of shunting of blood from the RV into the truncus. The mortality rate in the first year of life from CHF is high. Pulmonary branch stenosis and increased PVR may improve prognosis by decreasing the likelihood of CHF. Treatment consists of closure of the VSD, surgical separation of the pulmonary arteries from the truncus, and placement of a valved conduit to connect them to the RV. Late sequelae include progressive truncal valve regurgitation, progressive pulmonary vascular disease, and the need for conduit revision because of patient growth and valve degeneration.

In **total anomalous pulmonary veins**, the pulmonary venous flow enters the right atrium either directly or by one of many possible connections including the coronary sinus, superior vena cava, inferior vena cava, portal vein, hepatic vein, and ductus venosus. Because the venous blood mixes in the right atrium, cyanosis is present. There is an atrial communication, and the degree of cyanosis depends on the size of the ASD and the PVR. If left untreated, most (80%) die within the first year of life. The subdiaphragmatic anomalous veins are more likely to be associated with pulmonary venous obstruction. Surgical correction consists of connecting the common pulmonary venous channel to the left atrium. Obstruction may recur following surgery in those patients in whom obstruction was originally present, but the postoperative course is usually uncomplicated in those that are well repaired.

PALLIATIVE SURGICAL PROCEDURES

In cyanotic CHD associated with diminished pulmonary blood flow, palliative procedures have been aimed at increasing pulmonary blood flow by directly or indirectly shunting blood from the systemic veins or systemic circulation. These procedures have continued to evolve.

The **Fontan procedure** (with its many modifications), the final common pathway for single ventricle repair, obviates the need for an RV by rerouting the venous return from the superior and inferior vena cava directly to the pulmonary circulation, thus separating the systemic and pulmonary venous return. This operation was originally used in patients with tricuspid atresia but currently is the palliative procedure of choice for a variety of congenital heart defects, including hypoplastic left heart syndrome and morphologic single ventricle when the pulmonary bed has been protected by congenital or palliative (ie, pulmonary band) stenosis. The Fontan procedure performed in adulthood carries a relatively low perioperative risk and leads to relief of cyanosis and improved functional class. However, arrhythmias, protein-losing enteropathy, and progressive systemic ventricular dysfunction remain ongoing concerns. The extracardiac Fontan procedure (direct cavopulmonary anastomosis) may decrease the incidence of arrhythmias. Thromboembolic disease is also a major cause of morbidity and mortality among patients after the Fontan procedure, and this recognition has led some cardiologists to advocate prophylactic anticoagulation in these patients. However, insufficient data exist to support a blanket recommendation on this issue. The modified, or bidirectional, **Glenn procedure** (superior vena cava to confluent pulmonary artery) can be used as a staging procedure for a future Fontan procedure or as a palliative shunt that can increase pulmonary blood flow when a Fontan is contraindicated because of poor ventricular function. Because right atrial distention does not occur, atrial arrhythmias may be less common.

In cyanotic patients with inadequate pulmonary blood flow (eg, TOF, pulmonary and tricuspid atresia), early surgical **systemic-to-pulmonary shunts** are life-saving procedures. The **Waterston** (ascending-aorta-to-pulmonary-artery) and **Potts** (descending-aorta-to-pulmonary-artery) shunts have been largely abandoned because of the high frequency of pulmonary hypertension, stenosis distal to the shunt sites, and considerable difficulty with surgical take down, but adult patients with these types of shunts are still infrequently encountered. Pulmonary artery pressure can be estimated noninvasively using the brachial artery systolic cuff pressure and continuous wave Doppler echocardiography to measure the gradient between aorta and pulmonary artery across the shunt. The classic **Blalock-Taussig shunt** (subclavian artery anastomosed to the pulmonary artery) has a much lower risk of pulmonary vascular disease, with preferential blood flow into one lung (usually the left). Even when pulmonary vascular disease develops in the ipsilateral lung, the other lung is usually protected and late intracardiac repair may be possible. Because the subclavian artery is diverted, the ipsilateral arm is pulseless. The modified Blalock-Taussig shunt (now more commonly performed) uses a synthetic conduit and maintains perfusion to the arm. These shunts can become obstructed with recurrence of cyanosis, loss of the continuous murmur on physical examination, and decreased flow on Doppler echocardiography.

In the **Rastelli procedure**, extracardiac conduits from the right ventricle to the pulmonary artery may be used in pulmonary atresia and CC-TGA with PS, truncus arteriosus, and double-outlet RV with PS. They can be synthetic (heterograft) or cadaveric (homograft) and may or may not contain valves. Problems are caused by valvular obstruction or degeneration and obstruction of shunts, baffles, and conduits. Continued clinical and noninvasive follow-up is essential in this group of patients.

TRANSCATHETER RIGHT VENTRICULAR OUTFLOW TRACT INTERVENTIONS

TOF, pulmonary atresia, and double-outlet right ventricle are some of the CHD lesions with right ventricular outflow tract involvement that may require intervention for significant pulmonary stenosis or regurgitation. Previously these patients were offered surgery; however, with the advent of transcatheter options which minimize recovery time and avoid the risks of surgery, transcatheter interventions of the right ventricular outflow tract are now routinely considered in those at high risk for surgery as well as those with multiple prior sternotomies. The valves that are currently FDA approved are the Melody valve as well as the Edwards Sapien XT or S3 and are typically done in those with previously placed bioprosthetic pulmonary valves or those with right ventricular to pulmonary artery valved conduits which provide a landing zone for deployment. In native outflow tracts that are large, there are studies currently underway looking at valves that conform to the native anatomy. The important thing to consider in these patients with prior transcatheter interventions is the risk of endocarditis which warrants careful assessment if they are symptomatic such as obtaining blood culture before initiation of antibiotics. Also, thorough dental evaluation as well as antibiotic prophylaxis for certain dental procedures is recommended (Figure 31–32).

Abdelghani M, Nassif M, Blom NA, et al. Infective endocarditis after melody valve implantation in the pulmonary position: a systematic review. *J Am Heart Assoc.* 2018;7(13):e008163. [PMID: 29934419]

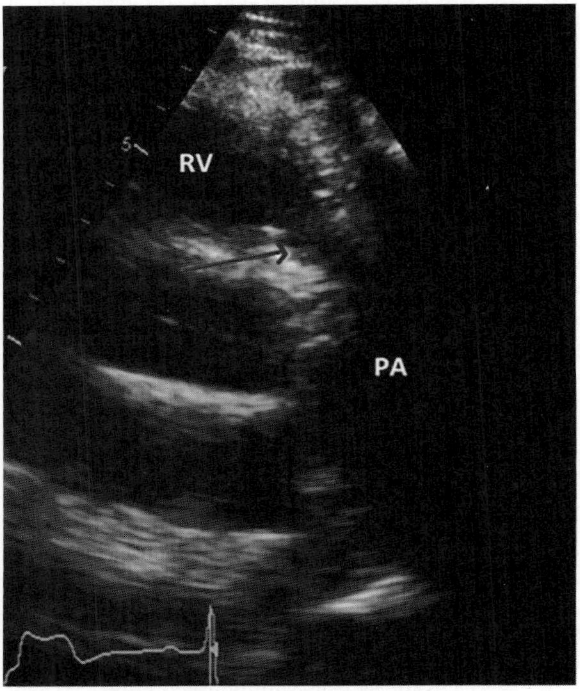

▲ **Figure 31–32.** (Arrow) Percutaneous stented bioprosthesis of the right ventricular outflow tract with a Melody valve. PA, pulmonary artery; RV, right ventricle.

Cheatham JP, Hellenbrand WE, Zahn EM, et al. Clinical and hemodynamic outcomes up to 7 years after transcatheter pulmonary valve replacement in the US melody valve investigational device exemption trial. *Circulation.* 2015;131(22):1960–1970. [PMID: 25944758]
Shahanavaz S, Zahn EM, Levi DS, et al. Transcatheter pulmonary valve replacement with the Sapien prosthesis. *J Am Coll Cardiol.* 2020;76(24):2847–2858. [PMID: 33303074]

HEART FAILURE IN THE ACHD POPULATION

With advances in the treatment of ACHD, patients are living longer. Recent data suggest that approximately 20% of adults affected with CHD present with heart failure. It has been noted that those hospitalized with heart failure are at a fivefold risk of death compared to those not admitted. The mechanisms of heart failure vary based on anatomy but are usually due to volume or pressure overload of a ventricle, either the sub pulmonary, the systemic ventricle, or single ventricle physiology because of pulmonary hypertension, myocardial injury, or ischemia. While the treatment for symptomatic heart failure typically mirrors that of acquired heart disease with systemic left ventricular dysfunction, there is no robust data for treatment in the asymptomatic individual with systemic right ventricular or single ventricular dysfunction. Device therapy may be considered in select patients with careful consultation with electrophysiology. These patients should be referred early to multidisciplinary teams consisting of ACHD, advanced heart failure and cardio-thoracic surgery specialists in high volume centers for evaluation for mechanical support and heart transplantation. Mechanical support unfortunately may not be an option in certain patients with ACHD due to their anatomy. In terms of transplantation, short-term 30-day and 1-year mortality is unfortunately worse in this group compared to those with acquired heart disease. While the absolute percentage of patients undergoing single or multiorgan transplants in the ACHD population is still low, this is a growing population, and it is relatively higher in younger groups with favorable 1-year mean conditional survival.

Budts W, Hesselink JR, Hurst TR, et al. Treatment of heart failure in adult congenital heart disease: a position paper of the Working Group of Grown-Up Congenital Heart Disease and the Heart Failure Association of the European Society of Cardiology. *Eur Heart J.* 2016;37(18):1419–1427. [PMID: 26787434]
Stout K, Broberg CS, Book WM, et al. Chronic heart failure in congenital heart disease: a scientific statement from the American Heart Association. *Circulation.* 2016;133(8):770–801. [PMID: 26787728]

PULMONARY VASODILATOR THERAPY IN THE ACHD POPULATION

In recent years, pulmonary vasodilators have been increasingly used in CHD. In patients with pre-tricuspid shunt lesions (ie, atrial septal defects and sinus venosus defects with partial anomalous pulmonary venous drainage) associated with pulmonary arterial hypertension, pulmonary vasodilators have been used in a "treat to close" approach. While previously labelled inoperable, those that significantly respond to vasodilator therapy may potentially be candidates for closure with therapy and close follow-up.

Pulmonary vasodilators have also been used in Eisenmenger patients demonstrating symptoms of heart failure and exercise intolerance. There is some data to suggest patients who are quite symptomatic can improve their functional class, oxygen saturation and 6-minute walk distance, and have improved survival.

The third group of patients these medications are used for, are in single ventricular physiology palliated with the Fontan circulation. While there has been no robust data to suggest a survival benefit, there are small studies including a recent randomized placebo controlled trial (FUEL) in teenagers which showed improved measures of exercise duration; however, there was no improvement in oxygen consumption at peak exercise.

Arnott C, Strange G, Bullock A, et al. Pulmonary vasodilator therapy is associated with greater survival in Eisenmenger syndrome. *Heart.* 2017;311876. [PMID: 28794135]

Bradley E, Ammash N, Martinez SC, et al. "Treat-to-close": Non-repairable ASD-PAH in the adult: Results from the North American ASD-PAH (NAAP) Multicenter Registry. *Int J Cardiol.* 2019;291:127–133. [PMID: 31031077]

Goldberg D, Zak V, Goldstein BH, et al. Results of the FUEL Trial. *Circulation.* 2020;141(8):641–651. [PMID: 31736357]

ARRHYTHMIAS IN CONGENITAL HEART DISEASE

Rhythm disturbances are a common source of morbidity among adult patients with CHD. In one cohort sudden death was noted on a quarter of patients with ACHD. Intra-atrial reentrant tachycardia (resembling atrial flutter) is particularly common in patients with prior atriotomies and atrial suture lines and is often poorly tolerated. Furthermore, the development of atrial flutter/intra-atrial reentrant tachycardia or atrial fibrillation may be a risk factor for sudden death. Modern interventional electrophysiologic techniques, using three-dimensional mapping and radiofrequency ablation, have expanded treatment options, and early electrophysiologic consultation should be considered for patients with complex CHD and recurrent atrial arrhythmias. Ventricular tachycardia is relatively common in patients with prior ventriculotomies (particularly for TOF repair) and with myopathic ventricles. Clinicians should have a low threshold to perform ambulatory ECG monitoring in these patients, and some advocate routine annual testing in patients with TOF. Sinus node dysfunction occurs frequently in patients with prior Fontan or atrial switch operations, and patients with atrial isomerism can be affected with either sinus node dysfunction or twin AV node-mediated reentrant tachycardias. The resultant bradycardia is associated with a higher rate of intra-atrial reentrant tachycardia or atrial fibrillation in these patients. AV node dysfunction is commonly seen in patients because of surgery and also in patients with AV septal defect and CC-TGA. The indications for pacing and defibrillation are similar to those in the general population, although an awareness of the patient's anatomy is important because patients with atrial switch procedures or single ventricles/Fontan circulations often require placement of epicardial pacing leads. Importantly, patients with adult CHD should be referred to electrophysiologists familiar with the ACHD spectrum.

Khairy P, van Hare GF, Balaji S, et al. ACES/HRS expert consensus statement on the recognition and management of arrhythmias in adult congenital heart disease: developed in partnership between the Pediatric and Congenital Electrophysiology Society (PACES) and the Heart Rhythm Society (HRS). Endorsed by the governing bodies of PACES, HRS, the American College of Cardiology (ACC), the American Heart Association (AHA), the European Heart Rhythm Association (EHRA), the Canadian Heart Rhythm Society (CHRS), and the International Society for Adult Congenital Heart Disease (ISACHD). *Can J Cardiol.* 2014;30(1):e1–e63. [PMID: 25262867]

PREVENTION OF INFECTIVE ENDOCARDITIS

The risk of infective endocarditis remains an issue of ongoing concern in many patients with congenital cardiac defects. The absolute magnitude of risk varies considerably from one lesion to another and is also dependent on whether the patient has been surgically treated. In 2007, the American Heart Association revised its guidelines regarding infective endocarditis prophylaxis. The revised guidelines suggest a much more conservative approach to the use of prophylactic antibiotics. Broadly speaking, infective endocarditis prophylaxis is now recommended in only three groups of patients with CHD: (1) those with unrepaired cyanotic CHD, including patients with palliative shunts and conduits; (2) those with a defect completely repaired (either surgically or by catheter-based intervention), using prosthetic material or device, during the first 6 months after the procedure; and (3) those with repaired CHD who have residual shunts at the site of or adjacent to the site of a patch or device. The risk of endocarditis in individual lesions is summarized in Table 31–2.

GENETIC COUNSELING & PREGNANCY

As many young adults with CHD have entered or are about to enter their reproductive years, genetic counseling and prepregnancy consultation are an important component of their care. The risk of congenital heart defects increases 5–10% (higher in specific disorders) in the offspring of patients with CHD. Preconception genetic counseling and genetic testing are indicated for patients with syndromic CHD as well as for patients with nonsyndromic CHD and a family history of CHD. In addition, testing for the 22q11 deletion is indicated in patients with TOF, truncus arteriosus, aortic arch anomalies, or VSD who display at least one

Table 31–2. Endocarditis in Adults with Congenital Heart Disease

Defect	M:F	Associated Defects	Risk of Endocarditis
Acyanotic			
Bicuspid AV	4:1	Coarctation	High
Valvar PS	1:1	VSD (see TOF), Noonan syndrome	Low (mild PS), intermediate (severe PS)
ASD secundum	1:2	Mitral valve prolapse	Low
ASD primum	1:1	Bridging AV valve leaflets, trisomy 21	Intermediate (with MR)
AV septal defect			
VSD	1:1	PS (see TOF), AR	Intermediate-high (unoperated or with AR)
			Low (operated without AR)
PDA	1:2–3	Coexists with many complex syndromes	Low (ligated), intermediate (patent)
Coarctation	2:1	Bicuspid AV	Low (operated[1]), intermediate (without treatment)
C-TGA	M > F	VSD, infundibular PS	Low (isolated C-TGA)
Ebstein anomaly	1:1	ASD	Low-intermediate
		PFO	
Coronary AV fistulae	1:1		Intermediate
Cyanotic			
TOF	1.5:1	RAA, ASD	Intermediate
Eisenmenger syndrome	M < F	VSD, ASD, PDA	Low
Tricuspid atresia	1:1[2]	Pulmonary atresia, ASD, VSD	?
Pulmonary atresia with intact septum	1:1		?
D-TGA	2–4:1	ASD, PFO, PDA, VSD, PS, RAA	Intermediate
Postoperative			
Fontan			Variable
Glenn			Variable
Blalock-Taussig			High
RV-PA conduit			High

[1]Unless there is associated bicuspid AV.
[2]In tricuspid atresia with transposition, M > F.
AR, aortic regurgitation; ASD, atrial septal defect; AV, aortic valve; C-TGV, congenitally corrected transposition of the great vessels; F, female; M, male; MR, mitral regurgitation; PA, pulmonary artery; PDA, patent ductus arteriosus; PFO, patent foramen ovale; PS, pulmonic stenosis; RAA, right-sided aortic arch; RV, right ventricle; TOF, tetralogy of Fallot; VSD, ventricular septal defect.

other feature of the 22q11 deletion syndrome (including dysmorphic facies, cleft palate, hypernasal speech, learning disabilities, behavioral or psychiatric disorders, thymic abnormalities, or hypocalcemia).

Most patients with acyanotic CHD can successfully carry a pregnancy to term. A small number of conditions place the patient and fetus at high risk during pregnancy. While there are many scoring systems that can be utilized, the ZAHARA score was the first that looked specifically at patients with CHD. Patients with unrepaired cyanotic heart disease, Eisenmenger syndrome with severe pulmonary vascular disease/pulmonary hypertension, Marfan syndrome with a dilated aortic root, severe LV outflow obstruction, and moderate to severe systolic dysfunction of the systemic ventricle are typically advised against pregnancy given that they are at exceptionally high risk. Other patients should be risk-stratified with respect to their tolerance of the anticipated hemodynamic changes of pregnancy and labor, namely expansion of intravascular volume, reduction of vascular resistance, and augmentation of cardiac output. It is therefore helpful to assess exercise tolerance prior to conception. Maternal and fetal mortality rates vary with functional class: in New York Heart Association (NYHA) class I, they are 0% and 0.4%, respectively; in NYHA class IV, the rates are 30% and 6.8%, respectively. The modified WHO classification is also useful to help risk stratify these patients. Although pulmonary edema occurs less commonly than in patients with acquired heart disease, it may be useful to assess ventricular function noninvasively prepartum and in the early months of pregnancy. Patients with significant CHD should receive close follow-up during pregnancy by a cardiologist familiar with their condition and should receive care in a high-risk obstetric clinic. Fetal echocardiography should be offered when the parent or a previous child is affected. Prophylaxis during vaginal delivery is generally recommended for those at high risk for endocarditis (see Table 31–1). For a complete discussion of pregnancy in patients with heart disease, please see Chapter 33.

Regitz-Zagrosek V, Hesselink JWR, Bauersachs J, et al. 2018 ESC Guidelines for the management of cardiovascular diseases during pregnancy. *Eur Heart J.* 2018;39(34):3165–3241. [PMID: 30165544]

RECOMMENDATIONS FOR EXERCISE & SPORTS PARTICIPATION

General recommendations regarding exercise should be individualized to the patient following a complete clinical and noninvasive evaluation. Exercise testing and ambulatory ECG monitoring should be included in this evaluation to define exercise capacity and detect significant asymptomatic arrhythmias. No exercise restrictions are recommended for patients with small or repaired ASDs, VSDs, or PDAs, repaired AV septal defects, repaired total or partial anomalous pulmonary venous connection, mild PS, repaired coarctation, or repaired congenital coronary artery anomalies, or patients with D-TGA who have had an arterial switch procedure. Patients with moderate PS, mild aortic stenosis, completely repaired TOF, or AV septal defect with moderate mitral regurgitation should be restricted to moderate dynamic and isometric exercise. Patients with Ebstein anomaly, D-TGA after atrial switch procedure, CC-TGA, or univentricular heart/Fontan circulation should be restricted to moderate dynamic exercise and mild isometric exercise. Patients with moderate aortic stenosis or TOF with residual disease should be restricted to mild dynamic and static exercise. Patients with Eisenmenger syndrome should be restricted to mild dynamic exercise.

ACQUIRED HEART DISEASE IN ADULTS WITH CONGENITAL HEART DISEASE

It is important not to ignore the presence of acquired heart disease in adults with CHD. Acquired and congenital heart lesions may interact in unexpected ways, for example, the association of rheumatic mitral stenosis causing increased shunting across an ASD in Lutembacher syndrome. Impaired diastolic function from hypertension or coronary artery disease in a patient with an ASD may also increase the magnitude of the left-to-right shunt. Similarly, increased systemic vascular resistance from hypertension in a patient with a VSD may worsen the shunt. The clinician must exclude coronary artery disease as a cause of chest pain in adults with congenital aortic stenosis and pulmonary hypertension. Also, the progression of atherosclerotic coronary disease (CAD) may be accelerated in association with aortic coarctation. In addition to associated risk factors as the CHD population ages, the traditional CAD risk factors affecting the general population such as obesity, hypertension, dyslipidemia, and diabetes mellitus may be amplified. It has been reported that at least 80% of CHD patients have at least one CAD risk factor. Hence, careful follow-up with a heightened awareness for these risk factors and institution of lifestyle modification and primary prevention needs to be implemented. Furthermore, a careful assessment of other comorbidities, neurocognitive decline, and extra cardiac organs involvement is also warranted.

Bhatt A, Foster E, Kuehl K, et al. Congenital heart disease in the older adult: a scientific statement from the American Heart Association. *Circulation.* 2015;131(21):1884–1931. [PMID: 25896865]

Cardiac Tumors

32

Shalini Dixit, MD
Rita F. Redberg, MD, MS

ESSENTIALS OF DIAGNOSIS

- A rare but critical diagnosis in the evaluation of cardiac masses.
- The history, physical examination, and imaging characteristics can yield valuable diagnostic clues.
- Diagnostic confirmation requires tissue biopsy.

General Considerations

Cardiac tumors, although considered a rare diagnostic entity, provide unique insight into the anatomic and pathophysiologic functioning of the heart. Reminiscent of benign, malignant, and metastatic neoplasms elsewhere in the body, theses tumors herald their presence by the secondary effects produced from enlarging within the confines of cardiac chambers and tissues. Because they rarely cause symptoms, cardiac tumors are generally unsuspected and may be discovered incidentally during evaluation of an unrelated condition. This chapter will help guide the astute clinician, focusing on when to consider this diagnosis and how to obtain the appropriate cardiovascular imaging studies. There are a wide variety of common cardiac tumors (Table 32–1).

Primary Cardiac Tumors

Primary tumors of the heart are rare, with a prevalence of 0.02% reported in combined data from multiple large autopsy series. Although cardiac myxoma has been traditionally reported as the most frequent tumor type in adults, increasing utilization of imaging studies has revealed a higher frequency of papillary fibroelastomas than previously known. In the pediatric population, rhabdomyomas represent the most common type of primary cardiac tumor (Table 32–2).

A. Benign Cardiac Tumors

The overwhelming majority of primary cardiac tumors, approximately 75% to more than 90%, are benign, and may arise from the endocardium, myocardium, or pericardium. Timely diagnosis is key because although the tumors themselves are generally curable, their obstructive and embolic effects can be catastrophic.

1. Myxoma: A stalked spherical tumor of the left atrium

A. Demographics—Approximately 50% of all benign primary cardiac tumors are myxomas. They are predominantly found in women, in the 30- to 60-year age group. The mean age at diagnosis is 51 years. Most commonly, myxomas are sporadic and isolated in occurrence; however, up to 10% are familial, typically transmitted in an autosomal dominant pattern. Familial myxomas tend to present earlier in life, with a mean age at diagnosis of 25 years. These patients also tend to have multiple (30–50%) and/or recurrent (12–22%) tumors.

B. Typical locations—Theoretically, myxomas can occur in any cardiac chamber or on any valve, but the most common site for a myxoma is the left atrium (74%), with 18% occurring in the right atrium and 4% each occurring in the right and left ventricles. The typical site of origin is near the region of the fossa ovalis with a stalk-like attachment to the interatrial septum (Figure 32–1). Ventricular myxomas almost always originate from the ventricular free wall.

C. Pathology—Myxomas vary in size, ranging from 1 to 15 cm in diameter, and are typically pedunculated. They are gelatinous in consistency, with a smooth or villous surface, and may be friable. Histologically, myxomas arise from multipotent mesenchymal cells and produce vascular endothelial growth factor. They are visualized as islands of tumor cells of variable shapes (round, elongated, or polyhedral), scattered within a pale-staining mucopolysaccharide matrix (Figure 32–2).

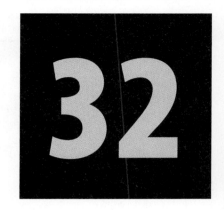

Table 32–1. Classification of Common Cardiac Tumors

Primary Cardiac Tumors
Benign Tumors
Myxoma
Papillary fibroelastoma
Lipoma
Fibroma
Hemangioma
Teratoma
Rhabdomyoma
Hamartoma (oncocytic cardiomyopathy)
Malignant Tumors
Sarcoma: includes angiosarcoma, rhabdomyosarcoma, fibrosarcoma, osteosarcoma, leiomyosarcoma, liposarcoma, synovial sarcoma
Lymphoma
Malignant fibrous histiocytoma
Epithelioid hemangioendothelioma
Benign or Malignant Tumors
Mesothelioma (includes cystic tumor of the atrioventricular node)
Paraganglioma
Secondary Cardiac Tumors
Metastasis to the heart and pericardium: commonly from malignant melanoma or neoplasms of the lung, hematopoietic system, gastrointestinal tract, kidney, breast, thyroid, and soft tissue

D. Associations—The Carney complex is an inherited autosomal dominant condition characterized by cardiac myxomas, myxoid fibroadenomas of the breast, and testicular and pituitary gland tumors. These occur in association with pigmented lentigines, blue nevi of the skin, and Cushing syndrome, due to primary pigmented nodular adrenocortical dysplasia.

The Carney complex appears to be a genetically heterozygous syndrome with gene localization to loci in 17q22-24, 2p16, and other regions. Inactivating mutations of *PRKAR1A*, a gene which maps to 17q22-24 and encodes the protein kinase A (PKA) regulatory subunit type 1a, are responsible for most cases of Carney complex. Carney complex should be considered in any patient with a diagnosis of myxoma, particularly if presenting early in life, with multiple tumors, or with a myxoma outside of the left atrium.

Bouys L, Bertherat J. MANAGEMENT OF ENDOCRINE DISEASE: Carney complex: clinical and genetic update 20 years after the identification of the CNC1 (PRKAR1A) gene. *Eur J Endocrinol.* 2021;184(3):R99–R109. [PMID: 33444222]. doi:10.1530/EJE-20-1120

2. Papillary fibroelastoma: A sea anemone on cardiac valves

A. Demographics—Papillary fibroelastomas have previously been designated the second-most common primary cardiac neoplasm in adults behind myxomas; however, recent work suggests they may, in fact, be the most common, likely related to the increase in cardiac imaging. While they have been reported in patients age 3–86 years, the typical age at diagnosis is 60 years. Papillary fibroelastomas are often discovered postmortem, with an autopsy incidence of 0.002–0.33%.

B. Typical locations—More than 80% of fibroelastomas are found on the valvular endocardium, typically of the

Table 32–2. Primary Cardiac Tumors: Location and Features

Cardiac Tumor	Typical Location	Interesting Features/Associations
Myxoma	Left atrium	Carney complex; constitutional symptoms
Papillary fibroelastoma	Cardiac valves	Can present with sudden death from coronary ostial obstruction
Fibroma	Left ventricular myocardium	Very large tumors that exert a mass effect
Rhabdomyoma	Cardiac chambers	Tuberous sclerosis
Angiosarcoma	Right atrium	Highly aggressive tumor
Rhabdomyosarcoma	Cardiac chambers	Commonest pediatric malignancy
Fibrosarcoma	Left atrium	White fish flesh tumor
Leiomyosarcoma	Smooth muscle cells of pulmonary veins and arteries	Epstein-Barr virus in immunosuppressed patients
Lymphoma	Right heart chambers	Immunocompromised patients
Paraganglioma	Pericardium; left atrial wall	Majority are hormonally inactive
Teratoma	Pericardium	Contain elements from all three germ cell layers

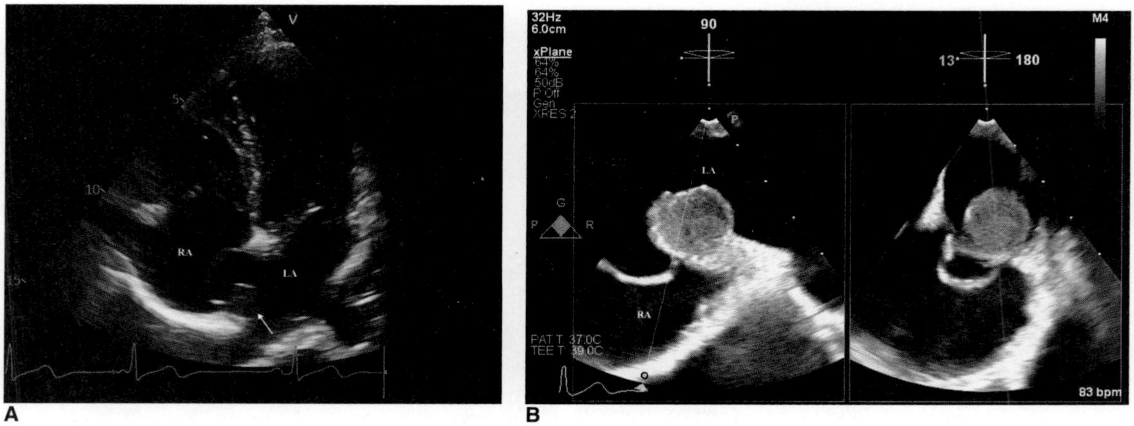

▲ **Figure 32–1.** Atrial myxoma. **A:** Transthoracic echocardiogram obtained in a 71-year-old woman who presented with palpitations. The apical four-chamber view shows an interatrial septal aneurysm with rightward bowing and an echogenic mass (*arrow*) near the superior portion of the interatrial septum, later found to be a left atrial myxoma. **B:** Bicaval view from preoperative transesophageal echocardiogram in the same patient depicts the left atrial myxoma with attachment site near the superior vena cava, while the corresponding biplane view on the right demonstrates rightward bowing of the interatrial septal aneurysm. LA, left atrium; RA, right atrium.

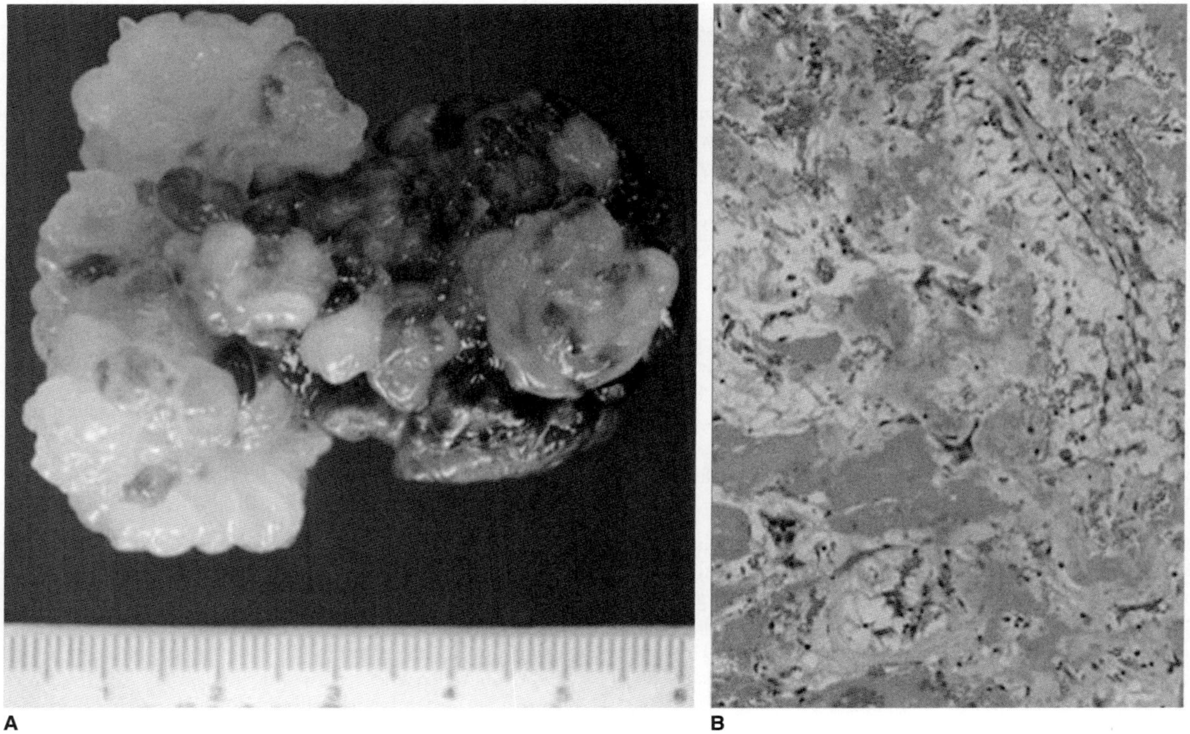

▲ **Figure 32–2.** Atrial myxoma. **A:** Gross pathology: The specimen shows a lobulated, gelatinous tumor with areas of hemorrhage resected from the left atrium of a 58-year-old female patient. The diagnosis was made incidentally on an echocardiogram, which the patient had preoperatively for an unrelated condition. **B:** Histology: Hematoxylin-eosin stain of the same mass reveals small, perivascular clusters of tumor cells scattered within a myxoid matrix rich in mucopolysaccharides and fibrin, consistent with a cardiac myxoma. (Reproduced with permission from Philip C. Ursell.)

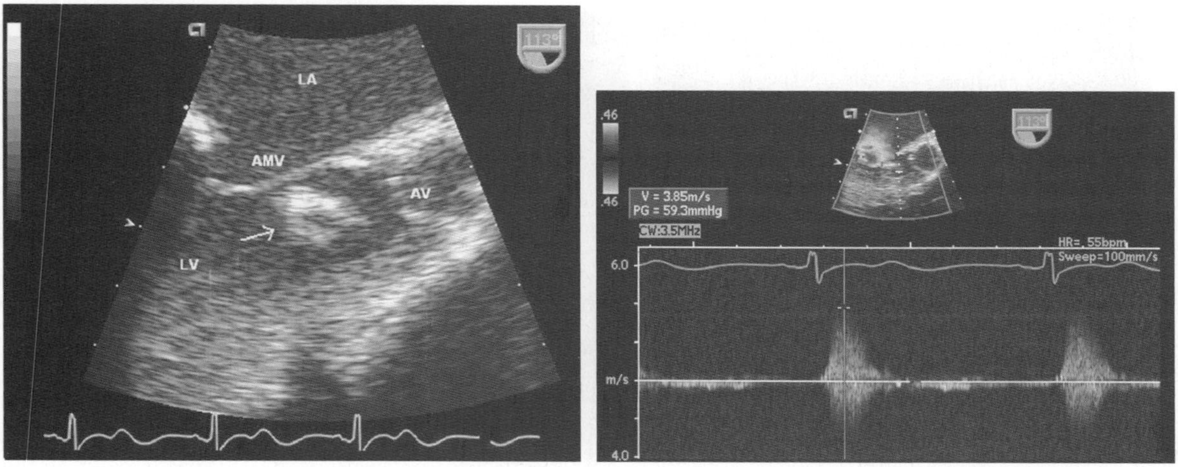

A B

▲ **Figure 32–3.** Papillary fibroelastoma. Transesophageal echocardiogram performed in a 75-year-old man presenting with dizziness. **A:** An irregular mass attached to the ventricular side of the anterior mitral leaflet is shown in this mid-esophageal long-axis view. The location on the downstream side of the valve and the frond-like surface are highly suggestive of a papillary fibroelastoma (*arrow*). **B:** Continuous wave Doppler flow demonstrates left ventricular outflow tract obstruction (59 mm Hg gradient) caused by the mass during systole. AMV, anterior mitral valve leaflet; AV, aortic valve; LA, left atrium; LV, left ventricle.

aortic and mitral valves, followed by the tricuspid valve. Unlike vegetations, fibroelastomas often occur downstream of the valve (ie, ventricular side of the mitral valve, aortic side of the aortic valve) and normally do not cause valvular dysfunction (Figure 32–3). The remainder of these tumors are located on the subvalvular apparatus as well as within the atria and ventricles.

C. PATHOLOGY—Known by different names, such as papillary endocardial tumor, cardiac papilloma, or giant Lambl excrescence, the papillary fibroelastoma has been likened to a sea anemone. The description arises from the multiple hair-like fronds of the tumor, which originate from a central core. Histologically, the papillary fronds are comprised of collagen and elastin tissue amid a mucopolysaccharide matrix with an endothelium lining.

D. ASSOCIATIONS—Iatrogenic papillary fibroelastomas, which often involve nonvalvular endocardial surfaces, have been reported in the literature after cardiac surgery and chest radiation, leading some to question whether these lesions may be reactive and not truly neoplastic. However, more recently r*KRAS* mutations were found in nearly 80% of analyzed tumors in one small cohort, arguing that at least a subset of papillary fibroelastomas is neoplastic in origin.

Tamin SS, Maleszewski JJ, Scott CG, et al. Prognostic and bioepidemiologic implications of papillary fibroelastomas. *J Am Coll Cardiol*. 2015;65(22):2420–2429. [PMID: 26046736] doi:10.1016/j.jacc.2015.03.569

3. Lipoma: An encapsulated adipose cell tumor of cardiac chambers.

A. DEMOGRAPHICS—Lipomas also account for about 8–12% of cardiac tumors, their incidence being slightly lower than that of the papillary fibroelastoma. They most commonly occur in middle-aged and older adults without a particular sex predilection.

B. TYPICAL LOCATIONS—Roughly 50% of lipomas originate from the subendocardial layer, protruding into the corresponding cardiac chamber, while the rest arise from the epicardial or myocardial layers and grow into the pericardial space. Rarely, lipomas can occur on cardiac valves.

C. PATHOLOGY—Lipomas are usually solitary, well-circumscribed encapsulated tumors with a wide spectrum of size and weight, with some measuring in kilograms! Histopathologically, they are composed of mature adipose cells that may be admixed with other cell types.

D. ASSOCIATIONS—Lipomatous hypertrophy of the interatrial septum can mimic a cardiac lipoma given its similar tissue characteristics. However, a primary distinguishing feature is the tendency of lipomatous hypertrophy to spare the interatrial septum in the region of the fossa ovalis, producing a characteristic "dumbbell" shape (Figure 32–4).

4. Fibroma: A giant tumor of the left ventricle

A. DEMOGRAPHICS—Fibromas are far more common in the pediatric population, being the second or third most common

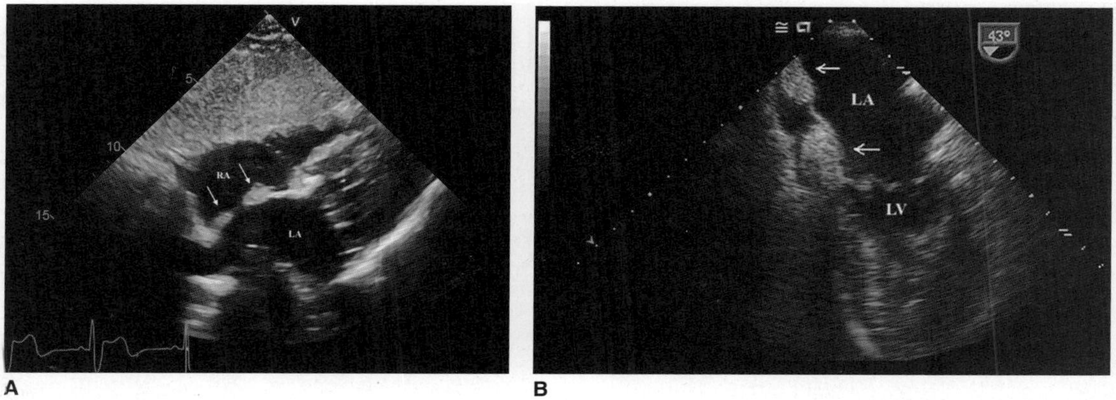

▲ **Figure 32–4.** **A:** Transthoracic echocardiogram in the subcostal view demonstrating a dumbbell-shaped mass consistent with lipomatous hypertrophy of the interatrial septum (*arrows*). **B:** Transesophageal echocardiogram in the mid-esophageal view showing lipomatous hypertrophy of the interatrial septum in a different patient (*arrows*). LA, left atrium; RA, right atrium.

benign cardiac tumor of childhood. Most cardiac fibromas are diagnosed in infants under 1 year of age; however, they have been reported in adults as well older than 50 years.

B. TYPICAL LOCATIONS—Fibromas typically arise from the ventricular myocardium, with a predilection for the left ventricle, particularly the left ventricular free wall and the interventricular septum, even at times mimicking hypertrophic cardiomyopathy (Figure 32–5).

C. PATHOLOGY—Typically solitary, fibromas are large tumors with diameters in the 1–10 cm range. As a result, they often exert a mass effect. Fibromas are not distinctly encapsulated though are clearly demarcated from surrounding myocardium and often contain small calcifications.

D. ASSOCIATIONS—A small subset of cardiac fibromas (3–5%) are associated with Gorlin syndrome (also known as nevoid basal cell carcinoma syndrome), an autosomal-dominant condition caused by mutations in the *PTCH1* gene and characterized by basal cell carcinomas, skeletal abnormalities, and ectopic calcification of the central nervous system. Fibromas have also been associated with familial adenomatous polyposis.

Baidoun M, Elgendy M, Loker J. Cardiac fibroma with cardiac arrest: a rare clinical presentation of Gorlin syndrome in an 8-month-old infant. *BMJ Case Rep*. 2021;14(6):e241519. Published 2021 Jun 23. [PMID: 34162607]. doi:10.1136/bcr-2020-241519.

5. Rhabdomyoma: The spontaneously regressing tumor of childhood

A. DEMOGRAPHICS—Rhabdomyomas are the most common benign cardiac tumor in children, accounting for 60% of all pediatric cardiac tumors, and are often detected in utero or in the first year of life.

B. TYPICAL LOCATIONS—Rhabdomyomas are frequently multiple, occurring predominantly in the right and left ventricular walls, though also found in the atria and occasionally on the atrioventricular valves (Figure 32–6).

C. PATHOLOGY—These tumors range in size from a few millimeters to several centimeters and grossly have a yellow or white appearance (Figure 32–7). Most rhabdomyomas spontaneously regress and are typically monitored with serial echocardiograms.

D. ASSOCIATIONS—More than 80–90% of rhabdomyomas are associated with tuberous sclerosis complex, an autosomal dominant genetic disorder caused by a pathogenic variant in one of two genes, *TSC1 or TSC2*, both of which lead to overactivation of mammalian target of rapamycin (mTOR) and thereby abnormal cell proliferation. TSC is characterized by the development of benign tumors in multiple organs, including the brain, heart, and, kidneys, as well as hypopigmented cutaneous macules.

6. Hemangioma: The benign vascular neoplasm

A. DEMOGRAPHICS—Hemangiomas account for about 5–10% of all benign cardiac tumors and can affect any age group, from newborns to older adults.

B. TYPICAL LOCATIONS—Hemangiomas can be isolated, but about one-third are found in multiple locations. These tumors can occur in any cardiac chamber (Figure 32–8).

C. PATHOLOGY—Hemangiomas are composed of mature blood vessels, and their gross appearance is that of a vascular lesion with reddish-purple coloration. Microscopically, they are composed of dilated vessels, bland endothelial cells, and fibrous connective tissue. There are three histologic subtypes: capillary, cavernous, or arteriovenous.

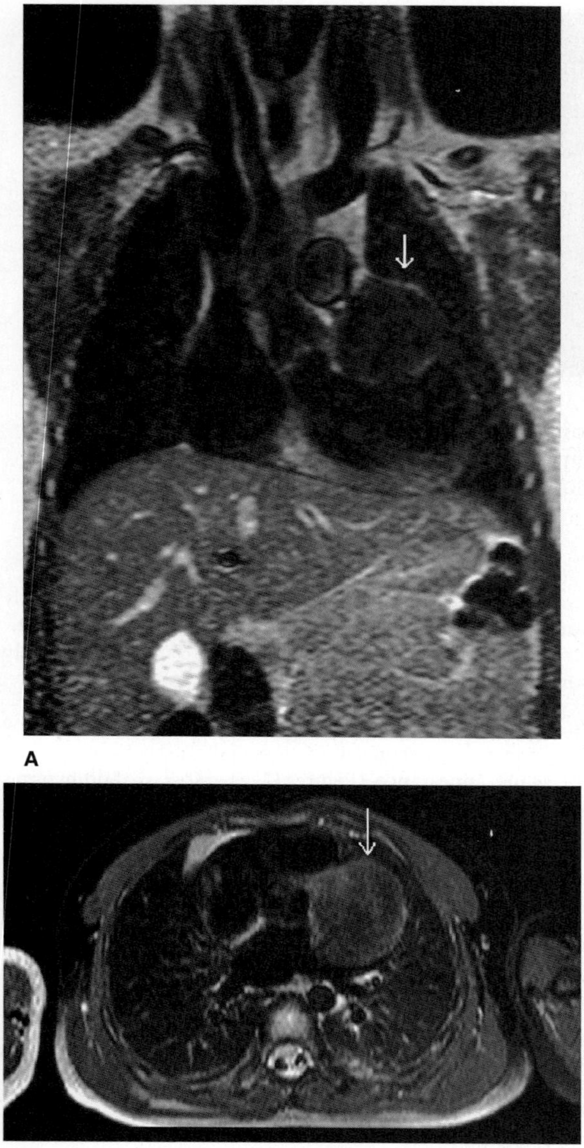

▲ **Figure 32–5.** Cardiac fibroma. **A:** Coronal T2-weighted spin-echo magnetic resonance image of the heart at the level of the left ventricular anterior wall and the aortic valve. A mass is visualized emanating from the anterior wall of the left ventricle (*arrow*). The mass is mildly heterogeneous with mild T2 hypointensity relative to the myocardium. **B:** Transaxial T2-weighted image demonstrates predominantly peripheral enhancement, suggestive of a cardiac fibroma. (Reproduced with permission from C. Higgins.)

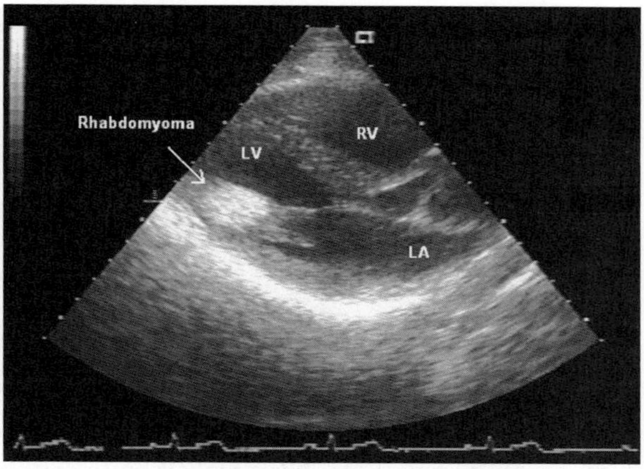

▲ **Figure 32–6.** Cardiac rhabdomyoma. Transthoracic echocardiogram in the parasternal long-axis view showing a rhabdomyoma in the inferolateral left ventricular wall of a patient with tuberous sclerosis. LA, left atrium; LV, left ventricle; RV, right ventricle.

Maleszewski JJ, Bois MC, Bois JP, Young PM, Stulak JM, Klarich KW. Neoplasia and the heart: pathological review of effects with clinical and radiological correlation. *J Am Coll Cardiol.* 2018;72(2):202–227. [PMID: 29976295]. doi:10.1016/j.jacc.2018.05.026.

Tyebally S, Chen D, Bhattacharyya S, et al. Cardiac tumors: JACC CardioOncology State-of-the-Art Review. *JACC CardioOncol.* 2020;2(2):293–311. [PMID: 34396236]. Published 2020 Jun 16. doi:10.1016/j.jaccao.2020.05.009

7. Cardiac hamartoma (histiocytoid cardiomyopathy): A tumor of Purkinje cells

A. DEMOGRAPHICS—Also known as oncocytic cardiomyopathy or Purkinje cell hamartoma, these tumors are rare with fewer than 150 reported cases and typically affect infants in the first year of life.

B. TYPICAL LOCATIONS—These tumors can arise on the endocardium or myocardium and may involve the sinoatrial and atrioventricular nodes, often producing arrhythmias and various conduction blocks.

C. PATHOLOGY—Grossly, cardiac hamartomas appear as multiple, small pale nodules. Histologically, they are composed of vacuolated, rounded myocytes with numerous mitochondria and evidence of disordered myofibrils.

Burke A, Tavora F. The 2015 WHO Classification of tumors of the heart and pericardium. *J Thorac Oncol.* 2016;11(4):441–452. [PMID: 26725181]. doi:10.1016/j.jtho.2015.11.009

Maleszewski JJ, Basso C, Bois MC, et al. The 2021 WHO classification of tumors of the heart. *J Thorac Oncol.* 2022 Apr;17(4): 510–518. [PMID: 34774791]. doi: 10.1016/j.jtho.2021.10.021. Epub 2021 Nov 10.

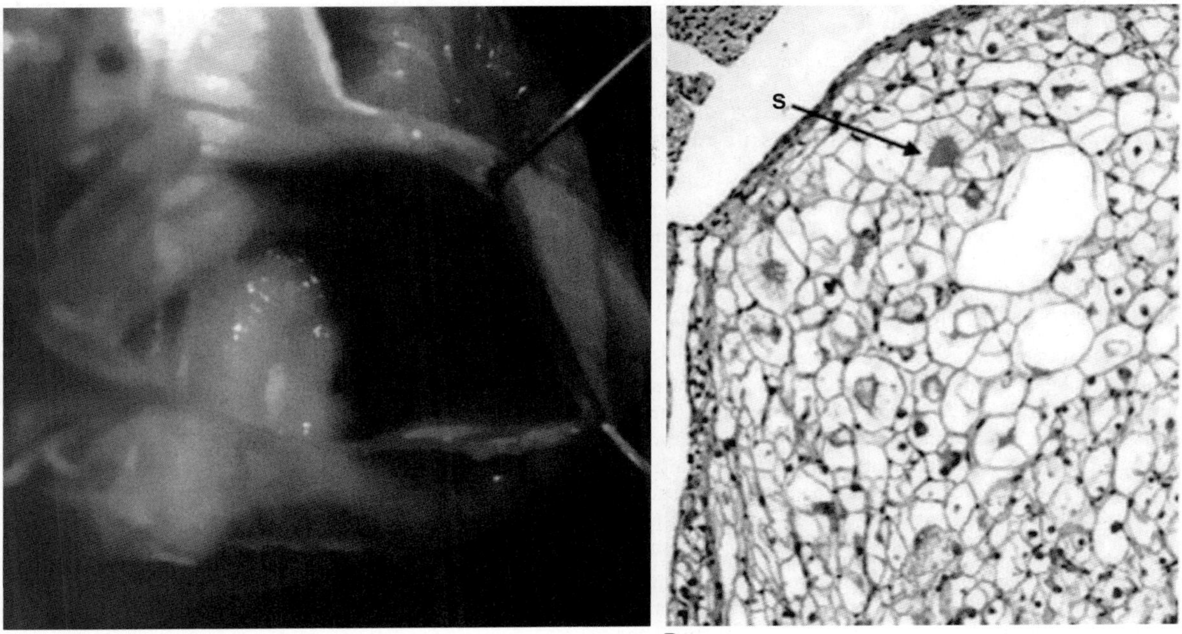

A B

▲ **Figure 32–7.** Cardiac rhabdomyoma. **A:** Gross pathology: The specimen shows a small, well-circumscribed grayish-white tumor seen at the right ventricular inlet in a newborn infant. **B:** Histology: Hematoxylin-eosin stain of the tumor reveals large round and polygonal cells with clear glycogen-rich cytoplasm and attenuated strands of cytoplasm, known as spider cells (*arrow*). Mitotic activity is absent, and these findings are consistent with the diagnosis of rhabdomyoma. (Reproduced with permission from Philip C. Ursell.)

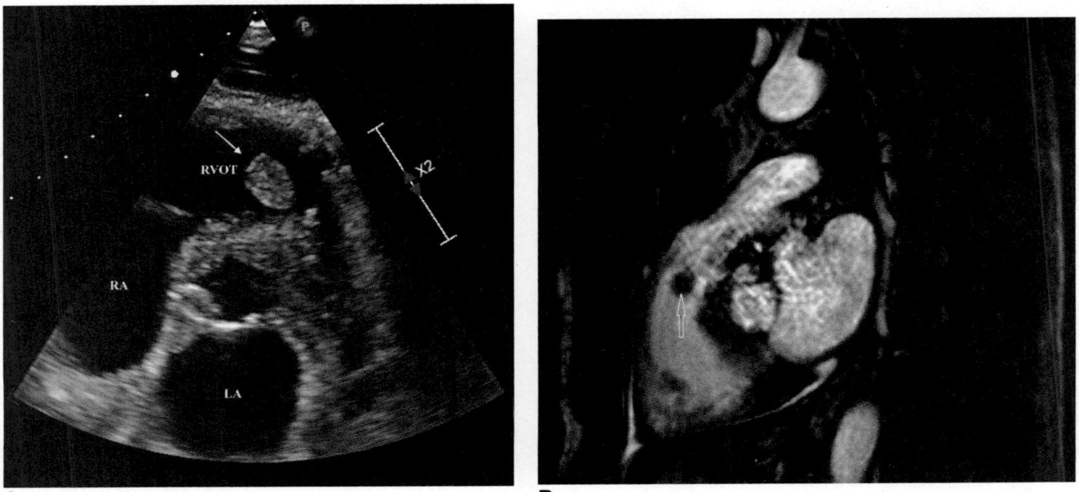

A B

▲ **Figure 32–8.** Cardiac hemangioma in a 59-year-old man presenting with new atrial flutter and heart failure found to have a mass in the right ventricular outflow tract. (**A**) Parasternal short-axis view demonstrates a smooth, mobile mass in the right ventricular outflow tract and subsequent (**B**) magnetic resonance images with steady-state free precession imaging show a mass (*arrow*) of intermediate intensity, slightly higher than that of the myocardium, with smooth contours and no evidence of ventricular invasion. LA, left atrium; RA, right atrium; RVOT, right ventricular outflow tract.

B. Malignant Cardiac Tumors

Up to a quarter of all primary cardiac tumors have malignant features.

1. Sarcoma: The invasive connective tissue tumor of the heart

A. DEMOGRAPHICS—Cardiac sarcomas are the most common malignant tumor of the heart in adults, comprising 50–75% of all primary cardiac neoplasms. They are typically diagnosed between the third and fifth decades of life, and metastatic spread at the time of diagnosis is common.

B. SPECIFIC TUMOR SUBTYPES—Cardiac sarcomas exist as various histologic subtypes, with angiosarcoma being the most common differentiated sarcoma, followed by rhabdomyosarcoma, myxofibrosarcoma, osteosarcoma, and leiomyosarcoma. However, undifferentiated pleomorphic sarcoma (UPS), previously referred to as malignant fibrous histiocytoma, is the most common primary malignant neoplasm of the heart and accounts for roughly 25% of cardiac sarcomas.

1. Undifferentiated pleomorphic sarcoma affects males and females equally and has a mean age of presentation of 44–47 years. These tumors typically arise from the posterior wall of the left atrium and are invasive with diffuse wall involvement. This group of sarcomas lacks specific histological patterns or immunohistochemical features, and pathology shows undifferentiated spindle cells with frequent mitotic activity.
2. Angiosarcomas characteristically arise from the right atrium or the right atrioventricular groove. They are composed of malignant cells that fashion into vascular channels and aggressively infiltrate surrounding structures (Figure 32–9), often demonstrating gross areas of hemorrhage.
3. Rhabdomyosarcoma: These malignant tumors of striated muscle are the most common pediatric cardiac malignancy, though remain rare, accounting for less than 5% of all primary cardiac sarcomas. They are large, invasive tumors which arise from the myocardium and often have valvular involvement. Due to their aggressive nature, they typically present with symptoms related to cardiac invasion or obstruction and are frequently metastatic at the time of diagnosis.
4. Myxofibrosarcomas generally arise in the left atrium and have a yellowish-white or grayish-white appearance on gross pathology. Histologically, myxofibrosarcomas demonstrate myxoid areas, often with curvilinear thin-walled blood vessels and spindle-shaped tumor cells. Unlike benign myxomas which typically arise from the interatrial septum, these tumors are often attached to the posterior wall of the left atrium and present due to symptoms of mitral valve obstruction.
5. Osteosarcomas may arise from any part of the heart but most commonly originate from the posterior wall of the left atrium, near the entrance of the pulmonary veins. They are highly invasive and often infiltrate into the adjacent myocardium or into the pericardium. These tumors exhibit a similar gross and microscopic appearance as osteosarcoma of the bone, demonstrating malignant spindle or ovoid cells mixed with osteoid or bone. Although cardiac osteosarcomas are predominantly osteoblastic, they often exhibit chondroblastic or fibroblastic differentiation as well, with areas resembling chondrosarcoma or myxofibrosarcoma. Osteosarcomas can metastasize to the thyroid, skin, lymph nodes, and lungs.
6. Leiomyosarcoma: These high-grade tumors are thought to arise from the smooth muscle cells of the pulmonary veins and arteries with subsequent myocardial infiltration and are most commonly seen in the posterior left atrium. Tumor pathology exhibits spindle or epithelioid cells arranged as compact bundles with regions of necrosis. Leiomyosarcomas are extremely aggressive with a high rate of local recurrence and systemic metastases.
7. Liposarcoma: Primary cardiac liposarcomas typically originate from the right-sided chambers, particularly the right atrium, though have also been reported on the mitral valve and other left-sided structures. Microscopic examination demonstrates fat cells mixed with fibrous tissue and lipoblasts.

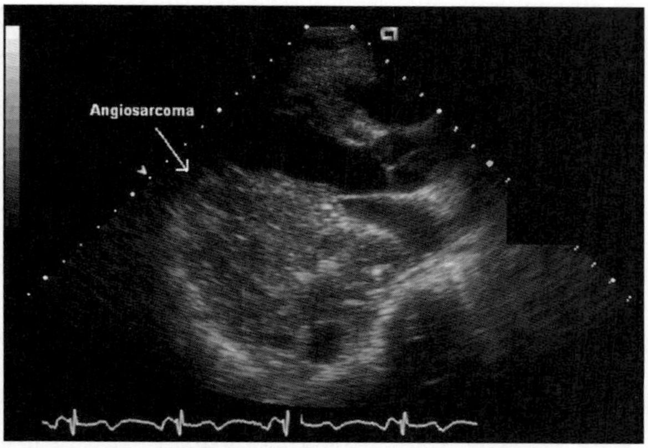

▲ **Figure 32–9.** Cardiac angiosarcoma. Transthoracic echocardiogram in a 60-year-old woman presenting with a 2-month history of dyspnea and palpitations. The parasternal long-axis view shows an infiltrating mass involving the left ventricular posterior wall and left atrium. Tumor biopsy confirmed the diagnosis of angiosarcoma.

C. ASSOCIATIONS—In the acquired immunodeficiency syndrome (AIDS), a specific type of cardiac angiosarcoma called Kaposi sarcoma has been well described. Another interesting association has been made between leiomyosarcomas and the Epstein-Barr virus in immunosuppressed patients, such as those with AIDS or after cardiac transplantation.

Sun D, Wu Y, Liu Y, Yang J. Primary cardiac myxofibrosarcoma: case report, literature review and pooled analysis. *BMC Cancer.* 2018;18(1):512. [PMID: 29720127]. Published 2018 May 2. doi:10.1186/s12885-018-4434-2.

2. Lymphoma: An infiltrative non-Hodgkin tumor of the right atrium

A. Demographic—Primary cardiac lymphoma is exceedingly rare, representing 1–2% of all cardiac tumors and comprising an even smaller percentage of all extranodal lymphomas. However, approximately 25% of patients with lymphoma will develop cardiac involvement.

B. Typical locations—Cardiac lymphoma can involve any area of the heart though has a predilection for the right-sided chambers, particularly the right atrium.

C. Pathology—Primary cardiac lymphoma belongs to the extranodal subtype of non-Hodgkin lymphoma. The majority of primary cardiac lymphomas are aggressive B-cell neoplasms with the most common being diffuse large B-cell lymphoma. Like extracardiac lymphoma, these tumors are infiltrative in nature, often involving the pericardium and encasing the vasculature, including the coronary arteries.

D. Associations—Primary cardiac lymphomas are predominantly found in immunocompromised individuals.

Asadian S, Rezaeian N, Hosseini L, Toloueitabar Y, Hemmati Komasi MM. The role of cardiac CT and MRI in the diagnosis and management of primary cardiac lymphoma: A comprehensive review [published online ahead of print, 2021 Aug 25]. *Trends Cardiovasc Med.* 2021;S1050-1738(21)00094-3. [PMID: 34454052]. doi:10.1016/j.tcm.2021.08.010.

Chen H, Qian S, Shi P, Liu L, Yang F. A presentation, treatment, and survival analysis of primary cardiac lymphoma cases reported from 2009 to 2019. *Int J Hematol.* 2020;112(1):65–73. [PMID: 32285360]. doi:10.1007/s12185-020-02881-2.

3. Mesothelioma: The pericardial tumor

A. Demographics—Primary cardiac mesothelioma is extremely rare though comprises half of all pericardial tumors. It typically affects adults with a slight male predominance.

B. Typical locations—These tumors are neoplasms of the mesothelial lining of the visceral or parietal pericardium and often invade the superficial myocardium. By definition, primary pericardial mesothelioma necessitates lack of pleural involvement or primarily pericardial disease.

C. Pathology—Cytology may be obtained from pericardiocentesis though is often unrevealing. On histology, mesotheliomas can be epithelial, sarcomatous, and biphasic subtypes.

D. Associations —Unlike pleural mesotheliomas, pericardial mesotheliomas have not been clearly linked to asbestos exposure.

C. Benign or Malignant Cardiac Tumors

1. Paraganglioma: A catecholamine-secreting neuroendocrine tumor of the heart

A. Demographics—Cardiac paragangliomas are exceedingly rare, neuroendocrine tumors that originate from the paraganglionic cells surrounding the great vessels, coronary arteries, and atria. They can be either secretory or nonsecretory, depending on whether or not they produce catecholamines. Only 1–2% of all paragangliomas, or extra-adrenal chromaffin cell tumors, occur in the chest, with primary cardiac paragangliomas comprising only a subset of these.

B. Typical locations—Most paragangliomas are secretory and tend to arise from the visceral autonomic paraganglia of the left atrial wall or adjacent to the pulmonary trunk and ascending aorta.

C. Pathology—Histologically, paragangliomas are composed of discrete small nests of tumor cells in a "Zellballen" pattern. A subset of paragangliomas produce a characteristic melanin pigment. Approximately 10% of these tumors are malignant; however, this is not determined by pathology or immunohistochemistry but rather by occurrence of tumor in tissues not typically affected by paragangliomas. As these are highly vascular tumors often involving critical structures, surgical resection is challenging.

Zubair MM, El Nihum LI, Haley SL, et al. Large, Hormonally Active Primary Cardiac Paraganglioma: Diagnosis and Management. *Ann Thorac Surg.* 2022;113(3):e167–e170. [PMID: 34111385]. doi:10.1016/j.athoracsur.2021.05.042

2. Teratomas: The germ cell neoplasm of childhood

A. Demographics—Approximately half of cardiac teratomas are diagnosed in utero with the other half typically diagnosed in children under 15 years of age. With a similar incidence as fibromas, cardiac teratoma is the second or third most common primary cardiac tumor in pediatric series. There are rare reported cases of cardiac teratomas manifesting in adults.

B. Typical locations—Teratomas typically arise within the pericardium but occasionally have an intramyocardial origin, with a few reports of teratomas occurring in the ventricular or atrial septum (Figure 32–10).

C. Pathology—Teratomas are germ cell neoplasms that contain endodermal, mesodermal, and ectodermal elements. The composition of each teratoma varies, but if more than half the tumor is comprised of well-differentiated germinal elements, it is designated a mature teratoma (Figure 32–11). Cardiac teratomas can be either benign or malignant in nature.

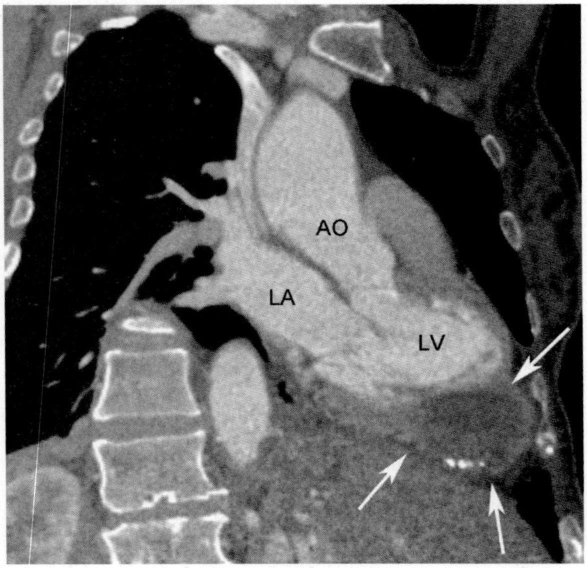

▲ **Figure 32–10.** Cardiac teratoma. Contrast-enhanced, multidetector computed tomography image of the heart in coronal section, performed in a 40-year-old woman with a history of ovarian cyst, presenting with chest pain. A cystic mass with areas of calcification involving the myocardium and pericardium was noted incidentally (*arrows*). The mass was resected and found to be a teratoma. AO, aorta; LA, left atrium; LV, left ventricle. (Reproduced with permission from Karen Ordovas.)

Tzani A, Doulamis IP, Mylonas KS, Avgerinos DV, Nasioudis D. Cardiac tumors in pediatric patients: a systematic review. *World J Pediatr Congenit Heart Surg*. 2017;8(5):624–632. [PMID: 28901236]. doi:10.1177/2150135117723904.

Yuan SM. Fetal primary cardiac tumors during perinatal period. *Pediatr Neonatol*. 2017;58(3):205–210.]PMID: 28043830]. doi:10.1016/j.pedneo.2016.07.004

D. Secondary Cardiac Tumors: The Far-Roaming Settlers

1. Demographics—Cardiac metastases are 20–40 times more common than primary cardiac tumors. Roughly 10% of patients with metastatic cancer have cardiac metastases. Secondary cardiac tumors affect a wide range of ages given the number and variety of cancers with a tendency toward secondary cardiac involvement.

2. Typical locations—Extracardiac malignancies can spread to the heart by one of four routes, including direct local invasion, lymphatic, hematogenous, and transvenous spread, as in the case of renal cell carcinoma which classically features extension of tumor thrombus into the inferior vena cava. Pericardial metastases are the most prevalent and often present with pericardial effusion and tamponade. Myocardial, coronary, and intracavitary involvement occur uncommonly, in order of decreasing frequency.

3. Common primary tumors associated with cardiac metastasis—Malignant melanoma has the highest predilection for cardiac spread, which is seen in as many as 50–65% of melanoma cases (Figure 32–12). Other neoplasms that commonly metastasize to the heart include carcinomas of the thorax such as breast, lung, and esophageal cancers, as well as hematologic tumors (eg, lymphoma and leukemia), renal cell carcinoma, and soft tissue sarcomas.

Clinical Findings

Cardiac tumors pose a significant challenge to diagnosis because they present with a wide array of signs and symptoms, many of which are nonspecific. Furthermore, it is often the size and anatomic location of the tumor, rather than its histopathologic features or malignant potential, that determine the clinical findings and the delay to presentation (Table 32–3).

A. Symptoms & Signs

Cardiac tumors present variably depending on their location within or around the heart. Tumors located in the pericardium often present with pericardial thickening, effusion, and/or tamponade and can manifest with pericardial constriction in the long term. Intracavitary tumors may obstruct blood flow or cause valvular obstruction or regurgitation ultimately leading to heart failure. Depending on the size and location of the intracavitary tumor, sudden cardiac death can be precipitated by obstruction, embolization into the coronary artery, or ventricular arrhythmias. Infiltrative cardiac tumors or those arising from the myocardium can cause heart failure symptoms from a restrictive or infiltrative cardiomyopathy. These tumors can also serve as a focus for atrial and ventricular arrhythmias, as well as create conduction system disturbances necessitating cardiac pacing.

Mechanical and obstructive manifestations of large cardiac tumors can produce effects on surrounding organs such as the respiratory and upper gastrointestinal tracts. Friable tumors, as a result of their unique tissue characteristics, are prone to causing both systemic and pulmonary emboli, and this can be further compounded by the presence of an atrial level shunt. Finally, like noncardiac malignancies, cardiac tumors can be associated with constitutional symptoms. Following are key examples of specific neoplasms and their typical presentations.

1. Heart failure—Malignant tumors or large-sized benign neoplasms like fibromas often present with heart failure from obstructive or restrictive pathology. Because angiosarcomas usually occur in the right atrium or pericardium, right-sided heart failure is often the presenting symptom. Cardiac lymphoma, due to its infiltrative nature, can lead to congestive heart failure symptoms from restriction.

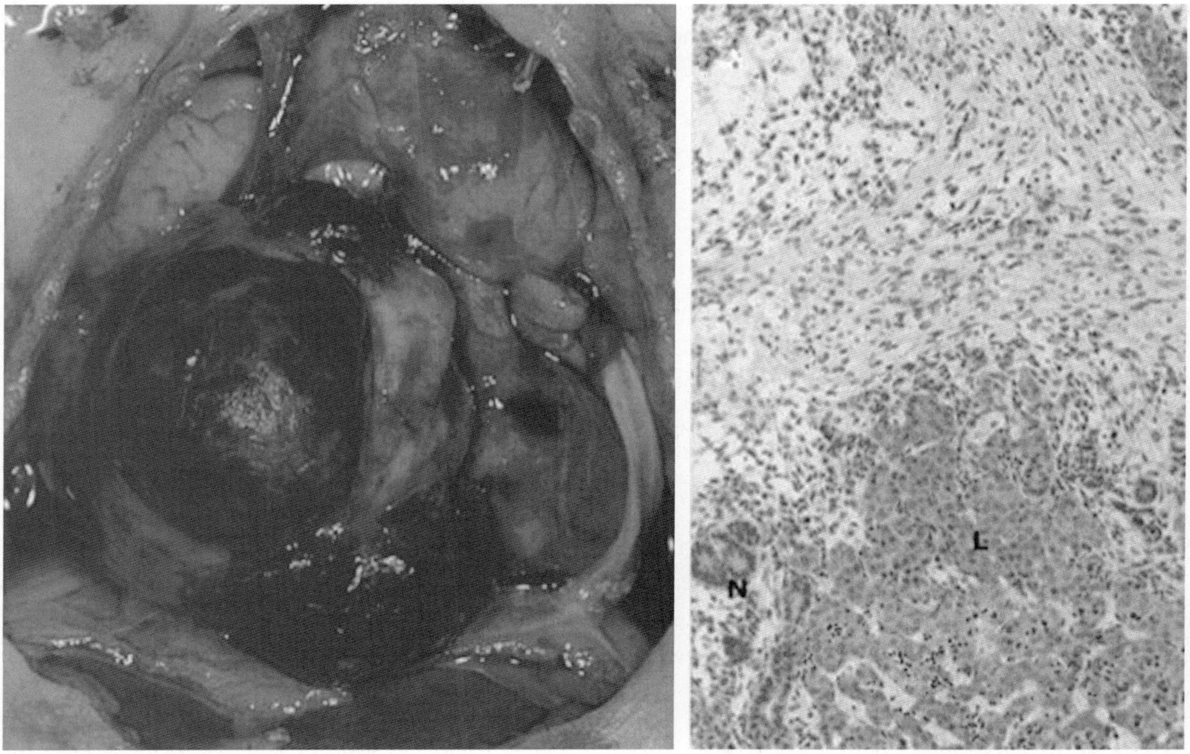

▲ **Figure 32–11.** **A:** Gross pathology: Postmortem specimen from a newborn infant with hydrops showing a large, encapsulated tumor arising from the pericardium and exerting a mass effect on the anterior cardiac chambers and the great vessels. **B:** Histology: Hematoxylin-eosin stain of the mass demonstrates liver (L) and neural (N) tissue, as well as glandular epithelium, consistent with a teratoma. (Reproduced with permission from Philip C. Ursell.)

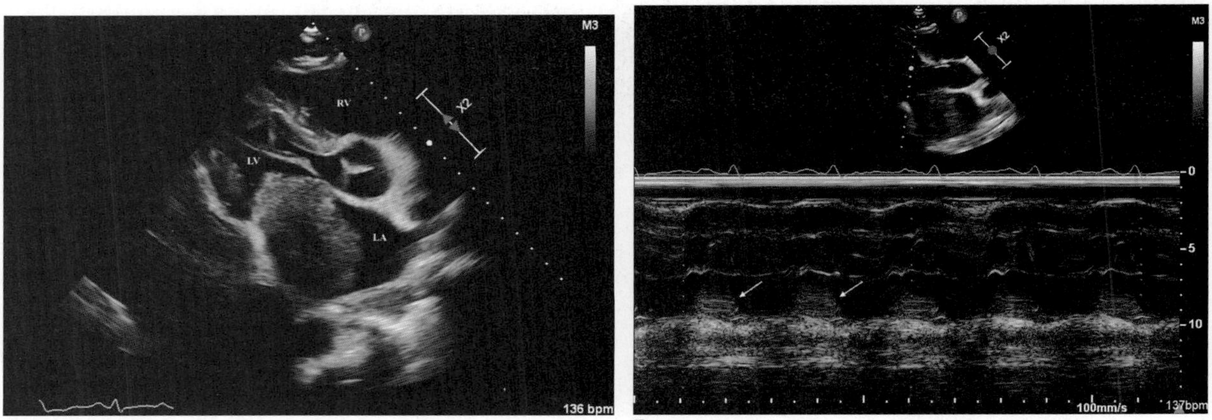

▲ **Figure 32–12.** Metastatic melanoma **A:** Transthoracic echocardiogram in a 35-year-old man with widely metastatic melanoma who presented with worsening respiratory distress. The parasternal long-axis view demonstrates a large, fairly homogenous left atrial mass, most likely representing metastatic melanoma, that occupies the majority of the left atrium and protrudes across the mitral valve during diastole. **B:** M-mode of the mitral valve showing the mass prolapsing into the left ventricle during diastole (*arrows*). LA, left atrium; LV, left ventricle; RV, right ventricle.

Table 32–3. Clinical Manifestations of Cardiac Tumors

Endocardial Involvement
Thromboembolism: cerebral, coronary, pulmonary, systemic
Cavity obliteration, outflow tract obstruction
Valve obstruction, valve damage
Myocardial Involvement
Arrhythmias: ventricular, atrial
Conduction abnormalities: sinus node, atrioventricular node, bundle branches
Left ventricular dysfunction: systolic, diastolic
Coronary artery involvement: angina, infarction
Electrocardiographic changes
Pericardial Involvement
Pericarditis
Pericardial effusion, tamponade
Pericardial constriction
Valvular Involvement
Valvular damage, obstruction, or regurgitation
Congestive heart failure
Sudden death or syncope
Vascular Involvement
Vessel dissection
Downstream embolism, infarction
Constitutional Symptoms
Fever
Night sweats
Anorexia
Weight loss

Cardiac or pericardial metastases may present with cardiomegaly, a new or changing murmur, or symptoms of heart failure.

2. Arrhythmia and sudden cardiac death—Left ventricular fibromas are associated with ventricular arrhythmias and can be associated with an increased risk of sudden cardiac death. Rhabdomyomas and cardiac hamartomas can also present with rhythm disturbances, such as heart block or ventricular tachycardia. Cardiac metastases may produce various arrhythmias and conduction delays depending on their location. Furthermore, an increased incidence of atrial arrhythmias has been noted in patients with atrial myxomas following surgical resection.

3. Angina/myocardial infarction—Papillary fibroelastomas can present with myocardial infarction and even sudden cardiac death if they obstruct a coronary ostium. In addition, any tumor that impinges on an epicardial coronary artery can predispose to anginal symptoms or frank myocardial infarction, as can be seen with cardiac lymphoma encasing the coronary arteries.

4. Obstructive and mechanical phenomena—Larger myxomas with smooth surfaces tend to present with obstructive cardiovascular symptoms, particularly at the level of the mitral valve, mimicking mitral stenosis. Fibromas exert a mass effect due to the large tumor burden, typically causing obstruction of left ventricular outflow. Similarly, rhabdomyomas may present with symptoms of obstruction. Most invasive cardiac malignancies and cardiac metastases can cause pericardial disease, often presenting with a pericardial effusion that may produce signs of tamponade and occasionally pericardial constriction. Malignant pericardial mesotheliomas can also present with pericarditis, tamponade, or constriction. Angiosarcomas, due to their predilection for the right atrium, can have vena caval obstruction as the presenting sign.

5. Embolic phenomena—Friable or villous cardiac myxomas are associated with a higher risk of embolization. Papillary fibroelastomas can form a nidus for platelet and fibrin aggregation and can present with embolic complications. Given the tumor's predilection for left-sided valves, papillary fibroelastomas more often lead to cerebrovascular and systemic emboli, though can also present with pulmonary embolism in the case of right-sided tumors.

6. Constitutional symptoms—Approximately 30% of patients with cardiac myxomas report constitutional symptoms such as fever, weight loss, arthralgias, and fatigue, which are thought to be secondary to various cytokines and growth factors secreted by the tumor such as interleukin-6 and tumor necrosis factor. Malignant primary cardiac tumors can produce constitutional symptoms such as cachexia, anorexia, and night sweats, similar to other noncardiac malignancies. However, these tumors usually present with heart failure, rhythm disturbances, or obstructive symptoms far before the onset of constitutional symptoms.

B. Physical Examination

The physical examination findings associated with cardiac tumors are generally nonspecific and often related to a secondary effect of the tumor, such as heart failure or an embolic complication. One of the characteristic physical examination findings ascribed to an intracardiac tumor, however, is the "tumor plop"—an auscultatory phenomenon resulting from the mechanical obstruction of the mitral valve orifice by the mass. The tumor plop should be heard in early diastole prior to the S_3 but after the opening snap, making it difficult to distinguish on auscultation. The coexistence of auscultatory features of mitral stenosis in the absence of a history of rheumatic fever should raise the possibility of an obstructive left atrial tumor.

Diagnostic Studies

Once limited to chest radiographs and angiography, the diagnostic armamentarium for cardiac neoplasms has grown expansively and continues to evolve with increasing sophistication of standard modalities like echocardiography, computed tomography (CT), cardiovascular magnetic resonance imaging (CMR), and positron emission tomography (PET). Advances in these noninvasive imaging techniques have

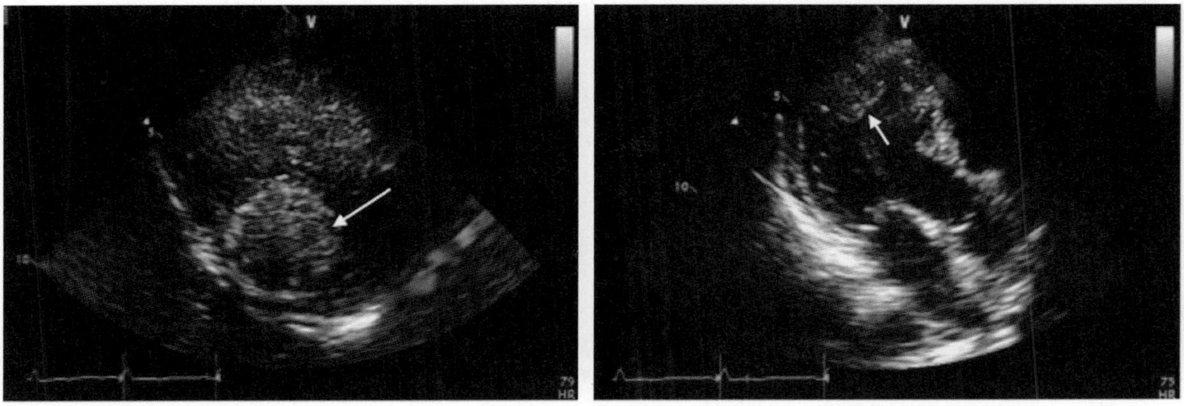

A B

▲ **Figure 32–13.** Cardiac fibroma. Transthoracic echocardiography parasternal short-axis view at the level of the cardiac apex (**A**) and apical three-chamber view (**B**) depicting an intramural mass in the left ventricle in a 57-year-old woman. Magnetic resonance imaging confirmed a T1 and T2 hypointense mass demonstrating delayed enhancement, consistent with the diagnosis of fibroma. (Reproduced with permission from Elyse Foster.)

facilitated the early, often incidental diagnosis of cardiac tumors. These imaging modalities can provide a wealth of information to both the cardiologist and the cardiac surgeon, aiding not only diagnosis but also therapeutic intervention and long-term surveillance. In many instances, particularly with benign cardiac tumors, a diagnosis can be reached without cardiac biopsy by using a structured imaging approach and relying on classic imaging features, location of the mass, and age at presentation to guide diagnosis.

A. Echocardiography

Due to the ease of image acquisition, lack of radiation, widespread availability, and relatively low cost, transthoracic echocardiography (TTE) is the favored initial diagnostic modality for cardiac tumors (Figure 32–13). TTE provides assessment of tumor size, location, and pericardial involvement. It has good spatial resolution making it the ideal imaging modality for assessing small, subcentimeter mobile masses or masses involving valves. Furthermore, TTE is crucial for understanding the hemodynamic consequences of a mass and any secondary valvular disease.

TTE is often followed by transesophageal echocardiography (TEE) when better characterization of atrial masses or valvular lesions is needed. Intraoperative TEE is crucial in aiding cardiac biopsy, guiding surgical intervention, assessing residual tumor burden, and detecting involvement of adjacent structures. TTE and occasionally TEE are also used as follow-up imaging modalities, both to look for recurrence after tumor resection and to monitor benign tumors that do not necessitate intervention.

In general, the sensitivity of both TTE and TEE is highest for endocardial lesions, as the mass is easily distinguished from the echolucent cardiac chamber. Their sensitivity is slightly lower for intramyocardial lesions and lowest for pericardial tumors. Despite high sensitivity, there are several important limitations of TTE, including poor acoustic windows, particularly in obese patients or those with chronic lung disease, difficulty in identifying tumor origin and extent given limited visualization of certain anatomy (eg, left atrial appendage, superior vena cava, extracardiac structures), and lack of tissue characterization. Although TEE offers improved spatial resolution and visualization of valves and posterior cardiac structures, it also remains the more invasive imaging modality (Figure 32–14).

Another valuable facet of echocardiography is the ability to perform real-time three-dimensional (3D) echocardiography, which is a volumetric method and thereby typically allows for visualization of the entire cardiac mass as opposed to a thin slice as seen in two-dimensional imaging. This leads to more accurate assessment of tumor size, shape, and anatomical relationships to adjacent structures. 3D echocardiography has been shown to be comparable to CMR for characterization of cardiac anatomy; however, unlike CMR, 3D echocardiography cannot delineate the vascularization of cardiac masses.

The use of ultrasound-enhancing agents, or echocardiographic contrast, allows for improved detection of smaller tumors and better visualization of intracavity masses, particularly in regard to their points of attachment and any invasion into surrounding cardiovascular structures (Figure 32–15). Perfusion contrast enhancement of cardiac masses can be used to help distinguish between vascular and nonvascular tumors. A mass demonstrating greater enhancement than the adjacent myocardium suggests a malignant, highly vascular tumor, while a poorly enhancing or nonenhancing mass suggests a benign tumor or a thrombus in the case of absent perfusion. However, this is not diagnostic.

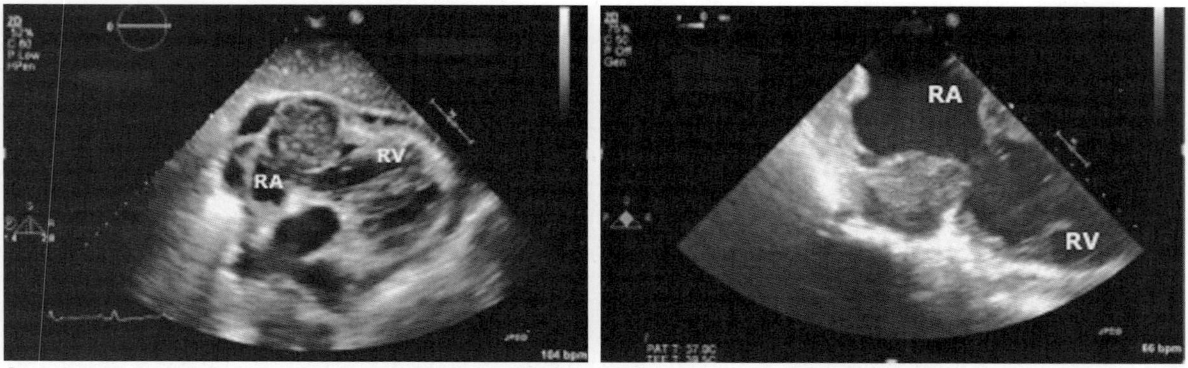

▲ **Figure 32–14.** Right atrial malignancy. **A:** Subcostal four-chamber view obtained on a transthoracic echocardiogram in a 54-year-old man with a malignant right atrial tumor. **B:** Transesophageal echocardiogram from the same patient; note the improved resolution of the tumor and the surrounding cardiac structures on this modality. RA, right atrium; RV, right ventricle.

Palaskas N, Thompson K, Gladish G, et al. Evaluation and management of cardiac tumors. Curr Treat Options Cardiovasc Med. 2018;20(4):29. Published 2018 Mar 20. [PMID: 29556752]. doi:10.1007/s11936-018-0625-z

Zaragoza-Macias E, Chen MA, Gill EA. Real time three-dimensional echocardiography evaluation of intracardiac masses [published correction appears in Echocardiography. 2012 May;29(5):i. Zaragosa-Macias, Elisa [corrected to Zaragoza-Macias, Elisa]]. *Echocardiography*. 2012;29(2):207-219. [PMID: 22283202]. doi:10.1111/j.1540-8175.2011.01627.x

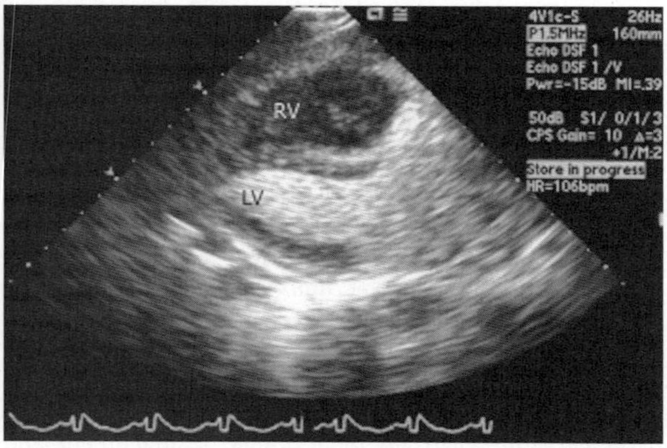

▲ **Figure 32–15.** Enhancement of intracardiac chambers using echocardiographic contrast agents. Transthoracic echocardiogram from a 59-year-old woman with endometrial cancer who presented with palpitations. Parasternal long-axis view using echocardiographic contrast demonstrates normal filling of the left ventricle (LV), with almost no filling of the right ventricle (RV), which is almost completely occupied by metastatic tumor from the endometrial cancer.

B. Cardiac Magnetic Resonance Imaging

CMR has emerged as an increasingly important diagnostic modality for cardiac tumors in recent years. Previously used to provide supplementary information to echocardiography and CT scans, CMR now plays a pivotal role in the primary diagnosis of neoplastic lesions of the heart. The high degree of natural contrast between the blood pool and cardiovascular structures permits clear delineation of cardiac masses. Furthermore, the direct multiplanar imaging capability of CMR is advantageous for demonstrating the complex relationships between cardiac masses and surrounding structures, while the lack of ionizing radiation is favorable. CMR can readily assess the dimensions, morphology, location, and extension of a cardiac mass; however, where it shines is its ability to provide tissue characterization.

Various signaling properties of a mass aid in histopathological characterization by indicating the presence of fatty infiltration, calcification, necrosis, hemorrhage, etc, which then can be correlated with specific diagnoses. For example, cardiac tumors demonstrate increased signal intensity on T2-weighted images, whereas fibrosis produces a low signal intensity. Delayed gadolinium enhancement with gadolinium in the context of a cardiac tumor indicates necrosis or nonviable tissue, often seen at the core of a tumor where cells have outgrown their blood supply. Gadolinium injection can also enhance highly vascular masses, as can the inversion recovery scouting sequence. The fat suppression technique on CMR can additionally detect adipose-rich tumors such as lipomas (Figure 32–16). Lastly, in patients with a suspected cardiac tumor, CMR has excellent diagnostic accuracy. In a large multicenter study of adult patients undergoing CMR for evaluation of suspected tumor, CMR diagnosis of pseudomass (ie, prominent normal structure or common variant), thrombus, benign tumor, and malignant tumor was accurate in more than 98% of patients. Accuracy of CMR for

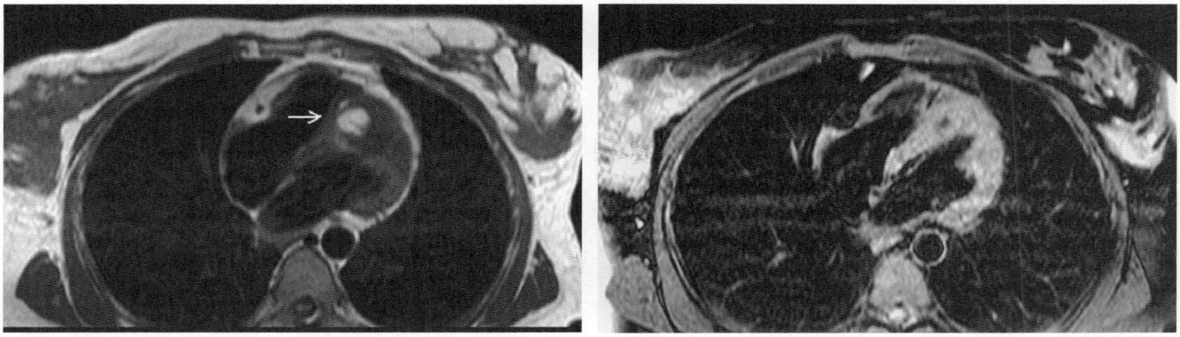

A B

▲ **Figure 32–16.** Cardiac lipoma. **A:** T1-weighted transaxial spin-echo magnetic resonance image of the heart through the level of the interventricular septum. A high-signal-intensity mass (*arrow*) is seen embedded in the distal anteroseptum. **B:** During application of fat saturation pulse, the mass loses its bright signal, suggesting the diagnosis of a cardiac lipoma. (Reproduced with permission from C. Higgins.)

diagnosis of cardiac masses has also been demonstrated in pediatric populations.

The main limitation of CMR compared with echocardiography is its lower temporal resolution. As such, it is not typically indicated for evaluation of valvular vegetations. Additional disadvantages include long acquisition times often requiring breath-holds, limited availability compared with echocardiography and CT, potential for claustrophobia, artifact from implantable cardiac devices, and contraindications such as older generation implantable cardiac devices.

Beroukhim RS, Ghelani S, Ashwath R, et al. Accuracy of Cardiac Magnetic Resonance Imaging Diagnosis of Pediatric Cardiac Masses: A Multicenter Study. *JACC Cardiovasc Imaging.* 2022; 8:1391–1405. doi:10.1016/j.jcmg.2021.07.010

Shenoy C, Grizzard JD, Shah DJ, et al. Cardiovascular magnetic resonance imaging in suspected cardiac tumour: a multicentre outcomes study. *Eur Heart J.* 2021;43(1):71–80. [PMID: 34545397]. doi:10.1093/eurheartj/ehab635fta

C. Computed Tomography

Cardiac CT is a rapid acquisition imaging technique that provides high-quality images with superior spatial resolution to CMR. Electrocardiographic (ECG) gating used with cardiac CT minimizes motion-related artifacts, resulting in improved image quality, and CT is an excellent option for patients with implanted devices who cannot undergo CMR. The superior spatial resolution of CT allows for accurate delineation of tumor size and location, degree of local invasion, and involvement of coronary arteries and other vasculature. In particular, CT is optimal for the evaluation of calcified masses and provides anatomic detail that is often crucial for preoperative planning.

In recent years, advances in multidetector CT hardware and post-processing software have made 3D reconstructions a useful tool in the evaluation of cardiac masses. These reconstructions can allow for better appreciation of tumor margins and relationships with surrounding structures, making them useful adjuncts in surgical planning. Finally, 3D printing of cardiac models is an emerging technology being used primarily for preoperative planning in patients with congenital heart disease, though its use has also been reported in cases of cardiac masses. While volumetric 3D echocardiography and CMR can also be used to generate 3D models, CT has been the predominant imaging modality for 3D printing largely due to its submillimeter spatial resolution.

Notable disadvantages of CT include radiation exposure, particularly in the pediatric population, a small risk of contrast-induced nephropathy, limited tissue characterization abilities, and lower temporal resolution as compared with CMR.

Al Jabbari O, Abu Saleh WK, Patel AP, Igo SR, Reardon MJ. Use of three-dimensional models to assist in the resection of malignant cardiac tumors. *J Card Surg.* 2016;31(9):581–583. [PMID: 27455392]. doi:10.1111/jocs.12812

Liddy S, McQuade C, Walsh KP, Loo B, Buckley O. The assessment of cardiac masses by cardiac CT and CMR including pre-op 3D reconstruction and planning. *Curr Cardiol Rep.* 2019;21(9):103. [PMID: 31367849]. Published 2019 Jul 31. doi:10.1007/s11886-019-1196-7

Vukicevic M, Mosadegh B, Min JK, Little SH. Cardiac 3D printing and its future directions. *JACC Cardiovasc Imaging.* 2017;10(2):171–184. [PMID: 28183437]. doi:10.1016/j.jcmg.2016.12.001

Wu CM, Bergquist PJ, Srichai MB. Multimodality imaging in the evaluation of intracardiac masses. *Curr Treat Options Cardiovasc Med.* 2019;21(10):55. [PMID: 314869926]. Published 2019 Sep 5. doi:10.1007/s11936-019-0756-x

D. Positron Emission Tomography

Whole-body ^{18}F-Fluorodeoxyglucose PET (^{18}F-FDG PET) is routinely used to look for distant metastases in patients with high-risk cancers, such as renal cell carcinoma or lung cancer. It can be useful in detecting cardiac metastases in an asymptomatic patient during staging of the primary malignancy. Moreover, ^{18}F-FDG PET can be helpful in differentiating benign from malignant cardiac masses on the basis of metabolic activity and can identify metastatic lesions which are more amenable to biopsy than cardiac masses.

Hybrid imaging using ^{18}F-FDG PET/CT has been shown to be both sensitive and specific for distinguishing benign from malignant tumors preoperatively in multiple small studies. More recently, integrated imaging with ^{18}F-FDG PET/CMR was demonstrated to be highly sensitive and specific for classification of benign versus malignant lesions in appropriately selected patients. While the role of ^{18}F-FDG PET in assessing response to chemotherapy or radiation and evaluating postoperative residual disease has been established for several malignancies and is commonly done in the case of secondary cardiac tumors (eg, lymphoma with cardiac involvement), there is a lack of data with regard to primary cardiac malignancies.

Martineau P, Dilsizian V, Pelletier-Galarneau M. Incremental value of FDG-PET in the evaluation of cardiac masses. *Curr Cardiol Rep*. 2021;23(7):78. [PMID: 34081218]. Published 2021 Jun 3. doi:10.1007/s11886-021-01509-z

E. Coronary Angiography

Coronary angiography can be useful in the workup of selected cardiac tumors. Cardiac neoplasms may have their own blood supply as a result of tumor angiogenesis, but they can also invade and involve epicardial coronary arteries. Evaluation of cardiac tumors frequently includes cardiac catheterization to evaluate coronary anatomy and to determine whether contrast enhancement, or "tumor blush," is present. The appearance of tumor blush has been described in many cardiac tumors such as myxomas, hemangiomas, rhabdomyomas, and angiosarcomas. Tumor blush itself is diagnostic of a cardiac tumor and can indicate which type of neoplasm is likely present. Since certain tumors characteristically appear in specific locations, the associated epicardial coronary blood supply to the lesion and the territory of the blush can aid substantially in tumor localization and identification.

Marok R, Klein LW. Tumor blush in primary cardiac tumors. *J Invasive Cardiol*. 2012;24(3):139–140. [PMID: 22388311]

Differential Diagnosis

Several normal and abnormal intra- and extracardiac structures can confound the diagnosis of cardiac tumors. Imaging features that favor a neoplastic process are a mobile, pedunculated appearance and an associated pericardial effusion. Masses that cross anatomic planes, from myocardium to pericardium or endocardium, are more likely to be tumors as well (Table 32–4).

Table 32–4. Differential Diagnoses of Cardiac Tumors

Intracardiac Structures, Normal Variants
Lipomatous hypertrophy of the interatrial septum
Eustachian valve
Chiari network
Septum spurium
Thrombus
Vegetation
Infective endocarditis
Nonbacterial thrombotic endocarditis
Libman-Sacks endocarditis
Caseous Calcification of the Mitral Annulus
Pericardial Cysts
Calcified Amorphous Tumor (CAT)
Extracardiac Structures
Diaphragmatic hernia
Loculated pleural effusion
Mediastinal mass/tumor

A. Normal Variant Structures

A sizable number of intracardiac structures that occur as anatomic variants can be mistaken for cardiac neoplasms. These include the Eustachian valve (Figure 32–17), seen at the junction of the inferior vena cava and the right atrium, and the Chiari network, a remnant of the sinus venosus, also encountered in the right atrium. The septum spurium is a superior fold at the coronary sinus opening, which can mimic an intracardiac mass, along with the Thebesian valve, which guards the opening to the coronary sinus. Lambl's excrescences have been described as filiform frond-like structures that are noted at sites of valve closure, particularly on the aortic and mitral valves.

Although lipomatous hypertrophy of the interatrial septum can imitate a tumor (Figure 32–18), it is easily distinguished by its characteristic location along the interatrial septum and its dumbbell-shaped appearance (See Figure 32–4). The shape is due to the thin fossa ovalis that separates the lipomatous atrial septum on either side. No intervention is required unless the hypertrophy causes arrhythmias or obstruction.

B. Thrombus

Intracardiac thrombi are fairly easy to differentiate from cardiac tumors if an astute assessment is made of the company they keep. For instance, left ventricular thrombi are associated with regional wall motion abnormalities and cardiomyopathies, particularly in the setting of an akinetic left ventricular apex (Figure 32–19). Left atrial thrombi may be associated with atrial fibrillation, left atrial enlargement, or mitral stenosis, whereas right atrial thrombi can be seen attached to indwelling catheters or pacemaker wires. Right ventricular thrombi, on the other hand, have been described

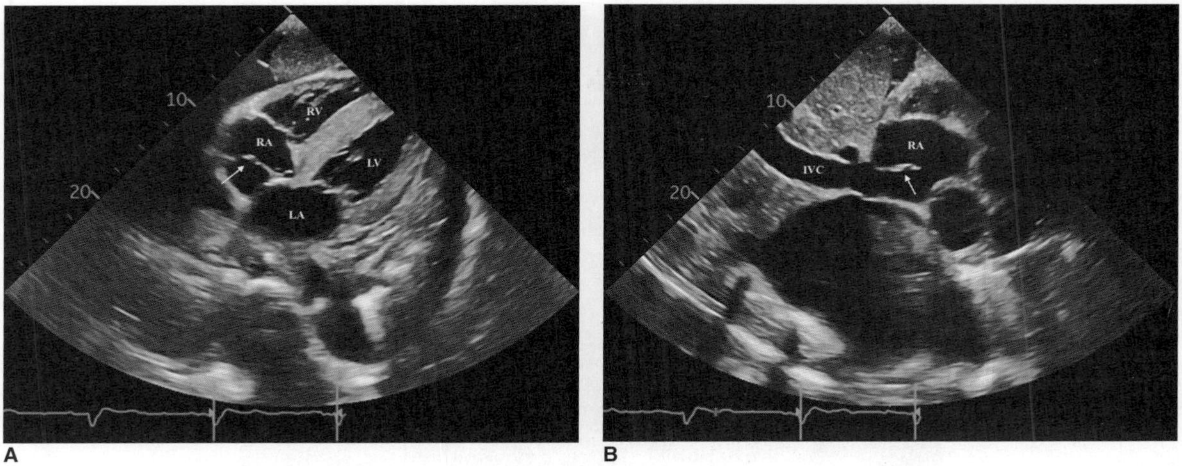

▲ **Figure 32–17.** Eustachian valve. **A:** Transthoracic echocardiogram in the subcostal view demonstrating a prominent Eustachian valve (*arrow*). This appearance has been erroneously called triatriatum dexter. **B:** Additional subcostal view showing the Eustachian valve (*arrow*) as a linear structure at the junction of the inferior vena cava and the right atrium. IVC, inferior vena cava; LA, left atrium; LV, left ventricle; RA, right atrium; RV, right ventricle.

in the setting of impaired right ventricular function and are often associated with pulmonary emboli.

C. Vegetation

A vegetation is defined on echocardiography as an independently mobile, oscillatory, echodense mass. Intracardiac vegetations can be infected or sterile and have certain imaging characteristics that can provide clues to their etiology. The vegetations associated with infective endocarditis are typically large and involve the valvular surface or endocardium in the trajectory of the regurgitant jet. These vegetations are associated with other clinical, laboratory, and

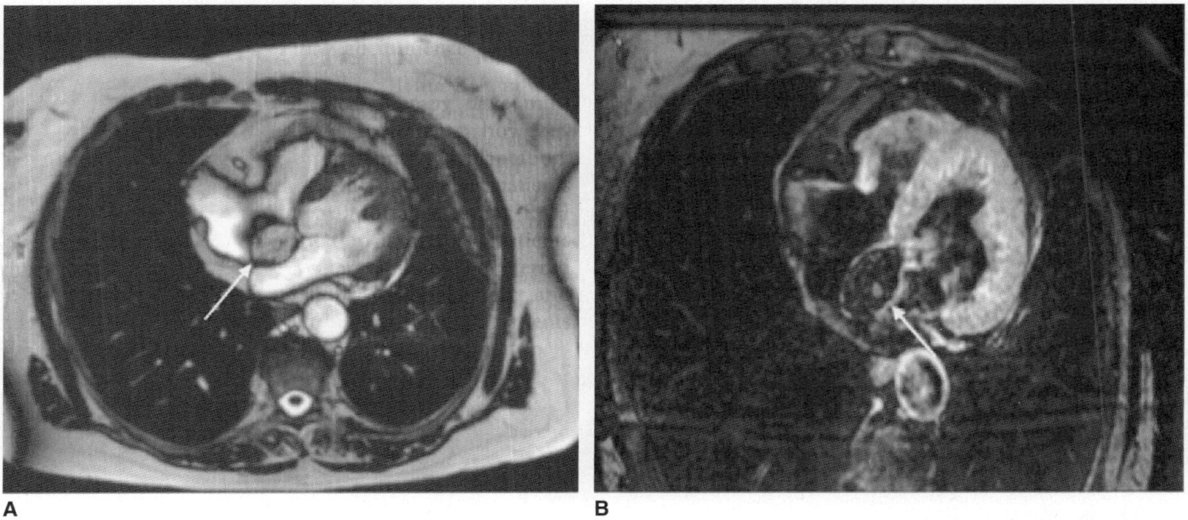

▲ **Figure 32–18.** Lipomatous hypertrophy of the interatrial septum. **A:** Steady-state free procession cine magnetic resonance image of the heart, demonstrating diffuse fatty infiltration of the right atrial wall, interatrial septum, and right ventricular free wall. There is sparing of the fossa ovalis, characteristic of lipomatous hypertrophy of the interatrial septum (*arrow*). **B:** After application of a fat saturation pulse, the infiltrative process in image A is no longer bright, indicative of fat content in the tissues. (Reproduced with permission from Kanae Mukai.)

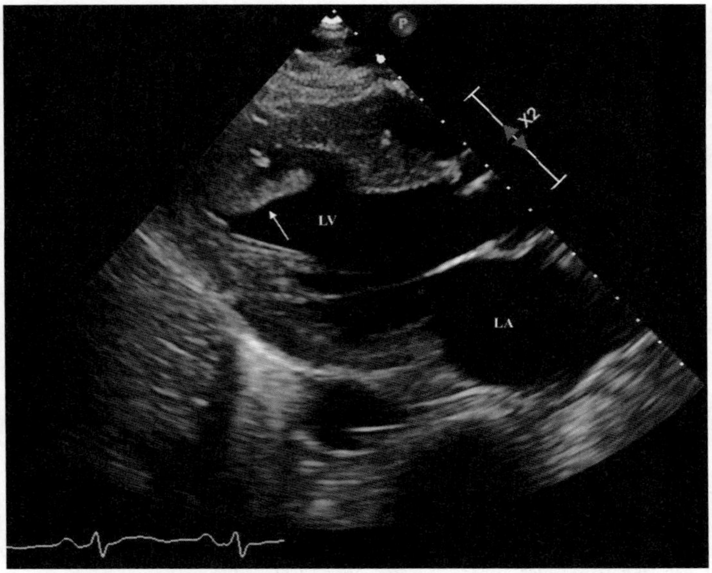

▲ **Figure 32–19.** Left ventricular thrombus. Transthoracic echocardiogram performed in a 67-year-old man with known coronary artery disease who presented with an embolic stroke shows akinesis of the left ventricular septal and anterior walls with a large, mobile echodense mass (*arrow*) at the left ventricular apex, consistent with thrombus. LA, left atrium; LV, left ventricle.

echocardiographic criteria for infective endocarditis and are more prevalent in certain demographic groups such as intravenous drug users, the immunocompromised, and those with prosthetic cardiac material. Nonbacterial thrombotic endocarditis (NBTE) and Libman-Sacks endocarditis are two distinct entities both comprised of sterile vegetations. The vegetations associated with NBTE, or marantic endocarditis, are small and located along the closure lines of valves; they are often associated with wasting conditions, such as cancer. Libman-Sacks endocarditis is one of the classic cardiovascular lesions associated with systemic lupus erythematosus, in which the sterile vegetations are located on both surfaces of involved cardiac valves.

D. Caseous Calcification of the Mitral Annulus

Caseous calcification of the mitral valve is a rare form of mitral annular calcification that typically affects the posterior mitral annulus (Figure 32–20). The condition, also referred to as liquefaction necrosis, usually runs a benign course, although it has been associated with valvular dysfunction and cerebral embolization of necrotic material. Differential diagnosis includes cardiac tumor and valvular abscess, warranting complementary imaging techniques for accurate assessment of this pathology.

Gulati A, Chan C, Duncan A, Raza S, Kilner PJ, Pepper J. Multimodality cardiac imaging in the evaluation of mitral annular caseous calcification. *Circulation*. 2011;123(1):e1–2. [PMID: 21200011]

E. Pericardial Cysts

Pericardial cysts are usually congenital abnormalities but can be acquired after cardiac surgery. They are typically located in the right or left costophrenic angles and can be identified on a chest x-ray or echocardiogram by their unilocular nature. Pericardial cysts are often asymptomatic or produce mild symptoms of chest pain and dyspnea. Occasionally, these cysts can rupture into the pericardial space resulting in cardiac tamponade.

F. Extracardiac Structures

A diaphragmatic hernia can mimic a left atrial mass on TTE. TEE, on the other hand, can help diagnose the hernia by showing an extracardiac structure indenting the left atrium posteriorly and the swirling heterogenous echodensities within this structure caused by the motion of the gastric contents. A loculated pleural effusion can also mimic a mass on echocardiography and, depending on its location, may indent either of the atrial chambers. Similarly, mediastinal masses and tumors can indent cardiac structures and produce a mass effect. This confusion can be readily mitigated, however, by using other imaging modalities, such as CT or CMR.

G. Calcified Amorphous Tumor

Calcified amorphous tumors (CATs) are nonneoplastic cardiac masses that consist of calcified nodules or flecks of calcification within a background of eosinophilic, amorphous, or fibrillary material. The true incidence of CATs is unknown,

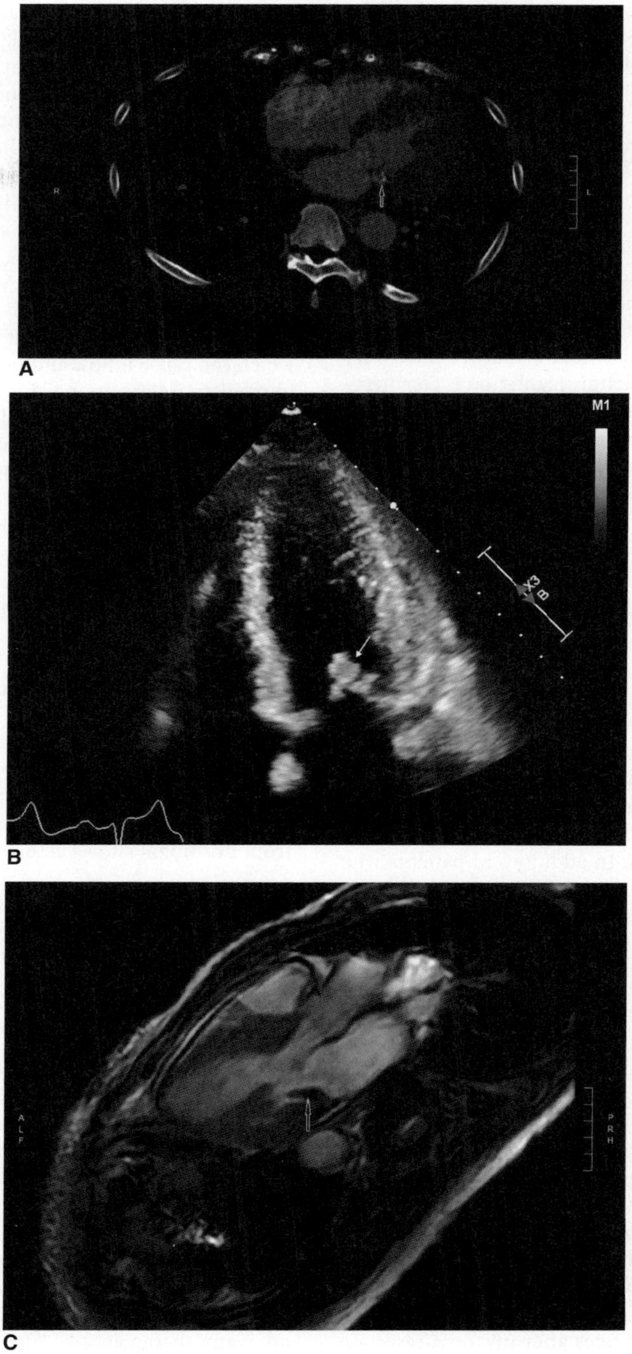

▲ **Figure 32–20.** Caseous mitral annular calcification. **A:** Contrast-enhanced axial cardiac computed tomography demonstrates heterogeneous calcification along the posterior mitral annulus (*arrow*). **B:** Transthoracic echocardiogram in the same patient shows a large echogenic lesion on the posterior mitral valve leaflet (*arrow*) with an area of central lucency. The lesion extends into the posterior subvalvular apparatus. **C:** Steady-state free precession cine magnetic resonance image in the three-chamber view demonstrates mass-like, low intensity thickening of the posterior mitral valve leaflet (*arrow*) and proximal posteromedial papillary muscle, compatible with caseous mitral annular calcification.

but they appear to compose only a very small portion of the nonneoplastic intracavitary cardiac masses, with approximately 30 cases reported in the literature.

Hussain N, Rahman N, Rehman A. Calcified amorphous tumors (CATs) of the heart. *Cardiovasc Pathol.* 2014;23(6):369–371. [PMID: 25123614]

Treatment

Cardiac neoplasms remain a rare group of entities with limited therapeutic options that mostly focus on tumor removal and debulking with a very limited role for chemotherapy and radiation. For certain cardiac tumors that are either very large or highly invasive, cardiac transplantation is an emerging option, with some data suggesting improved survival rates with orthotopic heart transplantation. However, given the concern for recurrence of the primary malignancy on the posttransplantation immunosuppression regimen, further research is warranted at this time.

A. Surgery

Surgical excision is typically the primary treatment option for all cardiac tumors. Surgery can often prove curative for benign tumors, and even for malignant tumors, it can significantly improve symptoms and quality of life. In patients who present with embolic complications or symptoms of obstruction, timely surgical intervention is required regardless of whether a tumor is benign or malignant. While most tumors will require open heart surgery, there have recently been case reports of minimally invasive resection of aortic valve papillary fibroelastomas. In addition, in patients who are exceedingly high risk for surgical excision, there have been reports of successful use of the AngioVac vacuum-assisted thrombectomy device for debulking or extraction of right atrial masses. However, further study is required to establish any clinical benefit.

1. Benign tumors—Although benign by definition, a significant portion of primary cardiac tumors may require expeditious surgical removal given the heart's limited ability to tolerate space-occupying lesions. Furthermore, tumors that appear large or friable on imaging studies should be considered for expedited surgery to mitigate the high pulmonary and systemic embolic risk, as well as the risk of sudden cardiac death from intracavitary lesions.

Myxomas and large (≥ 1 cm), left-sided, mobile papillary fibroelastomas are considered to have high embolic potential and should be removed expeditiously (Figure 32–21). Postoperatively, the mortality rates after myxoma resection are very good, although patients are at risk for atrial arrhythmias and atrioventricular nodal conduction abnormalities. Although there is a small but significant risk of myxoma recurrence after removal, recurrence of cardiac papillary fibroelastoma following surgical resection has not been reported in the literature.

Smaller papillary fibroelastomas and cardiac lipomas (< 1 cm), on the other hand, are often asymptomatic and do not warrant surgical therapy. Cardiac fibromas typically involve large areas of ventricular myocardium and can be a focus for life-threatening ventricular arrhythmias. For this reason, complete and prompt surgical resection is recommended, despite the fact that a large amount of ventricular tissue may be jeopardized in the process, necessitating reconstructive surgery with a synthetic patch.

Rhabdomyomas are best managed conservatively in the asymptomatic patient. Most rhabdomyomas regress spontaneously in childhood or early adolescence. However, symptoms often result from large rhabdomyomas, which can cause inflow and outflow obstruction, warranting immediate intervention. These lesions tend to be multiple, nonencapsulated, and embedded in myocardial tissue, often necessitating extensive surgical dissection. As resection usually involves large territories of myocardium, patients can require inotropic support postoperatively.

Cardiac teratomas, even when benign, can have serious mechanical complications very early in life. Therefore, appropriate treatment includes tumor resection in the fetus or cesarean section delivery and immediate surgical removal of the tumor in the infant.

Paragangliomas can be either benign or malignant, and a subgroup of these tumors are hormonally active, producing catecholamines that give rise to symptoms associated with heightened sympathetic activity. Although surgical excision is the treatment of choice for this tumor, perioperative α- and β-adrenergic blockade is warranted at the time of intervention to prevent catastrophic clinical outcomes from hormonal surges associated with tumor handling.

Enezate T, Alkhatib D, Raja J, Chinta V, Patel M, Omran J. AngioVac for minimally invasive removal of intravascular and intracardiac masses: a systematic review. *Curr Cardiol Rep.* 2022;24(4):377–382. doi:10.1007/s11886-022-01658-9.

Nisivaco SM, Patel B, Balkhy HH. Robotic totally endoscopic excision of aortic valve papillary fibroelastoma: The least invasive approach. *J Card Surg.* 2019;34(12):1492–1497. [PMID: 35129741]. doi:10.1111/jocs.14291.

2. Malignant tumors—Given that the prognosis of malignant cardiac tumors is extremely poor overall, surgery is often performed to relieve symptoms rather than to prolong life. Aggressive and invasive tumors such as cardiac sarcomas often present with mechanical symptoms from obstruction or compression but are not amenable to complete surgical resection. Debulking of the primary tumor can relieve symptoms though is typically only palliative unless adjuvant therapies are effective. Furthermore, given the propensity for primary malignant cardiac tumors to invade surrounding structures, including blood vessels, in-hospital mortality is high.

For metastatic cardiac lesions, surgery may occasionally be performed if there is a high likelihood of complete remission from the primary tumor. However, most commonly,

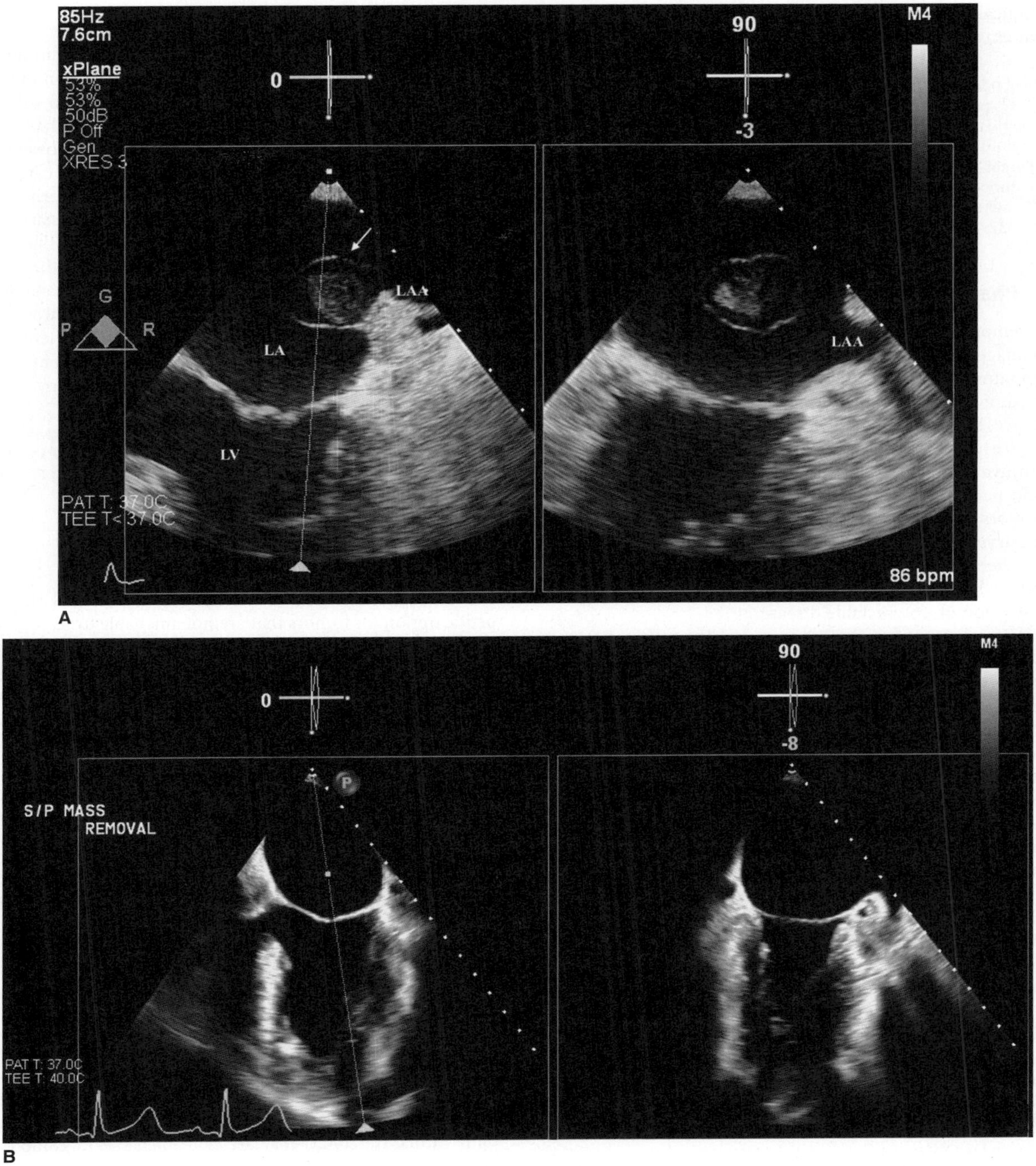

▲ **Figure 32–21.** Left atrial myxoma. **A:** Preoperative transesophageal echocardiogram in a 58-year-old woman referred for further work up after a left atrial mass was discovered incidentally on chest computed tomography scan shows a large, heterogeneous mass (*arrow*) attached to the lateral atrial wall, adjacent to the left atrial appendage. **B:** Postoperative transesophageal echocardiogram shows complete resection of the atrial myxoma following minimally invasive resection. LA, left atrium; LAA, left atrial appendage; LV, left ventricle.

surgical intervention is undertaken for palliative reasons in patients with cardiac metastases.

Svobodov AA, Glushko LA, Ergashov AY. Surgical treatment of primary cardiac tumors in children systematic review and meta-analysis. *Pediatr Cardiol.* 2022;43(2):251–266. doi:10.1007/s00246-022-02814-2.

Torabi S, Arjomandi Rad A, Vardanyan R, et al. Surgical and multimodality treatment of cardiac sarcomas: A systematic review and meta-analysis. *J Card Surg.* 2021;36(7):2476–2485. [PMID: 33797789]. doi:10.1111/jocs.15538

B. Pharmacologic Therapy

Chemotherapy does not have an established role in the management of benign tumors, where cardiac surgery remains the gold standard of treatment. However, in the case of rhabdomyomas associated with TSC, current evidence suggests that sirolimus, an mTOR inhibitor, can increase the regression rate of cardiac rhabdomyomas. Adjuvant chemotherapy regimens containing doxorubicin and paclitaxel have been used to treat malignant cardiac tumors such as sarcomas; however, the data to support a survival benefit with this approach are limited. Chemotherapy has also been used in this context for tumor cytoreduction in preparation for surgical resection and for palliation of unresectable disease.

Primary cardiac lymphoma, on the other hand, is considered more responsive to chemotherapy. A regimen using CHOP (cyclophosphamide, doxorubicin, vincristine, and prednisone), when combined with surgery, radiation, or both, has been shown to induce complete remission in one-third of patients, with a reported median survival of 1 year. This chemotherapy regimen has also been shown to effectively treat distant metastases from primary cardiac lymphomas. Therapy with the monoclonal CD20 antibody rituximab and autologous stem cell transplantation can also yield beneficial results. In patients with primary cardiac lymphoma, it is imperative to perform the first cycle of chemotherapy with close monitoring, as the infiltrative nature of the tumor and the potential brisk response to chemotherapy may result in tumor lysis syndrome.

Rhabdomyosarcomas have been shown to have a better outcome with chemotherapy when compared to other cardiac malignancies, and adjuvant chemotherapy regimens have been tried with varying degrees of success.

Chen XQ, Wang YY, Zhang MN, et al. Sirolimus Can Increase the Disappearance Rate of Cardiac Rhabdomyomas Associated with Tuberous Sclerosis: A Prospective Cohort and Self-Controlled Case Series Study. *J Pediatr.* 2021;233:150–155.e4. [PMID: 33631166]. doi:10.1016/j.jpeds.2021.02.040

Gyoten T, Doi T, Nagura S, et al. Primary cardiac malignant lymphoma: survival for 13 years after surgical resection and adjuvant chemotherapy. *Ann Thorac Surg.* 2015;99(3):1060–1062. [PMID: 25742830]

C. Radiation

The role of radiotherapy alone or as adjuvant is also limited. The high doses of radiation used to treat sarcomas in other locations are poorly tolerated by the heart, leading to short-term and long-term cardiac toxicity. Radiotherapy has not been shown to systematically prolong survival; however, there are anecdotal reports of its success in cases of cardiac sarcoma, in particular rhabdomyosarcoma. While primary cardiac sarcomas are relatively radio-insensitive, metastatic lesions associated with this tumor can be managed with radiation. With regards to primary cardiac lymphoma, the role of adjuvant radiotherapy remains controversial, with studies showing little to no improvement in overall survival when combined with systemic chemotherapy. However, there are reports of its successful use as salvage therapy in patients not achieving complete remission following chemotherapy.

Cichowska-Cwalińska N, Dutka M, Klapkowski A, Pęksa R, Maciej Zaucha J, Zaucha R. The role of radiotherapy in the management of primary cardiac lymphoma a case report and the literature review. *Leuk Lymphoma.* 2019;60(3):812–816. doi:10.1080/10428194.2018.1509321.

D. Cardiac Transplantation

Cardiac transplantation is emerging as a potential therapeutic option for tumors that are not amenable to resection, either because the tumor is too extensive or too infiltrative to allow for complete removal. Fibromas that involve large territories of the left ventricle have been successfully treated with cardiac transplantation, as have vastly invasive cardiac sarcomas in the absence of extracardiac disease. Cardiac transplantation has also been used for certain cases of recurrent atrial myxomas. This approach is limited by the potential for posttransplant recurrence, which may be accelerated by immunosuppressive therapy.

Rodriguez-Gonzalez M, Pérez-Reviriego AA, et al. Primary cardiac fibroma in infants: A case report and review of cases of cardiac fibroma managed through orthotopic heart transplant. *Ann Pediatr Cardiol.* 2021;14(2):224–227. [PMID: 25742830]. doi:10.4103/apc.APC_78_20.

E. Palliation

With newer and more scientific approaches to palliative care in the current medical milieu, terminal life-limiting cardiac neoplasms can be treated with palliation in cases where surgical outcomes are known to be poor. Specifically, in patients with cardiac sarcomas that are not amenable to complete resection, palliative surgery may be performed to relieve mechanical symptoms. In patients with malignant pericardial mesothelioma, a tumor with a poor response to chemotherapy and radiation, surgical pericardiectomy can serve as a palliative measure. In addition, in carefully selected patients with cardiac metastases, resection of metastatic lesions may provide symptomatic improvement and prolong life.

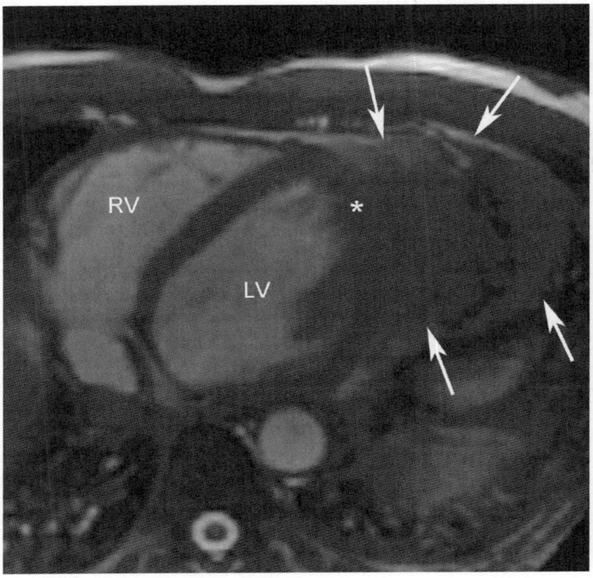

A

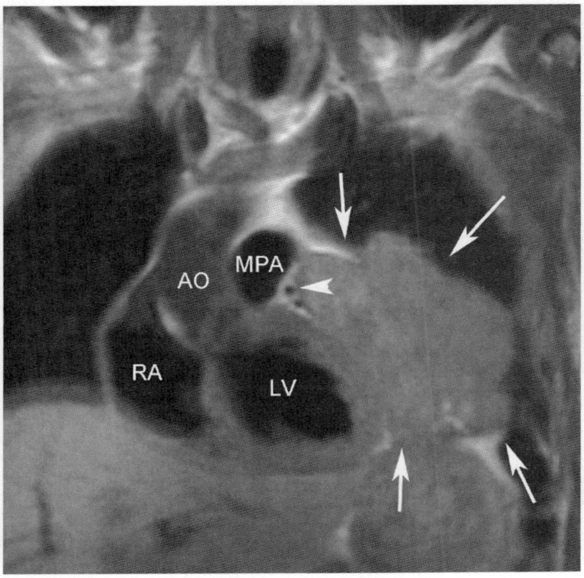

B

▲ **Figure 32–22.** Metastatic cardiac tumors. **A:** Magnetic resonance imaging of the heart in a 50-year-old man who presented with dyspnea on exertion 3 months after being diagnosed with a melanoma on his back. A large pericardial mass was demonstrated on this bright blood-cine steady-state free precession magnetic resonance image in the axial plane. The *arrows* show the extension of the mass into the pleural space and possibly lung parenchyma. The *asterisk* indicates different texture of the myocardial signal, suggesting myocardial invasion of the mass. **B:** Coronal black-blood T1-weighted image showing extension of the mass anteriorly and superiorly to impinge on the proximal left anterior descending artery (*arrowhead*). Biopsy of the mass confirmed metastatic melanoma. AO, aorta; LV, left ventricle; MPA, main pulmonary artery; RA, right atrium; RV, right ventricle.

Prognosis

The prognosis for cardiac tumors varies significantly with the nature of the neoplasm. For primary cardiac tumors, surgical resection usually results in complete cure if the tumor is benign. However, 1.5% of myxomas can recur within 10–15 years, usually in patients with familial or syndromic myxomas. For this reason, patients should be monitored with serial echocardiograms approximately every 5 years after resection.

Malignant primary cardiac tumors, in contrast, have a dismal long-term prognosis, most commonly because of early local invasion, metastatic spread, or recurrence after removal. Survival time, as expected, correlates inversely with tumor size and the degree of regional tumor extension at the time of surgery. In a large cohort of patients within the past decade, 1-, 3-, and 5-year survival rates were found to be 50%, 24%, and 19%, respectively.

The overall prognosis with cardiac sarcomas is very poor, with mean survival ranging from 9.6 to 16.5 months. Irrespective of histologic type, common features that predict a less aggressive disease course are location in the left atrium, low mitotic activity with scarce cellular pleomorphism on pathology, and absence of metastasis or necrosis. The survival of patients with primary cardiac lymphoma can be as long as 5 years with appropriate therapy but whittles down significantly if left untreated, to as low as 1 month. The median survival with cardiac lymphoma is just 7 months after initial diagnosis and is likely a result of distant metastasis, which can occur even after seemingly successful eradication of the primary cardiac tumor. When paragangliomas are completely resected, a 10-year survival rate as high as 84% has been reported in some series. However, postoperative recurrence rates for these tumors are in the 50% range, making routine surveillance imperative.

The prognosis for secondary cardiac tumors from metastases is uniformly poor, and long-term survival rates are similar to those quoted for the metastatic spread of each individual neoplasm (Figure 32–22).

Oliveira GH, et al. Characteristics and survival of malignant cardiac tumors: a 40-year analysis of over 500 patients. *Circulation.* 2015;132:2395–2402. [PMID: 26467256]

Padalino MA, Vida VL, Boccuzzo G, et al. Surgery for primary cardiac tumors in children: early and late results in a multicenter European Congenital Heart Surgeons Association study. Circulation. 2012;126(1):22–30. [PMID: 22626745]. doi:10.1161/CIRCULATIONAHA.111.037226

33 Cardiovascular Disease in Pregnancy

Kirsten Tolstrup, MD
Joyce N. Njoroge, MD

ESSENTIALS OF DIAGNOSIS

- Pregnancy.
- History of heart disease.
- Symptoms and signs of heart disease.
- Echocardiographic or other objective evidence of heart disease.

General Considerations

Cardiovascular complications occur in up to 4% of pregnancies and cause up to 27% of U.S. pregnancy-related deaths. The incidence is increasing due in part to (1) improved life expectancy of women with congenital heart disease who can pursue pregnancy and (2) a trend toward older maternal age. The unique hemodynamic changes associated with pregnancy make diagnosis and management of heart disease in pregnant patients a challenge to the physicians, who must consider not only the patient but also the risks to the fetus. This gap in medical progress has driven the increased appreciation and standardization of multidisciplinary approaches to managing cardiovascular disease in pregnancy with emerging Cardio-Obstetric programs worldwide. In addition, pregnancy risk scores, including the CARPREG II (Cardiac Disease in Pregnancy), mWHO (modified World Health Organization), and ZAHARA [Zwangerschap bij Aangeboren HARtAfwijking (Pregnancy in Women With Congenital Heart Disease)], have evolved over the past 2 decades. (Table 33–1)

In general, the normal hemodynamic changes associated with pregnancy are well tolerated by those who have a normal cardiovascular system, some valvular regurgitation, or left-to-right intracardiac shunts. The highest maternal and fetal morbidity and mortality is seen with severe obstructive valvular lesions, severe aortic disease (dilated thoracic aorta or uncorrected coarctation), New York Heart Association (NYHA) class III or IV heart failure and pulmonary hypertension, uncontrolled hypertension, and cyanotic congenital heart disease. As a rule, spontaneous vaginal delivery is preferred, often with the use of vacuum extraction or forceps to facilitate stage 2 of labor to avoid the hemodynamic stress associated with pushing. Cesarean section, with few exceptions should be reserved for obstetric indications.

ACOG Practice Bulletin No 212 Summary: Pregnancy and Heart Disease. *Obstet Gynecol.* 2019; 133(5):1067-1072. [PMID: 31022119]

Davis MD, Arendt K, Bello NA, et al. Team-based care of women with cardiovascular disease from pre-conception through pregnancy and postpartum: JACC Focus Seminar 1/5. *J Am Coll Cardiol.* 2021 Apr 13;77(14):1763–1777. [PMID: 33832604]

Silversides CK, Grewal J, Mason J, et al. Pregnancy Outcomes in Women With Heart Disease: The CARPREG II Study. *J Am Coll Cardiol.* 2018;71:2419–2430. [PMID: 29793631]

van Hagen IM, Hesselink JWR. Pregnancy in Congenital Heart Disease: risk prediction and counselling. *Heart.* 2020;106: 1853–1861. [PMID: 32611675]

Cardiovascular Physiology of Normal Pregnancy

Normal pregnancy is accompanied by significant physiologic changes, although the exact mechanisms remain virtually unknown (Table 33–2). This increased hemodynamic burden of pregnancy may unmask previously unrecognized heart disease. The normal signs and symptoms associated with pregnancy, such as shortness of breath, fatigue, and exercise intolerance, may obscure the diagnosis of heart disease. The clinician must, therefore, have a thorough knowledge of these normal changes and the aspects of the history and physical examination that suggest the presence of heart disease.

A. Blood Volume

The increase in maternal blood volume begins as early as the sixth week of pregnancy, peaks at approximately 32 weeks of gestation, and stays at that level (40–50% higher than pregestational levels) until delivery. A rapid rise in blood

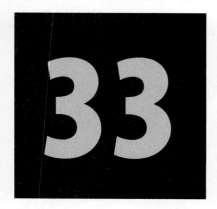

Table 33–1. Pregnancy Risk Scores

Risk Scores	Risk Factors	Points	Low Risk	High Risk	Prohibitive Risk
CARPREG II (2018)	Prior cardiac event or arrhythmia NYHA III or IV or cyanosis Mechanical Valve LVEF < 55% High-risk valve disease or LVOT obstruction Pulmonary Hypertension, RVSP > 49 mm Hg High-risk aortopathy Coronary artery disease No prior cardiac intervention Late pregnancy assessment	3 3 3 2 2 2 2 2 1 1	0–1 points … 5%	2 points … 10% 3 points … 15%	4 points … 22% 5+ points … 41%
ZAHARA (2010)	History of arrhythmia Prior Cardiac Meds NYHA III or IV Left-sided heart obstruction: - Peak gradient > 50 mmHg - AVA < 1 cm^2 Moderate/Severe AR or PR Mechanical valve Cyanotic heart disease	1.5 1.5 0.75 2.5 0.75 4.25 1	0 points … 2.9%	0.5–1.5 points … 7.5% 1.51–2.5 points … 7.5%	2.5–3.5 points … 43.1% > 3.5 points … 70%
mWHO (2006)	WHO I ***Low Risk*** Uncomplicated, small or mild: - Pulmonary stenosis - Patent ductus arteriosus - Mitral valve prolapse	WHO II ***Mild Increased Risk*** Unoperated ASD or VSD Repaired TOF Arrhythmias	WHO II-III ***Moderate Risk Depending on Individual*** Mild LV dysfunction HCM Other VHD Marfan's w/o aortic dilation Bicuspid aortic valve with aorta <45 mm	WHO III ***High Risk*** Mechanical valve Systemic right ventricle Fontan circulation Cyanotic heart disease (unrepaired) Other complex CHD Aortic dilation 40–45 mm in Marfan's Aortic dilation 45–50 mm in bicuspid aortic valve	WHO IV ***Pregnancy Contraindicated*** All PAH Severe LV dysfunction (LVEF < 30%, NYHA III-IV) Previous PPCM without recovery Severe MS Severe symptomatic AS Marfan's with aorta > 4.5 cm Bicuspid aortic valve with aorta > 5.0 cm Native severe coarctation

AR, aortic regurgitation; AS, aortic stenosis; ASD, atrial septal defect; AVA, aortic valve area; CHD, congenital heart disease; HCM, hypertrophic cardiomyopathy; LV, left ventricular; LVEF, left ventricular ejection fraction; LVOT, left ventricular outflow tract; MS, mitral stenosis; NYHA, New York Heart Association; PAH, pulmonary arterial hypertension; PPCM, peripartum cardiomyopathy; PR, pulmonic regurgitation; RVSP, right ventricular systolic pressure; TOF, tetralogy of fallot; VHD, valvular heart disease; VSD, ventricular septal defect.

Data from Silversides CK. *J Am Coll Cardiol*. 2018; 71:2419–2430; Balci A. *Eur Heart J*. 2010;31:615–616; Thorne S. *Heart*. 2006;92:1520–1525.

Table 33–2. Cardiovascular Changes in Normal Pregnancy

	First Trimester	Second Trimester	Third Trimester	At Term
Blood volume	+	+ +	+ + +	↑ 30–50%
Heart rate	+	+ +	+ + (+)	↑ 15–20 bpm
Stroke volume	+	+ + (+)	+	
Cardiac output	+	+ + (+)	+	↑ 30–50%
Systolic blood pressure	–	–	No change	↓ 5–10 mm Hg c/w mid-pregnancy
Diastolic blood pressure	–	– –	–	
Pulse pressure	+	++	+	
Systemic vascular resistance	–	– – –	– –	
Pulmonary vascular resistance	–	– –	–	
Left ventricular end-diastolic pressure	+	+ +	No change	
Venous compliance and volume	+	+ +	+	
Red blood cell mass	+	+	+	↑ 15–20%

Data from Fujitan S. *Crit Care Med*. 2005;33:S354.

volume is typically noted until mid-pregnancy, after which the rise plateaus. The plasma volume shows a more rapid and significant rise than the red blood cell mass, accounting for the appearance of physiologic anemia during pregnancy. The levels of hemoglobin and hematocrit may be as low as 11 g/dL and 33%, respectively. Iron supplementation may mitigate the drop in hemoglobin. The increased blood volume is maintained until after delivery when a spontaneous diuresis occurs. Simultaneously, there is increased venous return due to the relief of vena caval compression after delivery. These rapid postpartum changes in blood volume are critical for patients with underlying heart disease.

B. Cardiac Output

One of the most significant changes during pregnancy is the increase in cardiac output, which begins to rise during the first trimester and peaks around the 25th week of gestation before leveling off. Total cardiac output is the product of stroke volume and heart rate and increases up to 50% above pregestational levels. During early pregnancy, the increase in cardiac output is predominantly the result of an increase in stroke volume, augmented by increased intrinsic myocardial contractility. Numerous studies have shown a gradual increase in left ventricular systolic function attributed to left ventricular afterload reduction due to the low-resistance runoff of the placenta. The rise in left ventricular systolic function begins in early pregnancy, peaks in the 20th week, and then remains constant until delivery. As pregnancy advances, heart rate increases and stroke volume mildly decreases. The increased cardiac output in late pregnancy is maintained because of the increased heart rate. The heart rate increase typically peaks around 32 weeks gestation, reaching 15–20 bpm above the pre-pregnancy heart rates. There is a significantly greater increase in cardiac output in twin gestations compared with singletons.

A unique aspect of pregnancy is the hemodynamic changes induced by a change in a patient's position. When the patient is in the supine position, the gravid uterus induces profound mechanical compression of the inferior vena cava, decreasing venous return to the heart, and thus, cardiac output. A change from the supine to the left lateral position results in a 25–30% increase in cardiac output because of an increase in stroke volume.

C. Blood Pressure and Vascular Resistance

Systolic and diastolic pressures drop during pregnancy. A small decrease in systolic blood pressure begins in the first trimester, peaks at mid-gestation, and returns to or exceeds pre-pregnancy levels at term. The diastolic blood pressure decreases more than the systolic blood pressure, due to a significant fall in systemic vascular resistance (SVR), resulting in a wider pulse pressure. The systemic blood pressure increases during pregnancy with increased maternal age and parity. It also varies with the patient's position. The highest levels are recorded early in the pregnancy when the patient is upright, and the lowest levels occur when she is supine. During the latter part of pregnancy, the effect of position on systemic blood pressure depends on the relative degrees of inferior vena cava and aortic compression. It is recommended to use automated cuff measurements as there may be absence of the fifth Korotkoff sound in some pregnant women. Total vascular resistance, both systemic and the pulmonary, decreases during pregnancy. The mechanism for the fall in resistances is poorly understood but is attributed to the low-resistance circulation of the pregnant uterus and to hormonal changes (progesterone and prostaglandin among many) associated with pregnancy. The SVR drops approximately 10% in the first trimester and reaches a nadir around 20 weeks of gestation with SVR around 35% less than baseline. There is a small increase in SVR toward the end of pregnancy.

de Haas S, Doha CG, van Kuijk SMJ, van Drongelen J, Spaanderman MEA. Physiological adaptation of maternal plasma volume during pregnancy: a systematic review and meta-analysis. *Ultrasound Obstet Gynecol.* 2017;49:177–187. [PMID: 28169502]

Ramlakhan KP, Johnson MR, Hesselink JWR. Pregnancy and cardiovascular disease. *Nat Rev Cardiol.* 2020;17:718–731. [PMID: 32518358]

Regitz-Zagrosek V, Hesselink JWR, Bauersachs J, et al. 2018 ESC Guidelines for the management of cardiovascular diseases during pregnancy. *Eur Heart J.* 2018;39(34):3165–3241. [PMID: 30165544]

Etiology & Symptomatology

A. Congenital Heart Disease

Because the medical and surgical treatment of uncorrected or surgically corrected congenital heart disease (CHD) has improved, more women with CHD are surviving into adulthood and may seek pregnancy. It is recommended that patients with CHD consult with a cardiologist experienced in adult CHD and a maternal-fetal specialist before conception to risk stratify their pregnancy. The prevalence of cardiac complications greatly depends on the type of congenital lesion; regurgitant lesions are typically tolerated well, while stenotic lesions carry a higher risk. The risk for peripartum cardiovascular complication in this population is estimated to be up to 13%, predominantly with congestive heart failure/pulmonary edema and arrhythmias. Maternal mortality rates are highest among women with Eisenmenger syndrome and pulmonary arterial hypertension. Obstetric complications are not significantly increased, except in cases of hypertension and thromboembolic disease (2%). Premature delivery occurs in about 16%, and many of the infants are small for gestational age. Overall, offspring mortality is around 4%. The risk of recurrence of congenital malformations in the offspring depends on the type and ranges from 0.6% to 10%. While the rates of high-risk pregnancies have been increasing over the past decade, overall complication rates are slowly declining.

A few conditions place a patient at a high enough risk to advise against pregnancy (Table 33–3). These include high-risk patients with severe cyanotic CHD, markedly decreased functional capacity, symptomatic severe obstructive lesions, or Eisenmenger syndrome.

Lammers AE, Diller GP, Lober R, et al. Maternal and neonatal complications in women with congenital heart disease: a nationwide analysis. *Eur Heart J.* 2021;42:4252–4260. [PMID: 34638134]

Roos-Hesselink J, Baris L, Johnson M, et al. Pregnancy outcomes in women with cardiovascular disease: evolving trends over 10 years in the ESC Registry of Pregnancy and Cardiac Disease (ROPAC). *Eur Heart J.* 2019; 40: 3848–3855. [PMID: 30907409]

1. Acyanotic heart disease

A. Atrial septal defect—Secundum atrial septal defect is the most common congenital cardiac abnormality

Table 33–3. High-Risk Conditions That Warrant Advice Against Pregnancy

	Condition	Maternal Risk	Fetal Risk
1.	Cyanotic congenital heart disease	4–34% MI/stroke/death	12–40% miscarriage
2.	Eisenmenger syndrome	35% death	30% miscarriage, 15–20% fetal loss
3.	Severe pulmonary hypertension (> 75% of systemic blood pressure)	30–40% death	10% fetal loss
4.	NYHA class III/IV symptoms	10–56% death	30% fetal loss
5.	Severe symptomatic obstructive valvular lesions	56–78% CHF or pulmonary edema	11% death 33–66% preterm delivery
6.	Marfan syndrome with thoracic aorta > 4.0 cm	11–50% risk of dissection	50% risk of inheriting the syndrome 4–20% risk of fetal/neonatal death
7.	Loeys-Dietz syndrome	9% death in nonpregnant with aorta < 4.5 cm	50% risk of inheriting the syndrome

CHF, congestive heart failure; MI, myocardial infarction; NYHA, New York Heart Association.
Data from Crawford MH. *Cardiology.* 2001;95:25–30; Drenthen W. *J Am Coll Cardiol.* 2007;49:2303–2311; Hameed A. *J Am Coll Cardiol.* 2001;37:893–899; Silversides CK. *Am J Cardiol.* 2003;91:1382–1389; Elkayam U. *J Am Coll Cardiol.* 2005;46:223–230; Lind J. *Eur J Obstet Gynecol Reprod Biol.* 2001;98:28–35; Elkayam U. *Ann Intern Med.* 1995;123:117–122; Sliwa K. *Lancet.* 2006;368:687–693; Williams JA. *Ann Thorac Surg.* 2007;83:757–763.

encountered during pregnancy. Patients with uncomplicated atrial septal defects usually tolerate pregnancy with little problem. Patients may not be able to tolerate the acute blood loss that can occur at the time of delivery because of increased shunting from left to right caused by systemic vasoconstriction in response to hypovolemic hypotension. Patients with symptomatic or hemodynamically significant lesions should have these closed percutaneously or surgically prior to pregnancy to decrease the incidence of thromboembolism and arrhythmias. Percutaneous closure can be performed during pregnancy but is reserved for decompensated patients. The incidence of supraventricular arrhythmias may increase in older pregnant patients, and can result in right ventricular failure and venous stasis leading to paradoxical emboli. Low-dose aspirin, taken once daily after the first trimester until delivery, may help prevent clot formation. Patients should use compressive stockings, and all intravenous lines should have air filters. Pulmonary hypertension from an atrial septal defect usually occurs late in life, past the childbearing years. However, if there is severe pulmonary hypertension (Eisenmenger syndrome), pregnancy should be avoided. Bacterial endocarditis prophylaxis is not recommended. Vaginal delivery is preferred over cesarean section. Risk of CHD in the offspring is estimated to be 8–10%.

B. Ventricular septal defect—Most isolated ventricular septal defects have closed by adulthood. Women with ventricular septal defects generally fare well in pregnancy if the defect is small and pulmonary artery pressure is normal. Congestive heart failure and arrhythmia are reported only in patients with decreased left ventricular systolic function prior to pregnancy. Endocarditis prophylaxis during delivery is not recommended. Air filters should be used on intravenous lines to avoid paradoxical embolism. Large ventricular septal defects with pulmonary hypertension are a contraindication to pregnancy.

C. Atrioventricular septal defect (endocardial cushion defect)—This defect includes a large central defect that may lie above the valve (atrial septal defect) or may extend to variable degrees above and below the atrioventricular valve. The defect can therefore be small or large. Many of these are repaired in childhood. While most complete atrioventricular canal defects are seen in Down syndrome, most partial defects are seen in non–Down syndrome patients. Adult patients without repair range from asymptomatic to having symptoms of congestive heart failure, arrhythmias, and pulmonary hypertension with cyanosis. The key to good pregnancy outcome is exclusion of hemodynamically significant residual lesions, pulmonary hypertension, and cyanosis prior to conception. Trisomy 21 patients have a 50% risk of transmitting trisomy 21 and other genetic defects to their offspring.

D. Congenital aortic stenosis—This is most commonly caused by a congenital bicuspid aortic valve. The prevalence in the general population is 1–2% but may be as high as 9–21% in some families, where the condition appears to be autosomal dominant with reduced penetrance. The condition is usually more common in men (2:1 ratio). In patients with congenital aortic stenosis, the outcome during pregnancy depends on the severity of the obstruction. Pregnancy is usually well tolerated in mild-to-moderate aortic stenosis (aortic valve area [AVA] 1.0–2.0 cm^2). Patients with severe aortic stenosis with a valve area of less than 1.0 cm^2 and mean transvalvular gradients greater than 40 mm Hg may experience an increased risk of complications (from 10% to 44%). Although death is very rare, fetal morbidity is increased. The increased cardiac output and decreased SVR of pregnancy create an additional hemodynamic burden in these patients. Syncope, cerebral symptoms, dyspnea, angina pectoris, and even heart failure may occur for the first time during pregnancy. Ideally valve replacement should be performed before pregnancy in symptomatic patients with severe aortic stenosis or if the left ventricular ejection fraction is below 50%. Valvuloplasty, if needed, is preferred over surgery during pregnancy. As part of the bicuspid aortic valve syndrome, the aortic root often will be dilated, evidence that the condition is not only a disease of the valve but of the connective tissue as well. When the aortic root is dilated, there is an increased risk of aortic dissection during pregnancy, and such events have been reported when the aorta is greater than 40 mm, although the true incidence is unknown. The risk of aortic dissection is higher than in the general population but not as high as in Marfan syndrome. Current guidelines would advise counseling and consideration for prophylactic aortic root repair if the aorta exceeds 45 mm. Obtaining serial echocardiograms at least every 3 months to monitor progression of root dilatation appears prudent. Hemodynamic monitoring during labor and delivery should be performed in patients with moderate-to-severe aortic stenosis. Endocarditis prophylaxis is not recommended for vaginal delivery. Cesarean section is recommended in the presence of critical aortic stenosis, aortic aneurysm, or dissection. The risk for the condition in the offspring is variable but at least 4%.

E. Pulmonic stenosis—The natural history of pulmonic stenosis favors survival into adulthood even with severe obstruction to right ventricular outflow. Mild-to-moderate pulmonic stenosis (mean gradient < 40 mm Hg) usually presents no increased risk during pregnancy. Patients with severe pulmonic stenosis may occasionally tolerate pregnancy without the development of congestive heart failure. Vaginal delivery is tolerated well. Ideal treatment consisting of balloon valvuloplasty should be performed before conception but may be performed safely during pregnancy if necessary. The risk in the offspring is about 3.5%.

F. Coarctation of the aorta—In uncomplicated coarctation of the aorta, pregnancy is usually safe for the mother but may be associated with fetal underdevelopment because of the diminished uterine blood flow. The blood pressure may decrease slightly, as during normal pregnancy, but still remains elevated. Maternal deaths in these patients are usually the result of aortic rupture or cerebral hemorrhage from an associated berry aneurysm of the circle of Willis. Patients with the greatest risk during pregnancy are those with severe hypertension or associated cardiac abnormalities, such as bicuspid aortic valves. Treatment consists of limitation of physical activity and maintenance of systolic blood pressure around 140 mm Hg for fetal circulation; β-blockers are preferred and should be continued through delivery. Generally, vaginal delivery is recommended unless there are obstetric indications for a cesarean delivery. Good pain management for labor and delivery is very important to minimize maternal cardiac stress and help to control blood pressure. In cases of severe gradient across the coarctation or associated bicuspid valve with dilated aorta, cesarean section should be considered. Surgical treatment should be reserved for patients in whom complications develop (eg, aortic dissection, uncontrollable hypertension, and refractory heart failure).

G. PATENT DUCTUS ARTERIOSUS—Most patients with a patent ductus arteriosus undergo repair in childhood. A normal pregnancy can be expected in patients with small-to-moderate shunts and no evidence of pulmonary hypertension. Patients with a large patent ductus arteriosus, elevated pulmonary vascular resistance, and a reversed shunt are at greatest risk for complications during pregnancy. The decreased SVR associated with pregnancy increases the right-to-left shunt and may cause intrauterine oxygen desaturation. Patients in whom heart failure develops are treated with digoxin and diuretics. Closure of the patent ductus arteriosus may be done safely during pregnancy using a percutaneous ductal occluder device. The preferred mode of delivery is vaginal in most patients, with hemodynamic monitoring considered at the time of delivery. The risk of patent ductus arteriosus occurring in an offspring is about 4%.

Canobbio MM, Warnes CA, Aboulhosn J, et al. Management of pregnancy in patients with complex congenital heart disease: a scientific statement for healthcare professionals from the American Heart Association. *Circulation*. 2017;135:e50–87. [PMID: 28082385]

Ducas RA, Javier DA, D'Souza R, Silversides CK, Tsang W. Pregnancy outcomes in women with significant valve disease: a systematic review and met-analysis. *Heart*. 2020;106:512–519. [PMID: 32054673]

2. Cyanotic heart disease—Overall, outcomes in pregnancy among women with cyanotic heart disease have improved over the past decade.

A. TETRALOGY OF FALLOT—This is the most common cyanotic CHD found in pregnant patients. The syndrome consists of pulmonary stenosis, right ventricular hypertrophy, an overriding aorta, and a ventricular septal defect. The decrease in SVR, the increased cardiac output, and the increased venous return to the right heart augment the amount of right-to-left shunt and further decrease the systemic arterial saturation. Acute blood loss during postpartum hemorrhage is particularly dangerous because venous return to the right heart is impaired. The labile hemodynamics during labor and the peripartum period may precipitate cyanosis, syncope, and even death in surgically untreated women. Patients with uncorrected or partially corrected tetralogy of Fallot are advised against becoming pregnant because they have a high rate of miscarriages (12–40%) as well as a high risk of heart failure (15–25%), arrhythmias (5%) and stroke, myocardial infarction (MI), or death (4–34%). Patients who have had good surgical repair with no important hemodynamic residual lesions and good functional capacity may anticipate successful pregnancies, although the risk of arrhythmias may be increased. Pregnancy is usually well tolerated even in the setting of severe pulmonary regurgitation, if right ventricular function is no more than mildly depressed and sinus rhythm is maintained. Antibiotic prophylaxis is recommended for patients with uncorrected tetralogy of Fallot and those in whom prosthetic material has been placed within 6 months. Screening for 22q11.2 microdeletion should be considered in patients with conotruncal abnormalities before pregnancy to provide appropriate genetic counseling. In the absence of a 22q11 deletion, the risk of a fetus having CHD is approximately 4–6%. Fetal echocardiography should be offered to the mother in the second trimester.

B. TRANSPOSITION OF THE GREAT ARTERIES (TGA)—TGA implies that each great artery arises from the wrong ventricle. TGA is atrioventricular concordance with ventriculoarterial discordance, with the aorta arising from the systemic right ventricle while the pulmonary artery arises from the nonsystemic left ventricle. Most adults born with TGA will have had one or more operations in childhood. Comprehensive evaluation is recommended before pregnancy in all patients with TGA and prior repair. The risk of pregnancy depends on the type(s) of repair. For patients after atrial baffle, major prepregnancy concerns include ventricular function assessment, systemic atrioventricular regurgitation, and atrial arrhythmias. The physiologic stresses of pregnancy, although clinically well tolerated late after an atrial baffle procedure, carry an increased risk of right ventricular dysfunction that may be irreversible. Isolated reports are available on the outcome of pregnancy after the arterial switch procedure: In the absence of important cardiovascular residua, pregnancy is well tolerated. A comprehensive anatomic and functional assessment, including assessment of coronary artery anatomy, is recommended before a patient proceeds with pregnancy. Patients who had the atrial baffle should have antibiotic prophylaxis before vaginal delivery.

C. EISENMENGER SYNDROME—This syndrome may occur due to several types of CHD and is characterized by systemic-level pulmonary hypertension with right-to-left or bidirectional shunt with deoxygenation. The right-to-left shunt and deoxygenation will increase with the decrease in SVR occurring with pregnancy. The risk of maternal and fetal morbidity and mortality is so high that patients are advised against becoming pregnant. There is a 35% chance of death in the mother and 15–30% chance of fetal mortality. However, with advances in pulmonary vasodilators and pulmonary vascular remodeling agents, there have been modest improvements in outcomes of pregnancy with initiation of dual therapy early in pregnancy.

3. Surgically corrected congenital heart disease—The obstetric care of patients who have had surgical correction of a CHD requires an understanding of the type of surgical procedure, the sequelae, and the hemodynamic consequences. Although atrial flutter may occasionally develop following surgical closure, the successful closure of an uncomplicated atrial septal defect results in no increased maternal risk during pregnancy. Surgical closure of a patent ductus arteriosus that is not associated with pulmonary hypertension is also not associated with maternal complications during pregnancy. In pulmonary hypertension that develops before surgical closure, the decrease in the pulmonary vascular resistance may not be complete, and complications during pregnancy will depend on its severity. Correction of congenital pulmonary stenosis with either surgery or balloon dilatation that leaves little or no transvalvular gradient presents no difficulty to pregnant patients. Surgical correction of coarctation of the aorta with complete relief of the obstruction decreases the development of associated hypertension and the risk of aortic rupture during pregnancy. Successful repair of tetralogy of Fallot with little residual gradient across the pulmonary outflow tract and relief of the cyanosis should result, with careful management, in a normal pregnancy. Pregnancy after repair of complex CHD is increasingly encountered. In such patients, the outcome depends on the mother's functional status, the type of repair, the sequelae, and the cardiovascular response to an increase in stress.

Kearney K, Zentner D, Cordina R. Management of Maternal Complex Congenital Heart Disease During Pregnancy. *Curr Heart Fail Rep*. 2021;18:353–361. [PMID: 34783997]

Ladouceur M, Benoit L, Radojevic J, et al. Pregnancy outcomes in patients with pulmonary arterial hypertension associated with congenital heart disease. *Heart*. 2017 Feb 15;103:287–292. [PMID: 27511447]

Tutarel O, Ramlakhan KR, Baris L, et al. Pregnancy Outcomes in Women After Arterial Switch Operation for Transposition of the Great Arteries: Results From ROPAC (Registry of Pregnancy and Cardiac Disease) of the European Society of Cardiology EURObservational Research Programme. *J Am Heart Assoc*. 2020; 10:e018176. [PMID: 33350866]

B. Valvular Heart Disease

Many patients with valvular heart disease (VHD) can be treated successfully through their pregnancy with conservative medical treatment focused on optimization of intravascular volume and systemic load. Ideally, symptomatic patients should be treated before conception. Women with severe valvular disease should undergo prepregnancy counseling by a cardiologist with expertise in managing patients with VHD during pregnancy. Pregnant patients in stages C or D should be monitored in a tertiary care center by a heart valve team of cardiologists, surgeons, anesthesiologists, and obstetricians with expertise in managing high-risk cardiac patients. Drugs, in general, should be avoided whenever possible. Antibiotics for infective endocarditis prophylaxis for uncomplicated vaginal delivery are not indicated unless a prosthetic valve was placed within 6 months. Although there are few supportive data, antibiotic prophylaxis is often given for complicated vaginal deliveries.

1. Mitral valve disease

A. MITRAL STENOSIS—Mitral stenosis is the most encountered acquired valvular lesion in pregnancy and is almost always caused by rheumatic heart disease. Mitral stenosis may be first diagnosed during pregnancy and is the valvular disorder most likely to develop serious complications during pregnancy. Increased left atrial pressure and even pulmonary edema due to a decrease in diastolic filling time during the tachycardia of pregnancy may develop in women who were previously asymptomatic. In critical mitral stenosis, due to a large diastolic gradient (even at rest), any demand for increased cardiac output results in a significant elevation in the left atrial pressure and pulmonary edema. The most common symptoms include dyspnea, fatigue, orthopnea, and dizziness or syncope, symptoms that may be difficult to distinguish from the normal effects of pregnancy. The greatest danger is in late pregnancy and labor due to increased heart rate and cardiac output, blood volume expansion, and intensified oxygen demand. Pulmonary edema may occur immediately after delivery even after uncomplicated labor when the blood returns from the decompressed inferior vena cava. Mild-to-moderate mitral stenosis (mitral valve area > 1.5 cm^2) may be managed safely with the use of diuretics to relieve pulmonary and systemic congestion and β-blockers (metoprolol preferred) to prevent tachycardia to optimize diastolic filling. If diuretics are needed before the third trimester, then there is a high chance that additional measures such as balloon dilatation, commissurotomy, or early delivery may be needed, and close follow-up is needed. Diuretics, β-blockers, digoxin, or direct-current cardioversion for atrial fibrillation should be instituted in cases of hemodynamic compromise, taking into consideration maternal safety. Patients with mitral stenosis and atrial fibrillation should be anticoagulated. Refractory cases and patients with severe mitral stenosis with heart failure and those with significant pulmonary hypertension prompt mechanical relief, either by percutaneous balloon valvuloplasty or surgery, preferably before conception. Patients with a history of acute rheumatic fever and carditis should continue receiving penicillin prophylaxis.

B. MITRAL REGURGITATION—Mitral regurgitation (most commonly due to mitral valve prolapse) in the absence of

NYHA class III or IV heart failure symptoms is generally tolerated well during pregnancy, even if severe. The decrease in systemic blood pressure in pregnancy may reduce the amount of mitral regurgitation. Left ventricular dysfunction, if severe, may precipitate heart failure. Medical management includes use of diuretics; in rare instances, surgical management is necessary, preferably mitral valve repair, which is indicated for severe, acute regurgitation or ruptured chordae and uncontrollable heart failure symptoms. In the future, percutaneous mitral valve repair may be an option for severe, symptomatic mitral regurgitation during pregnancy.

C. MITRAL VALVE PROLAPSE—Mitral valve prolapse (MVP) is the most common heart disease encountered in pregnancy. Patients without comorbidity, such as a connective tissue, skeletal, or other cardiovascular disorders, tolerate pregnancy well. The click and murmur associated with MVP become less prominent during pregnancy due to the increased volume. No special precautions for isolated MVP are required although there is growing data regarding risk of sudden cardiac death and MVP. Antibiotic prophylaxis is not recommended. The incidence of complications of the MVP (3%) is similar in pregnant and nonpregnant patients.

2. Aortic valve disease

A. AORTIC STENOSIS—Aortic stenosis in pregnancy is usually caused by a congenital bicuspid aortic valve (see previous section).

B. AORTIC REGURGITATION—Isolated chronic aortic regurgitation without left ventricular dysfunction is usually tolerated well. Even if patients are symptomatic, they can often be treated medically with salt restriction, diuretics, and vasodilators. The most common causes are rheumatic disease, bicuspid aortic valve, endocarditis, and a dilated aortic root. Surgery is only indicated for patients with refractory (NYHA class III or IV) symptoms. Acute aortic regurgitation, as in nonpregnancy, is not well tolerated and should be regarded a surgical emergency.

3. Pulmonic and tricuspid valve disease

A. PULMONIC VALVE REGURGITATION—Pulmonic valve regurgitation may occur in isolation or in combination with other heart lesions. Isolated pulmonic regurgitation can be managed conservatively.

B. TRICUSPID VALVE DISEASE—Tricuspid valve disease may be congenital or acquired. Isolated tricuspid valve disease can be managed successfully with diuretics. Special care should be given to diuretic-induced placental hypoperfusion.

4. Prosthetic heart valves—Females with a prosthetic heart valve can usually tolerate the hemodynamic burden of pregnancy without difficulty. The function of the prosthesis can be evaluated and monitored throughout the pregnancy with noninvasive Doppler echocardiography. Two types of heart valves are available with their own distinct risks and advantages: tissue valves and mechanical prostheses. The main differences between the types are durability, risk of thromboembolism, valve hemodynamics, and effect on fetal outcome.

Tissue valves (bioprostheses) may be selected for a pregnant patient to avoid anticoagulation and risk of thromboembolism and should be considered in women of childbearing age who desire a pregnancy if there are no other indications for anticoagulation and if the patient accepts the eventual need for replacement of the prosthesis. Bioprostheses in young women in general are associated with an increased risk of structural valve deterioration. Recent data suggest that this risk is not further increased with pregnancy. The risk of failure is estimated to be at least 50% in 10 years and higher if in the mitral position. Therefore, most women of childbearing age will need reoperation, and the risk of a second open-heart surgery should be considered when discussing the risk with the patient. The newer pericardial bioprostheses may offer better durability, but not enough data are available at the moment to make an estimate of the risk. Homografts appear to have a very low risk of failure even in younger patients and also offer superior hemodynamic profiles over other valves and should therefore be considered when possible.

Mechanical valves are indicated in pregnant patients with other coexisting heart disorders requiring anticoagulation (eg, atrial fibrillation, apical thrombus, or history of thromboembolism). The risk of maternal thromboembolism is less than 4% when using warfarin throughout pregnancy, compared with up to 33% with the use of unfractionated heparin (UFH) throughout pregnancy, with a reported mortality of 1–4%. This complication is more likely in patients with the older generation valves (caged-ball, tilting disk) in the mitral position but is also reported in the newer bi-leaflet valves. Therefore, the choice of prosthetic valve and the safe method of anticoagulation are still of concern in pregnant patients and need further study.

The decision on the choice of anticoagulation should be made with both the patient and the physician after full discussion of potential risks and benefits, and the risk of pregnancy in patients with prosthetic heart valves should be discussed in detail with the patient and the family prior to conception. Women with mechanical heart valves and their providers should use shared decision-making to choose an anticoagulation strategy for pregnancy. Women should be informed that VKA during pregnancy is associated with the lowest likelihood for maternal complications but the highest likelihood of miscarriage, fetal death, and congenital abnormalities, particularly if taken during first trimester and if the warfarin dose exceeds 5 mg/day.

The incidence of warfarin embryopathy (nasal hypoplasia, hypoplasia of extremities, and mental retardation) has historically been estimated to be 5–30% when the fetus is exposed during the critical period of organogenesis between the fourth and eighth gestational weeks. The risk of miscarriage and still birth is estimated to be 15–56%, depending on the series. However, the risk of embryopathy is low (< 3%)

if the woman can be controlled on 5 mg or less of warfarin. UFH, which does not cross the placenta, is believed to be safe for use during pregnancy; however, due to increase in plasma volume and increased renal excretion, the drug needs to be administered in higher doses and with increased frequency. There is a small risk of osteopenia resulting in fractures and in heparin-induced thrombocytopenia. Low-molecular-weight heparin (LMWH) may provide an advantage in terms of less bleeding and a more predictable response. To adequately prevent thrombosis and prevent bleeding, both peak and trough anti-Xa levels should be measured (Table 33–4), and compliance with dosing is of utmost importance. LMWH has a lower risk of valve thrombosis than UFH when monitored. Anti-Xa activity should be measured once weekly for the first 4 weeks and later at least once every 2 weeks. Low-dose aspirin should be added in second and third trimesters for both mechanical and bioprosthetic valves. Table 33–4 shows a recommended regimen for anticoagulation in mechanical prosthetic heart valves considering the risk of the patient as well as the risk of side effects from the drugs. Patients with prosthetic heart valves should be monitored in a tertiary care center by a heart valve team of cardiologists, surgeons, anesthesiologists, and obstetricians with expertise in managing high-risk cardiac patients.

5. Infective endocarditis—Underlying structural abnormalities of the heart predispose patients to the development of infective endocarditis. The most common cause is rheumatic heart disease, with others being MVP, injection drug abuse, and medical procedures. The estimated incidence of infective endocarditis during pregnancy is 0.005–1.0% of all pregnancies. Although it is rare, the development of infective endocarditis during pregnancy can have devastating consequences, with maternal and fetal mortality rates estimated to be as high as 33% and 29%, respectively. The clinical diagnosis and the management of infective endocarditis in pregnancy are the same as for nonpregnant patients (see Chapter 22); however, special consideration must be given to the diagnostic and therapeutic approaches during pregnancy to reduce the risk to the fetus.

6. Rheumatic heart disease—Despite an overall decline in the incidence of rheumatic heart disease in Europe and North America, rheumatic valvular disease remains common world-wide in women of childbearing age.

The cardiac involvement in acute rheumatic fever often is a pan-carditis involving the endocardium, myocardium, and pericardium. It is the involvement of the endocardium, including the valvular and the sub-valvular apparatus, that gives rise to the acute manifestations as well as causes the development of chronic rheumatic VHD. The specific valvular conditions are described in previous sections. The mitral valve is most affected, followed by the aortic valve, and less frequently the tricuspid and pulmonic valves.

Mild rheumatic fever may be difficult to diagnose in pregnancy due to tachycardia, functional murmur, and anemia. The management of acute rheumatic fever is similar in pregnant and nonpregnant patients and consists of bed rest, anemia correction, and penicillin. In severe cases, vasodilators, positive inotropes, or even surgery may be required.

Table 33–4. Recommended Approach for Anticoagulation Prophylaxis in Women with Prosthetic Heart Valves During Pregnancy

	Higher Thromboembolic Risk	Lower Thromboembolic Risk
Conditions	Any mechanical mitral valve prosthesis Older-generation prosthetic (ball-in-cage) AVR Atrial fibrillation History of thromboembolism while receiving anticoagulation therapy Mechanical bileaflet or current-generation single-tilting disk AVR (lower INR OK) Mechanical On-X AVR (low INR (1.5–2) + aspirin	Bioprosthetic TAVI, SAVR without other indication for anticoagulation Bioprosthetic mitral valve without other indication for anticoagulation
Treatment	First trimester: LMWH (anti-Xa trough 0.8–1.2 U/mL) **THEN:** Warfarin (INR goal 3.0) until at least 1 week predelivery **THEN:** UFH (aPTT ≥ 2.5) **OR** LMWH (anti-Xa trough 0.8–1.2 U/mL)	Aspirin 75–100 mg daily monotherapy
	Of note, there is no anticoagulation strategy that is consistently safe for both Mother and Baby [Level 1] If therapeutic with warfarin ≤ 5 mg/day, can consider continuing therapy throughout pregnancy [Level 2a]	

aPTT, activated partial prothrombin time; AVR, aortic valve replacement; INR, international normalized ratio; LMWH, low-molecular-weight heparin; SAVR, surgical aortic valve replacement; TAVI, transcatheter aortic valve intervention; UFH, unfractionated heparin.
Data from Otto CM, et al. *Circulation*. 2020;143:e35–71.

Dagher MM, Eichenberger EM, Konadu KLA, et al. Maternal and fetal outcomes associated with infective endocarditis in pregnancy. *Clin Infect Dis*. 2021;73:1571–1579. [PMID: 34111290]
D'Souza R, Jackie O, Shah PS, et al. Anticoagulation for pregnant women with mechanical heart valves: a systematic review and meta-analysis. *European Heart J*. 2017;38:1509–1516. [PMID: 28329059]
French KA, Poppas A. Rheumatic heart disease in pregnancy: global challenges and clear opportunities. *Circulation*. 2018;137: 817–819. [PMID: 29459467]
Minhas AS, Rahman F, Gavin N, et al. Cardiovascular and obstetric delivery complications in pregnant women with valvular heart disease. *Am J Cardiol*. 2021;158:90–97. [PMID: 34452683]
Wilkie GL, Qureshi WT, O'Day KW, et al. Cardiac and obstetric outcomes associated with mitral valve prolapse. *Am J Cardiol*. 2022;162:150–155. [PMID: 34689956]

C. Myocarditis

This inflammatory process is either focal or diffuse and involves the heart musculature. Of all the infectious and noninfectious causes, viral infection with enterovirus, most commonly coxsackie B virus, accounts for most of the cases, but adenovirus, parvovirus B19, cytomegalovirus, Herpesviridae family, and more recently H1/N1 influenza virus have been implicated. Acute rheumatic fever is discussed in the previous section. Other important causes include acquired immunodeficiency syndrome (AIDS) and Chagas disease due to *Trypanosoma cruzi,* which is the most common cause in South and Central America. Most recently, the Severe Acute Respiratory Syndrome Corona Virus 2 (SARS CoV-2) has been associated with rare reports of clinical myocarditis although imaging studies have demonstrated cardiac inflammation and fibrosis in up to 78%. Only a few cases of myocarditis have been reported in pregnancy. Clinical manifestations range from incidental finding of silent myocarditis to overt heart failure with hemodynamic collapse. In the acute stage, the electrocardiogram (ECG) is almost always abnormal, showing Q waves with ST- and T-wave changes, which may mimic acute MI. The erythrocyte sedimentation rate (ESR) and cardiac enzymes are usually elevated. Viral cultures may or may not be helpful. Echocardiography may reveal regional wall motion abnormalities and cardiac MRI can be helpful in diagnosis. Although endomyocardial biopsy is the gold standard for the diagnosis of myocarditis, a negative result does not rule it out, and rarely does the biopsy aid in diagnosing the etiology or guide management. Therefore, endomyocardial biopsy is not routinely recommended. All pregnant women in whom myocarditis is suspected should be hospitalized. Therapy is supportive, with bed rest; avoidance of strenuous activity; and treatment of heart failure with digoxin, diuretics, and vasodilators. Angiotensin-converting enzyme (ACE) inhibitors should be avoided because of the risk of fetal anomalies. Administration of corticosteroids and immunosuppressive therapy has been controversial and has demonstrated no proven benefit. Potential complications of myocarditis include arrhythmia, heart blocks, and cardiogenic shock. Anticoagulation should be seriously considered, especially for patients with severe left ventricular dysfunction.

Mercedes BR, Serwat A, Naffaa L, et al. New-onset myocardial injury in pregnant patients with coronavirus disease 2019: a case series of 15 patients. *Am J Obstet Gynecol*. 2021;224:387.e1–9. [PMID: 33098814]

D. Cardiomyopathy

1. Peripartum cardiomyopathy (PPCM)—This rare but distinct form of heart failure with left ventricular dysfunction occurs during pregnancy or postpartum. Classically, it is described as occurring between the last month of pregnancy and 5 months postpartum, but cases that do not appear different have been reported from week 17 of pregnancy to 6 months postpartum. PPCM remains a diagnosis of exclusion. Its estimated incidence in the United States is about 1 in 1000 live births and is higher in other countries such as South Africa (1 in 1000), Haiti (1 in 300), and Nigeria (1 in 100) and rising. The increasing incidence is due in part to increased diagnosis with the frequent use of echocardiography as well as rising rates of advanced maternal age, pre-eclampsia, and multiparity. Its cause is unknown but is probably multifactorial with growing data demonstrating genetic predispositions such as with Titin mutations, among others. Risk factors include age greater than 30 years, patients with history of hypertension and preeclampsia, twin (or greater) pregnancies and multiparity. Black women in the United States experience PPCM rates up to four times higher than White women while also experiencing worse morbidity and mortality and lower rates of LV recovery. Histopathology reveals a dilated heart with pale myocardium, but myocardial biopsy is of little value and echocardiography is central to diagnosis. Because signs and symptoms of normal pregnancy resemble heart failure, PPCM is easily missed or diagnosed late in the course. PPCM usually presents with dyspnea, cough, orthopnea, paroxysmal nocturnal dyspnea, fatigue, palpitations, and chest pain. The echocardiogram demonstrates dilated left ventricle with marked overall impairment of systolic function. Right heart catheterization should be considered to optimize the treatment of these patients. Medical therapy is essentially supportive and like that for other forms of heart failure and includes salt restriction, diuretics, digoxin, and afterload reduction with hydralazine (the drug of choice). ACE inhibitors are contraindicated during pregnancy but can be used after delivery. There is no good evidence for the use of immunoglobulin, although it has been tried in some small trials. A possible promising specific treatment is the use of bromocriptine, a prolactin antagonist. It is believed that the increased oxidative stress as seen with PPCM transforms prolactin to an antiangiogenic and proapoptotic protein with harmful effects on the microvasculature. Further studies on this are still needed. Prophylactic low-dose UFH or LMWH should be considered for the prevention of thromboembolic phenomena when the diagnosis of PPCM is established. Warfarin is the drug of choice postpartum. In cases refractory to medical therapy, use of an intra-aortic balloon pump for temporary stabilization and a left ventricular assist device as a bridge to transplant are indicated.

Up to 50–80% of patients recover partially or even completely, typically within 2–6 months after delivery with improved mortality rates over the past few decades now as low as 4% at 12 months. There is distinct geographical variation in the rate of recovery, which appears to be at least 50% in the United States but no more than 20–40% in other countries and in women of African descent. Mortality rates also vary, and recent data from the United States estimate a mortality rate of 0–19%. Mortality in other regions appears higher (15–40%). There is an increased risk of death with increasing age, multiparity, African (Black) ethnicity, and when the diagnosis is delayed. An initial left ventricular ejection fraction less than 30% and left ventricular end-diastolic dimension ≥ 6.0 cm are associated with poor recovery at 1 year. Women with a history of PPCM have a significant risk of deleterious fetal and maternal outcome in subsequent pregnancies, even if their left ventricular function has returned to normal. The risk in subsequent pregnancies is around 20% if left ventricular systolic function is normal and around 45% if function has not recovered. Patients who have had fulminant courses and whose left ventricular function has remained depressed should be advised against becoming pregnant again. Women with severe symptoms refractory to medical therapy should terminate the pregnancy as this often results in improvement of symptoms and cardiac function. Recovery of left ventricular function may continue beyond 6 months, and repeat echocardiograms are recommended.

Goli R, Li J, Brandimarto J, et al. Genetic and phenotypic landscape of peripartum cardiomyopathy. *Circulation.* 2021;143:1852–1862. [PMID: 33874732]

Honigberg MC, Givertz MM. Peripartum cardiomyopathy. *BMJ.* 2019;364:k5287. [PMID: 30700415]

Sliwa K, Mebazaa A, Kleiner DH, et al. Clinical characteristics of patients from the worldwide registry on peripartum cardiomyopathy (PPCM): EURObservational Research Programme in conjunction with the Heart Failure Association of the European Society of Cardiology Study Group on PPCM. *Eur J Heart Fail.* 2017;19:1131–1141. [PMID: 28271625]

2. Hypertrophic cardiomyopathy—This primary myocardial disease shows a characteristic hypertrophy of the left or right ventricular myocardium. The hypertrophy is asymmetric and most commonly involves the intraventricular septum (asymmetric septal hypertrophy). Pathophysiologic mechanisms include presence of a hyperdynamic left ventricle, obstruction of left ventricular outflow tract, mitral regurgitation, and myocardial ischemia. Prevalence in the young population (age 23–35 years) is less than 1 per 1000. Many patients are asymptomatic. Severe illness is manifested by poor functional capacity, heart failure, and sudden death.

Dyspnea is the most common symptom, with others being chest pain (which may be postprandial), dizziness, syncope, and palpitations. In younger patients, sudden death may be the first manifestation, with an annual incidence in the population being 6%. Physical examination varies from normal to characteristic findings in patients with high gradients. The auscultatory hallmark is a diamond-shaped, grade 3–4/6 systolic murmur, heard best at the apex radiating to the left sternal border. The murmur increases in intensity during the strain phase of the Valsalva maneuver. Electrocardiogram shows ventricular hypertrophy, ST and T changes, and Q waves in inferolateral leads. Ventricular arrhythmias are commonly seen on ambulatory ECG monitoring. Echocardiography diagnostically demonstrates asymmetric septal hypertrophy (with a ratio of septum to posterior wall thickening exceeding 1.5) and decreased septal motion.

Most patients do well during pregnancy. High-risk pregnant patients with a higher likelihood of worsening symptoms during pregnancy include those who were symptomatic prior to pregnancy and asymptomatic patients with left ventricular dysfunction or severe left ventricular outflow track obstruction. Increased incidence of supraventricular as well as ventricular arrhythmia in pregnancy has been reported. Maternal hypertrophic cardiomyopathy does not influence fetal mortality, although the risk of premature birth is increased, and in about half of patients, it is familial with autosomal dominant inheritance and confers a 50% risk of affecting the child. Therefore, genetic counseling is recommended, and a detailed discussion regarding risks and a thorough evaluation of the patient are required prior to conception.

In asymptomatic patients, outcome is usually good, but close monitoring is recommended. Therapy needs to be individualized in symptomatic patients. β-Blockers have been used most frequently and are relatively safe in symptomatic patients but are not recommended for routine use. Of the calcium channel blockers, verapamil has been used sporadically in pregnant patients. Dual-chamber pacing for arrhythmia has been shown to be beneficial but is reserved for severely symptomatic cases refractory to medical therapy. Surgical myectomy has not yet been reported in pregnancy. Atrial fibrillation occurs in 10% of the patients, leading to an increased risk of systemic emboli and hemodynamic worsening. Sotalol, procainamide, and direct-current cardioversion have all been used to treat pregnant patients. Prophylactic placement of an implantable cardioverter-defibrillator should be considered in patients with high-risk features like in nonpregnant patients. Alcohol septal ablation may reduce symptoms but does not alter prognosis. Hemodynamic monitoring with a pulmonary catheter is recommended for clinical deterioration encountered during labor and delivery and should be considered even in asymptomatic patients. Fortunately, the strain of vaginal delivery is well tolerated in women with hypertrophic cardiomyopathy. Cesarean section is reserved for obstetric indications. Epidural anesthesia should be avoided. Magnesium should be used for tocolysis if needed.

Goland S, von Hagen IM, Greener GE, et al. Pregnancy in women with hypertrophic cardiomyopathy: data from the European Society of Cardiology initiated Registry of Pregnancy and Cardiac disease (ROPAC). *European Heart J*. 2017;38:2683–2690. [PMID: 28934836]

E. Coronary Artery Disease

Coronary artery disease is a leading cause of death in women in the United States. Coronary artery disease kills more women than the next 16 leading causes of death combined. The incidence of MI during pregnancy and postpartum is estimated to be 3–7 in 100,000. Because of a trend toward older childbearing age and increased metabolic syndrome, the incidence of coronary artery disease may be increasing. Earlier studies reported a mortality rate of 37–50% due to MI during pregnancy. However, recent data suggest the rate is much lower at 5–11%, possibly due to improved diagnosis and use of percutaneous coronary intervention in acute coronary syndromes during pregnancy. It is not clear if pregnancy itself increases the risk of MI. The known risk factors include age (30-fold increased if older than 40 years compared with younger than 20 years), hypertension, diabetes mellitus, smoking, and thrombophilia (Table 33–5). The causes of MI in pregnancy include atherosclerosis, congenital lesions (anomalous origin of coronary artery), inflammatory diseases of coronary arteries (Kawasaki disease), connective tissue (eg, Ehlers-Danlos) or vasospastic disorders, MI with nonobstructive coronary arteries (MINOCA), and spontaneous coronary artery dissection, which may account for up to 30% of cases. Only around 40% of the women who undergo coronary angiography will have atherosclerotic lesions as a cause of the MI. Coronary artery dissections may be seen at any time during the pregnancy but are much more common in the peripartum (50%) or postpartum period (34%). Most MIs that occur during pregnancy are anterior and transmural, involving the left anterior descending artery. Successful treatment of acute MI during pregnancy with thrombolytic therapy has been reported, but given the risk of placental and fetal bleeding, percutaneous coronary intervention is the preferred treatment for acute ST elevation MI in pregnancy. Fetal radiation protection should be attained with abdominal lead shielding. When percutaneous coronary intervention is indicated, bare-metal stents should be considered to minimize dual antiplatelet therapy duration. β-Blockers are the mainstay of medical therapy. Non-ST elevation acute coronary syndromes should be managed conservatively unless there are high-risk features where angiography may be considered. While coronary artery bypass grafting carries similar risk for the woman as in nonpregnancy, there is an increased risk of fetal mortality (10–19%). The most common presentation is angina pectoris. Patients with a high index of suspicion should undergo a stress test for risk stratification. Due to risk to the fetus, submaximal exercise at 70% of maximum predicted heart rate is recommended, preferably with fetal monitoring. Left ventricular function needs to be assessed to determine the choice of therapy and predict likelihood of survival. The normal physiologic changes of pregnancy may precipitate myocardial ischemia and heart failure in women with left ventricular impairment caused by an infarct. Troponin I remains the most useful marker for monitoring pregnant women for a myocardial injury because it is undetectable during normal labor and delivery, although women with preeclampsia and gestational hypertension may have mildly elevated levels. Lipid-lowering drugs of the statin type are contraindicated during pregnancy due to reported teratogenicity, and the risk clearly outweighs the potential benefit. Efforts should be made to limit myocardial oxygen consumption, particularly during late pregnancy and delivery, in women with known coronary artery disease.

Balgobin CA, Zhang X, Lima FV, et al. Risk factors and timing of acute myocardial infarction associated with pregnancy. *JAHA*. 2020;9:e016623. [PMID: 33106090]

Hayes SN, Kim ESH, Saw J, et al. Spontaneous coronary artery dissection: current state of the science: a scientific statement from the American Heart Association. *Circulation*. 2018; 137:e523–e557. [PMID: 29472380]

Mehta LS, Warnes CA, Bradley E, et al. Cardiovascular considerations in caring for pregnant patients: a scientific statement from the American Heart Association. *Circulation*. 2020;141:e884–903. [PMID: 32362133]

F. Arrhythmias

Most arrhythmias occurring during pregnancy are benign. Sinus tachycardia, sinus arrhythmia, sinus bradycardia, atrial premature beats, and ventricular premature beats are very common during pregnancy. These are easily diagnosed using standard diagnostic tools such as 12-lead ECG and ambulatory ECG monitoring. These arrhythmias are hemodynamically insignificant and require no treatment. The occurrence of more complex arrhythmias should, however, raise the suspicion of underlying cardiac disease. Symptomatic arrhythmias, which are rare during pregnancy, may develop during an otherwise uncomplicated pregnancy or in association with underlying cardiac disease. In fact, cardiac arrhythmias may be the first manifestation of cardiac disease during pregnancy.

Vaidya VR, Arora S, Patel N, et al. Burden of arrhythmia in pregnancy. *Circulation*. 2017;135:619–621. [PMID: 28154000]

1. Supraventricular arrhythmias

A. Paroxysmal supraventricular Tachycardia—Paroxysmal supraventricular tachycardia (PSVT), either atrioventricular nodal reentry tachycardia or resulting from an accessory pathway (see following discussion), has been

Table 33–5. Risk Factors for Acute Myocardial Infarction during Pregnancy

Risk Factor	Odds Ratio (95% CI)	*P* Value
Age		< 0.001
18–24	1 (Ref)	
25–29	1.7 (1.3–2.2)	
30–34	3.2 (2.5–4.1)	
35–39	5.1 (4.0–6.7)	
40–55	7.7 (5.7–10.3)	
Race		0.02
White	1 (Ref)	
Asian or Pacific Islander	0.8 (0.5–1.2)	
Black	1.3 (1–1.5)	
Hispanic	1.0 (0.8–1.2)	
Other or Unknown	1.2 (1–1.5)	
Insurance Source		< 0.0001
Private insurance	1 (Ref)	
Medicaid	1.0 (0.9–1.2)	
Medicare	0.3 (0.2–0.5)	
Other or Unknown	0.8 (0.6–1.1)	
Comorbid Conditions		
Coronary artery disease	517.4 (420.8–636.2)	<0.0001
Atrial fibrillation/Flutter	2.7 (1.5–4.7)	< 0.0001
Hyperlipidemia	4.3 (3.2–5.8)	< 0.0001
History of heart failure	8.2 (1.9–35.2)	0.0046
Obesity	1.9 (1.4–2.5)	< 0.0001
Substance abuse	2.1 (1.4–3.1)	0.0004
Prior MI	0.1 (0.0–0.1)	< 0.0001
Prior CABG	0.1 (0.0–0.4)	0.0002
Prior PCI	0.2 (0.1–0.4)	< 0.0001
Prior TIA or stroke	0.4 (0.2–1.0)	0.0373
Prior valve replacement	6.4 (2.4–17.0)	0.0002
Smoking	1.7 (1.4–2.1)	< 0.0001
Thrombophilia	1.7 (1.2–2.5)	0.0035

(*Continued*)

Table 33–5. Risk Factors for Acute Myocardial Infarction during Pregnancy (*Continued*)

Risk Factor	Odds Ratio (95% CI)	*P* Value
Hypertensive Disorders of Pregnancy		< 0.0001
Mild pre-eclampsia	1.5 (1–2.3)	
Pre-eclampsia or eclampsia superimposed on chronic hypertension	3.2 (2.5–4.2)	
Severe pre-eclampsia	2.0 (1.3–3.0)	
Eclampsia	6.0 (3.3–10.8)	
Other Complications of Pregnancy		
Abruptio placentae and placenta previa	1.6 (1.0–2.3)	0.0290
Preterm labor	0.6 (0.4–0.8)	0.0006
Premature rupture of membranes	0.4 (0.2–0.9)	0.0206
Thrombotic event	3.8 (2.3–6.2)	< 0.0001
Uterine rupture	4.2 (1.4–13.0)	0.0125
Laceration	0.3 (0.1–0.9)	0.0278
Postpartum hemorrhage	2.5 (1.9–3.2)	< 0.0001
Postpartum infection	4.0 (2.7–5.7)	< 0.0001

CABG, coronary artery bypass graft; CI, confidence interval; MI, myocardial infarction; PCI, percutaneous coronary intervention; TIA, transient ischemic attack.
Data from Balgobin CA, et al. *JAHA*. 2020;9;e016623.

estimated to occur in approximately 3% of pregnant patients. In patients with a previous history of PSVT, the frequency and severity of the episodes may increase during pregnancy. The symptoms of PSVT are dyspnea, lightheadedness, and anxiety in patients without underlying cardiac disease. In patients with underlying cardiac abnormalities, angina, heart failure, and syncope may occur as a result of myocardial ischemia and decreased cardiac output. Although there is concern about the effects of hypotension on the fetus during these episodes, women with PSVT do not have an increase in perinatal complications. Patients should have an echocardiogram to excluded structural heart disease. The Valsalva maneuver and carotid massage are less effective in pregnant women as compared with nonpregnant women. Intravenous adenosine, verapamil, or metoprolol are all effective in terminating the tachycardia. Maintenance therapy should only be considered if the arrhythmia is recurrent, and then verapamil or metoprolol may be a good choice. Ablation procedures should be avoided during pregnancy due to the radiation risk to the fetus. Theoretical concern for fetal effects of metoprolol have not been demonstrated in multiple studies and metoprolol and propranolol are considered safe; however, data for calcium channel blockers is limited.

B. Atrial flutter and atrial fibrillation—Atrial flutter, which is uncommon during pregnancy, and atrial fibrillation are usually found in patients with underlying cardiac disease. Atrial fibrillation is now the most frequent arrhythmia seen in pregnancy. The hemodynamic consequences and the associated symptoms depend on the underlying cardiac status and the ventricular rate during the tachycardia. During pregnancy, atrial fibrillation is most often found in association with mitral stenosis. The development of this arrhythmia in these patients may precipitate congestive heart failure and embolic events. Consideration should be given to anticoagulation therapy if persistent. β-Blockers, verapamil, and digoxin are preferred for long-term rate control, whereas verapamil or metoprolol usually will slow the heart rate acutely.

C. Wolff-Parkinson-White syndrome (WPW)—This preexcitation syndrome usually occurs in patients without underlying cardiac disease. Patients with WPW syndrome may have recurrent arrhythmias—most commonly, atrioventricular reentry tachycardia, atrial fibrillation, or atrial flutter. The hemodynamic effects of the associated arrhythmias are related to the type of arrhythmia and the ventricular rate. Many patients with WPW syndrome are asymptomatic, but pregnancy is associated with an increased incidence of arrhythmias in women with this syndrome. WPW may present with an irregular wide complex tachycardia, which is best treated with procainamide.

2. Ventricular arrhythmias

A. Premature ventricular complexes—Premature ventricular complexes (PVCs) are relatively common in pregnant women and may be associated with complaints of palpitations. Pregnant women with PVCs and no underlying cardiac disease have an excellent prognosis and require no treatment. Reassurance is frequently all that is required, along with avoidance of such aggravating factors as smoking and stimulants.

B. Ventricular tachycardia—Defined as the occurrence of three or more consecutive ventricular complexes, ventricular tachycardia is a serious cardiac arrhythmia that, if sustained, can lead to death. Ventricular tachycardia is rare during pregnancy, but when it occurs, it is usually associated with underlying cardiac disease. The most common cardiac abnormalities associated with ventricular tachycardia are MVP, other valvular diseases, and cardiomyopathy. The prognosis for patients with nonsustained ventricular tachycardia (< 30 seconds in duration) and no underlying cardiac disease is excellent. In such patients, the ventricular tachycardia is catecholamine-sensitive, and extreme exercise should be avoided. In some patients, therapy with β-adrenergic blocking drugs may be indicated. Sustained ventricular tachycardia (> 30 seconds in duration) or hemodynamically significant ventricular tachycardia is usually associated with underlying cardiac disease, and therapy with antiarrhythmics is usually indicated. Such patients should also undergo evaluation for such precipitating factors as myocardial ischemia, electrolyte imbalance, congestive heart failure, digoxin intoxication, stimulants, and hypoxia. Drugs that can be used are lidocaine, procainamide, or sotalol. Amiodarone should be avoided. In hemodynamically unstable patients, immediate direct-current cardioversion should be performed without concern for significant fetal risk. Patients with aborted sudden death, syncopal ventricular tachycardia, or ventricular fibrillation or flutter should have an implantable cardioverter-defibrillator implanted, preferably under echocardiographic guidance rather than fluoroscopy.

3. Heart blocks—First-degree heart block is evident as PR prolongation on the ECG and results from an increased time of conduction through the atrioventricular junction. First-degree heart block is primarily associated with rheumatic heart disease or digoxin therapy and does not usually require therapy. Second-degree heart block can be divided into two types: Mobitz type I (Wenckebach) and Mobitz type II. Mobitz type I is characterized by progressive lengthening of the PR interval until an impulse is blocked. It is a relatively benign disorder and occurs when vagal tone is increased. Treatment is seldom indicated. Mobitz type II is a sudden block of conduction without previous prolongation of the PR interval. It often precedes the development of complete heart block. It is rare during pregnancy but may occur in association with rheumatic heart disease or infections. If the ventricular rate is slow and the patient is symptomatic, treatment with permanent pacing is indicated.

Complete heart block can be congenital or acquired. Its onset is usually prior to the pregnancy, and it rarely progresses. Approximately half the cases of complete heart block occurring during pregnancy have an associated ventricular septal defect. Other causes include ischemic heart disease, myocarditis, and rheumatic heart disease. The need for pacemaker therapy depends on the ventricular escape rate. Symptoms are rare at a rate of 50–60 bpm; if the rate suddenly slows, however, syncope may develop. Permanent pacing is indicated in such patients.

G. Pericardial Diseases

Pericarditis is usually a mild, self-limited disease. Its incidence, diagnosis, and treatment are similar in pregnant and nonpregnant patients. Most pregnancies, even the complicated ones, may safely reach full term. Idiopathic pericarditis is the most common cause of pericardial disease, others being trauma, infections (viral, bacterial, fungal, tuberculosis), radiation, and collagen vascular diseases.

Sharp, stabbing chest pain that is exacerbated in the supine position and relieved by leaning forward is the most common complaint. Pathognomonic finding of pericardial friction rub is best heard with the diaphragm of the stethoscope over the second and fourth intercostal spaces in midclavicular line or the left sternal border, with the patient leaning forward and inspiring deeply. Characteristic diffuse ST-segment elevations with upward concavity and upright T waves have been reported in 80% of patients with acute pericarditis. Echocardiography is an important diagnostic modality and may reveal thickened pericardium, pericardial effusion, and, most importantly, cardiac tamponade.

Pregnant patients in whom pericarditis is suspected who present with ECG changes, tachycardia, and ill appearance should be hospitalized for complete bed rest. Nonsteroidal anti-inflammatory drugs (NSAIDs), aspirin, and indomethacin are effective analgesics that may be used safely before 20 weeks gestation. After 20 weeks gestation, prednisone not to exceed 25 mg/day is the preferred drug. Colchicine should be avoided although small case series have not seen significant fetal complications. Corticosteroids should be avoided in tuberculosis. Symptoms of a complicating pericardial effusion with cardiac tamponade mimic the symptoms of pregnancy and include shortness of breath, dyspnea on exertion, and fatigue. Echocardiogram will quickly establish the diagnosis. Treatment for symptomatic cardiac tamponade is percutaneous drainage with surgical pericardial window reserved for refractory cases.

Asymptomatic pericardial effusion is frequently encountered in all trimesters, most commonly in the third (up to 40%)

but resolves postpartum. Pericardial constriction has been rarely reported in pregnancy, although it could occur as a pericarditis sequel. Most patients have dyspnea, marked edema, and ascites in the latter half of pregnancy. Diuretics, corticosteroids, and pericardiectomy (reserved for refractory cases and associated with reasonable maternal and fetal risk) have all been used to treat pericardial constriction in pregnant patients. Preterm delivery and fetal death have been reported.

Lotan D, et al. Management and outcome of acute and recurrent pericarditis during pregnancy. *Eur Heart J.* 2020;41:ehaa946.2157. doi: 10.1093/ehjci/ehaa946.2157

H. Pulmonary Hypertension

1. Pulmonary arterial hypertension (World Health Organization class I)—This entity is defined as *mean* pulmonary artery pressure by right heart catheter of more than 25 mm Hg at rest, a pulmonary capillary wedge pressure or left ventricular end-diastolic pressure ≤ 15 mm Hg, and pulmonary vascular resistance more than 3 Wood units. Within this class is primary pulmonary hypertension, which poses a significant risk to pregnant women, with mortality approaching 40% when poorly controlled, warranting prevention of pregnancy or early therapeutic abortion (see Table 33–3). While rates of pulmonary hypertension during pregnancy are increasing as advances in therapies have improved overall prognosis and its diagnosis is no longer prohibitive of pregnancy, major adverse cardiac events are significantly higher in this population and risk stratification is crucial. The most common presenting symptoms are dyspnea, fatigue, chest pain, palpitations, syncope or near-syncope, and Raynaud phenomenon. Characteristic physical findings are a result of markedly increased pulmonary pressures, leading to right ventricular hypertrophy and failure with decreased cardiac output. The echocardiogram reveals elevated pulmonary artery pressures, right atrial enlargement, right ventricular hypertrophy, and tricuspid regurgitation. A new onset or worsening of symptoms is commonly seen in the second and third trimesters with increased circulating volume. The patients should be followed by a multidisciplinary team with experience in pulmonary hypertension and pregnancy. Patients should be followed monthly in the first and second trimesters and weekly in the third trimester, when the risk is highest.

Treatment options include oral calcium channel blockers or sildenafil in NYHA class I–II patients with normal right ventricular systolic function and epoprostenol (class B) or inhaled iloprost (class C) in NYHA class III patients. Parenteral prostaglandins are recommended for class IV patients if severe right ventricular dysfunction is present. Early initiation of dual therapy may support improved outcomes. Endothelin receptor blockers and soluble guanylate cyclase stimulators are class X and should be avoided and stopped at the time of pregnancy. Incidents of premature labor and delivery are high. Patients should lie in the left lateral decubitus position to improve cardiac output. Cesarean section is the preferred method of delivery. Epidural or spinal-epidural anesthesia is recommended. All patients should have central venous pressure monitoring, an arterial line, and careful attention to volume status. Swan-Ganz catheter is not recommended due to risk of complications. Patients should be monitored for 7–10 days postpartum prior to discharge to ensure stability. Patients with primary pulmonary hypertension should be considered for anticoagulation treatment with UFH or LMWH.

Martin SR, Edwards A. Pulmonary hypertension and pregnancy. *Obstet Gynecol.* 2019; 134:974–987. [PMID: 31599832]

2. Thromboembolic disease—Venous thromboembolic disease is a leading cause of morbidity and mortality during pregnancy and postpartum and accounts for 20% of maternal deaths in the United States. Venous thromboembolism affects pregnant women five times more frequently than nonpregnant women. It is estimated to complicate 2 in 1000 pregnancies. The diagnosis is complicated by symptoms like the usual pregnancy symptoms such as shortness of breath, tachycardia, and leg swelling. Up to 33% of deep venous thrombosis cases may occur in the first trimester, although the risk is highest postpartum (15 times higher than during the pregnancy). Risk factors for venous thromboembolism include age older than 35 years, body mass index more than 30 kg/m^2, a family or personal history of deep venous thrombosis or pulmonary embolism, varicose veins, smoking, or any known hypercoagulable state, as well as multiple previous pregnancies and cesarean section. Pulmonary embolism will occur in 15–24% of patients with untreated deep venous thrombosis and may be fatal in 15%. Diagnosis of deep venous thrombosis should be made with compression ultrasound or impedance plethysmography. Magnetic resonance imaging (MRI) can be performed to diagnose iliac thrombosis. The American Thoracic Society recommends initial screening chest x-ray and, if normal, to proceed to a ventilation-perfusion scan, which is considered safe throughout pregnancy. To further decrease radiation, consideration should be given to performing perfusion scan alone, or one may use dose-reduction techniques and use xenon-133 over technetium-99m. If there is no defect, then pulmonary embolism would be very unlikely. If the chest x-ray is abnormal, the test of choice would be a pulmonary angiogram. Except in the first trimester, pulmonary angiogram exposes the fetus to less radiation than a helical computed tomography (CT) scan, and the theoretical risk of exposing the fetus to iodine has not manifested in current studies. An echocardiogram may support the diagnosis of acute embolus by demonstrating right heart enlargement without hypertrophy and elevated pulmonary artery pressure. Hypokinesis with relative sparing of the right ventricular apex may be seen.

The main treatment for deep venous thrombosis during pregnancy consists of weight-based LMWH, although warfarin can be given after the first trimester until 35 weeks gestation. Treatment should be continued for at least 3 months or until 6 weeks postpartum. Pulmonary embolism, if stable, should be treated with intravenous heparin for at least 5 days. Oral anticoagulation should be continued for 6 months thereafter. In unstable pulmonary embolism, consideration of thrombolysis and embolectomy should be given. An inferior vena caval filter may also be needed.

ACOG: Thromboembolism in Pregnancy. Practice Bulletin 196, 2018.

I. Diseases of the Aorta

1. Marfan syndrome—Marfan syndrome is an inheritable autosomal dominant connective tissue disorder of the fibrillin gene on chromosome 15 with a prevalence of 1 in 3000–5000 individuals. It involves the ocular, skeletal, and cardiovascular systems. Patients are predisposed to aortic dissection or actual rupture of the aorta most commonly originating in the ascending portion during pregnancy, most likely in the third trimester. High-risk patients have significant associated cardiac abnormalities, such as MVP, mitral and aortic regurgitation, and an aortic root greater than 4.5 cm in diameter. Studies have demonstrated accelerated aortic root growth during pregnancy, therefore close monitoring is recommended. All women with Marfan syndrome planning to become pregnant should undergo a screening transthoracic echocardiogram. High-risk patients (aortic root > 4.5 cm or rapidly progressive dilatation) should have elective surgery before conception, preferably with valve-sparing surgery if no significant aortic regurgitation is present. Shared decision-making and discussion about risks should be pursued for women with aortic root 4–4.5 cm. If the diagnosis is made during pregnancy, β-blockers are strongly recommended, with some authorities advocating prompt termination of pregnancy with aortic repair. Close follow-up with echocardiography should be performed. Women at increased risk for complications during pregnancy should be advised against attempting a pregnancy that may be associated with a 50% maternal mortality rate (see Table 33–3). Patients with no dissection or aortic root enlargement can deliver vaginally with epidural anesthesia and facilitated stage 2 of labor. However, if there is aortic root enlargement, aortic regurgitation, or rapid progression of the aorta size, cesarean delivery is recommended. The risk of the offspring inheriting the disorder is 50%.

2. Loeys-Dietz syndrome—This syndrome is caused by genetic mutation in transforming growth factor (TGF)-β with autosomal dominant inheritance with variable clinical expression. The most common manifestations are aortic aneurysms with a high risk of dissection, hypertelorism, bifid uvula or cleft palate, generalized arterial tortuosity, and aneurysms throughout the arterial tree. Loeys-Dietz syndrome may be misdiagnosed as Marfan syndrome, but patients with Loeys-Dietz syndrome will have normal fibrillin gene. Women with this syndrome should be advised against pregnancy due to the risk of aortic dissection with normal aortic diameter and a risk for uterine rupture during pregnancy.

Cauldwell M, Steer PJ, Curtis S, et al. Maternal and fetal outcomes in pregnancies complicated by the inherited aortopathy Loeys-Dietz syndrome. *BJOG.* 2019;126:1025–1031. [PMID: 30811810]

Narula N, Devereux RB, Malonga GP, Hriljac I, Roman MJ. Pregnancy-Related Aortic Complications in Women with Marfan Syndrome. *J Am Coll Cardiol.* 2021;78:870–879. [PMID: 34446158]

J. Hypertension

Hypertension affects 12% of pregnancies and is responsible for 18% of maternal deaths in the United States, with rates that continue to rise and contribute to maternal and perinatal mortality. Risk factors include African-American ethnicity, age greater than 45 years, and women with diabetes. Hypertension in pregnancy causes increased rates of intracerebral hemorrhage, placental abruption, intrauterine growth retardation, prematurity, and intrauterine death. Hypertensive disorders in pregnancy can be divided into four groups: (1) chronic, persistent hypertension (blood pressure ≥ 140/90 mm Hg before pregnancy or before the 20th gestational week); (2) gestational hypertension (hypertension developing beyond the 20th gestational week, not associated with preeclampsia or eclampsia); (3) preeclampsia/eclampsia (de novo or superimposed hypertension beyond the 20th gestational week and coexistence with one or more of the following: proteinuria (> 300 mg protein/24 hours or spot protein/creatinine of ≥ 30 mg/mmol, or 2+ protein on dip stick [1 g/L]), renal insufficiency, liver involvement, neurologic or hematologic complications, uteroplacental dysfunction, or fetal growth restriction; eclampsia (includes presence of seizures); and (4) white coat hypertension. Proteinuria is no longer required for a diagnosis of preeclampsia with advanced disease occurring before protein is detectable in the urine. When present, proteinuria should be confirmed on two occasions, and the patient should be supine in the left lateral position and having rested for at least 10 minutes. The degree of blood pressure elevation does not correlate with risk for eclamptic seizures. Ambulatory blood pressure monitoring may be of value and improve risk prediction. Low-dose aspirin is the drug of choice for prevention of preeclampsia. The drug treatment of choice for mild hypertension is oral methyldopa, nifedipine, or hydralazine. Treatment should be initiated if blood pressure is more than 140/90 mm Hg (or ≥ 135/85 mm Hg at home). For severe hypertension (> 160/110 mm Hg), urgent initiation of intravenous therapies such as intravenous hydralazine or labetalol is important. Target diastolic blood pressure is 80–105 mm Hg depending on the risk.

Brown MA, Magee LA, Kenny LC, et al. Hypertensive disorders of pregnancy: ISSHP classification, diagnosis and management recommendations for international practice. *Hypertension*. 2018;72:24–43. [PMID: 29899139]

Clinical Findings

A. History

The evaluation of heart disease in pregnancy is difficult due to overlap seen with the normal anatomic and physiologic changes of pregnancy. Therefore, taking a careful history is very important and should include a history of rheumatic fever, valvular disorder, arrhythmia, CHD, coronary risk factors or established coronary artery disease, and cardiac surgery.

B. Symptoms & Signs

Reduced exercise tolerance and fatigue are the most common symptoms reported in pregnant women, probably due to increased body weight and anemia. Dizziness, lightheadedness, or even syncopal episodes may occur during the latter part of pregnancy caused by mechanical compression of the uterus on the inferior vena cava decreasing venous return and thus the cardiac output. Palpitations are also a frequent complaint but usually are not associated with a significant arrhythmia or may be associated with relative sinus tachycardia. Dyspnea and orthopnea, probably due to hyperventilation, are also reported.

C. Physical Examination

The physical examination of pregnant patients with normal cardiovascular systems changes because of the increased hemodynamic burden. The evaluation of patients with suspected heart disease during pregnancy requires a thorough knowledge of the normal physiologic changes (see Table 33–2).

A normal pregnant patient has a slightly fast resting heart rate, slightly widened pulse pressure, and warm extremities. Jugular venous distention is seen starting at the 20th week. Edema of the ankles and legs is commonly encountered in late pregnancy. A prominent but unsustained left ventricular impulse may be palpated in late pregnancy and may simulate the volume overload seen in aortic or mitral regurgitation. The auscultatory findings of normal pregnancy begin late in the first trimester and usually disappear 2–4 weeks after delivery. During cardiac auscultation, the first heart sound is loud and exhibits an exaggerated splitting. The second heart sound during late pregnancy is often increased and may exhibit persistent expiratory splitting, especially with the patient in the left lateral position. A third heart sound has been reported to be frequent in late pregnancy. However, because of its association with heart failure, the presence of a third heart sound should lead to further investigation of underlying heart disease, especially in women with symptoms and other signs suggestive of heart disease. A fourth heart sound is rarely heard during a normal pregnancy and may indicate hypertensive heart disease or presence of ischemia.

Systolic murmurs are common during pregnancy and result from the increased blood volume and hyperkinetic state. Most frequently, they are innocent early systolic murmurs, grade 1–2/6, that are best heard at the lower left sternal border and over the pulmonary area, radiating to the suprasternal notch or to the left of the neck. They usually represent vibrations created by ejection of blood into the pulmonary trunk. A cervical venous hum or mammary souffle heard best in the right supraclavicular area in a supine position is a benign systolic or continuous murmur occurring in late pregnancy (Table 33–6). Diastolic heart murmurs are unusual and usually represent valvular abnormalities.

D. Diagnostic Difficulties

Although systolic murmurs are common, the finding of a diastolic murmur is rare during a normal pregnancy and should warrant further diagnostic evaluation. Both systolic and diastolic murmurs associated with cardiac disease can increase or decrease in intensity during pregnancy. Innocent flow murmurs and benign vascular murmurs usually decrease in the sitting position. The systolic murmurs of aortic or pulmonic stenosis usually increase in intensity because of the increased cardiac output and blood volume. The diastolic murmur of mitral stenosis is also increased and may even be first detected during pregnancy. The augmented blood volume and the increased heart rate of pregnancy shorten the diastolic filling period and increase the rate of blood flow across the mitral valve. In contrast, murmurs of mitral or aortic regurgitation may soften or even disappear

Table 33–6. Cardiovascular Signs and Symptoms in Normal Pregnancy

Symptoms
Fatigue
Orthopnea
Dyspnea
Decreased functional capacity
Dizziness
Syncope
Physical signs
Jugular venous distention
Displaced left ventricular apical impulse
Right ventricular heave
Palpable pulmonary impulse
Increased intensity of the first heart sound
Persistent splitting of the second heart sound
Third heart sound
Systolic ejection murmur at the left lower sternal border or pulmonary area with radiation to the neck
Cervical venous hum, mammary souffle

during pregnancy as a result of the decrease in peripheral vascular resistance. The circulatory changes of pregnancy also affect the auscultatory findings in cardiac abnormalities, such as MVP and hypertrophic cardiomyopathy, which are dependent on volume. The increase in left ventricular volume during pregnancy may attenuate or abolish the click and late systolic murmur typical of MVP. The systolic murmur of hypertrophic obstructive cardiomyopathy may also decrease or disappear as the left ventricular volume increases during pregnancy.

E. Diagnostic Studies

1. Electrocardiography—The ECG is an important diagnostic technique that can indicate the presence of underlying cardiac abnormalities. Cardiac chamber hypertrophy, myocardial ischemia and infarction, pericarditis, myocarditis, conduction abnormalities, and the presence of atrial and ventricular arrhythmias may be detected by ECG. In patients with suspected cardiac arrhythmias, ambulatory ECG monitoring may be indicated. During normal pregnancy, sinus tachycardia, a shift of the axis to the left or right, may be observed, and transient ST abnormalities are common.

2. Echocardiography—Transthoracic echocardiography is an important diagnostic noninvasive study that can be performed safely in pregnancy. The intracardiac structures can be evaluated for abnormalities of the great vessels, cardiac chambers, and heart valves. Chamber sizes and ventricular function can also be measured.

During the echocardiographic examination, the normal physiologic changes that occur with pregnancy should be kept in mind. When the patient is evaluated in the left lateral position, an increase in the diastolic dimensions of the right and left ventricles is common because of volume increases that occur with a normal pregnancy. Because of the increase in the left ventricular dimensions, MVP may improve or disappear during pregnancy. Right and left atrial dimensions may also increase slightly; these changes increase as the pregnancy progresses. Small pericardial effusions are common throughout pregnancy in healthy women, but with highest incidence in the last trimester.

Doppler echocardiography provides reliable quantitative and qualitative information regarding the presence and severity of valvular stenosis and regurgitation. Doppler echocardiography can measure the valve area and gradients across stenotic valves. Small degrees of pulmonary, tricuspid, and mitral regurgitation have frequently been found in normal individuals, whether pregnant or not. In patients with CHD (corrected or uncorrected), Doppler echocardiography can detect the presence of intracardiac shunts and estimate the shunt ratios by determining the right and left cardiac outputs. It can measure pulmonary artery systolic pressure to assess the effects of the valvular lesions and intracardiac shunts on the pulmonary circulation.

Transesophageal echocardiography (TEE) provides superior images of the intracardiac structures and great vessels, providing the same detailed analysis of cardiac structure, function, and hemodynamic assessment possible with transthoracic echocardiography. TEE can be used for patients in whom the transthoracic examination is technically suboptimal and for those with suspected prosthetic or native valve dysfunction, infective endocarditis, CHD, or aortic dissection. Although experience with TEE during pregnancy has been limited, the procedure should be considered in pregnant patients for whom the risks are less than the possible benefit. The procedure should be performed by an experienced echocardiographer, and fetal monitoring, in addition to the routine monitoring of the patient, should be available (Table 33–7).

Table 33–7. Normal Diagnostic Test Findings in Pregnancy

Electrocardiogram
Sinus tachycardia
Increased incidence of arrhythmias
QRS axis deviation
Increased amplitude of R wave in lead V_2
ST-segment and T-wave changes
Small Q waves
Echocardiogram
Mildly increased biatrial size
Increased biventricular dimensions
Mildly increased left ventricular systolic function
Small pericardial effusion
Increased tricuspid valve diameter
Mild tricuspid, pulmonic, and mitral regurgitation
Chest roentgenogram
Increased lung markings
Horizontal positioning of the heart
Straightened left upper cardiac border

3. Exercise tolerance test—Little is known about the safety of an exercise test to establish ischemic heart disease in pregnancy. Fetal bradycardia, marked hypoxia, acidosis, and severe hypothermia at peak exercise have been reported. Considering these facts, the use of a submaximal stress test (approximately 70% of the maximal predicted heart rate) with close fetal monitoring is recommended, until more information regarding its safety is available. Maximal oxygen consumption, unchanged in pregnancy, could be used for the assessment of the functional status in cardiac patients during pregnancy.

4. Chest radiography—The usefulness of chest films during pregnancy is limited because of the potential hazard to the fetus from radiation exposure. Whenever a chest film is believed necessary, the abdominopelvic area should be shielded with lead to minimize exposure. The normal cardiac changes of pregnancy, such as chamber enlargement and the horizontal position of the heart because of the elevation of the diaphragm, should not be misinterpreted as cardiac disease. Newer and more accurate techniques such as Doppler echocardiography have largely replaced chest films in the evaluation of cardiac structure and function. Chest x-rays are recommended as part of the evaluation of the pregnant patient suspected of having acute pulmonary embolism.

5. Radionuclide studies—Myocardial perfusion scans and radionuclide ventriculography should be avoided, if possible, especially in the first trimester of pregnancy because of the risk of rare but possible fetal malformations. Also, in women of childbearing age, the incidence of coronary heart disease is low, and other noninvasive techniques, such as exercise echocardiography, can be used to assess coronary artery disease. In cases of suspected pulmonary embolism, a limited ventilation-perfusion scan (only performing the perfusion phase) may be performed weighing out the risks and the benefits. The minimal dose of isotope possible should be used, and xenon-133 is preferred over technetium-99m.

6. Computed tomography—CT scanning imposes ionizing radiation to the mother and in part to the fetus and should only be used if no other imaging modalities can provide the diagnostic information. Using specific low-dose protocols, the amount of radiation with a CT scan may be less than that of a radionuclide scan. For certain studies, iodine contrast is used, which may carry a small risk for hypothyroidism in the fetus, although newer studies have not been able to detect this. At present, it appears that the only time the benefit of CT angiography may outweigh the risk is in pregnant women suspected of pulmonary embolism. Aortic dissections should be evaluated by TEE or MRI.

7. Magnetic resonance imaging—MRI provides multiplanar images of the body with excellent soft-tissue contrast without the use of ionizing radiation. MRI is, in general, regarded as safe in pregnancy. However, safety data are limited. Therefore, MRI should be limited to cases where ultrasonography is inconclusive and where patient care depends on further imaging. Gadolinium contrast should be avoided.

8. Pulmonary artery catheterization—Bedside hemodynamic monitoring can be performed with a balloon-tipped pulmonary artery catheter. In most patients, inflating the balloon permits flotation of the catheter through the right heart without the need for fluoroscopy. With the catheter in the pulmonary artery, the balloon is inflated until it occludes a small vessel; the pulmonary artery wedge pressure obtained reflects the left ventricular end-diastolic pressure. Pulmonary artery pressures and cardiac output can also be measured. The placement of a balloon flotation catheter should be considered during the early stages of labor in any patient with cardiac disease who has been symptomatic during the pregnancy. Furthermore, because of postpartum hemodynamic changes, hemodynamic monitoring should be continued for up to 48 hours following delivery.

9. Cardiac catheterization—In some patients with cardiac disease who decompensate during pregnancy, complete diagnostic information cannot be obtained by noninvasive methods alone. This is particularly important when surgical intervention is contemplated. Cardiac catheterization in these patients may need to be performed during pregnancy. Because the radiation required for the performance of this technique has potentially adverse effects on the fetus, cardiac catheterization should be performed only if the needed information cannot be obtained by any other means. Whenever possible, cardiac catheterization should be performed after major organogenesis has occurred (> 12 weeks after the last menses). The radial approach is the preferred method to minimize the risk of radiation exposure to the abdomen, which should be lead shielded. The exposure to x-rays should be reduced to a minimum; catheter position can be guided in some cases by Doppler and contrast echocardiography.

Treatment

A. Pharmacologic Treatment

Treatment of the pregnant patient with cardiac disease requires the collaborative consultation of the obstetrician and cardiologist at regular intervals during gestation and careful planning for delivery with the anesthesiologist. All cardiovascular drugs during pregnancy should be avoided, if possible, especially in the first trimester. Most cardiovascular drugs cross the placenta and are secreted into the breast milk, mandating a detailed evaluation of risk-to-benefit ratio (Table 33–8).

1. Heart failure—Treatment of heart failure is more challenging in pregnant patients than in nonpregnant women. Salt restriction and activity limitation are extremely important. In patients with pulmonary congestion, medical therapy should begin with digoxin. Although digoxin has been safely used during pregnancy for many years, blood levels should be monitored to avoid toxicity. Diuretics, although not teratogenic, may cause impaired uterine blood flow and placental perfusion, and hence should only be used in severely symptomatic patients. Thiazide diuretics have been associated with neonatal thrombocytopenia, jaundice, hyponatremia, and bradycardia, and loop diuretic are preferred. Spironolactone should be avoided.

Afterload is already reduced during pregnancy; hence, further reduction in afterload may only be beneficial in selected cases. Hydralazine, the most frequently used afterload-reducing agent during pregnancy, is a direct arteriolar dilator and has not been associated with adverse fetal effects. ACE inhibitors are contraindicated in pregnancy due to their associated increased risk of premature delivery, low birth weight, fetal hypotension, renal failure, bony malformations, persistent patent ductus arteriosus, respiratory distress syndrome, and even death. Angiotensin II receptor blockers have similar adverse reactions and are thus rendered unsafe. Data on nitrates are limited and require further evaluation. β-Blockers may be used safely, although atenolol should be avoided.

Table 33–8. Alphabetical List of the Commonly Used Cardiovascular Medications, Their Potential Fetal Side Effects, and Overall Safety

Drugs	Potential Side Effects	Safety
Adenosine	Limited data (in first trimester only)	Safe
β-Blockers	Fetal bradycardia, hypoglycemia and apnea at birth, IUGR, uterine contraction initiation	Safe
Calcium channel blocker	Maternal hypotension leading to fetal distress, birth defects	Safe (Verapamil)
Digoxin	Low birth weight	Safe
Disopyramide	Uterine contraction initiation	Safe
Diuretics	Hyponatremia, bradycardia, jaundice, low platelets, impaired uterine blood flow	Safe (Likely)
Heparin	None reported	Safe (Likely)
Hydralazine	None reported	Safe
Lidocaine	CNS depression due to fetal acidosis with high blood levels	Safe
Mexiletine	IUGR, fetal bradycardia, neonatal hypoglycemia, and hypothyroidism	Safe
Nitrates	Fetal bradycardia	Safe (Likely)
Procainamide	None reported	Safe
Quinidine	Premature labor, fetal VIII cranial nerve damage with high blood levels	Safe
Sotalol	Limited data; bradycardia, reports of death	Safe (Likely)
Amiodarone	IUGR, prematurity, hypothyroidism, prolonged QT in the newborn	Unsafe
Nitroprusside	Thiocyanate toxicity	Unsafe (Likely)
Warfarin	Embryopathy, in utero fetal hemorrhage, CNS abnormalities	Unsafe (< 12 weeks, > 35 weeks)
ACE-I	IUGR, prematurity, low birth weight, neonatal renal failure, bony malformations, limb contractures, patent ductus arteriosus, death	Contraindicated
ARB	Same as ACE-I	Contraindicated

ACE-I, angiotensin-converting enzyme inhibitor; ARB, angiotensin receptor blockers; CNS, central nervous system; IUGR, intrauterine growth retardation.
Data from Halpern DG, et al. *JACC*. 2019;73:457–476.

2. Arrhythmias—During pregnancy, any precipitating factors for arrhythmias should be avoided or corrected. In general, conservative treatment of cardiac arrhythmias is indicated. Direct-current cardioversion is the treatment of choice in patients with hemodynamic compromise due to arrhythmia with minimal fetal risk. Although no antiarrhythmic is completely safe during pregnancy, most are tolerated well and are relatively safe. Drugs with the longest record of safety should be used as first-line therapy. Digoxin, although one of the safest drugs for treating arrhythmia during gestation, may cause increased risk of prematurity and intrauterine growth retardation. Adenosine has been reported safe and successful in terminating supraventricular tachycardias during pregnancy. Procainamide has been used safely and is the drug of choice in the treatment of wide-complex tachycardias. Amiodarone is associated with fetal hypothyroidism, smaller size at birth for date of gestation, and prematurity, and is also secreted in breast milk. Amiodarone is thus reserved only for treating life-threatening arrhythmias or those refractory to other medical therapy. Verapamil, although used during pregnancy, should be discontinued at the onset of labor to avoid dysfunctional labor and postpartum hemorrhage.

β-Adrenergic blocking agents are relatively safe and have frequently been used in pregnant patients to treat arrhythmia, hypertrophic cardiomyopathy, and hyperthyroidism. Metoprolol, a β_1-selective blocker, and propranolol and carvedilol, nonselective blockers, have been used frequently during pregnancy without significant side effects. Sotalol is used to treat supraventricular tachycardias in the fetus. Fetal and newborn heart rate, blood glucose levels, and respiratory status should be monitored closely. Data regarding fetal growth restriction with β-blocker therapy is conflicting.

Lidocaine may be used for ventricular tachycardia, especially in the setting of an acute MI, but it requires close monitoring of blood levels.

3. Thrombosis and thromboembolism—Even though increased concentrations of clotting factors, increased platelet adhesiveness, and decreased fibrinolysis in pregnancy result in an overall increased risk of thrombosis and embolism, the incidence is 2 per 1000 pregnancies, but the risk of pulmonary embolism is high if left untreated.

The major indications for anticoagulants during pregnancy include the presence of mechanical heart valves and prophylaxis for recurrent pulmonary thromboembolism. Some patients with rheumatic heart disease with atrial fibrillation and cardiomyopathies may also be candidates for anticoagulation during pregnancy. A recommended regimen for anticoagulation is suggested in Table 33–4.

Warfarin has been associated with fetal wastage due to spontaneous abortion and stillbirths, optic nerve atrophy and blindness, microcephaly, mental retardation, and even death due to intracranial hemorrhage. Its use in the first trimester is associated with warfarin embryopathy, a syndrome comprising of nasal bone hypoplasia and epiphyseal stippling. Warfarin poses significant risks to both the mother and the fetus during labor and delivery; however, breastfeeding women can be prescribed warfarin because it is not secreted in the breast milk. In the second trimester, warfarin is the treatment of choice, with international normalized ratio monitoring. Therefore, one recommendation is that warfarin should be given only after the 12th gestational week and should be stopped before delivery around the 35th week.

Heparin is generally the drug of choice for anticoagulation in pregnant patients unless there is a very high risk for thromboembolism (see section on prosthetic heart valves). As soon as pregnancy is diagnosed, oral anticoagulants should be discontinued, and subcutaneous heparin, with a goal partial thromboplastin time (PTT) of 2–2.5 times normal, should be initiated. If LMWH is used, anti-Xa levels (peak and trough) should be monitored. Complications of UFH administration include thrombocytopenia, alopecia, and osteoporosis. At the 36th week of gestation, subcutaneous heparin should be switched to intravenous route. To avoid the risk of bleeding during labor and delivery, heparin should be discontinued 24 hours prior. Anticoagulation should then be resumed 4 hours after delivery if there are no bleeding complications.

Low-dose aspirin has been safely used in pregnancy. Dipyridamole should not be used in a pregnant patient. Clopidogrel and prasugrel may be used if needed (avoid breastfeeding). Ticagrelor is not recommended. Direct oral anticoagulants are contraindicated during pregnancy. Thrombolytic therapy has been used safely and effectively but should be avoided whenever possible.

4. Endocarditis prophylaxis—The American Heart Association does not recommend prophylaxis for infective endocarditis in pregnant patients. However, many obstetricians do decide to administer antibiotics in high-risk patients at time of rupture of the membranes in patients undergoing vaginal delivery. The patients considered highest risk are those with mechanical prosthetic heart valves, those with a history of infective endocarditis, and those with uncorrected or recently corrected cyanotic CHDs or with residual defects. In addition, patients with a known infection should be treated.

Halpern DG, Weinberg CR, Pinnelas R, et al. Use of medication for cardiovascular disease during pregnancy: JACC State-of-the-Art Review. *J Am Coll Cardiol.* 2019;73:457–476. [PMID: 30704579]

B. Surgical Treatment

Ideally, most cardiac diseases requiring surgical correction are diagnosed and treated before the patient becomes pregnant. In general, cardiac surgery in pregnant patients is not associated with significant maternal risk but may cause fetal wastage. Fetal risk has been reported to be as high as 33%. Pregnant women requiring cardiac surgery need utmost care, adequate valve selection, and anticoagulation to ensure a good outcome.

Surgery should be reserved for severely symptomatic patients and those who are refractory to medical therapy, and it should be avoided in the first trimester, if possible. Procedures not involving cardiopulmonary bypass are preferred because of associated risks of fetal bradycardia and hypoperfusion.

C. Labor & Delivery

Labor and delivery are periods of maximal hemodynamic stress during pregnancy. Pain, anxiety, and uterine contractions all contribute to altered hemodynamics. Oxygen consumption is higher, and cardiac output is increased up to 50%. Both systolic and diastolic pressures are increased significantly during uterine contractions, especially in the second stage. Anesthesia and analgesia during labor and delivery may affect oxygen consumption, but they do not reduce increased cardiac output secondary to uterine contractions.

Acute decompensation may develop in patients with preexisting cardiac disease. This increase in preload and cardiac output can be devastating in a patient with limited cardiac reserve or an obstructive valvular lesion. Patients at greatest risk for complications during labor and delivery include those with significant pulmonary hypertension and those in NYHA functional class III or IV.

The preferred method of delivery is vaginal, with careful attention paid to pain control by regional anesthesia to avoid tachycardia. Postpartum hemorrhage and excessive fluid intake should be prevented. Invasive hemodynamic monitoring may be needed in some cases to guide treatment rapidly during labor and delivery. In these patients, the monitoring should be continued for at least 24–48 hours after delivery or until hemodynamic stability is ensured. Cesarean section, with few exceptions, should be performed only for obstetric indications because it can also create blood loss and fluid shifts. Regardless of the delivery method, however, effective pain control is essential.

Prognosis

Maternal mortality and morbidity rates during pregnancy depend on the underlying cardiac lesion and the functional status of the patient (see Table 33–3). The greatest risk of maternal mortality (25–50%) is for patients with pulmonary hypertension, Eisenmenger syndrome, NYHA class III and IV heart failure, and Marfan syndrome with a dilated aorta. Pulmonary vascular disease prevents the adaptive mechanisms of normal pregnancy and makes labor, delivery, and the early postpartum period particularly problematic. Moderate-to-severe mitral stenosis, aortic stenosis, the presence of mechanical prosthetic valves, uncomplicated coarctation of the aorta, uncorrected CHDs (without Eisenmenger syndrome), and Marfan syndrome with a normal aorta are associated with a 5–10% mortality rate. Left-to-right shunts, pulmonary valve disease, corrected CHD, bioprosthetic valves, and mild-to-moderate mitral stenosis have a mortality rate of less than 1%.

The functional status of a patient should be classified according to the NYHA classification system. Patients in class I or II can be expected to undergo pregnancy with a less than 0.5% risk of death.

Important Considerations

While the global maternal mortality rate has declined by 38% from 2000 to 2017, it has been steadily increasing in the United States from 7.2 deaths per 100,000 live births in 1987 to 17.4 deaths per 100,000 in 2018 with an increase of almost 200% in severe maternal morbidity between 1993 and 2014. These statistics are staggering and disproportionally affect Black and American Indian/Alaska Native women who are up to 2–3 times higher risk of experiencing peripartum mortality compared to White women. Important social determinants of health and structural racism in the United States contribute to these disparities and must be addressed.

The leading cause of death in pregnant women is acquired cardiovascular disease including cardiomyopathy, cerebrovascular disease, and hypertensive disorders of pregnancy. Growing collaborations between obstetricians and cardiologists have developed to address and prevent these concerning peripartum complications. Importantly, the presence of adverse pregnancy outcomes (APOs), such as hypertensive disorders of pregnancy, gestational diabetes, and preterm delivery or pregnancy loss, predicts future chronic cardiovascular disease including coronary artery disease, heart failure, stroke, and peripheral vascular disease.

Cardio-obstetrics is an expanding subspecialty within cardiology to improve prevention, early detection, and effective management of this patient population as well as to improve the transition from obstetrics care to chronic cardiology follow-up considering the long-term implications.

Grandi SM, Filion KB, Yoon S, et al. Cardiovascular disease-related morbidity and mortality in women with a history of pregnancy complications. *Circulation.* 2019;139:1069–1079. [PMID: 30779636]

Mehta LS, Sharma G, Creanga AA, et al. Call to action: maternal health and saving mothers: A policy statement from the American Heart Association. *Circulation.* 2021;144:e251–269. [PMID: 34493059]

O'Kelly AC, Michos ED, Shufelt CL, et al. Pregnancy and reproductive risk factors for cardiovascular disease in women. *Circ Res.* 2022;130:652–672. [PMID: 35175837]

Parikh NI, Gonzalez JM, Anderson CAM, et al. Adverse pregnancy outcomes and cardiovascular disease risk: unique opportunities for cardiovascular disease prevention in women: a scientific statement from the American Heart Association. *Circulation.* 2021;143:e902–916. [PMID: 33779213]

Sharma G, Lindley K, Grodzinsky A. Cardio-obstetrics: Developing a niche in maternal cardiovascular health. *J Am Coll Cardiol.* 2020;75:1355–1359. [PMID: 32192663]

Endocrinology & the Heart

34

René Baudrand, MD
Thomas Uslar, MD
Eveline Oestreicher Stock, MD

Endocrinology is the discipline that focuses on hormones, their interaction with specific receptors and related diseases. The endocrine system is involved in multiple functions such as growth, metabolic homeostasis, production and storage of energy, blood pressure regulation and reproduction. Hormones are defined as activated chemical signals secreted into the bloodstream that act on distant receptors in different tissues, regulated by precise feedback mechanisms.

In relation to the heart and the cardiovascular system, hormones produced in different glands (ie, cortisol and adrenal, triiodothyronine, and thyroid gland) or other organs (ie, renin and kidney or adiponectin and adipose tissue) will elicit indirect and direct biological effects depending on the localization of the receptors on target tissues. Furthermore, it is now clear that the heart is not just a target organ for different type of hormones but also is an "endocrine organ," by secreting natriuretic peptides that play a central role in fluid and electrolyte homeostasis. Since there are hundreds of different hormones and because receptors are so ubiquitous throughout the body, the effects of endocrine dysregulation on the cardiovascular system is frequently observed in clinical practice; many endocrine diseases are diagnosed due to cardiovascular manifestations. This chapter will update most of the endocrinopathies that can affect the heart, including the interplay of the endocrine system and the cardiovascular system, with special emphasis on evidence-based information from recent years.

THYROID & THE HEART

The thyroid gland is regulated by pituitary thyroid-stimulating hormone (TSH) and secretes mainly the pro-hormone thyroxine (T4) that is deiodated in peripheral tissues to active triiodothyronine (T3). Thyroid hormones are mostly bound to plasma proteins. Free T3 is the predominant inhibitor of the hypothalamus and pituitary to suppress further release of thyroid-releasing hormone (TRH) and TSH.

Thyroid diseases are quite common, affecting approximately up to 15% of the adult female population and a smaller percentage of males. This sex-specific prevalence likely results mainly from autoimmune diseases, however, with advancing age the incidence of thyroid disease in men reaches that of women. Thyroid hormone modulates oxidative and metabolic processes throughout the body by regulating, at the nuclear level, cellular protein synthesis. Thyroid hormones also regulate growth, central nervous system development, heart rate, gut motility, and thermoregulation. Nuclear thyroid receptors are widely distributed including the heart and cardiovascular system. Nongenomic actions of thyroid hormones have also been recognized based on rapid tissue responses outside of the nucleus, through regulation of ion transporter activity. Both overproduction and underproduction of thyroid hormone can disrupt normal metabolism and cardiovascular function.

The cardiovascular signs and symptoms of thyroid dysfunction are some of the most characteristic and clinically relevant signs and symptoms observed in clinical practice. Both hyperthyroidism or hypothyroidism induce changes in cardiac contractility, myocardial oxygen consumption, cardiac output, blood pressure, lipid parameters, systemic vascular resistance and thrombogenicity. For example, it is well known that hyperthyroidism can induce atrial fibrillation, although it is less recognized that hypothyroidism predisposes to ventricular dysrhythmias. Restoration of normal thyroid function usually reverses the abnormal cardiovascular effects.

Cardiovascular Effects of Thyroid Hormones

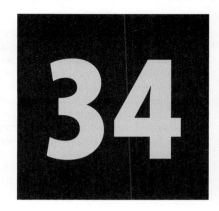

The mechanisms of thyroid hormone–induced dysfunction are multifactorial. It is well described that thyroid hormones have direct effects on cardiomyocytes via specific nuclear receptors. These genomic actions are mainly regulated by T3, which is predominantly produced in local tissues and has more than 10 times affinity of T4. The activation of thyroid receptors increases the number of β-adrenergic receptors in several tissues such as the heart, skeletal muscle, and even adipose tissue. They also amplify catecholamine action at a post-receptor level. Heart rate increases due to increased sinoatrial activity, a lower threshold for atrial activity and shortened atrial repolarization. These factors also create a favorable substrate for the generation of atrial fibrillation (AF) in hyperthyroidism. A similar effect on ventricular myocardium has been associated with ventricular arrhythmias. In addition, activation of the renin–angiotensin system and secondary increased sodium reabsorption in the kidney increase intravascular volume coupled with an increase in contractility due to increased metabolic demands and the direct effect of T3 on cardiac muscle. Moreover, systemic vascular resistance decreases because of T3-induced peripheral vasodilation leading to dramatic increases in cardiac output. Many of the clinical manifestations of thyrotoxicosis appear to reflect increased sensitivity to catecholamines. Consistently, **therapy with β-adrenergic blocking agents** requires higher doses than in routine cardiologic practice, but is very helpful in controlling sympathomimetic manifestations of thyroid hormone excess.

Regarding effects on coagulation, low levels of thyroid hormone are associated with higher incidence of acquired von Willebrand syndrome. On the other hand, hyperthyroidism increases levels of fibrinogen, factors VIII-X, and von Willebrand, increasing the risk for venous thromboembolism (Figure 34–1).

Clinical Approach to Thyroid Disorders

A. History and Medications

A family history of thyroid disease and goiter should be investigated, especially in female relatives. Presence of other immunologic polyglandular disorders increase the risk of developing autoimmune thyroid disease (hypothyroidism

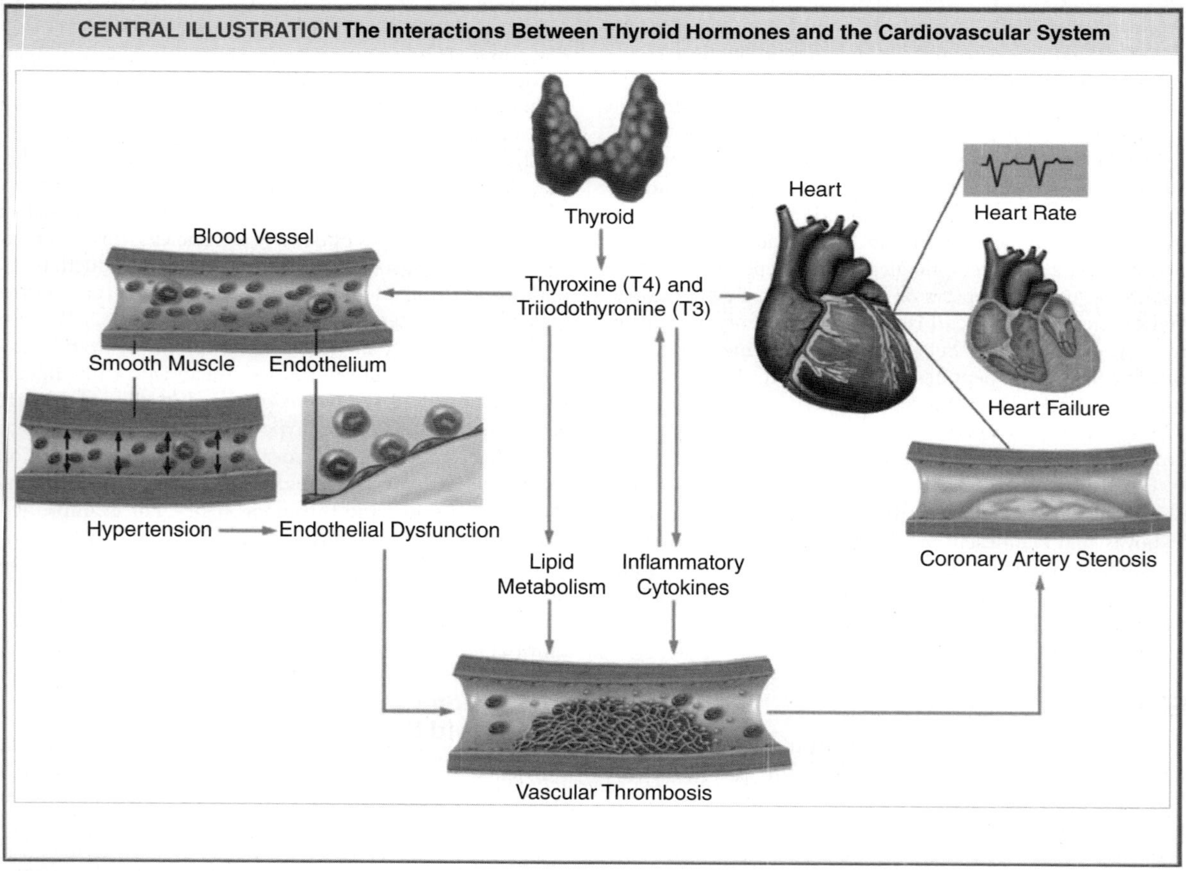

▲ **Figure 34–1.** Thyroid hormones (T4 and T3) have complex interactions with the CV system; mechanisms that include heart rate modulation, rhythm, myocardial contraction, coronary flow and blood pressure modulation (with the interaction of muscle tone and endothelial dysfunction). (Reproduced with permission from Razvi S, Jabbar A, Pingitore A, et al. Thyroid hormones and cardiovascular function and diseases. *J Am Coll Cardiol*. 2018;71(16):1781–1796.) [PMID: 29673469]

most frequently). Iodine ingestion in the form of amiodarone, an iodine-containing antiarrhythmic drug, or intravenous iodine-containing contrast media used in angiography and computed tomography (CT) scanning may induce transient hypothyroidism; excess iodide inhibits hormone synthesis (known as the Wolff-Chaikoff effect). Lithium carbonate, used in the treatment of mood disorders, can also induce hypothyroidism, goiter, and more rarely, hyperthyroidism. Many treatments used in oncology can lead to thyroid dysfunction including thalidomide/tyrosine kinase inhibitors (hypothyroidism), immunotherapy (silent thyroiditis), and alemtuzumab (autoimmune hyperthyroidism).

Long-term exposure to thyroid hormone excess may exert unfavorable effects on cardiac structure and function; may increase left ventricular mass, arterial stiffness, left atrial size and may induce diastolic dysfunction, thereby impairing left ventricle performance. However, since thyroid hormone excess does not induce cardiac fibrosis, these changes are usually reversed once euthyroidism is restored. In most instances, thyrotoxicosis is due to hyperactivity of the thyroid gland due to autoimmune activation (Graves disease) or nodules (toxic adenoma/multinodular goiter). Also, thyrotoxicosis can be transient (or subacute), secondary to viral or autoimmune injury. In these cases, thyroid hormone production is low, and increased circulation is secondary to tissue destruction and emptying of stored T4.

1. Hyperthyroidism

ESSENTIALS OF DIAGNOSIS

- TSH: low levels.
- T4 and/or free T4: high.
- T3 and/or free T3: high.
- Increased hormone production seen in Graves disease or toxic multinodular goiter.
- Decreased hormone production seen in transient/viral thyroiditis or exogenous cause.
- Autoimmune Graves disease: Diffuse goiter, exophthalmos and positive TSH receptor antibodies.

General Considerations

In general, thyrotoxicosis is the clinical syndrome that results from tissue exposure to high levels of circulating thyroid hormones. This clinical entity can be transient or chronic with a broad spectrum of severity.

The prevalence of hyperthyroidism in the United States has been reported in approximately 1.2% of the population (0.5% overt and 0.7% subclinical); with the most common causes diagnosed as Graves disease and toxic multinodular goiter.

The various forms of hyperthyroidism are summarized in Table 34–1.

Clinical Findings

A. Signs & Symptoms of Hyperthyroidism

Patients with hyperthyroidism often complain of weight loss despite increased appetite; this helps distinguish it from other wasting conditions such as cancer or chronic infections/inflammatory syndromes where appetite is usually diminished. Increased adrenergic activation leads to fine resting tremor of the extremities, anxiety, insomnia, and restlessness. Heat intolerance and diaphoresis are frequently seen. Proximal muscle weakness and muscle wasting may be prominent and affects usual activities like climbing stairs. An increased number of bowel movements or diarrhea may occur due to accelerated transit in the gut. Specific thyrotoxic eye signs (autoimmune orbitopathy) such as proptosis, periorbital edema, conjunctival redness, and extraocular muscle involvement are exclusively observed in Graves disease; these patients typically have a symmetric goiter (often with a bruit) with exophthalmos. In most conditions, a non-painful goiter is present. Painful goiter and fever are seen in viral thyrotoxicosis (subacute thyroiditis). Clinicians should always screen for hyperthyroidism in patients with persistent sinus tachycardia and AF, unexplained congestive heart failure, or unstable angina.

B. Cardiovascular Consequences of Hyperthyroidism

Patients with overt and subclinical hyperthyroidism are at increased risk of cardiac death, because of the increased risk of atrial arrhythmias and heart failure, especially in the elderly. Thyrotoxic atrial fibrillation (AF) has been associated with an increased risk of cerebrovascular and pulmonary embolism. Furthermore, autoimmune hyperthyroidism (Graves disease) has been associated with autoimmune cardiovascular involvement: pulmonary arterial hypertension, myxomatous valve disease, and cardiomyopathy.

AF is the most common cardiac complication of hyperthyroidism, occurring in an estimated 10–25% of overtly hyperthyroid patients compared with 0.4% of the general population. High-normal thyroid levels or even subclinical hyperthyroidism are associated with an increased risk of AF. Of note, ventricular arrhythmias usually indicate underlying cardiac disease and warrant further study.

Guideline recommendations for thromboembolic prophylaxis from the American College of Cardiology/American Heart Association (ACC/AHA) recommend anticoagulation; **because AF independently increases the risk for development of stroke or thrombosis, patients should receive anticoagulation during the hyperthyroid phase regardless of CHA2DS2-VASC score.**

Hyperthyroid patients most commonly complain of exercise intolerance and exertional dyspnea, due to inadequate

Table 34–1. Causes of Hyperthyroidism

Etiology	Comments
Graves disease (autoimmune)	Symmetric smooth goiter, ophthalmopathy, increased vascularization in Doppler US, TSH receptor antibodies, elevated ^{131}I uptake, homogeneous uptake on thyroid scintigraphy
Toxic multinodular goiter	Nodular goiter on Doppler US, nonhomogeneous uptake on thyroid scintigraphy
Autonomous thyroid nodule	Nodule on thyroid ultrasound (usually > 2 cm), single large "hot" nodule on thyroid scintigraphy, suppressing rest of thyroid tissue
Thyroiditis	
Subacute	Tender and painful goiter, decreased vascularization on ultrasound, low ^{131}I uptake, high ESR
Painless (silent)	Nontender goiter, low ^{131}I uptake, normal ESR, TPO antithyroid antibodies
Postpartum	Nontender goiter, antithyroid antibodies, low ^{131}I uptake, transient; may recur
Exogenous	
Amiodarone	Increased thyroid production (type 1) or low thyroid synthesis secondary to destruction (type 2)
Iatrogenic/Factitious	Absent goiter, low serum thyroglobulin, low ^{131}I uptake
Iodine induced	High 24-hour urinary iodide excretion; history of iodine ingestion or exposure (contrast agents)
Rare causes	
Struma ovarii	Hyperthyroidism with low TSH, low ^{131}I uptake in thyroid; positive uptake in the ovary
Trophoblastic tumors/Multiple pregnancy	Very high hCG
Metastatic follicular carcinoma	Usually obvious metastases on ^{131}I scan
TSH-producing adenoma	TSH not suppressed, tumor on MRI of pituitary; consider treatment with somatostatin analogs

CT, computed tomography; ESR, erythrocyte sedimentation rate; hCG, human chorionic gonadotropin; ^{131}I, radioactive iodine; MRI, magnetic resonance imaging; TPO, thyroid peroxidase; TSH, thyroid-stimulating hormone; US ultrasound.

increase in cardiac output during exercise (insufficient for the increase in cardiovascular demand during physical effort). Changes in loading conditions, loss of sinus rhythm, or a reduction in myocardial contractility may further impair the cardiovascular system in hyperthyroid patients, resulting in congestive heart failure (HF). Of note, overt hyperthyroidism has been associated with a 16% increase of CV events, predominantly HF.

Often, thyrotoxicosis precipitates exacerbation of angina when the increased demands placed on the heart present in a patient with underlying atherosclerotic coronary artery disease. Coronary symptoms rapidly improve once thyrotoxicosis is controlled.

C. Diagnostic Studies

1. Laboratory findings—Diagnosis is made by measurement of thyroid function tests (Table 34–2). TSH is suppressed in primary hyperthyroidism (usually well below the lower limit of detection in Graves disease), elevated total T4 and T3 confirm the biochemical diagnosis. If estrogen contraceptive/replacement therapy is used, measurement

Table 34–2. Laboratory Tests in Hyperthyroidism

Condition	T_4	T_3	TSH	Hormone Production
Graves disease	↑↑, N	N, ↑	↓↓	↑↑↑
Multinodular goiter	↑, N	N, ↑	↓	↑↑
Solitary nodule	↑, N	N, ↑	↓	↑
Early subacute and silent thyroiditis	↑↑	N, ↑	↓	↓
Exogenous T_4	↑	↓	↓	↓
Ectopic (Struma)	↑, N	N, ↑	↓	↑
TSH-producing pituitary tumor	↑	↑	↑, N (inappropriate)	↑

N, normal; T_3, triiodothyronine; T_4, thyroxine; TSH, thyroid-stimulating hormone.

of free T4 and T3 is warranted due to increase in thyroid-binding globulin. Measurement of total or free T3 is useful to rule out a condition known as **T3 thyrotoxicosis**, in which the serum T4 level is normal but T3 is elevated. If the only abnormality is a suppressed TSH level with normal peripheral hormones, subclinical hyperthyroidism must be considered. Thyroid function tests are not reliable during a period of illness, repeat testing is recommended after the illness resolves.

Antibody testing is helpful for diagnosis: TSH receptor antibody (TSAb), is specific for confirmation of Graves disease, avoids the need for radioiodine uptake scan, and predicts the risk of Graves ophthalmopathy. High titers of thyroid peroxidase antibodies (with negative TSAb) and elevated thyroglobulin are consistent with thyroid destruction observed in silent thyroiditis (eg, postpartum). Low TSH with suppressed thyroglobulin levels is observed in factitious or iatrogenic thyrotoxicosis.

2. Radiologic findings—Although only about one-third of patients have clinical evidence of eye involvement, enlarged extraocular muscles can be detected by CT imaging in up to 90% of patients. If eye findings are present, the diagnosis of Graves disease can be made without further testing. High thyroid hormone production can be inferred by increased thyroid vascularization on Doppler ultrasound. Consistently, elevated radioactive iodine uptake (RAIU) is seen in Graves disease, toxic multinodular goiter, and autonomously functioning thyroid nodule. By contrast, low vascularization in thyroid ultrasound and decreased RAIU is seen in transient thyroiditis and exogenous or factitious hyperthyroidism.

3. Electrocardiography & echocardiography—Sinus tachycardia is usually present, although any supraventricular tachycardia can be seen. AF occurs in 10–20% of hyperthyroid patients; its presence depends on the severity of thyroid excess and structural heart abnormalities. On echocardiography, a hypercontractile state is seen with rapid filling of a highly compliant left ventricle. Increased left ventricular mass and cardiac hypertrophy can also be seen.

Treatment

Treatment is directed at rapidly improving symptoms and reducing demands on the cardiovascular system. The mainstay of treatment is accomplished with antithyroid drugs that prevent thyroid hormone synthesis and release, usually followed by radioactive iodine thyroid ablation (Table 34–3). Surgery is reserved for hyperthyroidism with contraindications for radioactive iodine such as severe ophthalmopathy or giant goiter.

β-Blockers are most used to improve hyperadrenergic symptoms. The effect is observed in hours. If the tachycardia is severe, and is inducing cardiovascular dysfunction, esmolol may be given intravenously for rapid onset of action and short half-life with careful monitorization for signs of worsening HF. Peripheral adrenergic manifestations, such as tremor, sweating, nervousness, and tachycardia will improve almost immediately with β-blocker therapy, however systolic and diastolic contractile performance will not change due to direct effects of thyroid hormone on cardiac muscle not mediated by adrenergic receptors. Within the oral β-blockers, propranolol is a recommended because it also prevents the peripheral conversion of T4 to T3 helping

Table 34–3. Agents Used in the Treatment of Hyperthyroidism

Agent	Dose	Mechanism of Action
Thionamides		
Propylthiouracil (Pregnancy)	50–300 mg, PO three times daily	Inhibits thyroid hormone synthesis Inhibits T_4 conversion to T_3
Methimazole	5–40 mg, PO once daily	Inhibits thyroid hormone synthesis
β-Blockers		
Propranolol	10–80 mg, PO q6–8h	Decreases β-adrenergic activity; decreases T_4 conversion to T_3
Atenolol	50–200 mg/day PO	Decreases β-adrenergic activity
Nadolol	80–160 mg/day PO	Decreases β-adrenergic activity
Metoprolol	100–200 mg/day PO	Decreases β-adrenergic activity
Iodides		
Lugol	5 drops PO q6–8h	Prevents thyroid hormone release
Ipodate	3 g PO q2–3 days or 0.5 g/day	Prevents thyroid hormone release
Radioactive iodine	Calculated dose, usually 10–30 mCi	Destroys overfunctioning thyroid
Other agents		
Lithium	450 mg PO two times daily (monitor levels)	Prevents thyroid hormone release
Glucocorticoids	Hydrocortisone 50g IV q6–8h, prednisone 30–40 mg/day	Decreases peripheral conversion of T_4 to T_3; prevents thyroid hormone release

IV, intravenous; PO, oral; T_3, triiodothyronine; T_4, thyroxine.

reduce the levels of active hormone, despite its frequent posology, four times a day (20–80 mg qid). Other β-blockers with longer half-lives such as atenolol or bisoprolol can be used. The dose should be titrated to the patient's heart rate and control of adrenergic symptoms.

Thionamides are used in hyperthyroidism due to increased hormone production, such as Graves disease and toxic goiter. Thionamides prevent thyroid hormone release and synthesis, by blocking iodine oxidation, organification, and iodotyrosine coupling. To date methimazole is the preferred thionamide worldwide due to once-a-day dosing and lower incidence of side effects, such as the potential for severe hepatotoxicity with propylthiouracil (PTU). Because thionamides deplete intrathyroidal stores of thyroid hormone, they prevent radiation thyroiditis after radioactive iodine ablation. Doses of methimazole depend on the severity of thyrotoxicosis, usually between 5 and 30 mg daily. The effect of methimazole is observed only after 2–3 weeks of treatment and doses must be uptitrated frequently. Because of the teratogenic effects of methimazole, current guidelines recommend PTU in pregnant women during the first trimester; methimazole can be used subsequently during pregnancy.

Methimazole is typically withdrawn 5–7 days prior to radioactive iodine ablation. Secondary effects are extremely infrequent; rash/pruritus (< 5% of patients) is treated with antihistamines. The most concerning side effect is agranulocytosis (0.3–0.5% of patients), observed with higher doses and presents with severe sore throat and fever. Its presence alerts the clinician to immediate cessation of antithyroid drug therapy, evaluate need for hospitalization, and use of granulocyte colony-stimulating factor. Other drugs, including iodine-containing medications and corticosteroids, are usually reserved for the prevention of life-threatening conditions such as thyroid storm; occasionally, they are used for patients with severe congestive HF or unstable angina secondary to thyrotoxicosis.

In the case of severe hyperthyroidism or "thyroid storm," combination of treatment is used to decrease both, thyroid production and conversion. Parenteral corticosteroids are usually given in high doses to reduce peripheral conversion of T4 to T3. Doses are usually 50–100 mg of hydrocortisone every 6–8 hours. Since iodides abruptly prevent the release of thyroid hormone, they are used in conjunction with high doses of methimazole in thyroid storm (eg, Lugol solution).

Viral subacute thyroiditis can be treated with nonsteroidal anti-inflammatory drugs, and—occasionally—corticosteroids if pain control is an issue. Hormone excess is only transient due to destruction of stored T4-T3 and requires short-term β-Blockers therapy. Treatment of congestive HF and AF is essentially the same as for a euthyroid individual. Treatment should include use of a β-blocker to normalize the heart rate. The physician should be aware, however, that treatment of AF is limited to control of the ventricular rate because cardioversion will not be successful if thyrotoxicosis is present. Usually, sinus rhythm returns within 6 weeks with resolution of the thyrotoxic state in 60% of cases. Older patients, and those with underlying cardiac disease may not spontaneously convert and may require cardioversion. As described in the preceding discussion, anticoagulation should be considered until the patient is euthyroid and in sinus rhythm.

Prognosis

The prognosis is generally excellent for most hyperthyroid conditions. Transient hyperthyroidism due to autoimmune destruction or viral inflammation usually do not relapse. Graves disease and autonomously functioning thyroid nodules usually respond very well to radioactive iodine treatment (^{131}I) and only occasionally recur. As noted previously, giant multinodular goiters, especially if intrathoracic or close to the airway, are not candidates for ^{131}I and may ultimately require thyroidectomy.

Delitala AP. Subclinical hyperthyroidism and the cardiovascular disease. *Horm Metab Res.* 2017 Oct;49(10):723–731. doi: 10.1055/s-0043-117893. Epub 2017 Sep 15. [PMID: 28915531]

Kahaly GJ, Bartalena L, Hegedüs L, Leenhardt L, Poppe K, Pearce SH. 2018 European Thyroid Association Guideline for the Management of Graves' Hyperthyroidism. *Eur Thyroid J.* 2018 Aug;7(4):167–186. doi: 10.1159/000490384. Epub 2018 Jul 25. [PMID: 30283735]

Razvi S, Jabbar A, Pingitore A, et al. Thyroid hormones and cardiovascular function and diseases. *J Am Coll Cardiol.* 2018 Apr 24;71(16):1781–1796. doi: 10.1016/j.jacc.2018.02.045. [PMID: 29673469]

Yamakawa H, Kato TS, Noh JY, et al. Thyroid hormone plays an important role in cardiac function: from bench to bedside. *Front Physiol.* 2021 Oct 18;12:606931. doi: 10.3389/fphys.2021.606931. [PMID: 34733168]

2. Hypothyroidism

ESSENTIALS OF DIAGNOSIS

- TSH levels above normal range (primary hypothyroidism).
- Low total or free T4.
- Presence of thyroid peroxidase (TPO) antibodies: chronic thyroiditis/Hashimoto thyroiditis.
- Ultrasound characteristics can be used to aid in diagnosis of Hashimoto thyroiditis (pseudonodules, "lumpy, bumpy" thyroid).

General Considerations

Hypothyroidism is a clinical syndrome resulting from thyroid hormone deficiency, which results in a generalized slowing down of metabolic processes, slowed heart rate, diminished oxygen consumption, and deposition of glycosaminoglycans in extracellular spaces, particularly in skin and muscle; in extreme cases, the clinical syndrome of **myxedema** occurs, which is associated with altered consciousness, hypothermia, hypoventilation, and hypotension.

The prevalence of hypothyroidism has increased worldwide secondary to increased autoimmune disorders, changes in iodide access, age, and the inclusion of milder forms. Overt hypothyroidism, considered as low T4 and high TSH (> 10 mU/L) affects up to 2–4% of the adult population, mainly female patients. Subclinical hypothyroidism (SCH) is the clinical entity with normal total T4 (free T4 if estrogen use) and mildly elevated TSH (> 5 and < 10 mU/L). As expected, the incidence of SCH increases with age in women from 5% up to 10–15%. Overt hypothyroidism is associated with several cardiac manifestations including reduction in cardiac output and heart rate, and accelerated atherosclerosis, likely from the accompanying hyperlipidemia and diastolic hypertension seen in these patients. Hypothyroid patients have other atherosclerotic cardiovascular disease risk manifestations, such as increased C-reactive protein, homocysteine, and carotid intima-media thickness. The atherosclerosis is especially pronounced in the presence of hypertension; however, angina is uncommon, and the incidence of myocardial infarction is not increased. More commonly, angina is precipitated by rapid thyroid hormone replacement.

Even though it is clinically less evident, SCH has been associated with increased risk of heart failure, coronary artery disease events, and even increased mortality.

Finally, most cardiovascular manifestations of hypothyroidism are reversible with thyroid replacement therapy, especially milder cases.

Clinical Findings

A. Symptoms & Signs

1. Systemic symptoms & signs—Hypothyroidism is usually an insidious disease and may be subtle in its progression and presentation. Patients typically complain of weakness, lethargy, fatigue, weight gain (although increase is mild and obesity does not occur), depression (typically without insomnia), muscle cramps, constipation, cold intolerance, dry skin, and hair changes (both dry/coarse or hair loss). Women often have menstrual disorders or decreased fertility.

2. Cardiovascular pathophysiology—Classic cardiovascular findings are the opposite of those found in hyperthyroidism. There is a decrease in cardiac output because of reduced ventricular contractility, decreased heart rate, increased peripheral resistance, and reduced blood volume. The hemodynamic changes resemble those of congestive HF except that pulmonary congestion does not occur, and pulmonary artery and right ventricle pressures are often normal. In addition, cardiac output and systemic vascular resistance increase normally in response to exercise, unlike HF from other causes. Cardiac enlargement may occur due to a combination of interstitial edema, left ventricular dilatation, and pericardial effusion. Pericardial effusion in hypothyroidism is infrequent but can cause cardiac tamponade in severe cases. Interestingly, increased permeability of the epicardial vessels and decreased lymphatic drainage is the mechanism rather than autoimmunity.

B. Physical Examination

Because most hypothyroidism cases are diagnosed while the patient is asymptomatic and are subclinical, the classic cardiological signs are infrequent. Hypothermia, bradycardia with weak arterial pulses, and mild hypertension are characteristic vital signs in overt cases. Diastolic hypertension may be due to increased peripheral resistance and thyroid hormone replacement will normalize blood pressure in approximately one-third of these patients. In severe cases, pericardial/pleural effusion and anasarca may be present.

C. Diagnostic Studies

1. Laboratory findings—Asymptomatic hypothyroid individuals, such as the elderly, frequently go unrecognized. By far, the most common cause of hypothyroidism in the United States is Hashimoto thyroiditis. Other causes of hypothyroidism are listed in Table 34–4.

Table 34–4. Causes of Hypothyroidism

Causes	Comments
Destructive	
Radioactive iodine ablation	No palpable thyroid tissue (postactinic atrophy)
Thyroid surgery	Scar evident
External radiation to neck	History of malignancy
Autoimmune	
Hashimoto thyroiditis	Goiter, antithyroid antibodies
Following Graves disease	History of previous Graves; antibodies for TSH receptor; may have ophthalmopathy
Hereditary or congenital	
Congenital dyshormonogenesis	Goiter, usually diagnosed in childhood
Thyroid hormone resistance	Rare, familial
Iodine deficiency	Rare worldwide and in United States (iodine added to salt)
Drug-induced	
Lithium	Mild goiter, on lithium, usually with underlying predisposition to thyroid disease
Thionamides	History of hyperthyroidism
Iodines	Wolff-Chaikoff effect
Pituitary/hypothalamic failure	Low or inappropriate TSH. Other hormone deficiencies usually apparent

TSH, thyroid-stimulating hormone.

The combination of elevated serum TSH and low T4 (total or free) is diagnostic of primary hypothyroidism. Serum T3 levels are variable and may be within normal range or low, thus they should not be routinely measured in the screening or follow up of hypothyroidism. The absence of an elevated TSH level indicates either nonthyroidal illness or hypothalamic–pituitary dysfunction (secondary or central hypothyroidism). In SCH, TSH level is mildly elevated (usually < 10 mU/L) in the face of a normal T4 level. These patients are typically asymptomatic but although some studies have demonstrated lipid elevations in subclinical hypothyroidism, other studies did not confirm these data. Clinical trials have also demonstrated there is no clear evidence that levothyroxine therapy in subjects with milder form (TSH < 10 mU/L) of subclinical hypothyroidism could improve lipid status and the other cardiovascular risk factors. Prospective studies are necessary to clarify the cardiovascular risk in patients with mild subclinical hypothyroidism and to assess the importance of treating elderly people to improve or counteract the correlated risks. However, until clinical recommendations are updated, the decision to treat or not treat patients with SCH should be based on clinical judgment, practice guidelines, and expert opinion.

Antithyroid antibodies such as TPO (thyroid peroxidase) are elevated in autoimmune Hashimoto thyroiditis. Overt hypothyroidism is a common cause of hyperlipidemia; 95% of hypothyroid individuals will have elevated low-density lipoprotein (LDL) cholesterol due to slower metabolism of cholesterol, and 70% will have elevation in both LDL cholesterol and triglycerides. Anemia of chronic disease (normocytic) may be seen, as well as occasional hyponatremia from impaired free-water clearance.

2. Electrocardiography & echocardiography—Electrocardiographic (ECG) changes include low-voltage QRS complexes and flattened or inverted T waves, sinus bradycardia, and prolonged PR and QT intervals. Prolonged QT may increase ventricular arrhythmias and, rarely, may induce torsade de pointes that is reversible by treatment. Atrial, ventricular, and intraventricular conduction delays are three times as likely in patients with severe hypothyroidism when compared with the general population. Pericardial effusions occur in as many as 20% of overt hypothyroid patients. Because of the slow rate of fluid accumulation, cardiac tamponade is unusual.

Treatment

Treatment with T4, which is available in pure form and is stable and inexpensive, is recommended. Because T4 is converted to T3 in peripheral tissues, both hormones become available once T4 is administered. The half-life of T4 is 7 days, so it is given once daily. It is well absorbed, and blood levels and TSH are measured after 6 weeks of treatment. Replacement doses of T4 vary according to the TSH levels (as a proxy of T4 deficiency), patient's age, and body weight. Regarding cardiovascular effects of T4 supplementation, one of the most important considerations with thyroid hormone replacement therapy is the speed of rendering the patient euthyroid. Young patients without evidence of cardiac disease can be replaced with full doses of T4, usually 1.2–1.6 mcg per kg in overt hypothyroidism and 0.8 mcg per kg in subclinical hypothyroidism if indicated (infertility/peri-pregnancy, mood treatment, or dyslipidemia). Patients older than 55 years or patients with evidence or suspicion of cardiac disease require slow and judicious use of thyroid hormone replacement to prevent exacerbation of angina or precipitation of myocardial infarction. The typical regimen would begin with 0.5 mcg per kg and increase the dose gradually after 4- to 6-week intervals based on serum TSH/T4 measurements, targeting TSH to 2.0–3.0, avoiding low TSH levels to reduce potential cardiovascular complications and accelerated bone loss. Treatment of SCH in patients older than 70 years is not advised due to risk of iatrogenic hyperthyroidism.

Patients with unstable angina and hypothyroidism may be especially challenging to treat because of the risk of exacerbating the angina. Very small doses of hormone should be started, and the dosage increments must be made slowly over a longer-than-usual time. If necessary, angioplasty or coronary artery bypass grafting (CABG) should be recommended, after which—if revascularization is complete—thyroid hormone replacement can occur at the usual dosage and rate.

Treatment of myxedema coma is infrequent and multidisciplinary. Many authors recommend initial use of high-dose intravenous or intrarectal T4 (eg, 300–400 mcg) to overcome reduced intestinal absorption, to saturate thyroid receptors and replenish diminished stores, followed by 100 mcg/day. Others prefer a more conservative approach, but always preferring the intravenous route. **Stress doses of hydrocortisone should also be concomitantly administered** (50–100 mg intravenously every 6–8 hours) because hypothyroidism and adrenal insufficiency frequently coexist, and thyroid hormone replacement may precipitate adrenal crisis.

Prognosis

Most hypothyroid cases have an excellent prognosis, with complete reversal of symptoms and an excellent quality of life without affecting fertility or cardiovascular risk. In the absence of coexisting heart disease, treatment with thyroid hormone and restoration of a euthyroid status correct the hemodynamic, ECG, and serum enzyme alterations and restore heart size to normal. Therapy in chronic hypothyroidism is lifelong, with increasing doses over time due to progression of thyroid dysfunction.

Biondi B, Cappola AR, Cooper DS. Subclinical hypothyroidism: a review. *JAMA*. 2019 Jul 9;322(2):153–160. doi: 10.1001/jama.2019.9052. [PMID: 31287527]

Razvi S, Jabbar A, Pingitore A, et al. Thyroid hormones and cardiovascular function and diseases. *J Am Coll Cardiol*. 2018 Apr 24;71(16):1781–1796. doi: 10.1016/j.jacc.2018.02.045. [PMID: 29673469]

Table 34–5. Features of Amiodarone-Induced Thyrotoxicosis

	Type I	Type II
Pathogenesis	Excess hormone synthesis due to excess iodine in amiodarone molecule	Excess hormone release due to thyroid tissue destruction
Goiter	Often present; multinodular or diffuse	May be present if previous Hashimoto thyroiditis
Autoantibodies	May be present	Usually absent
Color-flow Doppler	Normal or increased flow	Decreased flow
Radioactive iodine uptake	Low or normal (in iodine deficient areas)	Suppressed or low
Thyroid ultrasound	Nodular, hypoechoic, large	Normal size, homogeneous thyroid tissue
Therapy	Methimazole, thyroidectomy unusual	Steroids
Subsequent hypothyroidism	Unusual	Frequent

3. Effect of Heart Disease on Thyroid Function

Acute or chronic illness, such as occurs with myocardial infarction, congestive HF, and during the postoperative period of cardiopulmonary bypass, can make the interpretation of thyroid function tests difficult. Levels of T3 and T4 can drop as much as 20–40% by decreased conversion and production, the so-called **euthyroid sick syndrome**. TSH is inhibited centrally and can be suppressed further by use of drugs, such as dopamine or corticosteroids. As recovery from the underlying illness occurs, the TSH level may rise above normal into the hypothyroid range. Consequently, patients with significant cardiovascular disease in the hospital are likely to have abnormal thyroid function tests with no evidence to support thyroid hormone replacement.

4. Cardiovascular Drugs & the Thyroid

The overall incidence of thyroid dysfunction in patients receiving amiodarone is estimated to be between 2% and 24%, and is mainly hypothyroidism. The prevalence depends on the dose of amiodarone, previous autoimmune injury, age, and iodine status. For example, amiodarone-induced thyrotoxicosis (AIT) is more common in countries with low iodine uptake whereas amiodarone-induced hypothyroidism is more common in areas that are iodine replete. Thyroid injury is also due to its metabolite, desethylamiodarone with direct cytotoxicity on thyroid cells. AIT may occur at any time during or even after amiodarone treatment, particularly in patients with an underlying predisposition to thyroid disease, such as those who have an autoimmune goiter (Hashimoto disease). Classic symptoms of thyrotoxicosis may be masked by the antiadrenergic effects of amiodarone. Pathogenesis of AIT is complex and can involve excessive thyroid hormone synthesis from the iodine load (so-called type I AIT, with high thyroid production) or destructive thyroiditis (type II AIT, with low thyroid production). Features of both types of AIT are listed in Table 34–5.

Therapy for AIT may be complex and requires knowledge of the underlying pathogenesis. In type I AIT, discontinuation of amiodarone is recommended to avoid the progression, close follow up, occasional radioactive therapy (with documented high iodine intake) or even thyroidectomy in selected cases. Type II AIT can be treated with moderate-dose of glucocorticosteroids (prednisone 20–40 mg/day) for 2 months with a gradual slow taper to minimize recurrence. Discontinuation of amiodarone is usually not necessary because destructive thyroiditis resolves within several weeks to months and rarely recurs. If the two types of AIT cannot be distinguished (usually thyroid vascularization seen on doppler ultrasound can be used as a proxy of thyroid production), then therapy with both corticosteroids and antithyroid drugs is recommended.

Ionidated products, such as amiodarone, radiologic contrast material containing iodine, such as that used in cardiac catheterizations, have the potential for causing transient thyrotoxicosis.

Ylli D, Wartofsky L, Burman KD. Evaluation and treatment of amiodarone-induced thyroid disorders. *J Clin Endocrinol Metab*. 2021 Jan 1;106(1):226–236. doi: 10.1210/clinem/dgaa686. [PMID: 33159436]

PARATHYROID & THE HEART

The parathyroid glands regulate the calcium in our bodies. Parathyroid hormone (PTH) is mainly responsible for the regulation of ionized calcium levels by concerted effects on three main target organs: bone, intestinal mucosa, and kidney. It participates in the regulation of calcium, phosphate, and magnesium homeostasis throughout the body. Hyperparathyroidism occurs when one or more parathyroid glands secrete excessive PTH and is classified as primary hyperparathyroidism if the unregulated overproduction comes from the parathyroid gland itself. Secondary hyperparathyroidism occurs in (relatively) hypocalcemic states in which the lack of negative feedback of calcium to the parathyroid glands results in overproduction of PTH and is usually seen in the setting of chronic hypocalcemia, vitamin D deficiency, or renal failure. Tertiary hyperparathyroidism can occur when chronic overstimulation of the parathyroid gland (as in renal failure) causes the autonomous release of PTH.

Patients with parathyroid disorders have increased cardiovascular morbidity and mortality, higher incidence of hypertension, arrhythmias, coronary microvascular dysfunction, left ventricular hypertrophy, and subclinical aortic valve calcification.

1. Primary Hyperparathyroidism

ESSENTIALS OF DIAGNOSIS

- Inappropriately normal or elevated PTH levels in the setting of elevated calcium levels.
- Serum calcium level above upper limit of normal (> 10.5 mg/Dl) corrected for serum albumin, or ionized calcium level higher than upper limit of normal.
- Increased 24-hour urine calcium excretion (calcium-to-creatinine clearance ratio > 0.02).
- Decreased serum phosphate level.
- Elevated alkaline phosphatase.

General Considerations

Primary hyperparathyroidism (PHPT) is most commonly due to overproduction of PTH from a parathyroid adenoma in about 80% of cases, and typically causes hypercalcemia. Rare causes include parathyroid hyperplasia in familial cases, often in the setting of a multiple endocrine neoplasia (MEN) syndrome and parathyroid carcinoma, accounting for 1–2% of cases. When hypercalcemia is detected in an outpatient setting, the most common diagnosis is primary hyperparathyroidism from a parathyroid adenoma. Although parathyroid hyperplasia is rare, it is usually found in the setting of the hereditary condition of MEN. MEN type I comprises hyperparathyroidism, pituitary adenoma, and neuroendocrine tumors; MEN II consists of hyperparathyroidism, medullary thyroid carcinoma, and pheochromocytoma. All patients with PTH-dependent hypercalcemia should be queried regarding lithium and thiazide diuretics intake, which should be discontinued if possible. Furthermore, a family history of hypercalcemia from an early age suggests familial hypocalciuric hypercalcemia (FHH). FHH is a highly penetrant disorder of the CASR (calcium-sensing receptor gene) that causes mild hypercalcemia and resembles primary hyperparathyroidism. However, In FHH, the 24-hour urinary calcium excretion will be very low (< 100 mg) and the calcium clearance/creatinine clearance ratio will be less than 0.01.

The hyperparathyroid state, by altering serum calcium and PTH, has the potential to adversely affect the cardiovascular system. Hypertension, left ventricular hypertrophy (LVH); hypercontractility; arrhythmias; and calcific deposits in the myocardium, aortic and mitral valves, and coronary arteries have all been described. Some but not all studies have demonstrated an increased incidence of cardiovascular death that seems to correlate with the degree and duration of disease.

Clinical Findings

A. Symptoms & Signs

1. Systemic symptoms & signs—Most patients with chronic hyperparathyroidism are asymptomatic and are detected through finding of hypercalcemia in routine laboratory testing. Nonspecific symptoms include fatigue, depression, difficulty in concentrating, personality changes, and vague aches and pains. Muscle weakness with characteristic electromyographic changes is also seen. Dyspepsia, nausea, and constipation can occur, likely secondary to hypercalcemia. No increase in the incidence of peptic ulcer disease has been demonstrated. Articular manifestations include chondrocalcinosis in up to 5% of patients.

2. Cardiovascular symptoms & signs—Acute elevation of calcium may cause hypertension, although this may be due to renal damage from nephrocalcinosis and elevated peripheral vascular resistance—a direct effect of calcium on the vascular smooth muscle cells. Arrhythmias are uncommon, but acute hypercalcemia can cause bradycardia and first-degree heart block. LVH is noted in as many as 80% of patients referred for parathyroidectomy and can be reversible, particularly in normotensive individuals. Valvular sclerosis, on the other hand, does not appear to improve after parathyroidectomy but also does not appear to progress. Several studies in Europe have reported increased cardiovascular morbidity and mortality in patients with otherwise asymptomatic hyperparathyroidism. However, the survival benefit was not observed until 15 years after parathyroidectomy in the largest study published to date. A population-based study from the United States did not find an increase in mortality in patients with PHPT. One explanation for the incongruent mortality data is that more patients in the U.S. studies had mild disease with lower serum calcium levels (mean calcium, 10.9 mg/dL [2.7 mmol/L]) and fewer symptoms than patients in the European studies, where average calcium levels were significantly higher.

B. Physical Examination

Calcium deposition in the cornea, or band keratopathy, may be noted. In hyperparathyroidism secondary to renal failure, calcium and phosphate may precipitate in the soft tissues and in and around joints. These precipitants are usually readily seen on radiograph and palpated on physical examination and, if severe, can limit mobility of the joints.

C. Diagnostic Studies

1. Laboratory findings—Typically, both serum calcium and ionized calcium are elevated, with an inappropriately normal or elevated PTH. Other causes of hypercalcemia are accompanied by a suppressed or low-normal PTH. The 24-hour urine calcium level is usually more than 200 mg. Phosphate levels are usually low or low-normal because PTH has a phosphaturic effect on the kidney, and a hyperchloremic metabolic acidosis is present because of the bicarbonaturic effect of PTH. Alkaline phosphatase levels may be elevated in the setting of hyperparathyroid bone disease.

2. Electrocardiography & echocardiography—Hypercalcemia decreases the plateau phase of the cardiac action potential, reflected by a shortened ST segment and a reduced QT interval. The QT interval corrected for heart rate is probably the most reliable ECG index of hypercalcemia. With severe hypercalcemia (calcium level > 16 mg/dL, or 4 mmol/L), the T wave widens, tending to increase the QT interval.

Echocardiography reveals a high incidence of LVH and calcification of aortic and mitral valves as well as the coronary tree and myocardium.

Treatment & Prognosis

Minimally invasive parathyroidectomy is the definitive treatment for hyperparathyroidism and is indicated in all patients with symptoms as well as patients believed to be at high risk for progressive disease. Localization studies to identify the diseased parathyroid gland(s) include ultrasonography, parathyroid scintigraphy, and multiphase or four-dimensional computed tomography. Reported success rate of parathyroidectomy exceeds 95% especially when expert hands and preoperative localization of the abnormal parathyroid tissue is possible and when parathyroidectomy is coupled with intraoperative PTH assay.

Successful parathyroidectomy normalizes calcium, phosphate, PTH, and alkaline phosphatase levels while improving bone density, decreasing the risk of kidney stones, slowing the progression of renal insufficiency, diminishing LVH, and improving symptoms. Hypertension may persist or progress in some patients, most likely the result of nephrocalcinosis and irreversible renal impairment. Postoperative hypocalcemia is common and if permanent, the patient will require lifelong calcium and vitamin D replacement.

Patients who meet the criteria for surgery but have medical contraindications or prefer not to undergo parathyroid surgery should be considered for medical treatment. They should adopt a normal calcium intake to avoid further increases in PTH levels. In patients in whom serum calcium is more than 1 mg/dL above normal or symptomatic hypercalcemia is present, a calcimimetic agent could be indicated. Cinacalcet activates the calcium-sensing receptor in the parathyroid gland, thereby inhibiting PTH secretion, and may normalize serum calcium in more than 70% of patients.

Bilezikian JP. Primary Hyperparathyroidism. *J Clin Endocrinol Metab*. 2018;103(11):3993–4004. [PMID: 30060226]

2. Hypoparathyroidism

Hypoparathyroidism usually occurs in the postoperative setting after neck or thyroid surgery. Acquired hypoparathyroidism not related to surgery is most often an autoimmune disease in the setting of Polyglandular Syndrome Type 1 in pediatric patients. Other causes of hypoparathyroidism due to parathyroid gland destruction, all very rare, include radiation and storage or infiltrative diseases of the parathyroid glands. Functional hypoparathyroidism can occur in patients with magnesium deficiency by inducing PTH resistance, which occurs when serum magnesium concentrations fall below 0.8 mEq/L (1 mg/dL or 0.4 mmol/L), or by decreasing PTH secretion, which occurs in patients with more severe hypomagnesemia. The hypocalcemia cannot be corrected with calcium; the patients must be given magnesium.

Symptoms include paresthesia, muscle spasms, cramps, tetany, circumoral numbness, and seizures. Cardiovascular manifestations are rare. The physical examination reveals positive Chvostek and Trousseau signs. Laboratory evaluation reveals a low serum calcium or ionized calcium with a low or inappropriately low normal PTH level. Hypoparathyroidism is associated with a prolonged QT interval on the ECG because of ST segment lengthening; the T wave is usually normal. Impaired left ventricular function has been reported. Restoration of eucalcemia may improve cardiac function. Acute management of hypocalcemia depends on calcium level and symptoms; urgent symptomatic hypocalcemia requires intravenous calcium in two steps: one ampule of 10% calcium gluconate, containing 90–180 mg elemental calcium in 50 mL of 5% dextrose, over 10 to 20 minutes followed by a slower infusion of calcium gluconate, 0.5 to 1.5 mg/kg/h over an 8- to 10-hour period. Conversely, chronic treatment for hypoparathyroidism consists of activated vitamin D (calcitriol) and calcium supplements.

Bilezikian JP. Hypoparathyroidism. *J Clin Endocrinol Metab*. 2020 1;105(6):1722–1736. [PMID: 32322899]

ADRENAL & THE HEART

The two adrenal glands are located above the kidneys and are the most active machinery of hormonal production of the whole body. This impressive capacity is elicited by their complex structure composed of an adrenal cortex and adrenal medulla. The adrenal cortex is separated into three layers. The outer layer, zona glomerulosa, produces aldosterone and regulates the arterial pressure and sodium balance. The zona fasciculata produces cortisol, which regulates the stress response and homeostasis. The inner zona reticularis is responsible for sexual differentiation and development. Interestingly, aldosterone is under control of the renin-angiotensin system, while the other hormones are regulated by the hypothalamus (CRH)-pituitary (ACTH)-adrenal axis. Conversely, the adrenal medulla has a different embryologic origin, from the neuroectoderm, is controlled by preganglionic sympathetic ganglia, and produces catecholamines which will enhance the stress response and survival.

Currently, adrenal disorders like primary aldosteronism are the leading cause of secondary hypertension. Nevertheless, other causes like cortisol, catecholamine excess, and specific enzymatic deficiencies cause cardiovascular complications.

1. Primary Hyperaldosteronism

ESSENTIALS OF DIAGNOSIS

- Screening is warranted in resistant hypertension, hypokalemia, adrenal incidentaloma, and personal/familiar history of young-onset cardiovascular complications.
- Inappropriate aldosterone production for sodium intake (> 6–9 ng/dL), independent of renin (plasma renin activity (PRA) < 1 ng/mL/h or direct renin concentration (DRC) < 8.5–10 μU/L).
- Imaging of the adrenals should be performed with CT to assess for adrenal hyperplasia versus adenoma.

General Considerations

Primary aldosteronism (PA) is a syndrome characterized by inappropriately high aldosterone production in relation to salt intake, independent of renin and other regulators, relatively insuppressible by salt loading. The importance of this condition lies in a high prevalence and a wide spectrum of clinical presentation that ranges from normotensive to refractory hypertensive patients. It is clinically important for three reasons: (1) it is the most frequent cause of "secondary" hypertension (between 12% and more than 24% in resistant hypertension); (2) it contributes to an excess risk of cardiovascular and renal morbidity and mortality independent of blood pressure; (3) it can be reversed and cured with targeted drug therapy or surgery. Despite its high prevalence, this condition remains significantly under-diagnosed, mainly attributed to low clinical suspicion of mild forms and a cumbersome diagnostic work-up.

Classically, the main causes of PA have been described as bilateral idiopathic hyperplasia in 60–70%, aldosterone-producing adenoma (APA) or Conn syndrome in 30%, and FH-2 (chloride channel, CLCN2 gene) are the most common forms of hereditary PA, currently estimated to account for approximately 6% of PA. FH-3 is a mutation of *KCNJ5* (potassium channel) and FH-4 is a mutation of CACNAIH (calcium channel). Several somatic mutations in the adrenal cortex have been discovered, accounting for approximately 50% of APA (potassium channel Kir 3.4), sodium/potassium and calcium ATPases (*ATP1A1* and *ATP2B3*), and voltage-dependent calcium channels (*CACNA1D*).

Clinical Findings

A. Symptoms & Signs

1. Systemic symptoms & signs—Consequences of excessive aldosterone production include sodium retention, with plasma volume expansion and hypertension; renal loss of potassium and bicarbonate, causing hypokalemia and metabolic alkalosis; and suppression of renin and angiotensin II synthesis. Patients usually come to medical attention because of hypertension, but currently the incidence of hypokalemia is very low. Hypertension may be moderate or severe, requiring several antihypertensives; malignant hypertension, however, is rare. Despite sodium retention, edema is not a feature of hyperaldosteronism; the kidney can presumably compensate for the excess sodium. Patients with PA, when matched for age, blood pressure, and the duration of hypertension, have greater left ventricular mass compared to patients with other types of hypertension. Overactivation of aldosterone receptor (MR) is thought to contribute to myocardial fibrosis (especially following myocardial infarction) and vascular fibrosis. Mineralocorticoid receptors are in the kidney, heart, blood vessels, immune system and brain. High dietary salt intake was shown to be an independent predictor for left ventricular wall mass in patients with PA. Randomized controlled trials have demonstrated improved survival in patients with HF treated with mineralocorticoid receptor antagonists spironolactone, and in patients with left ventricular dysfunction after a myocardial infarction treated with eplerenone (a selective mineralocorticoid receptor antagonist), providing further evidence for adverse cardiovascular effects of excess aldosterone.

Diagnostic Considerations

Current clinical practice guidelines recommend PA screening with a plasma aldosterone/renin ratio (ARR) in patients that meet "classic criteria," such as severe/resistant hypertension and/or hypokalemia, hypertension in the presence of adrenal mass, sleep apnea, or suspected personal and family history of early onset (< 40 years of age) hypertension. In this context, high plasma aldosterone (> 15–20 ng/dL) with suppressed renin and ARR more than 30 are confirmatory of PA. Nevertheless, this strategy seems to misdiagnose a large proportion of the spectrum of the disease. Missing cases of PA carries a risk of increased morbidity and excess costs related to cardiovascular disease.

Thus, the current recommendation is to maximize the detection of true positives by broadening the screening criteria and diagnostic cut-off values. The presence of hypokalemia is suggestive but not necessary, since less than 20% of severe cases have it. A positive screening is defined by the presence of suppressed renin, that is, plasma renin activity (PRA) less than 1 ng/mL/h or direct renin concentration (DRC) less than 8.5–10 μU/L in the presence of an unappropriated high plasma aldosterone (> 6–9 ng/dL).

For the correct interpretation of the results, samples should be collected in the morning, seated for 15 minutes and with unrestricted dietary salt intake before testing. Premenopausal women should be tested during the follicular phase of the menstrual cycle. Hypokalemia, if present, should be corrected prior to testing. In addition, it is also desirable to switch antihypertensive drugs involved in the aldosterone-angiotensin-renin axis 2–4 weeks prior to the study, especially mineralocorticoid receptor antagonists (MRAs) and diuretics.

Subjects with positive screening can undergo one of two strategies; the most practical one is to perform a therapeutic test with MRAs and evaluate blood pressure after 4–8 weeks. If it has decreased less than 10 mm Hg in systolic BP, the likelihood of PA is low. If it has fallen more than 10 mm Hg, PA is possible, and the higher the fall, the more likely the PA. The reduction of PA, number of medications that are stopped, and normalization of renin are outcomes used to continue MRA treatment. The second strategy is to undergo a confirmatory test: This is based on demonstrating the autonomy of aldosterone production through a suppression test. However, in patients with classic PA with plasma aldosterone more than 15 ng/dL and suppressed PRA, suppression tests should not be performed. The most used tests in tertiary centers are the saline infusion test and the oral sodium loading test. The former consists of the administration of an isotonic saline solution of 500 cc/hour during two to four hours. The persistence of plasma aldosterone levels above 5.8 ng/dL confirms the diagnosis of PA. In the oral sodium overload test, 2 g NaCl capsules are given every 8 hours for a period of 3 days and 24-hour urine is collected. The test is considered positive if urinary aldosterone is more than 12 μg/day, in the presence of urinary sodium more than 200 mmol/day. After confirmation of hyperaldosteronism or the clinical decision to try MR antagonists, imaging of the adrenals should be performed with CT to look for hyperplasia versus adenoma. In equivocal cases, adrenal vein sampling for aldosterone can be performed in tertiary centers.

Differential Diagnosis

Syndrome of apparent mineralocorticoid excess (AME): The renal MR has the same affinity for cortisol as for aldosterone, but cortisol circulates in concentrations 100–1000 times higher than aldosterone; the activation of the MR by cortisol is normally limited due to its conversion to inactive cortisone at the sites of aldosterone action by the enzyme 11-β-hydroxysteroid dehydrogenase type 2 (11-β-HSD2). This conversion may be impaired in AME by pathogenic variants of the *11-β-HSD2* gene, or by licorice ingestion, or by treatment with triazole antifungals that inhibit the enzyme. The resulting MR overactivation and renin suppression will give rise to hyporeninemic hypertension, premature hypertension, hypokalemia, and elevated cortisol/cortisone ratio. However, the clinical spectrum of AME is increasingly expanding, with partial mutations being described with mild hyporeninemic hypertension, which has been termed non-classic AME. Diagnosis is suspected with phenotype and confirmed with elevated serum or urine cortisol/cortisone ratio with or without 11β HSD type 2 sequencing. Other forms of low renin hypertension to include in the differential diagnosis: Liddle syndrome, congenital adrenal hyperplasia due to 11-beta-hydroxylase, and overt Cushing syndrome.

Treatment

Treatment for adrenal adenoma involves surgical resection. In as many as 70% of patients, this cures hypertension and hypokalemia. The blood pressure, however, may require several months following surgery to return to normal. Medical therapy for patients who are not surgical candidates or those with hyperplasia includes the aldosterone antagonists spironolactone in women (50–200 mg/day) or eplerenone, a selective MR antagonist with no anti-androgenic effects, in males and during pregnancy (50–200 mg/day). Importantly, to achieve a complete response and lower the enhanced cardiovascular burden of PA, it is mandatory to normalize renin (DRC > 10 μU/L, PRA>1 ng/mL/h) in addition to normal blood pressure.

Funder J. Primary aldosteronism. *Trends Cardiovasc Med.* 2022;32(4):228–233. [PMID: 33775861]

Vaidya A, Carey RM. Evolution of the primary aldosteronism syndrome: updating the approach. *J Clin Endocrinol Metab.* 2020;105(12):3771–3783. [PMID: 32865201]

Vaidya A, Mulatero P, Baudrand R, Adler GK. The expanding spectrum of primary aldosteronism: implications for diagnosis, pathogenesis, and treatment. *Endocr Rev.* 2018;39(6):1057–1088. [PMID: 30124805].

2. Cushing Syndrome

ESSENTIALS OF DIAGNOSIS

- Central obesity, muscle atrophy, amenorrhea, facial plethora, hypertension, hyperlipidemia, and hyperglycemia are classic clinical features in overt Cushing syndrome.
- A serum cortisol concentration of more than 1.8 μg/dL (50 nmol/L) at 08:00 a.m. after 1 mg dexamethasone given at 11:00 p.m., late night salivary cortisol above the upper limit of normal (ULN), or 24–hour urinary free cortisol above the ULN are needed for the diagnosis.
- Normal or elevated ACTH is observed in Cushing disease (Pituitary tumor), low ACTH in adrenal tumor or exogenous Cushing syndrome.

General Considerations

The term **Cushing syndrome** refers to excess cortisol in the systemic circulation. **Cushing disease** is the state of hypercortisolemia caused by an ACTH-producing pituitary adenoma (most frequent cause). Other causes of Cushing syndrome are ectopic ACTH production from tumors such as small-cell carcinoma of the bronchus or other neuroendocrine tumors; primary adrenal disease, secondary to glucocorticoid-secreting adrenal tumor, usually unilateral benign adenomas (increasing prevalence with incidentalomas observed in a radiologic image for another cause); or the exogenous use of corticosteroids, the most prevalent cause, since 1% of adults are on glucocorticoid treatment. **Pseudo-Cushing syndrome,** also described as non-tumoral hypercortisolism, refers to patients who, on screening, appear to have hypercortisolemia but have relatively few physical signs and no anatomical explanation. Causes include pregnancy, alcohol abuse, obesity, or some psychiatric conditions. Patients with Cushing syndrome typically have central obesity, hypertension, hyperlipidemia, and hyperglycemia. Thus, it is not surprising that they are at risk for coronary artery disease and increased cardiovascular mortality. The severity and the duration of the hypercortisolemia predicts greater risk of coronary disease and congestive HF. In the last decades, there are several studies that have shown that even mild Cushing syndrome (usually from an adrenal adenoma) is associated with increased CV morbidity and mortality.

Diagnostic Considerations

Screening and diagnostic tests for Cushing syndrome assess cortisol dysfunction related to tumor autonomy displayed as impaired glucocorticoid feedback with overnight 1 mg dexamethasone suppression test (DST), abnormal circadian rhythm evaluated by late–night salivary cortisol (LNSC), or increased cortisol daily production with 24–hour urinary free cortisol (UFC). Importantly, in case of mild adrenal Cushing syndrome, the most accurate test is DST (> 1.8 μg/dL) associated with low DHEA-S and ACTH. In clinical guidelines it is advised to use two different tests to confirm hypercortisolism and be aware that estrogen use contraindicates DST and renal failure contraindicates UFC. To determine cause and localization an image is needed and a baseline ACTH level should be performed. Elevated (or normal) ACTH indicates a pituitary tumor or less frequently ectopic production of ACTH. Low ACTH levels confirm adrenal disease and abdominal CT with adrenal protocol should be performed. All adrenal incidentalomas should be screened for hypercortisolism (even without phenotype), since up to 30% of cases have mild cortisol excess. Pituitary MRI is the imaging method of choice for detecting ACTH–secreting pituitary adenomas. However, in part because most lesions are very small, with use of standard 1.5T MRI only approximately 40% of microadenomas are clearly depicted. Therefore, when there is a small/equivocal adenoma (smaller than 6 mm), further testing should rule out an ectopic source of hypercortisolism. Inferior petrosal sinus sampling or desmopressin and CRH stimulation testing plus whole-body CT are commonly used for ACTH-dependent Cushing with no evident tumor. Imaging should be done only after the biochemical workup is completed and confirmed to localize the tumor.

Treatment

Treatment involves surgical removal of the pituitary tumor, usually without radiation, in Cushing disease; removal of the adrenal tumor; or removal of the ectopic source of ACTH production in Cushing syndrome. Recurrence is not infrequent in pituitary tumors; ectopic tumors may require adjuvant therapy. Adrenal adenomas managed with laparoscopic surgery have the best prognosis. Severe Cushing syndrome, as seen in adrenal carcinoma, has a poor prognosis and a multidisciplinary approach is needed. If surgical treatment is not feasible, medical treatment may be used for palliation of symptoms. Adrenal steroidogenesis inhibitors have been available for many years, including ketoconazole (mild effect), metyrapone, mitotane, and etomidate (infusion), as well as the recently approved osilodrostat. These drugs block one or more adrenal enzymes, decreasing glucocorticoid synthesis or adrenal androgen production and secretion, or both.

Fleseriu M, Richard A, Bancos I, et al. Consensus on diagnosis and management of Cushing's disease: a guideline update. *Lancet Diabetes Endocrinol.* 2021;9(12):847–875. [PMID: 34687601]

Isidori AM, Sbardella E, Zatelli MC, et al. Conventional and nuclear medicine imaging in ectopic Cushing's syndrome: a systematic review. *J Clin Endocrinol Metab.* 2015;100(9):3231–3244. [PMID: 26158607]

Nieman LK, Biller BMK, Findling JW, et al. Treatment of Cushing's syndrome: an Endocrine Society clinical practice guideline. *J Clin Endocrinol Metab.* 2015;100(8):2807–2831. [PMID: 26222757]

3. Adrenal Insufficiency

ESSENTIALS OF DIAGNOSIS

- Low cortisol and very high ACTH in primary insufficiency (Addison disease); low cortisol with normal or low ACTH in secondary insufficiency.
- Inability to acutely increase cortisol levels above 18 mg/dL in response to synthetic ACTH stimulation testing in both primary and secondary adrenal insufficiency.
- Hyperpigmentation, high ACTH, orthostatic hypotension, salt wasting, and hyperkalemia or low aldosterone are only observed in primary adrenal insufficiency (Addison disease).
- Hypovolemic shock, hypoglycemia, hyponatremia, and fever are observed in adrenal crisis.

General Considerations

Cortisol is essential for life and regulates gluconeogenesis, metabolism, immune response, circadian rhythm, and blood pressure. Adrenal insufficiency (AI) is deficient production of glucocorticoids. AI is classified into two types: primary AI, or Addison disease, in which the adrenal cortex is destroyed and there is deficiency of glucocorticoids, mineralocorticoids, and androgens; and secondary AI, in which pituitary adrenocorticotropic hormone (ACTH) inappropriate secretion leads to isolated decreased production of adrenal glucocorticoids. There is clinical evidence of increased mortality rates in patients with AI related to hormone deficiency, secondary effects of treatment, and adrenal crisis.

Currently, the most common cause of Addison disease is autoimmune destruction of the adrenal cortex. Classic adrenal hyperplasia (due to inborn defects in adrenal enzymes), metastasis, AIDS, and granulomatous diseases (such as tuberculosis and histoplasmosis) are other etiologic considerations. Adrenal hemorrhage usually occurs in the setting of anticoagulation or severe sepsis. The most common cause of secondary AI is withdrawal of corticosteroids, considering that up to 1% of adults are using chronic glucocorticoids (GC) for rheumatological diseases, autoimmune causes, or transplantation. GC suppresses the hypothalamic–pituitary–adrenal axis (low ACTH) and therefore causes adrenal cortex atrophy and glucocorticoid deficiency. It is important to be aware that GC withdrawal not only is observed after oral or parenteral use, but also with intraarticular or dermatological use. Primary AI is rare in the general population, with an incidence of less than 0.01%, but is increased with the presence of other autoimmune diseases. However, the overall risk of AI is increased in critically ill patients, especially those older or with partial response to pressors when hypotensive.

Clinical Findings

A. Symptoms & Signs

1. Systemic symptoms & signs—Glucocorticoid deficiency causes fatigue, anorexia, nausea, and vomiting. These lead to weight loss which is a cardinal symptom of AI. Hyperpigmentation of skin, palm creases, knuckles, and gums is pathognomonic of Addison disease secondary to increased ACTH through activation of melanocortin receptor type 1. Mineralocorticoid or aldosterone deficiency is also only observed in primary AI and causes renal sodium and bicarbonate wasting, resulting in orthostatic hypotension, craving for salt, hyponatremia, hyperkalemia, acidosis, and dehydration. Acute AI or crisis occurs when the patient is exposed to stresses such as treatment withdrawal, infection, trauma, and surgery, and cannot compensate adequately with augmented glucocorticoid release.

2. Cardiovascular symptoms & signs—Hypotension, often orthostatic, is usually present in patients with primary AI and occasionally causes syncope. Chronic AI is characterized by decreased systemic vascular resistance and decreased myocardial contractility. On the other hand, acute AI can have variable cardiac function with low, normal, or high systemic vascular resistance, cardiac output, and capillary wedge pressure. Thus, in acute AI—which can be superimposed on a setting of chronic AI—the patient may be in hypovolemic shock, accompanied by fever, volume depletion, depressed mentation, nausea, vomiting, abdominal pain, with hyponatremia, hyperkalemia, and occasional hypoglycemia. Shock and coma can rapidly progress to death, if untreated. Adrenal crisis should be considered in any patient with unexplained hypovolemic shock.

B. Physical Examination

The classic physical examination finding for chronic primary AI is hyperpigmentation of the skin and mucous membranes, especially over pressure points such as the knuckles, toes, elbows, and knees and in scars, palmar creases, nail beds, and areolae. Vitiligo is a clue that the AI is autoimmune in nature. In secondary AI, patients lack the hyperpigmentation; the presence of cushingoid features suggests recent glucocorticoid withdrawal used for nonendocrine indications such as atopy or immunologic disorders.

C. Diagnostic Studies

1. Laboratory findings—Hyponatremia, hyperkalemia, with occasional hypercalcemia, hypoglycemia, and acidosis, are observed in Addison disease. Patients with secondary AI will not have hyperkalemia because their renin (secreted by the kidney) and angiotensin system is able to stimulate aldosterone production. A normocytic, normochromic anemia with lymphocytosis and eosinophilia is seen on the blood smear.

The rapid ACTH stimulation test is used to diagnose AI, as a proxy of inappropriate acute response to a stress situation. Administration of synthetic ACTH (cosyntropin) causes an elevation of cortisol within 30–60 minutes. Failure to increase cortisol to 18 mg/dL confirms the insufficiency. ACTH level can help distinguish primary (high) from secondary causes (normal or low ACTH). High renin levels (due to aldosterone deficiency) and low DHEAS (due to reticular layer destruction of adrenal cortex), are also complementary lab tests to confirm primary AI.

In the setting of critical illness, the diagnosis of AI is more problematic. Although it is well known that stress such as that seen with hypotension, inflammation, sepsis, or surgery results in elevated cortisol levels, the definition of AI in this setting is less clear. Novel studies have shown a decrease in cortisol metabolism in the ICU setting. In the clinical setting of probable cortisol deficiency, supplementation is advised (150–200 mg/day).

2. Electrocardiography & echocardiography—ECG findings include sinus bradycardia, sinus tachycardia, nonspecific T-wave changes, peaked T waves if hyperkalemia is prominent, and low voltage and a shortened QT interval if hypercalcemia is present. Echocardiography reveals small cardiac chambers with normal function.

Treatment

The treatment of chronic Addison disease involves both glucocorticoid and mineralocorticoid replacement and is usually performed in tertiary centers. Treatment aims to normalize hyperpigmentation and intravascular volume status. Also, patients with other autoimmune diseases should be educated to increase GC doses in stress situations and to use emergency parental GC to avoid adrenal crisis. A medical alert bracelet is useful in such patients since the treatment of adrenal crises is lifesaving. If the patient is in serious shock, immediately use stress doses of corticosteroids, such as initial bolus of 100 mg of hydrocortisone intravenously and then 50 mg every 6–8 hours. Saline volume resuscitation along with glucose infusion is necessary to correct volume and electrolyte abnormalities. A search for the underlying precipitant, such as infection, coronary event, or glucocorticoid withdrawal should be undertaken and treated as necessary.

Betterle C, Presotto F, Furmaniak J. Epidemiology, pathogenesis, and diagnosis of Addison's disease in adults. *J Endocrinol Invest.* 2019 Dec;42(12):1407–1433. doi: 10.1007/s40618-019-01079-6. Epub 2019 Jul 18. [PMID: 31321757]

Laugesen K, Broersen LHA, Hansen SB, Dekkers OM, Sørensen HT, Jorgensen JOL. MANAGEMENT OF ENDOCRINE DISEASE: Glucocorticoid-induced adrenal insufficiency: replace while we wait for evidence? *Eur J Endocrinol.* 2021 Apr;184(4):R111–R122. doi: 10.1530/EJE-20-1199. [PMID: 33449912]

4. Pheochromocytomas and Paragangliomas

ESSENTIALS OF DIAGNOSIS

- Headache, palpitations, and sweating in conjunction with either hypertension (may be paroxysmal) or orthostatic hypotension.
- Biochemical evidence of excess catecholamines.
- Adrenal tumor or tumor along the sympathetic chain (paraganglioma).
- Pressor response to anesthesia induction or to antihypertensive or sympathomimetic drugs.

General Considerations

Catecholamine-secreting neoplasms, or pheochromocytomas and paragangliomas (PPGLs), can be life-threatening and cause hypertension, arrhythmia, and hyperglycemia. Annually 0.6 cases per 100,000 persons are diagnosed, accounting for 0.1–0.2% of underlying primary causes of hypertension. Eighty percent of pheochromocytomas are in the adrenals; 20% arise from extra-adrenal chromaffin tissue along the sympathetic chain and are known as paragangliomas. Most pheochromocytomas secrete predominantly norepinephrine; about 15% secrete mainly epinephrine. The majority of PPGLs occur sporadically, however, it has recently been estimated that the proportion of patients with hereditary tumors exceeds 40%. They are seen as part of a familial syndrome such as multiple endocrine neoplasia type 2 (hyperparathyroidism, medullary thyroid cancer, pheochromocytoma), or von Hippel-Lindau disease (cerebelloretinal hemangioblastomas, pheochromocytoma, pancreatic islet cell tumors, renal cell cysts, testicular cysts), or succinate dehydrogenase-deficient pheochromocytoma-paraganglioma syndrome (multifocal paraganglioma, renal cell carcinoma, GIST, pituitary adenoma), among others.

Despite the rarity of this condition, its importance cannot be overstated because of several reasons: (a) high morbidity and mortality due to inadvertent catecholamine hypersecretion (especially perioperative), (b) detection of familial disease requiring specialized follow-up, (c) malignant potential of 5–20% in pheochromocytoma and 15–35% in sympathetic paragangliomas. A correct diagnosis and treatment leads to cure and a missed diagnosis can be fatal.

Genetics

Current molecular classification encompasses PPGLs into three pathogenic clusters: those mediated by MAP kinase signaling pathway (gain-of-function mutation) with pathogenic variants in RET proto-oncogen causing multiple endocrine neoplasia type 2 (MEN2) and neurofibromatosis type 1 (NF1), along with others (TMEM127 and MAX); a cluster mediated by alterations in the Wnt signaling (somatic mutations in CSDE1 and UBTF-MAML3); and a cluster mediated by pseudohypoxia (mutations in von Hippel Lindau VHL, succinate dehydrogenase SHDx, and fumarate dehydrogenase FH). Up to 12–16% of PPGL have SHDx or FH mutations, including mainly paragangliomas (22–70%). The proportion of SHDx mutations among metastatic tumors is the highest among hereditary PPGLs, being estimated at 43–71% in adults.

Clinical Findings

A. Symptoms & Signs

1. Systemic symptoms & signs—The release of catecholamines from the tumor is unpredictable and usually causes paroxysmal attacks of headache, palpitations, and sweating. Patients may also complain of increased nervousness, irritability, and an impending sense of doom. Mild abdominal pain and constipation are relatively common. The clinician should suspect a pheochromocytoma/sympathetic paraganglioma in any patient in whom a sudden elevation of blood pressure develops during anesthesia induction.

In contrast, head and neck paragangliomas are manifested by a painless, slow-growing mass or by hearing loss and pulsatile tinnitus. Catecholamine hypersecretion (dopamine) is rare in these patients. Today, other forms of presentation have been increasing in frequency, being diagnosed earlier and smaller as incidentalomas due to increased use of imaging techniques, or in relation to the study of relatives with known germline mutations.

2. Cardiovascular symptoms & signs—The effects of catecholamines on the heart are mediated by β1-receptors and include increased heart rate, enhanced contractility, and augmented conduction velocity—all of which contribute to an increase in cardiac output. Eighty percent of patients will have hypertension, which can be either sustained, labile (with hypotension and hypertension), or paroxysmal. Orthostatic hypotension is often noted, whereas syncope occurs rarely.

Both dilated and hypertrophic cardiomyopathies and myocarditis have been described with pheochromocytoma, and exposure to high levels of catecholamines can cause contraction-band necrosis and fibrosis. Stress (Takotsubo) cardiomyopathy causes acute myocardial stunning and is reversible if the excessive catecholamine stimulus is removed early, before extensive replacement fibrosis takes place. Chest pain, angina, and acute myocardial infarction may occur in the absence of coronary artery occlusive disease. Catecholamine-induced increases in myocardial oxygen consumption, myocarditis, and coronary artery spasm likely contribute to the infarction. Cardiac arrhythmias such as atrial and ventricular fibrillation occur, especially in the setting of surgical resection of the tumor. Pulmonary edema and shock associated with myocarditis or infarction can be observed, or it may follow a hypertensive crisis.

B. Physical Examination

Sustained or paroxysmal hypertension is common. Orthostasis is also often seen, and noncardiogenic pulmonary edema of obscure origin has also been described. Retinal hemorrhage or papilledema is a rare occurrence. Interestingly, patients carrying PPGL-susceptibility genes may elicit specific clinical findings; Café-au-lait macules and skinfold freckling in neurofibromatosis type 1 (NF1), cutaneous amyloidosis, mucosal neuroma and marfanoid features in MEN2, blindness, hypoacusia, and focal neurologic deficits in VHL disease.

C. Diagnostic Studies

1. Laboratory findings—The diagnosis of pheochromocytomas and paragangliomas requires demonstration of excess catecholamine release and anatomical documentation of the tumor. Increased fractionated plasma metanephrines have the best performance (sensitivity 97% and specificity 93%) and must be at least two times the upper normal value. Urinary metanephrines have a similar performance, while plasma catecholamines lack sensitivity and specificity as it depends on the tumor secretion rate. LC-MS/MS is currently the preferred assay method because of its optimal analytical accuracy, cost-effectiveness, and minimal analytical interference from drugs (Table 34–6).

Hereditary pheochromocytomas and paragangliomas associated with pseudohypoxia lack the late enzymatic steps of catecholamine biosynthesis. For this reason, they elevate normetanephrines and not metanephrine. Up to 70% of SDHx carriers also elevate dopamine (or its metabolite 3-methoxytyramine). Occasionally, these tumors lack the initial catecholamine biosynthesis enzyme (tyrosine hydroxylase) and are biochemically silent. In those patients, the only potential biomarker is chromogranin A, a protein secreted in neuroendocrine cells. These are thought to be reasons for their often oligosymptomatic presentation, with larger tumors and worse prognosis.

2. Electrocardiography & imaging—ECG changes are common; nonspecific ST-T wave changes and prominent U waves may be seen. Sinus tachycardia, sinus bradycardia, and atrial and ventricular tachyarrhythmias have all been noted and may be associated with palpitations. Conduction disturbances, including right and left bundle branch block, and signs of LVH sometimes occur.

Clinically significant cardiomyopathy and increased left ventricular mass have been noted on echocardiography.

3. Localization studies—Initial localization is usually done either with CT or MRI of the abdomen, and these studies can detect approximately 95% of pheochromocytomas or paragangliomas. The tumors can be homogeneous or heterogeneous, including features of necrosis, hemorrhage, cystic changes, and calcifications. However, since paragangliomas may arise anywhere along the sympathetic chain, a whole body 68 Gallium DOTA PET/CT may be required in

Table 34–6. Drugs, Foods, and Conditions That Increase False Positive or Negative Tests for Pheochromocytoma

Test	Increase	Decrease
Catecholamines	Levodopa Severe stress Diseases: Guillain-Barré, lead poisoning, eclampsia, hypoglycemia, carcinoid, acute porphyria, amyotrophic lateral sclerosis, quinine, bretylium, methenamine, methocarbamine Ethanol, isoproterenol, methyldopa, MAO inhibitors, phenothiazines, α-methyl *p*-tyrosine, methenamine, bilirubin, labetalol	Fenfluramine Renal insufficiency Malnutrition, dysautonomia, quadriplegia
Metanephrines	Sympathomimetics: amphetamines, ephedrine, nasal decongestants, bronchodilators, methyldopa, MAO inhibitors, phenothiazines, "dual" antidepressants (venlafaxine, duloxetine)	Radiopaque media: Renografin, Hypaque–M, Renovist, Cardiografin, Urografin, Conray

MAO, monoamine oxidase.

selected cases. Functional imaging with 68Ga-DOTATATE PET scanning rather than 123I-metaiodobenzylguanidine (MIBG) is recommended for staging of metastatic/multifocal disease, presurgery staging of a pheochromocytoma ≥ 5 cm, or any suspicious paraganglioma specially in the setting of a germline mutation. In those cases, functional imaging adds value in improved specificity and sensitivity and links with targeted radionuclide therapy.

Treatment

Treatment of patients with paragangliomas and pheochromocytomas requires a multidisciplinary team of dedicated specialists in centers that have experience in management of these complex patients. Treatment involves the prevention of cardiovascular complications such as myocardial infarction, HF, hypertensive crisis and stroke, arrhythmias, and sudden death; it also involves surgical removal of the tumor. Recent advances in localizing imaging studies and the emergence of laparoscopic adrenalectomy along with proper preoperative medical preparation have reduced morbidity and mortality significantly. Patients need to be treated with oral antihypertensives and stabilized hemodynamically prior to surgery. Preoperative α blockade is used to reverse the effects of excessive catecholamines and prevent crises. Because most pheochromocytomas secrete norepinephrine, α-blockade should be given first to prevent aggravation of hypertension and precipitation of coronary spasm or pulmonary edema from unopposed α-receptor stimulation. The most used drugs are phenoxybenzamine, a nonselective and noncompetitive α1- and α2-adrenergic receptor blocker, and doxazosin, a selective and competitive α1-adrenergic receptor blocker. These drugs are initiated at least 7–14 days before surgery in gradually increasing dosages until blood pressure is less than 130/80 mm Hg and an upright systolic blood pressure more than 90 mm Hg have been suggested. Heart rate targets are 60–70 bpm and 70–80 bpm in seated and upright position, respectively. β-Blockers are added if reflex tachycardia or cardiac dysfunction is present. Hypotension occurs more frequently in patients who are normotensive between hypertensive paroxysms. However, normotensive patients with paragangliomas and pheochromocytomas with normal or elevated levels of catecholamines or metanephrines may also be at increased risk of intraoperative hemodynamic instability and should therefore receive presurgical α-blockade.

Patients are in general volume depleted and should be encouraged to hydrate well and increase sodium consumption. Ideally, patients should be admitted for administration of intravenous fluids at least 1 day prior to surgery. β-Blockade can be used to reduce β-adrenergic symptoms such as flushing, palpitations, or tachycardia. Nonselective β-blockers (β1 and β2 blockers), such as nadolol, propranolol, pindolol, and timolol, block the vasodilating arterial β2 receptors and should not be administered to patients with pheochromocytoma or paragangliomas. β-Blockers that selectively block β1-adrenergic receptors such as atenolol, bisoprolol, esmolol, and metoprolol induce reduced heart rate without an unopposed α-receptor–mediated rise in blood pressure. Extended-release metoprolol is the preferred oral preparation; esmolol is the preferred intravenous agent. Metyrosine is a drug that inhibits tyrosine hydroxylase, which catalyzes the first reaction in catecholamine biosynthesis (rate-limiting step). Because of side effects, it is usually reserved for treatment of hypertension in metastatic or inoperable pheochromocytoma.

Prognosis

Perioperative mortality overall has steadily decreased to about 2.4% due to improved medical preparation and surgical technique but reported morbidity rates can be as high as 25%. Surgical complication rates are higher in patients with severe hypertension and in patients undergoing reoperations. Surgical morbidity and mortality risks can be minimized by meticulous preoperative preparation, accurate tumor localization, and supportive intraoperative care.

Nonmetastatic surgically resected pheochromocytomas have a 5-year survival rate of 95%. Risk factors for death include large tumors (> 5 cm), metastatic disease, and local tumor invasion. In metastatic disease, the 5-year survival is less than 50%. If a surgical cure is achieved before the cardiovascular system has been irreparably damaged, cardiovascular health will be completely restored. In 25% of patients, hypertension persists due to underlying essential hypertension or irreversible vascular or renal damage but is usually well-controlled with standard antihypertensive agents. However, if severe hypertension persists, a search for a second or residual tumor should be considered.

Patients with a history of pheochromocytoma require long-term postoperative surveillance and aggressive treatment for cardiovascular risk factors. They have increased long-term risk of death from cardiovascular causes.

Lenders JW, Kerstens MN, Amar L, et al. Genetics, diagnosis, management and future directions of research of pheochromocytoma and paraganglioma: a position statement and consensus of the Working Group on Endocrine Hypertension of the European Society of Hypertension. *J Hypertens.* 2020;38(8):1443–1456. [PMID: 32412940]

Nölting S, Bechmann N, Taieb D, et al. Personalized management of pheochromocytoma and paraganglioma. *Endocr Rev.* 2022;43(2):199–239. [PMID: 34147030]

ACROMEGALY & THE HEART

ESSENTIALS OF DIAGNOSIS

- Frontal bossing, prominent cheeks and nose, thickened lips, prognathism, widely spaced teeth, and macroglossia, acral enlargement, and organomegaly.
- Elevated insulin-like growth factor -1 (IGF-1).
- Inability to suppress growth hormone to less than 1.4 ng/mL during glucose tolerance test.
- Pituitary adenoma found on magnetic resonance imaging.

General Considerations

Acromegaly is caused by an excessive secretion of growth hormone (GH), most commonly, by a pituitary adenoma in an adult, whereas gigantism occurs only in children. Characteristic clinical manifestations are due to the chronic effects of GH, mediated through insulin-like growth factor 1 (IGF-1 or somatomedin C) in the liver and the periphery. Bony overgrowth is the classic feature, particularly of the skull and mandible; they also present with organomegaly and premature death, often due to cardiovascular, cerebrovascular, and respiratory dysfunction.

Clinical Findings

A. Symptoms & Signs

1. Systemic symptoms & signs—Patients whose onset of disease precedes epiphyseal complete fusion develop increased linear growth, leading to gigantism. In contrast, patients whose tumors occur after epiphyseal maturation develop acromegaly, characterized by typical facial features (frontal bossing, prominent cheeks and nose, thickened lips, prognathism, widely spaced teeth, and macroglossia), acral enlargement, and organomegaly. Patients may also complain of symptoms related to the local expansion of the tumor such as headache or bitemporal hemianopsia. Impotence, galactorrhea, and amenorrhea may result from co-secretion of prolactin or the destruction of normal gonadotrophs by the tumor. Other symptoms include excessive sweating, hoarseness, carpal tunnel syndrome, polyuria, and polydipsia.

2. Cardiovascular symptoms & signs—The most frequent complications that these patients may encounter include cardiomyopathy, arrhythmias, hypertension, heart valve disease, atherosclerosis, and coronary artery disease. Cardiac dysfunction and HF are major causes of death in acromegalics. The older the patient and the longer the duration of disease, the more likely acromegalic cardiomyopathy will develop. The most striking clinical feature is concentric biventricular hypertrophy with inadequate filling leading to both systolic and diastolic dysfunction. Cardiomegaly occurs in about 15% of cases secondary to hypertension, atherosclerotic disease, or rarely due to acromegalic cardiomyopathy.

Other factors can potentially contribute to cardiac dysfunction. The coexistence of hypertension, diabetes, or both in this condition can accelerate the progression to cardiac hypertrophy and HF. The sinoatrial and atrioventricular nodes may also be affected, entailing cardiac arrhythmias and sudden death. Hypertension, the most common cardiovascular finding in acromegalics, occurs in about 35–50% of patients, is usually mild in nature, and is easily treated with antihypertensives. It is characterized by elevated diastolic blood pressure and a higher prevalence of non-dippers. The mechanism of hypertension may be due to increased sodium and extracellular fluid retention with increased plasma volume.

Because of the role of GH as a counterregulatory hormone for hypoglycemia, most acromegalics have either glucose intolerance or frank diabetes. Untreated acromegaly is associated with hypertriglyceridemia and elevated levels of apoprotein A-1, apolipoprotein E, fibrinogen, and plasminogen activator inhibitor-1 activity.

A rare disorder known as Carney syndrome involves GH-secreting pituitary tumors with multiple cardiac or cutaneous myxoma and pigmented nodular adrenocortical disease. The myxomas seen in Carney syndrome are usually multiple and may involve more than one chamber. Family members should be screened with echocardiography.

B. Physical Examination

Because acromegaly is such an insidious disease, changes in the body occur gradually and usually go unnoticed for many years until complications develop. Facial changes, including thick lips, macroglossia, bulbous nose, frontal bossing, prominent cheeks, hollow temporal fossa, and malocclusion with protrusion of the lower jaw, are usually seen. Synovial and periarticular swelling may be noted, and dorsal kyphosis, barrel chest, and spade-like hands with sausage-like digits are seen. The chest examination is most remarkable for gynecomastia and cardiomegaly.

C. Diagnostic Studies

1. Laboratory findings—Diagnostic tests should include GH levels, random and glucose suppressed, along with high IGF-1 levels. Because GH secretion is episodic, a random level alone is rarely helpful. Normally, GH is suppressed to less than 1.4 ng/mL in response to a glucose tolerance test (0.4 mcg/L when ultrasensitive GH-assays are available). Other findings often associated with acromegaly include hyperglycemia, hyperphosphatemia, and hypertriglyceridemia.

2. Electrocardiography & echocardiography—Cardiomegaly may be present, even in the absence of hypertension, suggesting a direct effect of GH on the myocytes. Both symmetric and asymmetric cardiac hypertrophy have been reported on echocardiography. In early stages of the disease, both ventricular dimension and wall thickness are increased; therefore, relative wall thickness remains unchanged. In later stages, impaired diastolic filling and cardiac dilatation occur, leading to congestive HF.

ECG abnormalities include ST depression and nonspecific T-wave changes, LVH, and intraventricular conduction defects. Cardiac arrhythmias often occur, with ventricular ectopy and atrial fibrillation or flutter being the most frequent.

Treatment

The goal in treating acromegaly is to normalize GH and IGF-1 concentrations to prevent early cardiovascular mortality. Treatment includes surgical removal of the pituitary adenoma with postoperative radiation therapy, or medical therapy with octreotide (200–500 mcg/day subcutaneously), a somatostatin analog, or cabergoline (to decrease prolactin) bromocriptine (5–30 mg/day) in selected cases. More recently, sustained-release somatostatin analogs with activities lasting up to 1 month, such as octreotide LAR and lanreotide acetate, are becoming more popular and are the treatment of choice for patients with residual GH hypersecretion following surgery. The dopamine agonist, cabergoline, may be added to somatostatin analog therapy to improve control of GH levels. Many authors have suggested that once control of the disease occurs, defined as a GH level of less than 1 μg/L and a normal age-adjusted IGF-1 level, the progression of cardiac disease can be arrested and cardiovascular mortality reduced.

Katznelson L, Jr Laws ER, Melmed S, et al. Acromegaly: an endocrine society clinical practice guideline. *J Clin Endocrinol Metab*. 2014;99(11):3933–3951. [PMID: 25356808]

Ramos-Leví AM, Marazuela M. Bringing cardiovascular comorbidities in acromegaly to an update. How Should We Diagnose and Manage Them? *Front Endocrinol (Lausanne)*. 2019 7; 10:120. [PMID: 30930848]

GROWTH HORMONE DEFICIENCY

Adult GH deficiency (GHD) is most often associated with damage to the hypothalamic-pituitary region as a result of tumors, congenital anomalies, and/or treatment with surgery and radiation. Unlike acromegaly, in which cardiac involvement has been appreciated for many decades, the cardiac abnormalities associated with GHD have only recently been recognized. GHD is associated with abnormal body composition due to increased fat mass, impaired capacity for exercise, decreased bone mineral density, decreased quality of life, and a risk of increased mortality from cardiovascular disease. Myocardial infarction, cardiac failure, and cerebrovascular accidents are the main causes of death.

The mechanisms responsible for the increase in cardiovascular disease are abnormalities in lipoprotein metabolism, premature atherosclerosis, impaired fibrinolytic activity, abnormal cardiac structure and function, and endothelial dysfunction. Characteristic hypokinetic syndrome has been described, composed of a decrease in left ventricular and septal wall thickness on echocardiography along with low heart rate and blood pressure.

Most commonly, adult GHD results from childhood onset of GHD that continues throughout life. Thus, the patient with a history of pituitary or hypothalamic disease, childhood-onset GHD, cranial irradiation, or trauma is a candidate for GHD testing. Testing consists of provocative stimulation with an insulin tolerance test. A biochemical diagnosis of adult GHD is determined by a subnormal response, for example, a peak level of GH less than 3–5 ng/mL. Testing should not be performed in patients with ischemic heart disease or seizure disorder. Treatment is initiated with a daily subcutaneous injection of 2–5 mcg/kg/day of GH and can be titrated to 10–12 mcg/kg/day. Side effects are dose-dependent and consist of fluid retention and carpal tunnel syndrome.

Lanes R. Cardiovascular risk in growth hormone deficiency: beneficial effects of growth hormone replacement therapy. *Endocrinol Metab Clin North Am*. 2016;45(2):405–418. [PMID: 27241971]

NEUROENDOCRINE TUMORS & THE HEART

General Considerations

Neuroendocrine tumors are rare malignancies that may arise from many locations, either from endocrine glands, from endocrine cells within secretory organs (thyroid C-cell and pancreas islets of Langerhans), but mainly from neuroendocrine cells allocated between exocrine cells throughout the digestive and respiratory tracts. Incidence of neuroendocrine tumors is rising and in the United States is second most frequent digestive neoplasia. Although these tumors can secrete several hormones, including ACTH (Ectopic Cushing syndrome) and GH-releasing hormone, they most commonly secrete serotonin and serotonin metabolites regulated by somatostatin. The presentation of the patient depends on the location of the neuroendocrine tumor and its secretion status. Symptoms include flushing and diarrhea, with liver metastases, and bronchospasm with pulmonary carcinoid. Hypoglycemia is observed in insulinoma and diarrhea with gastric ulcers in gastrinoma.

Determined by both mitotic count and Ki-67, neuroendocrine tumors are graded in low, intermediate and high, and is a very useful tool to select treatment and predict prognosis.

A unique cardiac manifestation occurring in patients with advanced neuroendocrine tumors is carcinoid heart disease (Hedinger syndrome). It consists of fibrotic plaque-like thickenings on the endocardium of the tricuspid and pulmonic valves, atria, and ventricles. Deposition may also be seen on the superior and inferior venae cavae, pulmonary artery, and coronary sinus. The right side of the heart is affected predominantly, and although left-sided heart disease may occur, it is of lesser significance because of the pulmonary deactivation of the hormonal substances. Thickening of the valves results in tricuspid regurgitation and pulmonic stenosis. Right ventricular dysfunction carries a poor prognosis and represents a major cause of morbidity and mortality, with death as a result of cardiac decompensation in as high as 43% in untreated patients. Elaboration of the variety of vasoactive substances secreted by the neuroendocrine tumor is believed to mediate the fibrosis.

To date, chromogranin A is the best biomarker in neuroendocrine tumors for both diagnosis and follow up. Diagnosis of carcinoid syndrome is made by documenting high 5-hydroxyindoleacetic acid (a serotonin metabolite) in a 24-hour urine collection, which helps identify individuals at risk of carcinoid heart disease, 30 mg of 5-hydroxyindoleacetic acid (a serotonin metabolite) in a 24-hour urine collection and an elevated NT-proBNP. Localization should be attempted with bowel series, CT, somatostatin receptor scintigraphy, and most recently, 68 Gallium DOTA PET/CT, since it is a somatostatin analog. All patients with carcinoid should undergo echocardiography to evaluate for heart involvement.

Treatment

Treatment is surgical removal of the tumor if it has not metastasized. Somatostatin analogues, octreotide and lanreotide, have been effective in controlling symptoms of carcinoid syndrome and have shown to shrink tumor metastases in addition to decreasing serotonin levels. Unfortunately, the heart disease does not improve with reduction of serotonin levels, and some patients will require valve replacement.

Jin C, Sharma AN, Thevakumar B, et al. Carcinoid heart disease: pathophysiology, pathology, clinical manifestations, and management. *Cardiology.* 2021;146(1):65–73. [PMID: 33070143]

DIABETES MELLITUS & THE HEART

General Considerations

Diabetes mellitus is a frequent, complex, and multifactorial disease that has increased dramatically in the past decades and will continue to be a serious global epidemic due to aging, obesity, sedentary lifestyle, and unhealthy habits.

Diabetes can be classified as (a) type 1 diabetes (autoimmune insulin deficiency, mainly in < 30 years), (b) type 2 diabetes (accounting for 90–95% of all cases with prevalence of up to 12% of US population) which has a heterogenous pathophysiology of insulin resistance leading to pancreatic β-cell failure), (c) gestational diabetes mellitus, or (d) others such as monogenic disorders.

Diagnostic criteria by the American Diabetes Association (ADA) are the following: A fasting plasma glucose higher than 126 mg/dL, a plasma glucose level more than 200 mg/dL random/2 hours after 75 g oral glucose tolerance test or glycosylated hemoglobin (HbA1c) more than 6.5%. In relation to the cardiovascular system, myocardial infarction is the leading cause of death in patients with type 2 diabetes. The incidence of coronary artery disease and myocardial infarction in diabetic patients is up to five times higher than in age-matched controls. Premature cardiovascular disease is also observed in patients with type 1 diabetes. Two types of vascular disease are seen: macrovascular disease, including atherosclerosis and microvascular disease, including retinopathy, nephropathy, neuropathy, and microangiopathy in the heart. Microangiopathy may explain the existence of congestive HF in diabetic patients without demonstrable coronary artery disease. Macrovascular disease develops prematurely in diabetic patients and is usually severe, with a striking predominance in diabetic women. Diabetics with no history of coronary heart disease (CHD) have risk for major cardiovascular events equal to that in established CHD. Consequently, the Adult Treatment Panel III in 2001 has designated diabetes as a "CHD risk equivalent," with a 10-year risk for major cardiovascular events (risk of myocardial infarction and coronary death) of more than 20%.

A large body of evidence now links the increased risk of atherosclerosis to a combination of factors present in diabetes such as hyperlipidemia, abnormalities of platelet adhesiveness, coagulation factors, hypertension, and oxidative stress and inflammation leading to endothelial dysfunction. The evidence is particularly striking in persons with type 1 diabetes with microalbuminuria and proteinuria; however, endothelial dysfunction also occurs in patients with type 2 diabetes and normal urinary albumin excretion as well as in patients with insulin resistance who are normoglycemic. Once established, endothelial dysfunction induces changes in vascular tone, reactivity, and function that contribute to the progression of vascular disease. Insulin sensitizers, hypolipidemic therapy, and angiotensin-converting enzyme inhibitors have all been shown to improve endothelial function.

Hyperinsulinemia and insulin resistance have been postulated to relate directly to both hypertension and CHD in type 2 diabetes. The so-called metabolic syndrome is a constellation of metabolic risk factors that includes obesity, insulin resistance, elevated triglycerides, low high-density lipoprotein, hypertension, and fasting hyperglycemia. It enhances the risk for CHD at any given LDL level. To achieve maximum benefit from risk factor modification, the underlying insulin-resistant state must be a primary target of therapy.

Clinical Findings

Angina and myocardial infarction in persons with diabetes are often manifested by atypical symptoms. Painless myocardial infarction may occur, and unusual pain patterns may delay diagnosis. Diabetic patients have a high mortality rate from myocardial infarction; recurrence is frequent, and the long-term prognosis is poor, with a higher incidence of congestive HF and ventricular rupture. Diabetic men have a 2.4-fold increase in HF, but diabetic women have a particularly high incidence: 5.1 times that of persons without diabetes. Of note, diabetic cardiomyopathy occurs even in the absence of epicardial vessel disease, causing some investigators to hypothesize a preponderance of small-vessel disease. Autonomic neuropathy frequently occurs and results in sympathetic denervation manifested by a fixed tachycardia with subsequent parasympathetic damage that results in lowering of the heart rate. Complete autonomic cardiac denervation eventually occurs, resulting in a heart rate that is no longer responsive to physiologic stimuli such as standing.

Echocardiographic studies may show abnormal systolic and diastolic function, with impaired diastolic filling (diastolic dysfunction) as one of the earliest manifestations of diabetic cardiomyopathy. Left ventricular dysfunction is likely multifactorial, reflecting the effects of hypertension, microvascular disease, and coronary atherosclerosis.

Treatment

Lifestyle modification in diabetes is a critical component of CV risk reduction and includes education, nutrition therapy, smoking cessation, psychosocial care and, importantly, physical activity. Obesity associated with diabetes must be treated by pharmacological treatment or even bariatric surgery. A body mass index (BMI) more than 30 kg/m^2 promotes and accelerates atherosclerotic CV disease, and increases left ventricular thickness and myocardial dysfunction.

The impact in reducing CV risk factors in diabetes have a synergic beneficial effect. For example, every 40 mg/dL decline in LDL cholesterol results in a 21% decrease in cardiovascular events. A decrease in systolic blood pressure by 10 mm Hg can decrease cardiovascular mortality by 20–40%. Similarly, the risk of acute myocardial infarction increases by 5.6% for every additional cigarette smoked per day.

Oral hypoglycemic agents such as sulfonylureas (insulin secretagogues), glibenclamide or glyburide, as well as insulin sensitizers (metformin the most widely used medication). Insulin injections or novel oral medications remain the mainstay of therapy for hyperglycemia. Over the last decades, new agents have demonstrated significant improvement in CV outcomes; GLP-1 receptor agonists (liraglutide, semaglutide), DPP4 inhibitors than increase GLP-1 (sitagliptin, vildagliptin) and sodium-glucose cotransporters 2 (SGLT2) inhibitors are becoming more widely used as primary medications for diabetes treatment and prevention in patients at increased CV risk for their improved outcomes and safety profiles. SGLT2 treatment, by reducing glucose reabsorption in renal tubule, is associated with significant improvements in patient's volume status, reducing hospitalizations and HF exacerbations, with significant cardiovascular risk reduction. The recent 2022 AHA/ACC guidelines for the management of heart failure strongly recommend that patients with HF with reduced ejection fraction receive treatment with four classes of medications including an SGLT2 inhibitor and weakly recommend use of an SGLT2 inhibitor in patients with HF with preserved ejection fraction.

Tight glucose control decreases the progression and development of diabetic microvascular complications in patients with both type 1 and type 2 diabetes. For the prevention of cardiovascular risk, ADA has recommended an individualized target for hemoglobin A1c level: of less than 7% in most adults, less than 6.5% for young patients, and less than 8% in subjects with hypoglycemia or short life expectancy. Intensive glycemic control aiming for near-normal levels has been shown to have beneficial effect (58% reduction in long term major cardiovascular disease events) on macrovascular outcomes in type 1 diabetes; however there is increased risk of hypoglycemia that is associated with poor outcomes, requiring specialized management and close follow up by diabetes specialist. Of note, a 1-unit higher HbA1c in subjects with diabetes increases the risk of myocardial infarction, stroke, or peripheral artery disease by almost 20%.

Clustered metabolic disorders in diabetes are associated with atherogenic dyslipidemia, low-level inflammation, and increased triglycerides, which also predicts CV risk in diabetic subjects. Thus, dyslipidemia therapy is a cornerstone treatment in diabetes. In most patients, drug therapy is indicated for reducing atherogenic lipid levels. Non-HDL cholesterol and Apolipoprotein B are better predictors of residual risk in diabetes than LDL cholesterol, as triglyceride-rich lipoproteins, such as very low-density lipoproteins (VLDL), are elevated and not quantified by LDL-C. Statins are generally initiated as first-line therapy. Ezetimibe can be added if non-HDL and LDL cholesterol levels are not reduced to the goal. Furthermore, human monoclonal antibodies directed against proprotein convertase subtilisin/kexin type 9 (PSCK9), alirocumab and evolocumab, as well as the newly FDA-approved inclisiran, a small interfering RNA- (siRNA-) based drug targeting PCSK9 are indicated to effectively reduce non-HDL cholesterol and LDL-C to goal. Pharmacologic therapy for hypertriglyceridemia includes fibrates, and omega-3 fatty acids; of note, only icosapent ethyl omega-3 formulation (EPA) has shown significant reductions in CV events, and CV death among patients with high TGs and either known CVD or diabetes, and who were already on statin therapy with relatively well-controlled LDL levels.

In relation to treatment indications, recent Cholesterol Guidelines (2018) highly recommended statin therapy for both primary and secondary prevention. In patients less than 75 years of age with diabetes, the target is to decrease LDL by 50%. In primary prevention, in adults 40–75 years with diabetes, effective lipid-lowering treatment is associated with an impressive reduction of 25% in CV risk.

In relation to hypertension, ADA and ACC/AHA guidelines recommend lowering blood pressure to 130/80 mm Hg or less; however, the more intensive target of less than 120 mm Hg does not appear to have consistent cardioprotective effects in patients with T2D, suggesting a U-shape relationship in diabetes between BP levels and CV outcomes.

Intensive antihypertensive therapy is often required to reach BP goals, the majority need two to three drugs. Early and vigorous antihypertensive therapy with angiotensin-converting enzyme inhibitors (ACE) or angiotensin receptor blockers (ARB) should be first-line therapy, especially if microalbuminuria is present. The novel MR antagonist finerenone (more powerful than eplerenone) has recently shown in RCT to decrease microalbuminuria when added to ARBs. Thiazide diuretics and calcium channel blockers are also considered first-line therapy by ACC/AHA and ADA.

Diabetes is considered a prothrombotic state secondary to altered coagulation, platelet dysfunction, and presence of kidney failure. Aspirin inhibits thromboxane synthesis by platelets and is effective in secondary prevention by reducing cardiovascular morbidity and mortality in patients who have a history of myocardial infarction or stroke. Recent trials have documented that aspirin has a modest but significant effect in primary prevention in diabetic adults with increased CV risks such as smoking, hypertension, dyslipidemia, family history of premature CHD, and albuminuria, but potential bleeding risks must be balanced.

A dedicated non-contrast heart CT may be used to quantify coronary calcium; coronary artery calcification (CAC), is considered a surrogate marker for endothelial damage and atherosclerosis. As expected, CAC is detected more commonly in diabetes (75%) than control subjects (50%). CAC more than 100 is indicative of increased risk of a major cardiac event and is helpful for adjusting lipid and aspirin treatment.

The Early Treatment Diabetic Retinopathy Study (ETDRS) showed that aspirin does not increase the incidence or severity of bleeding (vitreous/preretinal hemorrhages) in diabetic proliferative retinopathy or alter its course. Thus, it appears that there is no contraindication to aspirin use in patients with proliferative retinopathy. Treatment of CHD for diabetic patients is like that for nondiabetic persons with some important caveats. Endothelial dysfunction and the platelet and coagulation disturbances characteristic of type 2 diabetes have been proposed as mechanism contributing to the effects of diabetes on the morbidity and mortality in the setting of unstable angina, non–ST segment elevation myocardial infarction, and after percutaneous transluminal coronary angioplasty (PTCA), stenting, and CABG.

Diabetic patients have higher rates of adverse outcomes and restenosis in these settings. Early and midterm follow-up of diabetic patients after revascularization indicates that the incidences of myocardial infarction and repeat revascularization are reduced in patients undergoing CABG compared with those treated by percutaneous coronary intervention (PCI) alone. Antiplatelet agents have reduced the need for reintervention after PCI in the early–mid-term; however, repeat revascularization in diabetic patients continues to be substantially higher after PCI. Advances in PCI include the use of drug-eluting stents and adjunctive drug therapies, such as clopidogrel. Glycemic control is an important determinant of outcome after revascularization in diabetic patients. The impact of tight glycemic control after PCI was investigated in the Bypass Angioplasty Revascularization Investigation 2 in Diabetes (BARI-2D) study which found that there was little difference between insulin sensitization and insulin administration with respect to rates of death and cardiovascular events at 5 years. This trial also evaluated the effects of prompt revascularization by CABG or PCI versus medical therapy; patients who underwent CABG had better outcomes, especially those with diabetes and multivessel coronary artery disease. Results from the BARI-2D trial, combined with other randomized trials comparing PCI with CABG surgery, have so far shown that diabetics with multivessel coronary artery disease undergoing CABG have a survival advantage and reduced rates of subsequent cardiovascular events compared to PCI. Improvements in cardiovascular risk management are leading to better results in patients with diabetes, but future clinical trials are needed to answer many questions. Collective, multidisciplinary metabolic disease management is extremely important to evaluate and treat cardiovascular risk at an individual and population level. Until future trial results become available and new technologies and medical therapies emerge, aggressive secondary prevention and ongoing management of CHD in the setting of diabetes will continue to pose a challenge.

Heidenreich PA, Bozkurt B, Aguilar D, et al. 2022 AHA/ACC/HFSA Guideline for the Management of Heart Failure: A Report of the American College of Cardiology/American Heart Association Joint Committee on Clinical Practice Guidelines. *Circulation*. Epub 2022 Apr 1. 2022;145(18):e895–e1032. [PMID: 35363499]

Ho KL, Karwi QG, Connolly D, et al. Metabolic, structural and biochemical changes in diabetes and the development of heart failure. *Diabetologia.* 2022 Mar;65(3):411–423. doi: 10.1007/s00125-021-05637-7. Epub 2022 Jan 7. [PMID: 34994805]

Joseph JJ, Deedwania P, Acharya T, et al; American Heart Association Diabetes Committee of the Council on Lifestyle and Cardiometabolic Health; Council on Arteriosclerosis, Thrombosis and Vascular Biology; Council on Clinical Cardiology; and Council on Hypertension. Comprehensive Management of Cardiovascular Risk Factors for Adults With Type 2 Diabetes: A Scientific Statement From the American Heart Association. *Circulation.* 2022 Mar;145(9):e722–e759. doi: 10.1161/CIR.0000000000001040. [PMID: 35000404]

Schofield J, Ho J, Soran H. Cardiovascular risk in type 1 diabetes mellitus. *Diabetes Ther.* 2019 Jun;10(3):773–789. doi: 10.1007/s13300-019-0612-8. Epub 2019 Apr 19. [PMID: 31004282]; [PMCID: PMC6531592]

Effects of Diabetes on Peripheral Vascular Disease

Diabetes accelerates the rate of atherosclerosis in larger arteries; plaque formation is often diffuse, but tends to localize in areas of turbulent blood flow, such as at the bifurcation of the aorta or other large vessels. Clinical manifestations of peripheral vascular disease include ischemia of the lower extremities, erectile dysfunction and intestinal angina. Lower extremity arterial disease is clinically identified by intermittent claudication and/or the absence of peripheral pulses in the lower legs and feet. These clinical manifestations reflect decreased arterial perfusion of the extremity. However, there is evidence that a history of intermittent claudication and the palpation of peripheral pulses are unreliable techniques for the detection of peripheral arterial disease. Greater accuracy has been achieved with noninvasive testing using Doppler ankle-brachial pressure ratios, measurement of reactive hyperemia after exercise, pulse reappearance time, ultrasound duplex scanning, plethysmography, and CT/Magnetic resonance angiography. The American Diabetes Association and AHA recommend annual screening for peripheral arterial disease in patients with diabetes. Measurement of toe pressures has received a great deal of attention because of their predictability in defining individuals at high risk of gangrene, ulceration, and infection associated with occlusive arterial disease, even in patients with noncompressible vessels. Reduced toe pressures are highly associated with progression of lower extremity arterial disease to gangrene, ulceration, and the need for amputation.

The incidence and prevalence of peripheral arterial disease increase with age, smoking status, concomitant dyslipidemia, and with duration of diabetes. Concurrent peripheral neuropathy with impaired sensation makes the foot susceptible to trauma, ulceration, and infection. These factors contribute to progression to gangrene and osteomyelitis and, ultimately, to amputation. Critical limb ischemia and gangrene of the feet in patients with diabetes are 30 times more frequent than in age-matched controls. Diabetes accounts for approximately 50% of all nontraumatic amputations in the United States. A second amputation within a few years after the first is very common. PVD increases mortality, particularly if foot ulcerations, infection, or gangrene occur. Three-year survival after an amputation is less than 50%.

Prevention is critically important; by the time PVD becomes clinically evident, it may be too late to salvage an extremity or require costly resources. Currently, there are no randomized controlled trials comparing intensive or standard glucose-lowering therapy in patients with diabetes and PVD. However, there is evidence that glucose control is associated with an important reduction in microvascular and macrovascular complications. Treatment includes exercise, statins, antiplatelet therapy, and cilostazol (an oral phosphodiesterase type III inhibitor that causes vasodilation). Revascularization is only indicated if claudication impairs quality of life after pharmacotherapy and may include endovascular therapy or open surgery.

Soyoye DO, Abiodun OO, Ikem RT, Kolawole BA, Akintomide AO. Diabetes and peripheral artery disease: A review. *World J Diabetes.* 2021 Jun 15;12(6):827–838. doi: 10.4239/wjd.v12.i6.827. [PMID: 34168731]; [PMCID: PMC8192257]

ESTROGENS & THE HEART

1. Hormone Replacement Therapy

The importance of estrogen in the heart is highlighted by several studies that have shown an increased cardiovascular risk after menopause. Estrogen deficiency is associated with central adiposity, atherogenic dyslipidemia, glucose intolerance, sleep disorders and hypertension.

The use of estrogen or combined estrogen-progestin replacement therapy in postmenopausal women dramatically changed in the last decades. Initially, based on extensive observational data, estrogen was thought to be cardioprotective, and estrogen replacement therapy was routinely prescribed for both primary and secondary prevention of CHD even in women in the late seventies. However, prospective data from the Women's Health Initiative (WHI) combined estrogen-progestin trial reported an increase in CHD risk. Furthermore, the Heart and Estrogen/Progestin Replacement Study (HERS-I and II), other controlled trials, and two meta-analyses were unable to demonstrate a protective effect of estrogen replacement therapy on the heart. HERS demonstrated a 52% increased risk of major coronary events within the first year of the trial. During the second year, risk was equal in the two groups, and by years 4–5, risk was higher in the placebo group. The early increase in risk suggests that hormone replacement therapy (HRT) may predispose to thrombosis, arrhythmia, or ischemia. The WHI unopposed estrogen trial did not report an increase in CHD events, although stroke and venous thromboembolism were increased, as was seen in the combined estrogen-progestin trial. Further follow-up analysis has suggested that younger postmenopausal women taking postmenopausal hormone therapy (unopposed or combined) are *not* at increased risk for CHD. Collectively, these studies changed the indication, duration, and route of administration in hormone replacement therapy (HRT). Since rates of CHD, stroke, deep venous thrombosis, and pulmonary embolism were higher in women receiving HRT, the current recommendation is that postmenopausal HRT cannot be recommended solely for prevention of CHD.

The Effects of Estrogen Replacement on the Progression of Coronary Artery Atherosclerosis (ERA) trial demonstrated that postmenopausal HRT is not beneficial in the short term (3 years) in preventing progression or inducing regression of coronary atherosclerosis in women with established CHD who undergo angiography. It should be noted that both HERS and ERA were designed to examine the role of HRT in secondary prevention. The WHI is the first trial examining the effect of HRT in primary prevention and was terminated in early 2002 due to increased risk of invasive breast cancer. Rates of CHD, stroke, deep venous thrombosis, and pulmonary embolism were higher in women receiving HRT.

Most now agree that estrogen is a reasonable therapy when used short-term for menopausal symptoms, but it should not be prescribed for either primary or secondary prevention of CHD. In relation to treatment, transdermal estradiol should be preferred (alone for women without a uterus or in combination with progesterone), due to their neutral effect on CVD risk factors and coagulation parameters, mainly because it bypasses the liver. Also, HRT should be tried for vasomotor symptoms in selected patients, with the intention to be used for the shortest time possible and at the lowest effective dose.

Anagnostis P, Lambrinoudaki I, Stevenson JC, Goulis DG. Menopause-associated risk of cardiovascular disease. *Endocr Connect.* 2022 Apr 22;11(4):e210537. doi: 10.1530/EC-21-0537. [PMID: 35258483]; [PMCID: PMC9066596]

Flores VA, Pal L, Manson JE. Hormone therapy in menopause: concepts, controversies, and approach to treatment. *Endocr Rev.* 2021 Nov 16;42(6):720–752. doi: 10.1210/endrev/bnab011. [PMID: 33858012]

Oliver-Williams C, Glisic M, Shahzad S, et al. The route of administration, timing, duration and dose of postmenopausal hormone therapy and cardiovascular outcomes in women: a systematic review. *Hum Reprod Update.* 2019 Mar 1;25(2): 257–271. doi: 10.1093/humupd/dmy039. [PMID: 30508190].

2. Oral Contraceptives

Oral estrogen-progestin contraceptives have long been considered as risks for deep venous thrombosis, myocardial infarction, and stroke that occurred with the early high-dose pills. However, the reduction in estrogen content and the actual use of natural estradiol rather than ethinyl-estradiol has increased safety substantially. The reported increased risk in myocardial infarction and cardiovascular mortality reported in epidemiologic studies was seen among women older than 35 years who were cigarette smokers and used high doses of ethinyl estradiol and oral contraceptives. For women using contraceptive patch and vaginal ring, the numbers of myocardial infarctions have been too low to estimate risk. Of note, no excess risk has been noted with progestin-only formulations. The general consensus is that high-dose oral contraceptive use is not recommended for women older than 35 years who smoke, or who have elevated plasma TG levels, diabetes, or persistent hypertension. In them other options are preferred.

Oral contraceptives are associated with increased risk of hypertension and elevated blood pressure, especially those with synthetic estrogen. Women diagnosed with hypertension using estrogen-progestin pills should stop this contraceptive for 2 months and then reevaluate blood pressure. Progestin only contraceptives or intrauterine devices are preferred choices in young women with hypertension; of note, these treatments will not affect the potential study of the renin-angiotensin system to evaluate secondary hypertension.

Kalenga CZ, Dumanski SM, Metcalfe A, et al. The effect of non-oral hormonal contraceptives on hypertension and blood pressure: a systematic review and meta-analysis. *Physiol Rep.* 2022 May;10(9):e15267. doi: 10.14814/phy2.15267. [PMID: 35510324]; [PMCID: PMC9069167]

35 Connective Tissue Diseases & the Heart

Carlos A. Roldan, MD

The connective tissue diseases are immune-mediated inflammatory diseases, primarily of the musculoskeletal system; however, they frequently also involve the cardiovascular system. The most important of these diseases are systemic lupus erythematosus, rheumatoid arthritis, scleroderma, ankylosing spondylitis, polymyositis/dermatomyositis, and mixed connective tissue disease. They affect the endocardium including the valve leaflets, myocardium, coronary arteries, conduction system, and great vessels with different rates of prevalence and degrees of severity. Although heart involvement in patients with connective tissue diseases contributes significantly to their morbidity and mortality rates, there is a large discrepancy between clinically recognized heart disease, echocardiography studies, and postmortem series. Furthermore, their pathogenesis and natural history are still incompletely understood and their therapy is not yet standardized. Increased awareness and better understanding of the cardiovascular diseases associated with connective tissue diseases may lead to earlier recognition and treatment with consequent decreased morbidity and mortality. Finally, and of importance, patients with connective tissue diseases and associated heart disease should be consulted and managed by a heart team (including a cardiologist with imaging expertise, an interventional cardiologist, and in selected cases a cardiothoracic surgeon) and rheumatologists given the potential morbidity and mortality of their heart disease and the complexity and potential benefits, but also potential harm of their pharmacotherapy and cardiac interventions.

SYSTEMIC LUPUS ERYTHEMATOSUS

ESSENTIALS OF DIAGNOSIS

- Musculoskeletal and mucocutaneous manifestations of systemic lupus erythematosus (SLE).
- Libman-Sacks vegetations, atrioventricular (AV) valve regurgitation, intra- and extra-cardiac thrombosis, premature atherosclerosis, pericarditis, myocarditis, and SLE.
- Cardioembolism and SLE.
- Acute pericarditis with antinuclear antibodies detected in the pericardial fluid.

General Considerations

Systemic lupus erythematosus (SLE) is a multisystem chronically recurrent inflammatory disease that affects the musculoskeletal, mucocutaneous, visceral, and central nervous systems. Symptoms include fatigue, myalgias, arthralgias or arthritis, photosensitivity, and serositis. The prevalence of SLE varies widely, from 4 to 250 cases per 100,000 persons. It is more frequent in a patient's relatives than in the general population. SLE is predominantly seen in females, with a female-to-male ratio of 10:1. The pathophysiology of the disease is related to the multiorgan deposition of circulating antigen–antibody complexes and activation of the complement system, leading to humoral- and cellular-mediated inflammation.

SLE affects the cardiovascular system and is associated with two- to threefold higher incidence of major cardiovascular events than matched controls without SLE. Cardiovascular disease is the third most important cause of death in SLE patients (after infectious and renal diseases) during the earlier course of disease, but later, cardiovascular disease is a predominant cause of their death. The most significant SLE-associated heart diseases are valvular heart disease, arterial or venous thrombosis and systemic thromboembolism, premature coronary artery disease (CAD), and pericarditis. Myocarditis or cardiomyopathy and cardiac arrhythmias or conduction disturbances are less common. Independent predictors of their cardiovascular disease include duration, age of onset, and activity and severity of SLE, presence of antiphospholipid antibodies, and corticosteroid therapy.

Regarding the pathogenesis of SLE-associated cardiovascular disease, it is believed, as it is for the primary disease, that the immune complex deposition and complement activation lead to an acute, chronic, or recurrent inflammation of the endocardium and valve leaflets, vascular endothelium, pericardium, myocardium, or conduction system. The presence in these tissues of immune complexes, complement, antinuclear antibodies, lupus erythematosus cells, mononuclear inflammatory cells, necrosis, hematoxylin bodies, and deposits of fibrin and platelet thrombi support this theory. Many studies suggest that antiphospholipid antibodies (aPL) (immunoglobulin [Ig] A, IgG, or IgM anticardiolipin antibodies [aCL], lupus-anticoagulant [LA], or antibodies to plasma phospholipid-binding protein β_2-glycoprotein I) cause cardiovascular injury and thrombogenesis. These antibodies, present in as many as half of SLE patients, are directed against negatively charged phospholipids present in the membrane of endothelial cells causing endothelial dysfunction, endocardial and/or vascular injury, and increased endocardial, arterial, and/or venous thrombogenesis.

1. Valvular Heart Disease

General Considerations

Valvular heart disease is the clinically most important and frequent of the SLE-associated cardiovascular manifestations. Valvular heart disease is associated with an increased morbidity and mortality of SLE patients. It has been categorized as vegetations (Libman-Sacks endocarditis), leaflet thickening, valve regurgitation, and infrequently, valve stenosis. Although the true prevalence of clinically recognized valve disease is unknown, recent transesophageal echocardiography (TEE) series showed rates of at least 40%. Rates of valve disease are generally higher in patients with onset of the disease after age 25, in those who have had SLE for more than 5 years, in those treated with corticosteroids, in those with higher disease damage scores, in those with moderate to high levels of aPL, and in those older than 50 years.

The pathogenesis of SLE valve disease includes (1) an immune complex–mediated inflammation with subendothelial deposition of immunoglobulins and complement leading to an increased expression of α_3 β_1-integrin on the endothelial cells; (2) increased amount of collagen IV, laminin, and fibronectin; (3) proliferation of blood vessels; (4) inflammation and fibrosis; and finally, (5) commonly associated antiphospholipid antibodies with increased local or systemic thrombogenesis.

The proposed mechanisms of valve damage by aPL include (1) binding of aPL, which induces activation of endothelial cells and upregulation of the expression of adhesion molecules, secretion of cytokines, and abnormal metabolism of prostacyclins; (2) increased oxidized low-density lipoprotein (LDL) (LDL taken up by macrophages leads to macrophage activation and further damage to endothelial cells); (3) aPL interference with the regulatory functions of prothrombin and with the production of prostacyclin and endothelial relaxing factor, protein C, protein S, and tissue factor; and (4) a heparin-like–induced thrombocytopenia. All these factors lead to increased vasoconstriction, platelet aggregation, activation of the intrinsic and extrinsic coagulation systems, and thrombus formation.

A. Valve Vegetations or Libman-Sacks Endocarditis

Considered pathognomonic of SLE-associated valve disease, noninfective valve vegetations are almost exclusively seen on the mitral and aortic valves. Most vegetations are located on the coaptation portions of the leaflets, the atrial side for the mitral valve, and the ventricular side for the aortic valve. However, vegetations commonly extend through the leaflets into the opposite side (ventricular side for the mitral valve and aortic side for the aortic valve). The valve vegetations are usually sessile, are less than 1 cm^2 in size, have irregular borders and heterogeneous echodensity, and have no independent motion (Figures 35–1 and 35–2). Most valves with vegetations have associated thickening or regurgitation. Although valve vegetations have been seen more commonly in younger persons (< 40 years), their temporal association with SLE activity, severity, duration, and therapy has been variable.

Pathologic examination (see Figure 35–1) reveals that active Libman-Sacks vegetations have central myxoid degeneration, fibrinoid necrosis, and hemorrhages surrounded by predominant polymorphonuclear cellular infiltration, and peripherally by platelet or fibrin thrombus. Healed vegetations have central fibroblastic proliferation and fibrosis, neovascularization, minimal or no inflammatory cell deposition, and peripherally a hyalinized and endothelialized thrombus or not thrombus. Mixed vegetations, the most common type, are those with intermixed areas of activity and healing with peripherally superimposed thrombi with variable degrees of organization and endothelialization. Active, healed, and mixed vegetations can be seen in the same valve.

B. Valve Thickening

Leaflet thickening with or without abnormal mobility results from replacement of the normal spongiosum and endothelial layers by post-inflammatory fibrous tissue and infrequently by calcification. Valve thickening may be seen in up to half of patients; it is generally diffuse, with greater involvement of the middle and tip portions (see Figures 35–1 and 35–2). When leaflet thickening is localized, the basal, middle, and tip portions are equally affected. Valve thickening predominantly affects the mitral and aortic valves and is commonly associated with valve regurgitation, valve vegetations, or both. In contrast to rheumatic heart disease, mitral or aortic valve commissural fusion is seen in ≤ 30% of patients and is usually of mild degree. In young patients with no atherogenic risk factors, associated valve calcification is uncommon (< 5%). However, in middle-aged patients with traditional atherogenic risk factors, mitral annular and aortic valve calcifications are common (20%).

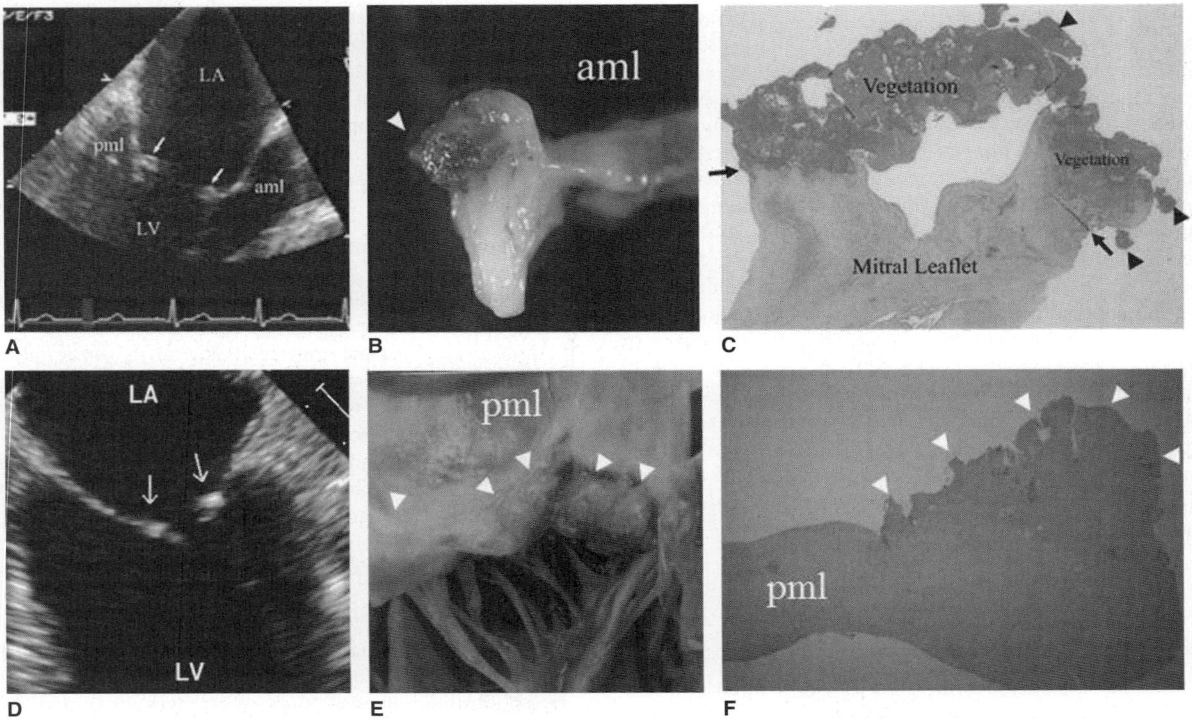

▲ **Figure 35–1. Libman-Sacks endocarditis: echocardiographic and histopathologic characteristics. A.** This two-dimensional (2D) long-axis TEE view of the mitral valve in a 28-year-old woman with SLE with acute confusional state and cognitive dysfunction demonstrates small, oval shape, and soft tissue echoreflectant Libman-Sacks vegetations (*arrows*) on the atrial side and tip portions of the anterior (aml) and posterior (pml) mitral leaflets with associated leaflet thickening and decreased mobility. Associated symptomatic severe mitral regurgitation was present. Therefore, patient underwent mitral valve replacement. **B.** Diffuse leaflet thickening with a Libman-Sacks vegetation on the atrial side and tip portion of the anterior leaflet is noted (*arrowhead*). **C.** Vegetation attached to the leaflets (*arrows*) shows amorphous eosinophilic fibrinous to granular deposits admixed with histiocytes, inflammatory cells, and superficial microthrombi (*arrowheads*). The mitral leaflet shows focal areas of myxoid degeneration and fibrinoid necrosis but no inflammation. **D.** This 2D-TEE view of the mitral valve in a 26-year-old woman with SLE with past stroke and acute TIA demonstrates small, sessile, and homogeneously hyperreflectant oval nodularities consistent with healed Libman-Sacks vegetations (*arrows*) on the left atrial (LA) side and distal portions of the anterior (aml) and posterior (pml) mitral leaflets associated with mild leaflets' thickening and severely decreased mobility, predominantly of the posterior mitral leaflet (pml). **E.** Photograph of the middle scallop of the posterior mitral leaflet (pml) demonstrates sessile, granular, protruding, grayish to brown discoloration, clustered, and coalescent Libman-Sacks vegetations (*arrowheads*) located on the coaptation point and predominantly on the LA side. **F.** This H&E histopathologic section of the posterior mitral leaflet (pml) demonstrates diffuse thickening predominant of the leaflet tip with a well adhered vegetation mainly on the LA side (arrowheads), but also extending to the LV side where appears organized and endothelialized.

C. Valve Regurgitation

This abnormality is predominantly mild in severity and therefore usually clinically silent. Although the prevalence of regurgitation is similar for the mitral, tricuspid, and pulmonic valves (about 50–75%) and the lowest for the aortic valve (25%), the mitral and aortic valves are those most associated with complications. Mitral or aortic valve stenosis mimicking rheumatic heart disease associated with respective valve regurgitation is uncommon.

Clinical Findings

A. Symptoms & Signs

Unless it is severe, valve disease is generally asymptomatic or overshadowed by the musculoskeletal and systemic inflammatory symptoms. However, clinical and subclinical embolic cerebrovascular disease is the most common manifestation of Libman-Sacks endocarditis. Multiple studies using different methodologies in different populations including a

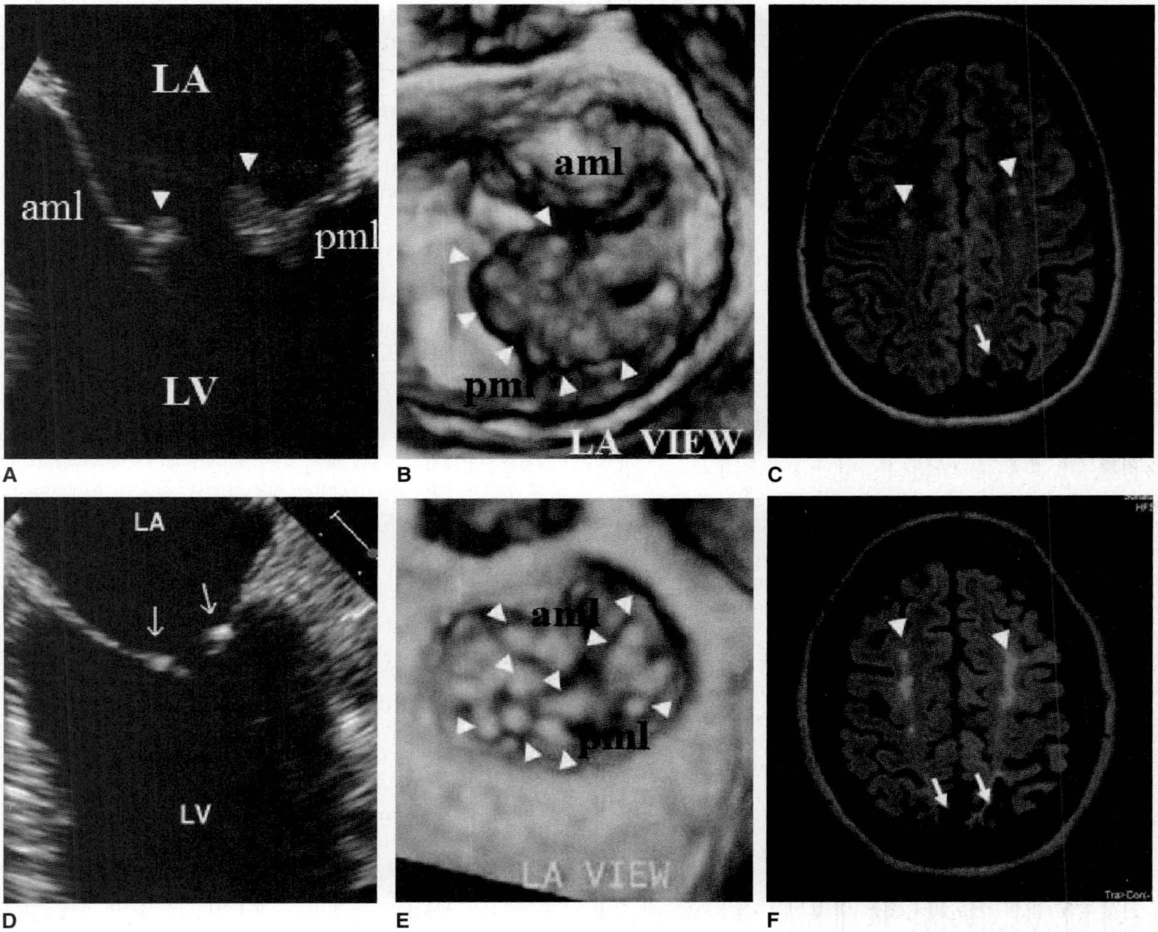

▲ **Figure 35–2. Libman-Sacks endocarditis of the mitral valve complicated with embolic cerebrovascular disease: Detection and characterization by two-dimensional and three-dimensional TEE. A.** This 2D-TEE close-up view of the mitral valve in a 29-year-old male with SLE and recurrent TIA demonstrates medium to large size, oval shape, sessile, and homogeneously soft tissue echoreflectant Libman-Sacks vegetations on the LA side and distal portions of the anterior (aml) and posterior (pml) mitral leaflets (*arrowheads*) associated with mild leaflets' tip thickening and decreased mobility. **B.** This 3D-TEE LA view during systole of the mitral valve demonstrates large, severely protruding, with irregular and nodular surface, tubular and multilobed shape, and with roll-like motion (move from LA to LV side during diastole) vegetations located on the LA side and tip of the entire anterior (aml) and posterior (pml) mitral leaflets (*arrows*) with associated decreased mobility and incomplete coaptation of the leaflets. Associated severe mitral regurgitation was demonstrated by color-Doppler. **C.** MRI of the brain demonstrates an old cerebral infarct (*arrow*) and multiple small deep white matter abnormalities (*arrowheads*). **D.** This 2D-TEE close view of the mitral valve in a 26-year-old woman with SLE with past stroke and acute TIA demonstrates small, sessile, and homogeneously hyperreflectant oval nodularities consistent with healed Libman-Sacks vegetations (*arrows*) on the left atrial (LA) side and distal portions of the anterior (aml) and posterior (pml) mitral leaflets associated with mild leaflets' thickening and severely decreased mobility. **E.** This three-dimensional (3D) TEE LA view of the mitral valve during systole demonstrates small to medium size, protruding, sessile, oval shape, and homogeneously echoreflectant nodularities (*arrowheads*) predominantly located at the tip of both leaflets and involving all scallops. **F.** Brain MRI demonstrates old cerebral infarcts (*arrows*) and multiple small white matter lesions (*arrowheads*). Both patients had cerebromicroembolic events by transcranial Doppler.

recent pathologic study correlating brain MRI with brain and cardiac pathology and a fully integrated, controlled, cross-sectional, and longitudinal study using 2D-TEE have demonstrated that patients with vegetations as compared to those without have more cerebromicroembolism per hour, lower cerebral perfusion, more stroke/TIA, greater neurocognitive dysfunction, and greater brain injury on magnetic resonance imaging (MRI) (see Figure 35–2); valve vegetations are strong independent risk factor for stroke/TIA, neurocognitive dysfunction, focal brain lesions, and all three outcomes combined; and patients with vegetations have reduced event-free survival time to stroke/TIA, cognitive disability, or death. These data support that Libman-Sacks vegetations generate platelet or fibrin macro-or-microemboli that occlude cerebral vessels resulting in ischemic brain injury, stroke/TIA, neurocognitive dysfunction or disability, and death. (See Figures 35–1 and 35–2). Also, left-sided vegetations may rarely embolize to the coronary arteries, and right-sided valve vegetations rarely embolize to the lungs or paradoxically embolize. In addition, severe valve regurgitation resulting from recurrent or acute native and bioprosthetic valvulitis, leaflet perforation, noninfective mitral valve chordal rupture, or superimposed infective endocarditis may occur in ≤ 4% of patients per year. Infective endocarditis can mimic, accompany, or trigger a flare of SLE and lead to severe valvular dysfunction, heart failure, and death from septicemia. Similarly, a flare of SLE can clinically and echocardiographically mimic infective endocarditis (pseudo-infective endocarditis). A low white count, elevated aPL and anti-DNA antibodies, depressed complements, and negative or low C-reactive protein support the diagnosis of active SLE with pseudo-infective endocarditis.

B. Physical Examination

The physical findings of musculoskeletal and mucocutaneous disease generally predominate in SLE patients, even in those with cardiovascular disease. If moderate-to-severe mitral or aortic regurgitation or stenosis is present, the auscultatory findings found on physical examination will be typical. Less significant degrees of regurgitation (these are the majority) may not be clinically detected or may be mistaken for functional murmurs related to fever, anemia, hypertension, or volume overload. In patients with focal (stroke and TIAs) and in those with nonfocal neurologic syndromes of seizures, confusional state, and cognitive dysfunction associated with focal brain injury on MRI, cardioembolism from Libman-Sacks vegetations should be strongly considered.

C. Diagnostic Studies

1. Electrocardiography—Results of electrocardiographic (ECG) studies are nonspecific. Left atrial abnormality and left ventricular (LV) hypertrophy can be seen in patients with chronic and severe aortic or mitral regurgitation.

2. Chest radiography—Cardiomegaly with LV and left atrial enlargement may be seen in the presence of significant mitral or aortic regurgitation.

3. Echocardiography—Transthoracic color-flow Doppler echocardiography (TTE) is the most applied technique for the diagnosis of SLE-associated valve disease. This technique accurately determines the presence and severity of valve regurgitation or stenosis and abnormal leaflet thickening, but not of vegetations. The prevalence of Libman-Sacks vegetations by TTE is less than 10%. This technique will also detect associated increased wall thickness, chamber enlargement, ventricular diastolic or systolic dysfunction, and associated left atrial and pulmonary hypertension. TEE is superior to TTE in detecting and characterizing SLE-associated valve masses and leaflet thickening. TEE detects valve vegetations in up to 35% of patients. Considering TEE as the standard, TTE has a low sensitivity (63% overall, 11% for valve vegetations), low specificity (58%), low negative predictive value (40%), and a moderate positive predictive value (78%) for detection of Libman-Sacks endocarditis. Three-dimensional as compared to 2D-TEE, detects more vegetations and determines larger sizes of vegetations; defines better the location, extent, shape, and appearance of vegetations; detects more often associated valve commissural fusion; and detects higher frequency of vegetations in patients with cerebrovascular disease (see Figure 35–2). By serial TEE, Libman-Sacks vegetations resolve, appear de novo, or change their morphology over time and may not be temporally related to SLE activity, severity, duration, or therapy. Therefore, TEE is indicated to exclude sources of cardioembolism in patients with a new or recurrent focal neurologic defect or in patients with a nonfocal neurologic deficit (moderate or worse cognitive dysfunction, seizures, or acute confusional state) and cerebral infarcts on MRI, in patients with moderate or worse valve regurgitation, and in patients with suspected complicating infective endocarditis. Although TEE is the most accurate diagnostic method for detecting Libman-Sacks endocarditis, it is semi-invasive and has potential risks. Therefore, identification of clinical variables with a high predictive value for Libman-Sacks endocarditis on TEE is clinically relevant. Preliminary data suggest that acute stroke/TIA or SLE duration of ≥12 years or SLE duration ≥ 5 years and age ≥ 32 years in those without stroke/TIA may provide high sensitivity (85%), specificity (81%), and positive and negative predictive values (both 83%) for detection of Libman-Sacks endocarditis on TEE.

Treatment

A. Specific Anti-inflammatory and Antithrombotic Therapy

In general, acute valvulitis complicated with valve vegetations and/or moderate or worse valve regurgitation is generally associated with active SLE disease, and therefore, treatment should focus on managing both active SLE disease and associated endocardial inflammation and thrombogenesis with anti-inflammatory and antithrombotic therapies. However, due to lack of randomized control studies, there are no expert consensus or guidelines about medical or surgical therapy of Libman-Sacks endocarditis. In a recent case series, combined anti-inflammatory (corticosteroids, disease-modifying antirheumatic drugs), or immunosuppressive therapy (eg, mophetil mycophenolate methotrexate, or cyclophosphamide), and antithrombotic (anticoagulant or antiplatelet agents) therapies resolved or significantly improved Libman-Sacks endocarditis and its associated embolic cerebrovascular disease (see Figures 35–3 and 35–4). It is anticipated that other antimetabolites (azathioprine,

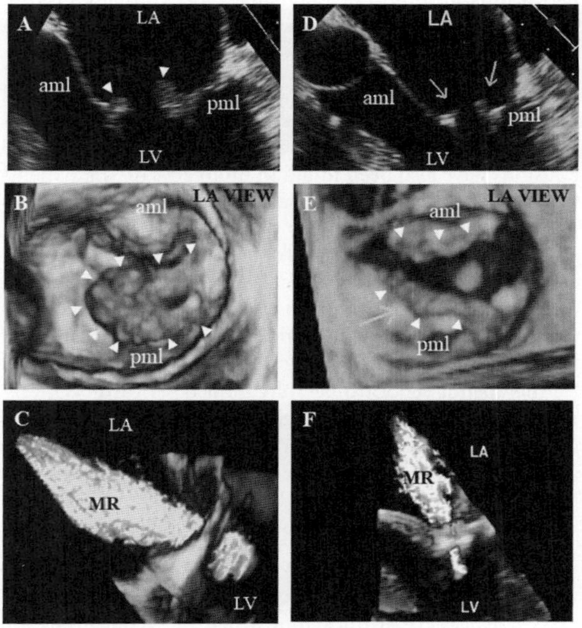

▲ Figure 35–3. Libman-Sacks endocarditis of the mitral valve complicated with embolic cerebrovascular disease and its response to medical therapy. **A.** This 2-DTEE view in a 29-year-old male with SLE and acute stroke demonstrates large, sessile, and oval-shaped Libman-Sacks vegetations (arrowheads) on the distal portions and atrial side of the anterior (aml) and posterior (pml) mitral leaflets (arrows). **B.** This 3-DTEE left atrial (LA) view of the mitral valve demonstrates large and protruding vegetations on the tip to mid portions and atrial side of the entire anterior and posterior mitral leaflets (arrowheads). **C.** Associated severe mitral regurgitation (MR) was demonstrated by 3D-TEE color Doppler. After 3 months of aspirin and clopidogrel, hydroxychloroquine, prednisone, and mycophenolate mofetil, mitral valve vegetations significantly decreased in size (arrows) by 2D (**D**) and 3D TEE (**E**). Mitral regurgitation also improved to mild (**F**). Abbreviations as in previous figures.

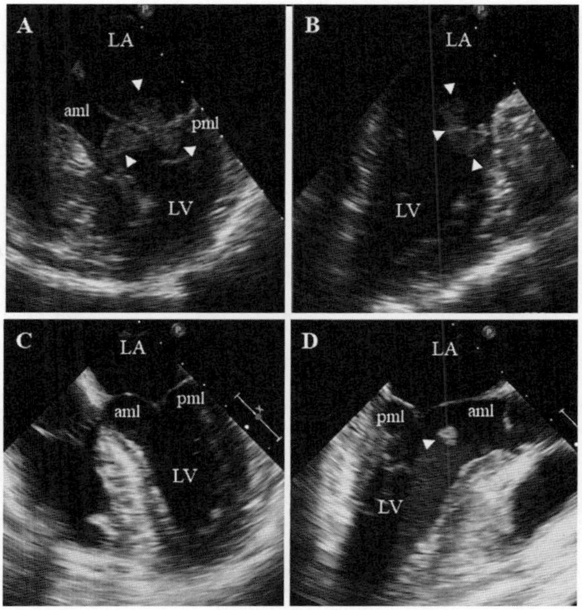

▲ Figure 35–4. Libman-Sacks endocarditis of the mitral valve complicated by embolic cerebrovascular disease and its response to medical therapy. A. This 2-D TEE view in a 31-year-old female with SLE and acute stroke demonstrates a large, tri-lobed, and soft tissue echoreflectant Libman-Sacks vegetation extending from the atrial side of both mitral leaflets into the subvalvular apparatus/chorda tendinea (arrowheads). **B.** An additional large, irregular shaped, and soft tissue echoreflectant vegetation is seen attached to the basal anterior wall of the LV (arrowheads). Despite the significant involvement with vegetations of the mitral valve and chordae tendinea, only mild mitral regurgitation was present. **C, D.** After 5 days of intravenous heparin and methylprednisolone, follow-up 2D-TEE demonstrates resolution of the mitral valve vegetations (**C**) and significantly smaller LV anterior wall vegetation (**D,** arrowhead). Abbreviations as in previous figures.

mercaptopurine, and leflunomide) and immunosuppressive monoclonal antibodies (belimumab, anifrolumab, rituximab, and obinutuzumab) used clinically or experimentally to treat active SLE may potentially be useful to treat and prevent SLE activity-associated cardiac complications.

B. Valve Surgery

Although valve surgery (valve replacement or repair) may be beneficial in highly selected cases, it is associated with 3–5 times higher morbidity and mortality as compared to non-SLE patients and therefore should be deferred until failure of medical therapy has been determined. Also, inflammation, thrombosis, damage, and accelerated degeneration of bioprosthetic valves by the underlying immune-mediated inflammation and thrombosis have been reported. However, medical versus surgical therapy for Libman-Sacks endocarditis needs to be studied in randomized controlled cross-sectional and longitudinal trials.

C. Other Therapy

Guideline-directed medical therapy including diuretics and vasodilators is indicated in severe symptomatic valve disease.

2. Pericarditis

General Considerations

Pericarditis, with or without effusion or pericardial thickening, is common in postmortem series. Also, about half of lupus patients suffer at least one episode of symptomatic pericarditis. In up to 20% of female patients less than 50 years old, acute pericarditis may be the initial manifestation of SLE. Most episodes are acute and are frequently associated with active SLE and valvulitis, myocarditis, pleuritis, or nephritis. Cardiac tamponade or constrictive pericarditis rarely occurs (< 2%).

Clinical Findings

A. Symptoms & Signs

The diagnosis of pericarditis is based on clinical manifestations rather than on the echocardiogram because an effusion or pericardial thickening is frequently absent. Symptomatic pericarditis is generally acute and uncomplicated and is most seen during flare-ups of the disease. Asymptomatic pericardial disease may be present in some patients. It is manifested by incidentally detected small effusions in most cases and far less frequently by pericardial thickening found on echocardiography. Asymptomatic pericardial disease is generally seen in patients with stable disease that is either mildly active or in remission. Occasionally, acute pericarditis, cardiac tamponade, or both may be the initial manifestation of SLE. Chronic constrictive pericarditis is rare. Infectious pericarditis is rare but catastrophic and most caused by *Staphylococcus aureus*. Finally, a pericardial effusion in SLE patients may also be secondary to severe uremia or nephrotic syndrome, hypoalbuminemia, or pulmonary hypertension with cor pulmonale.

Because it is frequently symptomatic, acute pericarditis is the SLE-related cardiovascular disease most often detected clinically. It may present with fever, tachycardia, pleuritic chest pain, and, on auscultation, the presence of a pericardial rub. If a large effusion is present, decreased heart sounds, jugular venous distention, and pulsus paradoxus may be noted.

B. Laboratory Findings

Pericarditis typically yields serofibrinous, fibrinous, or, rarely, serosanguineous exudative fluid containing low complement level and antinuclear antibodies. By immunofluorescence, the pericardium shows granular deposition of immunoglobulins and C3.

C. Diagnostic Studies

1. Electrocardiography—The ECG most frequently shows no abnormalities or nonspecific ST segment and T-wave changes. The characteristic diffuse ST segment elevation with upward concavity and PR segment depression of acute pericarditis are common. Low voltage or electrical alternans may also be seen if a large pericardial effusion is present.

2. Chest radiography—The chest radiography is generally of little diagnostic value because most patients with acute pericarditis have no—or only small—pericardial effusions. If a large pericardial effusion is present, cardiomegaly with a characteristic water-bottle shape may be seen.

3. Echocardiography—Echocardiography is the standard method to evaluate suspected SLE pericarditis and its associated complications. Small, asymptomatic pericardial effusions have also been found in up to 20% of SLE patients hospitalized with active disease. However, the absence of an effusion on echocardiography does not exclude a clinically suspected pericarditis. In cases of pericarditis with large pericardial effusion and clinically suspected cardiac tamponade, echocardiography may demonstrate right atrial or ventricular diastolic collapse and significant respiratory variability of the mitral or tricuspid Doppler inflows, indicating the need for therapeutic echocardiography-guided pericardiocentesis. In addition, serial follow-up echocardiography after pericardiocentesis or after anti-inflammatory therapy is helpful to guide the need of future interventions. Echocardiography is less useful in detecting pericardial thickening or calcification in cases of suspected chronic pericardial constriction.

4. Computed tomography and magnetic resonance imaging—These techniques are preferred methods for assessing pericardial thickening when the echocardiogram suggests constriction.

Treatment

A. Medical Therapy

Pericarditis is an indicator of serositis and of SLE disease activity. Therefore, for severe pericarditis, immediate immunosuppressive therapy with intravenous methylprednisolone or high-dose oral corticosteroids, followed by oral mycophenolate, intravenous cyclophosphamide, plasmapheresis, or in resistant cases off-label use of rituximab or obinutuzumab can be considered. For more indolent, recurrent, or chronic pericarditis, all SLE patients should be on baseline hydroxychloroquine or chloroquine, and additionally some combination of chronic colchicine, methotrexate, mycophenolate, azathioprine, mercaptopurine, or intravenous belimumab or anifrolumab can be considered. The use of nonsteroidal anti-inflammatory drugs (NSAIDs) is frequently limited by associated renal disease, hypertension, hypercoagulability, thrombocytopenia, or anticoagulation.

B. Surgical Therapy

In a patient with active SLE, a large pericardial effusion without indicators of tamponade should prompt an earlier diagnostic echocardiography-guided pericardiocentesis aimed to exclude infection and to prevent rapid progression or hemorrhagic transformation followed by aggressive immunosuppressive anti-inflammatory therapy. A pericardial window should be avoided in these patients due to their associated serositis with peritonitis and pleuritis and their high risk of infection. Pericardiectomy has been performed in isolated cases of SLE-associated chronic pericardial constriction.

3. Myocarditis or Cardiomyopathy

General Considerations

The most common form of myocardial disease in SLE is secondary subclinical and uncommonly clinical ventricular diastolic dysfunction due to four interrelated factors: (1) endothelial dysfunction–mediated microvascular CAD as determined by a decrease in coronary flow reserve by dipyridamole or adenosine Doppler TTE or directly by coronary fractional flow reserve; (2) a highly prevalent (25–35%) arterial hypertension; (3) premature peripheral arterial and aortic stiffness independent of or exacerbated by hypertension causing increased left ventricular (LV) afterload, LV mass and diastolic dysfunction; and (4) rarely, small vessel vasculitis or coronary arteritis. Although primary myocarditis can be frequently seen in autopsy series of patients with SLE; primary myocarditis is clinically evident in less than 10% of patients. Primary myocarditis can be associated with acute pericarditis (myopericarditis). Primary myocarditis manifests with LV diastolic and global or regional systolic dysfunction. Rarely, acute myocarditis complicated with heart failure may be the initial manifestation of active SLE. An association of cellular antigen Ro (SS-A) and La (SS-B) antibodies and this type of myocarditis has been established, but their primary pathogenic role is still undefined. Epicardial coronary arteritis as a cause of myocardial dysfunction is rare. Finally, a spontaneously reversible global cardiomyopathy similar to a stress cardiomyopathy, and hydroxychloroquine or chloroquine sulfate-induced dilated or restrictive cardiomyopathy have been reported.

Clinical Findings

A. Symptoms & Signs

About one-third of young patients with active SLE have asymptomatic diastolic dysfunction. Acute myocarditis or myopericarditis typically manifests with fever, tachycardia, chest pain, and, rarely, symptoms of heart failure, arrhythmias, or conduction disturbances. Acute myocarditis may clinically, electrocardiographically, and by laboratory mimic acute myocardial infarction. The myocarditis is generally mild and usually does not cause LV systolic dysfunction. Occasionally, severe dilated cardiomyopathy is seen. Characteristic manifestations of an acute coronary syndrome will also be present in those patients with myocardial dysfunction secondary to coronary arteritis, small-vessel vasculitis, acute coronary thrombosis without underlying atherosclerosis, or coronary embolism from aortic or mitral valve noninfective vegetations.

If significant diastolic or systolic dysfunction is present, tachycardia, fourth and third heart sounds, pulmonary rales, and edema may be found.

B. Diagnostic Studies

1. Electrocardiography—Nonspecific ST segment and T-wave abnormalities and atrial or ventricular ectopic complexes are common. Rarely, atrial or ventricular tachyarrhythmias can be detected.

2. Chest radiography—Cardiomegaly may be present if dilated cardiomyopathy has developed.

3. Echocardiography—Doppler echocardiography series, including tissue Doppler, strain, and strain rate in asymptomatic young patients without systemic or pulmonary hypertension and normal LV systolic function, have demonstrated up to one-third of LV and right ventricular (RV) diastolic dysfunction, predominantly of impaired relaxation. Diastolic dysfunction occurs three to four times more frequently in patients with active SLE. In unselected patients, the prevalence of asymptomatic LV systolic dysfunction is low (≤ 3%). These abnormalities are more commonly related to microvascular CAD or hypertension and less often to subclinical acute or recurrent myocarditis. When primary myocarditis is severe, diffuse, or regional wall motion abnormalities may be observed.

4. Radionuclide studies—Either first-transit or gated-acquisition radionuclide angiography also can be used to assess ventricular systolic and diastolic dysfunction, wall motion abnormalities, and chamber enlargement. In up to one-third of SLE patients, this technique has shown an abnormal ventricular function response to exercise, as evidenced by a fall or subnormal rise in ejection fraction and the appearance of new or worsened wall motion abnormalities indicative of myocarditis or CAD. Reversible, fixed, or mixed myocardial perfusion defects can be seen in patients with normal epicardial coronary arteries indicative of abnormal coronary flow reserve or microvascular disease or active or past myocarditis.

5. Magnetic resonance imaging—This technique improves the detection of subclinical and clinical myocarditis. Cardiac magnetic resonance imaging with T2-weighted imaging assesses myocardial edema (indicative of active inflammation) and gadolinium contrast enhancement assesses fibrosis and therefore differentiates better the pathogenesis of myocardial disease as vasculitis, myocarditis, or myocardial infarction.

6. Endomyocardial biopsy—Tissue samples may demonstrate SLE-associated myocarditis or cardiomyopathy when a clinical or serologic diagnosis cannot be made.

7. Cardiac biomarkers—Mild elevation of troponin I will be more common than elevation of creatine phosphokinase (CPK) and may occur in the absence of ECG or echocardiographic abnormalities.

Treatment

A. Specific Anti-inflammatory Therapy

As for pericarditis, primary myocarditis usually indicates severely active SLE disease, and therefore, in-patient intravenous pulse cyclophosphamide or oral mycophenolate in addition to intravenous methylprednisolone can be considered. Intravenous immunoglobulin therapy has also shown benefit in patients with acute myocarditis. Once patients are considered stable, outpatient therapy with antimalarials (hydroxychloroquine or chloroquine) supplemented with oral mycophenolate, methotrexate, mercaptopurine, azathioprine, or intravenous belimumab or anifrolumab can be considered, and in extremely resistant cases off-label use of rituximab or obinutuzumab while corticosteroids are gradually tapered. This therapy is usually continued for 6–12 months, and corticosteroids are titrated down based on overall SLE and cardiac clinical response. Finally, hydroxychloroquine therapy has been shown to decrease the development or prevent progression of SLE-associated myocarditis.

B. Other Therapy

Symptomatic therapy with NSAIDs or other analgesics, bed rest, and ECG monitoring for detection of arrhythmias are indicated. If symptomatic dilated cardiomyopathy is present, standard therapy of diuretics, vasodilators, and beta blocker therapy are used.

4. Thrombotic Diseases

General Considerations

Deep venous thrombosis, pulmonary embolism, and peripheral or cerebral arterial thrombosis are common in SLE patients. Acute coronary thrombosis or thromboembolism in the absence of angiographic CAD has also been reported. Both arterial and venous thrombotic events have been associated with aPL. Patients with SLE are subject to intracardiac thrombosis and cerebral or systemic thromboembolism independently of or exacerbated by aPL. Current data supports that Libman-Sacks endocarditis is the most common cause of clinical and subclinical embolic cerebrovascular disease. Multiple studies using different methodologies in different populations including a fully integrated, controlled, cross-sectional and longitudinal study using 2D-TEE demonstrated that patients with vegetations as compared to those without have more cerebromicroembolism per hour, lower cerebral perfusion, more stroke/TIA, greater neurocognitive dysfunction, and greater brain injury on MRI; valve vegetations are strong independent risk factor for stroke/TIA, neurocognitive dysfunction, focal brain lesions, and all three outcomes combined; and patients with vegetations have reduced event-free survival time to stroke/TIA, cognitive disability, or death. Retinal artery occlusion has also been associated with valvular heart disease. Therefore, Libman-Sacks vegetations may generate platelet or fibrin macro-or-microemboli that occlude cerebral vessels resulting in ischemic brain injury, stroke/TIA, neurocognitive dysfunction or disability, and death (see Figures 35–1 and 35–2).

Clinical Findings

A. Symptoms & Signs

Although acute pleuritic chest pain and tachycardia could be related to the presence of pericarditis, pleuritis, or pneumonitis, they should also prompt the suspicion of pulmonary embolism and deep vein thrombosis (DVT). Focal and nonfocal transient or permanent neurologic deficits are commonly due to cardioembolism from valvular disease and less often due to vasculitis or cerebritis or atherosclerosis.

B. Laboratory Findings

Antiphospholipid antibodies are highly associated with venous or arterial thrombotic events. However, these antibodies can be present in SLE patients without thrombosis and infrequently in patients who do not have SLE. Therefore, routine measurement of aPL to identify patients at high thrombotic risk and as a basis for prophylactic antiplatelet or anticoagulant therapy is appropriate, but their absence does not exclude underlying increased thrombogenesis.

C. Diagnostic Studies

1. Transesophageal echocardiography—TEE should be considered in SLE patients with acute or recent focal neurologic deficits, in those with nonfocal neurologic deficits and focal brain injury on brain MRI, and in those with peripheral arterial thrombosis to exclude cardioembolism from Libman-Sacks vegetations.

2. Plethysmography, scintigraphy, or venogram—These imaging methods of the lower extremities should be performed if DVT is suspected.

3. High-resolution computed tomography of the chest or pulmonary ventilation-perfusion scan—These methods should be considered if pulmonary embolism is clinically suspected.

Treatment

A. Specific Anti-inflammatory Therapy

Corticosteroids or immunosuppressive agents in combination with antithrombotic therapy (either warfarin alone or single or dual antiplatelet alone) may be beneficial in patients with active SLE and noninfective vegetations with or without thrombosis or thromboembolism. However, randomized controlled studies are not available comparing these therapeutic modalities.

B. Other Therapy

Anticoagulation with warfarin or new direct oral anticoagulants is the therapy of choice in patients with DVT and pulmonary embolism. In patients with Libman-Sacks vegetations and stroke or TIA or suspected embolic cerebral infarcts on MRI oral anticoagulation or single or dual antiplatelet therapy in combination with anti-inflammatory therapy provide a beneficial effect.

5. Coronary and Peripheral Artery Disease

General Considerations

Postmortem studies in SLE patients have demonstrated at least a 25% prevalence of CAD, but clinically evident disease and arteritis are less common. Clinical and subclinical (asymptomatic) functional small-vessel or microvascular CAD (defined as decreased myocardial flow reserve < 2) is twice more frequent than epicardial coronary disease in matched controlled clinical series. Correlates of underlying CAD include an increased prevalence (30–45%) of premature subclinical peripheral arterial disease in the form of aortic and coronary artery calcifications on CT (with two to three times higher rates in the aorta than in the coronary artery arteries), increased carotid and aortic intima media thickening, and plaques on carotid ultrasonography and TEE, respectively. Also, imaging and pathologic studies of the aorta and coronary arteries demonstrate that adventitial thickening is greater in SLE patients with atherosclerosis and abnormal arterial stiffness as compared to those without these abnormalities. These findings suggest that adventitial thickening is associated with and may be a pathogenic factor of atherosclerosis and arterial stiffness in SLE. Of importance, in SLE patients and in relation to age, atherosclerosis and stiffness within the aorta and within the carotid arteries progress in a parallel manner, but aortic atherosclerosis and stiffness progress at a two times higher rate than carotid atherosclerosis and stiffness.

After controlling for traditional risk factors for CAD, the risk of functional (abnormal coronary vasodilation or microvascular disease) or subclinical atherosclerotic epicardial CAD in the form of coronary artery calcifications in lupus patients is three to eight times higher than matched controls. This form of subclinical CAD portends a 35% increased risk of myocardial infarction, percutaneous coronary interventions (PCI), coronary artery bypass grafting (CABG), stroke, and death. Risk factors for CAD in SLE patients are a longer duration of the disease, a longer duration and dose of prednisone therapy, a high disease activity and damage score, lupus nephritis, and SLE-induced dyslipidemia (high levels of LDL phenotype B [the atherogenic phenotype], low levels of high-density lipoprotein [HDL], high levels of proinflammatory HDL, and high levels of triglycerides). Although, a high Framingham risk score is also an important predictor, this score by itself frequently underestimates these patients' cardiovascular risk. Patients with SLE, especially those ≤ 40 years old, have a two to threefold increased incidence of acute coronary syndrome as compared to those older than 40 years. Also, SLE patients with acute coronary syndromes have a twofold higher recurrence of events and 30-day mortality than controls with acute coronary syndromes without SLE.

The proposed pathogenetic mechanisms for CAD include activation of cellular and humoral immunity (including aPL) with activation of macrophages, $CD4^{+}CD28^{-}$ T cells, and dendritic cells. The cytotoxicity of these cells to the endothelium and vascular wall results in decreased production of prostacyclin and prostaglandin I and consequently in increased vasoconstriction. Also, vascular wall cytotoxicity results in an increased thrombosis via release of platelet-derived growth factor and thromboxane A_2. Cytotoxic cells also produce interferon-γ, which destabilizes atherosclerotic plaques by suppressing synthesis of collagen, increased proliferation of smooth muscle cells, and activation of macrophages to release free radicals and matrix metalloproteinases. Other proposed pathogenetic mechanisms for CAD include increased oxidation of LDL and increased production of inflammatory cytokines and chemokines such as heat shock proteins, C-reactive protein, rheumatoid factor, tumor necrosis factor-α, and interleukins. These cytokines are expressed on the endothelium of coronary arteries, recruit inflammatory cells, promote abnormal vascular smooth cell proliferation, and induce oxidative stress, endothelial apoptosis, and further upregulation of adhesion molecules and chemokines. A final proposed pathogenetic mechanisms for CAD are exacerbation of dyslipidemia (high levels of very-low-density lipoproteins and triglycerides and low levels of HDL), homocysteinemia, and insulin resistance. Uncommon pathogenetic factors include coronary arteritis, in situ coronary thrombosis, or embolization from a Libman-Sacks vegetation.

Clinical Findings

A. Symptoms & Signs

The presentation of CAD in SLE patients is not unique and involves stable or exertional angina, unstable angina, acute ST, or non-ST elevation MI, or, rarely, heart failure from ischemic LV dysfunction. In addition, fatal MI can occur in SLE patients, and some data suggest an increased risk of myocardial rupture after MI in SLE patients treated with corticosteroids. Coronary arteritis should be suspected in a young patient with an acute ischemic syndrome, active SLE, and evidence of vasculitis affecting other organs. Also, coronary embolism or in situ thrombosis warrants consideration when MI occurs in the presence of a cardioembolic substrate (valve vegetations), a recent cardioembolic event, or moderate to high levels of aPL.

B. Diagnostic Studies

Electrocardiography, exercise testing with or without perfusion scanning, and echocardiography can be used in SLE patients in whom CAD is suspected. However, the diagnostic value of these techniques is inferior to that in the general population due to their young age, female predominance, and lower prevalence of obstructive epicardial CAD. Positron emission tomography can demonstrate decreased myocardial blood flow and myocardial flow reserve indicative of coronary microvascular dysfunction in SLE patients without epicardial CAD at a rate twice more common than matched controls after adjusting for traditional atherogenic risk factors. Of clinical importance, microvascular dysfunction is predictive of major cardiovascular events and all-cause mortality. Electron-beam computed tomography (CT) has demonstrated a two to fivefold increased frequency of coronary calcification in asymptomatic patients as compared to matched controls without SLE after adjusting for traditional atherogenic risk factors. Cardiac MRI can detect subendocardial ischemia and small patchy areas of delayed contrast enhancement at rest and during exercise in up to 40% of patients with proven microvascular, but no epicardial CAD on coronary angiography. Also, contrast MRI in cardiac wise asymptomatic patients with active SLE demonstrates a more diffuse coronary vessel wall inflammation than in those without SLE (89% versus 24%, respectively), suggestive of subclinical coronary arteritis. A similarly high prevalence of perfusion abnormalities with normal coronary arteries has been reported using radioisotope myocardial perfusion imaging. Recent series in young SLE patients have also shown the development of premature carotid and aortic stiffness associated with intima media thickening and plaques, which may be markers of underlying premature epicardial or microvascular CAD. Therefore, contrast cardiac MRI or combined CTA with PET imaging may be necessary complementary imaging to coronary angiography to differentiate coronary arteritis from common coronary atherosclerosis. Also, suspected epicardial CAD may warrant coronary angiography because of the confounding clinical, echocardiographic, and myocardial perfusion features of functional or small-vessel CAD or lupus myocarditis. On coronary angiography, SLE patients with MI as compared with matched non-SLE patients with MI have more extensive and severe CAD.

Treatment

A. Specific Anti-inflammatory Therapy

Nonrandomized controlled studies have shown that hydroxychloroquine therapy may have a protective effect against the development and progression of atherosclerosis. If coronary arteritis is suspected, standard general medical therapy in combination with specific immunosuppressive anti-inflammatory therapy (intravenous cyclophosphamide or oral mycophenolate and high-dose or pulsed corticosteroids) may be considered before high-risk percutaneous or surgical revascularization procedures in patients with non-ST-elevation acute coronary syndrome or concomitantly with revascularization procedures in those with ST-elevation myocardial infarction. The duration of high-dose therapy is usually for several weeks and tailored based on overall SLE and cardiac clinical response, but in these cases, long-term immunosuppression and antimalarial therapy are necessary to prevent recurrent disease. Corticosteroids may have some additional danger for myocardial rupture in patients with recent transmural MI.

B. Other Therapy

Except for the use of immunosuppressive agents in suspected arteritis, the medical therapy of acute and chronic epicardial CAD is not different from that in the general population. Both percutaneous coronary intervention (PCI) and bypass surgery have been successfully performed in SLE patients. However, SLE patients have higher rate of post-PCI in-stent restenosis and more accelerated disease of bypass grafts. Also, PCI and bypass surgery pose higher morbidity and mortality in those with active SLE, and especially in those with coronary arteritis requiring aggressive immunosuppressive therapy.

6. Cardiac Arrhythmias & Conduction Disturbances

General Considerations

The prevalence of these abnormalities, including prolongation of the QT interval, is unknown. Although they are common with myocarditis and highly associated with the presence of anti-Ro/SS-A antibodies, no primary pathogenetic role of these antibodies has been demonstrated. Atrial fibrillation or flutter may be seen during episodes of acute pericarditis, myocarditis, pulmonary embolism, or pulmonary hypertension. Chronic or subacute conduction disturbances may be due to ischemia or inflammation and fibrosis of the conduction system due to associated atherosclerosis, vasculitis, or myocarditis. ECG is the most valuable technique for detecting arrhythmias and conduction disturbances.

Treatment

A. Specific Anti-inflammatory Therapy

Although experience is limited, acute high-degree atrioventricular (AV) blocks more commonly seen in association with acute myocarditis or myopericarditis may resolve with the use of intravenous immunosuppressives and high-dose corticosteroids, and therefore these drugs should be used before considering permanent pacing. Patients on hydroxychloroquine therapy have decreased incidence of atrial fibrillation. However, hydroxychloroquine and chloroquine can accentuate QT prolongation, especially in combination with other drugs known to have this effect; thus, these drugs must be dosed and monitored appropriately and used cautiously or avoided in the setting of established QT prolongation.

B. Other Therapy

Temporary pacing is an alternative treatment for acute AV blocks. Permanent pacemakers should be used in cases of symptomatic high-grade AV blocks that are unresponsive to immunosuppressives and corticosteroids. Hydroxychloroquine therapy has shown to decrease the development or prevent progression of SLE-associated cardiac arrhythmias.

Prognosis

The overall survival rate of SLE patients is about 75% over 10 years. If the heart, lung, kidney, or central nervous system is clinically involved, the prognosis is worse. Cardiovascular disease is the third major cause of mortality in SLE patients, after infectious and renal diseases early in the course of disease, but it becomes a predominant cause, especially CAD, at the later stage. Valvular disease, myocardial disease, and CAD are all known to decrease the survival of SLE patients.

Hussain K, Mariotti EG, Cattoni HM, et al. A meta-analysis and systematic review of valvular heart disease in systemic lupus erythematosus and its association with antiphospholipid antibodies. *J Clin Rheumatol.* 2021;27(8):e525–e532. [PMID: 32558678]

Manchanda AS, Kwan AC, Ishimoori M, et al. Coronary microvascular dysfunction in patients with systemic lupus erythematosus and chest pain. *Front Cardiovasc Med.* 2022;9:867155. [PMID: 35498009]

Martínez-Ceballos MA, Rey JCS, Granados JPA, et al. Coronary calcium in autoimmune diseases: a systematic literature review and meta-analysis. *Atherosclerosis.* 2021;335:68–76. [PMID: 34592584]

Restivo V, Candiloro S, Daidone M, et al. Systematic review and meta-analysis of cardiovascular risk in rheumatological disease: symptomatic and non-symptomatic events in rheumatoid arthritis and systemic lupus erythematosus. *Autoimmun Rev.* 2022;21(1):102925. [PMID: 34454117]

Roldan CA, Jr Sibbitt WL, Greene ER, et al. Libman-Sacks endocarditis and associated cerebrovascular disease: the role of medical therapy. PLoS One 2021;16(2):e0247052. [PMID: 33592060]

Roldan LP, Roldan PC, Jr Sibbitt WL, Qualls CR, Ratliff MD, Roldan CA. Aortic adventitial thickness as a marker of aortic atherosclerosis, vascular stiffness, and vessel remodeling in systemic lupus erythematosus. *Clin Rheumatol.* 2021;40(5): 1843–1852. [PMID: 33025269]

Roldan PC, Greene ER, Qualls CR, Jr Sibbitt WL, Roldan CA. Progression of atherosclerosis versus arterial stiffness with age within and between arteries in systemic lupus erythematosus, *Rheumatol Int.* 2019;39:1027–1036. [PMID: 30877372]

Slivka AP, Agriesti JE, Orsinelli DA. Natural history of nonbacterial thrombotic endocarditis treated with warfarin. *Int J Stroke.* 2021;16(5):519–525. [PMID: 33040698]

Weber BN, Stevens E, Barrett L, et al. Coronary microvascular dysfunction in systemic lupus erythematosus. *J Am Heart Assoc.* 2021;10(13):e018555. [PMID: 34132099]

Whittier M, Sanchez RB, Arora S, Manadan AM. Systemic lupus erythematosus and antiphospholipid antibody syndrome as risk factors for acute coronary syndrome in young patients: analysis of the national inpatient sample. *J Clin Rheumatol.* 2022;28(3):143–146. [PMID: 35293887]

Zagelbaum Ward NK, Koloffon CL, Posligua A, et al. Cardiac manifestations of systemic lupus erythematous: an overview of the incidence, risk factors, diagnostic criteria, pathophysiology and treatment options. *Cardiol Rev.* 2022;30(1):38–43. [PMID: 32991394]

RHEUMATOID ARTHRITIS

ESSENTIALS OF DIAGNOSIS

- Clinical evidence of rheumatoid arthritis.
- Pericarditis and myocarditis with granuloma on biopsy.
- Granulomatous valve disease, predominantly of the mitral and aortic valves.
- Premature atherosclerosis

General Considerations

Rheumatoid arthritis is an immune-mediated chronic inflammatory disease characterized by morning stiffness, arthralgias, or arthritis, predominantly of the metacarpophalangeal or proximal interphalangeal joints; rheumatoid nodules; serum IgM or IgG rheumatoid factor and anticyclic citrullinated peptide (anti-CCP) antibody; and articular erosions seen on a radiograph. The disease prevalence is about 1%, and it affects females more than males with a ratio of 2–4:1. The natural history of the disease is such that the median life expectancy is reduced by 7 years in men and 3 years in women. The most common causes of death are sepsis, cardiovascular disease, cardiopulmonary complications, and diffuse vasculitis.

Rheumatoid cardiovascular disease is produced by a nonspecific immune complex and cytokines (interleukin-6 and 1-β, tumor necrosis factor-α)–mediated inflammation, vasculitis, or granulomatous deposition on the pericardium, myocardium, heart valves, coronary arteries, aorta, or the conduction system. Clinically apparent rheumatoid heart disease occurs in 25–40% of patients, compared with up to 80% in autopsy series. Rheumatoid heart disease may appear as pericarditis, myocarditis, valvular heart disease, atherosclerotic CAD, coronary arteritis, aortitis, cor pulmonale, or conduction disturbances. The sole presence of rheumatoid arthritis is now considered an independent risk factor for premature development of atherosclerosis, especially CAD with also a three to fourfold increase in cardiovascular events at 10 years.

Predictors for clinical cardiovascular disease include active, long-standing (more than 10 years), and older age at onset of rheumatoid arthritis; elevated inflammatory markers (titers of rheumatoid factor, higher erythrocyte sedimentation, positive SS-A/SS-B, and anti-cyclic citrullinated peptide antibodies); elevated prothrombotic markers (higher levels of haptoglobin, von Willebrand factor, and plasminogen activator inhibitor); longer duration of corticosteroid therapy; active extraarticular, erosive polyarticular, and nodular disease; and systemic vasculitis. Epicardial adipose tissue thickness also correlates positively with cardiovascular disease. These findings suggest inflammatory and prothrombotic processes leading to cardiovascular disease. Heart disease is the third leading cause of death in patients with rheumatoid arthritis and accounts for nearly 50% of their mortality.

1. Rheumatoid Pericarditis

The prevalence of pericarditis is higher in hospitalized patients with active disease. Pericarditis generally follows the diagnosis of rheumatoid arthritis. There is a high association between pericarditis and IgG or IgM rheumatoid factor positivity, rheumatoid nodular disease, and ESR of more than 55 mm/h. Rheumatoid pericarditis occurs by three mechanisms: a nonspecific immune complex inflammatory process, vasculitis, and, less frequently, granulomatous, or nodular disease.

Clinical Findings

A. Symptoms & Signs

Rheumatoid pericarditis is generally uncomplicated and most commonly is evidenced by typical pleuritic pain. About one-third of patients are asymptomatic. On physical examination, most will have a pericardial rub. Rarely, pericarditis complicated with cardiac tamponade, large focal masses of fibrinous deposition causing focal tamponade, or constrictive pericarditis may occur, generally in adult patients with active and severe disease of a longer duration and in those with extra-articular involvement. Dyspnea and orthopnea, edema, jugular venous distention, rales, pulsus paradoxus, Kussmaul sign, and hepatojugular venous distention are common when cardiac compression is present.

B. Laboratory Findings

Findings commonly associated with rheumatoid pericarditis include an ESR more than 55 mm/h and high titers of rheumatoid factor. Pericardial fluid is exudative and serosanguineous, with a high protein content and high lactate dehydrogenase (LDH) but a characteristically low glucose level and may contain rheumatoid factor. The cellular content is usually more than 2000 cells/mL, predominantly neutrophils. On pericardial biopsy (by immunofluorescence), granular deposits of IgG, IgM, C3, and C1q are seen in the interstitium and blood vessel walls of the pericardium.

C. Diagnostic Studies

1. Electrocardiography—An ECG commonly shows nonspecific ST segment and T-wave changes; a classic diffuse ST segment elevation and PR depression can be seen. Low voltage or electrical alternans may be seen with large pericardial effusions.

2. Chest radiography—The chest radiography is generally normal. Cardiomegaly is seen in patients with large pericardial effusions. Pericardial calcifications are rarely seen.

3. Echocardiography—This is the most important diagnostic technique for rheumatoid pericardial disease. The most common findings are pericardial effusion and pericardial thickening. Right atrial or ventricular diastolic compression may be seen with large pericardial effusions and may indicate tamponade hemodynamics. The presence of pericardial thickening and calcification without significant effusion and the presence of symptoms or signs of cardiac compression suggest constrictive pericarditis, which can be confirmed by cardiac catheterization. However, absence of pericardial abnormalities on echocardiography does not exclude the presence of pericarditis in a patient with typical symptoms or a pericardial rub. Also, asymptomatic pericardial effusions are seen in about 25% of patients and are associated with renal disease, hypoalbuminemia, and pulmonary hypertension-cor pulmonale. Finally, echocardiography is commonly used to guide pericardiocentesis.

4. Computed tomography or magnetic resonance imaging—These imaging methods are superior to echocardiography in detecting the presence and extent of pericardial thickening and calcification in patients with suspected constrictive pericarditis.

Treatment

Since acute pericarditis indicates active disease in the setting of rheumatoid arthritis, high-dose oral or intravenous pulse corticosteroids are used acutely to control pericardial inflammation, followed by long-term rheumatoid-specific chronic therapy, including methotrexate, sulfasalazine, antimalarials, leflunomide, tumor necrosis factor-α receptor blockers (infliximab, adalimumab, etanercept, golimumab, certolizumab), anti–B-cell (CD20) therapy (rituximab),

T-cell stimulation inhibitors (abatacept), interleukin (IL)-6 receptor blocker (tocilizumab), or soluble IL-1 receptor antagonist (anakinra). Acute pericarditis complicated with a large pericardial effusion with or without clinical or echocardiographic evidence of tamponade can progress rapidly, can be potentially associated with, or caused by infection, and carry high morbidity and mortality. Therefore, an earlier diagnostic (aimed to exclude infection) or therapeutic echocardiography-guided pericardiocentesis followed by intensive immunosuppressive anti-inflammatory therapy are indicated. As in patients with SLE, pericardial window should be avoided due to commonly associated serositis (peritonitis and pleuritis) and increased risk of infection. For chronic constrictive pericarditis, high-risk pericardiectomy has been performed. The use of intrapericardial corticosteroids at the time of pericardiocentesis is controversial but may be effective.

Prognosis

The prognosis of rheumatoid arthritis in the presence of pericardial disease is unaltered when the pericardial involvement is mild. Large pericardial effusions with tamponade or chronic constrictive pericarditis, however, increase the morbidity and mortality rates among rheumatoid patients.

2. Rheumatoid Valvular Heart Disease

General Considerations

Rheumatoid valvular heart disease is produced by a nonspecific acute, chronic, or recurrent immune complex inflammatory process, vasculitis, or deposition of granulomata on the valve leaflets. The inflammatory process consists of infiltration with plasma cells, histiocytes, lymphocytes, and eosinophils that lead to leaflet fibrosis, thickening, and retraction. The valve granulomata, which resemble subcutaneous rheumatoid nodules and may result from focal vasculitis, are present inside any portion of the four valves, valve rings, papillary muscle tips, and atrial or ventricular endocardium. The aortic and mitral valves are most often affected. The granulomata are most located at the basal or mid portion of the valves, are usually focal, and generally produce none or mild valve dysfunction.

Rheumatoid valvular heart disease is more commonly subclinical and can manifest in five forms: (1) healed valvulitis with residual leaflet fibrosis and regurgitation and rarely stenosis; (2) rheumatoid valve nodules (Figure 35–5A); (3) acute or recurrent valvulitis with variable degrees of regurgitation and with Libman-Sacks–like vegetations (Figure 35–5, B–D); rarely, (4) aortitis with aortic root dilatation and aortic regurgitation; and (5) superimposed infective endocarditis. Acute and chronic valvulitis with resulting leaflet thickening and fibrosis is indistinguishable from that seen in SLE. In contrast, valve nodules appear to be unique to rheumatoid arthritis.

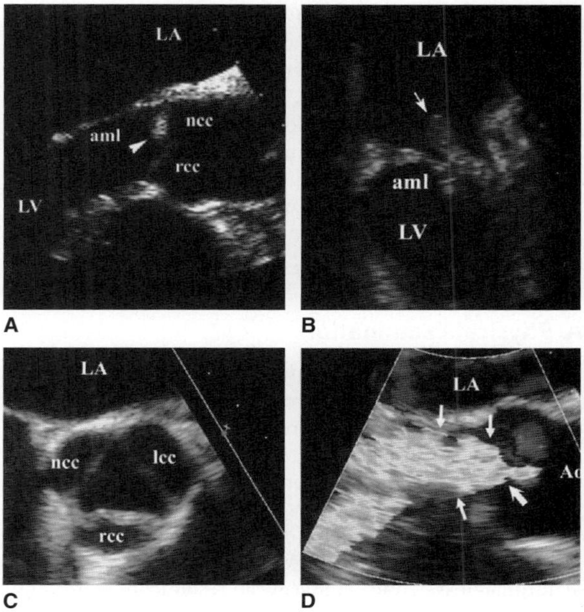

▲ **Figure 35–5. A: Rheumatoid aortic valve nodule in a 48-year-old woman with rheumatoid arthritis.** This transesophageal echocardiographic (TEE) longitudinal view of the left ventricular outflow tract demonstrates a well-defined nodule with oval shape and homogeneous soft tissue echoreflectance within the midportion of the aortic noncoronary cusp (ncc) (*arrowhead*). In contrast, the right coronary cusp (rcc) is normal. Aortic valve regurgitation was not demonstrated. aml, anterior mitral leaflet; LA, left atrium; LV, left ventricle. **B:** Severe mitral valvulitis with Libman-Sacks–like vegetations in a 52-year-old female with severe rheumatoid arthritis and recurrent transient ischemic attacks. This close-up four-chamber TEE view demonstrates marked thickening with soft tissue echoreflectance of the anterior and posterior mitral leaflets and a large and elongated soft tissue echoreflectant vegetation on the atrial side of the distal portion of the posterior mitral leaflet. After exclusion of infection, she was treated with warfarin, steroids, and tumor necrosis factor-α receptor inhibitors, and follow-up echocardiogram demonstrated remarkable improvement. **C and D:** Severe aortic valvulitis complicated by severe aortic regurgitation and subacute heart failure in a 47-year-old female with severely active rheumatoid arthritis. **C:** This basal short axis TEE view of the aortic valve shows diffuse thickening with soft tissue echoreflectance and decreased mobility of the non (ncc), left (lcc), and right (rcc) coronary cusps. **D:** Color Doppler longitudinal TEE view of the aortic valve (Ao) shows severe aortic regurgitation (*arrows*).

In previous series using TTE, rheumatoid valve disease has been reported in patients with long-standing rheumatoid disease and severe cases with erosive polyarticular and nodular disease, systemic vasculitis, and high levels of rheumatoid factor. In a TEE series, no correlation was found between valve disease and the duration, activity, severity, pattern of onset and course, extra-articular disease, serology, or therapy of rheumatoid arthritis. Therefore, a clinical or laboratory predictor or marker of rheumatoid valve disease is still undefined.

Clinical Findings

A. Physical Examination

The physical examination in rheumatoid valve disease may not be revealing because in most cases the degree of valve dysfunction is mild. In the rare cases of acute mitral or aortic valvulitis resulting in severe valve regurgitation or acute severe valve regurgitation from "rupture" of a nodule or a large nodule affecting leaflets coaptation, classic auscultatory findings and associated signs of rapidly evolving left ventricular failure may be present. Uncommonly, a clinical syndrome of systemic embolism can result from a thrombus or a valve strand superimposed on a valve nodule or from Libman-Sacks–like vegetations complicating acute valvulitis.

B. Diagnostic Studies

1. Electrocardiography and chest radiography—The ECG and chest radiography have limited diagnostic value. Both techniques may show chamber enlargement in cases of severe valve disease.

2. Color-flow Doppler echocardiography—TTE is the most used test for detecting and assessing the severity of rheumatoid valve disease. In a series using TEE in 34 patients with rheumatoid arthritis, 20 patients (59%) had mainly left-sided valve disease (valve nodules in 11 [32%], valve thickening in 18 [53%], at least moderate mitral or mild aortic regurgitation in 7 [21%], and valve stenosis in 1 [3%]). *Valve nodules* were generally single and small (4–12 mm), of homogenous echoreflectance, and of oval shape with regular borders, typically located at the leaflets' basal or mid portions, and equally affected the aortic and mitral valves (see Figure 35–5A). These nodules can also be seen on valve rings, papillary muscles tips, and atrial or ventricular endocardium. In some patients, mitral and aortic valve thickening is associated with mitral valve Libman-Sacks–like vegetations (see Figure 35–5B). *Valve thickening* was equally diffuse or localized. When the thickening was localized, it affected any leaflet portion, was usually mild, involved the mitral and aortic valves similarly, and rarely involved the annulus and subvalvular apparatus (see Figure 35–5).

Treatment

No specific anti-inflammatory therapy for rheumatoid valve disease has been established. The use of immunosuppressive agents or biologics including tumor necrosis factor-α receptor inhibitors in combination with corticosteroids, as noted earlier for pericarditis, in cases of acute severe valvulitis may result in significant improvement (see Figure 35–5, B–D). Also, in patients with Libman-Sacks–like vegetations, anticoagulation and anti-inflammatory therapy has resulted in improvement of valve masses and prevention of recurrent embolic events. Although no prospective trial data are available, prophylactic antiplatelet therapy may prevent cardioembolism in patients with valve nodules or thickening. Mitral valve repair and mitral or aortic valve replacement or homograft root-and-valve replacement have been successfully performed in acute or chronic severe valve regurgitation.

Prognosis

The short-term and long-term mortality rates of patients with rheumatoid arthritis with valve disease are significantly higher than those of matched controls. The 30-day and 1-year morbidity and mortality rates of patients with rheumatoid arthritis undergoing valve replacement or rarely valve repair are two to three times higher than those of patients without rheumatoid arthritis. Also, patients undergoing valve repair have higher rates of reoperation than patients without rheumatoid arthritis.

3. Rheumatoid Myocarditis

General Considerations

Secondary myocardial disease is more common than primary myocarditis in rheumatoid arthritis (about 50% versus ≤ 10%, respectively). The most common pathogenetic factors for secondary myocardial disease, more commonly manifested with diastolic dysfunction are similar to those described in SLE and include functional microvascular CAD, peripheral arterial stiffness, hypertensive heart disease, and epicardial CAD. Primary rheumatoid myocarditis is observed in as much as 30% of patients in postmortem series but is uncommon in clinical and echocardiographic reports. Rheumatoid myocarditis is more common in patients with active and extra-articular disease, highly positive rheumatoid factor, and systemic vasculitis. Rheumatoid myocarditis may result from autoimmunity, vasculitis, or granulomata deposition; rarely, it is due to amyloid infiltration. Patient with rheumatoid arthritis have a two to threefold increased risk of clinical heart failure, most commonly diastolic heart failure, as compared with matched controls without rheumatoid arthritis. Recently, a dilated or restrictive cardiomyopathy due to hydroxychloroquine therapy and characterized by myocyte enlargement due to perinuclear vacuolization and abundant myeloid figures within myocytes has been reported. Unless granulomata are present, rheumatoid myocarditis is difficult to differentiate on histopathology from other types of myocarditis.

Clinical Findings

The clinical presentation of primary rheumatoid myocarditis is similar to that for myocarditis from other causes. Most commonly, it is mild, asymptomatic, or overshadowed by other musculoskeletal disease manifestations and, therefore, often clinically unrecognized. When it is symptomatic, nonspecific symptoms of fatigue, dyspnea, palpitations, and chest pain may be present. The chest pain is usually pleuritic and probably reflects the presence of myopericarditis. Rarely, severe acute myocarditis with LV systolic dysfunction may present as congestive heart failure or symptomatic atrial or ventricular arrhythmias.

A. Physical Examination

The cardiovascular exam is usually normal. In severe cases, fever and sinus tachycardia are common. First and second heart sounds are normal; a third or fourth heart sound may rarely be present. Functional systolic murmurs may be present. If myopericarditis is present, a pericardial rub may be detected.

B. Laboratory Findings

Primary myocarditis with LV diastolic or systolic dysfunction has been associated with the presence of anti-SS-A/anti-SS-B and anti-CCP autoantibodies. In the majority of cases, mild elevation of myocardial isoenzymes, such as troponin I, and less often of CPK-MB may be seen.

C. Diagnostic Studies

1. Electrocardiography—The ECG is often normal. When abnormal, the ECG shows nonspecific ST segment and T-wave abnormalities. AV conduction disturbances and atrial or ventricular ectopy can be detected. As a result of residual interstitial myocardial fibrosis, patients have higher dispersion of repolarization as manifested by prolongation of the uncorrected and corrected QT intervals.

2. Echocardiography—Recent cross-sectional controlled Doppler echocardiography series, especially those including tissue Doppler, strain, and strain rate, have shown that patients with rheumatoid arthritis have a high prevalence rate of subclinical and clinical LV and RV diastolic dysfunction as compared with matched controls (30–76% and 25–45% versus less than 20%, respectively). The prevalence of subclinical LV systolic dysfunction is lower, but higher than matched controls (10–15% versus ≤ 6%). Also, longitudinal series have demonstrated a high incidence (40%) of clinical diastolic heart failure independent of traditional cardiovascular risk factors for diastolic dysfunction. As an indicator of global myocardial involvement, reduced LA contractility as determined by decreased global LA strain and increased LA volume index also occur. Less commonly, echocardiography may show segmental wall motion abnormalities or diffuse LV contractile dysfunction and chamber dilatation in cases of severe myocarditis. The echocardiographic features of amyloidosis due to rheumatoid arthritis are nonspecific but may coexist or mimic rheumatoid constrictive pericarditis.

3. Radionuclide scanning—Scanning with indium-111, gallium-67, or technetium-99 may show focal patchy or diffuse myocardial uptake indicative of active myocardial inflammation, necrosis, or both.

4. Magnetic resonance imaging—As in patients with SLE, cardiac magnetic resonance imaging detects subclinical and clinical myocarditis. T2-weighted imaging assesses myocardial edema (indicative of active inflammation) and gadolinium contrast enhancement assesses fibrosis. Therefore, magnetic resonance imaging differentiates better the pathogenesis of myocardial disease as myocarditis, vasculitis, or myocardial infarction.

Treatment & Prognosis

Limited data are available about the treatment of primary rheumatoid myocarditis, but control of the rheumatoid arthritis activity with disease modifying antirheumatic drugs (DMARDS) including biologics is important to prevent this condition. Acute in-patient treatment with intravenous immunosuppressive therapy and/or anti-rheumatoid biologics (tumor necrosis factor-α receptor blockers, rituximab, abatacept, tocilizumab, sarilumab) in combination with high-dose or pulse corticosteroids may be considered. This therapy may be continued orally on outpatient basis for several weeks and adjusted according to clinical course. Also, the incidence of new-onset heart failure in the setting of rheumatoid arthritis may decrease with tumor necrosis factor-α blocker therapy, although the use of these drugs in established heart failure is controversial. Nonspecific therapy includes bed rest, analgesics, and cardiac monitoring for at least 48–72 hours. In rheumatoid arthritis patients, diastolic heart failure doubles the mortality risk as compared with matched controls with diastolic heart failure but no rheumatoid arthritis. The mortality of those with systolic heart failure is significantly higher.

4. Rheumatoid Coronary Artery Disease

General Considerations

After controlling for traditional atherogenic risk factors, patients with rheumatoid arthritis have two to three times more epicardial and small-vessel CAD than matched controls after adjusting for traditional atherogenic risk factors. Therefore, rheumatoid arthritis is now considered an independent risk factor for CAD or CAD equivalent. Except for aPL, the pathogenetic factors for these two types of CAD in rheumatoid patients are similar to those described for patients with SLE. In unselected patients, functional microvascular CAD is the predominant type (~50%), followed by nonobstructive (~25%)

and obstructive epicardial CAD (~25%). Also, in patients with established rheumatoid disease a high prevalence rate (up to 60%) of subclinical coronary artery calcification by CT is seen as compared with those with recent onset of the disease (43%) and matched controls (38%). By age 65–70 years, 75–80% of patients with rheumatoid arthritis have evidence of CAD on angiography (one-third of them with three vessels CAD) and a high incidence of myocardial infarction (4.8–5.9 events per 1000 person-years). The prevalence and incidence rates of CAD in patients with rheumatoid arthritis are similar to those of type 2 diabetic patients and are correlated with carotid or aortic atherosclerosis or stiffness. Coronary arteritis, in-situ coronary thrombosis in the absence of atherosclerosis or arteritis, or coronary embolism are rare. Coronary arteritis is rare and occurs in patients with rheumatoid nodules, overt vasculitis, rapidly progressive rheumatoid disease, and high titers of rheumatoid factor (Figure 35–6). Traditional atherogenic risk factors and Framingham and Reynolds scores underestimate the risk of CAD. Older age at onset of rheumatoid arthritis, longer duration of corticosteroid therapy, disease duration more than 10 years; active extraarticular, erosive polyarticular, and nodular disease; vasculitis; and positive rheumatoid factor or anti-CCP antibody are better predictors of CAD and commonly associated carotid and aortic atherosclerosis and stiffness. These clinical features also predict a higher incidence of acute coronary syndromes. Mitral valve calcification on echocardiography is also predictive of coronary artery calcification on CT, and a coronary calcification score more than 100 Agatston units on CT is predictive of future cardiovascular events (MI, congestive heart failure, stroke, and death). Patients with parameters of active and chronic inflammation have reduced small- and large-artery elasticity or associated plaques and have a twofold independent risk of MI, heart failure, stroke, and cardiovascular mortality compared with matched controls. Also, rheumatoid patients with acute coronary syndromes have a twofold higher recurrence rate of events and mortality than matched controls.

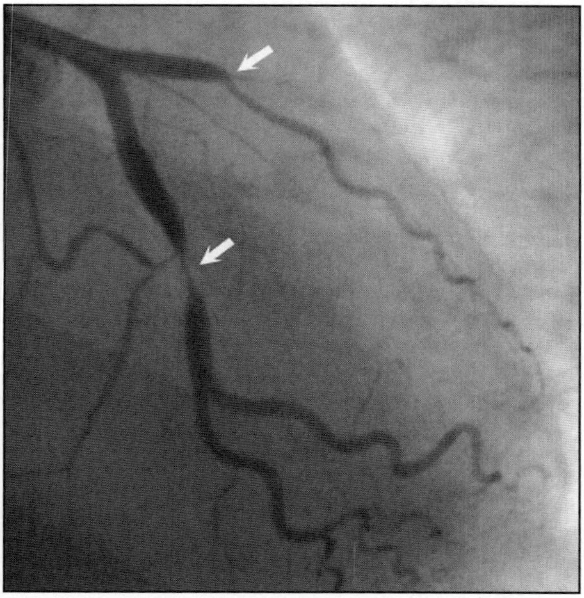

▲ Figure 35–6. Coronary arteritis complicated by a non–ST elevation myocardial infarction in a 47-year-old female with severely active rheumatoid arthritis. This left coronary artery angiogram demonstrates an occluded left anterior descending coronary artery (*upper arrow*) and a 90% stenosis of the circumflex artery (*lower arrow*). Successful stent placements on the anterior descending and circumflex arteries were performed. Since the patient also had associated severe aortic valvulitis (described in Figure 35–5, C and D) and clinical and serology data consistent with severely active rheumatoid arthritis, in addition to standard care for an acute coronary syndrome, the patient was also successfully treated with intravenous pulse corticosteroids and cyclophosphamide.

Clinical Findings

A. Symptoms & Signs

Patients with rheumatoid arthritis with active CAD may frequently have atypical chest pain mimicking pericarditis, myocarditis, pleuritis, or osteochondritis. Atherosclerotic CAD will manifest as chronic stable angina, unstable angina, or acute MI, whereas coronary arteritis is more commonly seen as unstable angina or acute non-ST elevation or ST-elevation MI.

Tachycardia, third or fourth heart sounds, and pulmonary rales, if LV failure is present, are seen during acute ischemic syndromes.

B. Diagnostic Studies

1. Electrocardiography—An ECG will show diagnostic Q waves indicative of previous MI, T-wave inversion suggestive of ischemia, or ST elevation or depression suggestive of epicardial or subendocardial ischemic injury.

2. Echocardiography—Resting and stress echocardiography are useful in the detection of wall motion abnormalities in those with obstructive CAD but have decreased sensitivity for microvascular disease or coronary arteritis. Dipyridamole or adenosine Doppler TTE has also been used to assess coronary flow reserve in those with microvascular disease. During severe ischemia, echocardiography may show segmental wall motion abnormalities or myocardial scars if previous infarction has occurred. This technique will also determine the presence (or absence) of LV dysfunction and its severity.

3. Other tests—Patients with high ESR (≥ 60 mm/h), C-reactive protein, serum amyloid, soluble vascular adhesion molecule-1, and interferon-γ have abnormal small- and large-artery vasodilatory response and are at increased risk for cardiovascular events and mortality. Electron-beam CT detects subclinical coronary artery calcification in patients with established disease. Computed coronary tomography angiography may detect early CAD, identify, quantify, and characterize high-risk plaque morphology and its response to medical therapy.

Myocardial isoenzymes, such as troponin I (the most sensitive) and CPK-MB may be elevated if myocardial necrosis has occurred. Exercise treadmill testing, with or without radionuclide scanning can also be used to detect suspected CAD. Coronary angiography should be considered when there is a high suspicion of CAD, an abnormal exercise treadmill test, or incapacitating symptoms. The diagnosis of coronary arteritis can be suspected if multiple stenotic lesions and aneurysmal lesions are found in the epicardial coronary arteries in a patient with severely active disease (see Figure 35–6).

Treatment

In general, control of inflammation with DMARDS including hydroxychloroquine, tumor necrosis factor-α blockers, other biologics, methotrexate therapy, leflunomide, and statins may reduce the development or progression of endothelial dysfunction, arterial stiffness, and premature atherosclerosis. DMARDs have shown to decrease the risk of myocardial infarction, heart failure, cardiovascular death, and all-cause mortality. Statins have shown to decrease the formation and prevent progression of coronary plaque formation, decrease the incidence of acute coronary syndromes and cardiovascular disease in general, and reduce all-cause mortality. The JAK (Janus kinase) inhibitors used to treat rheumatoid arthritis have recently received a black box warning regarding the use in established cardiovascular or thrombotic disease; thus, for the time being these drugs should be avoided in patients with established or suspected coronary artery disease. Although experience and controlled studies in this area are limited and according to a specific clinical scenario, suspected severe and symptomatic coronary rheumatoid arteritis can initially be treated acutely with high doses of corticosteroids and, if refractory, with rituximab, plasmapheresis, or intravenous cyclophosphamide in conjunction with heparin, aspirin, β-blockers, nitrates, and less often calcium channel blockers (see Figure 35–6). Limited data are also available about PCIs or CABG in coronary arteritis, but if clinical circumstances allow it, it is reasonable to treat patients medically, and then reassess the need for PCI as the blood vessel may spontaneously heal and remodel. Symptomatic atherosclerotic CAD should be treated medically or ultimately with coronary revascularization as deemed necessary and appropriate. Amelioration of inflammation with low-dose corticosteroids, tumor necrosis factor-α blockers, other biologics, or statins may decrease the effects of vascular inflammation and dysfunction and consequently of coronary events. Furthermore, cyclooxygenase-2 selective inhibitors, which inhibit prostaglandin I-2 (a vasodilator and inhibitor of platelet aggregation), and NSAIDs increase the risk of acute coronary syndromes in rheumatoid patients. Finally, discontinuation of statin therapy may increase the risk of acute coronary syndromes.

Prognosis

Patients with rheumatoid arthritis as compared with matched controls, have a twofold increased risk for myocardial infarction, congestive heart failure, stroke, and cardiovascular mortality. Also, the presence of ischemia on exercise echocardiography portends a three times higher mortality rate than in matched controls with negative studies. In addition, those with an acute coronary syndrome have a higher recurrence rate of events and mortality than matched controls (58% versus 30% and 40% versus 15%, respectively). Furthermore, in rheumatoid patients PCI or CABG carry two to four times higher related morbidity and mortality rates than those of matched controls. Preoperative corticosteroid use and longer disease duration are associated with higher mortality in patients undergoing CABG.

5. Conduction Disturbances & Arrhythmias

General Considerations

The prevalence and incidence of atrial arrhythmias, especially of atrial fibrillation, and consequently of stroke are 30% higher in rheumatoid arthritis patients than in matched controls. The prevalence of sinus or AV nodal or intraventricular conduction disturbances in patients with rheumatoid arthritis may be higher than in age-matched controls in the general population. Possible mechanisms include premature CAD, acute inflammation of the sinus or AV node or His bundle (related to pancarditis), vasculitis of the arterioles supplying the conduction pathway, granulomata deposition in the conduction system, and amyloid infiltration.

Clinical Findings

The mean age of patients with conduction disturbances is generally more than 60 years, and most of these patients have severe forms of rheumatoid arthritis with nodular disease, requiring chronic corticosteroid therapy. The conduction disturbances are generally mild, asymptomatic, and incidentally diagnosed by ECG.

A. Symptoms & Signs

In rare cases, high-degree AV block may be evidenced with tiredness, dizziness, presyncope, or syncope. Although it is uncommon, high-degree AV block may be asymptomatic because the joint disease severely limits the patient's activity. Rarely, AV block is transient and may reverse with anti-inflammatory therapy.

B. Diagnostic Studies

The best diagnostic methods are routine ECG complemented by 24-hour or longer ECG monitoring.

Treatment

The treatment of severe and symptomatic high-degree AV or intraventricular blocks associated with acute myocarditis or valvulitis consists of temporary pacing and intravenous immunosuppressive therapy in combination with high-dose corticosteroids followed by chronic antirheumatoid therapy. Patients who are unresponsive to this therapy within 7–10 days should be considered for permanent pacemakers.

6. Rheumatoid Pulmonary Hypertension

General Considerations

The causes of pulmonary hypertension with normal pulmonary venous pressure (types I and III) including serum hyperviscosity, interstitial fibrosis, obliterative bronchiolitis, pulmonary vasculitis, or thromboembolism are more common than that from left heart disease (type II). Since patients with pulmonary arterial hypertension (defined as mean pulmonary artery pressure ≥ 25 mm Hg, pulmonary capillary wedge pressure or LV end-diastolic pressure ≤ 15 mm Hg, and a pulmonary vascular resistance of ≥ 240 dyn/cm^{-5} or ≥ 3 Wood units) have poor prognosis unless recognized and treated early with vasodilator therapy, it is essential to establish this diagnosis as accurately and as early as possible. The prevalence of these diseases is uncertain, but low. Since the mortality rate is high within 1 year of diagnosis, prompt diagnosis is vital. Lung biopsy or bronchoalveolar lavage may confirm pulmonary vasculitis and bronchiolitis obliterans, both of which are responsive to immunosuppressive therapy. Interstitial lung disease, CHF, and valvular heart disease are independent predictors of pulmonary hypertension.

Severe pulmonary hypertension may lead to RV hypertrophy, enlargement, and diastolic followed by systolic dysfunction (cor pulmonale) and produce the symptoms and signs of right-sided heart failure.

Clinical Findings

A. Symptoms & Signs

Dyspnea is a common manifestation of pulmonary hypertension and cor pulmonale. However, moderate pulmonary hypertension with or without mild cor pulmonale can be asymptomatic.

Findings on physical examination include a parasternal heave, split second heart sound with loud pulmonic component, tricuspid regurgitation, right-sided S_3 gallop, and rarely, hepatomegaly and edema.

B. Diagnostic Studies

1. Electrocardiography—An ECG may show right atrial and ventricular enlargement, right axis deviation, and/or right bundle branch block.

2. Color-flow Doppler echocardiography—This technique may show right atrial and ventricular enlargement, hypertrophy or diastolic (most commonly) or systolic dysfunction, tricuspid and pulmonic regurgitation, and evidence of high pulmonary artery systolic and diastolic pressures. Pulmonary hypertension may not be accompanied by echocardiographic evidence of cor pulmonale, especially if the pulmonary artery pressure is less than 50 mm Hg. In controlled series of asymptomatic patients, the prevalence of pulmonary hypertension on echocardiography is five times higher in rheumatoid patients than in controls (21% versus 4%). Echocardiography can rule out left-sided heart disease as a cause of pulmonary hypertension. Echocardiography can also assess response to therapy.

3. Open-lung biopsy and bronchoalveolar lavage—These methods should be done if severe pulmonary vasculitis or bronchiolitis obliterans is suspected as the cause of pulmonary hypertension.

Treatment & Prognosis

The treatment of pulmonary hypertension from pulmonary vasculitis or active inflammatory interstitial disease is intravenous immunosuppressive agents as noted previously in combination with high-dose corticosteroids, but the prognosis is poor, and most patients die within 1 year of diagnosis. However, newer antirheumatoid therapies should be considered and may improve survival if the rheumatoid arthritis process can be controlled. The treatment of pulmonary arterial hypertension includes endothelin receptor antagonists, prostacyclins, and/or phosphodiesterase inhibitors.

Azpiri-Lopez JR, Delgado DAG, Pedraza IJC, et al. Echocardiographic evaluation of pulmonary hypertension, right ventricular function, and right ventricular-pulmonary arterial coupling in patients with rheumatoid arthritis. *Clin Rheumatol.* 2021;40(7):2651–2656. [PMID: 33443606]

Cacciapaglia F, Spinelli FR, Piga M, et al. Estimated 10-year cardiovascular risk in a large Italian cohort of rheumatoid arthritis patients: Data from the Cardiovascular Obesity and Rheumatic DISease (CORDIS) Study Group. *Eur J Intern Med.* 2022;96:60–65. [PMID: 34657778]

Chen HH, Lin CH, Hsieh TY, Chen DY, Ying JC, Chapo WC. Factors associated with incident severe pulmonary arterial hypertension in systemic autoimmune rheumatic diseases: a nationwide study. *Rheumatology* (Oxford). 2021;60(11): 5351–5361. [PMID: 33547781]

Huang S, Cai T, Weber BN, et al. The association between inflammation, incident heart failure, and heart failure subtypes in patients with rheumatoid arthritis. *Arthritis Care Res* (Hoboken). 2021;10:1002. [PMID: 34623035]

Karpouzas GA, Ormseth SR, Hernandez E, Budoff MJ. The impact of statins on coronary atherosclerosis progression and long-term cardiovascular disease risk in rheumatoid arthritis. *Rheumatology* (Oxford). 2021;61(5):1857–1866. [PMID: 34373923]

Kim GH, Park YJ. Accelerated diastolic dysfunction in premenopausal women with rheumatoid arthritis. *Arthritis Res Ther.* 2021;23(1):247. [PMID: 34560895]

Malmberg M, Palomaki A, Sipilaa JOT, Rautava P, Gunn J, Kyto V. Long-term outcomes after coronary artery bypass surgery in patients with rheumatoid arthritis. *Ann Med.* 2021;53(1): 1512–1519. [PMID: 34461789]

Malmberg M, Palomaki A, Sipilaa JOT, Rautava P, Gunn J, Kyto V. Long-term outcomes of surgical aortic valve replacement in patients with rheumatoid arthritis. *J Clin Med.* 2021 Jun 4; 10(11):2492. [PMID: 34199991]

Ozen G, Aniello SD, Pedro S, Michaud K, Suissa S. Reduction of cardiovascular disease and mortality versus risk of new onset diabetes with statin use in patients with rheumatoid arthritis. *Arthritis Care Res* (Hoboken). 2022. doi: 10.1002/acr.24866. [PMID: 35119769]

Park E, Griffin J, Bathon JM. Myocardial dysfunction and heart failure in rheumatoid arthritis. *Arthritis Rheumatol.* 2022;74(2):184–199. [PMID: 34523821]

Roldan CA, DeLong C, Qualls CR, Crawford MH. Characterization of valvular heart disease in rheumatoid arthritis by transesophageal echocardiography and clinical correlates. *Am J Cardiol.* 2007;100(3):496–502. [PMID: 17659935]

SYSTEMIC SCLEROSIS

ESSENTIALS OF DIAGNOSIS

- Sclerotic skin, esophageal dysfunction, Raynaud phenomenon.
- Functional or structural small-vessel CAD.
- Multisegmental myocardial perfusion abnormalities in the absence of epicardial CAD.
- Diastolic heart failure.
- Pulmonary hypertension and cor pulmonale.

General Considerations

Systemic sclerosis or scleroderma is a generalized disorder characterized by excessive accumulation of connective tissue; fibrosis; and degenerative changes of the skin, skeletal muscles, synovium, blood vessels, gastrointestinal tract, kidney, lung, and heart. Raynaud phenomenon, esophageal dysfunction, and sclerotic skin characterize the disease and are present in more than 90% of patients. The two major clinical variants are diffuse cutaneous (20% of cases) and limited cutaneous disease (80%). The less common diffuse type is characterized by skin thickening of the distal and proximal extremities and the trunk, with frequent involvement of the kidney, lung, or heart. In the more common limited type, which includes the CREST syndrome (calcinosis, Raynaud phenomenon, esophageal dysfunction, sclerodactyly, and telangiectasia), the skin changes are limited to the face, fingers, and distal portions of the extremities. A third, uncommon variant is the overlap syndrome, which includes systemic sclerosis in association with other connective tissue disease.

The incidence of systemic sclerosis is 10–20 per million populations per year. The disease affects all races, is three times more common in women than in men, and usually occurs between the ages of 30 and 50 years. The diffuse cutaneous type has a poorer prognosis than does the limited type. The overall cumulative survival rates after 3, 6, and 9 years are 86%, 76%, and 61%, respectively. The prognosis is worst for males who are older than 50 years with lung, heart, or kidney disease. Pulmonary disease, including pulmonary hypertension and interstitial lung disease, and heart diseases are the major causes of death; these are followed by kidney disease, with a cumulative survival of only 20% at 7 years. Subclinical and symptomatic cardiovascular disease occurs in as many as 60% of patients with systemic sclerosis. The predominant conditions are functional and structural microvascular CAD, myocarditis, pulmonary and systemic hypertension-related heart disease, and pericarditis. Atrial and ventricular arrhythmias and conduction abnormalities are less common but clinically relevant. Cardiovascular disease is associated with duration and severity of systemic sclerosis, severity and duration of peripheral Raynaud phenomenon, positive anti-Scl-70, RNA polymerase III and anticentromere antibodies, higher levels of inflammatory markers, overlap syndrome, and peripheral myositis. Cardiovascular disease is generally less common and less severe in the limited type than in the diffuse type. African Americans have higher prevalence rate of diffuse systemic sclerosis, more prevalent and severe pulmonary hypertension, and overall higher mortality than Americans of European descent.

1. Coronary Artery Disease

Pathophysiology

Patients with systemic sclerosis alone, independently of traditional atherogenic risk factors, have three times higher risk of developing CAD. In systemic sclerosis, the intramyocardial coronary arteries and arterioles are predominantly affected. The two main mechanisms by which the intramyocardial arteries are affected are: (1) abnormally increased small-vessel vasoconstriction due to an immune-mediated endothelial cell injury and increased production of platelet-derived growth factor impairing the endothelial response to vasodilation. The intramyocardial coronary arteries and arterioles are also affected by mast cell degranulation of histamine, prostaglandin D_2, and leukotrienes C_4 and D_4, leading to further coronary vasoconstriction. In these patients, high levels of asymmetric dimethylarginine, an endogenous inhibitor of nitric oxide synthase, have been reported. Increased avascularity and capillary ramifications on nailfold video capillaroscopy correlate with decreased coronary flow reserve and support a diffuse microvascular remodeling process. The common finding on autopsy of myocardial contraction-band necrosis (necrotic myocardial cells with dense eosinophilic bands) resulting from ischemia and reperfusion is likely related to intermittent intramyocardial coronary spasm or intramyocardial Raynaud phenomenon. Furthermore, almost all patients with evidence of intramyocardial CAD have peripheral Raynaud phenomenon. (2) Obstructive microvascular disease due endothelial proliferation, intimal hypertrophy, intimal smooth muscle cell migration, fibrinoid necrosis, fibroblasts stimulation and proliferation, fibrosis, and ultimately, vessel narrowing. In contrast, the prevalence of epicardial CAD in patients with systemic sclerosis is lower than microvascular CAD. Increased carotid artery and aortic stiffness is frequently associated with microvascular CAD and is indicative of a systemic microcirculatory disease.

Clinical Findings

A. Symptoms & Signs

Typical anginal chest pain is uncommon; when present, it is related more commonly to pericarditis, pulmonary hypertension, or commonly associated esophageal disease than to myocardial ischemia. In fact, typical acute coronary syndromes are uncommon in these patients (< 2%). Most patients, even with resting or stress-induced myocardial perfusion imaging defects or wall motion abnormalities, are asymptomatic. Although functional or structural microvascular CAD is the rule, severe vasospasm of the epicardial coronary arteries leading to transmural ischemia or MI has rarely been reported. Ischemic heart disease in these patients is most manifested as subacute or chronic diastolic and uncommonly systolic congestive heart failure. However, typical acute coronary syndromes due to epicardial CAD are still more common in these patients than in matched patients without systemic sclerosis. Acute ischemic heart failure and related sudden cardiac death are also more common in these patients than in matched controls with ischemic heart disease but no systemic sclerosis. In addition, the in-patient mortality in patients with STEMI or NSTEMI is twofold higher than matched controls without systemic sclerosis.

B. Diagnostic Studies

1. Electrocardiographic exercise testing—This method has limited sensitivity because the prevalence of epicardial CAD in patients with scleroderma is low.

2. Radionuclide studies—Resting or exercise-induced multisegmental perfusion abnormalities are common; they are frequently reversed or improved with nifedipine or dipyridamole, which suggests microvascular dysfunction or recurrent vasospastic episodes leading to myocardial ischemia or fibrosis since coronary angiography most commonly shows no significant epicardial coronary stenosis. Cold-induced reversible or partially reversible myocardial perfusion defects further support microvascular dysfunction or coronary vasospasm. On myocardial perfusion, most patients show fixed defects and some show reversible defects or both fixed and reversible defects (Figure 35–7A). Most patients have normal LV function at rest despite the high frequency of perfusion defects, but almost half have an abnormal LV response (a failure to increase the ejection fraction > 5% from baseline) during exercise radionuclide ventriculography.

3. Echocardiography—Due to the predominant involvement of the intramyocardial coronary arteries, echocardiographic findings typical of transmural ischemia or MI are uncommon. In controlled series in asymptomatic young patients using dipyridamole or adenosine Doppler TTE, dobutamine stress echocardiography, and multidetector CT, reduction in coronary flow reserve (< 2.5) and wall motion abnormalities, but no epicardial CAD on coronary angiography have been detected in 30–50% of patients as compared with less than 5% of matched controls. Reduction in coronary flow reserve is more common in the diffuse form of scleroderma and is related to the duration and severity of the disease. As a result of functional and, later, of obliterative microvascular disease, LV and RV diastolic and uncommonly systolic dysfunction can occur. Occasionally, a transmural MI due to epicardial coronary vasospasm can occur, and its echocardiographic diagnosis relies on the same findings as those of atherosclerotic disease. The cold pressor test with simultaneous echocardiography demonstrates transient wall motion abnormalities in patients with angiographically normal or mild epicardial CAD.

4. Cardiac magnetic resonance imaging, positron emission tomography, and non-contrast cardiac computed tomography—In controlled studies using cardiac MRI have demonstrated lower myocardial perfusion reserve indicative of microvascular dysfunction, late gadolinium enhancement indicative of focal myocardial fibrosis, and increased extracellular volume suggestive of diffuse fibrosis. These last two findings may result from microvascular disease-related ischemic or healed myocarditis. Similar reductions in myocardial flow reserve have been shown using PET. In these controlled series, reduction in myocardial flow reserve was an independent predictor of myocardial infarction, heart failure, or death. Finally, non-contrast computed tomography demonstrates 3–4 times higher presence and extent of coronary calcium deposition in systemic sclerosis patients as compared with matched controls.

5. Coronary angiography—This diagnostic study usually shows normal epicardial coronary arteries, a slow dye flow indicative of increased intramyocardial coronary resistance, and impaired coronary sinus blood flow indicative of abnormal coronary flow reserve (Figure 35–7B–E). In patients with typical or atypical angina, epicardial CAD, is more

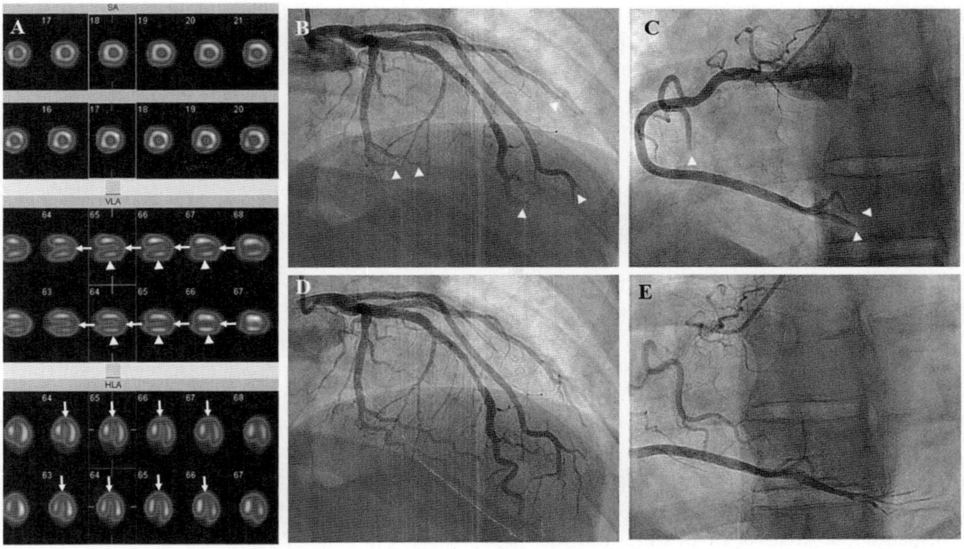

▲ **Figure 35–7.** Microvascular coronary artery disease in a 42-year-old woman with systemic sclerosis, angina pectoris, and active Raynaud phenomenon. **A:** This pharmacologic stress test with technetium-99-sestamibi SPECT myocardial perfusion imaging demonstrate when comparing stress (top images) with rest (bottom images), especially on the vertical and horizontal long-axis views, an anteroapical myocardial infarction with mild peri-infarct ischemia (arrows) and mild inferior ischemia (arrowheads) **B–E:** Therefore, patient underwent coronary angiography which demonstrated no epicardial coronary artery disease. However, microvascular coronary artery disease was evident by very sluggish epicardial antegrade coronary flow. Note the incomplete filling of the left coronary arteries (arrowheads in **B**) and right coronary artery (arrowheads in **C**) after four cardiac cycles. By the 6th cardiac cycle, the left (**D**) and right (**E**) epicardial coronary arteries were nearly fully visualized. Patient was treated with calcium channel blockers with significant improvement of symptoms.

commonly non-obstructive and is seen in less than 50% of patients. Finally, in patients with myocardial infarction, normal epicardial arteries are seen in more than 30% of patients.

Treatment

Nifedipine and nicardipine have demonstrated short- and long-term improvement in the frequency and severity of angina and perfusion defects. Nitrates and captopril have shown similar beneficial effects. If coronary vasculitis is suspected, oral mycophenolate or intravenous cyclophosphamide is used. Rituximab may be a salvage therapy that can be considered.

2. Myocarditis

General Considerations

Two types of systemic sclerosis-related myocardial disease have been described. The most common is due to functional or structural microvascular CAD causing recurrent intramyocardial ischemia leading to myocardial stunning, hibernation, necrosis, or fibrosis; the second and much less common is an acute inflammatory myocarditis. Patients with systemic sclerosis who have skeletal myopathy have twice the prevalence of myocardial disease, compared with patients without peripheral myopathy. Myocardial disease is also more common and severe in patients with diffuse cutaneous disease, anti-Scl70 antibodies, anticentromere antibodies, overlap syndrome with vasculitis, Raynaud phenomenon, and who are older than 60 years.

Clinically apparent myocarditis is rare. Postmortem series report a high prevalence of ischemic myocardial disease. Focal or diffuse myocardial fibrosis and contraction-band necrosis are common. Contraction-band necrosis typical of transient coronary occlusion and reperfusion is common but not pathognomonic. These pathologic findings differ from atherosclerotic myocardial disease by their lack of relation to coronary arteries and frequent involvement of the RV and subendocardium.

Clinical Findings

A. Symptoms & Signs

Focal or diffuse myocardial fibrotic disease may result in significant LV diastolic or systolic dysfunction, arrhythmias, and conduction disturbances. Patients with skeletal myopathy and those with myocarditis more commonly have clinical heart failure. Insidious symptoms are most common, and the physical findings of heart failure are similar to those of other conditions. Acute symptoms of heart failure and sudden death rarely occur.

B. Diagnostic Studies

Elevation of troponin I and NT-proBNP in asymptomatic or symptomatic patients may support intermittent myocardial ischemia, myocarditis, or fibrosis. Also, serum anti-heart and anti-intercalated disk autoantibodies, both specific serum markers of autoimmune myocarditis, are higher in systemic sclerosis patients with myocardial disease as compared to controls without systemic sclerosis and non-inflammatory myocardial disease.

1. Electrocardiography—A septal infarction pattern, ventricular arrhythmias, or conduction abnormalities seen in some patients correlate with septal or anteroseptal thallium perfusion abnormalities or areas of myocardial fibrosis on gadolinium-enhanced MRI in the presence of normal epicardial coronary arteries. This may represent septal fibrosis.

2. Echocardiography—LV systolic dysfunction is uncommon in asymptomatic patients, but when associated with heart failure, it portends an 80% mortality rate at 1 year. In contrast, a high prevalence (30–50%) of LV diastolic dysfunction using tissue Doppler echocardiography and especially using myocardial longitudinal, circumferential, and radial strain and strain rate is seen in patients with either diffuse or limited cutaneous disease, compared with less than 10% in controls. Type I LV diastolic dysfunction is twice more common than type II, and type III is rare. Similarly, a high prevalence (40%) of RV diastolic dysfunction independently of pulmonary hypertension has been reported. LV diastolic dysfunction correlates with high levels of soluble vascular cell adhesion molecule-1 and ESR as well as the duration and severity of Raynaud phenomenon. Also, RV dysfunction in patients with normal pulmonary artery pressure improves with nicardipine therapy. These data support functional microvascular CAD as the cause of LV and RV diastolic dysfunction. However, a decreased and heterogeneous integrated backscatter in the subendocardium by ultrasonic video densitometry in young, nonhypertensive patients support interstitial collagen deposition and fibrosis as another cause of myocardial dysfunction.

3. Radionuclide studies—Radionuclide angiography demonstrates abnormal resting ejection fraction in 15% of patients. Myocardial perfusion scanning is a sensitive method for diagnosis and follow-up of the ischemic myocardial disease and for assessing therapeutic responses.

4. Magnetic resonance imaging and angiography—This technique can accurately detect myocardial inflammation, myocardial infarction or fibrosis, and aneurysms of the coronary arteries. T2-weighted imaging with myocardial hyperintensity is indicative of active myocardial inflammation, and delayed gadolinium enhancement is indicative of increased interstitial collagen deposition and myocardial fibrosis.

5. Endomyocardial biopsy—This technique has been used occasionally to diagnose systemic sclerosis-related myocardial disease; however, the heterogenous and nonspecific pattern of involvement limits the sensitivity and specificity of this technique.

Treatment

Calcium channel blockers may abolish or decrease the frequency and severity of episodes of ischemia and thereby of myocardial fibrosis, but this hypothesis has not been longitudinally tested. Although oral mycophenolate and less commonly intravenous immunosuppressive therapy (especially cyclophosphamide) and/or methylprednisolone in acute inflammatory myocarditis may be beneficial, supportive data are limited. Prednisone 30 mg/day and above has been associated with acute systemic sclerosis renal crisis; thus, generally, if prednisone or methylprednisolone is used, the dose should be restricted to ≤ 25 mg/day. Recently, rituximab has been used for chronic systemic sclerosis conditions, including myocarditis, with some success in case reports. Otherwise, symptomatic LV systolic or diastolic dysfunction is treated with current standard therapy.

Prognosis

The presence of an S_3 gallop is indicative of LV systolic dysfunction and portends an increased risk of death. Patients with clinical heart failure have a 100% mortality rate at 7 years, with the highest number (80%) occurring during the first year after diagnosis.

3. Conduction Disturbances & Arrhythmias

General Considerations

Conduction defects occur in up to 20% of patients with scleroderma; the highest prevalence is seen in those patients with demonstrated myocarditis or myocardial perfusion defects. Fibrous replacement of the sinoatrial and AV nodes, bundle branches, and surrounding myocardium is seen on postmortem series of patients with conduction disturbances.

Clinical Findings

A. Symptoms & Signs

Arrhythmias are common and frequently associated with active myocarditis. Atrial or ventricular premature contractions, supraventricular tachycardias, and nonsustained ventricular tachycardia are also common. Ventricular and supraventricular arrhythmias are more common in patients with diffuse cutaneous disease than in those with the limited type. Palpitations occur in 50% of patients. Syncope can occur and is related to either high-degree AV block or ventricular arrhythmias; it may occasionally be the primary manifestation of systemic sclerosis. Syncope can also occur in patients with severe pulmonary hypertension. Forty percent to 60% of cardiac deaths in patients with scleroderma who have active myocarditis may be sudden and related to ventricular arrhythmias.

B. Diagnostic Studies

1. Electrocardiography—Most patients have a normal ECG, which is highly predictive of normal LV function. The presence of left or right bundle branch block or bifascicular block generally correlates with resting or exercise-induced LV systolic dysfunction. Also, LV potentials on signal-averaged ECG, complex atrial and ventricular arrhythmias, or conduction abnormalities on ECG are common and correlate with LV dysfunction or myocardial perfusion defects.

2. Electrophysiologic studies—These studies show a high prevalence of abnormal sinoatrial and AV nodes and His-Purkinje function and conduction. However, electrophysiologic studies are recommended only for patients with syncope of undefined origin in whom sustained ventricular tachycardia is suspected, or in survivors of sudden cardiac death.

▶ Treatment

A pacemaker is indicated for symptomatic high-grade conduction disturbances, and antiarrhythmic or implantable cardioverter-defibrillator therapy is appropriate for symptomatic ventricular arrhythmias.

▶ Prognosis

The presence on ambulatory ECG of frequent ventricular and supraventricular arrhythmias predicts a mortality risk two to six times higher than that of patients without arrhythmias. Because these arrhythmias are strong independent predictors of sudden cardiac death, 24-hour ambulatory ECG monitoring may be considered in patients with systemic sclerosis to identify patients at high risk for significant arrhythmias and sudden cardiac death. Cardiac conduction defects on the resting ECG also indicate a poor prognosis with a mortality rate of 50% by 6 years following diagnosis.

4. Pericarditis

▶ General Considerations

The pathogenesis of systemic sclerosis pericardial disease is unknown and is usually clinically silent. A low clinical prevalence of pericardial disease contrasts with that of postmortem and echocardiographic series (~50%). Fibrinous pericarditis, chronic fibrous pericarditis, pericardial adhesions, and pericardial effusion are the pathologic types described.

▶ Clinical Findings

A. Symptoms & Signs

Pericardial disease is rarely the initial manifestation of systemic sclerosis. Symptomatic pericardial disease occurs in less than 20% of patients. The most common clinical presentation is a chronic pericardial effusion with dyspnea, orthopnea, and edema; it is less frequently seen as an acute pericarditis with fever, pleuritic chest pain, dyspnea, and pericardial rub. Cardiac tamponade or pericardial constriction is rare. Symptomatic pericardial disease is two to four times more common in patients with the diffuse form of systemic sclerosis than in those with the limited cutaneous form of the disease. Asymptomatic pericardial effusions are common in patients with cor pulmonale and hypoalbuminemia.

B. Diagnostic Studies

1. Echocardiography—Echocardiography commonly shows asymptomatic small pericardial effusions and uncommonly pericardial thickening. It can also confirm clinically suspected cardiac tamponade.

2. Computed tomography and magnetic resonance imaging—These imaging studies are important diagnostic adjuncts to echocardiography. They aid in the assessment of pericardial thickening or calcification in patients with suspected chronic constriction.

3. Other tests—Pericardial fluid aspirates are usually exudative without autoantibodies, immune complexes, or complement depletion. Antiphospholipid antibodies may be associated with pericardial disease.

▶ Treatment

Symptomatic pericarditis or significant pericardial effusions can be treated acutely with NSAIDs. NSAIDS may be hazardous in systemic sclerosis due to gastroesophageal disease and hypertension. Therefore, colchicine has become standard for acute pericarditis in systemic sclerosis. Patients with chronic or recurrent pericarditis patients can be treated with mycophenolate, and in resistant cases with rituximab. The role of immunosuppressive therapy and especially pulse corticosteroid therapy is less defined in these patients, and as noted earlier, if prednisone ≥ 30 mg/day is used, the risk of systemic sclerosis renal crisis markedly increases. If tamponade is suspected, pericardiocentesis is usually successful. Corticosteroids alone are not effective in patients with large, chronic pericardial effusions.

▶ Prognosis

Patients with pericarditis and moderate pericardial effusion have a cumulative survival of only 25% after 6–7 years, with the highest mortality rates the first year after diagnosis. This high mortality rate is believed to be related to complicating or accompanying progressive renal failure in patients with chronic pericardial effusions and to sudden death in those with associated acute myopericarditis or myocarditis.

5. Valvular Heart Disease

The true prevalence of valvular heart disease in patients with systemic sclerosis is unknown but is most commonly non-specific and mild in severity. Clinically significant valvular heart disease is low (≤ 10%), but higher than in matched controls without systemic sclerosis. The overall incidence of valvular heart disease is also higher than matched controls. Postmortem series report a prevalence of up to 18%. Rarely, systemic embolism from noninfective mitral valve vegetations, similar to those of SLE, has been described. One echocardiographic series reported a 67% frequency of mitral regurgitation in systemic sclerosis patients, compared with only 15% in controls. Nonspecific thickening of the mitral or aortic valves without significant regurgitation also can be seen. In addition, a disproportionately high clinical and echocardiographic prevalence of mitral valve prolapse has been described in patients with either diffuse or limited scleroderma. Functional tricuspid regurgitation of mild to moderate degree is commonly due to pulmonary hypertension and cor pulmonale.

6. Pulmonary Hypertension

Resting (pulmonary artery pressure ≥ 40 mm Hg) and exercise-induced (pulmonary artery pressure ≥ 50 mm Hg) pulmonary hypertension using Doppler echocardiography or right heart catheterization is detected in 10–20% and 35–50% of patients, respectively. The frequency of pulmonary hypertension may be similarly related to left heart disease (~40%) and pulmonary arterial hypertension (~30–40%), but less often to lung disease/hypoxia (~20–30%). From the time of diagnosis of systemic sclerosis, the incidence of pulmonary hypertension over a median follow-up of 3 years is about 25%. Pulmonary arterial hypertension from inflammatory vasculopathy or pulmonary vasospasm is more often associated with the limited cutaneous type, Raynaud phenomenon, parameters of endothelial dysfunction, anticentromere antibodies, NT-proBNP and endothelin-1 levels, digital ulcers, pulmonary diffusion capacity less than 60%, and abnormal lung uptake of gallium and technetium-99m Sestamibi. Serum proteins such as collagen IV, endostatin, insulin-like growth factor binding protein, matrix metallopeptidase-2, neuropilin-1, N-T-proBNP, and RAGE (receptor for advanced glycation end-products) may discriminate with high accuracy patients with systemic sclerosis and pulmonary arterial hypertension. Abnormal pulmonary function tests, abnormal lung uptake of gallium and technetium-99m sestamibi, and radiographic abnormalities often precede cor pulmonale on echocardiography (Figure 35–8). In patients with pulmonary hypertension, a higher prevalence and severity of RV diastolic dysfunction independently of age and LV mass has been reported. An RV tissue Doppler E velocity of less than 11 cm/s

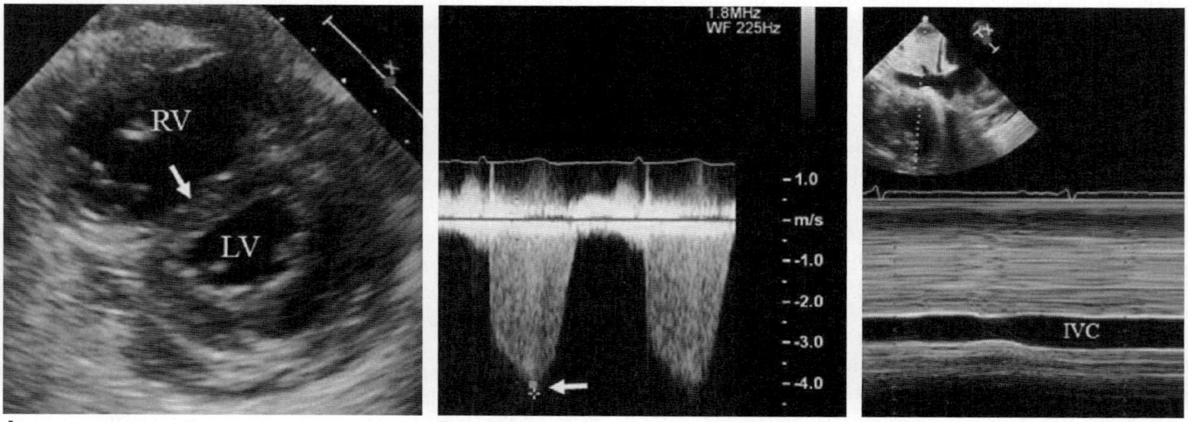

A B C

▲ Figure 35–8. A 48-year-old female with scleroderma and CREST syndrome and severe pulmonary hypertension, cor pulmonale, and right-sided heart failure due to severe interstitial lung disease. A: This parasternal transthoracic echocardiographic (TTE) short axis view demonstrates severe right ventricular (RV) dilatation and systolic dysfunction with associated abnormal interventricular septal motion of pressure and volume overload (flattening or inversion of the septum during late systole and early diastole and during mid to late diastole, respectively) (*arrow*). LV, left ventricle. **B:** Continuous wave Doppler shows a tricuspid regurgitation peak velocity of 4.1 m/s, equivalent to an RV systolic pressure of 67 mm Hg. **C:** Dilated inferior vena cava (IVC) with minimal diameter change with a sniff indicating a right atrial pressure of ≥ 15 mm Hg. Therefore, this patient's estimated pulmonary artery systolic pressure is 67 + 15 mm Hg = 82 mm Hg, which is consistent with severe pulmonary hypertension.

selects patients with pulmonary artery pressure more than 35 mm Hg. The sensitivity of Doppler echocardiography for detection of pulmonary hypertension as compared with right heart catheterization is moderate (about 60%) but highly specific (98%). Therefore, in patients with suspected pulmonary hypertension, the ultimate diagnosis and therapeutic decisions are best determined with right heart catheterization. Expert consensus for performing right heart catheterization include the combination of progressive dyspnea over 3 months, unexplained dyspnea, worsening of WHO dyspnea functional class; any finding on physical examination of elevated right heart pressures or right heart failure; pulmonary artery systolic pressure more than 45 mm Hg and RV dilation on echocardiography; and diffusion lung capacity for carbon monoxide less than 50%.

In patients with pulmonary arterial hypertension, endothelin receptor antagonists, prostacyclins, and/or phosphodiesterase inhibitors should be considered. Oxygen, calcium channel blockers, and angiotensin-converting enzyme inhibitors may provide additional long-term benefits in these patients, but randomized controlled data are limited. Selected patients with severe systemic sclerosis-related lung disease can undergo lung transplantation with higher morbidity and mortality to that of patients without systemic sclerosis. In patients with active inflammatory interstitial lung disease, mycophenolate is the drug of choice and in resistant cases rituximab has been used with some success. For progressive interstitial lung disease in systemic sclerosis, both tocilizumab and nintedanib have also been effective especially when used in conjunction with mycophenolate.

The severity of pulmonary hypertension, independently of its cause is a powerful independent predictor of death over 2 years follow-up. Patients with a pulmonary artery systolic pressure of ≥ 36 mm Hg have decreased survival rates of 81%, 63%, and 56% at 1, 2, and 3 years, respectively, from the diagnosis. Also, using a pulmonary artery systolic pressure of less than 30 mm Hg as reference, the hazard ratio for death is 1.67 for a pressure of 30–36 mm Hg, 2.37 for 36–40 mm Hg, 3.72 for 40–50 mm Hg, and 9.75 for a pressure more than 50 mm Hg.

Afifi N, Khalifa MMM, Ananny AA, Hassan HG. Cardiac calcium score in systemic sclerosis. *Clin Rheumatol.* 2022;41(1):105–114. [PMID: 34495426]

Colaci M, Schinocca C, Bosco YD, et al. Heart valve abnormalities in systemic sclerosis patients: a multicenter cohort study and review of the literature. *J Clin Rheumatol.* 2022;28(1):e95–e101. [PMID: 33252390]

Dumitru RB, Bissell LA, Erhayiem B, et al. Predictors of subclinical systemic sclerosis primary heart involvement characterized by microvasculopathy and myocardial fibrosis. *Rheumatology* (Oxford). 2021;60(6):2934–2945. [PMID: 34080001]

Glynn P, Hale S, Hussain T, Freed BH. Cardiovascular imaging for systemic sclerosis monitoring and management. *Front Cardiovasc Med.* 2022;9:846213. [PMID: 35433887]

Haque A, Kiely DG, Kovacs G, Thompson AAR, Condliffe R. Pulmonary hypertension phenotypes in patients with systemic sclerosis. *Eur Respir Rev.* 2021;30(161):210053. [PMID: 34407977]

Hinze AM, Perin J, Woods A, et al. Diastolic dysfunction in systemic sclerosis: risk factors and impact on mortality. *Arthritis Rheumatol.* 2022;74(5):849–859. [PMID: 34927390]

Kurmann RD, El-Am EA, Radwan YA, et al. Increased risk of valvular heart disease in systemic sclerosis: an underrecognized cardiac complication. *J Rheumatol.* 2021;48(7):1047–1052. [PMID: 33452164]

Ross L, Costello B, Brown Z, et al. Myocardial fibrosis and arrhythmic burden in systemic sclerosis. *Rheumatology* (Oxford). 2022:keac065. [PMID: 35136975]

Ross L, Paratz E, Baron M, Gerche AL, Nikpour M. Sudden cardiac death in systemic sclerosis: diagnostics to assess risk and inform management. *Diagnostics* (Basel). 2021;11(10):1781. [PMID: 34679479]

ANKYLOSING SPONDYLITIS

ESSENTIALS OF DIAGNOSIS

- Characteristic lumbar spine and sacroiliac arthritis.
- Positive HLA-B27 assay.
- Aortic root sclerosis and dilation, leaflet thickening, and subaortic bump on echocardiography.
- Aortic regurgitation.

General Considerations

Ankylosing spondylitis, also known as axial spondyloarthritis, Marie-Strümpell or Bekhterev disease, is an inflammatory disorder that affects predominantly the vertebral and sacroiliac joints. It manifests itself as chronic low back pain and limitation of back motion and chest expansion. Less frequently, it affects the peripheral joints and extra-articular organs such as the heart. The disease is estimated to affect 1 in 2000 of the general population, and predominantly white men less than 40 years old with a male-to-female ratio of 3–12:1. More than 90% of patients are positive for the histocompatibility antigen HLA-B27. Although the manifestations of the cardiovascular disease generally follow the arthritic syndrome by 10–20 years, they rarely precede it. The most important cardiovascular manifestations of the disease are aortitis, with or without aortic valvulitis or regurgitation; conduction disturbances; mitral regurgitation; myocardial dysfunction; and pericardial disease. The clinical prevalence of cardiovascular disease in ankylosing spondylitis varies widely. The rates are higher in patients with more than 20 years of disease duration, older than age 50, with peripheral articular involvement, with active disease, and in those with increased epicardial adipose tissue thickness.

1. Aortitis & Associated Valve Disease

General Considerations

The pathogenesis of aortitis is still undefined. Increased platelet-aggregating activity and platelet-derived growth factor are believed to be pathogenetic factors in the characteristic proliferative endarteritis of aortic root disease. The inflammatory process also is mediated by plasma cells and lymphocytes. It occurs in the intima, media, and adventitia of the proximal aortic wall and sinus of Valsalva and results in a marked fibroblastic reparative response, fibrous thickening, and calcification. This process extends proximally to the aortic annulus, valve cusps, and adjacent commissures. The consequent dilatation, thickening, and stiffness of the aortic root and annulus and the thickening or retraction of the aortic valve cusps cause aortic regurgitation generally of mild to moderate degree. Severe aortic regurgitation is rare. The mitral valve is frequently involved by downward extension of the aortic root fibrosis into the intervalvular fibrosa and base of the anterior mitral leaflet. This often results in localized fibrotic thickening at the base of the anterior mitral leaflet forming the characteristic "subaortic bump," which may cause anterior mitral leaflet retraction with decreased mobility and asymmetric or incomplete mitral leaflets' coaptation and mitral regurgitation.

Clinical Findings

The most common and characteristic manifestation of ankylosing spondylitis–associated heart disease is proximal aortitis, with or without aortic valvulitis or regurgitation. Associated mitral valve disease is also common. Aortitis and aortic regurgitation are generally mild to moderate, clinically silent, and chronic. In rare cases, severe aortic regurgitation from severe acute or chronic aortitis or valvulitis or complicating infective endocarditis occurs. Clinically silent aortic root or valve disease, with or without aortic regurgitation, can be present in one-third of patients before the joint disease manifests itself. Although it happens rarely, severe aortic regurgitation may present with mild or no articular disease.

A. Physical Examination

The most common and salient clinical findings in patients with ankylosing spondylitis will be those of the articular disease because cardiac disease, when present, is generally mild to moderate and asymptomatic.

B. Diagnostic Studies

1. Chest radiography—The appearance of the cardiac silhouette and great vessels is usually normal. If severe aortic root disease or aortic regurgitation is present, the ascending aorta may appear dilatated or elongated, and LV and atrial enlargement may be noted.

2. Color-flow Doppler echocardiography—By TEE, aortic root thickening, increased stiffness, and dilatation are seen in 60%, 60%, and 25% of patients, respectively. Aortic valve thickening detected in 40% of patients is manifested mainly as nodularities of the aortic cusps. Using speckle-tracking echocardiography, decreased transverse strain of the anterior and posterior walls of the proximal aorta may be an early manifestation of aortic root disease. Associated aortic regurgitation is common and ranges from 20% to 40% of moderate degree in up to 25% and of severe degree in less than 5% of patients. Mitral valve thickening seen in 30% of patients manifests predominantly as basal thickening of the anterior mitral leaflet, forming the characteristic "subaortic bump" (Figure 35–9).

Associated mitral regurgitation, seen in almost half of patients, is moderate in one-third of them. The described aortic root and valve abnormalities by TEE are less common and nonspecific appearing when using TTE.

3. Radionuclide ventriculography—This method can assess LV systolic or diastolic function and LV enlargement.

Treatment

A. Medical Therapy

1. Specific anti-inflammatory therapy—Although limited data are available, immunosuppressives and corticosteroids should be considered in acute aortitis and valvulitis associated with ankylosing spondylitis. Corticosteroids, methotrexate, sulfasalazine, tumor necrosis factor-α blockers, and IL-17 blockers have been used with some success. JAK inhibitors have recently been approved for ankylosing spondylitis but should be used cautiously in preexisting cardiovascular disease.

B. Surgical Therapy

Due to the absence of multiorgan disease and infrequent need of immunosuppressive therapy in these patients, their mortality rate during aortic valve replacement is probably similar to that of the general population. However, aortic valve replacement during active aortitis is associated with higher risk of prosthetic valve dehiscence.

2. Conduction Disturbances

Conduction disturbances occur in 30–35% of patients and are the second most common associated heart disease. Conduction disturbances result from the subaortic fibrotic process extending to the basilar septum, leading to dysfunction of the AV node, the proximal portion of the bundle of His, bundle branches, and fascicles. In fact, echocardiographic studies have demonstrated an association of conduction disturbances with aortic root thickening and subaortic bump. Although the prevalence of HLA-B27 is increased in patients with ankylosing spondylitis who have implanted pacemakers for heart block, it may be absent in these patients. Furthermore, because HLA-B27 may be present in 6% of normal patients, it cannot be implicated as a primary

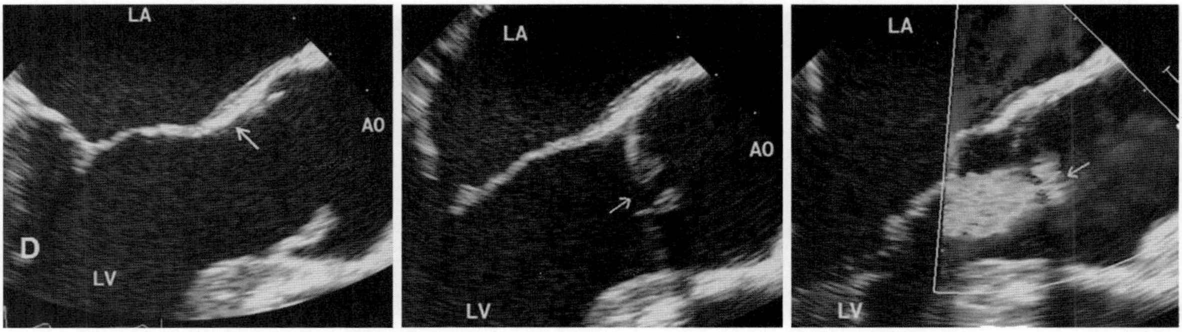

A B C

▲ **Figure 35–9. Aortitis and valvulitis in a 37-year-old man with ankylosing spondylitis. A.** This 2D-TEE long-axis view of the aortic root (Ao) and valve during systole demonstrates aortic root walls thickening and sclerosis, predominantly of the posterior wall, extending to the base of the anterior mitral leaflet creating the characteristic subaortic bump (*arrow*). Also, note the thickening, retraction, and decreased doming mobility of the aortic valve cusps, predominantly of the right coronary cusp. **B.** This 2D-TEE long-axis view during diastole shows thickening predominantly of the tip portions and retraction of the aortic cusps leading to an incomplete coaptation (*arrow*). Also note the decreased mobility of the basal and mid portions of the anterior mitral leaflet. **C.** This 2D-TEE long-axis view with color Doppler imaging shows moderate to severe aortic regurgitation (*arrow*). Associated mild mitral regurgitation was also present.

pathogenetic factor in ankylosing spondylitis–associated conduction disturbances.

Clinical Findings

The prevalence of conduction disturbances varies greatly but is at least 20%. AV blocks (first, second, and, rarely, third degree) are most frequent, followed by sinus node dysfunction (sinus arrhythmias, sinoatrial block, sinus arrest, and sick sinus syndrome) and bundle branch or fascicular block.

Patients with conduction disturbances are generally asymptomatic, and disturbances can be detected before clinically manifested in less than one-fifth of patients. The conduction disturbances can occasionally be transient during active inflammation, and therefore symptomatic patients can be treated with temporary pacing. The prevalence of aortic root disease and valve regurgitation is high in the presence of conduction disturbances, in contrast to the small number of cases of aortic regurgitation in patients without conduction disturbances. Occasionally, severe conduction disturbances associated with symptoms requiring cardiac pacing may precede the diagnosis of ankylosing spondylitis. Therefore, unrecognized ankylosing spondylitis should be considered in patients with unexplained conduction disturbances or aortic regurgitation.

A. Physical Examination

Severe bradyarrhythmias will be clinically detected if patients are symptomatic; otherwise, conduction disturbances are generally incidentally detected with ECG.

B. Diagnostic Studies

ECG, including 24-hour ambulatory and event monitoring, can detect the described conduction disturbances.

Treatment

A. Specific Anti-inflammatory Therapy

The role of anti-inflammatory therapy in patients with conduction disturbances is undefined, although both NSAIDS and corticosteroids have been used successfully. In patients with active disease a trial of high-dose prednisone to determine reversibility can be considered before proceeding with permanent pacing. If reversible, the patient should be placed on an anti-TNF biologic or IL-17 blocker to prevent future episodes.

B. Other Therapy

Permanent pacing has been successfully performed. The most common indications for pacing are complete heart block and sick sinus syndrome.

3. Myocardial Disease, Atherosclerosis, & Pericardial Disease

Although the frequency of myocardial disease in patients with ankylosing spondylitis is higher than in the general population and is associated with aortic root and valve disease, it is generally subclinical and therefore commonly incidentally detected. Primary myocardial disease is rare. Although its pathogenesis is unknown, it is caused by a diffuse increase in the myocardial interstitial connective tissue and reticulum fibers. Secondary myocardial disease is more common, is predominantly manifested as subclinical diastolic dysfunction, and related to underlying microvascular CAD or aortic stiffness leading to increased LV afterload and LV mass. Controlled Doppler and speckle-tracking echocardiography series in patients younger than 50 years old with no clinical heart disease have reported LV diastolic dysfunction in about one-third of patients, predominantly impaired relaxation. Diastolic dysfunction is unrelated to age, disease duration, or disease activity. Rarely, cardiac amyloidosis with diastolic heart failure has been reported. LV systolic dysfunction is uncommon. If significant LV systolic or diastolic dysfunction is present, third or fourth heart sounds and pulmonary rales may be present. Although in general no specific therapy for primary myocardial disease has been defined, immunosuppressive and/or high-dose corticosteroid therapy may be considered in those with primary myocarditis if acute, and methotrexate or sulfasalazine chronically. Since tumor necrosis factor-α blockers may exacerbate congestive heart failure, only patients with normal LV systolic function should be treated with these agents.

Patients with ankylosing spondylitis have a twofold increase in CAD, which is more commonly subclinical and in the form of microvascular CAD and coronary calcifications. These patients also have a higher prevalence of subclinical and clinical atherosclerosis as compared to matched controls and manifested as carotid intima-media thickening or plaques and increased carotid and aortic stiffness. Patients with anterior uveitis have higher risk for development of acute coronary syndromes.

Although the true prevalence of **pericardial disease** is unknown, it is rare in ankylosing spondylitis, and its pathogenesis is also undefined. It is generally asymptomatic and usually incidentally detected by echocardiography as pericardial thickening or small pericardial effusions. No specific therapy has been defined.

Prognosis

The overall prognosis of patients with ankylosing spondylitis is good and almost comparable to that of a general population. In the past, the presence of severe cardiovascular disease significantly decreased the survival of these patients. Currently, improved diagnostic and therapeutic technologies have allowed early diagnosis, appropriate follow-up, and proper timing of valve replacement, pacemaker implantation, and treatment of atherosclerosis in patients with cardiovascular disease. These factors have made the prognosis of ankylosing spondylitis with cardiovascular disease more benign.

Lai YF, Lin TY, Chien WC, et al. Uveitis as a risk factor for developing acute myocardial infarction in ankylosing spondylitis: a national population-based longitudinal cohort study. *Front Immunol.* 2022;12:811664. [PMID: 35087531]

Park HS, Laiz A, Vega JS, et al. Valve abnormalities, risk factors for heart valve disease and valve replacement surgery in spondyloarthritis. a systematic review of the Literature. *Front Cardiovasc Med.* 2021;8:719523. [PMID: 34631824]

Tański W, Gac P, Chachaj A, Sobieszczanska M, Poreba R, Szuba A. Selected clinical parameters and changes in cardiac morphology and function assessed by magnetic resonance imaging in patients with rheumatoid arthritis and ankylosing spondylitis without clinically apparent heart disease. *Clin Rheumatol.* 2021;40(11):4701–4711. [PMID: 34173901]

Tennenbaum J, Abisror N, Sellam J, et al. TNF inhibitors for the management of inflammatory heart disease in spondyloarthritis: French multicentre case-series and literature review. *Rheumatology* (Oxford). 2021;60(7):e247–e249. [PMID: 33502470]

POLYMYOSITIS/DERMATOMYOSITIS

ESSENTIALS OF DIAGNOSIS

- Muscle weakness, characteristic skin lesions.
- Myocarditis and arrhythmias or conduction disturbances.
- Pericarditis, coronary arteritis, and valve disease.

General Considerations

Polymyositis or dermatomyositis is an acquired, chronic, inflammatory myopathy that presents clinically as symmetric proximal muscle weakness of the extremities, trunk, and neck. Dermatomyositis differs from polymyositis by the presence of a rash on the face, neck, chest, and extremities, most commonly over the extensor surfaces, especially the dorsum of the hands and fingers. The incidence of polymyositis and dermatomyositis is estimated to be one to five new cases per million population per year in the United States. Overlap syndrome is the association of polymyositis/dermatomyositis with other connective tissue diseases, such as systemic sclerosis, SLE, and rheumatoid arthritis. Rarely, polymyositis or dermatomyositis can be associated with the aPL syndrome. Adults in the fourth to sixth decades are most affected. Both childhood polymyositis/dermatomyositis and that with malignancy are less common. Females, especially black females, are predominantly affected. A cumulative survival rate of 50–75% after 6–8 years has been reported. The major causes of death (in descending order) are malignancy, sepsis, and cardiovascular disease. Polymyositis or dermatomyositis portends a twofold increased risk for ischemic heart disease, heart failure, ischemic stroke, and cardiovascular mortality. Poor prognostic indicators of the disease include an age older than 45 years, cardiopulmonary disease, and cutaneous necrotic lesions.

Clinical Findings

Myocarditis, pericarditis, and functional or structural microvascular CAD are the most common cardiac manifestations of polymyositis and dermatomyositis. Conduction disorders and arrhythmias, epicardial atherosclerotic CAD, coronary arteritis, valve disease, and pulmonary hypertension are uncommon. Although clinically manifested heart disease may occur in less than 25% of patients, it accounts for at least 10% of mortality. Pericarditis, coronary vasculitis, pulmonary hypertension with cor pulmonale, mitral valve prolapse, and hyperkinetic heart syndrome have also been reported. Clinically overt heart disease is less common than that found in postmortem series. Clinical heart disease is more common in polymyositis and overlap syndrome than in dermatomyositis or in malignant and childhood polymyositis/dermatomyositis. The presence of heart disease may not correlate with age or disease activity, severity, or duration and does not differ between men and women.

1. Myocarditis

Myocarditis is characterized at postmortem by diffuse interstitial and perivascular lymphocytic infiltration, contraction-band necrosis, and fibrosis. In postmortem series, myocarditis can be seen in half the patients, manifested equally as active myocarditis or focal myocardial fibrosis. Myocarditis more commonly (25–40%) lead to subclinical or clinical LV diastolic dysfunction and less often to cardiomyopathy with LV systolic dysfunction and arrhythmias or conduction disturbances (in about 10% of cases). Acute myocarditis as the principal manifestation of polymyositis has been reported as a mimicker of acute MI, fatal cardiac arrhythmias, or heart failure. A high correlation has been demonstrated between myocarditis and active myositis. About half of patients with peripheral myositis, as indicated by uptake of technetium-99m pyrophosphate, also have myocardial uptake. Increased myocardial uptake frequently associated with depressed ejection fraction and abnormal wall motion is indicative of active myocardial inflammation. Myocarditis may manifest itself clinically as congestive heart failure or as dilated cardiomyopathy. However, series using cardiac MRI in asymptomatic patients have shown late gadolinium-enhanced patchy epicardial and intramyocardial areas (predominantly in the septum and lateral walls) typical of postinflammatory myocardial fibrosis in almost half of patients. These findings suggest a high prevalence of subclinical myocarditis. Myocarditis and cardiomyopathy are associated with anti-mitochondrial autoantibodies, elevation of CPK and CRP, and pulmonary hypertension. With 2D and 3D Doppler and speckle-tracking echocardiography, subclinical LV and RV diastolic dysfunction, predominantly impaired relaxation, and reduction in LV and RV longitudinal systolic strain, ranges from 12% to 76%, but decreased ejection fraction is uncommon. Patients with polymyositis/dermatomyositis have higher incidence of heart failure and higher mortality than matched controls without polymyositis/dermatomyositis.

2. Pericarditis

Acute uncomplicated pericarditis with small-to-moderate pericardial effusions has been described; acute pericarditis with cardiac tamponade and chronic constrictive pericarditis are rare. Pericarditis affects less than 20% of adults and is more frequent in patients with the overlap syndrome and in children. Echocardiography, however, shows a prevalence of pericardial effusion, usually small, in up to 25% of adults and up to 50% of children. Only rarely does pericarditis form part of the initial clinical presentation of polymyositis/dermatomyositis.

3. Coronary Artery Disease

Epicardial CAD with angina has been reported in 20–25% of patients. Microvascular disease may be as prevalent, but coronary arteritis is rare. Postmortem series demonstrated the presence of coronary arteritis in 30% of patients, manifested as active vasculitis with intimal proliferation or as medial necrosis with calcification.

4. Arrhythmias & Conduction Disturbances

Right bundle branch block, left anterior fascicular block, bifascicular block, nonspecific intraventricular conduction block, left bundle branch block, and AV block can occur. Occasionally, conduction disturbances can progress to more severe forms, despite remission of the disease, and permanent pacing is required.

The prevalence of arrhythmias varies. The most common arrhythmias are premature ventricular and atrial beats. Supraventricular tachyarrhythmias and ventricular tachycardia are rare. Patients with supraventricular and ventricular arrhythmias have higher in-patient and out-patient mortality than those without them. Ventricular arrhythmias are associated with the presence of anti-mitochondrial autoantibodies. Sudden cardiac death may occur in a small number of patients. Active myocarditis or residual myocardial degeneration and fibrosis extending to the sinoatrial, AV nodal, and bundle branches explain the arrhythmias and conduction abnormalities.

5. Valvular Heart Disease

Except for a higher prevalence of mitral valve prolapse, no other specific valve disease has been reported. The cause of mitral prolapse has not been determined. Noninfective valve vegetations and severe valvulitis with severe regurgitation similar to those seen in SLE have been rarely reported.

6. Pulmonary Hypertension, Cor Pulmonale, & Hyperkinetic Heart Syndrome

Both pulmonary hypertension secondary to interstitial lung disease and primary pulmonary vasculopathy leading to cor pulmonale have been found. Pulmonary arterial hypertension is highly associated with interstitial lung disease, congestive heart failure, and valvular heart disease. In hyperkinetic heart syndrome, abnormally increased LV performance has been demonstrated in up to one-third of patients with polymyositis. The cause of this asymptomatic abnormality is unknown, but can be associated with troponin I elevation, and evidence of active myocarditis on gadolinium-contrast cardiac MRI.

Treatment & Prognosis

The consideration of immunosuppressive and corticosteroid therapy in patients with severely active disease complicated by myocarditis, pericarditis, or conduction disturbances is similar to that previously described for other connective tissue diseases. Usually high-dose corticosteroids are used acutely, and if the patient does not improve, intravenous immunoglobulin, cyclophosphamide, plasmapheresis, or rituximab can be considered. For chronic therapy, some combination of oral methotrexate, azathioprine, mycophenolate, or leflunomide, intravenous immunoglobulin, or rituximab can be considered. In patients with pulmonary arterial hypertension, endothelin receptor antagonists, prostacyclins, and/or phosphodiesterase inhibitors have been used.

Huang Y, Liu H, Wu C, et al. Ventricular arrhythmia predicts poor outcome in polymyositis/dermatomyositis with myocardial involvement. *Rheumatology* (Oxford). 2021;60(8):3809–3816. [PMID: 33369674]

Lin CY, Chen HA, Hsu TC, Wu CH, Su YJ, Hsu CY. Time-dependent analysis of risk of new-onset heart failure among patients with polymyositis and dermatomyositis. *Arthritis Rheumatol.* 2022;74(1):140–149. [PMID: 34180158]

Naaraayan A, Meredith A, Nimkar A, Arora G, Bharati R, Acharya P. Arrhythmia prevalence among patients with polymyositis-dermatomyositis in the United States: an observational study. *Heart Rhythm.* 2021;18(9):1516–1523. [PMID: 34048962]

Sabbagh SE, Fernandez IP, Dominguez MC, et al. Anti-mitochondrial autoantibodies are associated with cardiomyopathy, dysphagia, and features of more severe disease in adult-onset myositis. *Clin Rheumatol.* 2021;40(10):4095–4100. [PMID: 33851273]

Xiong A, Hu Z, Xhou S, et al. Cardiovascular events in adult polymyositis and dermatomyositis: a meta-analysis of observational studies. *Rheumatology* (Oxford). 2021 Nov 16:keab851. doi: 10.1093/rheumatology/keab851. [PMID: 34791063]

Zhang L, Zhu H, Yang P, et al. Myocardial involvement in idiopathic inflammatory myopathies: a multi-center cross-sectional study in the CRDC-MYO Registry. *Clin Rheumatol.* 2021;40(11):4597–4608. [PMID: 34184155]

MIXED CONNECTIVE TISSUE DISEASE

ESSENTIALS OF DIAGNOSIS

- Raynaud phenomenon, sclerodactyly.
- Myopathy.
- Pericarditis, pulmonary hypertension.
- High ribonucleoprotein antibody titers.

General Considerations

Patients with mixed connective tissue disease are those with clinical findings of SLE, rheumatoid arthritis, scleroderma, and polymyositis. Characteristically, these patients have high titers of antibodies to nuclear ribonucleoprotein (RNP) and speckled antinuclear antibodies. Rheumatoid agglutinins also occur in more than half of patients. The disease occurs at all ages, affecting predominantly females (80%). Its prevalence is similar to that of systemic sclerosis; it is more common than polymyositis, but less common than SLE. This disease has no racial or ethnic predominance. Primary cardiac involvement in mixed connective tissue disease may be less common than in other connective tissue diseases.

Clinical Findings

A. Symptoms & Signs

Pericardial disease manifested as pericarditis, small pericardial effusions, or pericardial thickening is the most common. Pericarditis is more common in children, affecting one-third to almost half of patients. In rare cases, pericarditis complicated with cardiac tamponade can be the initial presentation of the disease (Figure 35–10). Mitral valve prolapse has also been reported in this disease, with an unusually high prevalence (30%). Verrucous thickening of the mitral valve and regurgitation have been rarely detected and are indistinguishable from those of SLE. Infrequently, supraventricular, or ventricular arrhythmias and conduction disturbances have been reported. Functional or microvascular disease is the most common type of associated CAD. Acute coronary syndromes may also result from coronary vasospasm, in situ thrombosis, coronary embolism from a valve vegetation, and rarely from coronary aneurysmal disease or arteritis. Myocarditis is characterized on histology by interstitial lymphocytic infiltrates and variable degrees of myocardial fibers necrosis and, when acute, can be reversible with corticosteroids and intravenous pulse cyclophosphamide. On echocardiography, the spectrum of the disease ranges from diastolic dysfunction to global or regional LV systolic dysfunction and heart failure. Acute myocarditis may mimic an MI and can be complicated by congestive heart failure and death. Because of the high frequency of pulmonary disease (80%) in patients with mixed connective tissue disease, pulmonary hypertension associated with pulmonary fibrosis or proliferative pulmonary vasculopathy of the small and medium-sized pulmonary arteries can occur, especially in patients with features of systemic sclerosis. Pulmonary thromboembolism is rare.

The clinical manifestations of primary cardiac disease, pulmonary hypertension, and cor pulmonale associated with mixed connective tissue disease do not differ from the other connective tissue diseases.

B. Diagnostic Studies

The methods used to diagnose cardiac disease associated with mixed connective tissue disease are the same used for other connective tissue diseases.

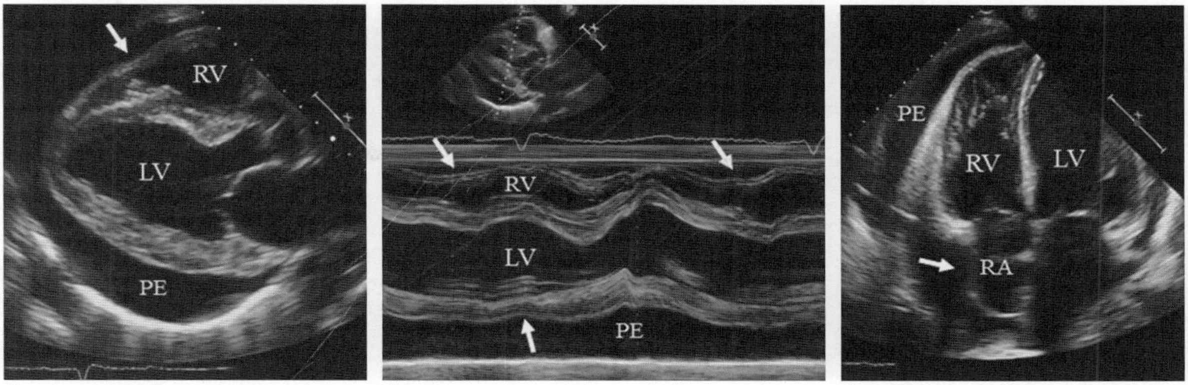

A B C

▲ **Figure 35–10. A 70-year-old male with active mixed connective tissue disease with predominant features of diffuse scleroderma with a large pericardial effusion complicated with clinical and echocardiographic evidence of cardiac tamponade. A:** This parasternal long axis transthoracic echocardiographic view demonstrates a large pericardial effusion (PE) predominantly posteriorly located and associated with right ventricular (RV) diastolic compression (*arrow*). **B:** This two-dimensional guided M-mode image from the parasternal long-axis view demonstrates significant RV diastolic compression (*upper arrows*) and some degree of posterior left ventricular (LV) diastolic compression (*lower arrow*). **C:** This apical four-chamber transthoracic echocardiographic view demonstrates right atrial (RA) diastolic collapse (*arrow*). Therefore, the patient underwent urgent pericardiocentesis, and after all cultures returned negative, the patient was successfully treated with pulse corticosteroids and cyclophosphamide.

Treatment

Although limited data are available, the treatment of heart disease associated with active mixed connective tissue disease is similar to that described for other connective tissue diseases, and in particular, the immunosuppression closely parallels the therapy of heart and systemic disease in SLE, although therapy for vasospasm (Prinzmetal-type angina) is used more frequently. Endothelin receptor antagonists, prostacyclins, phosphodiesterase inhibitors, and less often calcium channel blockers including levosimendan, have demonstrated both acute and sustained reduction in pulmonary vascular resistance with improvement in RV systolic function and hemodynamics in patients with pulmonary arterial hypertension with or without clinical right heart failure.

Prognosis

The overall mortality rate of patients with mixed connective tissue disease is 13% at 6–12 years. The prognostic implications of cardiac disease associated with mixed connective tissue disease are unknown.

Qu C, Feng W, Zhao Q, et al. Effect of levosimendan on acute decompensated right heart failure in patients with connective tissue disease-associated pulmonary arterial hypertension. *Front Med* (Lausanne) 2022;9:778620. [PMID: 35308558]

Tan S, Moir S, Seneviratne S. Connective tissue disease associated myocarditis on computed tomography coronary angiogram. *Heart Lung Circ.* 2021;30(12):e121–e122. [PMID: 34332890]

Ungprasert P, Wannarong T, Panichsillapakit T, et al. Cardiac involvement in mixed connective tissue disease: a systematic review. *Int J Cardiol.* 2014;171(3):326–330. [PMID: 24433611]

36 The Athlete & the Heart

Antonio B. Fernandez, MD
Stephanie Saucier, MD

ESSENTIALS OF DIAGNOSIS

- The patient has an extensive history of exercise training.
- There may be profound sinus bradycardia, sinus arrhythmias, or atrioventricular conduction delays at rest that disappear with exertion.
- The athlete's heart may demonstrate four-chamber enlargement and mild left ventricular hypertrophy, but normal diastolic function and B-natriuretic peptide levels. The diastolic wall-to-volume ratio should be < 0.15 mm/m^2/mL by magnetic resonance imaging.
- Most morphologic changes reverse with detraining.

General Considerations

The salutary physiologic effects of exercise training on the cardiovascular system have been studied extensively, but intense exercise training can produce cardiac adaptations that mimic pathological conditions. Consequently, clinicians should be aware of the normal cardiac structural and functional responses to exercise training to distinguish these changes from clinical diseases that could also affect athletes.

A. Physiology of Exercise Training

The "athlete's heart" refers to the normal structural and physiologic cardiac adaptations to exercise training. Clinical characteristics of the athlete's heart include resting sinus bradycardia (occasionally profound), sinus arrhythmia, atrioventricular (AV) conduction delays, systolic flow murmurs, four-chamber enlargement, and an increase in cardiac mass, but usually normal or augmented ventricular systolic function.

The magnitude of these cardiac changes depends on a variety of factors including the duration and intensity of the exercise training, the body size of the athlete, the sport, and the physiologic demands of the exercise used to train for that sport. Sports can be roughly classified according to the type and intensity of the exercise performed and the degree of static and dynamic exercise required, but such classifications are innately flawed because they do not consider exercises used in training. Dynamic (isotonic) exercise and sports primarily involve changes in muscle length and joint movement with rhythmic contractions and small intramuscular force. Static (isometric) exercise and sports mainly involve large intramuscular force with little or no change in muscle length or joint movement. Most sports require elements of both.

The acute cardiovascular response to dynamic (aerobic) exercise includes a decrease in peripheral vascular resistance and increases in heart rate, stroke volume, cardiac output, systolic blood pressure, the arteriovenous oxygen difference, and oxygen consumption. Endurance exercise training increases maximal exercise capacity as measured by maximal oxygen uptake. This increase in exercise capacity is produced by increases in the arteriovenous oxygen difference and cardiac output due to increased stroke volume.

Endurance (aerobic) sports, such as long-distance running, and their required training produce the greatest reductions in heart rate and the largest increases in maximum oxygen consumption, cardiac output, stroke volume, and cardiac chamber dimensions. Endurance exercise predominantly produces a volume load on the left and right ventricles. Static or strength sports, such as weightlifting, in contrast, produce only small increases in oxygen consumption and minimal changes in cavity size, but may be associated with mild to modest increases in wall thickness, some of which may be due to increased body mass in such athletes. These changes in wall thickness with little change in chamber dimensions mimic the changes produced by pressure load.

B. Chamber Morphologic Adaptations to Endurance Training

The morphologic adaptations to endurance training have been characterized by echocardiography and

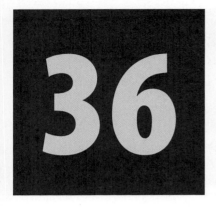

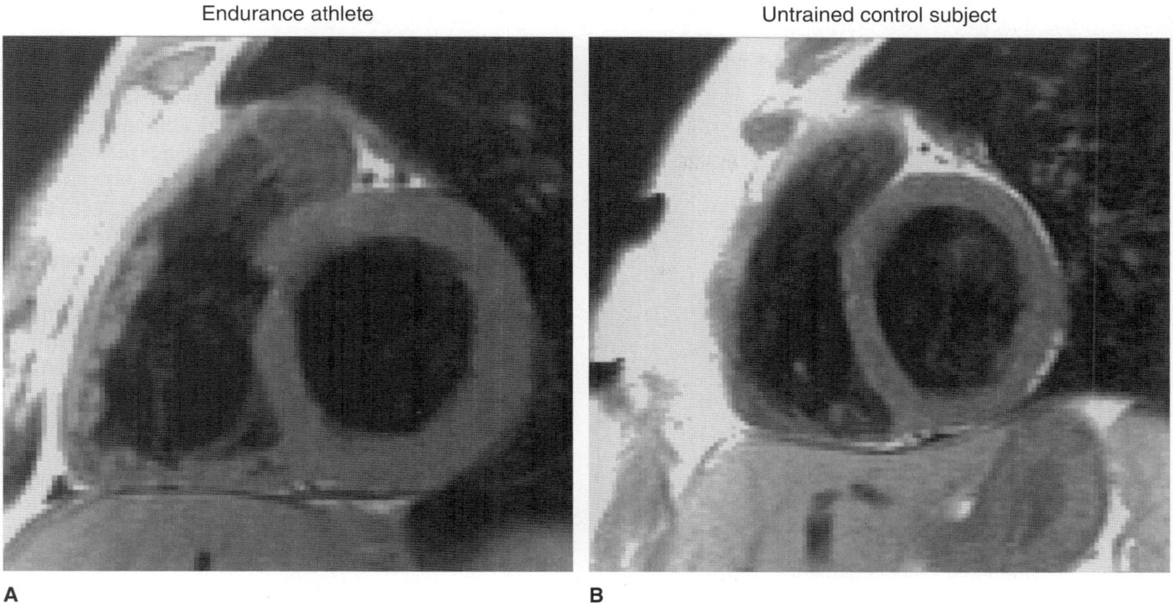

▲ **Figure 36–1.** End-diastolic, T1-weighted, short axis slice from an endurance athlete (**A**) and an untrained control subject (**B**). Compared with the heart of the control subject, the endurance athlete's heart is characterized by an enlarged volume and a greater myocardial mass of both ventricles, while the proportions of the left and right heart are the same as in the untrained control subject. (Reproduced with permission from Scharhag J, et al. *J Am Coll Cardiol.* 2002;40:1856. Copyright © American College of Cardiology Foundation.)

magnetic resonance imaging. Cardiac remodeling occurs in approximately one-half of trained athletes. It consists of increases in left and right ventricular and left atrial cavity dimensions and volumes almost always associated with normal systolic and diastolic function (Figure 36–1). Few studies have examined right atrial size, but this may also be increased.

There can be an overlap between the athlete's heart and mild forms of cardiac disease such as hypertrophic cardiomyopathy (HCM; Figure 36–2). The morphologic features of the athlete's heart are reversible with cessation of training in most individuals. Therefore, cessation of exercise can help distinguish these two conditions. Many athletes resist the idea of detraining, however, so other approaches are often required. In addition, the effect of long-term, high-intensity endurance exercise on the increased left atrial size can persist in some athletes after exercise cessation, and it is thought to increase the long-term risk of atrial arrhythmias.

C. Sudden Cardiac Death in Athletes

Clinicians require knowledge of the athlete's heart primarily because vigorous exertion increases the risk of sudden cardiac death (SCD) during exercise in individuals with known or occult heart disease. Consequently, clinicians need to know what cardiac findings in athletes are normal and how to advise individuals with diagnosed cardiac disease concerning exercise.

The frequency of SCD in young athletes is not clearly defined, although the largest registry of such events estimates a rate in the United States of only 66 deaths per year. Other estimates have ranged from 1 in 23,000 to 1 in 300,000 deaths in athletes per year. This variance is likely attributable to collection bias, incomplete identification of cases, and an imprecise denominator. A study of SCD in a defined population of American collegiate athletes suggested an incidence of SCD as high as 1 in 43,000 athletes. Ultimately, a large-scale case registry will be needed to better understand the prevalence, causes, and risk factors for sudden death in the young in the United States.

The most common cause of SCD in athletes younger than 35 years of age in the United States is HCM, accounting for up to one-third of sport-related deaths. Other frequent causes include congenital coronary artery anomalies, myocarditis, and aortic rupture, and less commonly, arrhythmogenic right ventricular cardiomyopathy, coronary artery disease, and conduction system abnormalities. In contrast, the most common cause of exertion-related SCD in the Veneto region of Italy is arrhythmogenic right ventricular cardiomyopathy, either because mandatory Italian screening has detected and eliminated athletes with HCM

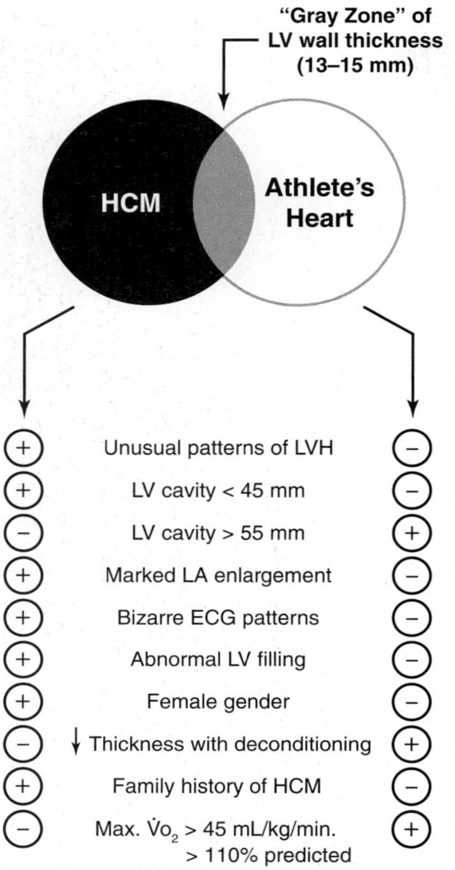

▲ **Figure 36–2.** Clinical criteria used to distinguish non-obstructive hypertrophic cardiomyopathy (HCM) from athlete's heart when maximal left ventricular (LV) wall thickness is within shaded gray area of overlap, consistent with both diagnoses. ECG, electrocardiogram; LA, left atrium; LVH, left ventricular hypertrophy. (Reproduced with permission from Maron BJ, et al. Cardiac disease in young trained athletes. Insights into methods for distinguishing athlete's heart from structural heart disease, with particular emphasis on hypertrophic cardiomyopathy. *Circulation*. 1995;91(5):1596–1601.)

or because of population differences in the prevalence of disease. In contrast to young athletes, SCD in athletes older than 35 years is most frequently due to occult coronary artery disease (CAD), and multiple studies have documented an increase in acute myocardial infarction (MI) and SCD among older adults during vigorous exertion.

Maron BJ, Haas TS, Murphy CJ, Ahluwalia A, Ramos SR. Incidence and causes of sudden death in U.S. College athletes. *J Am Coll Cardiol*. 2014;63:1636–1643. [PMID: 24583295]

Clinical Findings

A. Medical History & Physical Examination

As with all of medicine, the most important element of evaluating athletes and their clinical findings is the medical history, and in the medical history, the most important element is what prompted the athlete to obtain medical evaluation. Abnormalities found on screening examinations in an asymptomatic athlete have far less import than abnormalities found during the evaluation of a symptomatic individual. In our clinical experience, most clinical abnormalities found during screening ultimately turn out to be normal variants of the athlete's heart syndrome. Consequently, dividing athletes into those with and without symptoms is an important initial approach to their evaluation.

The other key elements of the history are the athlete's exercise training history and his or her exercise performance. Marked changes in cardiac dimensions require considerable amounts of exercise training so that cardiac findings in an athlete with a short or low-level training history are of more concern than similar findings in an athlete with high volumes of training. It is also extremely useful to be able to assess the athlete's level of performance. Excellent endurance exercise performance requires a large cardiac stoke volume, so that excellent exercise capacity is reassuring but does not absolutely exclude important disease. Family history of cardiac disease or unexpected or unexplained sudden death (including drowning, unexplained car accidents, or sudden infant death syndrome) is also useful in evaluating young athletes since most conditions causing SCD during exercise in this group are congenital or inherited.

The evaluation of both symptomatic and asymptomatic athletes should include a thorough physical examination. Vital signs are usually notable for training bradycardia with a resting heart rate as low as 30 bpm in highly trained aerobic athletes. Asymptomatic adolescent athletes with heart rates in this range can participate without further evaluation. Athletes may also have an S_3 and S_4 gallop. Athletes frequently have classical flow murmurs related to their slower heart rates and concomitant increased stroke volume. These functional murmurs typically are systolic and less than IV/VI in intensity. They are typically present supine because of enhanced venous return in this position and absent with the athlete upright; they have no diastolic component and are associated with a normal physiologic split of the second heart sound. Because HCM is the most frequent cause of SCD in young athletes, auscultation during the Valsalva maneuver or after arising from the squatting position, either of which should decrease cardiac dimensions and increase the murmur of HCM, is useful.

Syncope is a common problem among athletes and a frequent reason for referral to a cardiologist. Syncopal events are significant if judged to be not neurocardiogenic (vasovagal) and if they occur during exercise. Post-exertional syncope is a common phenomenon in athletes. It is usually benign and does not require further workup. Under normal circumstances, exercise increases cardiac output and decreases peripheral vascular resistance due to vasodilation. Syncope after exercise can occur because the increases in cardiac output and heart rate decrease more rapidly than does the peripheral vasodilation. The net effect when the individual stops exercising is an increase in vasodilation without the compensatory increase in heart rate and cardiac output, thus explaining post-exertional syncope. In contrast, syncope during exercise usually suggests a cardiac origin, such as anomalous coronary artery anatomy or cardiac arrhythmias.

The American Heart Association (AHA) position on screening athletes before competition recommends a 12-element history and physical examination. The historical elements are important, but young athletes often respond positively to many of these queries, again highlighting the importance of separating the evaluation of athletes with abnormalities found on screening from those presenting with symptoms.

B. Diagnostic Studies

1. Electrocardiogram—Many clinical and electrocardiographic (ECG) findings of concern in the general population are normal for athletes. The accuracy of the ECG interpretation is particularly difficult in young athletes due to ECG evolutionary changes that are related to age. Furthermore, there are inconsistencies in the definitions of ECG abnormalities and definite criteria for the diagnosis of several diseases. While the routine use of ECG for preparticipation screening remains controversial in young adults, its use remains a cornerstone of any cardiac evaluation in athletes with cardiac complaints. It is recommended as part of a routine evaluation for all master athletes more than 40 years of age since it occasionally identifies a prior MI. It is also prudent to emphasize that patients with symptoms or an abnormal cardiac examination require further evaluation even if the ECG is normal.

Sinus bradycardia as low as 30 bpm, sinus arrhythmia, prolonged PR interval up to 300 ms, sinoatrial block, junction rhythms, and Wenckebach phenomenon are common in athletes due to a high resting parasympathetic tone and should not prompt further workup if the athlete is asymptomatic, has good exercise capacity, and the abnormalities disappear during exercise. Approximately 80% of athletes exhibit a resting heart rate between 45 and 60 bpm, but only 5% show a heart rate less than 40 bpm. Resting pulse less than 35 bpm is rare and usually only seen in endurance athletes. Mobitz type 2 AV block usually denotes cardiac conduction disease but cannot be differentiated from Mobitz type 1 when conduction is 2:1. Two-to-one AV block in an asymptomatic athlete should be considered type 1 or Wenckebach until proven otherwise. Third-degree AV block at rest is extremely rare in athletes but can be observed by prolonged monitoring during sleep. Any cardiac conduction abnormalities should raise concern if the subject has symptoms, if the block persists or develops during exercise, or if the heart rate does not increase appropriately with exertion. QRS axis varies with age, but in athletes, mild right or left axis deviations should not trigger further evaluation unless there is history of pulmonary disease or systemic hypertension. An acceptable rage is between −30 and +115 degrees.

Incomplete right bundle branch block is extremely common in athletes. In contrast, complete block of either bundle, even in asymptomatic athletes, should prompt further investigation. Increased QRS amplitude is present in up to 80% of the athletes, but if the increased voltage is not accompanied by axis changes, repolarization changes, atrial abnormalities, increased QRS width, or a family history of HCM, it does not warrant further evaluation.

Manifest preexcitation (delta waves) is sometimes found on 12-lead surface ECGs of athletes, but it has been associated with only a small fraction (< 1%) of the cardiovascular sudden deaths among young competitive athletes in a U.S. registry. The exact number, however, remains unclear due to possible unrecognized preexcitation in unscreened athletes. Most individuals with Wolff-Parkinson-White syndrome demonstrate normal cardiac anatomy. Nonetheless, athletes with preexcitation should undergo standard echocardiography to exclude concomitant HCM or Ebstein anomaly. There is no clear consensus regarding the asymptomatic athlete with an ECG that demonstrates preexcitation. There is concern regarding the increased risk of SCD, most notably among athletes with accessory pathways having short refractory periods that allow very rapid ventricular rates during atrial fibrillation. Therefore, athletes with short refractory period bypass tracts capable of antegrade conduction and a history of atrial fibrillation should undergo an ablation of the accessory pathway before participating in competitive sports (Class I; Level of Evidence B). The Heart Rhythm Society and the Pediatric and Congenital Electrophysiology Society recommend that people age less than 21 years undergo initial stress testing to determine whether there is sudden and complete loss of preexcitation during exercise, which would denote low risk because of an accessory pathway with a long refractory period. If a person cannot be determined to be at low risk by stress testing, then an invasive electrophysiologic study is recommended, with ablation if the bypass tract has a high risk for SCD because of an effective refractory period less than 250 ms (Class IIa; Level of Evidence B). Small q waves may be present in athletes. The ECG in patients with HCM may also show q waves, but these "septal q's" are often seen in the inferior and/or lateral leads and suggest HCM if they are more than 3 mm in depth and/or more than 40 ms duration in at least two leads. Athletes with pathologic Q waves should be referred for further evaluation to exclude HCM (Table 36–1).

Early repolarization in V_3–V_6 with an elevated J point and peaked upright T waves is common in athletes and especially in male endurance athletes of African/Afro-Caribbean descent. The repolarization pattern may also include a domed ST segment followed by a biphasic or inverted T wave. These benign repolarization changes must

Table 36–1. Electrocardiogram Abnormalities That Require Further Evaluation

LBBB RBBB IVCD	Any QRS >120 ms	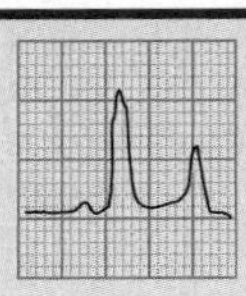
QRS axis deviation	More leftward than −30° More rightward than 115°	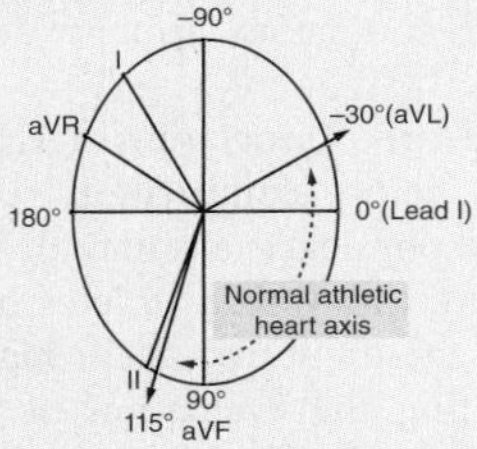
QTc interval	> 470 ms in males > 480 ms in females < 340 ms in any athlete	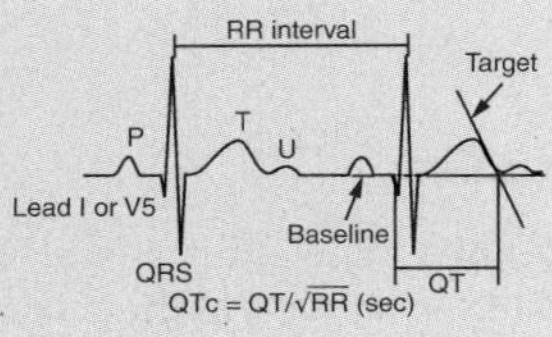
Brugada pattern	Presence of Type 1 pattern: coved ST segment in V1 and V2 gradually descending into inverted T wave	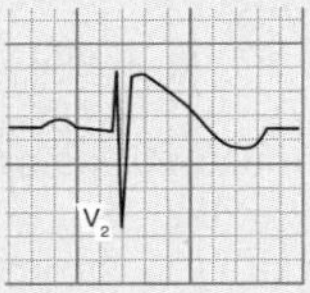
Pre-Excitation	Delta wave and PR interval < 120 ms	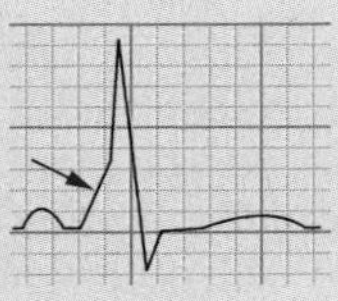
Ventricular extrasystoles, heart block, and supraventricular arrhythmia	Atrial fibrillation/flutter, supraventricular tachycardia, complete heart block or ≥ 2 PVCs in one 12-lead ECG	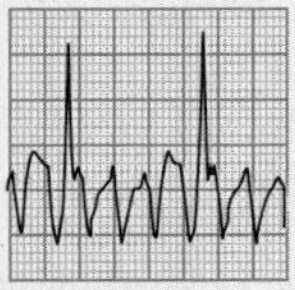

ECG, electrocardiogram; IVCD, intraventricular conduction delay; LBBB, left bundle branch block; PVCs, premature ventricular contractions; RBBB, right bundle branch block.
Reproduced with permission from Uberoi A, Stein R, Perez MV, et al. Interpretation of the electrocardiogram of young athletes. *Circulation.* 2011;124(6):746–757.

be distinguished from the Brugada ECG pattern which commonly present in leads V_1–V_2.

2. Other noninvasive cardiovascular evaluations—ECG and echocardiography are indicated when clinical, historical, or physical findings suggest the possibility of structural heart disease (valvular disease, HCM, arrhythmogenic right ventricular cardiomyopathy, or prior MI). Tilt table testing is often positive in athletes because of their resting bradycardia and large venous capacitance and thus should not be used or should be used cautiously in athletes to evaluate lightheadedness, syncope, or presyncope.

Echocardiography in highly trained endurance athletes may show evidence of four-chamber cardiac enlargement. Left ventricular end-diastolic dimensions can exceed 60 mm in 15% of athletes. Left ventricular wall thickness can occasionally exceed the upper normal limit of 12 mm. Values of 13–15 mm may be seen in normal athletes, although marked wall thickening of more than 16 mm is unusual, and the ratio of the septal to posterior wall thickness does not exceed 1.2. The left ventricular cavity in HCM typically has asymmetric wall thickening, although symmetric wall enlargement may occur, and the cavity dimensions are usually small (< 45 mm). In contrast, the athlete's heart typically has symmetric mild increases in left ventricular wall thickness and an increase in left ventricular chamber size of 55 mm or greater.

Left atrial enlargement in athletes is also common, and anterior-posterior diameters more than 40 mm, the upper limit of normal, exist in 20% of high-performance athletes. This increased atrial size may contribute to the observation that atrial fibrillation is more common in older athletes than in age-matched nonathletes.

Left ventricular diastolic function measured by tissue Doppler is normal in most athletes despite the hypertrophy, and normal diastolic function can help distinguish the athlete's heart from pathologic hypertrophy. The systolic anterior motion (SAM) of the mitral valve and mitral leaflet elongation can help with the diagnosis of HCM. These changes could happen in HCM even when the walls are not severely thickened. Stress echocardiography could provoke SAM and can provide more information than at rest.

Cardiac MRI can also help distinguish athlete's heart from HCM. A left ventricular diastolic wall thickness–to–cavity volume ratio of less than 0.15 mm/m^2/mL is useful in diagnosing athlete's heart. In HCM, intravenous gadolinium used in contrast-enhanced MRI is taken up by areas of myocardium with extra expanded cellular space indicating areas of fibrosis and scarring, also referred to as "late gadolinium enhancement" (LGE). LGE is not typical of the athlete's heart, especially in young athletes, but has been observed in older athletes with a history of lifelong, intense exercise training. This LGE could represent myocardial fibrosis induced by high-intensity, prolonged endurance exercise, but its significance is unknown. The fibrosis has a predilection for the interventricular septum at the right ventricular insertion points, suggesting that it could relate to the constant flexing at this "hinge" point produced by exercise and the right ventricular enlargement that occurs acutely after prolonged exercise and with long-term endurance exercise training.

Finally, detraining is another approach that could help to distinguish the athlete's heart from HCM. Three months of detraining should be sufficient to reverse the left ventricular hypertrophy of the athlete's heart and to distinguish this condition from HCM, although some studies suggest 6 months may be required. A decrease of more than 2 mm in left ventricular wall thickness with detraining relative to peak training is more consistent with athlete's heart since patients with HCM should not demonstrate a change with deconditioning.

Corrado D, Pelliccia A, Heidbuchel H, et al. Recommendations for interpretation of 12-lead electrocardiogram in the athlete. *Eur Heart J.* 2010;31:243–259. [PMID: 19933514]

Uberoi A, Stein R, Perez MV, et al. Interpretation of the electrocardiogram of young athletes. *Circulation.* 2011;124:746–757. [PMID: 21824936]

Zaidi A, Ghani S, Sharma R, et al. Physiological right ventricular adaptation in elite athletes of African and Afro-Caribbean origin. *Circulation.* 2013;127:1783–1792. [PMID: 23538381]

Integrating the Clinical Findings in Evaluating Athletes

Evaluating athletes, just like evaluating any patient, requires a careful integration of all aspects of the history, physical examination, and imaging findings. Clinicians should be careful of overreacting to borderline abnormalities found in asymptomatic athletes during screening. These often lead to "diagnostic creep" in which one borderline abnormality, such as a flow murmur, leads to other borderline abnormalities, with no clinician willing to diagnose normalcy. Such cases often are best handled by clinicians who have extensive experience dealing with athletes.

A. Preparticipation Screening

To prevent SCD in athletes, Italy has mandated by law the screening of all athletes ages 12 through 35 prior to participation in organized competitive sport. This is a state-subsidized national program that includes a history and physical, an ECG, and a 3-minute step test. The evaluation is performed by accredited sports medicine doctors specifically trained for this task. Further testing is done for abnormal findings or if there is a family history of sudden death or MI or a personal history of syncope or palpitations. The incidence of SCDs in 12- to 35-year-old athletes in one region of Italy, Veneto, has decreased since the implementation of this law due to decreases in deaths from arrhythmogenic right ventricular hypertrophy. No changes in the nonathlete population mortality rate occurred over the same time period.

Based on this single-center data, the European Society of Cardiology (ESC) and the International Olympic Committee (IOC) recommended the addition of an ECG to preparticipation screening. In contrast to the Italian experience, mandated preparticipation ECG and exercise testing in Israel has had no effect on the incidence of SCD in athletes. The AHA has also proposed guidelines for screening athletes prior to participation, but the AHA guidelines do not recommend routine ECG screening. Consequently, whether athletes require a routine ECG prior to athletic participation is controversial, and preparticipation ECG is not presently recommended in the United States. Clinicians should perform such ECG screening in individual athletes when the clinical situation warrants such testing or to reassure anxious parents. In such screening, however, the clinician should be wary of the diagnostic creep noted earlier.

In 2001, the AHA also published recommendations for preparticipation medical evaluations for master athletes.

These are individuals older than 35 years who are involved in masters sports training programs and participate in organized competitions designed for older athletes. Exercise testing is recommended for master athletes who have a moderate-to-high cardiovascular risk profile for coronary heart disease; this risk profile includes men older than 40 years and women older than 50 years (or postmenopausal) with one or more independent coronary risk factors (hypercholesterolemia or dyslipidemia, hypertension, current or recent cigarette smoking, diabetes mellitus, or a history of MI or sudden death in a first-degree relative < 60 years old). An exercise test is also recommended for master athletes of any age with symptoms suggestive of coronary heart disease or those ≥ 65 years of age even in the absence of risk factors or symptoms. A positive test requires further evaluation to determine the coronary anatomy. Although these are the current AHA guidelines, we also regard the recommendation for routine exercise testing in asymptomatic individuals as controversial since athletes frequently have false-positive ECG responses to exercise testing and there is limited clinical evidence to justify the routine revascularization of asymptomatic individuals, especially those with excellent exercise tolerance.

B. Recommendations for Sport Participation

Based on the routine history and physical examination prior to sport participation, the athlete should be either given clearance for participation, clearance to participate with activity limitations, or exclusion from participation pending further evaluation. If a cardiac diagnosis is made, limitations or exclusion might be warranted. In 2015, the AHA and American College of Cardiology published a scientific statement regarding eligibility and disqualification recommendations for competitive athletes with cardiovascular abnormalities. These recommendations are helpful once a diagnosis is made. This document summarizes experts' opinion regarding the type of sports the athlete can perform based on the cardiac pathology. Guidelines for sports participation for children with medical conditions have also been published and can assist in determining the level of sport recommended. Decisions should be individualized for each athlete since there are no definite data to determine the exercise risk for every cardiac condition, and guidelines are necessarily restrictive since they will be used by clinicians of varying ability. The decision to restrict sports participation should involve the athlete, the parents, and the coach.

Lampert R, Olshansky B, Heidbuchel H, et al. Safety of sports for athletes with implantable cardioverter-defibrillators: results of a prospective, multinational registry. *Circulation.* 2013;127: 2021–2030. [PMID: 23690453]

Maron BJ, Zipes DP, Kovacs RJ. Eligibility and disqualification recommendations for competitive athletes with cardiovascular abnormalities: Preamble and general considerations. *J Am Coll Cardiol.* 2015;66:2343–2355. [PMID: 26542655]

Novel Coronavirus Disease 2019 (COVID-19) & Return-to-Play Considerations

As in many aspects of health care, the COVID-19 pandemic has challenged the return to play (RTP) after a COVID-19 infection. An ACC expert panel convened during the pandemic to provide insight and guidance regarding the cardiovascular sequelae of the disease and the potential for myocarditis. The ACC 2022 Consensus Decision Pathway on Cardiovascular Sequelae of COVID-19 in adults highlights that the prevalence of clinical myocarditis in athletes following COVID-19 is low and close to 0.5–0.7%. The document also emphasizes that cardiac testing is not required for every competitive athlete. Athletes should abstain from exercise during the acute symptomatic period. The cardiac triad testing (ECG, cardiac troponin, and echocardiogram) prior to RTP (recommended in the initial phases of the pandemic) is now only recommended in those athletes with cardiopulmonary symptoms (eg, chest tightness, worsening exertional shortness of breath, palpitations, lightheadedness/syncope) regardless of initial or recurrent infection. In addition, it could also be used for athletes with new cardiopulmonary symptoms after RTP or those requiring hospitalization for a suspected cardiac cause. For athletes who are asymptomatic or have non-cardiopulmonary symptoms, no cardiac testing is recommended prior to RTP. Routine cardiac magnetic resonance (CMR) screening in athletes after COVID-19 infection is not recommended. However, it could be used as a diagnostic tool when there is a strong suspicion of myocarditis or other myocardial or pericardial involvement or when one of the cardiac triad tests are abnormal in the setting of a high pretest probability of myocarditis. If the CMR is concerning for myocardial injury, then the RTP guidelines on myocarditis from the ACC/AHA should be followed. These guidelines recommend that athletes with myocarditis should be restricted from exercise for 3–6 months.

They may RTP once the systolic function has normalized, serum biomarkers of myocardial injury have normalized, and any clinically relevant arrhythmias on ECG monitoring or exercise stress testing have resolved. Notably, the clinical significance of persistent LGE in asymptomatic athletes with prior myocarditis is unknown, so these athletes should continue to be monitored.

The 10-day recommendation for exercise abstinence is no longer necessary. The Centers for Disease Control and Prevention (CDC) self-isolation guidelines recommend 5 days. Nonetheless, asymptomatic athletes could resume training after 3 days of exercise abstinence. For those with mild-moderate, non-cardiopulmonary symptoms, training can resume after symptom resolution (this excludes anosmia and ageusia which may have a more prolonged course). Regardless of the symptomatology, all athletes with prior COVID-19 should implement a graded and personalized RTP regimen with diligent surveillance for new or recurrent cardiopulmonary symptoms. If an athlete had a remote infection (> 3 months) and no longer has any cardiopulmonary symptoms, no further cardiac testing is required. Post-vaccination myocarditis following COVID-19 vaccination is rare and athletes who received a COVID-19 mRNA vaccine do not require routine screening for myocarditis prior to RTP in the absence of suggestive symptoms.

Gluckman TJ, Bhave NM, Allen LA, et al. 2022 ACC expert consensus decision pathway on cardiovascular sequelae of COVID-19 in adults: myocarditis and other myocardial involvement, post-acute sequelae of SARS-CoV-2 infection and return to play: a report of the America College of Cardiology Solution Set Oversight Committee. *J Am Coll Cardiol.* 2022; Mar14:[Epub ahead of print]. {PMID: 35307156]

Maron BJ, Udelson JE, Bonow RO, et al. Eligibility and disqualification recommendations for competitive athletes with cardiovascular abnormalities: task force 3: hypertrophic cardiomyopathy, arrhythmogenic right ventricular cardiomyopathy and other cardiomyopathies, and myocarditis: a scientific statement from the American Heart Association and American College of Cardiology. *J Am Coll Cardiol.* 2015;66:2362–236271. [PMID: 26542657]

37 Thoracic Aortic Aneurysms & Dissections

John A. Elefteriades, MD

ANEURYSMS

ESSENTIALS OF DIAGNOSIS

- Ascending aortic diameter > 4 cm on imaging study.
- Descending aortic diameter > 3.5 cm on imaging study.

General Considerations

In the *ascending* aorta, aneurysms tend to take on three common patterns, as indicated in Figure 37–1. These include the supracoronary aortic aneurysm, annuloaortic ectasia (Marfanoid), and tubular diffuse enlargement.

The most common pattern is that of supracoronary dilatation of the ascending aorta. In this pattern of disease, the short segment of aorta between the aortic annulus and the coronary arteries remains normal in size. Sinuses are "preserved," meaning that the aorta indents normally, forming a "waist," just above the level of the coronary arteries. For this type of aneurysm, a supracoronary tube graft suffices.

In the second type, annuloaortic ectasia, the aortic annulus itself becomes dilated, giving a shape to the aorta like an Erlenmeyer chemistry flask. In this type of disease, the segment of aorta between the annulus and the coronary arteries is diseased, dilated, and thinned. The sinuses of Valsalva are "effaced," meaning that the normal indentation, or waist, is lost. When surgery is required, the entire aortic root must be replaced.

In the third type of ascending aortic disease, the configuration is midway between the previous two patterns; that is, there is some dilatation of the annulus and root and some effacement of the sinuses, but these elements are not dramatic. The overall appearance is that of a large tube, rather than a flask. For such aortas, either supracoronary tube grafting or aortic root replacement may be appropriate.

The Crawford classification (Figure 37–2) is used to categorize the appearance of an aneurysm in the *descending* aorta and *thoracoabdominal* aorta. This classification, based on the longitudinal location and extent of aortic involvement, has implications for surgical strategy and affects the risk of perioperative complications.

Type I aneurysms involve most of the thoracic aorta and the upper abdominal aorta. Type II aneurysms, the most extensive and most dangerous to repair, involve the entire descending and abdominal aortas. Type III aneurysms involve the lower thoracic and abdominal aortas. Type IV aneurysms are predominantly abdominal but involve thoracoabdominal exposure because of the proximity of the upper border to the diaphragm.

Etiology

The genetics of Marfan disease, a well-known cause of aneurysms of the thoracic aorta, have been well delineated, with over 1300 mutations identified on the fibrillin gene.

Increasingly, it is being appreciated that patients who do not have Marfan disease also manifest familial clustering of thoracic aortic aneurysms and dissections. Patients with aneurysms often answer one or both of the following questions affirmatively: "Do you have any family members with aneurysms anywhere in their bodies? Did any of your relatives die suddenly or unexpectedly of apparent cardiac causes?" Detailed construction of family trees on over 500 patients with thoracic aneurysm has indicated that 21% of aneurysm probands have a first-degree relative with a known or likely aortic aneurysm. The true number is certainly much higher, as these estimates are based only on family interview and not on head-to-toe imaging of relatives. Figure 37–3 shows the 21 positive family trees of 100 families analyzed. The most likely pattern of inheritance appears to be autosomal dominant with incomplete penetrance. A more recent analysis has shown that the location of the proband's aneurysm largely influences the location of the aneurysms in the family members. If the proband

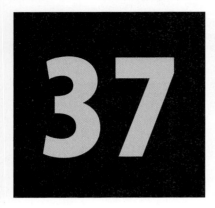

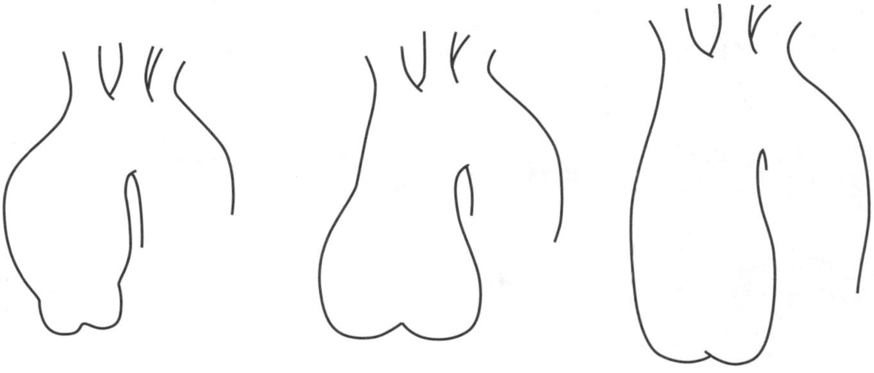

▲ **Figure 37–1.** The three common patterns of ascending aortic aneurysm.

has an ascending aneurysm, the likelihood is that the family members have ascending aneurysms. If, however, the proband has a descending aneurysm, it is likely that the family members have abdominal aortic aneurysms. These proband–family member observations are in keeping with the general concept that aneurysm disease divides at the ligamentum arteriosum: Ascending and arch aneurysms represent one disease, largely nonatherosclerotic, while

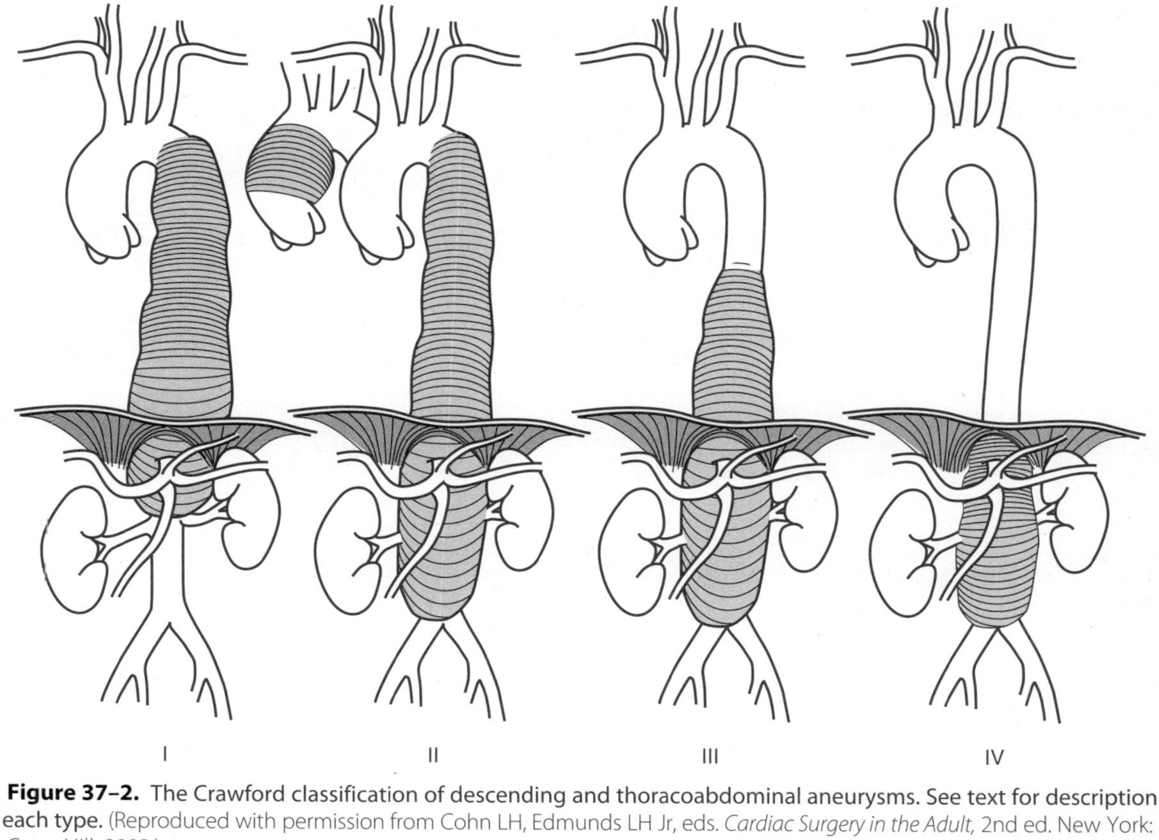

▲ **Figure 37–2.** The Crawford classification of descending and thoracoabdominal aneurysms. See text for description of each type. (Reproduced with permission from Cohn LH, Edmunds LH Jr, eds. *Cardiac Surgery in the Adult,* 2nd ed. New York: McGraw-Hill; 2003.)

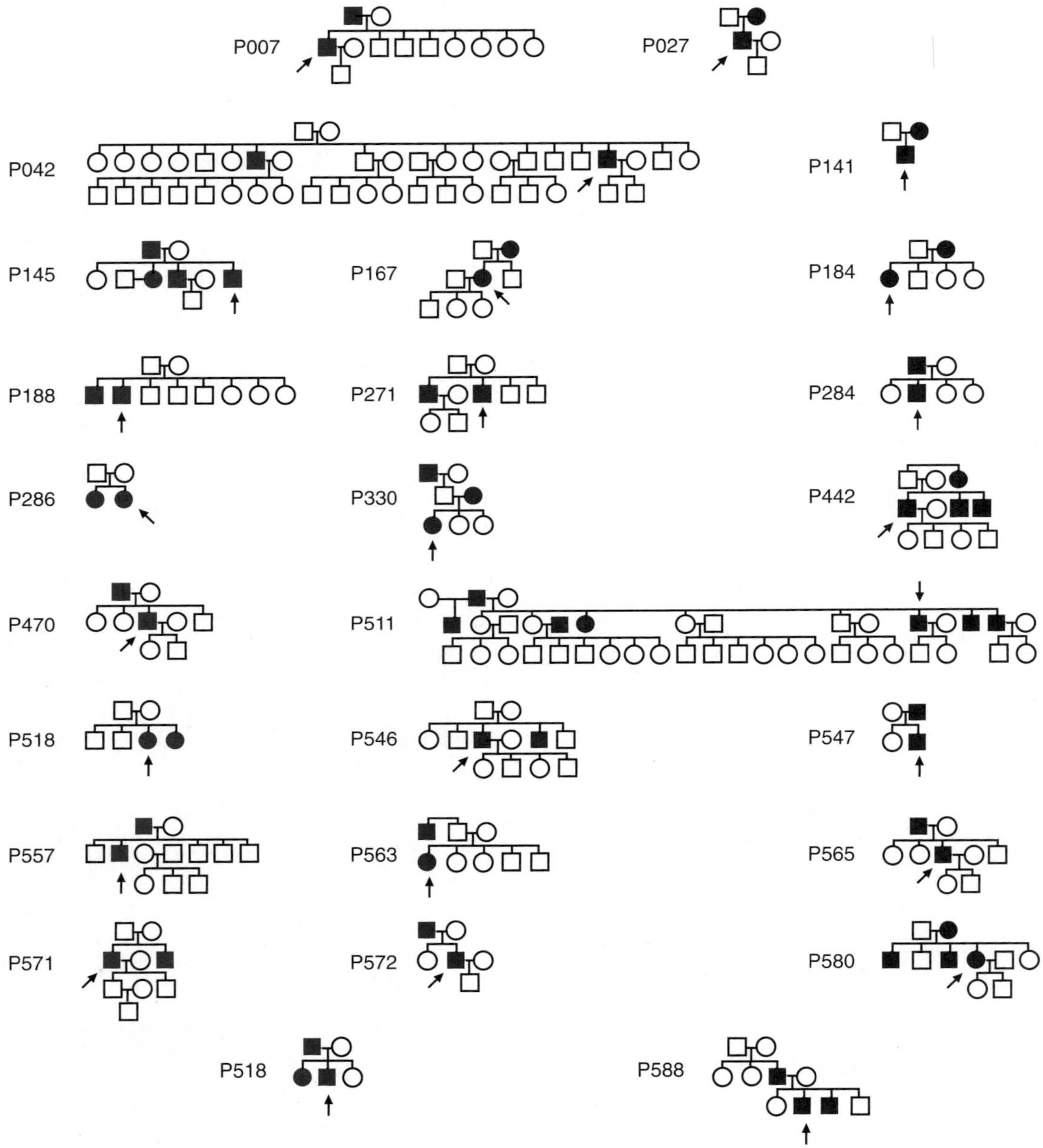

▲ **Figure 37–3.** The 21 positive family trees among the first 100 families assessed for genetic patterns of thoracic aortic disease.

descending and abdominal aneurysms represent another disease, largely atherosclerotic.

This concept of two diseases separated at the ligamentum arteriosum correlates perfectly with recent evidence that the ascending and descending aortic smooth muscle cells arise from different embryologic layers (neural crest and mesoderm, respectively).

Application of modern molecular genetic techniques is successfully making progress toward determining the specific genetic aberrations responsible for family clustering and for thoracic aneurysms in general. Original progress was made largely by linkage analysis of large families with multiple members affected. Now, as automated genomic analysis has become feasible and affordable, much scientific discovery has been made by direct exome sequencing. Milewicz, Dietz, Loeys, and others have succeeded in identifying specific familial aneurysm patterns and their underlying mutations. Nearly all these familial aortic disorders are transmitted in an autosomal dominant fashion (with decreased penetrance). The ACTA2 disorder presents with aortic dissection at small diameters and the MYLK disorder may dissect without prior aneurysmal enlargement. These mutation-specific categorizations have led to the advent of personalized medicine based on the specific underlying mutation and its accompanying rupture and dissection patterns. Specialized centers have begun routine whole exome sequencing (WES) in all patients with thoracic aortic aneurysm and dissection. Figure 37–4 shows the distribution of variants found at one high-volume center.

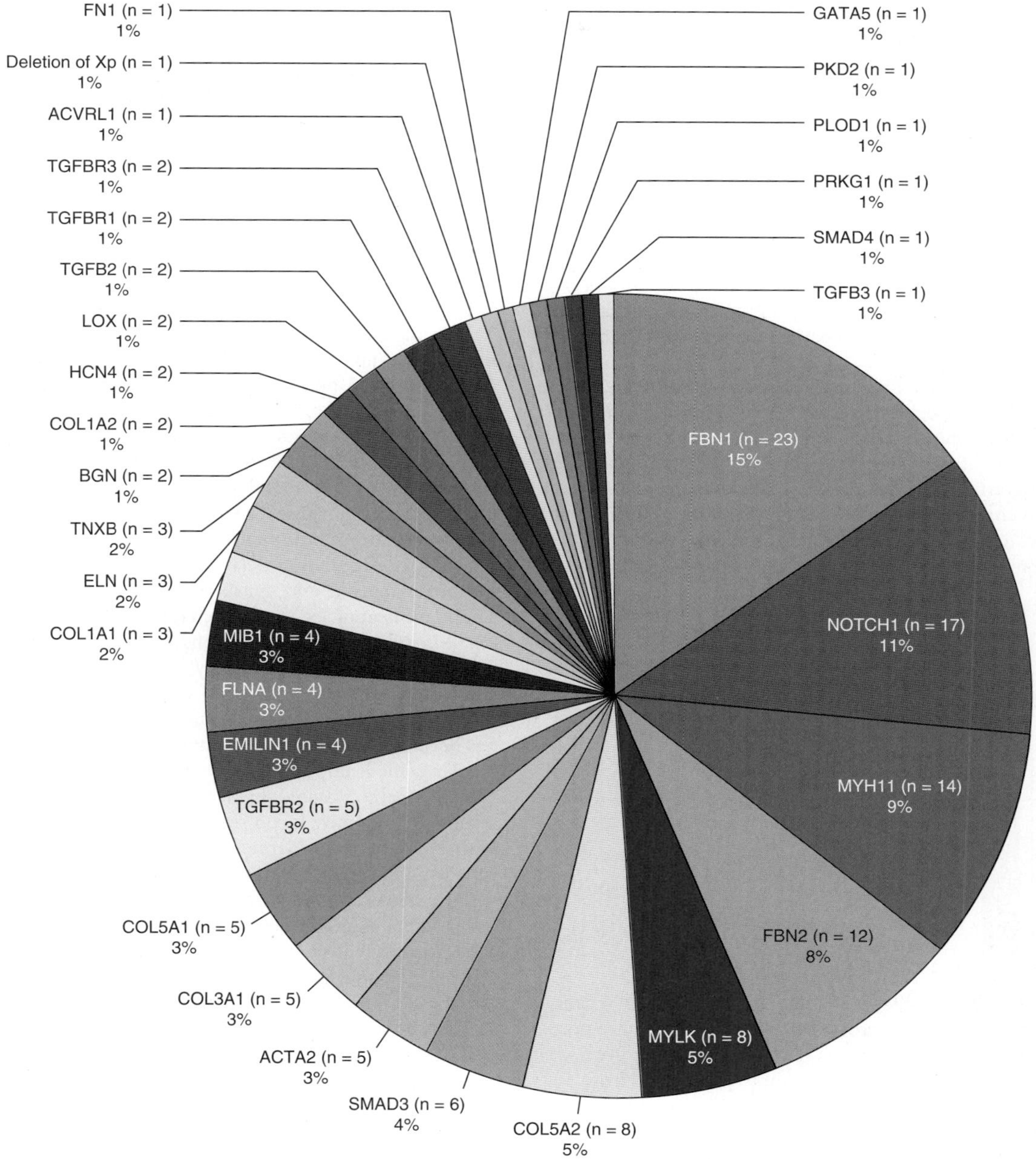

▲ **Figure 37–4.** Frequency distribution of genetic defects in genes implicated with thoracic aortic disease, identified via whole exome sequencing.

It is important to recognize that most genetically triggered thoracic aortic aneurysms are "single gene, single letter" diseases. That is to say, not only are these aneurysmal diseases caused by a single gene, but also by only a single change in a single "letter" (nucleotide or base) among the 2.2 billion letters that comprise the human genome. This stands in contradistinction to many other diseases, which are genetically multifactorial (eg, dozens of genes are known to contribute to coronary artery disease). This single-letter causation is crucially important—providing opportunities for precise diagnosis and, hopefully, future genetically based treatment.

Examination of single nucleotide polymorphisms (SNPs) in the blood of hundreds of patients with thoracic aortic aneurysms via genome-wide surveys using large (> 30,000) SNP libraries has been accomplished. An "RNA signature" in the blood of patients with thoracic aortic aneurysm was found, which can predict with about 85% accuracy from a blood test alone whether the patient harbors a thoracic aortic aneurysm. This "signature" is composed of specific RNAs that are either markedly upregulated or markedly downregulated in aneurysm patients, compared with healthy controls.

Patients who have a genetic predisposition for aneurysm development, specifically those patients with annuloaortic ectasia or ascending aortic aneurysm, are significantly protected from atherosclerosis (Figure 37–5). Remarkably, they have less arterial medial thickness and less calcification than normal controls—and myocardial infarction is very rare in these patients. It appears likely that the same mutations that promote lysis of the aortic wall also prevent plaque build-up.

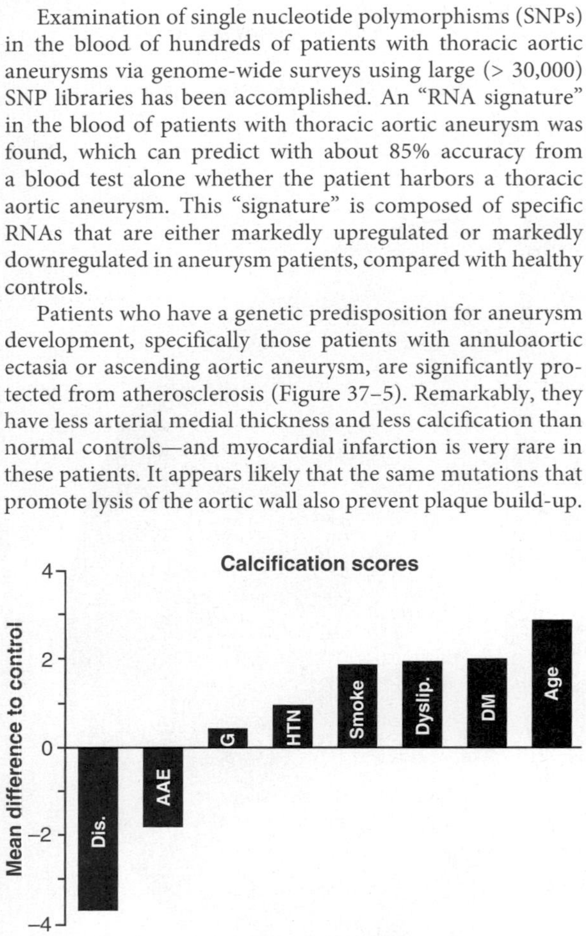

▲ **Figure 37–5.** Difference in overall calcification scores relative to the control group for all risk factors analyzed. Note that patients with ascending aortic dissection or annuloaortic ectasia are significantly "protected" from arteriosclerosis, manifesting lower calcification scores. AAE, annuloaortic ectasia; Age, age (in 10-year intervals); Dis, ascending aortic dissection; DM, diabetes mellitus; Dyslip, dyslipidemia; G, male gender; HTN, hypertension; Smoke, smoking history.

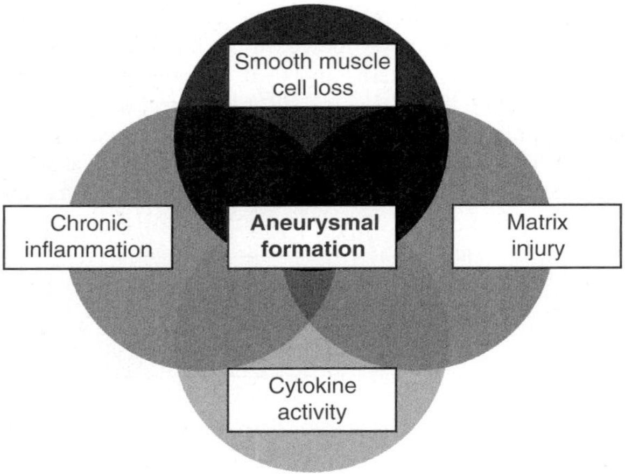

▲ **Figure 37–6.** Diagram illustrating the overlapping cellular and molecular processes that contribute to aortic aneurysm formation.

Accepting that most patients with thoracic aortic aneurysms have an underlying genetic predisposition to the condition, how does this genetic programming lead to the development of an aneurysm? Rapid progress is being made in elucidating these mechanisms. Aneurysm formation is currently thought to involve the following processes (Figure 37–6): extracellular matrix proteolysis, chronic inflammation, cytokine activity, and smooth muscle cell loss. A recent recognition is that abnormal mechanosensing and mechanoregulation between smooth muscle cells and the aortic lamellae and matrix also play an important role. The identification of these mechanisms raises the intriguing possibility of interfering pharmacologically with this pathophysiology, so that aneurysm formation or progression can be stopped. The importance of the transforming growth factor-β (TGF-β) pathway in aneurysm formation has been demonstrated; the ability of angiotensin receptor–blocking medications (ARBs) (eg, losartan) to interfere with this pathophysiologic mechanism is being tested, and results of randomized, controlled studies are now becoming available. One recent large study failed to show any clinical advantage of ARBs. At this time, it may be said that no specific pharmacologic strategy exists for delaying aneurysm progression. Results of trials of proteolytic antagonists and β-blockers have been underwhelming. The potential roles of statin medications, anti-inflammatory agents (cyclooxygenase [COX]-2 inhibitors), immunosuppressants (sirolimus), and antibiotics (doxycycline) are being investigated.

The proteolytic enzymes called matrix metalloproteinases (MMPs) are receiving extensive attention in aneurysm pathophysiology. These powerful enzymes are found in excess in thoracic aortic aneurysms (Figure 37–7) and are thought to play a major role in destroying the substance of the aortic wall, leading to decreased wall strength and, ultimately, dilatation and rupture.

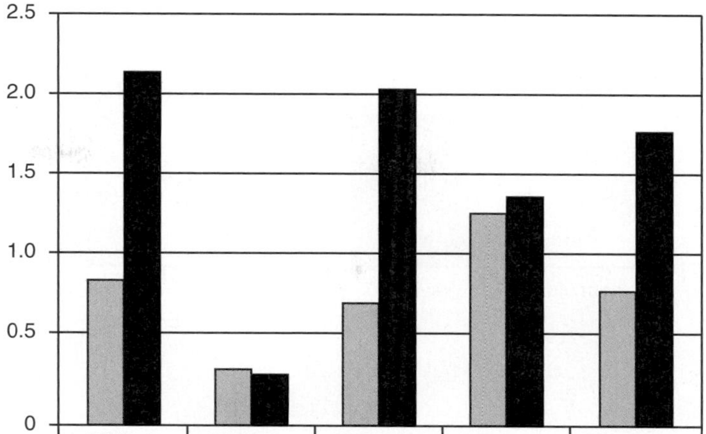

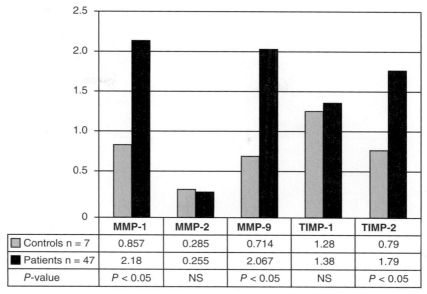

	MMP-1	MMP-2	MMP-9	TIMP-1	TIMP-2
■ Controls n = 7	0.857	0.285	0.714	1.28	0.79
■ Patients n = 47	2.18	0.255	2.067	1.38	1.79
P-value	$P < 0.05$	NS	$P < 0.05$	NS	$P < 0.05$

▲ **Figure 37–7.** Note overabundance of matrix metalloproteinase (MMP)-1 and MMP-9 and TIMP-2 in aortas of patients with thoracic aortic aneurysm, compared with controls. This information suggests an important role for MMP enzymes in the pathophysiology of aneurysm disease. NS, not significant; TIMP, tissue inhibitor of metalloproteinases.

The biologic changes in the aortic wall discussed earlier are vitally important, but hemodynamic forces need to be considered as well. As the ascending aorta reaches a diameter of 6 cm, its distensibility vanishes, so that the aorta becomes essentially a rigid tube (Figure 37–8). Because of this rigidity, the force of systole can no longer be beneficially dissipated by elastic expansion of the aorta, and this translates into increased wall stress. Especially at high blood pressures, this wall stress becomes excessive, setting the stage for disruption of the aortic wall via rupture or dissection. It is instructive to note how closely this mechanical data dove-tails with the clinical behavior of the aorta: The mechanical properties deteriorate at 6 cm diameter, and that is precisely the hinge point for clinically manifest rupture and dissection.

Clinical Findings

A. Incidence & Prevalence

It is generally acknowledged, based on data from the Centers for Disease Control and Prevention, that aneurysm disease is the 15th most common cause of death for human beings. The incidence of aortic dissection is estimated to be 30 per million population per year. However, new studies are confirming the long-standing suspicion that these figures represent gross underestimates. Very recent data show that, on computerized tomography (CT), aortic dilatation exceeding 4.0 cm is found in 2.8% of individuals older than 50 years. It has been rightly presumed that many individuals dying with chest pain after presenting to an emergency department may have aortic dissection rather than myocardial infarction. Now, evidence is accumulating that substantiates this presumption. Clinical series that have applied routine postmortem computed tomography in patients succumbing to out-of-hospital cardiac arrest have confirmed that 2–7% of such patients actually have died of Type A aortic dissection, with intrapericardial rupture.

B. Natural History

The Yale computerized database now contains information on nearly 4500 patients with thoracic aortic aneurysm, including many thousands of tabulated serial imaging studies and tens of thousands of patient-years of follow-up. This database and these methods of analysis have permitted assessment of multiple fundamental topics and questions regarding the natural behavior of the thoracic aorta and have shed light on appropriate criteria for surgical intervention.

1. How fast does the thoracic aorta grow?—Via specifically developed statistical methods designed to account for important potential sources of error, the annual growth rate of an aneurysmal thoracic aorta has been determined to be, on average, 0.12 cm. The descending aorta grows faster than the ascending aorta, at 0.19 cm/year. Also, the larger the aorta becomes, the faster it grows.

2. At what size does the aorta dissect or rupture?—Critical to decision-making in aortic surgery is an understanding of when complications occur in the natural history of unrepaired thoracic aortic aneurysms. In the case of

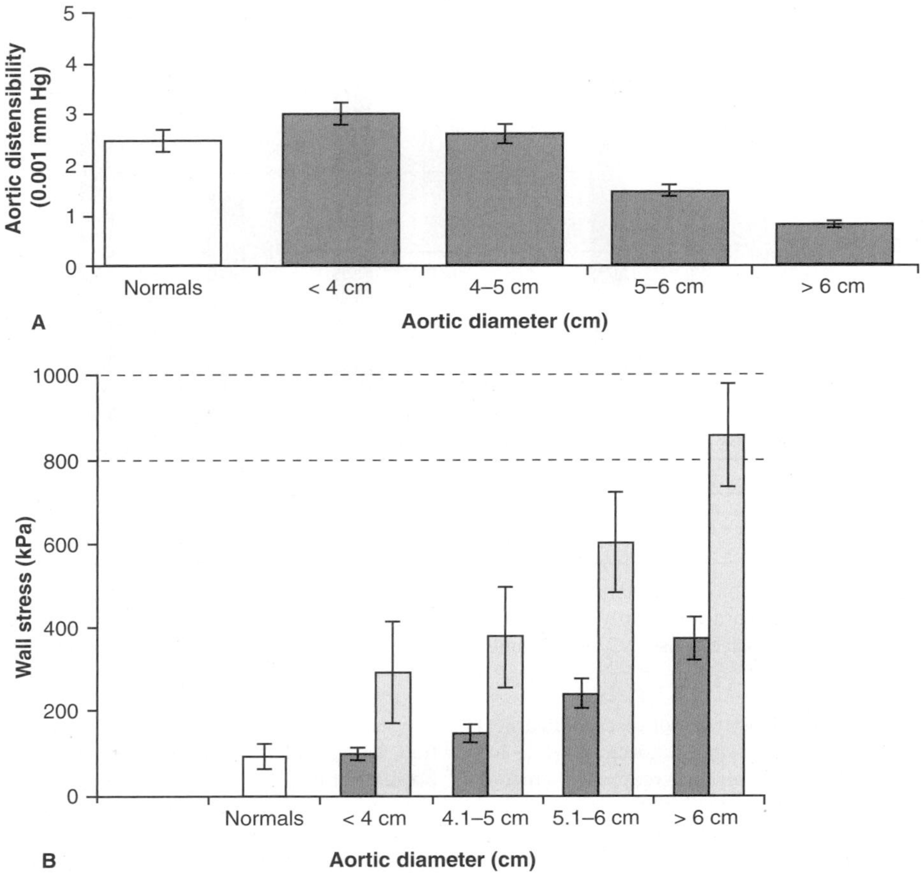

▲ **Figure 37–8. A:** Distensibility values in normal aortas and aortic aneurysms of different diameters. Distensibility of ascending aortic aneurysms decreases rapidly as diameter increases, to very low values at dimensions > 6 cm. At 6 cm, the aorta is essentially a rigid tube, unable to dissipate the force of systole by expanding phasically during the cardiac cycle. **B:** Exponential relationship between wall stress and aneurysm size in ascending aortic aneurysms. The dark columns represent a blood pressure of 100 mm Hg, and the light columns represent a blood pressure of 200 mm Hg. The lines at 800–1000 kPa represent the range of maximum tensile strength of the human aorta. Note that a patient with a 6-cm aneurysm and a blood pressure of 200 mm Hg (as during stress or extreme exertion) "flirts" with the limits of the ultimate strength of his or her aorta wall.

the thoracic aorta, the two complications that are vitally important are rupture and dissection. Knowing when these complications are likely to occur permits rational decision-making regarding elective, preemptive surgical intervention to prevent their occurrence.

Size criteria apply only to asymptomatic aneurysms. We are learning increasingly that the aorta can indeed "communicate" with us—via pain. Symptomatic (painful) aneurysms should be resected regardless of size. For ascending aneurysms, this pain is usually felt anteriorly, under the breastbone. For descending thoracic aneurysms, the pain is usually felt in the interscapular region of the upper back. For thoracoabdominal aneurysms, the pain is usually felt lower in the back or in the left flank. Other symptoms may occasionally be produced by thoracic aortic aneurysms, including bronchial obstruction, esophageal obstruction, and phrenic nerve dysfunction; these symptoms also constitute indications for surgical intervention.

Very recent statistical analysis reveals two sharp "hinge points" (Figure 37–9) in ascending aortic size at which rupture or dissection occurred: at 5.25 and 5.75 cm. An aortic size of 6.0 cm was associated with an 8-percentage point increase in the probability of rupture and dissection relative to the 4.0–4.4 cm reference group.

If a surgeon were to wait for the aorta to achieve the median size at the time of complications to intervene, by definition, rupture or dissection would have occurred in half of the patients (Figure 37–10). Accordingly, it is important to

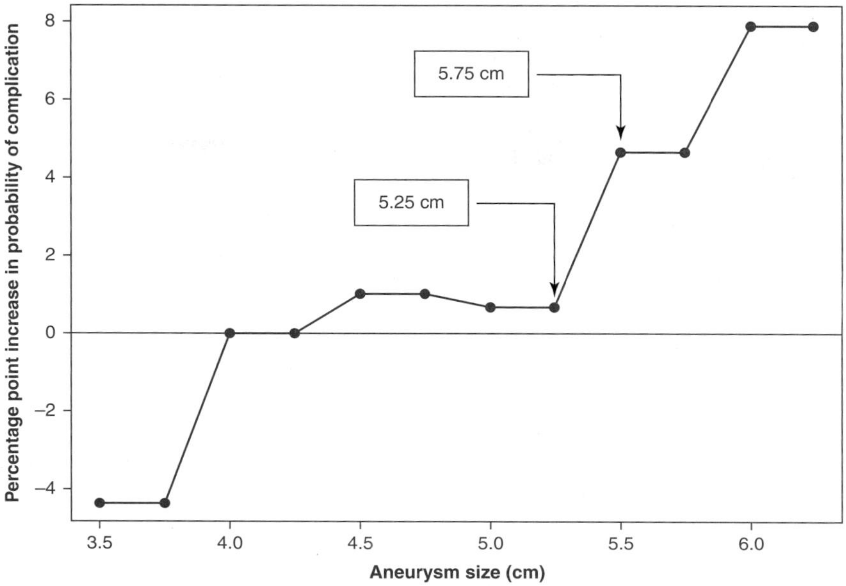

▲ **Figure 37–9.** The "hinge points" (*arrows*) in the cumulative, lifetime incidence of complications (rupture or dissection) of thoracic aortic aneurysms, based on size. By the time the ascending aorta reaches the dimensions on the *x*-axis, the percentage of patients shown on the *y*-axis have already incurred rupture or dissection.

intervene before the median value is attained. The following recommendations take this factor into account, permitting preemptive surgical extirpation before rupture or dissection in most patients.

Current recommendations, listed in Table 37–1, are based on the hinge points noted in Figure 37–9. Specifically, prophylactic extirpation of the aneurysmal ascending aorta is recommended when the aneurysm measures 5.5 cm; for the descending aorta, which does not rupture until a larger size, surgical intervention is recommended when the aneurysm measures 6.5 cm. At institutions with a large experience in thoracic aortic surgery, where such operations can be accomplished at low risk, it is appropriate to intervene even earlier, at smaller aortic sizes than indicated earlier. Application of these criteria will prevent most ruptures and dissections, without prematurely exposing the patient to the risks and inconveniences of surgery. The efficacy of this management algorithm has recently been documented in a large cohort of prospectively followed patients. As WES progresses, we will develop patient-specific criteria for intervention that are based not only on size, but also on the specific mutation carried by an individual patient.

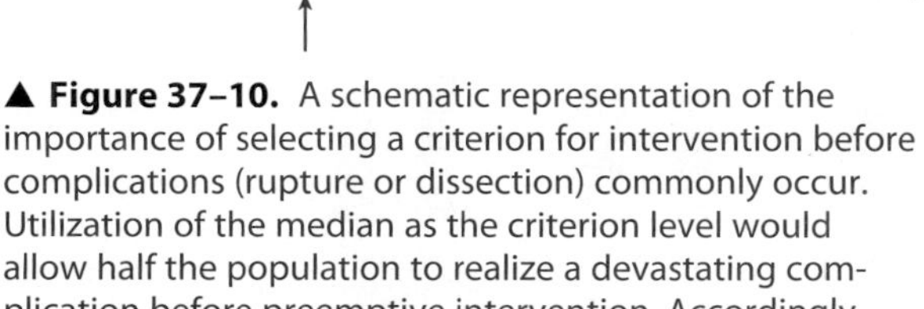

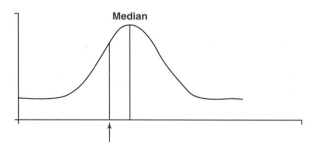

▲ **Figure 37–10.** A schematic representation of the importance of selecting a criterion for intervention before complications (rupture or dissection) commonly occur. Utilization of the median as the criterion level would allow half the population to realize a devastating complication before preemptive intervention. Accordingly, a criterion below the median is selected (*arrow*) to allow preemptive intervention before a large proportion of patients have suffered a complication.

It is well-known that patients with Marfan disease are prone to unpredictable dissection at an early size. For this reason, earlier intervention is recommended for patients with Marfan disease as indicated in Table 37–1.

For patients with a positive family history, but without Marfan disease, the same criteria are applied as for Marfan

Table 37–1. Size Criteria for Surgical Intervention for Asymptomatic Thoracic Aortic Aneurysm

	Marfan	Non-Marfan
Ascending	5.0 cm	5.5 cm
Descending	6.0 cm	6.5 cm

disease, because malignant early behavior of the aneurysm in these patients may be seen as well.

If the patient has a positive family history, or if an afflicted family member has suffered rupture, dissection, or death, preemptive surgical extirpation is carried out earlier than otherwise.

Studies of aortic anatomy increasingly recognize that patients with a bicuspid aortic valve also have inherently deficient aortas. About 5% of bicuspid patients will dissect the aorta during their lifetimes. Therefore, although controversial, lower intervention dimensions have often been applied for patients with bicuspid aortic valve, as for Marfan disease. Bicuspid aortopathy was considered, so to speak, as "Marfan's light." However, recent data indicate that bicuspid patients are not quite as vulnerable as initially thought, so traditional, non-Marfan criteria can be applied. The inherent propensity of the bicuspid aorta to dissect must also be taken into account in planning surgical management of the ascending aorta in a patient who requires aortic valve replacement for stenosis or regurgitation. In such circumstances, the ascending aorta should usually be resected if it is 4.5 cm or greater in diameter, thus preventing future dissection events. In fact, experienced aortic surgeons, if they are in the chest to perform aortic valve replacement, will often replace the ascending aorta even at 4 cm diameter—to avoid the need for a later operation.

3. What is the yearly rate of rupture or dissection for thoracic aortic aneurysms?—The preceding data indicate the cumulative lifetime rates of dissection or rupture by the time the aorta reaches a certain size. Determining the yearly risk of complications from the natural history of thoracic aortic aneurysm is more challenging because it requires extremely robust data. Such data must produce enough hard endpoints to permit analysis within a year's time for different size strata. Calculations of yearly rates of rupture or other complications based on size of the aorta have been produced. These yearly rates are expressed based simply on the size of the aorta (Figure 37-11).

These data all point to a diameter of 6 cm as a very dangerous size threshold. At or above this size, the yearly risk for rupture is about 4%, the yearly risk of dissection is about 4%, and the risk of death is about 11%. (Death is often directly related to catastrophic complications from the aneurysm. In fact, recent studies from Japan, based on routine postmortem CT scan "autopsies," show that a staggering 8% of all sudden deaths are due to Type A aortic dissection.) The chance of any one of these phenomena occurring—rupture, dissection, or death—is 14%/year. As a mnemonic point of reference, a 6-cm aneurysm can be equated to about the diameter of a soft drink can. When a thoracic aortic aneurysm reaches the diameter of a soda can, it has certainly reached the point where it poses a major risk to the patient. All current societal guidelines recommend a general criterion for prophylactic surgery of 5.5 cm for the ascending aorta (for individuals of average body size).

These analyses should permit accurate decision-making when seeing a patient during an office visit and considering preemptive surgical extirpation of thoracic aneurysms. These data allow the physician to form a reasonable estimate of the individual patient's risk of dissection, rupture, or death for each future year of life, if the aorta is not resected. The risk of rupture, dissection, or death based on aortic size is presented graphically in Figure 37–11.

The question arises whether the same surgical intervention criteria should apply for a small woman as for a large man.

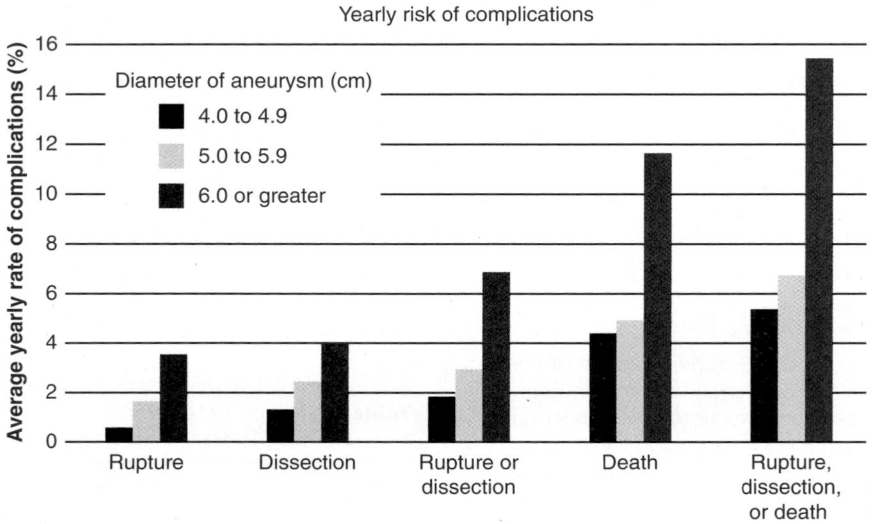

▲ **Figure 37–11.** Probabilities that rupture, dissection, or death will occur have been calculated for aortic aneurysms in the chest. The likelihood of these events jumps sharply for aneurysms that reach 6 cm or higher.

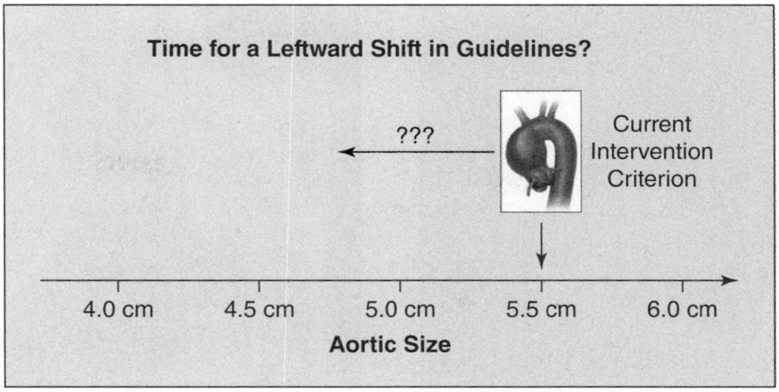

▲ **Figure 37–12.** Consideration is currently being given as to whether the general criterion for intervention for ascending aortic aneurysm (in individuals of normal body size) should be "shifted-left" on the aortic size chart—to 5.5 cm.

It is true that a larger individual can be "allowed" a larger aorta, generally speaking. Conversely, even a moderate-sized aneurysm can be quite threatening in an individual of small stature. For this reason, adverse event rates (rupture or dissection) based on aortic size corrected for body surface area (BSA) have been analyzed. By plotting the aneurysm size along the horizontal scale and the BSA along the vertical scale, each particular patient can be classified into low-, medium-, or high-risk categories—thus taking account of the aneurysm size in relation to the patient's physical size.

Two important recent developments regarding aortic prediction have occurred. First, it has been found that ascending aortic length (measured from the aortic annulus to the leading margin of the innominate artery) predicts adverse aortic events a bit more accurately than diameter. Elongation, it appears, is another sign of a damaged, vulnerable aorta. Secondly, it has been found, based on CT scans obtained fortuitously just *before* aortic dissection, that the dissection process itself produces an instantaneous 8-mm enlargement of the aorta. So, the aorta is actually smaller at the moment of dissection than previously appreciated on *post-dissection* scans. This argues that we should consider shifting our general criterion for intervention to 5.0 cm instead of 5.5 cm (Figure 37–12.) The next iteration of societal guidelines may endorse this "left-shift" to smaller sizes for intervention.

Very recent studies have shown that enlargement of the aortic root is more "malignant" than similar degree of enlargement of the ascending aorta itself.

C. Symptoms & Signs

Most thoracic aortic aneurysms are asymptomatic and are detected fortuitously during imaging of other thoracic structures. When they are symptomatic, deep visceral pain in the upper anterior chest or interscapular back can occur. The aorta can "talk" to the patient via ascending sympathetic fibers that reach pain centers in the brain. Aortic pain differs from angina pectoris because it is not necessarily precipitated by exertion nor relieved by rest or nitroglycerin. Often, it is rather constant and not influenced by body motion or position. All patients with chest pain should have a screening chest radiograph. Rupture of a thoracic aneurysm usually causes excruciating pain, accompanied by profound dyspnea as the chest fills with blood, and quickly results in shock. A large ascending aortic aneurysm occasionally may result in dysphagia or stridor due to esophageal or large airway obstruction. Rarely, a large aneurysm may cause bone pain due to pressure against thoracic skeletal structures.

D. Physical Examination

Physical examination is usually unremarkable. The presence of a murmur of aortic regurgitation should raise the suspicion of ascending aortic aneurysm, as should features suggestive of Marfan syndrome or related conditions. The thumb-palm sign, in which the tip of the thumb can be extended beyond the edge of the flat palm, can be a useful indicator of connective tissue laxity, raising the specter of associated aneurysm disease (Figure 37–13). Rarely, an abnormal pulsation will be felt due to a large aneurysm contacting the chest wall.

E. Diagnostic Studies

The remarkable strides made in recent decades in three-dimensional body imaging have dramatically advanced the diagnosis and treatment of thoracic aortic aneurysm. Echocardiography (especially transesophageal), computed tomography (CT), and magnetic resonance imaging (MRI) scans all yield images that clarify the presence, location, size, and extent of aneurysmal disease. An example of the precise imaging afforded by MRI is indicated for a specific, very extensive aneurysm in Figure 37–14. Proper interpretation of CT and MRI scans is essential; specifically, axial sections for aortic measurements must be selected carefully so that the aorta is vertical at the chosen site (oblique measurements will be exaggerated by an oblong rather than circular aortic

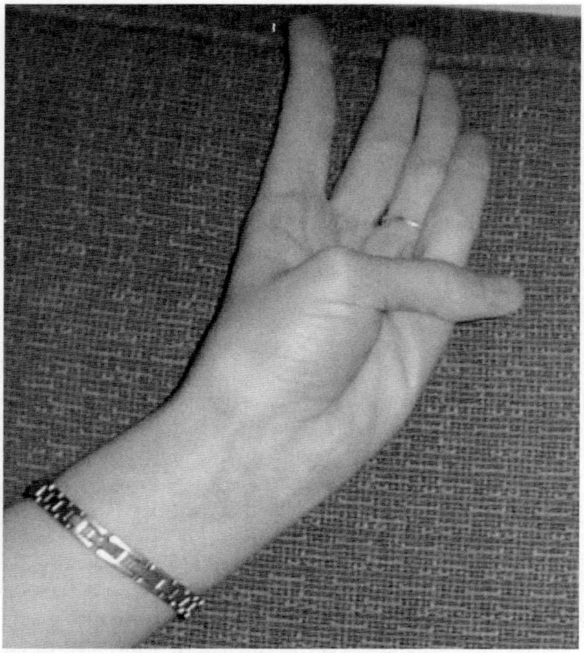

▲ **Figure 37–13.** Patient with a positive "thumb-palm" sign for connective tissue disease. Being able to cross the thumb beyond the edge of the palm indicates that the long bones are excessive and the joints are lax. (Reproduced, with permission, from Elefteriades JA, et al. Guilt by association: paradigm for detecting a silent killer [thoracic aortic aneurysm]. *Open Heart*. 2015;2:e000169. With permission from BMJ Publishing Group Ltd.)

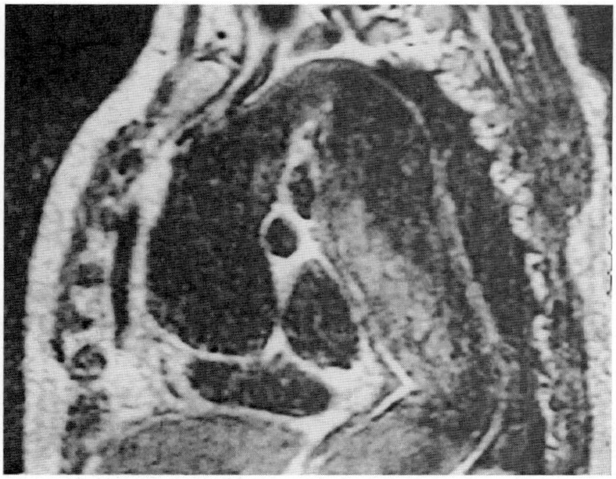

▲ **Figure 37–14.** Magnetic resonance scan of a massively dilated aorta, which extends from the aortic valve to the iliac bifurcation. Note that the heart is compressed to a small shadow crushed between the elongated aorta and the diaphragm. This aneurysm was successfully resected in two stages.

contour). The "centerline method" applies automatic computerized assessment of diameter perpendicular to the long axis of the aorta, thus avoiding obliquity issues.

It is easy to make errors in measurement of aorta on CT or MRI imaging. Potential sources of errors are indicated in Figure 37–15.

In this era of specialized three-dimensional imaging, it is important not to forget the chest radiograph, which can often yield significant information about the thoracic aorta. An example is provided in Figure 37–16. Ascending aortic aneurysm presents as a bulge beyond the right hilar border. Arch aneurysm produces enlargement of the aortic knob. Descending thoracic aneurysm is often easily seen as a deviation of the stripe of the descending aorta, which normally runs parallel to and just left of the vertebral column.

Many if not most thoracic aortic aneurysms are found incidentally on three-dimensional imaging studies done for another, unrelated purpose. Most thoracic aneurysms remain undiagnosed in the general population. Recently, a paradigm called "guilt by association" has been proposed for uncovering hidden aneurysms in the general public based on the close association of thoracic aortic aneurysm with a group of related conditions (Figure 37–17). These related conditions include various medical conditions (intracranial aneurysm, abdominal aortic aneurysm, temporal arteritis, autoimmune disorder, renal cysts), certain aortic anatomic variants (bovine aortic arch, direct origin of left vertebral artery from aortic arch, bicuspid aortic valve), and family history of aneurysm disease. The presence of one of these associated conditions warrants imaging to rule out concurrent silent aortic aneurysm.

Treatment

A. Risks of Aortic Surgery

It is certainly helpful to know numerically and statistically the cumulative and yearly rates of rupture, dissection, and death imposed by an aortic aneurysm of a specific size. On the other hand, the equation is incomplete without the consideration of the risks inherent in elective, prophylactic surgical extirpation of the thoracic aorta. Certainly, these are major operations, and the surgical risks most feared include death, stroke, and paraplegia. However, these operations have become safer, reflecting increased surgical experience, improved perfusion techniques, improved (nonporous) grafts, effective antifibrinolytic agents for perioperative use, improved methods of spinal cord preservation, and the advent of centers specializing in aortic care and surgery. Several contemporary reports emphasize the "safety of thoracic aortic surgery in the present era." Mortality rates and rates of other complications after aortic surgery are quite low, especially for operations performed electively on stable patients, in whom the safety of ascending aortic and aortic

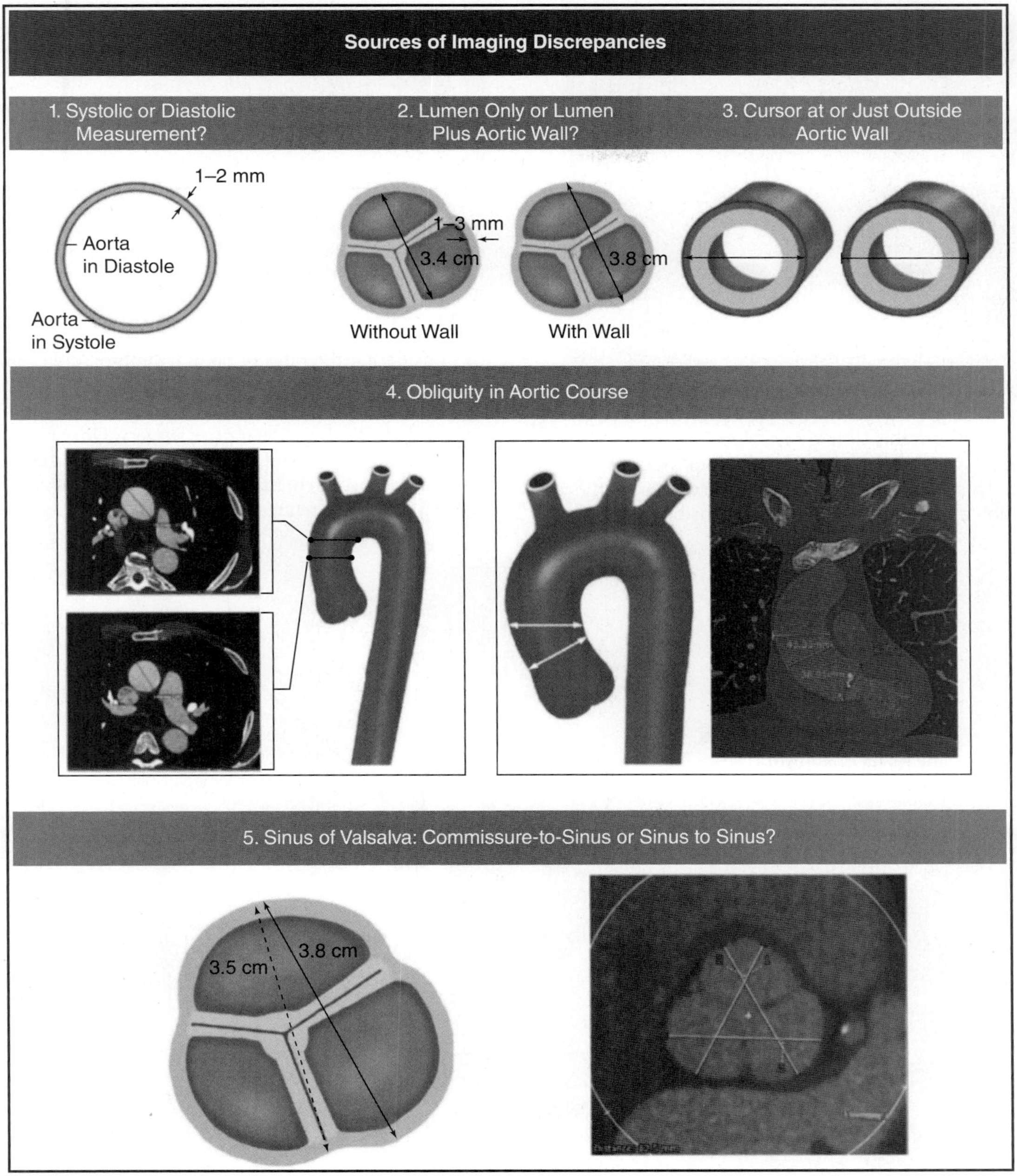

▲ **Figure 37–15.** Potential sources of error in measurement of the aorta on CT images. These errors plague everyday practice and impede accurate assessment of growth over time. These sources of error include: systole vs. diastole, with or without aortic wall, cursor on or just outside of aortic wall, obliquity of the measuring line relative to the aorta, and sinus-to-commissure or sinus-to-sinus for the aortic root (sinuses of Valsalva). (Reproduced with permission from Elefteriades JA, Mukherjee SK, Mojibian H. Discrepancies in Measurement of the Thoracic Aorta: JACC Review Topic of the Week. *J Am Coll Cardiol.* 2020;76(2):201–217.)

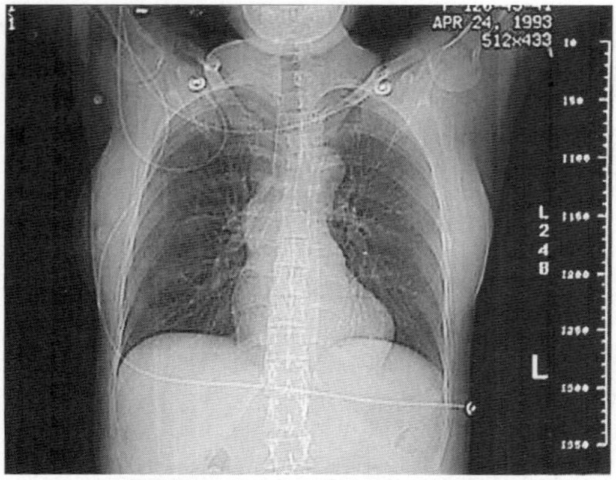

▲ **Figure 37–16.** An exemplary chest radiograph indicating that significant information about the aorta can be gleaned from this simple test. Note the bulge of the ascending aorta to the right of the upper mediastinal border. This young patient with Marfan disease suffered dissection at an ascending aortic dimension of 4.8 cm.

Table 37–2. Current Risks of Thoracic Aortic Surgery

	Mortality (%)	Stroke (%)	Paraplegia (%)
Ascending/arch	2.9	3.0	0.5
Descending/ thoracoabdominal	2.9	4.2	5.3

arch surgery is as high as 98%. Table 37–2 shows the pertinent rates of morbidity and mortality.

B. Indications & Contraindications

By considering the rates of natural rupture, dissection, and death from the thoracic aneurysm itself versus the risks of operation, the physician can make an informed recommendation about elective, preemptive surgery. Once patients and their families are provided the natural history and surgical risk data, they often have strong opinions of their own. Some patients are reluctant to undergo major surgery, with

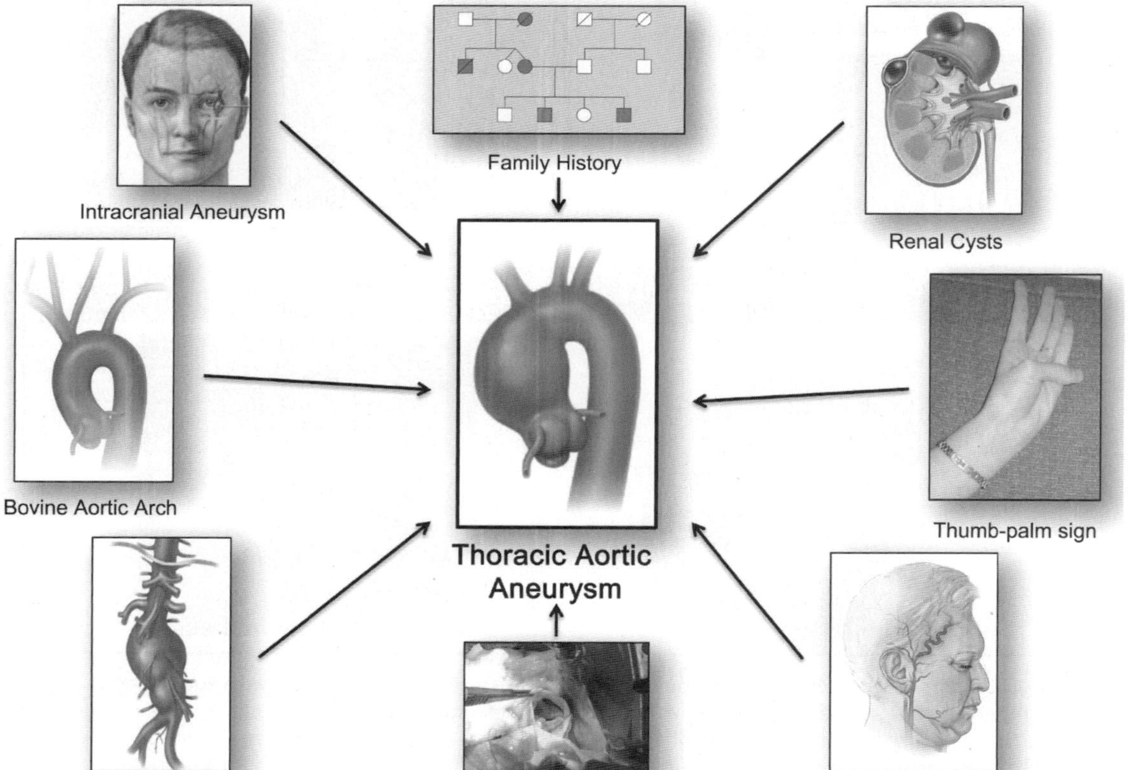

▲ **Figure 37–17.** Paradigm of "guilt by association" for detection of silent thoracic aortic aneurysms. (Reproduced with permission from Elefteriades JA, et al. Guilt by association: paradigm for detecting a silent killer [thoracic aortic aneurysm]. *Open Heart*. 2015;2:e000169. With permission from BMJ Publishing Group Ltd.)

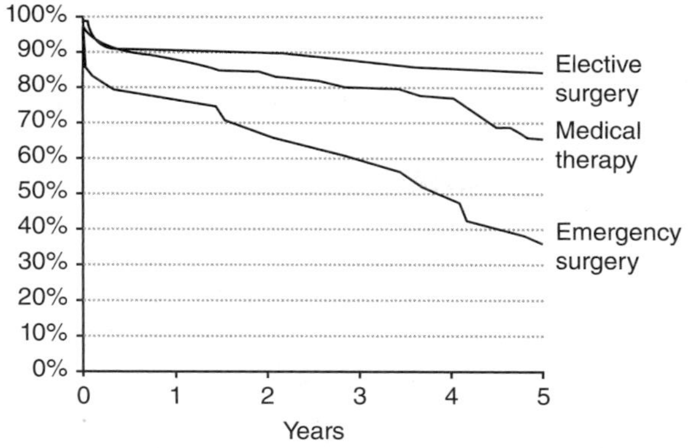

▲ **Figure 37–18.** Long-term survival rates based on treatment. Medically treated patients had, of course, smaller and less symptomatic aneurysms. Note particularly that patients having emergent surgery not only manifested a higher likelihood of perioperative mortality, but also had a poorer long-term outlook. On the other hand, patients who received elective surgery showed excellent survival rates, comparable to an age- and sex-matched normal population. These data argue for elective, prophylactic extirpation of the aneurysmal aorta, before rupture or dissection can occur.

its significant attendant risks, for an asymptomatic problem. Most patients, however, seem to feel they will never be comfortable until the threatening aneurysm is resected.

One more very important general point needs to be considered. Once the aorta has dissected, the prognosis is forevermore adversely affected (Figure 37–18). Patients who required emergency surgery not only had a higher rate of early mortality, but their survival curve was dramatically poorer. Patients who elected for planned, nonemergent procedures showed a survival rate very similar to that of a normal population. The poor long-term outlook for patients who required emergency surgery is due largely to the fact that, even after surgical replacement of portions of the aorta, the remainder of this vital organ will always remain dissected. Because the aortic wall was deficient to start with, at half-thickness, after dissection, it is rendered even more vulnerable to subsequent enlargement and rupture.

C. Surgical Techniques

As discussed earlier, the type of operation for the ascending aorta is based on the pattern of aneurysmal pathology. For many patients, a supracoronary tube graft suffices (Figure 37–19A). For others, a composite graft, including both a valve and a graft, with obligate coronary artery reimplantation, is appropriate (Figure 37–19B). Newer valve-sparing aortic replacement procedures (eg, David procedure) have been developed and validated in large clinical series. Although these valve-preserving operations are becoming increasingly popular, the long-term fate of the preserved valve remains somewhat controversial.

The main debate regarding the conduct of ascending aortic operations and those on the aortic arch concerns the optimal means of protecting brain function during the time that anastomoses in the vicinity of the aortic arch are performed. Deep hypothermic circulatory arrest—a state of suspended animation, which is generally safe for 30–45 minutes or longer—is preferred by many surgeons because of its simplicity and effectiveness. In a study on 500 patients, the effectiveness of this remarkable technique as a sole means of brain preservation was confirmed. Retrograde cerebral perfusion—via the superior vena cava—has its advocates, although the actual amount of effective brain perfusion achieved by this means has been questioned. Direct perfusion of the head vessels—usually via a cannula in the innominate artery or cannulas in both the innominate and the left carotid artery—also has its supporters, despite its added complexity. Direct perfusion is gaining in popularity, and it does provide a margin of protection, especially for very complex arch reconstructions or for surgical teams relatively inexperienced with arch replacement. However, very recent evidence has demonstrated a sobering 100% rate of cerebral embolic events (often subclinical) with antegrade perfusion. No technique has been demonstrated as conclusively superior over the others.

For descending and thoracoabdominal operations, the technique of left atrial to femoral artery bypass has become extremely popular. This method takes strain off the heart by diverting blood away from the left ventricle. This approach mitigates the effect of high aortic cross-clamping on cardiac afterload. It also perfuses the lower body, especially the extremely vulnerable spinal cord. Despite decades of concerted attention, paraplegia from descending and thoracoabdominal aortic replacement continues to be a major clinical problem. The cause is multifactorial, with clamp time, air and particulate embolism, and disconnection of critical intercostal branches all playing a role. Besides the benefits of left atrial to femoral artery perfusion, most authorities feel that routine spinal fluid drainage and deliberate maintenance of a strong postoperative blood pressure (to encourage collateral blood flow) are also effective adjuncts against the complication of postoperative paraplegia.

D. Specific Clinical Scenarios & Issues

1. Patient with pain, but aneurysm smaller than criteria—The answer to whether such an aorta should be replaced is a resounding yes. The dimensional criteria are specifically intended for asymptomatic patients. Any and all symptomatic aneurysms need to be resected because symptoms are a precursor to rupture. Aneurysm pain represents stretching or irritation of the aortic adventitia, the adjacent chest wall, the mediastinal pleura, or some other structure impinged on by the expanding aneurysm. Even an aorta smaller than the criterion can rupture or dissect. The size

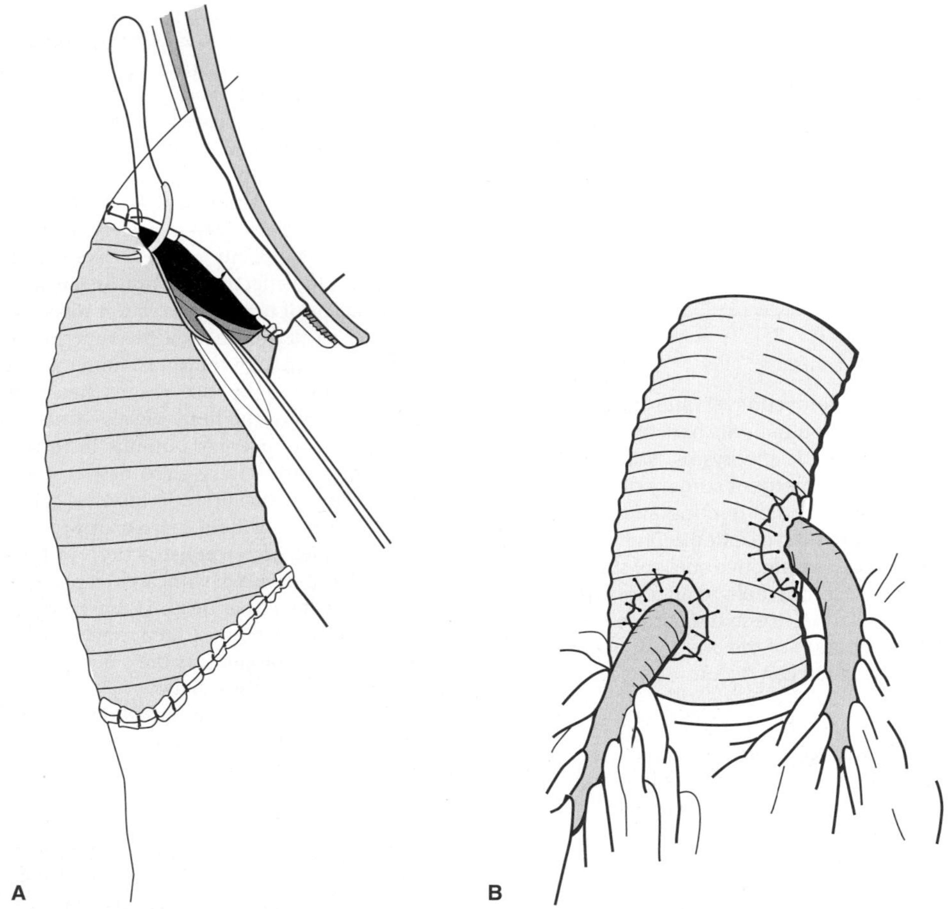

▲ **Figure 37–19. (A)** Supracoronary tube graft replacement and **(B)** composite graft replacement. (**A**: Reproduced with permission from Cooley DA, Wukasch DC. *Techniques in Vascular Surgery*. Philadelphia: WB Saunders; 1979.)

criteria are "fuzzy" lines, not sharp demarcations. A patient with pain but a relatively small aneurysm is of great concern, and preemptive resection is needed. In one case, a patient complained of pain typical of an ascending aortic aneurysm. The aorta was 5.0 cm. Because the medical team thought this was too small for resection, they underestimated the symptoms at presentation. The aorta subsequently ruptured, and the patient died within 48 hours. This point cannot be overemphasized: The size criteria are explicitly intended only for asymptomatic patients; all symptomatic aneurysms need to be resected.

2. Differentiating aneurysm pain from musculoskeletal pain—This very important point is not always easy to determine, even in the most experienced hands. The patient usually has a good sense of whether the pain is originating from muscles and joints. The clinician usually gets an additional understanding by asking the following questions:

a. Is the pain influenced by motion or position? (If so, it is probably musculoskeletal.)
b. Do you have a history of lumbosacral spine disease or chronic low back pain? (If so, the symptoms may not be aortic in origin.)
c. Do you feel the pain in the interscapular back? (An affirmative answer indicates an almost certain relationship to thoracic aortic aneurysm.) The interscapular region corresponds to the upper descending aorta.

Presume that the pain is aortic in origin if no other cause can be conclusively established. This is the only approach that can prevent rupture.

3. Appropriate interval for serial aortic imaging—Patients with a thoracic aortic aneurysm should be monitored indefinitely. Stable, asymptomatic patients can undergo imaging about once every 2 years, remembering that the aneurysmal aorta grows at a relatively slow 1 mm/year. In case of new onset of symptoms, imaging should be done promptly, regardless of the interval from the prior scan. For new patients, for whom only one size data point is available, imaging should be done at shorter intervals until the behavior of aorta is understood. Imaging may be done every 3–6 months for new patients with moderately large aortas. Remember to compare the present scan with the patient's first scan, not with the last prior scan. That is the way to detect growth. Many patients have suffered because scans were only compared with the last prior scan, and major growth went undetected.

4. Choice of imaging modality for serial follow-up—Three quality imaging techniques are currently available: echocardiography, CT scan, and MRI. If echocardiography is chosen, it is important to remember that a standard transthoracic echocardiogram cannot see the distal ascending aorta, the aortic arch, or the descending aorta with conclusive accuracy because of intervening air-containing bronchi and lung tissue. Supplement such studies with a periodic CT scan or MRI, which can visualize the entire aorta. The choice between CT and MRI may depend on ease of availability and radiologic expertise in a particular environment. Both modalities can image the entire aorta extremely well. Elevated creatinine or contrast allergy may contraindicate CT and instead favor MRI. The need to evaluate complex aortic lesions in multiple imaging planes would also favor MRI (although very recently, concerns have been raised about the risk to the kidneys of gadolinium contrast agents used for MRI scanning). Of course, indwelling metallic foreign objects, such as pacemakers or metal artifacts from previous surgery, may make CT the necessary choice instead of MRI. The advantages and limitations of echocardiography are shown in Figure 37–20. Both echocardiography and CT are required for complete evaluation of the entire aorta.

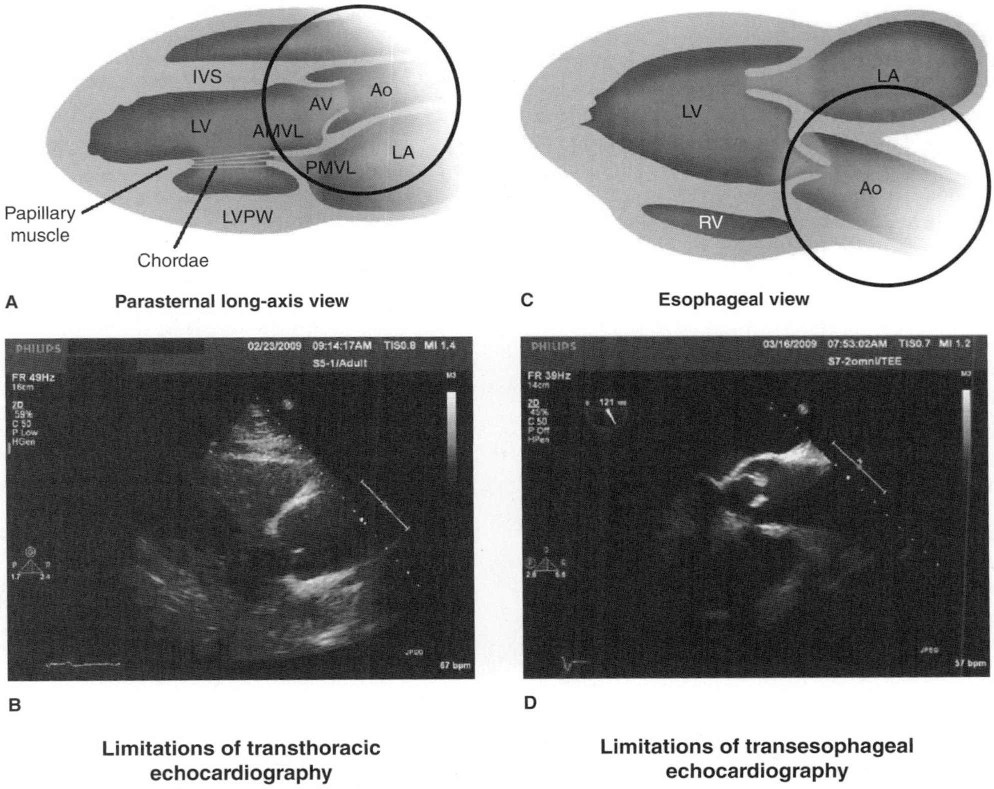

▲ **Figure 37–20. A and B:** Limited distance above the aortic valve (AV) for which the ascending aorta (Ao) can be seen on transthoracic echocardiography. Schematic **(A)** and actual echocardiographic **(B)** image. AMVL, anterior mitral valve leaflet; IVS, interventricular septum; LA, left atrium; LV, left ventricle; LVPW, left ventricular posterior wall. **C and D:** Limited distance above the aortic valve for which the ascending aorta can be seen on transesophageal echocardiography. The tracheal air column interferes with visualization of the upper ascending aorta. Schematic **(C)** and actual echocardiographic image **(D)**. RV, right ventricle. (**A and C:** Reproduced with permission from Mr. Rob Flewell. **B and D:** Reproduced with permission from Elefteriades JA, et al. Thoracic aortic aneurysm clinically pertinent controversies and uncertainties. *J Am Coll Cardiol.* 2010;55:841. Copyright © 2010 by the American College of Cardiology Foundation.)

5. Evaluation of family members—The data on familial inheritance has become strong enough that the treating physician is obligated to recommend that family members be evaluated. Physicians of family members should be made aware that aneurysm disease has been diagnosed in the family. A CT scan is recommended for adult males and for females beyond childbearing age. For children and for females of childbearing age, echocardiography of the ascending aorta and abdominal aorta is recommended. Investigators hope to identify humoral markers or genetic aberrations that can be used for familial screening of the aneurysm trait in the very near future. Routine genetic testing via Whole Exome Sequencing, while somewhat controversial and inconsistently approved by insurers, is becoming more and more widespread. We now offer and encourage screening of patients and family members by WES for nearly all of our patients. (See Figure 37–4, which presents, in pie diagram form, the most recent specific genetic findings from WES for thoracic aortic aneurysm.)

6. Activity restrictions—Continuation of any and all aerobic activities, including running, swimming, and bicycling, is recommended. Serious weight lifters, at peaks of exertion, can elevate systolic arterial pressure to 300 mm Hg or higher. This type of instantaneous hypertension is, of course, not prudent for aneurysm patients. Weight lifters should limit themselves to one-half their body weight. The evidence for effort-induced aortic dissection is mounting. Participation in contact sports or those that might produce an abrupt physical impact, such as tackle football, snow skiing, water skiing, and horseback riding, is proscribed.

7. Role of stent grafting—A word of caution is appropriate concerning stent grafts. Stent therapy has become routine for many patients (especially those with abdominal or descending aortic aneurysms). It is certainly less invasive and more easily tolerated than open surgical techniques. Specialists, however, must avoid "irrational exuberance." Owing to the high need for subsequent conventional surgery after abdominal aneurysm stent placement, the large, multicenter Eurostar study questioned the very efficacy and advisability of stent grafting. Endoleak, stent dislodgement, and aneurysm expansion or rupture were disturbingly widespread in medium-term follow-up. It should be remembered that stents were originally designed to keep tissue from encroaching on the vessel lumen, not to keep the vessel from expanding. One noted authority believes that the aneurysmal aorta essentially "ignores" the stent graft, dilating regardless of the stent, at its own pace (personal communication, Dr. L. Svensson). Also remember that the natural history of the thoracic aorta is that aneurysms grow slowly and that hard endpoints (rupture, dissection, and death) take years to be realized. For this reason, short-term stent studies are nearly meaningless. Long-term studies are needed. This newer modality of treatment should be approached with enthusiasm tempered by caution. Its advent should not at this point influence the decision about whether or not to intervene for a specific aneurysm; criteria (see earlier in chapter) should be met before any intervention, including stent therapy, is undertaken. Stent therapy appears especially well suited for patients with traumatic rupture of the descending aorta, in which setting a stent can be acutely life-saving. Those cautions having been stated, it is important to recognize that stent therapy is proliferating rapidly and that incremental improvements in the stent hardware are being made on a regular basis.

Blumel R, Patel K, Rizzo JA,. Accuracy of the "Thumb-Palm Test": for detection of ascending aortic aneurysm. *Am J Cardiol.* 2021 Jul 1;150:114–116. doi: 10.1016/j.amjcard.2021.03.041. Epub 2021 May 18. [PMID: 34020772].

Erbel R, Aboyans V, Boileau C, et al. 2014. ESC guidelines on the diagnosis and treatment of aortic diseases: document covering acute and chronic aortic diseases of the thoracic and abdominal aorta of the adult. The Task Force for the Diagnosis and Treatment of Aortic Diseases of the European Society of Cardiology (ESC). *Eur Heart J.* 2014;35(41):2873–2926. [PMID: 25173340]

Humphrey JD, Schwartz MA, Tellides G, Milewicz DM. Role of mechanotransduction in vascular biology: focus on thoracic aortic aneurysms and dissections. *Circulation Research.* 2015;116:1448–1461. [PMID: 25858068]

Kalogerakos P, Zafar MA, Li Y, et al. Root dilatation is more malignant than ascending aortic dilatation. *J Am Heart Assoc.* 2021;10(14):e020645. [PMID: 34238012]

Leshnower BG, Rangaraju S, Allen JW, Stringer AY, Gleason TG, Chen EP. Deep hypothermia with retrograde cerebral perfusion versus moderate hypothermia with antegrade cerebral perfusion for arch surgery. *Ann Thorac Surg.* 2019;107:1104–1110. [PMID: 30448484]

Mansour AM, Peterss S, Zafar MA, et al. Prevention of aortic dissection suggests a diameter shift to a lower aortic size threshold for intervention. *Cardiology.* 2018;139:139–146. [PMID: 29346780]

Mori M, Mahmood SUB, Yousef S, et al. Prevalence of incidentally identified thoracic dilatations: insight for screening criteria. *Can J Cardiol.* 2019; Jul;35(7):892–898. [PMID: 31292088]

Ostbereg NP, Zafar MA, Ziganshin BA, Elefteriades JA. The genetics of thoracic aortic aneurysms and dissection. *Biomolecules.* 2020;10:182. [PMC7072177] [PMID: 31991693]

Wu J, Zafar MA, Li Y, et al. Ascending aortic length and risk of aortic adverse events: The neglected dimension. *J Am Coll Cardiol.* 2019;74:1883–1894. [PMID: 31526537]

Ziganshin BA, Bailey AE, Coons C, et al. Routine genetic testing for thoracic aortic aneurysm and dissection in a clinical setting. *Ann Thorac Surg.* 2015;100(5):1604–1611. [PMID: 26188975]

AORTIC DISSECTION

ESSENTIALS OF DIAGNOSIS

- Usually middle-aged or elderly hypertensive men; occasionally, young patients with history of Marfan syndrome or other connective tissue disorder. Rarely, young women in late pregnancy or labor.
- Acute chest pain, frequently with hemodynamic instability.

- Possible appearance of shock but normal or elevated blood pressure.
- Various neurologic symptoms, such as Horner syndrome, paraplegia, and stroke.
- Absent or unequal peripheral pulses.
- Aortic regurgitation.
- Widened mediastinum on chest radiograph.
- Confirmatory aortic imaging study.

General Considerations

A. Terminology

Aortic dissection refers to a splitting of the layers of the aortic wall (within the media) permitting longitudinal propagation of a blood-filled space within the aortic wall. Aortic dissection is thought to be the most common cause of death related to the human aorta (Figure 37–21).

Three related but distinct entities—acute aortic transection, rupture of aortic aneurysm, and aortic dissection—are commonly confused, both in substance and in terminology (Figure 37–22). **Acute aortic transection** is a traumatic phenomenon, with disruption of the wall of the aorta, without a propagating dissection. The aortic wall is intrinsically normal and resistant to the dissection process. **Rupture** of aortic aneurysm is self-explanatory; however, confusion in terminology may arise if an acute aortic transection or an acute aortic dissection happens to rupture—a common eventuality. **Acute aortic dissection** refers to the very specific process of separation of layers of the aortic wall, discussed fully in this chapter. For dissection to occur, the aortic wall must nearly always be affected by structural disease of the media.

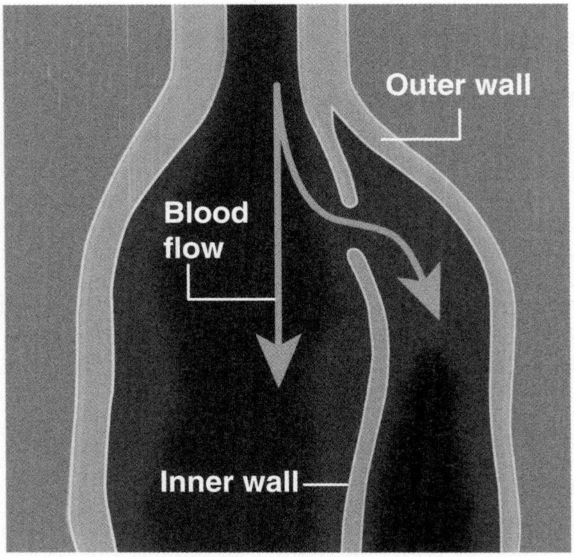

▲ **Figure 37–21.** Schematic depiction of aortic dissection.

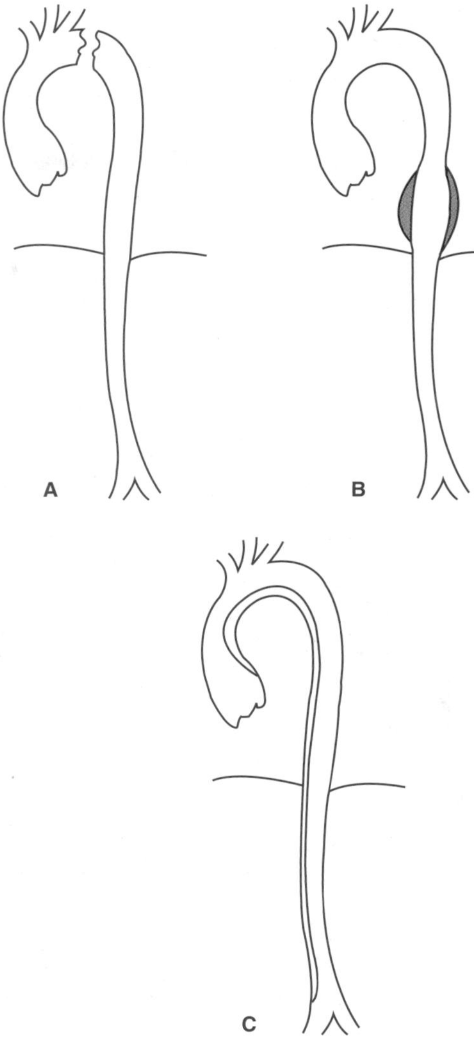

▲ **Figure 37–22.** Frequently confused terminology. See text for a description of the very different disorders of acute aortic transection **(A)**, ruptured aortic aneurysm **(B)**, and acute aortic dissection **(C)**.

Recent years have brought recognition of two important variants of aortic dissection: intramural hematoma (IMH) and penetrating aortic ulcer (PAU) (Figure 37–23).

IMH of the aorta differs from typical dissection in that there is no flap defining a true and a false lumen, and the hematoma (on axial imaging) is located circumferentially around the aortic lumen, rather than obliquely oriented across the aortic lumen. Whether the IMH arises from a small intimal tear (not detected radiographically) or from rupture of a vasa vasorum within the aortic wall remains

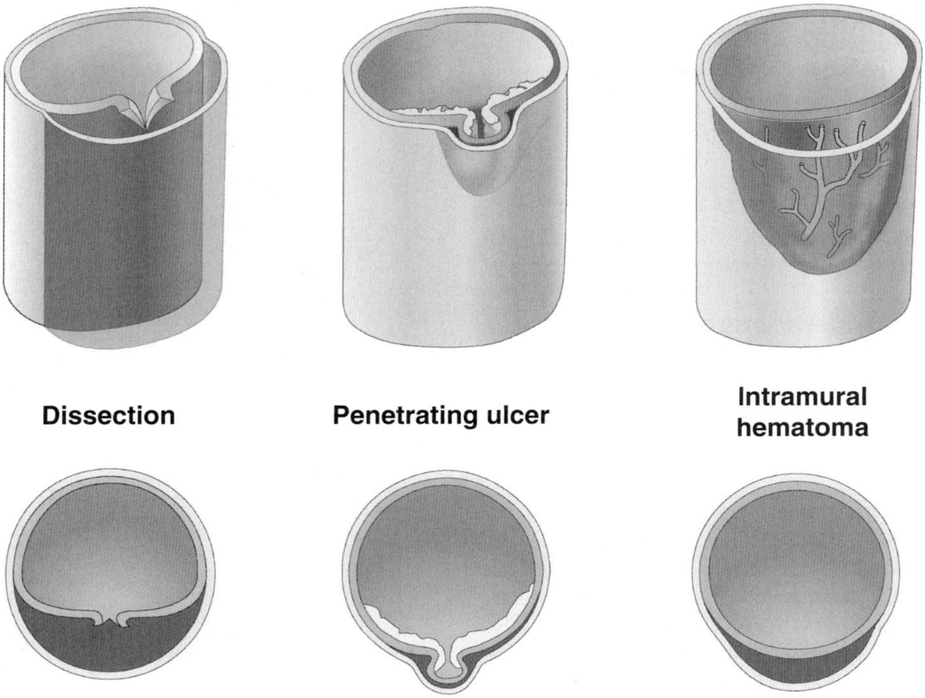

▲ **Figure 37–23.** Schematic of variant forms of aortic dissection: typical dissection, penetrating ulcer, and intramural hematoma. A true dissection has to have a flap.

controversial. The clinical course is variable; the hematoma may persist, reabsorb (returning the aorta to a normal appearance), lead to aneurysm with the possibility of rupture, or convert to dissection. PAU involves a local penetration deep into the wall of the aorta, resembling a penetrating ulcer of the stomach. This lesion disrupts the internal elastic lamina and erodes into the media, which in some cases may mimic or initiate aortic dissection, pseudoaneurysm formation, IMH, or rupture. Extensive arteriosclerosis is a common accompaniment of PAU (see Figure 37–23).

It is important to recognize that IMH and PAU are diseases of advanced age. In addition, it is important point to mention that, although branch vessel occlusion is part and parcel of typical aortic dissection, the variants of aortic dissection PAU and IMH never occlude branch vessels.

The general management of these lesions is still a matter of debate. Most authorities believe that descending aortic IMH and PAU can be managed medically, with "anti-impulse" therapy (see Treatment section). However, early (but not immediate) surgical intervention is preferred in suitable operative candidates to preempt rupture due to a high incidence of death from rupture. Some of the discrepancy in recommendations also has to do with regional differences: In Japan, IMH behaves in a more benign fashion than in the Western world, perhaps reflecting fundamental genetic differences in the aortic wall or differences in body size and aortic dimension. Stent therapies are often applied for IMH or PAU and are proliferating progressively in the Western world.

For ascending aorta IMH and PAU, most authorities agree on aggressive immediate surgical intervention, although Japanese experience challenges the need for routine surgery, even in this anatomic location.

B. Anatomic Classification

Aortic dissections may be ascending (type A) or descending (type B). The two patterns are determined by the location of the inciting intimal tear. Tears occur in two very specific locations: (1) in the ascending aorta, 2–3 cm above the coronary arteries, and (2) in the descending aorta, 1–2 cm beyond the left subclavian artery. The first type of tear produces ascending dissection and the second, descending dissection. Please note that ascending dissections usually go around the aortic arch to involve the descending and abdominal portions of the aorta (Figure 37–24).

Clinical Findings

A. Symptoms & Signs

Aortic dissection produces intense, severe pain, often described as tearing or shearing in quality. This pain is sudden in onset (a differentiating feature from the pain of

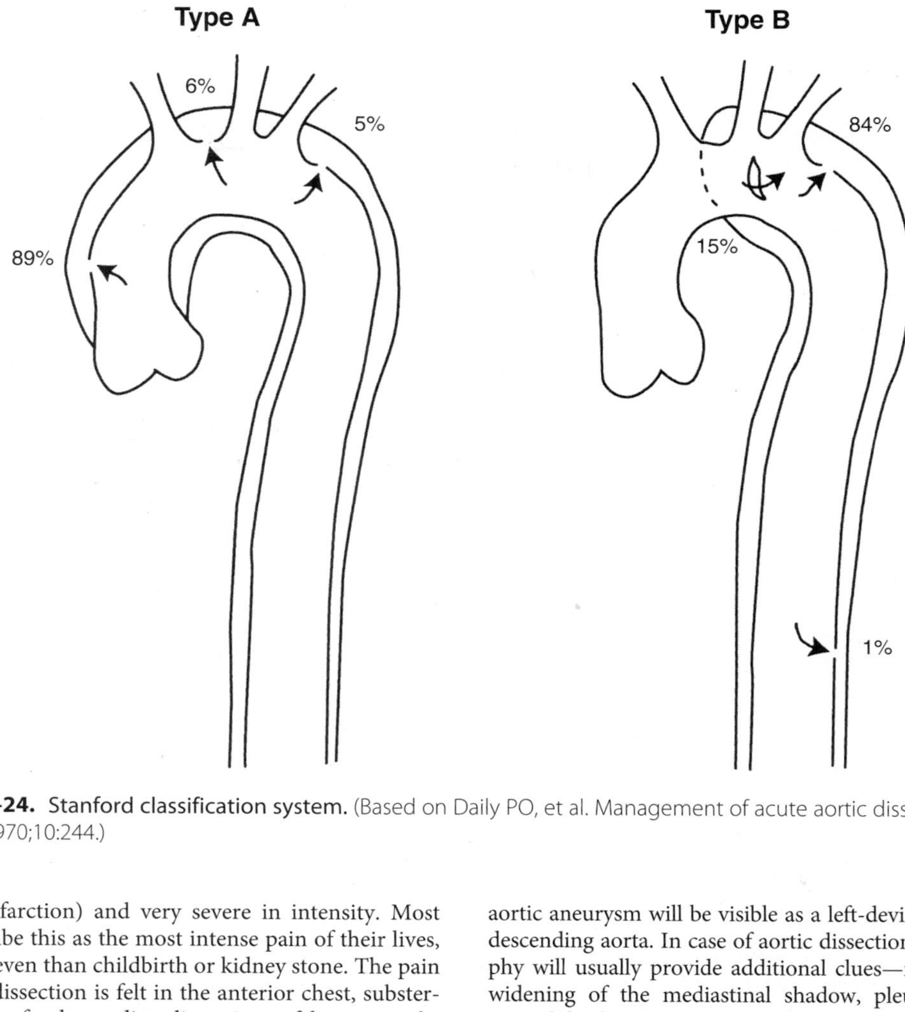

▲ **Figure 37–24.** Stanford classification system. (Based on Daily PO, et al. Management of acute aortic dissections. *Ann Thorac Surg*. 1970;10:244.)

myocardial infarction) and very severe in intensity. Most patients describe this as the most intense pain of their lives, more intense even than childbirth or kidney stone. The pain of ascending dissection is felt in the anterior chest, substernally, and that of a descending dissection is felt posteriorly, between the scapulae. The "tearing," "shearing," "knife-like" quality of the pain is quite consistent with the pathophysiology. The pain can migrate downward, into the flank or pelvis, as the dissection process propagates distally. Impending aortic rupture should be considered when pain subsides and later recurs. On occasion, painless dissection does occur, perhaps as often as in 15% of patients; this is usually picked up later, on a routine imaging study done for another reason.

B. Diagnostic Studies

1. Chest radiography—Chest radiography is a useful screening test. Many, if not most, aortic dissections occur in the setting of a chronic aortic aneurysm. To the astute observer, chronic thoracic aneurysms can be visualized on a chest radiograph. The enlarged ascending aorta will protrude to the right of the upper mediastinal border, an arch aneurysm will show as an exaggerated aortic knob, and a descending aortic aneurysm will be visible as a left-deviated stripe of the descending aorta. In case of aortic dissection, chest radiography will usually provide additional clues—most commonly, widening of the mediastinal shadow, pleural effusion, or inward displacement of aortic medial calcification.

2. Three-dimensional imaging methods—Multiple types of three-dimensional imaging modalities are pertinent in aneurysm disease and aortic dissection, and all have excellent sensitivity and specificity: transesophageal echocardiography (TEE), CT scanning, and MRI. Many patients undergo a TEE and either a CT or an MRI. The CT or MRI shows the three-dimensional structure of the entire aorta. The TEE, while partially blinded to the aortic arch and abdominal aorta, provides information about pericardial effusion and tamponade, valve function, and left ventricular function. TEE images both ascending and descending aortas well.

The primary diagnostic criterion for aortic dissection by CT or MRI is demonstration of two contrast-filled lumens separated by an intimal flap. Sensitivity and specificity of CT and MRI for diagnosis of aortic dissection are approaching 100%. TEE does not lag far behind in accuracy. Contrast aortography, once the gold standard, has fallen by the wayside for diagnosis of aortic dissection, being more invasive and not offering nearly the amount of three-dimensional anatomic information afforded by CT, MRI, and TEE.

Differential Diagnosis

The imaging studies discussed earlier provide specific information that rules in or out the presence of aneurysm or dissection. The main diagnostic issue involves (1) maintaining a high index of suspicion for aneurysm disease and (2) being aware of the protean presentations of aneurysm disease. In particular, aortic dissection has been called "the great masquerader" because it can produce symptoms related to virtually any organ. A high index of suspicion is required to establish the diagnosis promptly, since the presentations of aortic dissection are so myriad and mimic a wide array of other diseases. Specifically, all patients admitted with chest pain without obvious cause should have their thoracic aorta imaged. Patients with a ruptured or dissected thoracic aorta often "masquerade" as heart attacks. It is especially important to rule out aortic dissection in patients about to be treated for myocardial infarction, as administration of thrombolytic drugs in patients with acute aortic dissection is associated with a high mortality.

Among conditions for which aortic dissection can be confused are myocardial infarction, musculoskeletal chest pain, pericarditis, pleuritis, pneumothorax, pulmonary embolism, cholecystitis, ureteral colic, appendicitis, mesenteric ischemia, pyelonephritis, stroke, transient ischemic attack, and primary limb ischemia. Especially troublesome to clinicians in emergency departments are patients with abdominal symptoms and signs without apparent abdominal cause; aortic dissection must be considered in such patients.

Given the extensive differential diagnosis, aggressive, objective diagnostic testing is necessary when the possibility of aortic dissection is considered. The diagnosis is most strongly suggested when migratory chest and back pain of less than 24 hours in duration arises in a patient with a history of hypertension. The following recommendations are made for the physicians who are the first to evaluate such patients: (1) Keep aortic dissection (and ruptured thoracic or abdominal aneurysm) in the differential diagnosis. (2) Image freely and liberally to rule out aortic pathology. A CT scan can exclude all three major chest diagnoses likely to result in death: coronary artery disease, pulmonary embolism, and aortic aneurysm or dissection (thus the name "triple rule-out CT"). Modern CT scanners are ideal for this purpose. (3) Remember the D-dimer test. A negative D-dimer, which is most commonly applied to rule out pulmonary embolism, also rules out aortic dissection. The clot that forms in the false lumen of an aortic dissection liberates D-dimer quite strikingly. This simple blood test is nearly 100% sensitive in picking up aortic dissection. If the D-dimer is not elevated, your patient has not suffered an acute aortic dissection. (4) Remember to look at the aorta, even if the CT scan is ordered for other, especially abdominal, examination.

Attention to these recommendations will also serve to discourage litigation for failure to diagnose aortic dissection.

Treatment

A. Pharmacotherapy

Most patients will require intensive medical therapy for acute aortic dissection, either as sole treatment or as a stabilizing measure until appropriate surgical therapy is undertaken.

It has been recognized that aortic dissection propagates more vigorously when either blood pressure or force of cardiac contraction is excessive. Accordingly, blood pressure needs to be controlled in patients with acute aortic dissection or other acute aortic syndromes, including aortic rupture or impending rupture. Nitroglycerin and nitroprusside are usually used for this purpose, because of their effectiveness, their rapid onset of action, and their quick cessation of action on discontinuation. (Nicardipine, a calcium channel blocking agent, has recently become popular for acute control of hypertension, largely because the cost of nitroprusside has increased.) Blood pressure should be reduced as low as possible without producing neurologic dysfunction or oliguria. Usually, the severity of general occlusive vascular disease determines how low the blood pressure can safely be taken. The blood pressure may be lowered to 90–100 mm Hg initially, until the patient's response can be evaluated. Depressed mental status or oliguria may indicate that the blood pressure has been lowered too far for a specific patient. For older patients with extensive end-organ vascular disease, lowering the blood pressure pharmacologically to 120–130 mm Hg may need to suffice.

However, to lower blood pressure by afterload reduction alone would actually increase the sheer stress on the aortic wall (*dp/dt*). It is crucial to also decrease the force of cardiac contraction (Figure 37–25). The morphology of the arterial pulse wave must be blunted by decreasing the force of cardiac contraction. The *dp/dt*, reflected in the upslope of the initial portion of the aortic pulse wave, must be decreased, usually by administering a short-acting β-blocker, such as esmolol. Another approach is administration of the α- and β-adrenergic antagonist labetalol by intravenous infusion. When β-blocking drugs are contraindicated, calcium channel blockers offer a reasonable substitute.

Together, the afterload reduction and the β-blockade are referred to as "anti-impulse" therapy for acute aortic dissection. Regardless of whether the dissection is ascending or descending, or whether or not the patient will be taken emergently to the operating room, such therapy must be instituted to discourage rupture or extension of the dissection.

Anti-impulse therapy is the appropriate initial response once the diagnosis of any type of acute aortic dissection or related process is made. Often, such therapy is undertaken even while imaging studies are being performed to confirm the diagnosis of aortic dissection and define the anatomic type, location, and extent of the process. Definitive therapeutic decisions and treatments will follow.

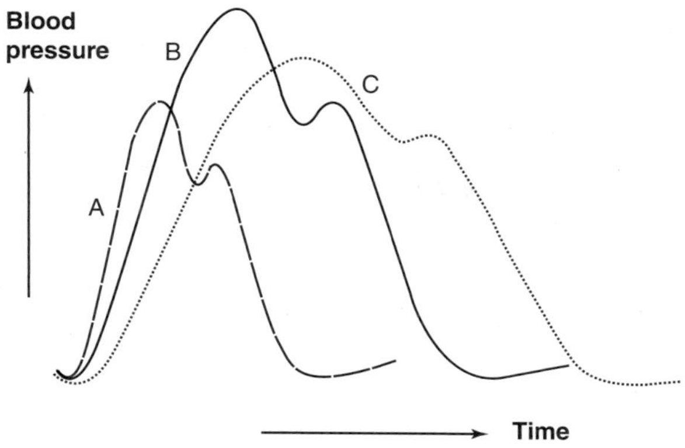

▲ **Figure 37–25.** Diagram of aortic pressure curves under various conditions. The continuous line **(B)** represents the baseline state. Administration of a vasodilator agent such as nitroprusside is represented by the dashed curve **(A)**. There is significant decrease in pressure levels and acceleration in heart rate, but this is accompanied by a steepest slope of the ascending portion of the curve (increased dp/dt_{max}). β-Blockade administration is represented by the dotted line **(C)**. Although the degree of pressure lowering is usually smaller, the drug negative inotropic and chronotropic effects result in decreased impulse and dp/dt_{max}.

B. Surgical Treatment

For acute aortic dissection, the following guidelines regarding definitive therapy apply.

Ascending aortic aneurysms require urgent surgery because death from intrapericardial rupture, aortic regurgitation, or myocardial infarction from coronary artery involvement usually occurs in patients who do not undergo surgery. The dissection layers are reapproximated as a "sandwich" between layers of Teflon felt (Figure 37–26). Overall survival at experienced centers is about 85% for patients with acute type A aortic dissection. The exact surgical procedure performed, vis-à-vis the proximal aortic root and the coronary arteries, varies depending on the circumstances. For patients in whom dissection occurs in the setting of Marfan disease or other cause of annuloaortic ectasia (proximal root enlargement), the aortic valve, aortic root, and ascending aorta are replaced with a prefabricated "composite graft" including both a valve and a graft (see Figure 37–19B). Another option is a valve-sparing aortic root replacement, which is becoming progressively more popular, even in the setting of an acute ascending aortic dissection. In this procedure, the aorta is replaced down to the aortic annulus, but the native aortic valve is reimplanted inside the new aortic graft.

Descending dissections, in the absence of specific vascular complications, do well with medical management (short- and long-term "anti-impulse" therapy with β-blockers and afterload-reducing medications). If a specific complication occurs, this is addressed directly by surgery ("complication-specific" approach to descending aortic dissection). Ninety-one percent of patients survived the initial hospitalization (type B aortic dissection is "milder" than type A dissection), and about 66% had a completely uncomplicated course while receiving anti-impulse medical therapy alone. The majority of complications were related to vascular malperfusion of specific organs. Stent therapy for acute or chronic type B dissection is controversial. The INSTEAD study of routine stent grafting for (late) acute type B dissection demonstrated some mid-term survival benefit, at the cost of substantial early stent-related complications, but methods of analysis have been questioned. There is growing enthusiasm for routine stent therapy of all acute type B aortic dissections, even uncomplicated cases, to prevent later complications.

The subacute and chronic stages of aortic dissection are managed differently from acute dissection. Once the patient with type A dissection has been brought safely through surgery, or the type B patient has been stabilized with anti-impulse therapy, the patient is observed closely for the first month, with repeat aortic imaging. After that point, it is uncommon for the dissection to extend, cause symptoms, or rupture in the short-term to mid-term. The patients are then monitored similarly to those with chronic aneurysm. Over years, enlargement of the dissected aorta will develop in some patients and require resection. The same dimensional criteria for surgical intervention can be applied as for nondissected aneurysms. It is usually the most proximal portion of the descending aorta, just beyond the subclavian artery, that dilates first and requires surgical replacement.

▶ Prognosis

Aortic dissection is often fatal without early diagnosis and aggressive treatment. The presenting symptoms and signs are so myriad and nonspecific (see earlier in chapter) that dissection may be overlooked initially in up to 40% of cases; in fact, the diagnosis is not made until postmortem examination in a disturbingly large fraction of patients. This can be a frequent cause of litigation, and guidelines have recently been outlined so litigation can be avoided. Few other conditions demand such prompt diagnosis and treatment, since the mortality rate of untreated dissection approaches 1–2% per hour during the first 48 hours, 89% at 14 days, and 90% at 3 months.

Aortic dissection can result in death in four ways: (1) intrapericardial rupture (of an ascending dissection), (2) acute aortic regurgitation (from an ascending aortic dissection), (3) free rupture into the pleural space (of a descending dissection), and (4) occlusion of any branch of the aorta (with consequent organ ischemia).

Branch vessel occlusion comes about via impingement on the true lumen of any branch vessel (coronaries to iliacs) by the distended false lumen (Figure 37–27).

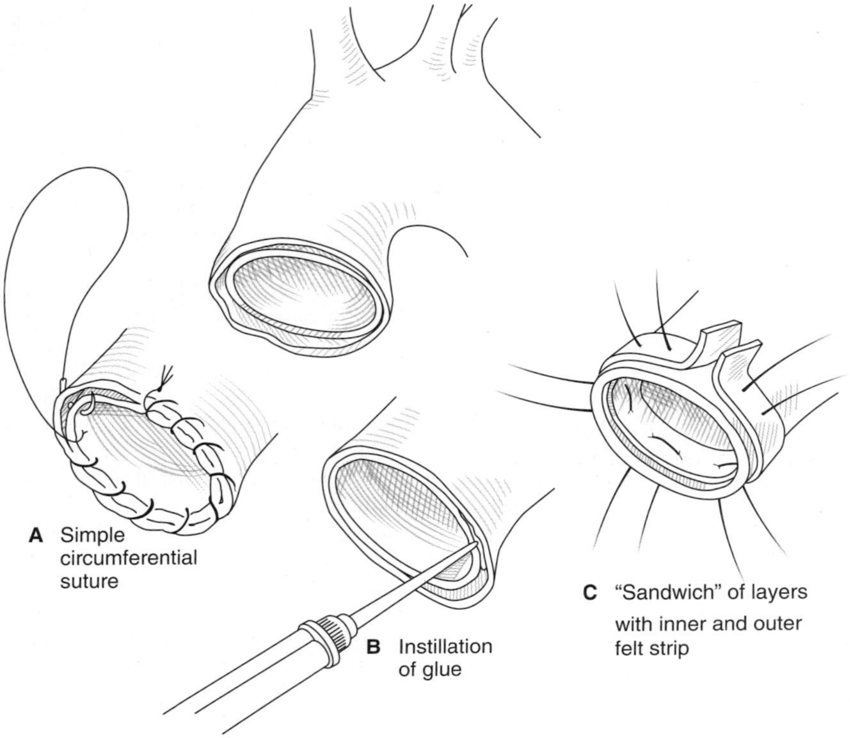

▲ **Figure 37–26.** Alternate methods of dealing with the dissection prior to anastomosis.

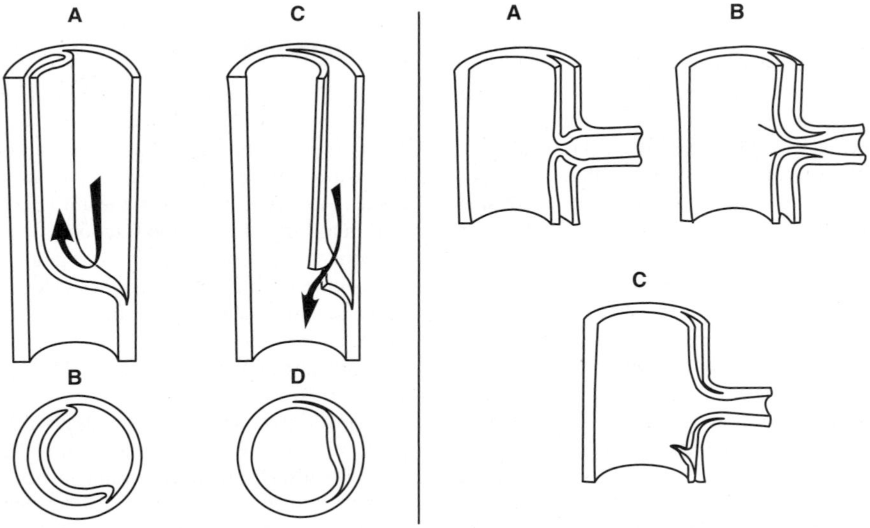

▲ **Figure 37–27.** Depiction of means by which the dissected lumen can compromise the true lumen, seen in various planes. The figures on the left look at the aorta itself. Note the relief of impingement when the flap fenestrates (images left, C and D, and right, C).

The acute aortic regurgitation of an ascending dissection may be very poorly tolerated, compared with chronic aortic regurgitation, because the sudden nature allows no time for cardiac adaptation. Cardiogenic shock may result.

Several general advances promise to mitigate the scourge of aortic diseases on society. Aortic aneurysms are diagnosed more frequently (incidentally) due to widespread application of imaging techniques for other reasons (echocardiography, CT, MRI). Aortic aneurysms are diagnosed more frequently (deliberately) due to increasing recognition that these are inherited diseases, and family members are screened. Advances in genetics are increasingly facilitating the recognition of specific mutations underlying aortic diseases in specific patients and their families. Personalized therapy, based on individual molecular genetics, is now feasible. Advances in genetics hold promise for effective screening tests for the general population. Concurrently, surgical therapies have become extremely safe.

Appropriate intervention criteria have been developed that permit evidence-based preemptive surgical intervention to prevent rupture and dissection. Gene-specific criteria for surgical intervention are indicated in Figure 37–28 for many important causative genes. Near-normal prognosis can be achieved for affected patients, provided that surgery is carried out before onset of aortic dissection. Public awareness of aneurysm disease has increased (eg, via the John Ritter Foundation) but needs to be promoted more fully.

Charilaou P, Ziganshin BA, Peterss S, et al. Current experience with acute type B aortic dissection: validity of the complication-specific approach in the present era. *Ann Thorac Surg.* 2016; 101(3):936–943. [PMID: 26518373]

Chou AS, Ziganshin BA, Charilaou P, Tranquilli M, Rizzo JA, Elefteriades JA. Long-term behavior of aortic intramural hematomas and penetrating ulcers. *J Thorac Cardiovasc Surg.* 2015;151(2):361–373.e1. [PMID: 26496809]

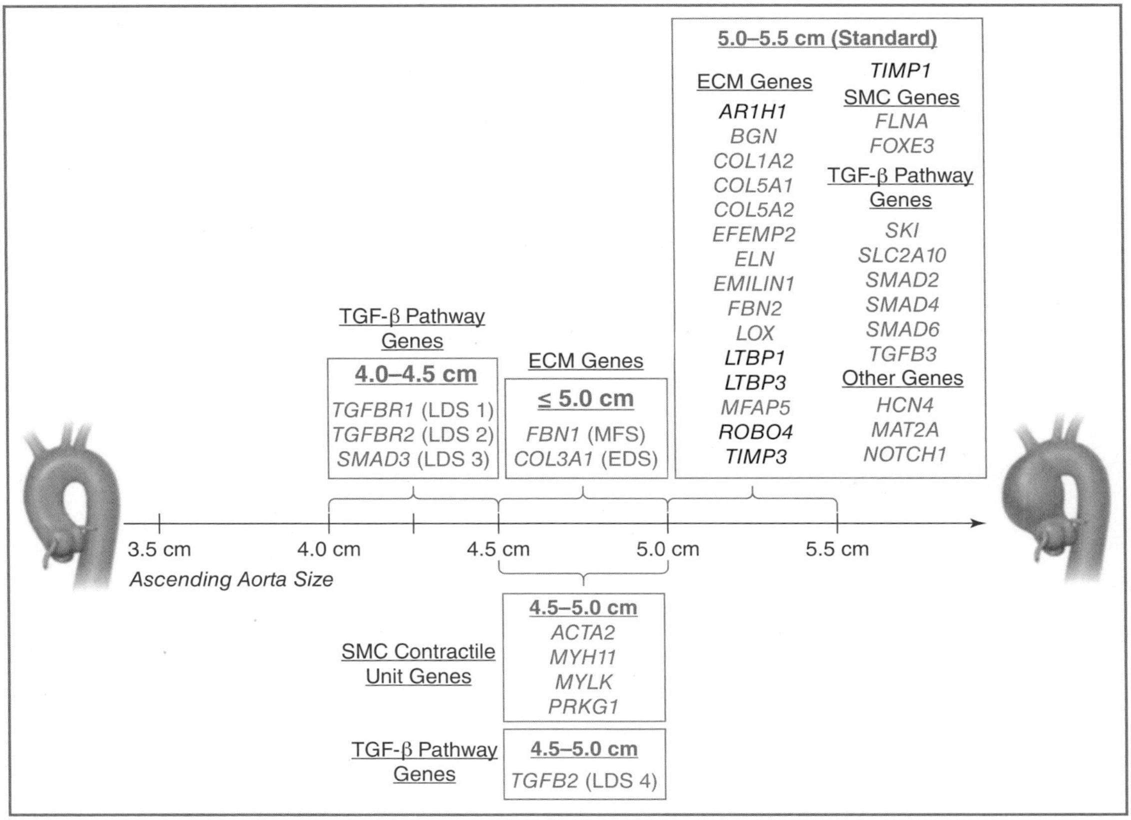

▲ **Figure 37–28.** Recommended intervention criteria (aortic diameter) for aneurysms caused by 38 genes currently known to be associated in the causation of thoracic aortic aneurysm. (Reproduced from Faggion Vinholo T, Brownstein AJ, Ziganshin BA, et al. Genes associated with thoracic aortic aneurysm and dissection: 2019 Update and Clinical Implications. Aorta (Stamford). 2019;7(4):99–107.)

Clough RE, Nienaber CA. Evidence for and risks of endovascular treatment of asymptomatic acute type B aortic dissection. *J Cardiovasc Surg (Torino)*. 2017;58:270–277. [PMID: 28045241]

Lau C, Leonard JR, Iannacone E, Gaudino M, Girardi LN. Surgery for acute presentation of thoracoabdominal aortic disease. *Semin Thorac Cardiovasc Surg*. 2019 Spring;31(1):11–16. [PMID: 26496809]

Spinelli D, Benedetto F, Donato R, et al. Current evidence in predictors of aortic growth and events in acute type B aortic dissection. *J Vasc Surg*. 2018 Dec;68(6):1925–1935.e8. [PMID: 30115384]

Index

Note: Page numbers followed by *t* indicate tables; those followed by *f* indicate figures.

I